FOOD, NUTRITION and DIET THERAPY

MARIE V. KRAUSE, B.S., M.S., R.D.

Formerly Dietitian in Charge of Nutrition Clinic and Associate
Director of Education, Department of Nutrition, New York Hospital.
Therapeutic Dietitian and Instructor in Dietetics, Mount Sinai
Hospital, Philadelphia, Pa. Therapeutic Dietitian and First
Assistant to Instructor in Nutrition, Department of Medicine,
University of Chicago Clinics.

L. KATHLEEN MAHAN, M.S., R.D.

Nutritionist, Clinical Training Unit, Child Development and Mental
Retardation Center; Lecturer, School of Home Economics, University
of Washington; Consulting Nutritionist in Private Practice, Seattle,
Washington; Formerly Assistant Professor and Director, Program in
Clinical Nutrition, College of Nursing and Allied Health Sciences,
Rush University, Chicago, Illinois.

Sixth Edition – Illustrated

1979   W. B. SAUNDERS COMPANY   Philadelphia • London • Toronto

W. B. Saunders Company: West Washington Square
                           Philadelphia, Pa. 19105

                           1 St. Anne's Road
                           Eastbourne, East Sussex BN21 3UN, England

                           1 Goldthorne Avenue
                           Toronto, Ontario M8Z 5T9, Canada

Listed here is the latest translated edition of this
book together with the language of the translation
and the publisher.

5th Edition (French) Les Editions HRW Ltee. Montreal, Quebec, Canada

Library of Congress Cataloging in Publication Data

Krause, Marie V

Food, nutrition and diet therapy.

1. Diet therapy.   2. Nutrition.   3. Food.   I. Mahan, L.
   Kathleen, joint author.   II. Title.   [DNLM: 1. Diet
   therapy.   2. Nutrition. WB400 K91n]

RM216.K74 1978   615'.854   77–11341

ISBN 0–7216–5513–0

Food, Nutrition and Diet Therapy   ISBN 0–7216–5513–0

Last digit is the print number: 9   8   7   6   5   4   3   2   1

To

HILDA S. WHITE, Ph.D.

Give me neither poverty nor riches;
feed me with food convenient for me.

Proverbs 30:8

FOREWORD

Textbooks and reference manuals are periodically revised to incorporate new knowledge and to discard out-of-date information. This text, now in its sixth edition, has undergone an extensive revision. The timing of the revision coincides with a period during which clinical nutrition is experiencing great advances. There has been an explosion of knowledge about the biochemical basis of life processes and about the changes that occur with disease. Newer medical research methods have made it possible to exploit the latest advances in biochemistry for the improved nutriture of the ill patient. Knowledge of intermediary metabolism is being applied to accommodate, correct or override the metabolic changes that occur with disease.

Nutritional maintenance of the ill patient is recognized by the health professions as a primary therapeutic regimen. Techniques for nourishing by vein have made possible the most exquisite metabolic studies, unencumbered by the processes of digestion and absorption. The metabolic stresses of trauma are better understood and, as a result, patients who previously would have succumbed to malnutrition and starvation can now be kept alive. Information obtained by the application of the newest techniques has direct pertinence for the patient who can be fed by mouth. It is still preferable to use conventional approaches to patient nourishment when the gastrointestinal tract is intact. When it becomes necessary to provide nourishment by tube feeding, chemically defined formulations that meet known nutrient requirements can also be used. There is a new confidence, a new nutrition.

While not every nurse and dietitian will have the opportunity to work directly with total parenteral nutrition teams, it is important to have some appreciation of the advances that have been made in this area. The ability to provide measured quantities of essential nutrients and adequate sources of energy directly by vein is making it possible to estimate the requirements for absorbed nutrients, that is, the true measure of metabolic requirements for nutrients in various disease states as well as in the normal state of good health. Studies of requirements for nutrients taken by mouth must always allow for variations in intestinal absorption and in the availability of nutrients for

absorption, as influenced by the nutrient interactions and plant fiber adsorption that occur during the digestive process. In addition, a better appreciation of requirements for trace minerals has evolved. It has been stated that nutritional science has moved from the epoch of the discovery and understanding of vitamins to an era of trace minerals nutrition. If that is true, we are in for exciting times because the research and analytical methods are available to hasten such intricate research.

Research and clinical experience in the nutritional management of the various disease states has required the restructuring of therapeutic diets and other systems for nutritional care. This sixth edition of *Food, Nutrition and Diet Therapy* is clinical in its approach while incorporating the newer knowledge of nutrition. Dietary regimens have been restructured when appropriate to be in keeping with the most recent clinical research and experience.

Nurses and dietitians are not necessarily restricted to therapeutic diets. As professionals on the health care team, they may find themselves working in the area of preventive medicine or public health or counseling patients who have recovered from their illnesses but need information on adequate diets. Thus, a sound knowledge of normal nutrition is required. Some patients, through genetic errors or because of allergies or for other reasons, will require nutritional management that is a slight departure from the usual; for them, of course, this will be "normal nutrition." A thorough knowledge of a patient's dietary practices obtained from the dietary history, along with awareness of the condition to be treated, forms the true foundation of diet therapy.

All that we have discussed is brought together in the three major parts of this text. Part One, Science of Nutrition, provides the background necessary for the material that follows. Included is a discussion of the nutrients: which ones are needed, how they are digested and absorbed and what happens to them when they enter the metabolic processes of the cells. Interwoven in the discussion is the treatment of the energetics of reactions, which in reality is the study of metabolic motivation—why reactions go one way and not another, why protein is synthesized or broken down.

The requirement for nutrients to sustain growth, or maintenance in the case of adults, is treated in the Unit called Nutrition in the Life Cycle. This important section of the book provides a valid appreciation of the wonderful thing that is the human machine. Here we learn that, although we are endowed with considerable latitude in our utilization of and need for the nutrients in food, the greatest efficiency is realized when nutrient intake and energy balance are optimal—optimal in this sense meaning the proper amounts and balance of nutrients and an energy intake that meets but does not exceed requirements. After this review of human nutrient needs through the life cycle, we come to a unit that describes people's individual dietary habits and what these mean when put together in the com-

munity with all of the cultural and geographic variations that define society.

Part One leads quite logically to the next section of the book, Diet Therapy and Nutritional Care in Disease. The approach is as clinical as possible so that the student is constantly aware of what is to be accomplished with each condition being treated. The metabolic changes and stresses that accompany disease or that are manifest as a result of departure from normal are presented and discussed, for this information also is necessary for the development of the appropriate nutritional care.

Part Three, Foods, discusses ways that foods can be combined into nutritious meals for proper nourishment. Nutrition, being an extremely personal matter, lends itself to all sorts of individual expressions. These can take the form of vegetarianism, esoteric meal patterns, meal skipping, gorging or abstinence from food as suits the individual. The student, then, should know about the composition of foods and what happens during processing (which includes cooking) in order to be able to evaluate the nutritional significance of any given dietary pattern and to know when to leave well enough alone and when to introduce changes to assure adequate nutrition. In the long run, that is what nutrition is all about—the provision of foods to meet nutrient and caloric needs regardless of physiological demands. This book forms a sound foundation for understanding and meeting that challenge.

PHILIP L. WHITE, Sc. D.

PREFACE

Much of today's training of the health professional takes place in an interdisciplinary setting, and this is particularly evident in dietetics and nutrition. Increasingly, the student of dietetics is receiving clinical experience in the same setting as the nursing student. The sixth edition of *Food, Nutrition and Diet Therapy* reflects this multidisciplinary training and provision of health care. We felt the need for a text that recognizes the broad area nutrition occupies in the care of patients and the fact that much nutritional care is provided by non-dietetic professionals. We also felt the need for a text that would be at the level of professional nursing and dietetic students and, in some cases, of medical students. Accordingly, this edition has been extensively revised and expanded.

Health care professionals are concerned with the mental and social well-being of their patients as well as with their physical well-being. Discussions throughout this text deal with the individual as a member of the community, but they also take into consideration the individual's uniqueness in terms of nutritional needs, life style and goals; of the meaning of food and eating; of the stage of growth and development; and particularly of the behavioral changes needed to improve dietary habits and the processes through which learning takes place.

The first part of the book is an introduction to the basic science of nutrition and deals with normal nutrition, or nutrition in the healthy individual. Woven throughout, however, are references to clinical situations that the health student is likely to meet in practice.

An important addition to this first section is Chapter 11, The Assessment of Nutritional Status, one of the chapters prepared by the new co-author. The concept of assessment is discussed along with the accepted techniques and standards for measurement of nutritional status. This chapter should arouse particular interest because it contains practical tools for measuring nutritional status in the hospital environment or in the health care agency.

Unit Three, Nutrition in the Life Cycle, discusses human growth and development and the role played by nutrition.

Added to Chapter 14, Nutrition in Infancy, is an expanded discussion of breast feeding and its advantages for the human infant. Chapter 16 has an added discussion of a newly developing area—the ways nutrition affects longevity and the aging process.

Chapter 18, Food and Nutrition in the Community, brings together in one chapter much of the information that in previous editions was covered separately. Topics of particular interest to public health practitioners, such as nutrition surveys, food budgeting, planning of inexpensive meals, food assistance programs and food legislation, are covered here. Combining this information in one chapter allows for its easy integration into a public health curriculum and also makes the chapter a very good reference.

Part Two has been retitled Diet Therapy and Nutritional Care in Disease to indicate that the concept of nutrition in health and disease is broader than a simple manipulation of the diet. Nutritional care includes education, economic support, meal planning, family planning, drug therapy, medical treatment and nursing care. The first chapter in this section, The Nutritional Care Process, describes the process of assessing the individual's nutritional status, identifying nutritional needs or problems, planning the objectives of care to meet these needs, implementing nutritional care activities and evaluating the care. Step by step the reader is taken through the process as it is applied to a specific patient. The next chapter, also new, covers the important topic of the interactions between drugs, nutrients and nutritional status. This aspect of nutritional care is particularly significant for those patients whose treatment includes many different drugs.

Beginning with Unit Six, chapters on the nutritional care for patients with various diseases are grouped according to organ systems. Chapter 32, which discusses patients who have diseases of the nervous system and mental illness, has had extensive revision to include discussions of hyperactivity and orthomolecular psychiatry and the new knowledge about the effects of certain amino acids on the level of neurotransmitters in the brain and the possible effects of this on mental functioning.

An entirely new unit on Physiological Stress includes two chapters: Chapter 34, Nutritional Care for Patients Having Surgery, Trauma or Burns, and Chapter 35, The Metabolic Stress Response and Methods for Providing Nutritional Care to Stressed Patients. Besides describing the appropriate nutritional care, this latter chapter explores the body's response to starvation as well as the effects of infection on nutritional status. Methods of nutritional support, including tube feedings, elemental diets and total parenteral nutrition, are explained in detail.

Two additional authors have contributed new chapters to this edition. Dr. Dorice Narins, Associate Professor, Clinical Nutrition, Rush University, Chicago, discusses in Chapter 36 the role of nutrition in the etiology as well as in the therapy of cancer. She also revised Chapter 7, Minerals. Deborah Roland,

Assistant Professor, Clinical Nutrition, Rush University, writes about nutrition in the care of children with inborn errors of metabolism in Chapter 39, an important addition to the book. This chapter includes a number of exchange lists to help make this information practical and useful.

Nutritional care of the high-risk or premature neonate is presented in Chapter 37, a new part of Unit Sixteen, Diseases of Infancy and Childhood. We felt this chapter was necessary because, as more of these small infants survive owing to improved methods of respiratory assistance, health professionals are faced with the need to develop techniques for feeding them. Nurses are taking more responsibility for this management in intensive care nurseries and are in need of guidelines in this rapidly expanding field.

Part Three, Foods, has been streamlined considerably in this edition. It is not meant to be the basis for a food preparation course, since nurses and dietitians in most cases are no longer responsible for the preparation of diet foods and meals and since there is a plethora of fine cookbooks to meet these needs. Basic information on foods, food purchasing and labeling is still included, for use as a reference for the student and for answering patients' questions about food preparation.

We are indebted to a number of people for help in the development of this sixth edition. Very deep appreciation goes to Sue Gentry, R.D., who gave considerable information and advice regarding the nutritional care for patients with renal disease. Kathleen Lamos, R.N., Judy Marlette, Ph.D., and Emilie Beck, R.N., deserve thanks for their critical evaluation of certain sections of the book. Other thanks go to Therese Mondeika, R.D., Dorothy Pringle, Ph.D., Donna Weihoffen, R.D., Jennifer Karr, R.D., Myra Levine, R.N., Arthur Rosoff, M.D., Paul Wong, M.D., and Kim Michaels, R.D. Sheila Henderson, R.D., Linda Brown, R.D., and the nutrition staff at Lutheran General Hospital, Des Plaines, Illinois, deserve special thanks for many of the photographs added to this edition. We would also like to thank Helen L. Dietz, Senior Nursing Editor at W. B. Saunders, for her unfailing "reminders" and tireless effort to keep us moving. Janis Moore deserves special thanks for her flexibility, persistence and cooperation in preparing the book for production. Lastly, Kathleen would like to thank her husband, Robert Raab, for his support and incredible patience throughout the process of this revision.

Marie V. Krause

L. Kathleen Mahan

CONTENTS

Part One

SCIENCE OF NUTRITION

This section of the book deals with the information relative to normal nutrition and the foods that supply it. Special emphasis is given to the principles of optimum nutrition and their application to the life cycle; appreciation of the importance of nutrition in providing and maintaining health; background and knowledge for the application of nutrition to the student's personal needs; and principles of learning and application for teaching nutrition. Stress is placed on selection of foods required to meet the physiological and psychological needs of an individual and to conform to his or her socioeconomic background.

Chapter 1

INTRODUCTION— NUTRITION IN THE HEALTH OF INDIVIDUALS AND POPULATIONS

The volume of scientific knowledge in nutrition is in the process of translation into action with a speed unparalleled in history. Much progress has been made to date in the understanding of foods and their relation to health. Most people concern themselves with food several times daily, and there is undoubtedly no practice or habit which can influence the health of an individual as much as the decisions that are made with regard to the kinds and amount of foods consumed. The body is made up of many materials. These can be supplied by a wide variety of foods to insure good health. The body is, broadly speaking, the product of its nutrition. You are what you eat. Therefore, it is important that daily decision-making on this important aspect of health be properly guided and not conditioned by pseudoscientific or faddist influences.

NUTRITION

Good nutrition is necessary for good health, and concern with food is important if certain illnesses are to be prevented. What is *nutrition?* It has different meanings. Many people identify it with that portion of nutrition that arouses their own interest. To some nutritionists, the subject is only biochemistry. To nurses, dietitians, nutritionists and physicians, nutrition may mean meals for the sick in terms of calories, protein, carbohydrate, fat, minerals and vitamins. To the layman, it represents food or it may mean a "special diet." By one definition, nutrition is "the combination of processes by which the living organism receives and utilizes the materials (food) necessary for the maintenance of its functions and for the growth and renewal of its components."[20]

Sir Harold Himsworth proposed that "nutrition is the analysis of the effect of food and its constituents on the living organism."[7] The science of nutrition is a young and dynamic biological science. It is based on the fundamental principles of chemistry and biology, biochemistry, microbiology, anatomy and physiology. The practice of nutrition is dependent upon the application of the principles of many sciences and the correlation of many disciplines, some of which include agriculture, food technology, anthropology, psychology, sociology, economics, religion, communications and education.

Nutrition, in the concept of this book is food and its relationship to the well-being of the human body. It includes (1) the metabolism of foods, (2) the nutritive value of foods, (3) the qualitative and quantitative requirements of food at different age and developmental levels to meet physiological changes and activity needs, and (4) the economic, psychological, social and cultural factors that affect the selection and eating of foods. The science and practice of nutrition exist for and attempt to contribute to a more secure life, relatively free of disease and retarded mental and physical development.

NUTRITIONAL STATUS

Sometimes the term nutrition is used to refer to the nutritional status of an individual. "The condition of the body resulting from the utilization of the essential nutrients available to the body"[1] is termed the *nutritional status*. It may

be good, fair or poor, depending on the intake of dietary essentials, on the relative need for them, and on the body's ability to utilize them.

Good nutritional status is noted when a man or woman benefits from the intake of a well-balanced dietary and there are body reserves of many of the nutrients. *Optimum* nutrition means that the essential nutrients, namely carbohydrates, proteins, fats, minerals, vitamins and water, are supplied and utilized to maintain health and well-being at the highest possible level, which is still vague and undefined.

Good nutrition is essential for normal organ development and function; for normal reproduction, growth and maintenance; for optimum activity and working efficiency; for resistance to infection; and for the ability to repair bodily damage or injury. *Poor* nutritional status exists when man is deprived of an adequate amount of the essential nutrients over an extended period of time. This is relative, because the body stores of some nutrients last longer than others. At times demands may go up, and intake, being constant, may become inadequate. The result is poor nutritional status.

Nutritional deficiencies result whenever inadequate amounts of essential nutrients are provided to tissues which require them for normal functioning. The deficiency may be primary or secondary. A *primary deficiency* may occur when the dietary is lacking in a particular nutrient or nutrients. Scurvy is due to a lack of ascorbic acid in the dietary. An adequate amount of the vitamin will correct the condition.

A nutritional deficiency disease may occur as a result of conditioning factors in persons consuming diets considered adequate. If the deficiency is caused by bodily states that interfere with digestion, absorption, or utilization of essential nutrients, or by stress factors that increase the requirements for or cause destruction or abnormal excretion of nutrients, it is referred to as a *secondary deficiency*.

Pernicious anemia, caused by a deficiency of vitamin B_{12}, is considered a secondary deficiency because individuals with this disorder cannot absorb vitamin B_{12}, even though it may be present in the food ingested. The absorption depends on the presence of an intrinsic factor, a mucoprotein enzyme secreted in the stomach.

A clear distinction between primary and secondary malnutrition in population surveys is important. False conclusions can be drawn when the conditioning factors associated with secondary malnutrition are not recognized. All examples of malnutrition are not caused by dietary inadequacies or primary deficiencies.

The first step in evaluating a person's nutritional status is to obtain a dietary history. A history of a previously inadequate diet is often the first clue to a nutritional deficiency influencing the disease process. The correlation of the information from the dietary history, medical history, physical examination, anthropometric measurements and appropriate laboratory tests is used to determine the nutritional status of an individual or group. (See Chapter 11, Assessment of Nutritional Status.)

Table 1–1 illustrates various clinical findings, which are grouped with the deficiencies or syndromes which they suggest. (Clinical deficiency signs are discussed further in Chapter 11.) Many of these clinical findings are related to deficiencies of one or more of the vitamins or minerals. Although these signs are important, their presence in tabular form does not indicate that vitamin deficiencies in nutrition are the only ones of importance. Other serious forms of malnutrition* are as prevalent, but their clinical signs are less specific. Less than normal weight and height for a certain age, for example, are important clinical indicators of calorie and protein undernutrition. These findings will be discussed in detail in subsequent chapters.

APPLIED NUTRITION

The objective of *applied nutrition* is to adapt the principles of the science of nutrition to meet the needs of an individual or group.

Dietetics is the science and art of utilizing food and the fundamental knowledge of nutrition and metabolism in various conditions of health and disease. The science consists of a knowledge of food composition and nutrient requirements in different states of health and disease, and the art consists of knowing how to plan and prepare the necessary foods, so that the individual, well or ill, will be persuaded to eat and adhere to the dietary program. This means that economic factors, individual eating patterns and cultural influences all must be considered. If the individual is ill and has little appetite, or if he has well-established food habits, the task of fulfilling the dietary prescribed may be more difficult. This calls for knowledge of the relationship of the disease

---

*Malnutrition can mean either *under-* or *over*nutrition. The prefix "mal" means bad.

process and medical therapy to appetite and the ability to apply the principles of the teaching and learning processes in order to implement a therapeutic change in the food habits of an individual.

Diet therapy is the use of food as a factor in aiding recovery from illness, relating the art and science of nutrition to the symptoms of the disease.

Nutritional care includes diet therapy but goes further to include all the services needed to apply the scientific principles of nutrition to benefit the health of an individual. It also includes food consumption information, nutritional status assessment, nutrition counseling and education, economic assistance to promote better dietary intake, and monitoring and evaluation of the individual's and community's health.

The dietary regimens are *classified* according to nutrients, fiber, texture and consistency, qualitative and quantitative restrictions, and management programs, or a combination of these factors. The high protein, high vitamin, high calorie regimen is an example of a diet concerned with nutrients. Low residue and high residue modifications are examples of diets classified according to fiber. The soft diet and liquid diet are types of dietaries prescribed for texture and consistency. Restricted or quantitative designations are the diabetic diet, the 1000 kcalorie diet and the 500 mg. sodium diet. A diet given in consecutive stages for the treatment of gastric ulcer or the therapy following massive small bowel resection is considered a type of therapeutic management program. All diets overlap in some respects. The goal is to modify the customary dietary pattern of an individual as little as possible for the therapy indicated. The nutritional care may well be, quite simply, an adequate diet.

HISTORY

Man has always been concerned about food, along with the two other factors basic to living, namely, shelter and clothing. He apparently began his life as a carnivorous animal; he was a hunter of game and a fisherman. Only at the end of the Stone Age did he begin to cultivate grains for food and add berries and honey to his staple, meat.

Archeological evidence reveals that the development of communities, towns and cities came through the settling of groups of people to cultivate foods. Learned men of ancient times offered theories about the health values of specific foods. Some of their wisdom is recorded in historical philosophical treatises and in chapters of the Bible.

During the eighteenth century when scientific discoveries were changing concepts and causing intellectual ferment, the French chemist Antoine Laurent Lavoisier recognized the relationship of the process of respiration (intake of oxygen and output of carbon dioxide) to the metabolism of food. He had discovered the role of oxygen in combustion and investigated the relation of the burning flame to the metabolism of organic foods. Lavoisier is called the "father of nutrition." He, with the physicist Laplace, used guinea pigs for the first quantitative studies on respiration, and animals have continued to play a major role in nutritional studies. These early investigations were followed by intense interest in the energy value or calorie value of foods, particularly the carbohydrates, fats and proteins.

In 1896 W. O. Atwater, who has been called "the father of American nutrition," published the first extensive table of food values ever published in this country. At that time, only proteins and calories were generally considered to be of nutritional importance. It was not until 20 years later that E. V. McCollum, one of the principal early workers in the field of accessory food factors, popularized the concept of "protective foods"—those primarily useful for their content of vitamins and minerals. Shortly after World War I, this resulted in a marked increase in the consumption of leafy vegetables, citrus fruit and milk.

At the same time Graham Lusk was exerting his far-reaching influence on dietary habits. An expert on calorie needs, it was he who first secured popular acceptance of the fact that adolescents required as much food as did adults. Space does not permit a comprehensive listing of all the other nutritionists who have contributed to our knowledge of the science of nutrition during the past century. Many men and women, ideas and equipment, along with the sciences of chemistry, physiology, biology and medicine, have contributed to the development of the science of nutrition. Some of the various pathways that have been used to accrue present knowledge in this field are summarized in Figure 1–1.

An abundance of reading material on the history of nutrition is available for exploration by

Table 1–1   CLINICAL FINDINGS AND SUGGESTED DEFICIENCY OR SYNDROME

FINDINGS	SUGGESTED DEFICIENCY OR SYNDROME
General	
Underweight (T)*	Calories, protein, calcium, phosphorus, vitamins
Underheight	Iron, zinc, folic acid, vitamin B_{12}, ascorbic acid, thiamin,
Pallor (T)	B complex
Hair	
Dry, staring hair, usually with pediculi (N)	Unknown
Skin	
Perifolliculosis (N)	Ascorbic acid, unknown
Follicular hyperkeratosis	Vitamin A, unknown
Xerosis (N)	Vitamin A, unknown
Dermatitis of pellagra (N)	Niacin
Erythematous	
Intertriginous	
Hyperkeratotic	
Ichthyotic	
Dyssebacea, especially in nasolabial folds, external canthi, behind ears and in body folds (N)	Riboflavin, unknown
Intertrigo (N)	Niacin, riboflavin, unknown
Acne (T)	
Acne vulgaris	Unknown, riboflavin, pyridoxine, vitamin A
Acne rosacea	Unknown, riboflavin
Acne varioliformis	Unknown
Palmar erythema	Unknown, B complex, riboflavin, amino acids
Spider telangiectasis	Unknown
Suborbital pigmentation (T)	Unknown
Hemorrhagic manifestations (N)	Ascorbic acid, vitamin K, unknown
Eyes	
Bitot's spots	Vitamin A
Corneal vascularity	Unknown, riboflavin
Circumcorneal injection	Unknown, riboflavin
Rosacea keratitis	Unknown, riboflavin
Follicular conjunctivitis	Vitamin A, unknown
Scarlet conjunctivitis	Niacin
Blepharitis (T)	Unknown, vitamin A, riboflavin
Canthi fissures (T)	Riboflavin, unknown
Night blindness	Vitamin A
Photophobia (T)	Vitamin A, riboflavin

*Teachers (T) or nurses (N) may be instructed to detect appearance of these signs.

the interested student. Not only is it pleasant reading, but it is essential to present and future knowledge.[9, 11, 16–19]

NATIONAL AND INTERNATIONAL NUTRITIONAL PROGRESS

In the history of nutrition science, one major trend is outstanding: the application has become ever broader. Prior to World War I, available knowledge was used mainly for the prevention and alleviation of dietary deficiency diseases in the individual or in small groups. The next step, an organized health approach, was planned distribution of preventive foods, such as butter (vitamin A), iodized salt and cod liver oil (vitamin D). Meanwhile, the isolation of vitamins progressed; and just before World War II, it became practical to improve staple foods with synthetic nutrients as a means of attacking deficiency diseases in large populations. Vitamin D was added to milk, vitamin A to margarine. White flour and bread were enriched with thiamin, riboflavin, niacin and iron. Nationwide control of specific dietary diseases was now feasible, and a program was launched. Better nutrition education, a national school lunch program, improvements in agriculture practices, advances in food handling, preservation and distribution were included in the program.

In today's atmosphere of consumerism, nothing, including nutrition, has escaped attention.

Table 1–1   CLINICAL FINDINGS AND SUGGESTED DEFICIENCY OR SYNDROME (*Continued*)

FINDINGS	SUGGESTED DEFICIENCY OR SYNDROME
Lips	
Cheilosis	Riboflavin, B complex, pyridoxine
Chapping (N)	Unknown
Increase in vertical fissuring	
Atrophic cheilosis	
Angular stomatitis (N)	Riboflavin, B complex, iron
Angular fissures (N)	Riboflavin, B complex, iron
La perleche (N)	Riboflavin, B complex, iron
Tongue	
Scarlet red glossitis (N)	Niacin, folic acid, vitamin B_{12}, protein
Beefy red glossitis (N)	Niacin, B complex, folic acid, vitamin B_{12}, protein
Magenta glossitis (N)	B complex, riboflavin
Chronic glossitis of malnutrition (N)	Niacin, folic acid, vitamin B_{12}, B complex, protein, unknown
Edema of the tongue (N)	Niacin, unknown
Oral Mucous Membranes	
Scarlet stomatitis (N)	Niacin
Lichen planus	Unknown
Leukoplakia	Unknown
Teeth and Gums	
Caries (N)	Unknown
Malocclusion (T)	Vitamin D, unknown
Scorbutic gums (N)	Vitamin C
Gingivitis	Vitamin C, unknown
Skeletal	
Rachitic deformities (N)	Vitamin D, calcium, phosphorus
Osteomalacia	Vitamin D, calcium, phosphorus
Nervous	
Nutritional polyneuropathy	Thiamin, B complex
Retrobulbar neuritis	Thiamin, unknown
Central ophthalmoplegia	Thiamin
Encephalopathic states	Thiamin, niacin, B complex, unknown
Combined system disease	B complex, vitamin B_{12}
Organic reactive psychoses	Thiamin, niacin, B complex, unknown
Circulatory	
Beriberi heart disease	Thiamin
Edema (T)	Protein, thiamin
Endocrine	
Simple goiter	Iodine

From Jolliffe, N. (ed.): Clinical Nutrition. 2nd ed. New York, Harper & Brothers, 1962.

People are becoming interested in nutrition and want to know more about their food and what is in it. We now have nutritional labeling of foods, efforts by the food companies to provide nutritionally fortified foods, and methods of dating food which allow the consumer to know how long it has been on the shelf. These changes and more, all resulting from consumer interest, result in better food and nutrition for the American people.

INTERNATIONAL NUTRITION AGENCIES

The League of Nations planted the seeds for international cooperation in nutrition by publication of a document entitled "The Relation of Nutrition to Health, Agriculture, and Economic Policy." This famous report drew attention to the connections between food and health. Although World War II prevented the cooperative plans of the League of Nations from being put into full-scale use, a series of notable events insofar as nutrition was concerned took place in the United States during this period. In 1940, the Food and Nutrition Board of the National Research Council was established and accepted the responsibility of studying nutrition on a world-wide scale. This organization studied the substantial material on nutrition published by the League of Nations and published the first recommended daily dietary allowances in 1941. These allowances have been updated and revised approxi-

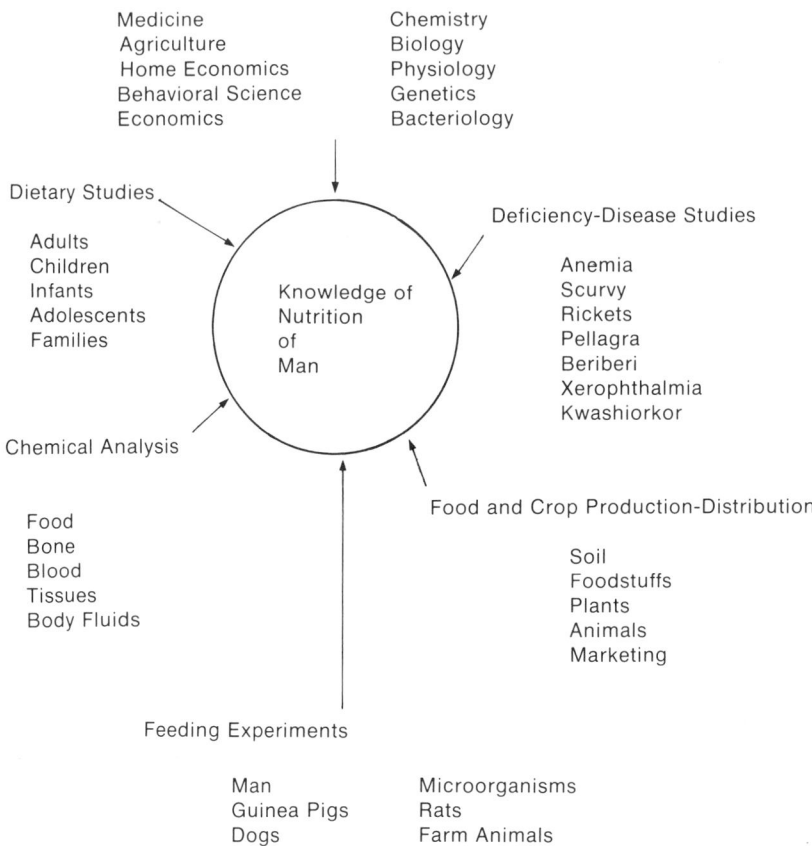

Contributing Fields:

Medicine   Chemistry
Agriculture   Biology
Home Economics   Physiology
Behavioral Science Genetics
Economics   Bacteriology

Dietary Studies

Adults
Children
Infants
Adolescents
Families

Knowledge of
Nutrition
of
Man

Deficiency-Disease Studies

Anemia
Scurvy
Rickets
Pellagra
Beriberi
Xerophthalmia
Kwashiorkor

Chemical Analysis

Food
Bone
Blood
Tissues
Body Fluids

Food and Crop Production-Distribution

Soil
Foodstuffs
Plants
Animals
Marketing

Feeding Experiments

Man   Microorganisms
Guinea Pigs Rats
Dogs   Farm Animals

Figure 1–1 Methods and areas of investigations that lead to the development of the science of nutrition. (After Lowenberg, M. E.: Food and Man. New York, John Wiley & Sons, Inc., 1967.)

mately every five years, the most recent revision being published in 1974.[3] These recommended goals can be used in planning and in evaluating food supplies for healthy people from the nutritional point of view and are discussed in detail in Chapter 10. In 1952 the amounts of nutrients adjusted to cover the additional requirements created by disease and injury as outlined by the Committee on Therapeutic Nutrition were published.[14]

After World War II, the Food and Agricultural Organization (FAO) and the World Health Organization (WHO) were created as divisions of the United Nations. FAO is dedicated to raising world-wide levels of nutrition and standards of living by securing improvement in the efficiency of production and distribution of food and agricultural products. To tackle this huge task, many sub-units of FAO were created, such as the Divisions of Nutrition, Economics, Forestry, Fisheries and Agriculture. As an example of a broad effort that one way or another involves all these specialties, one can point to the FAO-sponsored development of fish-farming. Dr. Shao Wen-ling, FAO's Chinese authority on fish-farming, helped to develop fish-farming projects in Thailand, Burma, Indonesia and Ceylon. The king of the cultivatable fishes is the common carp. Several varieties of this fish are reared in ponds, particularly in Southeast Asia, and make significant contributions to the protein content of the national dietaries. Such FAO experts as Dr. Wen-ling (seen in action in Fig. 1–2) are asked to visit a country for a given period of time. There they establish centers for

fish culture and train local personnel so that when they leave the country the work continues.

The World Health Organization (WHO) is the medically oriented unit of the United Nations. The Nutrition Division of WHO concerns itself primarily with the medical aspects of malnutrition as part of an overall effort to raise levels of nutrition throughout the world (Fig. 1–3). As might be expected, much of the work of WHO and FAO overlaps. Indeed, it has been customary during the past few years for these two organizations to convene joint committees to prepare authoritative reports on some pressing nutrition subjects, such as nutritional requirements.

Still another subdivision of the United Nations is the United Nations Children's Fund. This was originally called the United Nations International Children's Emergency Fund (UNICEF) and is still known by these initials. UNICEF is principally a supply agency and has been active in bringing relief to children of the "have-not" nations through food distribution programs using surplus foods from the "have" nations. In recent years this agency has been primarily concerned with eradication of widespread protein malnutrition and was awarded a Nobel Prize in 1965 for its great contributions to child health.

In the early seventies the three agencies—FAO, WHO and UNICEF—began combining their efforts in the form of a new program—Applied Nutrition Program (APN). With a coordination of these agencies, there can be a multifaceted, interspecialty approach.

Another United Nations Organization subdivision that sometimes works tangentially in nutrition is the United Nations Educational Scientific and Cultural Organization (UNESCO).

The International Education and Health Act of 1966, the Foreign Aid Program and the Food for Freedom Program were set up to include combating malnutrition as a major objective in their programs. The efforts of these United States programs are closely coordinated with FAO, WHO and UNICEF.

To this list of international agencies should be added the Agency for International Development, a U.S. government agency. Variously known in the past as the "Interdepartmental Committee for Nutrition in National Development (ICNND)" and the "Nutrition Section of the Office of International Research," this agency once had nutritional responsibilities principally at the

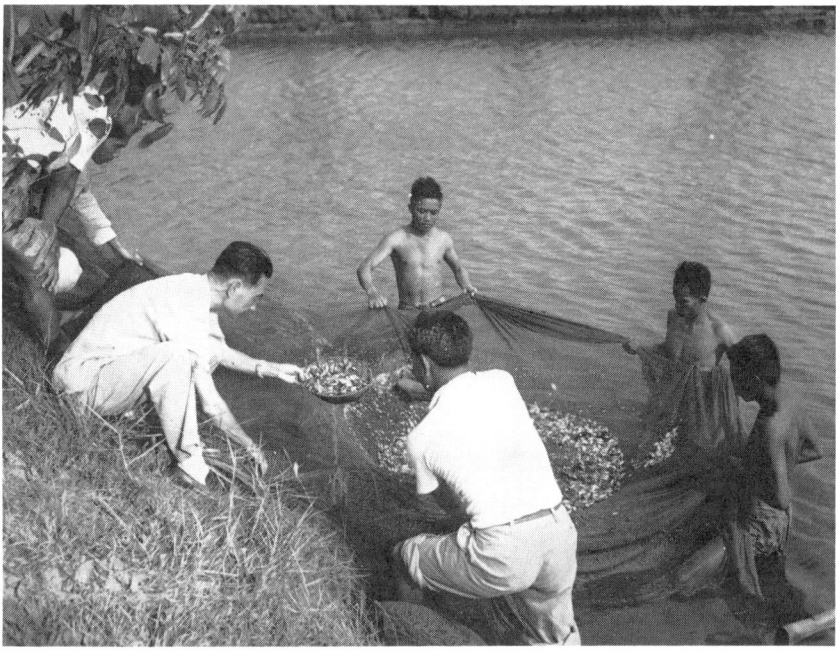

Figure 1–2 Dr. Shao Wen-ling, FAO fisheries expert, giving fish culture instruction in Thailand. This education resulted in adding much needed protein to the diet. (Courtesy of the Food and Agriculture Organization of the United Nations.)

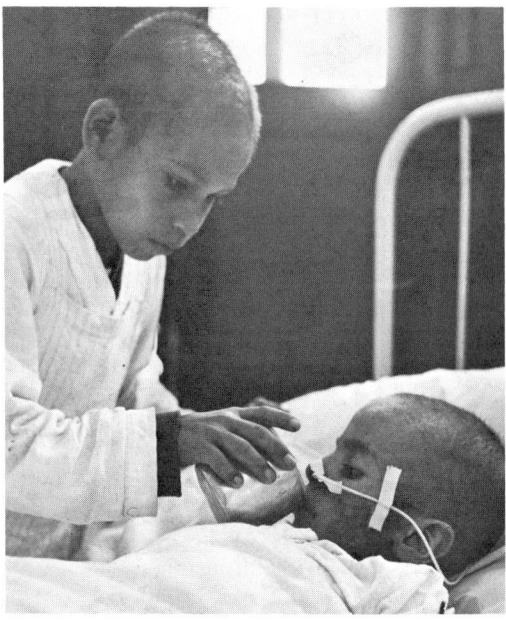

Figure 1–3 General Hospital, Guatemala City, Guatemala. Two victims of malnutrition—one recovering, the other one with a long way to go. There is almost a daily arrival of malnutrition cases at hospitals in Central America where, either because of ignorance or insufficiency, children's diets are often found to be extremely low in protein, vitamin A, and riboflavin. Eggs, meat and citrus juices are not considered foods for children. The task of nutrition education undertaken by the Institute of Nutrition of Central America and Panama is a tremendous one when it is realized that these people have used the same low nutritive value foods for generations, have seen the ravages of resulting disease without determining the cause, and have made little change in their eating habits. (Photo by Maxine Rude. Courtesy of the World Health Organization.)

international level. Its nutrition survey programs in more than 25 countries serve as models of excellence and its introduction of nutrition into long-range government planning will continue to bear fruit for years to come.

UNITED STATES NUTRITION AGENCIES

The principal agencies of the federal government of the United States involved in public health nutrition programs are the Department of Health, Education and Welfare and the Department of Agriculture. In the former department, the agencies dealing primarily with public health nutrition are the Public Health Service, the Children's Bureau and the Food and Drug Administration.

The Public Health Service provides some nutrition services for native Indians and the general population and also trains qualified candidates in public health nutrition. The Division of Medical Care Administration, concerned principally with Medicare, also deals with public health nutrition.

The National Institutes of Health not only has a program of nutrition research in its facilities in Bethesda, Maryland, but supports nutrition research through its grants program.

The Children's Bureau is principally a service agency concerned with the practical aspects of maternal and child care.

The Nutrition and Consumer Research Institute of the U.S. Department of Agriculture (USDA) coordinates nutrition services available to the public through federal, state, and other agencies. This organization works through the research and education programs of the State Land Grant Universities. The Agricultural Research Service also conducts research in its laboratories in Beltsville, Maryland, and cooperates with State Experiment Stations research programs. The standard food composition tables result largely from the food analysis data compiled and assembled by the USDA laboratories. Of great importance are the dietary surveys of the household consumption of foods in the United States performed by the USDA. The results of these studies have been published every 10 years since 1935, except in 1975. The sixth nationwide survey was started in 1977 and should be completed by 1978. These surveys show trends in food and nutrient consumption in the United States.

The Food and Drug Administration has a division of nutrition that is assigned the responsibility of insuring the safety of the national food supply. To this end it has developed analytical methods, established food standards and examined the safety of food additives. Its activity best known to the public is its constant campaign against nutrition quackery.

PRIVATE NUTRITION GROUPS

In addition to these international and federal agencies, numerous private organizations devote some or all of their energies to nutrition—both basic and applied. Among these are three professional organizations, members of which have carried on research and teaching in all aspects of nutrition. These are the American Home Economics Association (1909), the American Dietetic Association

(1917) and the American Institute of Nutrition (1933).

The Nutrition Foundation (1941) is supported by food and related industries. This organization makes funds available for nutrition research. Also, it summarizes and interprets current research in nutrition through the monthly publication, *Nutrition Reviews.*

The Department of Foods and Nutrition of the American Medical Association (A.M.A.) is an extremely active organization whose primary purpose is the dissemination of sound nutrition information to physicians. To this end it publishes scholarly articles on nutrition in the Journal of the American Medical Association and sponsors nutrition conferences and symposia. Another organization concerned primarily with nutrition education of the public is the Society for Nutrition Education.

In 1974 four private nutrition agencies formed the National Nutrition Consortium, Inc.* Concerned about the problems of the unusually low U.S. food production at the time and rising food costs and inflation, they formulated Guidelines for a National Nutrition Policy and presented them to the U.S. Senate Select Committee on Nutrition and Human Needs. This report identifies the considerations necessary for effective long-range governmental planning and implementation of food and nutrition programs in relation to the nation's health and other national responsibilities.[12] It is still speculation whether a national nutrition policy will be developed and implemented, but it certainly is needed.

WORLD NUTRITION PROBLEMS

In 1960, FAO intensified its efforts to resolve the nutrition problems by launching a 5-year Freedom from Hunger Campaign to dramatize the world's need for food. Attention was focused on information concerning research and national action programs. The United States, Canada and Australia, among other nations, contributed a great deal of financial and technical help and material toward providing food and other services to developing countries.

In May, 1966, FAO issued a statement to the effect that more babies were born in 1965 than the world can feed. Consequences of this situation, which usually means insufficient calories and protein, are far-reaching. Severe shortage of protein lowers resistance of infants and young children to most infective agents, results in the syndromes of kwashiorkor and marasmus and causes physical and mental retardation.

Iron deficiency affects millions of people in the world, augmenting the degree of anemia already caused by intestinal and blood parasites. Low levels of calcium intake, especially in children and pregnant and lactating women, and of iodine are causes for concern. In practically every nutrition survey made, vitamin A deficiency has been found in some groups of the child population. Populations which use corn as the staple food often develop pellagra. Beriberi results when polished rice constitutes 80 to 90 per cent of their diet. Ascorbic acid deficiencies occur in such countries as Ethiopia, Libya, Iran, Turkey and Chile.

The widespread suffering from undernutrition, especially in the undeveloped countries, shows that a large segment of the world's population has not yet escaped the fear of malnutrition and hunger. The effective application of the developments in agriculture, animal husbandry, and food science and technology is needed to increase food production in the developing countries. However, without limitation of the present rate of increase of the population, these efforts can achieve only limited success in combating malnutrition. The world's population and especially the population of the developing countries grew more rapidly in the decade 1962–1972 than any time previously for which we have records, and there is no indication that this rate of growth will diminish. While food production in these countries increased 2.7 per cent, population increased 2.4 per cent, leaving little real gain in food production.[13]

Another problem is the inability of governments to mount a continual, long term effort against hunger. In a lecture in 1975, Adekke Boerma, Director-General of FAO of the United Nations made the following statement in reference to the lack of progress against world hunger by the FAO since its inception over 30 years ago:

The fact is that, for most of the 30 years, the international community has been fighting the war against hunger in piecemeal fashion, without the over-all sense of commitment and integrated purpose which alone can win wars. Having failed to accept the necessary kind of general master strat-

---

*American Institute of Nutrition, American Society for Clinical Nutrition, American Dietetic Association, and the Institute of Food Technology.

egy that John Boyd Orr (first Director-General) offered, it was unable or unwilling to replace it with anything comparable. And the reason for all this, as I indicated earlier, has quite simply been the lack of political will on the part of governments. So long as no major world food crisis threatened, they felt no need for the kind of massive, concerted action that is required to overcome the world food problem once and for all. So the war drifted on, some advances being made here and there but with no frontal assault on the more difficult areas, with the result that the over-all shape of the struggle did not fundamentally change.[1]

What basically bothered the governments involved was the giving up of national sovereignty and control in order to come together and cooperate in feeding people who are hungry.

Another food crisis like a World War was needed to bring out the spirit of cooperation. Just such a crisis happened in the early seventies after several years of bad weather and the realization that the North American grain reserves were dangerously low. In 1974 a United Nations World Food Conference met in Rome with the purpose of mounting a new attack against hunger. The achievements of the Conference were the following:

1. Adoption of a comprehensive series of resolutions for increasing agricultural production in developing countries.

2. Adoption of methods for increasing the flow of external financial resources to these countries to support their efforts.

3. Endorsement of an internationally coordinated system of nationally held grain reserves involving all countries who are in a position to participate.

4. Endorsement of a Global Information and Early Warning System on food and agriculture to be operated by FAO.

5. Recommendation of an improved policy of food aid with a minimum target of 10 million tons of grain per year.

6. Recommendation of the establishment of a World Food Council as an organ of the UN General Assembly, serviced within the framework of FAO, and headquartered in Rome with political authority for carrying out the other recommendations.

Although nothing new to FAO was presented at the conference, a very valuable outcome was the "concerted thrust of political will on the part of governments" against world hunger.[1] It remains to be seen what the long-term effects of this conference will be. The UN World Food Council, created as an outcome of this meeting to promote the implementation of the resolutions, has met yearly since the first Rome conference in 1974.

In 1969 a White House Conference on Food, Nutrition and Health was held to explore what needed to be done in the United States (1) to improve the nutrition of the most vulnerable groups of people—the very poor, pregnant and nursing mothers, children and adolescents, and the aging; (2) to develop new technologies of food production, processing and packaging; (3) to improve nutrition teaching in the schools—from Head Start to nursing and medical schools; and (4) to improve Federal programs that affect nutrition such as food stamp, commodity distribution and school lunch programs. Surveys indicate considerable malnutrition (both undernutrition and overnutrition), anemia and degenerative disease in the United States. (See Chapter 18.)

Assistance is needed in areas where the problem of nutrition is of crucial importance for the development of individuals to their full potential, mentally and emotionally as well as physically. How to make enough food of the right kind available to all people everywhere and how to teach all people of the world to choose and enjoy foods for nutritive value is a great challenge.

Preventive Medicine and Nutrition

In the last half century medical care, public health and scientific research have brought about dramatic progress in the betterment of health. Perhaps nothing is more indicative of this improvement than the increase in longevity. In 1900 the average span of life in the United States was about 49 years. Today the figure is over 70.

Much of this progress has been due to the control of preventable diseases, particularly those affecting the young, and nutrition has played a large part. Malnutrition adversely affects the life, development and health of more people in the world than any disease. It kills millions of infants and small children, especially in the technically underdeveloped areas. More and more attention is being focused on preventive medicine or productive health than on curative measures. Prevention is far more effective than therapy, for what can be prevented does not need to be treated. The World Health Organization defines health as "a state of complete physical, mental, and social well-

being, and not merely the absence of disease infirmity.''[21] Nutrition is one of the most important environmental factors affecting the state of an individual's or nation's health.

A dietary *inadequate in calories* will bring about an impairment of physical efficiency, and production output diminishes in direct proportion to the caloric insufficiency. Muscle strength and muscle endurance are diminished in prolonged semistarvation.

Vitamin deficiency impairs physical fitness, affects mental well-being, and will also affect the capacity for work.

Protein deficiency causes muscular weakness, easy fatigability and, as a result, impaired work performance.

A controlled study, as well as observation during and following World War II, demonstrated clearly that poorly fed people are affected mentally as well as physically. Changes of personality and outlook were observed. As a result of inadequate nutrition, people become irritable, morose, depressed, and lacking in initiative and ambition. Sufficient kinds and amounts of food prevent or correct these changes.

Studies of industrial workers in various sections of the United States reveal that many people consume inadequate diets with resulting poor nutritional status. Poor nutrition is costly in both time and money to industry since poorly nourished workers frequently show more fatigue and less efficiency and have a higher absenteeism record due to illness than workers whose food habits are good. Nutrition education programs in work, school and health settings can be successful in improving nutritional status and learning and working efficiency.

FOOD HABITS

Food habits have been with us a long time. They are as old as yesterday, as contemporary as today, as modern as tomorrow. Food habits are the response of individuals or groups to social and cultural pressures in selecting, consuming, and utilizing portions of the available food supply.

History. Food habits, the foodways of cultures, are influenced by social organization. Through the study of habits of primitive tribes, it was found that the role of food was related to the social status as well as to the physical status of the members of the tribe. During pregnancy women received favorite foods, the implication being that a prospective warrior might be born. Children were well fed, either from the milk of the mother or from the milk of animals. The aged were nourished because they were the ones who could provide wisdom to the younger generation.

Today's social structure of rural and urban groupings has developed from yesterday's primitive tribes. In this country, since the beginning of the twentieth century, changes have occurred in social organization, with movement from rural to urban and metropolitan areas where jobs are located. With the increasing urbanization in the United States during the past generation, breakfast and lunch have become skimpier and dinner larger.

Urban food supply includes variety in food and variety in food service, while the characteristics of rural food supply are home-grown products which are home-processed, home-cooked, and home-served. However, present shipping and shopping centers throughout the country give urban and rural dwellers equal opportunities of choice in most sections of the United States. Ready to eat foods are available and utilized in both the urban and rural areas, thus replacing many of the home-prepared foods.

Development of Food Habits. The American dietary is continually changing. Changes in food habits are motivated by moral dictation, social desirability, scientific sanction or forced changes which are stimulated by physical circumstances, such as pressure for time, crop failures, or lowering of economic status of individuals, groups or nations, which may follow as the result of war. The most notable changes are those which have resulted from improvement in transportation. At the beginning of the twentieth century, the United States was largely agricultural and a considerable proportion of the food was grown by the consumer or his neighbors. With the present elaborate system of transportation, perishable foods are available the year round, as refrigeration, automated processing and packaging conspire to defy seasons and banish spoilage. Technological advancements have made it possible for innumerable new items to appear on grocery shelves and, ultimately, on the family table.

Attitudes toward foods are influenced by the geographical location. Groups residing along the seacoast where fish is available like to eat fish, while inland groups eat available grains and the flesh of animals.

Changes in food habits are also motivated by the bodily state of individuals during pregnancy, illness, aging and obesity. An illness which imposes dietary restrictions or an unpleasant experience with food may result in a lifelong avoidance of some particular food or foods. Food used as a punishment for children may result in a permanent dislike of the food the child is forced to eat.

The baby is taught to eat foods which the mother likes and which the mother had been taught to eat by her mother. If the mother likes sweetened cereal, the baby will establish a habit of eating sweetened cereal. (See page 316, eating habits and the psychology of infant and child feeding.) The growing child is influenced by the environment and habits of the family group (see page 332, adolescent food habits), the social group, the school group and, later, the work or professional group. If there is an intermarriage of cultures, an adjustment or blending of the eating habits of the wedded nationalities occurs. The offspring from this intermarriage are influenced by the food habits of each parent.

Each nationality has characteristic food patterns. The food patterns are developed from available foods. For example, cereal or rice is the basic core of the food pattern of Orientals, while meat is the principal core of the Eskimo's food pattern. A mixture of food is the basis of our food pattern. Characteristic beverages, supplementary foods, and ceremonial or festival foods are added to the food plans. (Consult Chapter 17.)

Food also has social and ceremonial significances. Many business transactions are conducted at the dining table in a club or restaurant. To maintain social position, women's clubs hold their meetings at a luncheon in a desirable hotel. Holidays are celebrated with special meals. Religious festivities are designated with feasts or banquets, and decisive moments in life, such as christenings, weddings, and funerals, are honored with serving of special food.

Food habits are largely established during early childhood and can be changed later only by gradual introduction of new foods and new ideas. The enlarged dietary of many Americans shows that new food will be accepted. Europeans and others came to America with their national foods. Now many people, and not only in large urban centers, enjoy Italian spaghetti, Chinese specialties, German sauerkraut, Mexican tacos and many others.

Poor food habits account for a large number of the nutritional deficiencies which are prevalent today. Persons who skip meals, those who are grossly overweight, and poorly nourished teen-age girls are groups who have acquired poor food habits. Studies in the United States reveal that many Americans have low nutritional standards, and poor food habits through the years ultimately take a toll. A poor diet is the first step toward poor nutrition. To improve the nutritional status and health of the masses, better food habits are needed. The changes an individual will make in his or her dietary depend on the motivation he or she develops. The nutritionist or nutrition counselor is in a position to identify that motivation and to determine whether the individual's dietary provides the essential nutrients. In this way, the nutritionist or nurse identifies the group of foods supplying the nutrients that the individual must include or restrict in order to improve nutritional intake. Thus the individual may adhere to his customary pattern and be encouraged to select foods providing the necessary nutrients from those known to him.

FOOD FADS, FALLACIES AND QUACKERY

There are always faddists who insist there is some magic quality in some peculiar kind of food or diet. Examples are the grapefruit diet, or use of large amounts of seaweed or of blackstrap molasses. Various fad diets have caught the fancy of the overweight populace who try to lose poundage by "not counting calories," consuming extra protein foods, or adhering to formula diet routines. There are the self-styled "experts"—food quacks—who have a smattering of knowledge or are promoting some patented product they want to sell. Food faddists and food quacks are closely related. The psychosomatic manifestations of food dislikes are numerous, adding to food fallacies and symbolism.

The mere fact that a diet sounds extraordinary is no reason for condemning it if it is adequate in nutrients. In fact various native diets may sound strange to an American but provide nutrients as well as or better than the pattern to which he or she is accustomed. The type of fad diet which is not recommended is one which is inadequate in nutrients or recommends replacing wholesome foods with expensive so-called "health foods."

Television and radio advertising are often

misleading. Facts of minor importance are built up to suit advertising purposes. The same is true of popular or unreliable literature. The information may not necessarily be harmful but may lead to use of the fad food, which is expensive, at the sacrifice of relatively inexpensive, basic foods that are needed.

The promotion of the use of vitamin concentrates has been overworked in the field of advertising. There is a definite need for these products, but they should be taken under the advice of a physician, not because they are recommended on the radio or television. It is the general consensus that the natural foodstuffs rich in the various vitamins are the best source. The American people have been made exceedingly "diet-conscious." "Diet" usually means a specific hard-to-follow regimen. Clever advertising through the radio, television, the press, drug store windows, and the mail has done much to convince the public that it needs to buy, at high prices, products which actually could be supplied from ordinary foodstuffs at little additional cost. This is especially true regarding the vitamins. (See Fig. 1–4.) As Gifft and associates stated: "They (Americans) know enough to be concerned but not enough to differentiate between legitimate and spurious causes for concern or to recognize when claims and warnings are based on misinformation or on valid information erroneously applied."[5]

The Food and Drug Administration is particularly concerned about the promotion of "food supplements" as cure-alls for conditions which require medical attention. In 1958 the Food and Drug Administration[4] outlined the following four basic "myths" of nutrition used by practically all food-fad promoters:

Myth No. 1. *Most disease is due to faulty diet.* It is implied that it is virtually impossible for the average person to obtain an adequate dietary without use of a food supplement. False claims for prevention or cure of many serious diseases are made in favor of the preparation being promoted.

Myth No. 2. *Soil depletion causes malnutrition.* It is claimed that crops grown on poor soil or where chemical fertilizers are used are nutritionally inferior. The true story is that genetic make-up of the seed, not soil fertility, primarily affects the nutritional composition of a food.[8] The *quantity* may be reduced on poor soil but there will be very little if any effect on the *quality*.

Myth No. 3. *Foods are overprocessed.* The faddists claim that much nutritive value is lost in processed foods such as white flour, milled cereals, canned foods, and even pasteurized milk. This is very much exaggerated.

Myth No. 4. *Subclinical deficiencies are a constant danger.* It is claimed that anyone with a tired feeling, an ache or a pain in any part of the body is using a faulty diet and needs a supplement of some kind. This is an especially appealing argument for the hypochondriac who is looking for just such a "cure." Diseases caused by dietary deficiencies are relatively rare in the United States, and the food supply is unsurpassed in volume, variety and nutritional value. Any normal person will experience occasional worn-out, dragged-down feelings. If such feelings persist, the advice of a competent physician should be sought, not that of a food quack.

Certain food superstitions have been brought down through the ages with no basis of truth. For example, one will hear that "milk products and fish cannot be eaten at the same meal"; that "fish and celery are brain foods"; that "whole wheat bread is low in calories"; that "honey has no calories"; that "tomato juice makes acid"; that "starch and protein

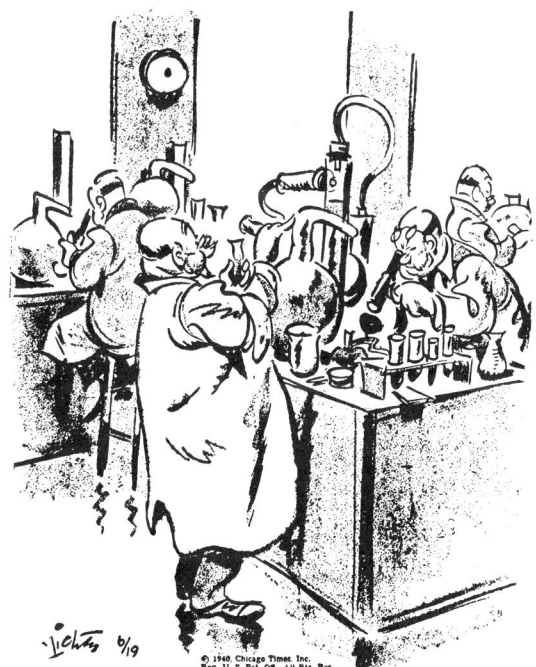

Figure 1–4 "I've worked on vitamins for years and I've discovered that the three most important elements necessary to life are breakfast, lunch and dinner!" (Courtesy of George Lichty and the Chicago Sun-Times Syndicate.)

cannot be eaten together,'' and many other ''facts'' equally as ridiculous.

Combating Food Faddism. Whenever an individual is persuaded to eat a food or group of foods for a health reason, it is the health benefit as *perceived* by the individual and not the actual benefits or lack of them that is important. The motive of using food to promote health is present, but it needs to be redirected through more nutrition education. The most effective means of combating food faddism and misinformation is through nutrition education. A properly informed population will not succumb to false propaganda. The health professional has many opportunities to clarify the information and to present sound facts, as well as to set an example through good food attitudes and food habits, including weight control. The American Medical Association, the American Dietetic Association, and other related groups have extensive programs and available material to combat food fallacies and quackery.

THE NUTRITIONAL CARE OF PATIENTS

While the nurse does not plan menus or prepare foods served to patients in the hospital or in the home, assistance in meeting their nutritional needs is given by her or him in many ways. With the help of the dietitian he or she can devise ways and means of feeding those who have to be fed and encourage those who need to consume an adequate amount of food. It is important to know whether the patient eats the food served and how much he eats. The nurse consults with members of the team concerning the nutritional welfare of the patients and takes the necessary steps to revise the dietary regimen or resolve the problems presented. She or he implements the knowledge of nutrition principles and understanding of the eating practices of people in the nursing care that is given to patients in the hospital or in the home. Nutritional care should always be part of the total care plan for a patient. (See Chapter 20, The Nutritional Care Process.)

A patient's eating habits are influenced largely by his economic status, food idiosyncrasies, nationality or ethnic group, religion and social environment. During his or her hospitalization, especially if it is prolonged, the nurse and dietitian/nutritionist have an opportunity to assist the person to improve his customary dietary where indicated. Many patients utilize their hospitalization as a learning experience and are motivated to make changes in their food habits. Objectives for nutrition education in the care plans for these patients are especially useful. Often times, individuals on the regular dietary of the hospital offer as much of a challenge for teaching as those on therapeutic regimens. The extent to which they will adjust to or adopt the change in their customary pattern will depend largely on how they perceive the task. An individual may find the choice of food and the regimen unsatisfactory, and if the nurse or dietitian has not explored with him his usual selections, he will not have benefited by his hospitalization from a nutritional viewpoint.

To change deep-seated food habits is usually a slow process. Extensive changes must be made as gradually as possible, with complete understanding on the part of the patient as to why the change is being made. In certain circumstances, while giving a bath, making an assessment, or delivering the food tray, the nurse has an excellent opportunity to teach good food habits. He or she can discuss or make suggestions to guide the patient toward good habits.

Nutrition is considered one of the important medical sciences and has an important place in health care today. It is vital in the attainment and maintenance of good health, as well as in the treatment of disease. Research in nutrition is being carried on in many colleges and universities throughout the world, and clinical nutrition research is expanding rapidly. It is a comparatively new science. Thus, many of the concepts and much of the knowledge gained so far must be considered as subject to modification when still more knowledge is obtained. The nutrition picture is constantly changing. Progress lies in research, investigation, and new knowledge.

The study of nutrition fulfills the twofold purpose of education: (1) it provides knowledge useful in personal living, and (2) it provides knowledge useful for professional practice. It is the responsibility of every student of health to apply personally the principles of nutrition and to pass on to others the knowledge gained in order to keep a far-reaching nutritional improvement program alive.

PROBLEMS AND SUGGESTED TOPICS FOR DISCUSSION

1. What do the following terms mean: nutrition, optimum nutrition, dietetics, science of nutrition, nutritional status, health, diet, diet therapy, and applied nutrition? Explain the difference between food and nutrition.

2. How are nutrition and health related?
3. Explain the importance of food habits. How are food habits developed? Analyze your food habits, and decide which ones need to be improved.
4. From the list of references select those pertaining to the history of nutrition and prepare a short report on some historical event in nutrition.
5. List at least ten "food fads and fallacies," and state what is wrong with each one.
6. Analyze the community where you live and describe an example in which a community agency has fostered improved nutrition.
7. Explain how nutrition becomes an aspect of total nursing care.

CITED REFERENCES

1. Boerma, A. H.: The 30 years' war against world hunger. Proc. Nutr. Soc., *34*:145, 1975.
2. Elvehjem, C. A.: A forty year look at nutrition research. J. Am. Diet. Assoc., *38*:236, 1961.
3. Food and Nutrition Board, National Research Council: Recommended Dietary Allowances. 8th ed. Washington, D.C., National Academy of Sciences, 1974.
4. Food Facts Vs. Food Fallacies. Washington, D.C., Food and Drug Administration, 1958.
5. Gifft, H., Washbon, M. and Harrison, G. G.: Nutrition, Behavior, and Change. Englewood Cliffs, New Jersey, Prentice-Hall, Inc., 1972.
6. Goldblith, S. A. and Joslyn, M. A.: Milestones in Nutrition. Westport, Connecticut, AVI Publishing Co., 1964.
7. Himsworth, H.: What nutrition really means. Nutr. Today, *3*(3):18, 1968.
8. Janssen, W. F.: Food quackery—a law enforcement problem. J. Am. Diet. Assoc., *36*:110, 1960.
9. Lowenberg, M. E., et al.: Food and Man. 2nd ed. New York, John Wiley & Sons, 1974.
10. Lusk, G.: In Nutrition. Clio Medica Series, Paul B. Hoeber, New York, 1933.
11. McCollum, E. V.: A History of Nutrition—The Sequence of Ideas in Nutrition Investigations. Boston, Houghton Mifflin Co., 1957.
12. National Nutrition Consortium, Inc.: Guidelines for a National Nutrition Policy. U.S. Senate Select Committee on Nutrition and Human Needs, Washington, D.C., U.S. Government Printing Office, 1974. (Also in Nutr. Rev., May, 1974.)
13. Panel on Nutrition and the International Situation to the Senate Select Committee on Nutrition and Human Needs: National Nutrition Policy—Report and Recommendation VI. Washington, D.C., U.S. Government Printing Office, 1974.
14. Pollack, H. and Halpern, S. L.: Therapeutic Nutrition. Washington, D.C., National Research Council, National Academy of Sciences, Publ. No. 234, 1952.
15. Roe, D. A.: A Plague of Corn: The Social History of Pellagra. Ithaca, New York, Cornell University Press, 1973.
16. Todhunter, E. N.: Development of knowledge in nutrition, Part I: animal experiments and Part II: human experiments. J. Am. Diet. Assoc., *41*:328 and 335, 1962.
17. Todhunter, E. N.: Some classics of nutrition and dietetics. J. Am. Diet. Assoc., *44*:100, 1964.
18. Todhunter, E. N.: The evolution of nutrition concepts—perspectives and new horizons. J. Am. Diet. Assoc., *46*:120, 1965.
19. Todhunter, E. N., Darby, W. J., and McNutt, K. W.: A Bedside Library for Nutrition Scholars in Present Knowledge in Nutrition. 4th ed. New York, The Nutrition Foundation, Inc., 1976, pp. 557–574.
20. Turner, D.: Handbook of Diet Therapy. 5th ed. Chicago, University of Chicago Press, 1970.
21. World Health Organization—What It Is, What It Does. How It Works. Geneva, Switz., WHO, 1956.

ADDITIONAL REFERENCES

Arrington, L. R.: Foods of the Bible. J. Am. Dietet. A., *35*:816, 1959.
Bell, J. N.: Let 'em eat hay. Today's Health, Sept., 1958.
Bengoa, J. M.: Nutrition activities of the World Health Organization. J. Am. Dietet. A., *55*:228, 1969.
Bogert, L. J., Briggs, G. M. and Calloway, D. H.: Nutrition and Physical Fitness. 9th ed. Philadelphia, W. B. Saunders Company, 1973, Chapters 1 and 16.
Bruch, H.: The allure of food cults and nutrition quackery. J. Am. Dietet. A., *57*:316, 1970.
Darby, W. J. (ed.): Food—The Gift of Osiris. 2 volumes. London: Academic Press, 1977.
Food and Agriculture Organization: Nutrition and Working Efficiency. Pamphlet. Rome, 1962.
Food and Agriculture Organization: World Food Problems. No. 2: Man and Hunger. Pamphlet. Rome, 1957.
Food and Nutrition. Science, *188*:501, 1975.
Food Facts Talk Back. Chicago, American Dietetic Association, 1957.
Hegsted, D. M.: Food and nutrition policy—now and in the future. J. Am. Diet. Assoc., *64*:367, 1974.
Holt, L. E.: Perspective in nutrition—Nutrition in a changing world. Am. J. Clin. Med., *11*:543, 1962.
Joint FAO/WHO Ad Hoc Expert Committee: Energy and Protein Requirements. Technical Rep. No. 522, Geneva, Switz., WHO, 1973.
Jukes, T.: Down the primrose path with "organic" foods. School Foodservice J., *28*:52, 1974.
King, C. G.: America's role in world nutrition. Review of Nutrition Research. New York, Borden, Inc., *30*(1):1, 1969.
— — —: Notes on history of nutrition in America. J. Am. Dietet. A.: *56*:188, 1970.
McHenry, E. W.: Foods Without Fads. Philadelphia, J. B. Lippincott, 1960.
Mead, M.: Food Habits Research: Problems of the 1960's. Washington, D.C., National Academy of Sciences—National Research Council, Publ. No. 1225, 1964.
Moore, H. B.: The meaning of food. Am. J. Clin. Nutrition, *5*:77, 1957.
National Academy of Science: Role of Nutrition in International Programs. Pamphlet. Washington, D.C., National Research Council, 1961.
Nutrition misinformation and food faddism. Nutr. Rev., *32* (Suppl.), July, 1974.
Paddock, W., and Paddock, P.: Famine—1975. America's decision: Who will survive? Boston, Little, Brown and Company, 1967.
Schaefer, A. E., et al.: Are we well fed? Nutrition Today, *4*:2, Spring, 1969.
Schafer, R. and Yetley, E. A.: Social psychology of food faddism. J. Am. Diet. Assoc., *66*:129, 1975.

Senate Select Committee on Nutrition and Human Needs: National Nutrition Policy Study—Report and Recommendation—IV. Washington, D.C., U.S. Government Printing Office, 1974.

Simoons, F. J.: Eat Not This Flesh: Food Avoidances in the Old World. Madison, Wisconsin, University of Wisconsin Press, 1961.

Stiebeling, H. K.: Our share in better world nutrition. J. Am. Dietet. A., *45*:315, 1964.

Stiebeling, H. K.: Improved use of nutritional knowledge—Progress and problems. J. Am. Dietet. A., *45*:321, 1964.

Swaminathan, M.: Nutrition and the world food problem. Review of Nutrition Research, New York, Borden Inc., *28*(1):1, 1967.

UNIT ONE

NUTRIENTS IN FOOD— THEIR DIGESTION, ABSORPTION AND METABOLISM

INTRODUCTION

Foods constitute all the solid and liquid materials taken into the digestive tract that are utilized to maintain and build body tissues, regulate body processes and supply heat, thereby sustaining life.

Foods are composed of various compounds, both organic and inorganic, so that any food is a chemical compound or mixture of chemical compounds. These compounds and elements of which foods are composed are proteins, lipids, carbohydrates, minerals, vitamins and water, and can be grouped as organic and inorganic compounds and elements.

Organic Compounds. Proteins, lipids, carbohydrates, vitamins.

Inorganic Elements. Water and minerals: calcium, phosphorus, sodium, potassium, sulfur, chlorine, iron, iodine, copper, magnesium, manganese, cobalt, zinc and others.

The constituents in food are known as nutrients. For all the nutrients essential to normal functioning, the body must depend on the wise selection of foods. If food is not properly chosen, there will be an inadequacy of one or more of the essential nutrients. An essential nutrient is one that must be provided to the body by food. It cannot be synthesized by the body. The nutrients that must be supplied in food and are essential for growth and normal functioning of the body are as follows:

Proteins as sources of the following amino acids:

      isoleucine
      leucine
      lysine
      methionine
      phenylalanine
      threonine
      tryptophan
      valine

Minerals:

      calcium
      phosphorus
      iron
      sodium
      potassium
      iodine
      magnesium
      sulphur
      chlorine
      manganese
      copper
      zinc
      cobalt
      molybdenum

Carbohydrate as source of:
      glucose

Fat as source of:
      linoleic acid

Fat-soluble Vitamins:
      A
      D
      E
      K

Water-soluble Vitamins:
      thiamin
      riboflavin
      niacin
      pyridoxine
      ascorbic acid
      folic acid
      cobalamin

All the food constituents enumerated above and their specific functions in human nutrition will be more fully discussed in later chapters under their respective headings.

METABOLISM

Metabolism comes from a Greek word, "metaballein," meaning to change or alter. Broadly speaking, metabolism may be defined as tissue change. It is the chemical process of transforming foods into complex tissue elements and of transforming complex body substances into simple ones, along with the production of heat and energy. See Figure 2–1 for an illustration of where the metabolic processes take place within a cell. The two main phases of metabolism are (1) *anabolism,* the synthesis of cellular materials for growth, maintenance and repair of body tissues and (2) *catabolism,* the breaking down of cellular materials into simpler constituents for energy production or excretion.

The anabolic processes are the chemical changes whereby simple substances are combined to form more complex substances with the net result that new cellular materials are produced and energy is stored. The catabolic processes are concerned with the breaking down of the complex substances, which results in the release of energy and a wearing out and using up of cellular materials. These processes occur constantly and simultaneously in the body. When anabolism exceeds catabolism, growth occurs. If catabolism exceeds anabolism, the breakdown is faster than the building up processes, making the body lose substance and weight. In health, a balance is maintained between these two constantly operating opposing processes so that body weight and tissue substance are maintained, or added to if desired.

The amount of food consumed can have a profound effect on whether anabolism or catabolism will predominate in a given situation. The person who consumes less food than he requires loses weight because the catabolic state predominates. The person who consumes more food than required and gains adipose tissue is in an anabolic state.

Some factors that increase anabolism are increase in the supply of raw materials (food) to the body, rest and certain endocrine secretions such as insulin and some adrenal and sex hormones (for example, during adolescence increased secretions of sex hormones stimulate growth). Some factors that increase catabolism are fever, bacterial toxins, fractures, burns and certain endocrine secretions (for example, thyroxine and cortisone).

Chapter 2

ENERGY

Energy is defined as the capacity to do work or to produce a change in matter. When used in nutrition, energy deals mostly with the chemical energy locked in foodstuffs by reason of the chemical bonding present in the nutrients.

The ultimate source of all energy in living organisms is derived from the energy of the sun. Plants transform heat and light, through the action of chlorophyll with sunlight (photosynthesis), into energy which is stored as po-

tential chemical bond energy within different foodstuffs, principally as carbohydrates, proteins and fats. (See Chapter 3, Fig. 3–1.) This chemical energy is used by animals which are unable to use the energy of the sun directly.

The comparisons often drawn between a steam engine and the human body, while useful, may be misleading. The steam engine relies upon the combustion of fuel to yield heat to generate steam to perform work required. Al-

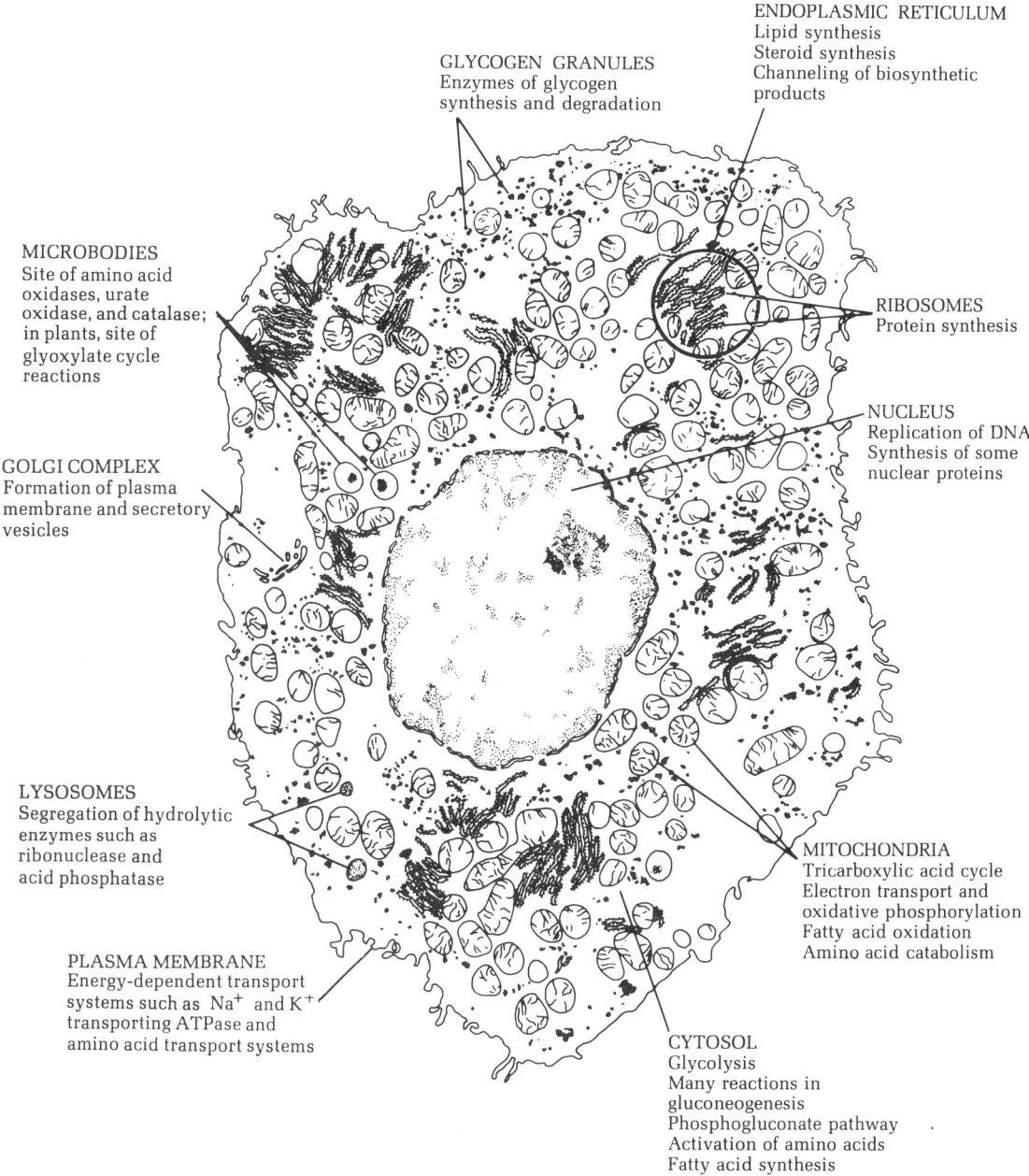

ENDOPLASMIC RETICULUM
Lipid synthesis
Steroid synthesis
Channeling of biosynthetic
products

GLYCOGEN GRANULES
Enzymes of glycogen
synthesis and degradation

MICROBODIES
Site of amino acid
oxidases, urate
oxidase, and catalase;
in plants, site of
glyoxylate cycle
reactions

RIBOSOMES
Protein synthesis

NUCLEUS
Replication of DNA
Synthesis of some
nuclear proteins

GOLGI COMPLEX
Formation of plasma
membrane and secretory
vesicles

LYSOSOMES
Segregation of hydrolytic
enzymes such as
ribonuclease and
acid phosphatase

MITOCHONDRIA
Tricarboxylic acid cycle
Electron transport and
oxidative phosphorylation
Fatty acid oxidation
Amino acid catabolism

PLASMA MEMBRANE
Energy-dependent transport
systems such as Na^+ and K^+
transporting ATPase and
amino acid transport systems

CYTOSOL
Glycolysis
Many reactions in
gluconeogenesis
Phosphogluconate pathway
Activation of amino acids
Fatty acid synthesis

Figure 2–1 Compartmentation of some important enzymes and metabolic sequences in the liver cell of the rat. Traced from an electron micrograph. (From: Lehninger, A. L.: Biochemistry, 2nd ed. Worth Publishers, 1976.)

though foods undergo combustion in the body and eventually yield heat, that heat is not productive. It is largely a by-product of metabolism generated by the mechanical activity of muscles (mechanical energy). It is useful in that it does maintain body temperature. The chemical energy available from foods is used for muscular work (kinetic energy), for brain and nerve activity (electrical energy) and in synthesis of body tissue (chemical energy). Man's source of energy is released by the metabolism of food and it must be supplied regularly to meet the energy needs for the body's survival.

Production of ATP for Storage of Energy

The foods from which energy is available (carbohydrate, fat and protein) are converted in the body to glucose, fatty acids and amino acids before they reach the cell. Within the cell these nutrients react with oxygen to form carbon dioxide and water. This over-all reaction proceeds through a long series of steps, with the rates of reaction controlled by various enzymes. The energy produced is used to form *adenosine triphosphate (ATP)*. ATP is a nucleotide composed of adenine (nitrogen base), ribose (pentose sugar) and three phosphate radicals. The last two phosphate radicals in this compound are attached through an *energy-rich bond*. These bonds contain several times the energy of other chemical bonds and are very labile. ATP can release its energy instantly for mechanical work (muscle contraction), transport of material through cell walls and syntheses of chemical compounds. In the reaction ADP (adenosine diphosphate) is formed, which can be phosphorylated to ATP by the oxidative reactions. This process is continuous. ATP has been referred to as the energy currency of the cell, for it can be spent and remade again and again.[7] (See Fig. 2–2.)

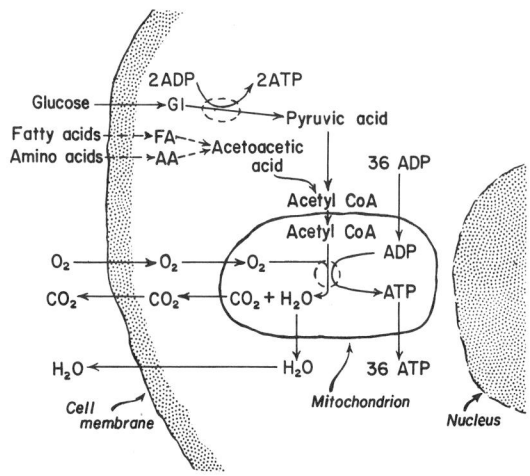

Figure 2–2 Formation of adenosine triphosphate in the cell, showing that most of the ATP is formed in the mitochondrion. (From: Guyton, A. C.: Textbook of Medical Physiology, 5th ed. W. B. Saunders Co., 1976, p. 22.)

Enzymes in Metabolism

The rapid chemical changes are brought about by the action of enzymes, coenzymes and hormones. They control biologic oxidation of the cells. Every cell synthesizes the thousands of enzymes required for its metabolic processes. They are proteins of high molecular weight. Those enzymes concerned with metabolism of the cell are usually retained within the cell and are called *endoenzymes*. Those enzymes which are released by the cell and catalyze reactions in the environment of the cell are called *exoenzymes*. These are the digestive enzymes, a small group but very important to nutrition. They are liberated by special cells in the salivary glands, liver, pancreas and intestinal mucosa and pass into the digestive tract where they reduce foodstuffs to simpler, readily absorbed compounds.

Enzymes show a great deal of *specificity* in that each enzyme is so constructed that it will catalyze only one particular reaction. The compound being acted on by an enzyme is called the enzyme's *substrate*. It is thought that the enzyme and its substrate fit together like lock and key during the catalytic process. The enzyme and substrate must fit together or the reaction will not take place. They first combine in a complex, then break apart, producing the new reaction products and the original enzyme. Evidence suggests that the enzyme attaches to its substrate at two points on the substrate surface. This attachment places a strain upon the substrate molecule, so that it becomes reactive; the enzyme breaks away unchanged and is ready to repeat the process.

Some enzymes (pepsin, for example) consist entirely of protein, while others may contain a non-protein portion. The protein part is called the *apoenzyme* and the non-protein part is called a *coenzyme*. Coenzymes are usually small, organic molecules (of which the B vitamins are a part) and almost always contain a phosphate group. The reactions involved in cellular oxidation and formation of ATP require a series of enzymes with their coenzymes to effect the combination of hydrogen with oxygen to form water. These with all the other enzymes of the oxidative process are believed to be arranged in an orderly fashion on the inner surface of the mitochondria (Fig. 2–3), thus facilitating rapid procession of the chemical reactions.

Hormones in Metabolism

Hormones, which are secretions of the endocrine glands, act as *chemical messengers* in energy production to *initiate or control* enzyme action. Thyroxine from the thyroid gland controls the body's metabolic rate; production of

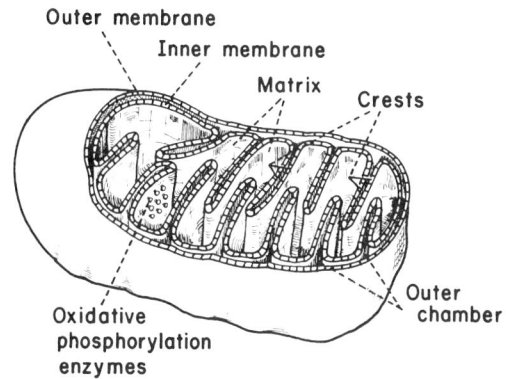

Figure 2–3 Structure of a mitochondrion. (Modified from: De Robertis, Saez, and De Robertis: Cell Biology, 6th ed. 1975. In Guyton, A. C.: Textbook of Medical Physiology, 5th ed. W. B. Saunders, 1976.)

thyroxine, in turn, is controlled by thyrotropic hormone from the anterior pituitary gland. Steroid hormones regulate the ability of the cell to synthesize enzymes. Insulin secreted by the pancreas gland controls the rate of glucose utilization in the tissues.

THE CALORIE

The unit of energy commonly used in human nutrition is the *kilocalorie* (kcalorie or 1000 calories). Although kilocalorie is the proper term, *calorie* is commonly used interchangeably. The *calorie* is the standard unit for measure of heat. Since heat is one result of energy generated by the body, the calorie can serve as a measure of energy production. *One kcalorie* is the heat energy required to raise the temperature of 1 kilogram of water 1 degree Centigrade.

MEASUREMENT

The total caloric content (total energy) available from a food can be measured by means of a device called a bomb calorimeter. (See Fig. 2–4.) This consists of a closed steel container in which the food is burned while the container is immersed in a known volume of water. The weighed food sample is burned in an oxygen atmosphere by igniting it with an electric spark. The rise in temperature of the water after ignition of food can be used to calculate the heat energy or calories generated. Each food has a specific caloric value; that is, a given amount of food will yield a certain number of calories when metabolized, and the caloric yield depends on the composition of the food in terms of protein, fat and carbohydrate.

The amount of heat produced per gram of purified samples of protein, fat and carbohydrate burned in the bomb calorimeter is as follows:

1 gm. of protein	5.65 kcalories
1 gm. of fat	9.45 kcalories
1 gm. of carbohydrate	4.10 kcalories

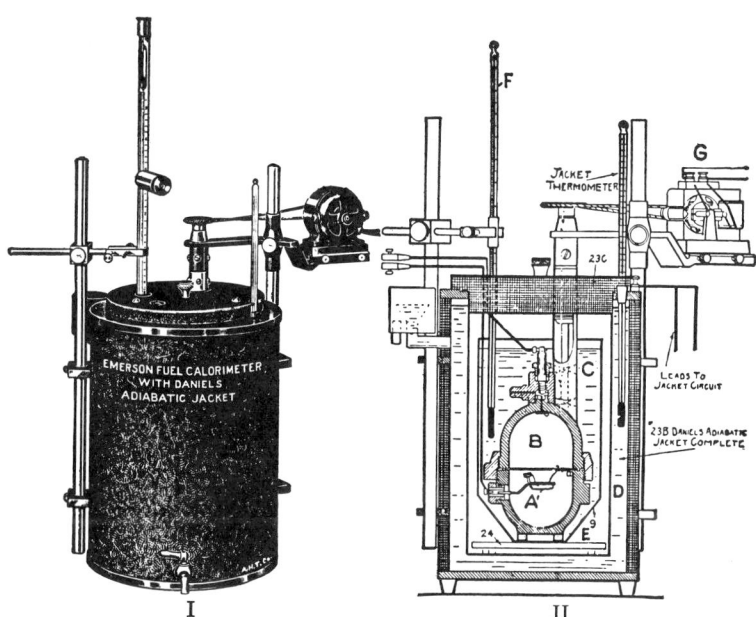

I   II

Figure 2–4 Bomb calorimeter as seen from the outside (I) and in longitudinal section (II). The water in the inner chamber (C) changes in temperature when the food in the food pan (A) is burned. The water in the outer chamber (D) acts as insulation, with the intervening air in the air space (E). The amount of heat produced is measured at F by the change in temperature of a measured amount of water. B is an oxygen chamber, and G is an electric motor for stirring the water.

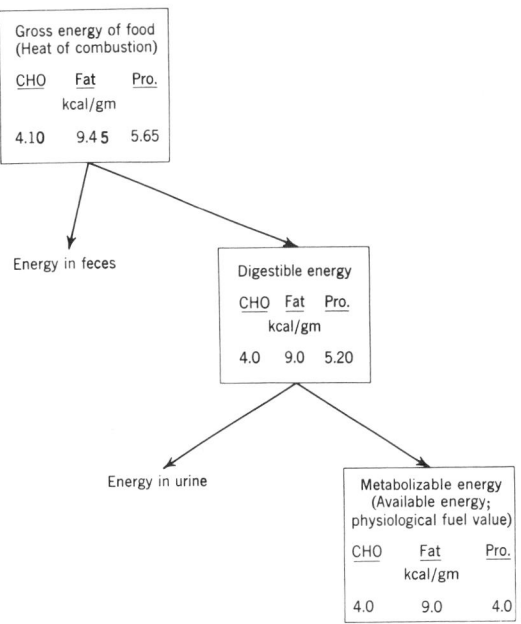

Figure 2–5   Energy value of food. (From: Pike, R. L., and Brown, M. L.: Nutrition: An Integrated Approach, 2nd ed. John Wiley and Sons, 1975.)

Calculation of Food Value. The energy value of one tablespoon of oil (14 grams of fat) is approximately 126 kcalories (14 × 9). Most foods, however, are complex and contain protein, fat and carbohydrate. For example, 2 eggs (100 grams) contain approximately:

13% protein or	
13 gm. × 4 kcal./gm.	= 52 kcalories
12% fat or	
12 gm. × 9 kcal./gm.	= 108 kcalories
1% carbohydrate or	
1 gm. × 4 kcal./gm.	= 4 kcalories
Total	164 kcalories

Research in food values has repeatedly demonstrated that the composition of foods is variable because of factors beyond control, such as climate, soil, variety, degree of maturity, storage, methods of handling and analyzing.

More precise calorie values of foods based on analysis of samples reported by chemists may be found in *The Agriculture Handbook*, No. 8, 1963 revision, *Agriculture Handbook No. 456*, 1975, and *Bulletin (Home and Garden)*, No. 72, 1970, published by the United States Department of Agriculture (see Appendix Table 2). These tables are useful in calculating the specific nutritive value of each food. The values in Handbook No. 8 are given for 100-gram portions of food and those in Bulletin No. 72 and Handbook No. 456 are listed for average servings of foods. Another source in which composition is given for common serving sizes of foods is *Bowes and Church Food Values of Portions Commonly Used*, 12th edi-

In the body some food is not completely digested and absorbed. Since the body is not completely efficient in this process, the extent to which the ingested nutrient is available to the cells, or its *digestibility*, is of importance. Normally about 98 per cent of the carbohydrate, 95 per cent of the fat and 92 per cent of the protein is absorbed. However, there is a rather large variation in the digestibility of proteins.

As far as utilization by the cells is concerned, the calorie yield of carbohydrate and fat in the body is almost the same as in the bomb calorimeter because they are completely oxidized to carbon dioxide and water. This is not true of proteins. The amino (NH_2) group of the amino acids is not oxidized in the body as it is in the bomb calorimeter but is excreted in the urine, chiefly as urea, with smaller amounts of creatinine, uric acid and other compounds. The potential energy value of the energy-yielding nutrients in food is summarized in Figure 2–5.

The approximate caloric values 4, 9, 4 per gram of protein, fat and carbohydrate respectively can be used for all practical purposes to estimate the caloric values of foods in the average American mixed diet. Alcohol contains 7 kcal./gm. (See Table 2–1.)

Table 2–1   CALCULATION OF CALORIC CONTENT OF LIQUOR

To calculate the kcaloric content of an amount of liquor, the following equation can be used:

.8 kcal./proof/oz. × proof × ounces = kcal.

.8 kcal./proof/oz. = the factor necessary to account for the kcaloric density of alcohol (7 kcal./gm.) and the fact that not all of the alcohol in liquor is available for energy.

proof = 2 × the percentage of alcohol in the liquor and is necessary because not all of the liquor is alcohol.

ounces = the amount of liquor consumed.

For example, to calculate the kcaloric content of two 4-oz. glasses of wine (12% alcohol):

.8 kcal./proof/oz. × 24 proof × 8 oz. = 154 kcal.

(From Gastineau, C. F.: Alcohol and Calories, Mayo Clin. Proc., *51*(2):88, 1976.)

tion, 1975, by Charles and Helen Church. From such tables of caloric values of foods (Appendix, Tables 1, 2, and 3), the approximate caloric value of any diet can be calculated.

THE JOULE

The International Organization for Standardization (ISO) recommended the adoption of the joule (J.) as the preferred unit for energy measurements in all branches of science. The recommendation was adopted by the National Bureau of Standards in the United States in 1964.

The nutritional kilocalorie is a measure of thermal energy and cannot be as precise as the joule, which is a measure of mechanical energy. To convert kilocalories to kilojoules, one multiplies kilocalories by 4.184 (4.2). This is the conversion factor recommended by the Committee on Nomenclature, International Union of Nutritional Sciences. The Committee on Nomenclature of the American Institute of Nutrition in 1970 recommended that replacement of the kilocalorie (kcal.) by the kilojoule (kJ.) be effected as soon as the mechanics of the transition can be established.[1] The conversion factor 4.184 is used in Table 2–2 to express the 1974 RDA's for energy for adults. The final values have been rounded off after conversion to the closest 50 kJ.

The figures of 4 kcal. per gram of carbohydrate and of protein, 9 kcal. per gram of fat and 7 kcal. per gram of alcohol, converted to kilojoules and rounded off, would be 17 kJ. per gram for carbohydrate and protein, 38 kJ. per gram for fat and 29 kJ. per gram for alcohol.[8]

MEASUREMENT OF HEAT PRODUCED BY THE BODY

The amount of heat produced by the body can be measured by direct or indirect methods.

Direct Calorimetry. With the direct method a human subject is placed in a special calorimeter, and the amount of heat produced is measured. This method is very expensive, and there are few such large calorimeters available.

Indirect Calorimetry. The indirect method is a much simpler technique whereby the rate of metabolism is measured by determining with a respiration apparatus the oxygen consumption or carbon dioxide production of the body in a given period of time. Using the *respiratory quotient* $\left(RQ = \dfrac{\text{moles } CO_2 \text{ expired}}{\text{moles } O_2 \text{ consumed}} \right)$, these determinations are then converted into calories of heat produced per square meter of body surface per hour and expressed as caloric expenditure. This method is much more widely used and has the added advantage of mobility and low equipment cost. (See Fig. 2–6.)

Table 2–2 FOOD AND NUTRITION BOARD 1974 ENERGY ALLOWANCES FOR ADULTS IN KCALORIES AND KJOULES

AGE	WEIGHT	KCAL.	KJ.
MALES			
11–14 yr.	44 kg.	2800	11750
15–18 yr.	61 kg.	3000	12600
19–22 yr.	67 kg.	3000	12600
23–50 yr.	70 kg.	2700	11350
51+ yr.	70 kg.	2400	10100
FEMALES			
11–14 yr.	44 kg.	2400	10100
15–18 yr.	54 kg.	2100	8800
19–22 yr.	58 kg.	2100	8800
23–50 yr.	58 kg.	2000	8400
51+ yr.	58 kg.	1800	7550

Conversion factor of 4.18 was used and the kjoules rounded off to the nearest 50 kjoules.

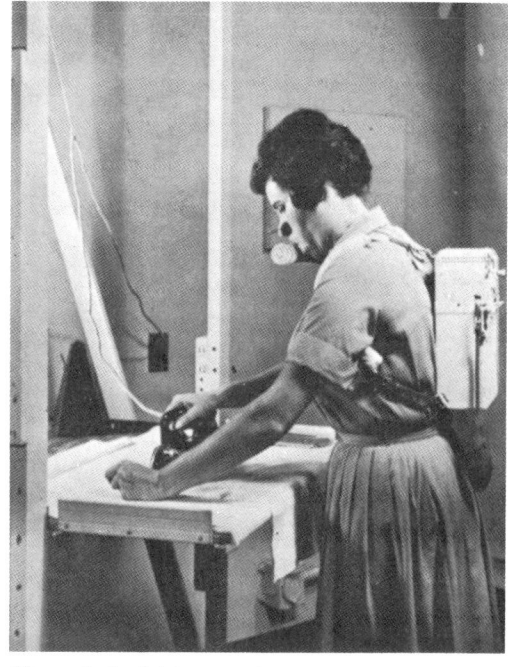

Figure 2–6 Subject standing at a work table ironing and wearing a respirometer, which measures the caloric expenditure. (Courtesy of U.S. Department of Agriculture, Office of Information.)

This method may be applied when the body is lying at rest or engaged in various activities. To determine the caloric expenditure for various activities, the subject would carry the respirator apparatus with him.

BASAL METABOLISM

The *basal metabolism* is the minimum amount of energy needed by the body at rest in the fasting state. It indicates the amount of energy needed to sustain the life processes: respiration, cellular metabolism, circulation, glandular activity and the maintenance of body temperature. It is usually measured by indirect calorimetry, with a tank type respiration apparatus, with the body at complete physical and mental rest, relaxed, but not asleep, at least 12 hours after the last meal and several hours after any strenuous exercise or activity and in a comfortable temperature and environment.

Resting metabolism is the energy expenditure under similar conditions except at any interval after eating. In other words, SDA is included. (See p. 31 for discussion of SDA.)

Factors that Affect the Basal Metabolic Rate. It is generally accepted that a variation of from 10 to 15 per cent above or below the normal metabolic rate per square meter of body surface at each age for each sex is within normal limits. Factors that influence the basal metabolic rate are outlined below.

SURFACE AREA. The greater the body surface or skin area, the greater will be the amount of heat loss and, in turn, the greater the necessary heat produced by the body. It is surprising to find that a tall thin person has a larger surface area and, consequently, a higher basal metabolism, than a short stout individual of the same weight.

SEX. Women, in general, have a metabolism about 5 to 10 per cent lower than men even when of the same weight and height. This may be accounted for by a difference in body composition between the male and female. Generally speaking, women have a little more fat and less muscular development than men. Another reason for the difference in basal metabolic rate may revolve around the effects of the male and female hormones on metabolism. During menstruation metabolism increases somewhat.

PREGNANCY. During pregnancy the adult female has an increased metabolism which is thought to be due to increases in muscle development of the uterus, placenta and fetus,

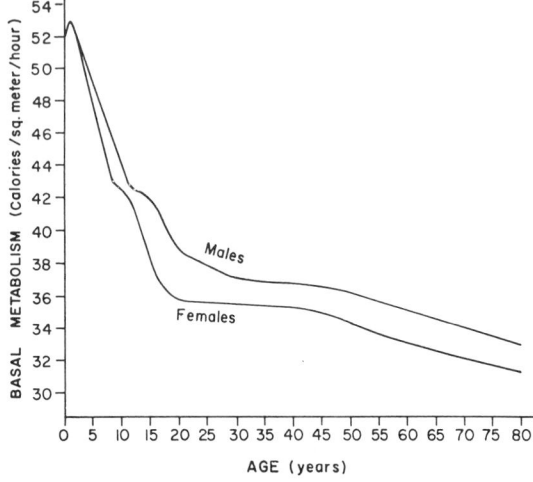

Figure 2–7 Normal basal metabolic rates for each sex at different ages. (From: Guyton, A. C.: Textbook of Medical Physiology, 5th ed. W. B. Saunders Co., 1976.)

and to respiration rate and cardiac work. The percentage of increase was recently reported by Blackburn and Calloway to be 13 per cent when calculated on a per kg. basis. Because of increased weight, though, the total BMR increase was 28 per cent.[2]

AGE. The metabolic rate is highest during the periods of rapid growth, chiefly during the first and second years, and reaches a lesser peak through the ages of puberty and adolescence in both sexes. The BMR declines about 2 per cent per decade during adult life probably owing to lower muscle tone from lessened activity.[5] (See Fig. 2–7.) The increased BMR in childhood results in greater heat production and accounts for the fact that a child will often refuse a jacket when his mother is chilly.

BODY COMPOSITION. A large proportion of inactive adipose tissue lowers the basal metabolic rate since adipose tissue requires less oxygen and thus has a lower metabolic rate than muscle tissue. Athletes with greater muscular development show about a 5 per cent increase in basal metabolism over nonathletic individuals.

ENDOCRINE GLANDS. The secretions of the endocrine glands are the principal regulators of the metabolic rate, particularly those of the thyroid gland. When the supply of *thyroxine* is inadequate, the basal metabolism may fall 30 to 50 per cent of the normal rate. If it is hyperactive, the basal metabolic rate may increase to almost twice the normal amount. In fact, an abnormal basal metabolic rate has been used as an indicator of thyroid function and malfunc-

tion. The BMR test is a good test which unfortunately is being used less because of its expense in both time and equipment.

The male sex hormones increase the basal metabolic rate about 10 to 15 per cent and the female sex hormones a little less.

The growth hormone can increase the BMR as much as 15 to 20 per cent, resulting from the stimulation of cellular metabolism.

Stimulation of the sympathetic nervous system, as during emotional excitement, increases cellular activity by the release of the hormone *epinephrine* (adrenaline), which acts directly to cause glycogenolysis and increase basal metabolic rate. Other hormones, such as cortisol and insulin, may influence metabolic rate.

NUTRITIONAL STATUS. In marked undernourishment or starvation conditions, an individual will demonstrate a lowered metabolism, often as much as 50 per cent below normal. This decrease in metabolism has been postulated to be due to an adaptive mechanism of the body that conserves energy and possibly to a decrease in mass of active tissue.

SLEEP. During sleep the metabolic rate falls approximately 10 to 15 per cent below that of waking levels. This drop is due to muscular relaxation and decreased activity of the sympathetic nervous system. This usually amounts to 40 to 80 kcalories less per day, depending upon the number of hours of sleep, the degree of relaxation and the size of the body.

CLIMATE. Differences in metabolic rates have been noted between individuals living in the tropical regions and those living in cold regions. Those living in the tropics exhibit about a 10 per cent decrease in metabolic rates compared with those in cold climates. This is largely a result of the increased secretion of thyroxine in cold climates. Human beings moving to arctic regions have been known to have basal metabolic rates as much as 15 to 20 per cent above normal.[7] However, man is usually able to keep his environment fairly constant by using clothing, heated homes or air conditioning, so that usually climate does not affect BMR.

FEVER. Infections or fevers increase the BMR about 7 per cent for each degree rise in body temperature above 98.6°F. or 13 per cent for each degree (C.) above 37°C.

TOTAL ENERGY REQUIREMENT

The energy requirement of an individual takes precedence over all other needs. Many individuals throughout the world are not meeting their requirements to supply the total energy needs of their bodies. The minimum calorie needs must be met first and other specific nutrients can be acquired later.

The three factors that determine the total energy requirement of an adult are:
1. Basal metabolism
2. Physical activity
3. Specific dynamic action of food

The growth requirements during childhood, pregnancy or lactation must also be considered.

Basal Energy Requirement. The basal metabolic needs (involuntary activity) constitute approximately 50 per cent to 70 per cent of the total daily caloric requirements for many individuals, especially those engaged in sedentary or moderately active activities. The standard basal energy requirement for individuals of average height and weight is 1 kcalorie (4.184 kjoules) per kilogram of body weight per hour. (See Table 2–3.) For a young adult male whose ideal weight is 70 kilograms, the basal require-

---

Table 2–3   CALCULATION OF BASAL ENERGY REQUIREMENT

Example: 20-year-old woman, 165 cm. in height, 55 kg. in weight (ideal body weight for this woman).

Method 1:   1 kcal./kg. IBW/hr. × IBW in kg. × 24 hr. = basal energy requirements per day.
　　　　　　　1 kcal./kg. IBW/hr. × 55 kg. × 24 hr. = *1320 kcal./day*

Method 2:   Using the nomogram in Figure 2–8:
　　　　　　　a. place the end of a ruler at 55 kg. on the bottom of graph I, which measures weight in kg.
　　　　　　　b. place the other end of the ruler at 165 cm. on the bottom of graph II, which measures height in cm.
　　　　　　　c. the point 1.6 m.² at which the ruler intersects graph III is the surface area of this woman.
　　　　　　　d. starting over again, place one end of a ruler at 1.6 m.² on graph III.
　　　　　　　e. place the other end of the rule at 20–29 years on the bottom half of graph IV, which measures the age of females.
　　　　　　　f. the point at which the ruler now intersects graph V is the basal energy requirement per day for this woman.
　　　　　　　　　1380 kcal./day

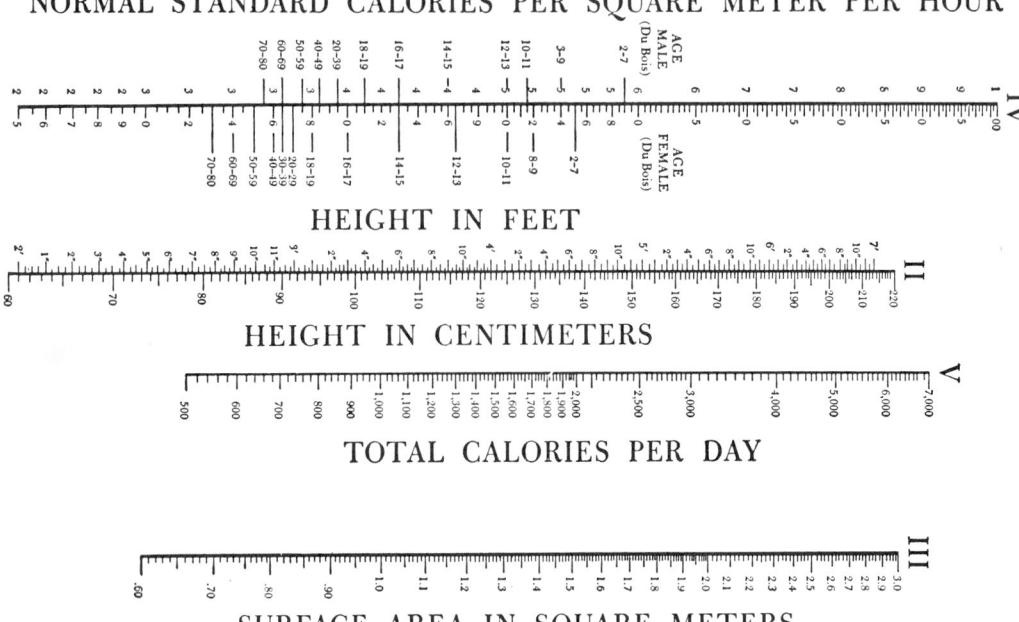

NORMAL STANDARD CALORIES PER SQUARE METER PER HOUR

HEIGHT IN FEET

HEIGHT IN CENTIMETERS

TOTAL CALORIES PER DAY

SURFACE AREA IN SQUARE METERS

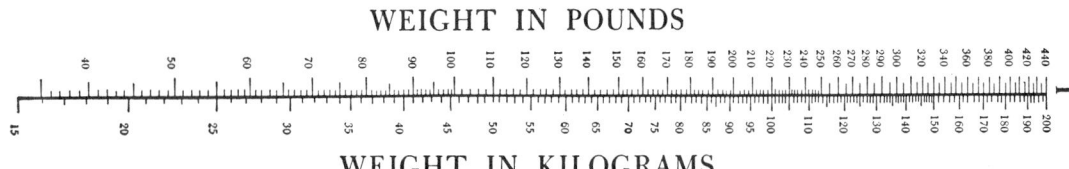

WEIGHT IN POUNDS

WEIGHT IN KILOGRAMS

Figure 2–8 Place the chart on a flat, smooth table. Use only a ruler with a true straight edge. Do not draw lines on the chart but merely indicate their positions by the straight edge of the ruler. Locate the various points by means of needles (pin stuck through the eraser of a lead pencil). Locate the patient's normal weight on Scale I and his height on Scale II. The ruler joining these two points intersects Scale III at the patient's surface area. Locate the age and sex of the patient on Scale IV. A ruler joining this point with the patient's surface area on Scale III crosses Scale V at the *basal* energy requirement. To convert Calories (kcal) to kJ, multiply by 4.184. (Nomogram of Boothby and Sandiford, adapted by the Mayo Clinic and reprinted with their permission. In Bogert, L. J., Briggs, G. M., and Calloway, D. H.: Nutrition and Physical Fitness. 9th ed. W. B. Saunders, 1973.)

ment would be 1680 kcalories (70 kg. × 1 kcal./kg. × 24 hr.) or 7030 kjoules. For a young adult female whose ideal weight is 58 kilograms, the basal requirement would be approximately 1400 kcalories (5850 kjoules).

The ideal or desired weight for height and age is used in determining the energy requirement instead of actual weight because the present weight of an individual may be abnormal— overweight or underweight. (See Table 15 in Appendix for men and women, and Tables 16 and 17 for children.)

To be more exact in calculating basal energy requirements, one can use the nomogram in Figure 2–8, which in addition to body weight,

considers surface area, age and sex. (See Table 2–3.)

No person could exist for very long if he received only sufficient calories to cover his basal metabolic needs. The ordinary activities of life which require moving about and the various forms of muscular activity and the ingestion of food increase the energy needs of the body.

Physical Activity. Next to basal needs, physical activity is the greatest single factor influencing the energy needs of an individual. Besides the *size of the body* doing the exercise (more energy required for a heavier person), the kind and speed of the work or exercise are

Table 2–4 EXAMPLES OF DAILY ENERGY EXPENDITURES OF MATURE WOMEN AND MEN IN LIGHT OCCUPATIONS*

| Activity Category | Time (hr.) | MAN, 70 K G. | | WOMAN, 58 K G. | |
		Rate (kcal./min.)	Total [kcal. (kJ.)]	Rate (kcal./min.)	Total [kcal.(kJ.)]
Sleeping, reclining	8	1.0–1.2	540(2270)	0.9–1.1	440(1850)
Very light Seated and standing activities, painting trades, auto and truck driving, laboratory work, typing, playing musical instruments, sewing, ironing	12	up to 2.5	1300(5460)	up to 2.0	900(3750)
Light Walking on level, 2.5–3 mph, tailoring, pressing, garage work, electrical trades, carpentry, restaurant trades, cannery workers, washing clothes, shopping with light load, golf, sailing, table tennis, volleyball	3	2.5–4.9	600(7520)	2.0–3.9	450(1890)
Moderate Walking 3.5–4 mph, plastering, weeding and hoeing, loading and stacking bales, scrubbing floors, shopping with heavy load, cycling, skiing, tennis, dancing	1	5.0–7.4	300(1260)	4.0–5.9	240(1010)
Heavy Walking with load uphill, tree felling, work with pick and shovel, basketball, swimming, climbing, football	0	7.5–12.0		6.0–10.0	
TOTAL	24		2740(11,500)		2030(8,530)

*Figures include BMR and SDA
Data from Durnin, J. V., and Passmore, R.: Energy, Work and Leisure, London, Heinemann Educational Books, 1967, p. 166. (From Food and Nutrition Board, Recommended Dietary Allowances, 8th ed., Washington, D.C., National Research Council, NAS, 1974, p. 27.)

factors of concern in determining the total energy requirement. The *more vigorous the physical work,* the greater the calorie cost. A man doing heavy work (e.g., a miner) may need 4800 or more kcalories per day, while an individual of the same body build and age and height living in the same climate but doing sedentary work (e.g., a bank clerk) may require only 2500 kcalories. In general the food intake should meet the energy output except in individuals who need to gain or lose weight. Modern living with its many labor-saving devices and electronic equipment is conducive to less activity. A discussion of overweight and underweight is given in Chapter 27.

The inactive or sedentary person usually requires approximately 30 per cent additional calories above basal, while a lightly active person might need 50 per cent above basal, a moderately active person 75 per cent, and a very active person 100 per cent above basal. See Table 2–4 for descriptions of various levels of activity.

Individual energy expenditure varies considerably in a given activity. Most people have characteristic habits of motion or twitches. One person will sit quietly relaxed while another will unconsciously be making many habitual motions. The same is true in performing a task. One person will be very efficient and make few motions while another individual will expend much more energy making many un-

Table 2–5   ENERGY COST OF ACTIVITIES EXCLUSIVE OF BASAL METABOLISM AND INFLUENCE OF FOOD*

ACTIVITY	KCAL./KG./HR.	ACTIVITY	KCAL./KG./HR.
Bicycling (century run)	7.6	Piano playing (Liszt's	
Bicycling (moderate speed)	2.5	"Tarantella")	2.0
Bookbinding	0.8	Reading aloud	0.4
Boxing	11.4	Rowing in race	16.0
Carpentry (heavy)	2.3	Running	7.0
Cello playing	1.3	Sawing wood	5.7
Crocheting	0.4	Sewing, hand	0.4
Dancing, foxtrot	3.8	Sewing, foot-driven machine	0.6
Dancing, waltz	3.0	Sewing, motor-driven machine	0.4
Dishwashing	1.0	Shoemaking	1.0
Dressing and undressing	0.7	Singing in loud voice	0.8
Driving automobile	0.9	Sitting quietly	0.4
Eating	0.4	Skating	3.5
Fencing	7.3	Standing at attention	0.6
Horseback riding, walk	1.4	Standing relaxed	0.5
Horseback riding, trot	4.3	Stone masonry	4.7
Horseback riding, gallop	6.7	Sweeping with broom, bare floor	1.4
Ironing (5-pound iron)	1.0	Sweeping with carpet sweeper	1.6
Knitting sweater	0.7	Sweeping with vacuum sweeper	2.7
Laundry, light	1.3	Swimming (2 mph)	7.9
Lying still, awake	0.1	Tailoring	0.9
Organ playing (30% to 40%		Typewriting rapidly	1.0
of energy hand work)	1.5	Violin playing	0.6
Painting furniture	1.5	Walking (3 mph)	2.0
Paring potatoes	0.6	Walking rapidly (4 mph)	3.4
Playing Ping-Pong	4.4	Walking at high speed	
Piano playing (Mendelssohn's		(5.3 mph)	9.3
songs)	0.8	Walking downstairs	†
Piano playing (Beethoven's		Walking upstairs	‡
"Apassionata")	1.4	Washing floors	1.2
		Writing	0.4

*From Taylor, C. M., and McLeod, G.: Rose's laboratory handbook for dietetics, 5th ed., New York, The Macmillan Co., 1949, p. 18.

†Allow 0.012 kcal. per kilogram for an ordinary staircase with 15 steps without regard to time.

‡Allow 0.036 kcal. per kilogram for an ordinary staircase with 15 steps without regard to time.

necessary motions. If these two individuals are eating the same number of calories, the efficient one will expend less energy and is more apt to store calories not used or needed. Each individual has a characteristic capacity to utilize and store calories. See Table 2–5 for a list of caloric expenditures for various activities.

Mental work does not appreciably affect the energy requirement. Fatigue after studying results not from the mental work but from the physical activities or muscle tension that accompany the study habits.

In highly *emotional states* the physical activity of restlessness, muscle tension and aggravated motions of the body expend energy.

The *state of health* may have a marked effect on physical activity. Such physiological and psychological stresses as fatigue, tension and lack of sleep may influence the physical activity and total caloric requirement.

A very low *environmental temperature* or a very high environmental temperature may increase slightly the caloric needs. These additional calories are required to cover the work cost of maintaining body temperature at 37° C. The energy cost of work in cold weather is slightly greater than in warm weather. However, in extreme heat (greater than 98° F or 37° C) heavy activity or work requires greater energy expenditure. Nature, however, regulates heat loss very effectively in the various climates by enabling human beings to shiver or sweat as the temperature dictates.

With *increased age and decreased activity* people need to adjust their eating habits and caloric intake to maintain the desired weight. It has been proposed by The Food and Nutrition Board National Research Council (see Table 2–2) that kcalorie allowances be reduced to 90 per cent of the amount required as a mature adult for persons above 50 years of age in order

to compensate for decreased activity and decreased BMR.

Specific Dynamic Action of Food. All foods give a stimulus to metabolism but not all foods have the same effect on metabolism. This stimulus is called the *specific dynamic action* or *calorigenic effect* of food. Carbohydrate or fat increases the heat production by about 5 per cent of the total calories consumed. If the food intake is composed solely of protein, the increase may be as much as 30 per cent. If the food intake is very high in protein, about 15 per cent should be added.[10] This specific dynamic action effect of food is not due to the energy needed for digestion of food since nutrient substances injected into a vein still cause this effect. The mechanism of specific dynamic action (SDA) is still not completely understood, but for a liberal mixed diet, about 10 per cent of total energy requirements for basal metabolism and muscular activity should be added to cover SDA. For some ill understood reason, SDA is enhanced by exercise.[4, 11]

Growth. In the growing child, energy must be provided over and above that required for the basal metabolic rate, physical activity and specific dynamic action. This additional energy is required to cover the cost of increasing body weight and height. Growing infants may store as much as 12 to 15 per cent of the energy value of their food intake in the form of new tissue. As a child becomes older, the rate of growth diminishes and the caloric requirement for growth is reduced. (See Table 10–1.) The kcaloric allowances in the Table are proposed as average and approximate amounts for feeding groups of children. The needs of an individual child are governed by his growth and physical activity. (See Chapters 14 and 15.)

Additional calories are required to meet the energy costs of pregnancy and lactation, which are also periods of growth. (See Chapter 13.)

Estimation of Daily Energy Requirement of an Adult. The total daily energy requirement is commonly estimated by adding together the requirement for basal metabolism, physical or muscular activity and the specific dynamic action (SDA) of food.

The method used depends on the degree of accuracy desired. For research purposes the individual has a basal metabolism determination. The energy cost of the daily activities is determined by the respirometer which the individual carries around with him (Fig. 2–6). The results of all activities added together would give the total energy requirement for physical activity. An additional 10 per cent would be

Table 2–6 RULE OF THUMB DETERMINATION OF IDEAL BODY WEIGHT

Females: 100 lb. (45 kg.) for the first 5 ft. (152 cm.)
plus
5 lb. (2.2 kg.) for every inch (2.54 cm.) of height over 5 ft. (152 cm.)

Males: 110 lb. (45 kg.) for the first 5 ft. (152 cm.)
plus
5 lb. (2.2 kg.) for every 1 inch (2.54 cm.) of height over 5 ft. (152 cm.)

Example: female, 165 cm. 45 kg. for 152 cm.
plus
2.2 kg. × 13 cm./2.54 cm. = 11.4 kg.
45 kg. + 11.4 kg. = 56.4 kg.
To adjust for frame size, 10 lb. (4.5 kg.) would be added in the case of a large frame or subtracted in the case of a small frame.

added to account for the SDA and the total would be the energy requirement.

Another method involves estimating the basal metabolism requirements from surface area measurements and the activity needs from accurate records of all activities during the waking hours plus the additional factor of the effect of food in metabolism (SDA). The activity records would be translated into energy expended since the cost of each activity is known and a total energy requirement could be determined. See Table 2–5 to determine the approximate energy cost of activities during the day.

A less precise procedure but accurate enough for many purposes is as follows:

1. *Determine the ideal body weight (IBW) of the individual in kilograms.* This can be determined from a record of the person's constant weight, the Metropolitan Life Insurance Tables (see Appendix Tables 14 and 15) or from the rule of thumb presented in Table 2–6.

2. *Determine basal needs:*
male = 1.0 kcalorie (4.18 kJ.)/kg. of ideal body wt./hour × 24
female = 0.95 kcalorie (4.0 kJ.)/kg. of ideal body wt./hour × 24

3. *Subtract* 0.1 kcalorie (.42 kJ.)/kg. of ideal body wt./*hours of sleep.*

4. *Add activity increment.*

5. *Add specific dynamic action* (10 per cent of basal needs plus activity increment).

6. *Sum* equals the *approximate daily calorie requirement.*

An even cruder method for estimating total energy requirements for the person at his or her ideal body weight is the following:

Multiply the IBW in kg. by one of these

Table 2–7   CALCULATION OF TOTAL ENERGY REQUIREMENT*

Example: 20-year-old female, 165 cm. tall and weighing 55 kg.
          Activity: light.

Method 1:   a. Determine IBW—55 kg. is IBW for this woman.
            b. Basal needs = .95 kcal./kg. IBW/hr. × 55 kg. × 24 hr. = 1254 kcal. (5250 kJ.).
            c. Sleep = .1 kcal./kg. IBW/hr. × 55 kg. × 8 hr. = 45 kcal.
                 1254 kcal. – 45 kcal. = 1209 kcal.
            d. Activity: light = 50% above basal = 625 kcal. (2600 kJ.).
                 1209 kcal. + 625 kcal. = 1834 kcal. (7850 kJ.).
            e. SDA = 10% above energy requirement = 184 kcal.
                 1834 kcal. + 184 kcal. = *2022 kcal./day (8500 kJ/day)*

Method 2:   Factor for sedentary = 30 kcal./kg. IBW.
            Factor for moderately active = 35–40 kcal./kg. IBW.
            This woman has light activity, so let's use the factor of 33 kcal./kg. IBW/day.
            55 kg. × 33 kcal./kg. IBW/day = *1815 kcal./day (7600 kJ./day)*

*The difference of 207 kcal./day between these two calculations is a minor one. It is only a guideline and should be adjusted depending on whether the individual maintains her weight on this level of caloric intake.

factors, which include basal, activity and SDA requirements:

          sedentary: 30 kcal. (125 kJ.)/kg.
moderately active: 35–40 kcal.
            (145–170 kJ.)/kg.
      very active: 45 kcal. (190 kJ.)/kg.

The disadvantages of this method are that (1) no correction is made for sex or age, and (2) the estimation of activity is a rough one. (See Table 2–7.)

Activities may be classified as sedentary or light, moderate, heavy and very heavy work. The sedentary person expends very few calories daily in work. He may spend most of his time sitting, reading and talking. The person who engages in light physical activity sits, walks and stands. The person who exercises moderately may stand, walk, do housework, gardening or carpentry and spends little time sitting. The person with strenuous or heavy work is constantly active. His least strenuous exercise is standing and walking. He may participate actively in outdoor games, skating, swimming, tennis, and so on for significant lengths of time and engage in work activities involving considerable expenditure of energy (e.g., a construction worker). See Table 2–4 for a description of a typical day's activities and caloric expenditure.

ENERGY STORES

When a person is exercised or when he is fasting, he is relying on his body energy stores. At first the energy comes from stored ATP and creatine phosphate. When this source is de-pleted after a few minutes, anaerobic glycolysis takes over, reconstituting ATP (see Chapter 6). The third and final source is oxidative phosphorylation of body nutrients—glycogen, fat and eventually protein. Then oxygen uptake is the limiting factor. Fat is carried as the primary energy store because it provides over twice as many calories per gram as glycogen or tissue protein. See Figure 2–9 for the difference between energy stores of a normal weight individual and an obese individual.

RECOMMENDED CALORIE ALLOWANCES

The calorie recommendations for adults, revised in 1974 by the Food and Nutrition Board, National Research Council, National Academy of Sciences, are based on the degree of activity of a reference man and woman, both aged 22, living in a temperate climate and weighing 70 and 58 kilograms, respectively.[6] (Weight gained after this age is likely to be adipose tissue.) The physical activity of these individuals is considered to be "light" with occupations that could be described neither as sedentary nor as heavy physical labor. The man could be employed as a delivery man, a teacher or a laboratory worker. The woman could be an active homemaker, or a saleswoman in a shop. Thus the daily kcaloric allowances for the reference man and woman are 2700 and 2000 kcal. (11,300 and 8,360 kJ.), respectively. These are lower calorie allowances than were recommended in the previous standards (1958, 1963 and in the case of men, 1968), based on changes in the American way of life, new research information and concern for the

Table 2–8 1974 RECOMMENDED ALLOWANCES FOR ENERGY ADJUSTED FOR AGE AND SEX

AGE CATEGORY	MEN	WOMEN
15–18 yr.		
kcal./kg.	49	39
kJ./kg.	205	161
19–22 yr.		
kcal./kg.	45	36
kJ./kg.	188	151
23–50 yr.		
kcal./kg.	39	34
kJ./kg.	161	144
51+ yr.		
kcal./kg.	34	31
kJ./kg.	143	130

large segment of the population which is now overweight. As previously stated, the report recommends a decrease in calories needed for each decade after the age of 22. See Table 2–8.

It is understood that calorie allowances must be adjusted to meet the specific needs of an individual and to maintain body weight at the desired level.

The daily allowances for infants and children, different age groups, and for pregnancy and lactation are listed in the table of Recommended Dietary Allowances (Chap. 10). In order to better understand the use of the material, it is strongly advised that every student read and become familiar with the scientific basis for the allowances as revised in 1974.[6]

The calorie allowances for pregnancy, lactation, infants and children will be discussed in Chapter 13, Nutrition for Pregnancy and Lactation; Chapter 14, Nutrition in Infancy; and Chapter 15, Nutrition in Childhood and Adolescence.

REGULATION OF ENERGY INTAKE AND EXPENDITURE

The ability of the healthy, normal adult human being to control his energy intake in order to match his energy output is most remarkable. Body weight, the indicator of this balance, is quite stable. For instance, during a single year the average adult will ingest one million kcalories of which over 99 per cent will be expended. If only 1 per cent of these million kcalories (10,000 kcal.) was stored, this would result in a 3 lb. (1.4 kg.) weight gain for that year.[3] Thus the body's energy balance control is extremely sensitive.

This balance between intake and expenditure depends on the control of activity and hunger. Hunger, the desire to eat and consume energy in the form of food, is controlled by a multiplicity of factors, most of which are believed to be integrated in the hypothalamus of the brain. A final message then goes out from the hypothalamus saying "eat" or "stop eating."

Even more fascinating is the situation of obesity in which this controlling system has

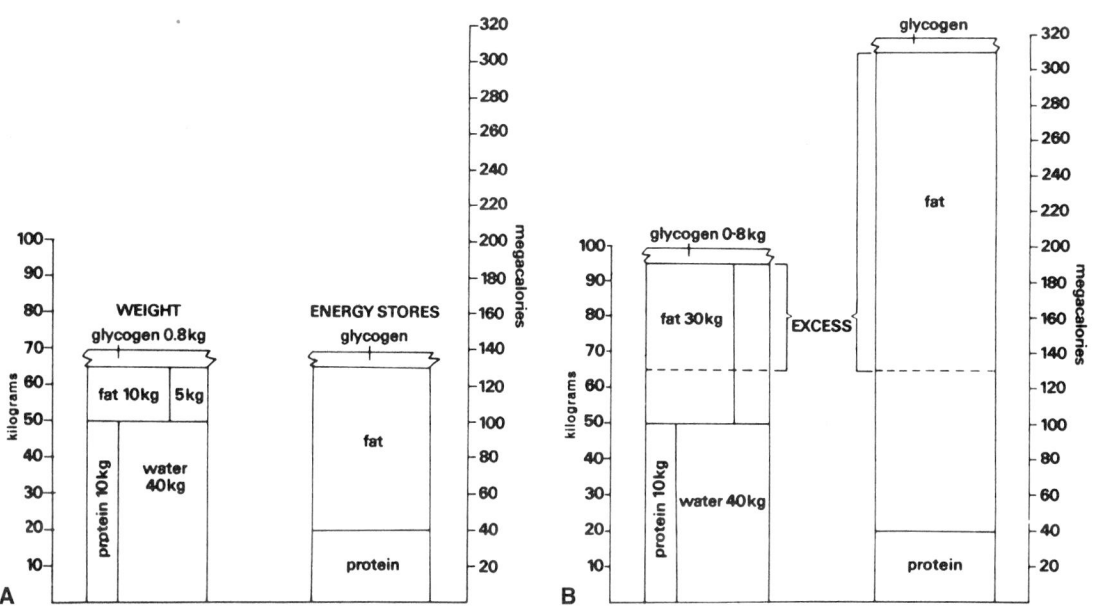

Figure 2–9 *A*, Body weight and energy stores of a normal adult weighing about 69 kg. *B*, Obese adult weighing 99 kg. Excess fat would supply total energy for three months. (From: Garrow, J. S.: The regulation of body weight. In Silverstone, T. (ed.): Obesity: Its Pathogenesis and Management. Publishing Sciences Group, 1975.)

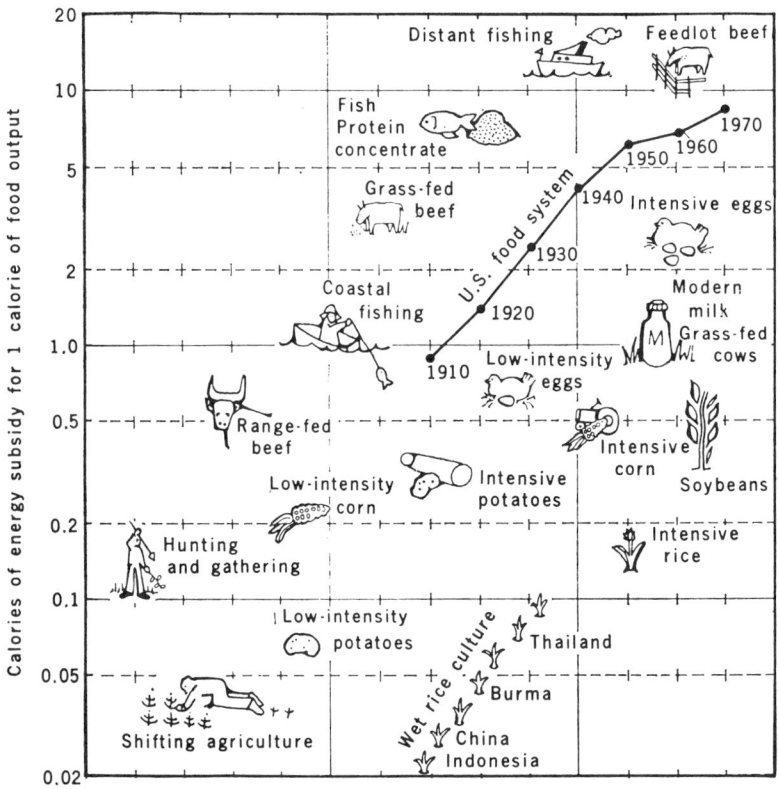

Figure 2–10   Energy subsidies for various food crops. The energy history of the U.S. food system is shown for comparison. (From: Steinhart, J. S., and Steinhart, C. E.: Energy use in the U.S. food system. Science, *184*:307, 1974.)

"failed." There has been too much hunger and either not enough activity to warrant the hunger or too little satiety. Why does this happen? A complete discussion of hunger and satiety, to the extent that we understand them, will be presented in Unit 8—Imbalance of Body Weight.

CHOICE OF FOODS TO PROVIDE ENERGY

After the number of calories needed for daily activity is determined, the raw materials to provide the calories are supplied in the form of food in various proportions of proteins, fats and carbohydrates. A great variety of common foods are available for supplying the necessary minerals and vitamins, in addition to furnishing fuel. In this country there is an abundance of food for the majority of the population, and the problem is one of wise selection based on nutrition education, rather than one of availability. In many parts of the world there are extreme calorie shortages.

People's ideas about the caloric value of specific foods are often incorrect. For example, there are approximately 60 kcalories in an average slice of bread—slightly *less* than in a medium apple. A cup of whole milk contains about 170 kcalories, as does one small scoop (⅛ qt.) of orange water ice.

A common rule in building a suitable diet is to include first the necessary protective foods, then complete the calorie allowance by adding any foods desired. This procedure will be discussed in detail in Chapter 10.

ENERGY IN THE PRODUCTION OF FOOD

Just as the human body is dependent on the energy content of food for its own energy, so the production of that food is dependent on energy. A most simplistic example of food production requiring low energy is that of a plant such as a carrot, which through photosynthesis utilizes solar energy to form chemical energy in the form of carbohydrates, vitamins, minerals, and protein in its tissue. This is then consumed directly as a raw, fresh carrot by man. But if one cans, freezes, dices, cooks or packages this carrot, the energy for the carrot production

has increased. In fact, the more processing performed on this carrot, the further it is transported or the fancier its package, the more energy of production it represents.

About 13 per cent of the U.S. total energy consumption is used to bring food from the farm to the consumer, and meat processing makes up the largest segment of this energy cost. Animal protein is a very energy-expensive item because only 10 per cent of the plant protein fed to raise the animal is returned as animal protein.[9] To summarize, we use about 8 kcalories of energy to obtain a single kcalorie of food energy, compared with primitive cultures which obtained 5 to 50 kcalories of food energy for every kcalorie used in its production.[12] (See Fig. 2–10.)

Unfortunately the energy used in our food production is increasing as we continue to eat fabricated foods and convenience foods. Our food supply is becoming more "energy intensive," which is questionable in a world in which millions of people do not have enough to eat and whose requirements could be met by low energy foods such as grains and vegetables.

In addition much nonrenewable energy is wasted in the home storage and preparation of food where electrical or gas refrigerators do not have proper insulation, electrical appliances are used unnecessarily or heating appliances are inefficient. For instance, mixing by hand instead of with an electric mixer uses *renewable* human energy instead of nonrenewable electric energy. By using human energy one would expend additional kcalories and help prevent gaining that extra pound! We must become more conscious of our personal use of nonrenewable energy in food preparation and make necessary changes to reduce that use if possible. To reduce the energy intensiveness of our food production will require changes on the farm and in the home.

PROBLEMS AND SUGGESTED TOPICS FOR DISCUSSION

1. What does "calorie" in nutrition mean? How is it used?
2. (a) Consult food composition tables for the calorie values of food and list those which have 500 kcalories per serving, 200 kcalories per serving, 100 kcalories per serving and 50 kcalories per serving. (b) On the basis of the protein, fat and carbohydrate value, determine the energy value (kcalories) of:

> 23 gm. whole wheat bread
> 244 gm. whole milk
> 190 gm. grapefruit sections
> 150 gm. raw tomato

3. What is meant by basal energy expenditure and total energy expenditure?
4. List the foods you have consumed during one 24-hour period and compute the total calorie value. Compare with the calorie allowance recommended by the Food and Nutrition Board of the National Research Council.

CITED REFERENCES

1. Ames, S. R.: The joule-unit of energy. J. Am. Diet. Assoc., *57*:415, 1970.
2. Blackburn, M. W., and Calloway, D. H.: Basal metabolic rate and work energy expenditure of mature pregnant women. J. Am. Diet. Assoc., *69*:24, 1976.
3. Bray, G. A., and Campfield, L. A.: Metabolic factors in the control of energy stores. Metabolism, *24*:99, 1975.
4. Bray, G. A., Whipp, B. J., and Koyal, S. N.: The acute effects of food intake on energy expenditure during cycle ergometry. Am. J. Clin. Nutr., *27*:254, 1974.
5. Durnin, J. V., and Passmore, R.: Energy, Work and Leisure. New York, William Heinemann Educational Books, Ltd., 1967.
6. Food and Nutrition Board, Recommended Dietary Allowances. 8th ed. Washington, D.C., National Research Council, NAS, 1974.
7. Guyton, A. C.: Textbook of Medical Physiology. 5th ed. Philadelphia, W. B. Saunders Co., 1976, pp. 23 and 1012.
8. Harper, A. E.: Remarks on the joule. J. Am. Diet. Assoc., *57*:416, 1970.
9. Hirst, E.: Living off the fuels of the land. Natural History, *82*:21, 1973.
10. Latner, A. L.: Cantarow and Trumper Clinical Biochemistry. 7th ed. Philadelphia, W. B. Saunders Co., 1975, p. 451.
11. Miller, D. S., and Mumford, P.: Obesity: physical activity and nutrition. Proc. Nutr. Soc., *25*:100, 1966.
12. Steinhart, J. S., and Steinhart, C. E.: Energy use in the U.S. food system. Science, *184*:307, 1974.

ADDITIONAL REFERENCES

Bogert, L. J., Briggs, G. M., and Calloway, D. H.: Nutrition and Physical Fitness. 9th ed. Philadelphia, W. B. Saunders Company, 1973, Chapter 2.

Davidson, S., Passmore, R., and Brock, J. F.: Human Nutrition and Dietetics. Baltimore, Williams & Wilkins Co., 1976, Chapters 2 and 3.

Joint FAO/WHO Ad Hoc Expert Committee, Energy and Protein Requirements. World Health Organization, Technical Report No. 522, Geneva, Switzerland, 1973.

Konishi, F.: Food energy equivalents of various activities. J. Am. Dietet. A., *46*:186, 1965.

Nutritive Value of Foods. Home and Garden Bulletin No. 72. United States Department of Agriculture, 1970.

Pike, R. L., and Brown, M. L.: Nutrition: An Integrated Approach. New York, John Wiley & Sons, Inc., 1975, pp. 814–854.

Review: Variability in metabolic rate. Nutr. Rev., *25*:12, 1967.

Walsingham, J. M.: Dependence of food supply on non-solar energy. Nutrition, *29*:337, 1975.

Watt, B. K., and Merrill, A. L.: Composition of Food: Raw, Processed and Prepared. Agriculture Handbook Number 8, U.S. Department of Agriculture, revised, 1963.

Chapter 3

CARBOHYDRATES

CARBOHYDRATES AROUND THE WORLD

Carbohydrates furnish most of the energy which is needed to move, perform work, and live; they are the starches and sugars. In the form of grains they furnish the major source of food for the people of the world and have the highest yield of energy per acre of land. However, the consumption of carbohydrates throughout the world is highly variable. In America about 45 per cent of the diet is composed of them, and an even higher proportion is used in other countries.[17] In the Orient, for example, where rice is a dietary staple, a higher proportion of calories is provided by carbohydrates. In the tropics carbohydrates may furnish as much as 90 per cent of the energy. See Chapter 17, Geographic and Cultural Dietary Variations, for grains used in the various countries. They are the cheapest, most easily obtainable, and most readily digested form of fuel. Since many of the foods which are high in carbohydrate content, such as bread, cereals, potatoes and other root vegetables are relatively inexpensive, the proportion of carbohydrates in the diet is greater at the lower economic levels. The chief sources of carbohydrates are grains, vegetables, fruits, syrups and sugars. That grains supply only carbohydrates is a popular misconception. Grains also supply a major portion of the protein for much of the world's population.

DEFINITION AND COMPOSITION

Carbohydrates are an important group of organic compounds that are composed of the three elements of carbon, hydrogen and oxygen. In their simplest form the general formula is $C_nH_{2n}O_n$. The hydrogen and oxygen are present in the same proportion as in water, H_2O, and there is one molecule of water for each carbon. From this comes the term carbohydrate, but this simple relationship gives no indication of the structure. More accurately the carbohydrates are defined as polyhydroxy aldehydes and ketones. They vary from simple sugars containing from three to seven carbon atoms to very complex polymers. Only the hexoses (6-carbon sugars) and pentoses (5-carbon sugars) and polymers built up from them play important roles in nutrition.

Photosynthesis. Plants store carbohydrates as their chief source of energy. Water, minerals and nitrogen in the soil are taken by the plant roots, trunk and branches to the leaves. The leaves absorb carbon dioxide (CO_2) from the air. The energy of sunlight acting on water (H_2O) and carbon dioxide in the presence of chlorophyll (the green coloring matter of leaves) enables the leaves to make sugar and release oxygen (O_2).

$$CO_2 + H_2O \xrightarrow[\text{plant enzymes}]{\underset{\text{chlorophyll}}{\text{sunlight}}} \text{Carbohydrate } (CH_2O) + O_2$$

This process is photosynthesis (Fig. 3–1). It involves the hydration of carbon dioxide to yield carbohydrate, and is nature's first step in the manufacture of all foods. The carbohydrate made in the leaves will be used in the growth of the plant (or tree) and be stored in its leaves, stems, roots, seeds, pods and fruits. Thus, it can be said that the sun furnishes the energy for all living matter. To recover the locked-in energy of sunlight, the carbohydrate in plants is burned in the body and yields carbon dioxide and water. Not all the potential energy in sunlight is captured by photosynthesis.

CLASSIFICATION

Carbohydrates are classified as monosaccharides, disaccharides, oligosaccharides and polysaccharides. Monosaccharides (the simple sugars) cannot be hydrolyzed to a simpler form. Disaccharides may be hydrolyzed to give 2 molecules of the same or different monosaccharides. Oligosaccharides yield 3 to 10 monosaccharide units and polysaccharides more than 10 units—up to 10,000 or more.

Monosaccharides. The principal monosac-

charides which occur free in foods are glucose, an aldohexose, and fructose, a ketohexose. They may exist in either an open-chain or a ring structure, as shown on facing page. When they are linked together as di- or polysaccharides they are held in the cyclic form. Galactose and mannose, two other aldohexoses which occur in bound form in food, have the same structure as glucose except for the orientation of the hydroxyl groups around the six carbon atoms.

Glucose (dextrose, grape sugar) is abundant in fruits, sweet corn, corn syrup, certain roots and honey. Glucose is the principal product formed by hydrolysis of more complex carbohydrates in the process of digestion. It is the form of sugar normally found in the blood stream. Glucose is oxidized in the cells to give energy and is stored in the liver and muscles as *glycogen,* a complex carbohydrate known as "animal starch." Under normal conditions the central nervous system can utilize only glucose as a major source of fuel. It is the best form of sugar to use when an immediate supply of sugar is needed, for it requires no changes in order to be utilized. It is relatively inexpensive and may be added to liquid foods to increase carbohydrate intake without seriously affecting the flavor of the food since it is only 3/5 as sweet as cane sugar.

Sorbitol and mannitol, hexahydric alcohols derived from glucose and mannose respectively, have a sweetening power similar to glucose (Table 3–1). *Sorbitol* is absorbed slowly and it serves to keep blood sugar levels high following a meal. It has been used in weight reduction as an aid to delay the onset of hunger sensations. It has the same calorie value as glucose and is found in many fruits, vegetables and dietetic products.

Mannitol is poorly digested and yields about

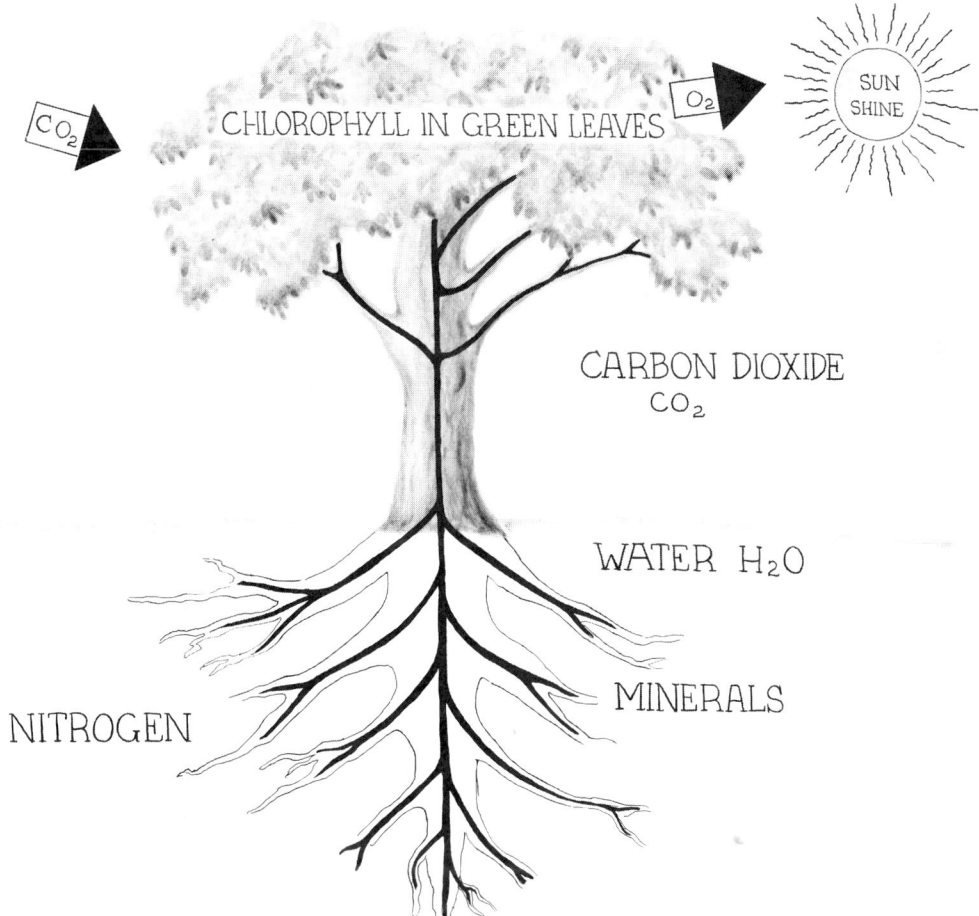

Figure 3–1 Synthesis of carbohydrates in plant life. Light from the sun is harnessed by the green chlorophyll of plant leaves. Cells in green leaves utilize this energy in synthesizing carbohydrates from the carbon dioxide in the air and the water in the soil. Carbohydrates are the chief form in which plants store potential energy.

Glucose

Glucose   Fructose   Fructose

one-half the calories per gram as glucose. It has been added to some foods for use as a drying agent. Pineapples, olives, asparagus, sweet potatoes and carrots, as well as sugarless gum and other dietetic products, contain some mannitol.

Fructose (levulose, fruit sugar) is found together with glucose and sucrose in honey and fruit. It is the sweetest of the sugars. Technology has advanced to the point where levulose can be made from glucose. Now sweeteners containing glucose and levulose can be made from grains rather than only from the sugar beet and sugar cane.

Galactose is not found free in nature but is produced from lactose (milk sugar) by hydrolysis in the digestive process. It is found in nerve tissue.

Mannose is not found free in foods but is derived from mannosans which are found in manna and some legumes. (See Table 3–2.)

Several *pentoses* (5-carbon sugars) occur in bound form in food. *Ribose* and *deoxyribose* are derived from the nucleic acids of meat. They are essential components of nucleic acids and some coenzymes but are not essential nutrients since they can be synthesized in the body. *Arabinose* and *xylose* are constituents of the pentosans in fruits.

Xylitol, an alcohol of xylose with the sweetness of sucrose, is poorly absorbed and is also being considered as a non-nutritive sweetener.

Disaccharides. Disaccharides, or double sugars, are exemplified by sucrose (cane or beet sugar), maltose (malt sugar) and lactose (milk sugar). Each of the three double sugars is made up of two hexose molecules:

Sucrose = glucose and fructose
Maltose = glucose and glucose
Lactose = glucose and galactose

Table 3–1   SWEETNESS OF SUGARS

SUGAR OR SUGAR PRODUCT	SWEETNESS VALUE
Levulose, fructose	173
Invert sugar	130
Sucrose	100
Glucose	74
Sorbitol	60
Mannitol	50
Galactose	32
Maltose	32
Lactose	16

From Freed, M. Food Product Development, February-March, 1970.

They are hydrolyzed by digestive enzymes to the constituent monosaccharides before absorption into the body.

Sucrose is ordinary table sugar. It is found mainly in sugar cane, sugar beets, molasses, maple syrup and maple sugar. When sucrose is hydrolyzed a 50:50 mixture of glucose and fructose forms. This mixture is called invert sugar and frequently is seen on labels of foods. Sucrose is a very inexpensive and common form of sugar in the diet.

Maltose or malt sugar does not occur free in nature. It is a so-called "derived" sugar, since it is a product of the digestion of starch by diastase, a plant enzyme obtained from sprouting grain. (This occurs in the manufacture of beer.) Maltose is formed during digestion by the action of enzymes called amylases. The reaction begins with salivary amylase; other amylases are present in the intestine and pancreatic juice. Another enzyme, *maltase,* in the intestine hydrolyzes maltose to two molecules of glucose, in which form it is absorbed. Maltose is not readily fermented by bacteria in the colon. Because fermentation frequently leads to diarrhea, this property makes maltose useful in combination with dextrin in infant formulas.

Lactose is the principal sugar found in milk; 4 to 6 per cent in cow's milk and 5 to 8 per cent in human milk. It is not found in plants and is limited almost exclusively to the mammary glands of lactating animals. It is less soluble than the other common disaccharides and is only about one-sixth as sweet as sucrose. It yields glucose and galactose upon hydrolysis and is digested more slowly than the other disaccharides. Some individuals have a deficiency of the enzyme *lactase* which hydrolyzes lactose. Under such circumstances, some of this unhydrolyzed sugar passes into the large intestine where it is fermented by intestinal bacteria and may have a laxative action. An excess amount may cause diarrhea, flatulence and abdominal cramping. Because it is less sweet than sucrose, it is often used to increase the calorie content of a liquid feeding without making it taste too sweet. However, it is difficult to dissolve and therefore not very practical. In the process of making cheese, some of the lactose in milk is converted to lactic and other acids which contribute to the flavor. Lactose remains in the whey and is obtained commercially as a by-product of the manufacture of cheese. As a consequence most cheese contains little or no lactose and thus can usually be tolerated in the lactase-deficient individual.

Lactulose, a new synthetic disaccharide, is composed of one molecule of galactose and one molecule of fructose. It is not metabolized by man and can possibly be used as a laxative.

Polysaccharides. The chief polysaccharides of interest in nutrition—starch, dextrin, cellulose, and glycogen—are assembled from glucose units. Other important plant and animal structures contain other monosaccharides. In some cases several different monosaccharides are combined in the polysaccharide molecule. As a group, polysaccharides are far less soluble and more stable than the monosaccharides. Starch and glycogen are completely digestible; other polysaccharides are partially or completely indigestible.

Starch occurs in two forms, namely, *amylose* (long straight-chain glucose units) and *amylopectin* (branched arrangement of glucose units). It is found in grains, roots, vegetables and legumes. Starches are encased within the plant cells by cellulose walls in the form of granules of varying sizes and shapes and are typical for each starch. The composition of each starch differs, but all contain both amylose and amylopectin. Starches are insoluble in cold water and must be cooked. Cooking causes the granules to swell and the mixture to thicken or gel. Amylopectin in the starch granules participates in this process. Cooking softens and ruptures the cell to make the starch available for the enzymatic digestive processes in the intestine.

The food industry also modifies food starch. The natural starch structure is changed by a chemical process to make it a better thickening agent in foods such as salad dressing, pie filling, canned soup or gravy, canned pudding or baby food. Although structurally different, the caloric value of the *modified food starch* is the same as for the natural starch—4 kcal./gram.

Dextrins are the intermediate products in the hydrolysis of starch to maltose and finally to glucose. This is accomplished by the action of dry heat (toasting of bread) or by enzymes during digestion. Dextrin is more soluble and sweeter than the original starch. Another commonly used product in the degradation of starch is *corn syrup*. Made from corn starch, corn syrup has the functions of giving sweetness or adding body or viscosity and is used in many food products from bakery products and confections to ice cream, beer and canned fruits.

Glycogen is a polysaccharide branched very much like amylopectin. Figure 3–2 illustrates the structure of glycogen. It is a very large molecule with a molecular weight from one

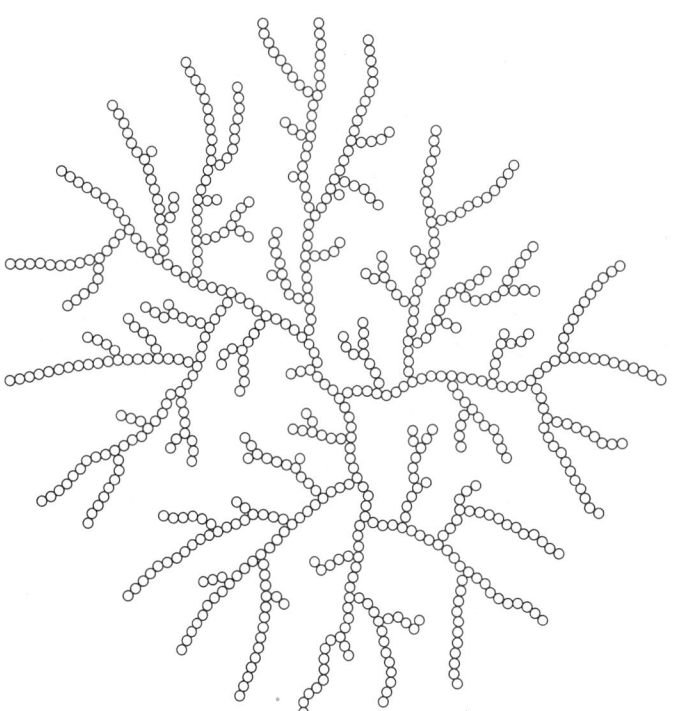

Figure 3–2 The structure of glycogen. (From: McGilvery, R. W.: Biochemistry: A Functional Approach. Philadelphia, W. B. Saunders Company, 1970.)

million to four million. Glycogen is the storage form of carbohydrate in man and animals and is the primary and most readily available source of glucose and energy. Normally about ¾ pound or 340 grams of glycogen is stored in liver and muscle. Muscle glycogen is used directly for energy. Liver glycogen may be converted to glucose and carried by the blood to the tissues for their use. Very little glycogen is found in food. The small amounts in meat and seafood are largely converted to lactic acid at the time the animals are slaughtered. Since the amount of glycogen stored at any time is very small, a constant supply of carbohydrate should be available to the body. Most of the carbohydrates consumed daily are in excess of the immediate energy needs and limited glycogen storage capacity. They are quickly converted into fats and stored in the adipose tissues.

Cellulose and *hemicellulose* are the cellular framework of plants. Cellulose resembles starch in that it is made up of many glucose molecules. The molecules are unbranched and resemble amylose. It is not soluble in ordinary solvents, and the angle of attachment between the glucose molecules in starch and cellulose is different. Whereas starch is readily digested by humans, cellulose is not. Humans do not have the enzyme needed to hydrolyze cellulose rapidly enough to be of any use. An econom-

ically feasible process for the conversion of cellulose to a carbohydrate form utilizable for energy production has not yet been developed. Ruminants can make use of cellulose, since it is digested by bacteria in the rumen.

The principal function of cellulose in human nutrition is to furnish indigestible "bulk" which promotes efficient intestinal function. This is commonly referred to as *roughage* or *fiber* in the diet. Cellulose occurs in fruit, vegetable pulp and skin, stalks and leaves and the outer coverings of grains, nuts, seeds, and legumes.

Hemicelluloses differ chemically from cellulose in that they may consist of hexoses, pentoses and acid forms of these compounds. They are also readily broken down by dilute acid. Pectin and agar-agar are typical hemicelluloses. *Pectin* is made up of units of a derivative of galactose whereas agar is composed of galactose units. These compounds are not energy sources because they are not hydrolyzed in the gut to yield simple sugars. Their nutritional function resides in the fact that they absorb water, form a gel and increase bulk which gives them a laxative property. Pectins, found in partially ripe fruit and fruit seeds and commercial preparations, are widely used for making jelly. *Agar-agar* is extracted from a seaweed, is used as a thickening agent, and can be seen on the labels of many foods. Many other

carbohydrate and noncarbohydrate gums are also used in food processing for the same functions of thickening and stabilizing.

Additional types of insoluble carbohydrates occurring in the cell walls of plants are *lignin*, *algin* and *gums*. These are used in food processing to give body and smooth consistency or to serve as a stabilizer in the product. *Inulin*, a polysaccharide composed of fructose units, is found in onions, garlic, artichokes and mushrooms. It has little dietary significance.

Synthetic fiber products, *methyl cellulose* and *carboxymethylcellulose*, besides being used in laxatives, are used in the production of low-calorie foods because of their ability to produce bulk and a feeling of satiety. The use of synthetic celluloses is increasing rapidly in a society that demands satisfying but low-calorie foods.

DEFINITION OF FIBER IN THE HUMAN DIET. The long-standing inattention to dietary fiber has resulted in a confusion about what actually is "dietary fiber." It is different from *crude fiber*, which is mainly lignin and cellulose and is the material in food remaining after a vigorous standardized treatment with acid and alkali. The USDA Handbook and other tables of food composition list the crude fiber of foods. *Dietary fiber*, the significant substance for man's digestive tract, contains two to five times more substances than just crude fiber.[16] In addition to lignin and cellulose, dietary fiber also includes hemicellulose, gums, pectin, and other carbohydrates not normally digested by man.[19]

Other Polysaccharides.[10, 15] The *mucopolysaccharides* occur in combination with protein in body secretions and structures and are responsible for the viscosity of body mucous secretions. They are not found in significant quantity in food. Some of the common mucopolysaccharides are *hyaluronic acids,* part of intercellular material; *chondroitin sulfate,* found in cornea, cartilage, skin, aorta and heart valves; *heparin,* present as a naturally occurring anticoagulant in blood; *keratosulfate,* related to blood group substances; and *dermatan sulfate,* present in the skin.

Table 3–2 summarizes briefly the types, sources and end products of carbohydrates. It also indicates the particular carbohydrates in the American diet and the quantitative importance of each carbohydrate to the total intake.

The increasing awareness that specific carbohydrates play roles in metabolic processes not previously suspected prompted the preparation of a table of the simple as well as the more complex sugars found in foods.[11] (See Appendix Table 12.) Such a table is useful in comparing the intake of specific carbohydrates in dietaries.

FUNCTION OF CARBOHYDRATES IN THE BODY

The body tissues require a constant daily supply of carbohydrate in the form of glucose in all metabolic reactions. Comparatively little is stored. The amount of glycogen stored in the liver is approximately 110 gm. and in the muscles about 225 gm. and there is about 10 gm. of glucose in the blood. For some individuals, the supply available from the storage depots would be insufficient for one day's need.

1. The principal function of carbohydrate is to serve as a major source of energy for the body. It must be supplied regularly and at frequent intervals in order to meet the energy needs of the body. Each gram of carbohydrate yields approximately 4 kcalories regardless of the source—monosaccharide, disaccharide or polysaccharide.

2. Carbohydrates exert a protein-sparing action. If insufficient carbohydrates are available in the diet, the body will convert protein to glucose in order to supply energy (gluconeogenesis). The energy needs of the body take precedence over all other needs. It has been found that for optimum utilization of amino acids for protein formation, carbohydrates must be supplied simultaneously with the essential amino acids. Protein utilization seems to be favorably affected by the presence of carbohydrates in the same meal, and nitrogen balance is improved.

3. The presence of carbohydrates is necessary for normal fat metabolism. If there is insufficient carbohydrate, larger amounts of fat are used for energy than the body is equipped to handle and oxidation is incomplete. There is an accumulation of acidic intermediate products (the ketone bodies) and acidosis results. Sodium combines with these acids so that they are excreted as sodium salts in the urine. This could lead to severe losses of sodium and cause sodium imbalance.

4. In the liver, glucuronic acid, a metabolite of glucose, has an important function in combining with chemical and bacterial toxins, as well as some normal metabolites, and converting them into a form in which they may be excreted.

Table 3–2   TYPES, SOURCES AND END-PRODUCTS OF THE CARBOHYDRATES

CARBOHYDRATES	APPROXIMATE PERCENTAGE OF TOTAL CARBOHYDRATE INTAKE*	CHIEF FOOD SOURCES	END-PRODUCTS OF DIGESTION	REMARKS
POLYSACCHARIDES:				
a) Indigestible	3			
1. Celluloses and hemicelluloses		Stalks and leaves of vegetables; outer covering of seeds	0	May be partially split to glucose by bacterial action in large bowel
2. Pectins		Fruits	0	Chemical hydrolysis yields galactose and arabinose
b) Partially digestible	2			
1. Inulin		Jerusalem artichokes, onions, garlic	Fructose	
2. Galactogens		Snails	Galactose	Digestion incomplete; further splitting by bacteria may occur in large bowel; may be production of flatus from raffinose and stachyose
3. Mannosans		Legumes	Mannose	
4. Raffinose		Sugar beets, kidney beans, lentils, navy beans	Glucose, Fructose and galactose	
5. Stachyose		Beans		
6. Pentosans		Fruits and gums	Pentoses	
c) Digestible				
1. Starch and dextrins	50	Grains; vegetables (especially tubers and legumes)	Glucose	The most important group quantitatively; usually accompanied by some maltose
2. Glycogen	Negligible	Meat products and seafood	Glucose	
DISACCHARIDES:				
1. Sucrose	25	Cane and beet sugars, molasses, maple syrup	Glucose and fructose	
2. Lactose	10	Milk and milk products	Glucose and galactose	

	Amount*	Food sources	Digestion/absorption products	Remarks
3. Maltose	Negligible†	Malt products, infant formulas	Glucose	
4. Trehalose		Mushrooms, insects, yeast	Glucose	
MONOSACCHARIDES:				
a) Hexoses:				
1. Glucose	5	Fruits; honey; corn syrup	Glucose	In fruits and vegetables the contents of glucose and fructose depend on species, ripeness, and state of preservation
–Sorbitol		Fruits, vegetables, dietetic products		
2. Fructose	5	Fruits; honey	Fructose	
3. Galactose	0	0	Galactose	These monosaccharides do not occur in free form in foods; see under lactose and mannosans
4. Mannose	0	0	Mannose	
–Mannitol		Pineapples, olives, asparagus, sweet potatoes, carrots, dietetic products		
b) Pentoses:				
1. Ribose	0	0	Ribose	These monosaccharides do not occur in free form in foods
2. Xylose	0	0	Xylose	They are derived from pentosans of fruits and from the nucleic acids of meat products and seafood
3. Arabinose	0	0	Arabinose	
CARBOHYDRATE DERIVATIVES:				
1. Ethyl alcohol	Variable	Fermented liquors	Absorbed as same	These substances are the products of natural or induced carbohydrate breakdown
2. Lactic acid	Negligible	Milk and milk products		
3. Malic acid	Negligible	Fruits		
4. Citric acid	Negligible	Fruits		

*Calculated from the average dietary of the middle-income group in the United States.

†Except in infant formulas.

(Adapted from Duncan, G. G. (ed.): Diseases of Metabolism. 5th ed., Philadelphia, W. B. Saunders Company, 1964, p. 106.)

5. Glucose has a specific influence in that it is indispensable for the maintenance of the functional integrity of the nerve tissue and is the sole source of energy for the brain. Thus a constant supply of glucose from the blood is essential for the proper functioning of these tissues. Any lack of glucose or the oxygen for its oxidation may cause irreversible damage to the brain.

6. Lactose remains in the intestines longer than the other disaccharides and thus encourages the growth of beneficial bacteria, resulting in a laxative action. One of the functions of these bacteria is believed to be the synthesis of certain vitamins (B-complex vitamins and vitamin K).

7. As previously described, cellulose and the closely related insoluble, indigestible carbohydrates aid in normal elimination. They stimulate the peristaltic movements of the gastrointestinal tract and absorb water to give bulk to the intestinal contents.

8. Carbohydrates or products derived from them serve as precursors to such compounds as nucleic acids, connective tissue matrix and galactosides of nerve tissue.

9. Foods which we tend to think of primarily for their carbohydrate content (e.g., cereals) also supply significant quantities of protein, minerals, and B-vitamins.

METABOLISM OF CARBOHYDRATES

The digestion, absorption and metabolic breakdown of carbohydrates are discussed in Chapter 6. Figure 3–3 briefly summarizes and reviews the digestion products of carbohydrates in the gastrointestinal tract and their subsequent fate, demonstrating the interrelations among carbohydrates.

Carbohydrates are absorbed through the intestinal mucosa as monosaccharides, primarily glucose with minor quantities of other sugars. All carbohydrate is then carried in the portal blood to the liver, after which it will be utilized in one of five ways. First, much of the glucose is used for immediate energy needs via oxidation *(tricarboxylic acid cycle)* to CO_2 and H_2O. This takes place in all tissues. Second, part is stored as glycogen in liver and muscle tissue. Third, some is converted to fatty acids and possibly stored as triglycerides in fat tissue (unfortunately an unlimited ability of the human body!). Fourth, a small amount is converted to

other necessary carbohydrates, such as ribose, fructose (for spermatozoa), deoxyribose, glucosamine and galactosamine. Fifth, some becomes the carbon skeletons for the production by the body of the nonessential amino acids.

The utilization of glucose for energy involves a complex series of reactions (each one catalyzed by its specific enzyme and in many cases a B vitamin coenzyme) in which the energy is released, part of it as heat and part in the form of ATP *(adenosine triphosphate)*, a special "high energy phosphate" or storage form of energy, which can be used as needed for muscular work, synthetic processes and other needs of the body. The first step in glucose metabolism is conversion of glucose to glucose-6-phosphate. From this point it may be broken down anaerobically to two 3-carbon units, with release of a small amount of energy, and then via an active 2-carbon unit, called *acetyl coenzyme A,* to carbon dioxide and water, with liberation of a much larger amount of energy. These reactions occur in all tissues. Refer to the discussion on cell metabolism in Chapter 6.

Glycogen synthesis *(glycogenesis)* also starts by way of glucose-6-phosphate which one may envision as sitting astride the crossroads of carbohydrate metabolism. Figure 3–5 gives an abbreviated schematic outline of these reactions.

Fructose and galactose are converted to glucose in the liver and possibly to some extent in the intestinal mucosal cell. Some individuals lack the specific enzymes required for one or the other of these transformations. Mild to severe abnormalities in metabolism may result. The amount of glucose available is not limited to that supplied by the carbohydrates in the food. Glucose may be synthesized from amino acids, from protein and from the glycerol portion of fat. This process is known as *gluconeogenesis*. It is linked to the level of glucose in the blood and is under hormonal control. Refer to the discussion on cell metabolism in Chapter 6.

Blood Sugar Regulation

The blood sugar is held at a remarkably constant level, 70 to 100 mg. per 100 ml. under fasting conditions. Some of the factors which influence the level of blood sugar are listed in Table 3–3. After a meal the sugar level increases but returns to the normal level as the glucose is utilized and stored. As glucose in the blood is taken up by the tissues, liver glycogen

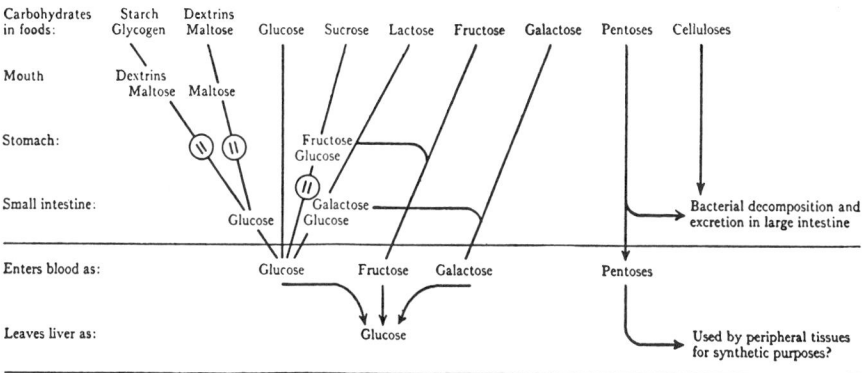

Figure 3–3 Products of carbohydrate digestion at various levels of the gastrointestinal tract and their subsequent fate. The ringed "ditto" signs indicate that the same products as at the preceding level continue to appear. (From: Duncan, G. G. (ed.): Diseases of Metabolism, 5th ed. Philadelphia, W. B. Saunders Company, 1964.)

is continually converted to glucose *(glycogenolysis)* and diffuses into the blood. (See Figure 3–4.) Muscle glycogen is used only for energy and cannot be returned to the blood as glucose; however, lactic acid produced from muscle glycogen oxidation is carried to the liver where it can be converted to glucose and glycogen *(Cori cycle)*. If fasting is prolonged, gluconeogenesis occurs and amino acids and glycerol are converted to glucose.

A battery of hormones is involved in the regulation of these reactions. *Insulin* is produced by the beta cells of the islets of Langerhans in the pancreas and affects carbohydrate metabolism by inducing the synthesis of certain enzymes. It has been called the "feasting hormone" because its liberation is enhanced by a high glucose level in the blood and to a lesser extent by the ingestion of protein

or infusion of amino acids (particularly arginine), or ketone bodies. Hormones such as glucagon and the gastrointestinal hormones, stimulation of the vagus nerve, and certain drugs such as tolbutamide (an oral hypoglycemic agent) also stimulate its release. Insulin works to lower blood glucose by (1) increasing the facilitated diffusion of glucose into muscle and adipose cells, (2) promoting storage of glucose as glycogen in the liver and muscle cells and (3) enhancing the uptake of glucose by adipose and liver cells for conversion into fat. In summary then, insulin increases the rate of glucose utilization for all three purposes—oxidation, glycogenesis and lipogenesis.

Glucagon, produced by the alpha cells of the islets of Langerhans, has an effect exactly opposite to that of insulin. It causes a rise in the amount of sugar in the blood by increasing

Table 3–3 FACTORS INFLUENCING THE LEVEL OF BLOOD SUGAR

FACTORS THAT LOWER BLOOD SUGAR	FACTORS THAT INCREASE BLOOD SUGAR
Prolonged undernutrition	Excessive carbohydrate intake
Decreased absorption of glucose	Increased absorption of glucose
Increased exercise	Reduced exercise
Liver damage	Liver damage
Kidney abnormalities (renal glycosuria)	Hyperactivity of anterior pituitary
	Hyperactivity of adrenal cortex
Anterior pituitary deficiency	Diabetes mellitus
Hypothyroidism	Epinephrine
Adrenal insufficiency	Anesthesia
Insulin	Toxemias
Sulfonylureas (stimulate insulin release)	Head injuries
Biguanides	Fright and anger
	Glucagon
	Glucocorticoids
	Growth hormone
	Thyroxine

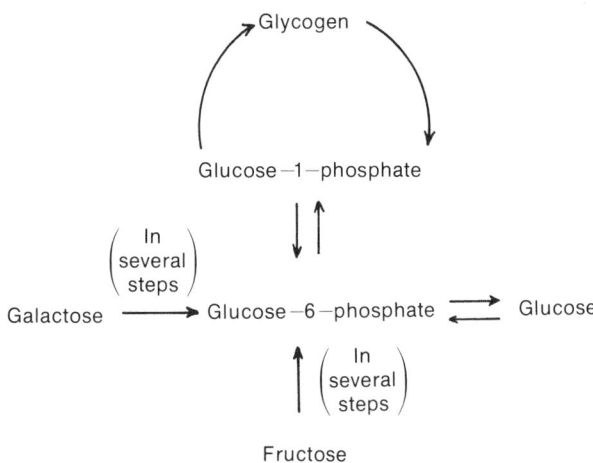

Figure 3–4 Summary of the overall process of glycogen formation and hydrolysis. Glycogen synthesis involves uridine diphosphate (UDP) and uridine triphosphate (UTP) as well as ADP and ATP.

glycogenolysis and gluconeogenesis and stimulates the release of insulin from the pancreas. A similar form produced by the intestine (enteroglucagon) also stimulates the release of insulin but does not have glycogenolytic activity and appears to be under a different control than pancreatic glucagon. Thus, insulin and glucagon may be considered to be antagonists, and it is at least in part through their opposing efforts that carbohydrate metabolism is maintained in a steady state.

Epinephrine, a hormone derived from the amino acid tyrosine and produced by the adrenal medulla gland, tends to favor the breakdown of liver and muscle glycogen to yield blood glucose (glycogenolysis) and decreases the release of insulin from the pancreas, thereby raising the blood sugar. The secretion of epinephrine is increased during anger or fear, and the increased formation of glucose which follows presumably serves as a source of extra energy to permit the body to respond more rapidly to the crisis.

Glucocorticoids, steroid hormones elaborated by the adrenal cortex, also influence blood glucose levels by stimulating gluconeogenesis. These hormones apparently reduce the utilization of glucose by the tissues and also increase the rate at which protein is converted into glucose. The net result of these two actions is to increase blood glucose; i.e., these steroid hormones counteract the action of insulin. Glucocorticoids also influence protein and fat metabolism which will be discussed in subsequent chapters.

When the blood glucose concentration is severely decreased, *thyroxine* secretion by the thyroid gland is increased. It stimulates hepatic glycogenolysis and gluconeogenesis and the blood glucose concentration rises. Thyroxine also increases the rate of hexose absorption from the intestine.

The *growth hormone,* also called *somatotropin* and *adrenocorticotropin,* elaborated by the anterior pituitary gland, also raises the blood glucose. Growth hormone increases amino acid uptake and protein synthesis by all cells, diminishes cellular uptake of glucose and increases the mobilization of fat for energy. It spares both protein and carbohydrate. *Adrenocorticotropin* increases glucocorticoid secretion by the adrenal cortex.

For a summary of the processes adding glucose to the blood and the processes removing glucose from the blood refer to Figure 3–5.

Metabolism of Ethyl Alcohol (Ethanol). Ethyl alcohol yields approximately 7.0 kcal./gm. when completely metabolized. It is rapidly absorbed from the stomach and small intestine; uniformly distributed throughout the body water; and rapidly oxidized with little or none stored. Small amounts are lost into the urine and into the respired air by diffusion. The "breath test" to determine driver intoxication is a practical application of this physiological fact.

In the liver, ethyl alcohol is converted to acetaldehyde, and then to acetyl-CoA which, as has been discussed, may readily be utilized for energy. The rate of metabolism of alcohol is increased by fructose, but the effect varies with the individual. This is a possible reason for mixing alcohol with fruit juices or sugar-containing (fructose and glucose) mixers.

Experimental animals fed appreciable amounts of ethanol will grow about as efficiently as animals fed isocaloric quantities of carbohydrate or fat, if the protein, vitamin,

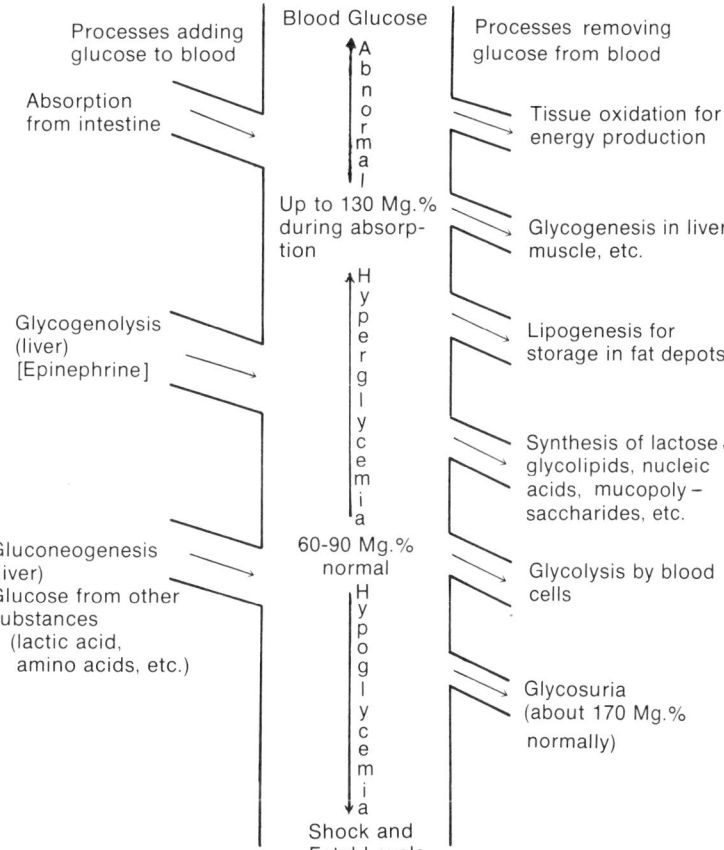

Figure 3–5 Blood glucose maintenance. (Adapted from: West, E. S., et al.: Textbook of Biochemistry, 4th ed. The Macmillan Company, 1966.)

essential amino acid and fatty acid requirements are met. Apparently, a high ethanol diet can provide the major portion of the calorie needs of an individual; however, such a diet would be inadequate in all other respects.

This has been of necessity a very brief outline of carbohydrate metabolism. (The details of this very complex subject are presented in biochemistry texts listed at the end of this chapter.) Common abnormalities of carbohydrate metabolism are presented in Part 2 of this volume.

DAILY DIETARY ALLOWANCE

The body can utilize protein or fat for energy if carbohydrate is limited. However, if fat is serving as the main source of energy, intermediates in the oxidative process are formed faster than they can be completely oxidized. Accumulation of these products causes acidosis. Utilization of protein for energy is wasteful because protein foods are expensive, the part burned for energy cannot be used for building body proteins, and the nitrogen is excreted in the urine and wasted. Approximately 58 per cent of the amino acids in the body proteins and approximately 10 per cent of the fat can be converted to glucose.

Adequate nutrition is possible at extremes of either high or low carbohydrate intake, provided that the calories and essential nutritional needs of the body are met. An active adult consumes about 50 per cent (200 to 400 gm.) of his daily calories in carbohydrates. According to the Food and Nutrition Board of the National Research Council in the 1974 revision,

Carbohydrate can be made in the body from some amino acids and the glycerol moiety of fats; there is therefore no specific requirement for this nutrient in the diet. However, it is desirable to include some preformed carbohydrate in the diet to avoid ketosis, excessive breakdown of body protein, loss of cations, especially sodium, and involuntary dehydration. Fifty to 100 gm. of digestible carbohydrate a day will offset the undesirable metabolic responses associated with high fat diets and fasting.[6]

Table 3–4   CARBOHYDRATE AVAILABLE PER PERSON PER DAY AND PER CENT FURNISHED BY STARCH AND SUGARS

YEAR	GRAMS CARBO- HYDRATE	PER CENT STARCH[1]	PER CENT SUGARS[2]	PER CENT OF TOTAL KCALORIES
1909–1913	492	68.3	31.7	56.2
1925–1929	476	58.7	41.3	54.4
1935–1939	436	56.8	43.2	52.8
1947–1949	403	52.4	47.6	49.4
1957–1959	374	49.6	50.4	47.3
1965	374	48.8	51.2	47.0
1971	380	47.1	52.9	46.8
1974	385	46.5	53.5	45.9

[1] Grains and starch vegetables.
[2] Fruits and sugar.
(Adapted from Friend, B.: Nutrients in United States food supply. Am. J. Clin. Nutr. *20*:911 and 912, 1967. Sugar, 1975, The Sugar Assoc., Inc., Washington, D.C., 1975. Figures from USDA, 1974. Friend, B., and Marston, R.: Nutritional Review. Consumer and Food Economics Institute, Agricultural Research Service, November, 1974.)

CARBOHYDRATE IN THE AMERICAN DIET

Trends in Consumption of Carbohydrates

Today's average American consumes a diet in which 45 per cent of the calories come from carbohydrate—two-thirds of which is sugar (see Table 3–4). Thus, a total of about 15 to 17 per cent of the calories come from sugar, which is a per capita sugar consumption of 80 to 100 pounds per year.[17] Although there was a 25 per cent increase from 1909–1913 to 1925, since then the consumption of sugars and sweeteners has remained fairly stable at this level; however, the form has changed.[13] Whereas in 1949 the majority of sugar was eaten from the 5 or 10-pound bag of sugar, today the majority is eaten in processed foods to which sugar or sweetener has been added in the processing.

While consumption of simple sugars has remained stable since 1925, the consumption of complex carbohydrates (starch) has decreased (see Fig. 3–6). Thus, there has been a decrease in the total carbohydrate consumption within the past 65 years from about 500 grams per person per day in 1909–1913 to about 380 grams in 1974 (see Fig. 3–7). The decrease in complex carbohydrate consumption is reflected in less consumption of grains, breads, cereals and potatoes. A decreased consumption of fiber and roughage, which are usually contributions of complex carbohydrates, also comes with this trend. In summary, the trend is overwhelmingly in favor of continued U.S. consumption of simple sugars and refined carbohydrates in processed foods as compared with fresh foods.[18]

Sugar and Health

The consumption of sugar (sucrose) has been postulated by several investigators to be a factor in the development of coronary heart disease.[8] A problem with making a definitive statement is that in the typical American diet it is difficult to separate the influence of dietary sucrose from dietary fat in the development of CHD. The evidence now is not strong enough to say that sugar consumption is a causative factor in the development of coronary heart disease.[8] (See Chapter 28—Nutritional Care for Patients with Cardiovascular Diseases.)

Sugar consumption has also been implicated in the increasing incidence of obesity. Again, though, there is no evidence to implicate sucrose any more than alcohol, fat or protein. Obesity results from an excess of calories regardless of the source. There can be the occasion, however, when similar to the alcoholic, the "carboholic" loses all control after the first bite of concentrated carbohydrate and goes on a binge with a resulting large intake of calories and eventual overweight.[2] (See Chapter 27—Nutritional Care in Conditions of Overweight and Underweight.)

The case for sugar, particularly sucrose, in the etiology of dental caries is stronger. It has been found that all forms of carbohydrate, including starch, can cause caries in the presence of the proper bacteria. Interestingly, the total amount of sugar consumed does not seem to be

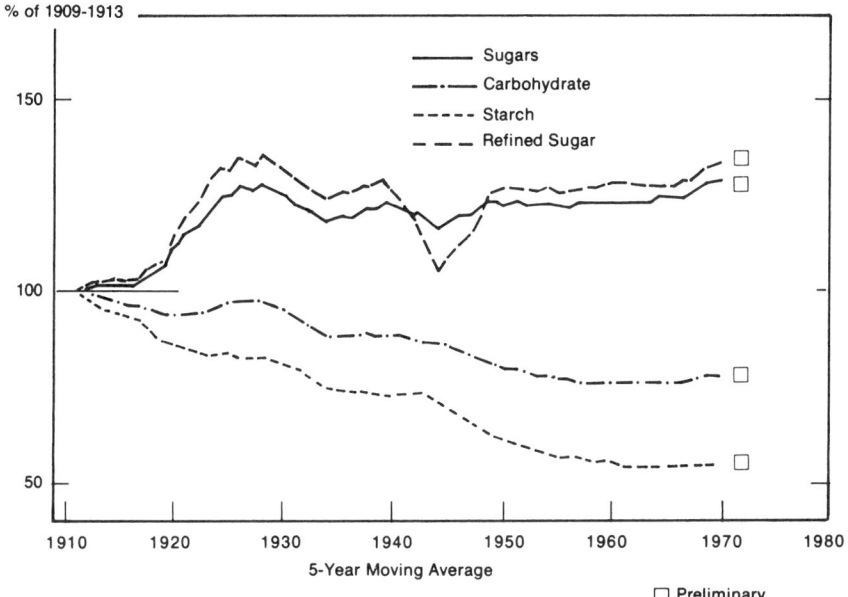

Figure 3–6 Carbohydrate consumption in the United States, 1910–1970. Note: There is a decline (about 25 per cent) in total carbohydrate consumption, a severe drop in starch consumption (approximately 50 per cent) and a rather static consumption for sugars and refined sugar with the exception of the growth phase following World War I and the sharp drop during World War II. (From: Agricultural Research Service, U.S. Department of Agriculture.)

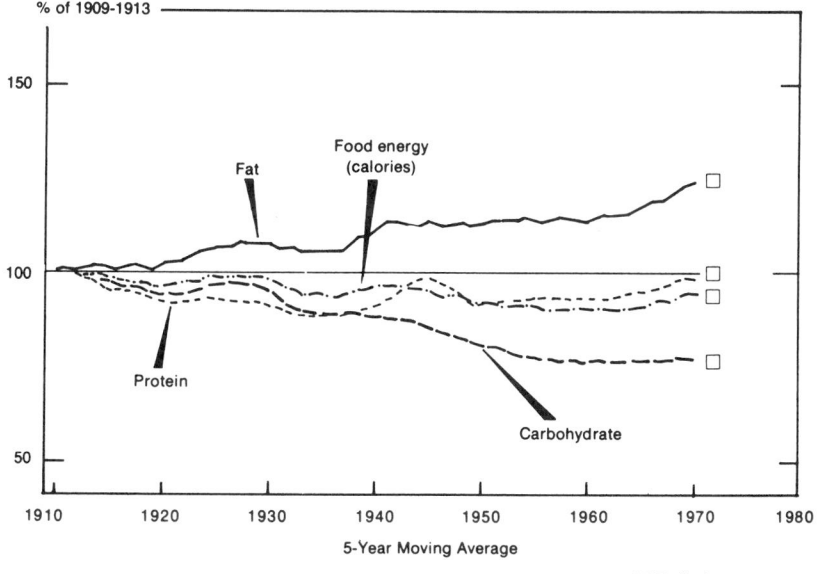

Figure 3–7 Consumption of protein, fat, carbohydrate and calories in the United States, 1910–1970. Note: Trends for protein and carbohydrate consumption apparently are plateauing, while the slight upturn in total calories appears to be a result of an increase in fat consumption. (From: Agricultural Research Service, U.S. Department of Agriculture.)

the deciding factor in the development of caries, but rather the physical form (sticky vs. liquid) and manner and frequency (a between-meal snack vs. part of a meal) with which it is eaten.[9] Bibby concludes that the increasing frequency of eating or snacking and the popularity of mixtures of sugar and flour as snack items (e.g., pastries, cookies, cakes) may be the most important reasons for the increased incidence of dental caries in this country.[1] (See Chapter 33—Nutritional Care for Patients with Diseases of the Musculoskeletal System.)

Dietary Fiber and Health

No longer can fiber avoid the attention of nutritionists. Its appearance, or rather disappearance, from the diet of Western man is being scrutinized as a factor in the etiology of common noninfective diseases of the colon, such as constipation, diverticulosis, cancer, hyperlipoproteinemia, and diabetes.[4, 5] Several protective qualities have been attributed to dietary fiber. By affecting stool bulk, softness, and transit time, it is thought to be a factor in (1) lessening colonic pressure that may lead to diverticula[14] (see Chapter 23—Nutritional Care for Patients with Intestinal Diseases), (2) reducing the exposure of the gut mucosa to possible carcinogenic substances in the feces[3] (see Chapter 36—Nutrition, Diet and Cancer), and (3) lowering blood cholesterol by binding

with bile acids, thus leading to an increased cholesterol degradation and excretion via the bile acid pathways (see Chapter 28 on cardiovascular disease). However, the findings are not definitive enough yet to define an adequate or recommended level of fiber intake. Much of the evidence is epidemiological, comparing disease incidence in countries with high fiber intakes with the incidence in Western countries where the fiber intake is relatively low, but where a number of other factors are also different. Nelson estimates that the fiber intake of the average American adult is low at .8–3.2 gm. of crude fiber per day.[12]

COMMON SOURCES OF STARCHES AND SUGARS

The groups of food providing appreciable amounts of carbohydrate in the dietary are (1) grains, (2) fruits, (3) vegetables, (4) milk, and (5) the concentrated sweets. (See Table 3–5.) Most of these foods provide other nutrients as well as carbohydrate.

Refined sugar, syrups and cornstarch are examples of pure carbohydrates, and many of the sweets such as candy, honey, jellies, molasses and soft drinks contain little, if any, of other nutrients. These are referred to as "empty calories" because they contribute nothing except calories to the dietary of an individual. An excessive intake of these empty calories tends to reduce the intake of the

Table 3–5   CARBOHYDRATE CONTENT* OF SOME TYPICAL FOODS

SUGAR	CARBO-HYDRATE (PER CENT)	STARCH	CARBO-HYDRATE (PER CENT)
Concentrated Sweets		*Grain Products*	
Sugar: Cane, beet, powdered,	99.5	Starches: Corn, tapioca, arrowroot	88–86
brown, maple	96–90	Cereals (dry): Corn, wheat, oat, bran	85–68
Candies	95–70	Flour: Corn, wheat-sifted	80–70
Honey (extracted)	82	Popcorn (popped)	77
Syrup: Table blends, molasses	75–55	Cookies: Plain, assorted	71
Jams, jellies, marmalades	70	Crackers, saltines	72
Carbonated, sweetened beverages	10–12	Cakes: Plain, without icing	56
Fruits		Bread: White, rye, whole wheat	52–48
Prunes, apricots, figs (cooked, unsweet)	31–12	Macaroni, spaghetti, noodles, rice (cooked)	30–23
Bananas, grapes, cherries, apples, pears	23–15	Cereals (cooked): Oat, wheat, grits	16–10
Fresh: Pineapples, grapefruits, oranges,		*Vegetables*	
apricots, strawberries	14–8	Boiled: Corn, white and sweet potatoes, lima,	
Milk		dried beans, peas	26–15
Skim	6	Beets, carrots, onions, tomatoes	7–5
Whole	5	Leafy: Lettuce, asparagus, cabbage, greens,	
		spinach	4–3

*From Composition of Foods, Agriculture Handbook No. 8. Agricultural Research Service, U.S. Department of Agriculture, Washington, D.C.

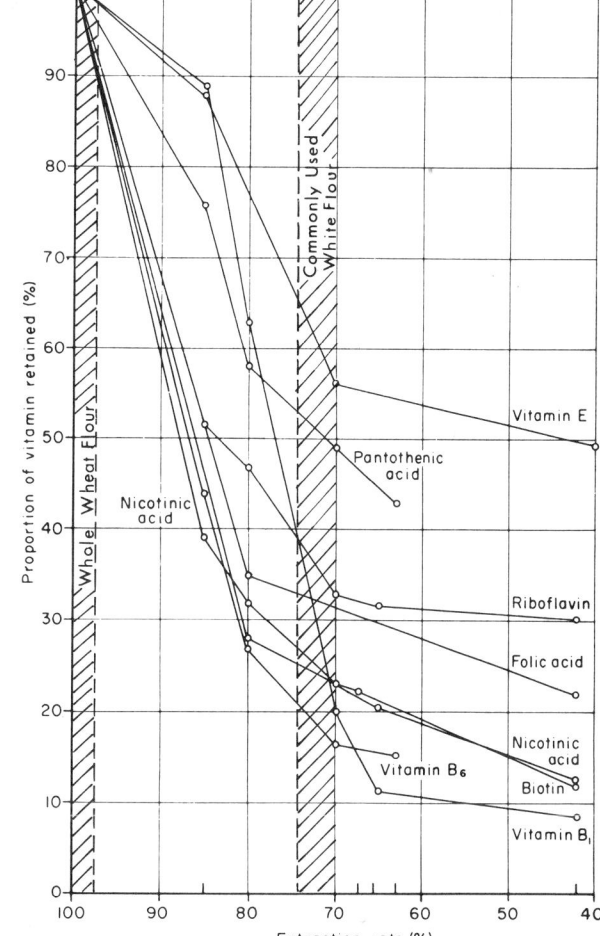

Figure 3–8 Relationship between extraction rate and proportion of total vitamins of the grain retained in flour. (Adapted from: Proposed Fortification Policy for Cereal-Grain Products. Washington, D.C., National Academy of Sciences, 1974.)

health-protecting foods, largely by taking away one's appetite for them.

Most carbohydrate foods contain more than one nutrient. For example, the whole grains, wheat, corn, rice and to a lesser degree oats, rye, barley, buckwheat and millet, contain in addition to starch varying amounts of proteins (incomplete), minerals and vitamins.

The carbohydrates in fruits are principally the monosaccharides glucose and fructose (sucrose if sweetened). They contribute vitamins, minerals, cellulose, hemicellulose, pectin and water, in varying amounts. (Fruits such as avocados and olives contain considerable fat.)

Vegetables have a varying amount of glucose. The leafy vegetables are high in water and cellulose content and many contribute minerals and vitamins. The root tubers and seed variety (potatoes, beets, carrots, turnips, peas, beans) have a higher starch content.

They, too, contribute some protein, minerals and vitamins, water and cellulose, in varying amounts. Legumes (dried beans and peas, soybeans, nuts) contain appreciable amounts of protein as well as minerals and vitamins. Soybeans and nuts contribute good quality protein and fat (soybean oil, peanut oil).

Milk, though generally listed with the protein foods, supplies the disaccharide lactose. It is the only animal food contributing appreciable quantities of carbohydrate to the dietary. As mentioned, the glycogen in meat is usually broken down before the meat reaches the market.

THE ENRICHMENT OF BREAD, FLOUR AND CEREALS

Because the American diet was considered to be short in certain essential nutrients, the Council on Foods and Nutrition of the Ameri-

a Kernel of Wheat

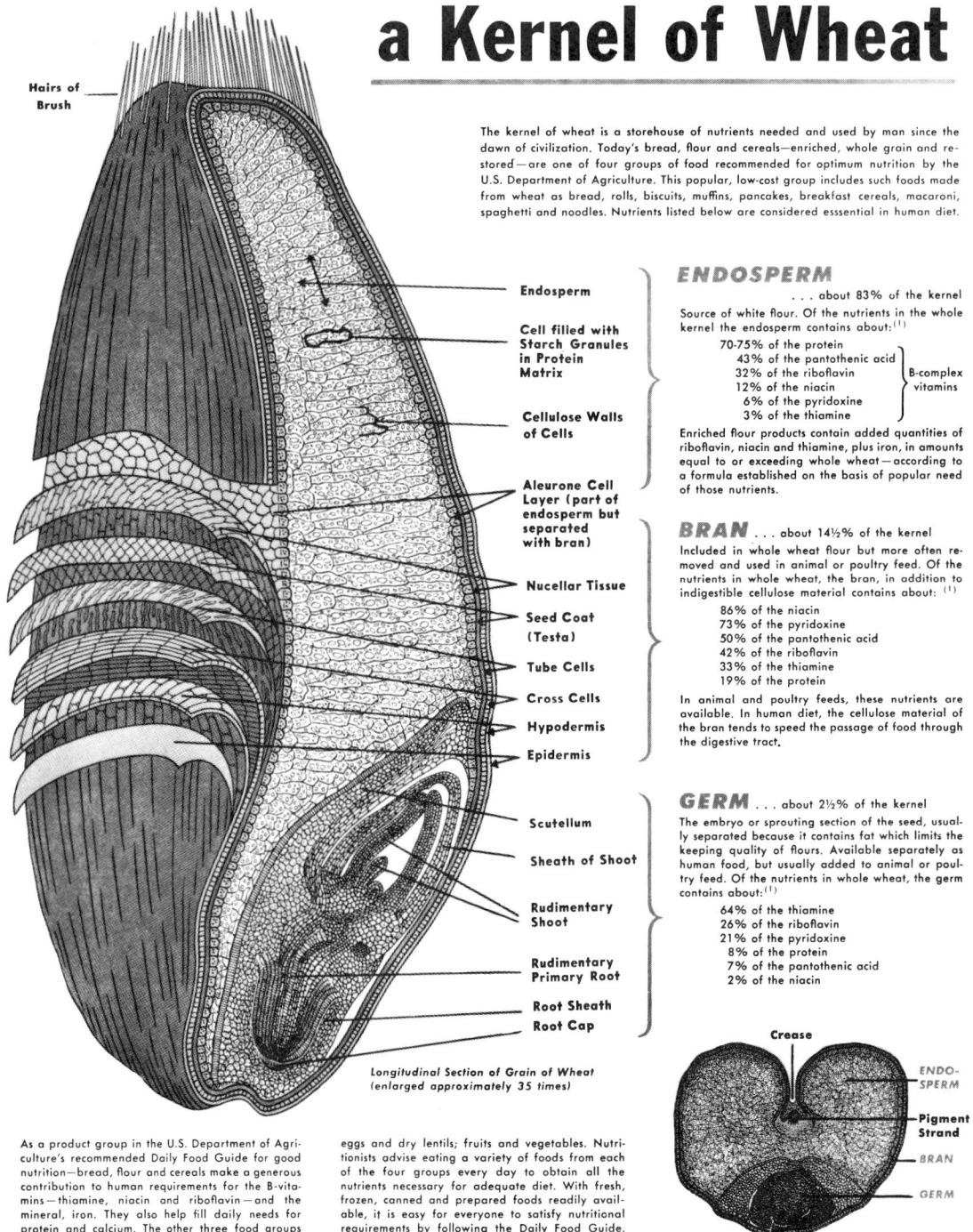

The kernel of wheat is a storehouse of nutrients needed and used by man since the dawn of civilization. Today's bread, flour and cereals—enriched, whole grain and restored—are one of four groups of food recommended for optimum nutrition by the U.S. Department of Agriculture. This popular, low-cost group includes such foods made from wheat as bread, rolls, biscuits, muffins, pancakes, breakfast cereals, macaroni, spaghetti and noodles. Nutrients listed below are considered esssential in human diet.

Hairs of Brush

Endosperm

Cell filled with Starch Granules in Protein Matrix

Cellulose Walls of Cells

Aleurone Cell Layer (part of endosperm but separated with bran)

Nucellar Tissue

Seed Coat (Testa)

Tube Cells

Cross Cells

Hypodermis

Epidermis

Scutellum

Sheath of Shoot

Rudimentary Shoot

Rudimentary Primary Root

Root Sheath

Root Cap

Longitudinal Section of Grain of Wheat (enlarged approximately 35 times)

ENDOSPERM

. . . about 83% of the kernel

Source of white flour. Of the nutrients in the whole kernel the endosperm contains about:[1]

70-75% of the protein
43% of the pantothenic acid
32% of the riboflavin   } B-complex
12% of the niacin   } vitamins
6% of the pyridoxine
3% of the thiamine

Enriched flour products contain added quantities of riboflavin, niacin and thiamine, plus iron, in amounts equal to or exceeding whole wheat—according to a formula established on the basis of popular need of those nutrients.

BRAN . . . about 14½% of the kernel

Included in whole wheat flour but more often removed and used in animal or poultry feed. Of the nutrients in whole wheat, the bran, in addition to indigestible cellulose material contains about: [1]

86% of the niacin
73% of the pyridoxine
50% of the pantothenic acid
42% of the riboflavin
33% of the thiamine
19% of the protein

In animal and poultry feeds, these nutrients are available. In human diet, the cellulose material of the bran tends to speed the passage of food through the digestive tract.

GERM . . . about 2½% of the kernel

The embryo or sprouting section of the seed, usually separated because it contains fat which limits the keeping quality of flours. Available separately as human food, but usually added to animal or poultry feed. Of the nutrients in whole wheat, the germ contains about:[1]

64% of the thiamine
26% of the riboflavin
21% of the pyridoxine
8% of the protein
7% of the pantothenic acid
2% of the niacin

Crease

ENDO-SPERM

Pigment Strand

BRAN

GERM

Cross Section View

As a product group in the U.S. Department of Agriculture's recommended Daily Food Guide for good nutrition—bread, flour and cereals make a generous contribution to human requirements for the B-vitamins—thiamine, niacin and riboflavin—and the mineral, iron. They also help fill daily needs for protein and calcium. The other three food groups are: milk and milk products; meats, poultry, fish, eggs and dry lentils; fruits and vegetables. Nutritionists advise eating a variety of foods from each of the four groups every day to obtain all the nutrients necessary for adequate diet. With fresh, frozen, canned and prepared foods readily available, it is easy for everyone to satisfy nutritional requirements by following the Daily Food Guide.

(1) Flour Milling And Baking Research Association, Chorleywood, Hertfordshire, England.

Figure 3–9   Diagram shows the structure, composition and nutritive values of a kernel of wheat. © 1976, Wheat Flour Institute, Washington, D.C.

Table 3–6 COMPARISON OF THREE B-VITAMINS AND IRON IN WHEAT BREAD (POUND LOAVES)

BREAD	THIAMIN (mg.)	RIBOFLAVIN (mg.)	NIACIN (mg.)	IRON (mg.)
Whole wheat made with 2% non-fat dry milk	1.17	0.56	12.9	10.4
White enriched* with 3 to 4% non-fat dry milk	1.8	1.1	15.0	11.3
White unenriched with 3 to 4% non-fat dry milk	0.31	0.39	5.0	3.2

*Enriched bread may also furnish, as an optional ingredient, added harmless calcium salts in such quantity that each pound of the finished bread will contain 600 milligrams of calcium. (From Standards of Identity for Bakery Products, U.S. Dept. HEW, FDA, Federal Register 36:23074 (1971), 38:28558 (1973), 39:5188 (1974).)

(From Composition of Foods, Agriculture Handbook No. 8 Agricultural Research Service, U.S. Department of Agriculture, Washington, D.C.)

can Medical Association and the Food and Nutrition Board of the National Research Council approved several staple foods as carriers of additional nutrients. They have issued statements regarding the addition of specific nutrients to foods from time to time, and in 1953 issued a joint statement to serve as a valuable guide. This will be more fully discussed in Chapter 18.

Among the common staple foods selected or approved as carriers of added nutrients are bread, flour and cereals. The highly refined grains are more resistant to spoilage, but have become deprived of the most protective elements, such as essential amino acids (proteins), vitamins and minerals (see Fig. 3–8).

When the whole grain is used, minerals and vitamins are present in appreciable amounts. When the bran layers and germ (see Figure 3–9) are removed by the process of refining, most of the thiamin, riboflavin, niacin and iron are lost. Since people have become accustomed to the refined products, enrichment to replace the elements removed in the milling process has been accepted as the best solution.

The result of the enrichment of bread is seen in Table 3–6. Bread and flour enrichment is mandatory in 37 states (also Puerto Rico, Canada and other countries). It is widely practiced in those states without legal requirements. Almost 95 per cent of the white bread sold in the United States is enriched.[7] There also are federal standards for the enrichment of rice and corn grits. Nutrition scientists are in general agreement that this improvement in the nutritive quality of food has made a significant contribution to the improvement of nutrition and health.

PROBLEMS AND SUGGESTED TOPICS FOR DISCUSSION

1. List the amounts of the various carbohydrate foods you consume during a period of 24 hours and a period of 3 days.
2. Evaluate the list of carbohydrate foods. Classify them into "sugars" and "starches." List the monosaccharides.
3. What per cent of the daily dietary should be normally consumed in the form of carbohydrate foods? When might it be increased? Decreased?
4. Keep a record of your diet for one day. Calculate the carbohydrate and calorie content. What percentage of the calories were derived from carbohydrates? What percentage of the carbohydrate calories were derived from fruits, vegetables, breadstuffs and cereal foods? What percentage of the carbohydrate calories were derived from sugars, candy, soft drinks, cake and pie? List any changes you could make in carbohydrate content to improve your diet, and give reasons.
5. Why do you like to eat carbohydrate foods?
6. What factors tend to raise and to lower the blood sugar? What is the form of carbohydrate in the circulating blood? What is the normal concentration?
7. List the functions of carbohydrates in the body. What becomes of the carbohydrate eaten in excess of the body's daily need for energy?

CITED REFERENCES

1. Bibby, B. G.: The cariogenicity of snack foods and confections. J. Am. Dent. Assoc., 90:121, 1975.
2. Bloom, W. L., and Clark, M. S.: Diagnosis and treatment of the obese carboholic. Obesity, 1:10, 1964.
3. Burkitt, D. P.: Epidemiology of cancer of the colon and rectum. Cancer, 28:3, 1971.
4. Burkitt, D. P.: Some diseases characteristic of modern western civilization. Br. Med. J., 1:274, 1973.

5. Burkitt, D. P., Walker, A. R., and Painter, N. S.: Dietary fiber and disease. JAMA, *229*:1068, 1974.
6. Calloway, D. H.: Dietary components that yield energy. Environ. Bio. Med., *1*:175, 1971.
7. Enriched Bread. Am. Instit. of Baking, Chicago, 1976.
8. Grande, F.: Sugar and cardiovascular disease. In Stare, F. J. (ed.): Sugar in the Diet of Man. World Rev. Nutr. Diet., Karger, Basel, *22*:248, 1975.
9. Gustafsson, B. E., et al.: The Vipeholm dental caries study: the effect of different levels of carbohydrates intake or caries activity in 436 individuals observed for 5 years. Acta. Odontol. Scand., *11*:232, 1954.
10. Guthrie, H. A.: Introductory Nutrition. 3rd ed. St. Louis, C. V. Mosby Company, 1975.
11. Hardinge, M. G., Swarner, J. B., and Crooks, H.: Carbohydrates in foods. J. Am. Dietet. A., *46*:197, 1965.
12. Nelson, R. A.: Role of unavailable carbohydrate (UC) in digestion. In White, P. L., Fletcher, D. C., and Ellis, M., (eds.): Nutrients in Processed Foods—Fats, Carbohydrates. Acton, Mass., Publishing Sciences Group, Inc., 1975.
13. Page, L., and Friend, B.: Level of use of sugars in the United States. In Sipple, H. L., and McNutt, K. W. (eds.): Sugars in Nutrition. New York, Nutrition Foundation Inc., Academic Press, 1974.
14. Painter, N. S., Almeida, A. Z., and Colebourne, K. W.: Unprocessed bran in treatment of diverticular disease of the colon. Br. Med. J., *2*:137, 1972.
15. Pike, R. L., and Brown, M. L.: Nutrition: An Integrated Approach. 2nd ed. New York, John Wiley & Sons, Inc., 1975.
16. Scala, J.: J. Food technology, *28*:34, 1974.
17. Stare, F. J. (ed.): Sugar in the Diet of Man. World Review of Nutrition and Diet, Karger, Basel, *22*:237, 1975.
18. Toscano, V. A.: Sugars and other carbohydrates. In White, P. L., Fletcher, D. C., and Ellis, M. (eds.): Nutrients in Processed Foods—Fats, Carbohydrates. Acton, Mass., Publishing Sciences Group, Inc., 1975.
19. Trowell, H.: Dietary fibre, coronary heart disease and diabetes mellitus. Plant Foods for Man, *1*:11, 1973.
20. White, P. L., Fletcher, D. C., and Ellis, M. (eds.): Nutrients in Processed Foods—Fats and Carbohydrates. Acton, Mass., Publishing Sciences Group, Inc., 1975.

ADDITIONAL REFERENCES

Antar, M. A., et al.: Changes in retail market food supplies in the United States in the last 70 years in relation to the incidence of coronary heart disease, with special reference to dietary carbohydrate and essential fatty acids. Am. J. Clin. Nutr., *14*:169, 1964.

Bogert, L. J., Briggs, G. M., and Calloway, D. H.: Nutrition and Physical Fitness. 9th ed. Philadelphia, W. B. Saunders Company, 1973.

Bondy, P. K., and Rosenberg, L. E. (eds.): Diseases of Metabolism. 7th ed. Philadelphia, W. B. Saunders Company, 1974.

The dietary iron controversy/the experts debate. Nutr. Today, *7*:2, 1972.

Friend, B.: Nutrients in United States food supply. Am. J. Clin. Nutr., *20*:987, 1967.

Gray, G. M.: Carbohydrate digestion and absorption—role of small intestine. N. Engl. J. Med., *292*:1225, 1975.

Green, D. E.: The mitochondrion. Sci. Am., *210*:63, 1964.

Guyton, A. C.: Textbook of Medical Physiology. 5th ed. Philadelphia, W. B. Saunders Company, 1976.

Harper, H. A.: Review of Physiological Chemistry. 15th ed. Los Altos, California, Lange Medical Publications, 1975.

Holum, J. R.: Principles of Physical, Organic and Biological Chemistry. New York, John Wiley & Sons, 1969.

Levine, R.: Carbohydrates. In Goodhart, R. S., and Shils, M. C. (eds.): Modern Nutrition in Health and Disease. Philadelphia, Lea and Febiger, 1973.

Mazur, A., and Harrow, B.: Textbook of Biochemistry. 10th ed. Philadelphia, W. B. Saunders Company, 1971.

McGilvery, R. W.: Biochemistry: A Functional Approach. Philadelphia, W. B. Saunders Company, 1970.

Mendeloff, A. I.: A critique of fiber deficiency. Am. J. Dig. Dis., *21*:109, 1976.

Present Knowledge in Nutrition. 3rd ed. The Nutrition Foundation Inc. 1967, Chapter 3, Present knowledge of carbohydrate.

The role of fiber in the diet. Dairy Council Digest, *46*:1, 1975.

Sugar:1975. Washington, D. C., The Sugar Association, Inc., 1975.

Chapter 4

LIPIDS

The term lipid, which is often used interchangeably with the term fat, was created to include a heterogeneous group of compounds related actually, or potentially, to the fatty acids. They have in common the properties of being (1) insoluble in water, (2) soluble in organic solvents such as ether and chloroform and (3) utilizable by living organisms. The group thus includes the ordinary fats and oils, waxes and related compounds. The principal foods contributing fat to the diet are butter, margarine, lard, vegetable oil, salad dressing, the visible fat of meat, the skin of chicken and the invisible fat found in cream, homogenized milk, milk products, egg yolk, meat, fish, nuts, olives, avocados and in whole-grain cereals.

CLASSIFICATION AND COMPOSITION

The principal groups of lipids important in nutrition are listed and classified in Table 4–1.

Most natural fats are composed of about 98 to 99 per cent triglycerides and the vast majority of these are *long chain* triglycerides. The 1 or 2 per cent remaining include traces of mono- and diglycerides, free fatty acids, phospholipids and unsaponifiable matter containing sterols.

TRIGLYCERIDES

Like carbohydrates, triglycerides (the main component of ordinary fats and oils) are composed of carbon, hydrogen and oxygen. Structurally they are esters of a trihydric alcohol (glycerol) and fatty acids. (See top of facing page.) The fatty acids can have from 4 to 30 carbon atoms and make up the bulk of the triglyceride. One hundred grams of fat will contain 95 grams of fatty acids.

Fatty Acids: Saturated and Unsaturated. A fatty acid or hydrocarbon chain is described with regard to two characteristics: chain length and degree of saturation with hydrogen. The *length* is defined as the number of carbon atoms

Table 4–1 CLASSIFICATION OF LIPIDS IMPORTANT TO NUTRITION

I. *Simple Lipids*
  A. Fatty acids
  B. Neutral fats: Mono-, di-, triglycerides (esters of fatty acids and glycerol)
  C. Waxes (esters of fatty acids with high molecular weight alcohols)
    1. Sterol esters
    2. Nonsterol esters

II. *Compound Lipids*
  A. Phospholipids: Compounds of fatty acids, phosphoric acid and nitrogenous base
    1. Phosphoglycerides
      a. Lecithin
      b. Cephalin
      c. Sphingomyelins
  B. Glycolipids: Compounds of fatty acid combined with carbohydrate and a nitrogenous base
      a. Cerebrosides
      b. Gangliosides
  C. Lipoproteins: Lipids in combination with protein

III. *Derived Lipids*
  A. Fatty acids: Mono- and diglycerides
  B. Glycerol: Water-soluble component of triglycerides and interconvertible with carbohydrate
  C. Sterols
    1. Cholesterol, ergosterol
    2. Steroid hormones
    3. Vitamin D
    4. Bile salts
  D. Fat-soluble vitamins
    1. Vitamin A
    2. Vitamin E
    3. Vitamin K
    4. Coenzyme Q (ubiquinone)

in the chain. For example, C_{16} denotes 16 carbons in the chain. Frequently, the terms "short" (6 or less carbons), "medium" and "long" (12 or more carbons) are used to describe the chains of fatty acids in triglycerides. The *degree of hydrogen saturation* is defined by the number of double bonds between the carbon atoms in the chains. A chain may contain all the hydrogen it can hold and have no double bonds, in which case it would be called a *saturated fatty acid*. It may contain one

$$\begin{array}{ccc}
\text{H} & & \text{H} \\
| & & | \\
\text{H}-\text{C}-\text{OH} & & \text{H}-\text{C}-\text{OOC}-\text{R}_1 \\
| & & | \\
\text{HO}-\text{C}-\text{H} & \text{R}-\text{COOH} & \text{R}_2-\text{COO}-\text{C}-\text{H} \\
| & & | \\
\text{H}-\text{C}-\text{OH} & & \text{H}-\text{C}-\text{OOC}-\text{R}_3 \\
| & & | \\
\text{H} & & \text{H}
\end{array}$$

Glycerol   Fatty Acid   Triglyceride

double bond and be called a *monounsaturated fatty acid,* or it may be a *polyunsaturated fatty acid* and contain several double bonds. (See figure below.)

The whole series of saturated fatty acids has been found in natural fats. However, the only unsaturated fatty acids that naturally occur in large amounts contain 18 carbons, although there are small amounts of 16- and 20-carbon unsaturated fatty acids.

IDENTIFICATION. A convenient shorthand gives the number of carbon atoms (chain length) and the number of double bonds (chain saturation). For example, linoleic acid is designated as $C_{18:2}$ because it has 18 carbons and 2 double bonds. Besides this form of identification, fatty acids also have common names that usually indicate the fat from which they were isolated, e.g., linoleic—linseed oil, butyric—butter.

The diversity of natural fats is influenced by the properties of triglycerides in each fat, and the triglycerides are related to their fatty acids. The physical properties of the fatty acids are related to their chemical structure. The shorter and more unsaturated the fatty acids, the more liquid or soft the fat or oil is at room temperature. Solid fats such as mutton tallow contain large amounts of palmitic ($C_{16:0}$) and stearic ($C_{18:0}$) acids. Oils (fats that are liquid at room temperature) usually have a high proportion of oleic ($C_{18:1}$) and linoleic acids ($C_{18:2}$).

Complete separation and identification of the fatty acids in a fat was an almost impossible task using the older chemical procedures. By means of gas-liquid chromatography it is now possible to get a complete profile. At least 60 different fatty acids have been found in butter fat.

Synthetic Fats. *Medium chain triglycerides* are unnaturally occurring forms of fat that are absorbed and metabolized differently from long chain triglycerides. They are triglycerides composed of fatty acids with lengths of 8 and 10 carbon atoms and were made to provide a source of dietary fat for people with fat malabsorption problems. The principal fatty acid is octanoic acid ($C_{8:0}$).

Polyglycerol esters are synthetic hybrid fats made by the esterification of fatty acids. Although they look and taste like fat, they have fewer calories—6.5 to 8.5 kcal./gram instead of 9 kcal./gram for traditional fats. Food processors are using them to make low-calorie, palatable foods.

Characteristics of Animal and Vegetable Fats. There is considerable species variation in fats from animal sources. The major components of the fats of land animals are palmitic, stearic and oleic acids, with smaller amounts of linoleic acid and traces of arachidonic acid ($C_{20:4}$). The fat of the herbivorous animals (beef and mutton tallow) is harder (more saturated) than pork and poultry fats. The degree of un-

$CH_3(CH_2)_{16}COOH$ Stearic Acid (Saturated)

$CH_3(CH_2)_7CH=CH(CH_2)_7COOH$ Oleic Acid (Mono-unsaturated)

$CH_3(CH_2)_4CH=CHCH_2CH=CH(CH_2)_7COOH$ Linoleic Acid (Polyunsaturated)

$CH_3CH_2CH=CHCH_2CH=CH-CH_2-CH=CH(CH_2)_7COOH$ Linolenic Acid (Polyunsaturated)

18 Carbon Acids

saturation of pork, beef and chicken fat may vary, depending on the diet. In fact, in response to pressure from associations concerned with heart disease and from consumers conscious of saturated fat intake, the beef industry is experimenting with different feeds which will result in meat and fat with fewer saturated fatty acids. The problems at present are with safety and cost. Fish have softer fat than land animals and unsaturated fatty acids with 20 and 22 carbons predominate. The flavors of all meats are distinguished from each other by the flavor of their respective fats.

Vegetable oils are predominantly unsaturated. About 85 per cent of the fatty acids of the common food oils is oleic and linoleic, although the proportions of the two vary widely, from 15 per cent linoleic in olive oil to 75 per cent in safflower oil. An exception is coconut oil. It is almost completely saturated but has a low melting point because of a high content of medium chain fatty acids (8 to 12 carbons). Table 4–2 lists the analysis of some oils and fats of animal and plant origin.

Reactions of Fats. Enzymes of the digestive tract act as catalysts for the hydrolysis of triglycerides to their component fatty acids and glycerol. If the fat is hydrolyzed with alkali (*saponification*), salts of the fatty acids or soaps are formed. Formation of insoluble soaps in the intestinal tract may be of concern

Table 4–2 RELATIONSHIP OF IODINE VALUES TO POLYUNSATURATION*

OIL SOURCE	APPROXIMATE PER CENT POLYUN-SATURATION	IODINE VALUE
Safflower	78	140–150
Soybean (S/B)	62	125–135
Corn oil	58	110–128
Cottonseed (C/S)	54	100–115
Peanut (P/N)	33	85–100
Lard	10	55–70
Palm	10	45–55
Butterfat	4	25–40
Cocoa butter (C/B)	4	30–40
Palm kernel (P/K)	2	15–25
Coconut oil (C/N)	2	5–15

*Iodine value is a measure of the degree of unsaturation of a lipid.

(From White, P. L., Fletcher, D. C., and Ellis, M. (eds.): Nutrients in Processed Foods—Fats and Carbohydrates, Acton, Mass., Publishing Sciences Group, Inc., 1975, p. 18.)

in some abnormal conditions characterized by poor fat absorption.

HYDROGENATION.   Unsaturated fatty acids may add hydrogen to the double bonds. So oleic acid, linoleic acid and linolenic acid when completely hydrogenated become stearic acid. Vegetable oils may be converted to solid fats by hydrogenation. Complete hydrogenation would produce a very hard and unpalatable fat. When the process is controlled, fat of any desired consistency can be prepared, and commercially hydrogenated vegetable oils such as Crisco and Spry are creamy solids at room temperature, similar to lard and butter fat.

$$-\underset{\underset{H}{|}}{\overset{\overset{}{|}}{C}}=\underset{\underset{H}{|}}{\overset{\overset{}{|}}{C}}- \; + \; H_2 \; \rightarrow \; -\underset{\underset{H}{|}}{\overset{\overset{H}{|}}{C}}-\underset{\underset{H}{|}}{\overset{\overset{H}{|}}{C}}-$$

Hydrogenation

Margarine is also made by hydrogenating oils but with additional processing to produce a product that will melt readily and simulate butter. It is emulsified with milk that has been cultured with a microorganism to add flavor. A yellow vegetable dye and vitamins A and D are added to give the margarine the appearance and nutritive value of butter.

A serious disadvantage of hydrogenation is that it lowers the polyunsaturated fatty acid content of the fat and may form some trans-isomers of the unsaturated acids. A product of the same consistency but of higher linoleic acid content may be prepared by mixing a portion of almost completely hydrogenated fat with some of the original oil. This procedure is used for some margarines, as some of the labels on "tub" or "soft" margarines show. See Table 4–3.

In 1964 the Food and Drug Administration moved to prohibit manufacturers from branding vegetable oil products as "polyunsaturated." The action was taken following a consumer survey on public understanding of current labeling of such products. The survey revealed that label terms such as "polyunsaturated," "unsaturated," "low in cholesterol," and similar statements misled many people to believe that these foods will reduce blood cholesterol and thus be effective in treating or preventing atherosclerotic diseases. It is believed they play no significant part in reducing

Table 4–3   FATTY ACID COMPOSITION OF FATS AND OILS IN TABLE GRADE MARGARINES

| | % of Total Fatty Acids | | | |
| | Unsaturated Fatty Acids | | | Saturated Fatty Acids |
Margarine Type	Monoenoic	Dienoic	Trienoic	
Stick—All Vegetable	35–66	12–48	0.5–4	17–25
—Animal Fat	52–57	2–11	0–0.5	36–41
Tub—All Vegetable	22–48	25–65	0.5–3	15–23
Liquid—All Vegetable	14–36	42–75	0.5–5	10–17

FATTY ACID COMPOSITION OF BUTTERFAT

| | % of Total Fatty Acids | | | | |
| | Unsaturated Fatty Acids | | | | Saturated Fatty Acids |
	Oleic	Linoleic	Linolenic	Arachidonic	
Butterfat	28–31	1.0–2.5	0.2–0.5	0.2–0.4	63–70

(From Food Fats and Oils. 4th ed. Institute of Shortening and Edible Oils, Inc., Washington, D.C., 1974, p. 16.)

blood cholesterol unless the diet is changed in other respects.

RANCIDITY. When fats and oils are exposed to warm, moist air over a period of time, chemical changes occur which produce unpalatable flavors and disagreeable odors, commonly called rancidity. Hydrolysis of butter fat in the presence of oxygen, airborne bacteria and heat releases butyric acid and other products with very strong taste. The oxygen of the air can attack the double bonds of the polyunsaturated fatty acids, forming peroxides which may be toxic in large amount. Rancid fat has a toxic effect on rats given low-fat diets.

The oxidative process destroys vitamin A and vitamin E. Vitamin E is present in rather large amounts in vegetable fats. It is an antioxidant and protects against rancidity but in the process is, itself, inactivated. Fortification of fats or fatty foods with antioxidants such as butylated hydroxyanisole (BHA) and butylated hydroxytoluene (BHT) extends the storage time and protects essential nutrients. Precautions should be taken to lessen the danger of rancidity by storage of fat-containing foods at low temperature and limiting the storage time of susceptible foods such as butter and lard.

FUNCTIONS

FUNCTIONS OF TRIGLYCERIDES

Energy. Fats serve as a concentrated source of energy. Each gram of fat supplies 9 kcalories, which is more than twice the amount of energy supplied by each gram of carbohydrate. The main source of this energy is the fatty acids, which supply 40 to 50 carbon atoms for oxidation as compared with 3 from glycerol. Because of the high energy density and low solubility of fats, they are used as a storage form of energy. Not only ingested fat but carbohydrate and amino acids not immediately used by the tissues are converted to fat and stored in the adipose tissue. Up to two-thirds of the total energy of the cells may be supplied by triglyceride rather than carbohydrate. Fat spares protein for tissue synthesis.

Other Functions. Adipose tissue helps to hold the body organs and nerves in position and to protect them against traumatic injury and shock. The subcutaneous layer of fat insulates the body, which serves to preserve body heat and maintain body temperature. Fats aid in transport and absorption of the fat-soluble vitamins. Fats spare thiamin since they can be metabolized for energy, as compared with carbohydrate, whose metabolism requires thiamin. In the stomach they depress gastric secretions and slow the emptying time of the stomach, thus providing a pleasant feeling of satiety after a meal. Fats also retard the rapid development of hunger which occurs after a carbohydrate meal. Fats add to the palatability of food as well as to the flavor of the diet.

Essential Fatty Acids (EFA). Three polyunsaturated fatty acids, namely, linoleic, linolenic and arachidonic acids, have essential fatty acid activity. However, only two—linoleic and arachidonic—have been desig-

nated as essential fatty acids for the human.[7] They have important roles in fat transport and metabolism and in maintaining the function and integrity of cellular membranes. They also are a part of the fatty acids of cholesterol esters and phospholipids in plasma lipoproteins and mitochondrial lipoproteins. Serum cholesterol has been shown to be lowered by EFA, but the mechanism is not entirely clear.[10] Fatty acids with EFA activity are also precursors of a group of hormone-like compounds, *prostaglandins*, which participate in the regulation of blood pressure, heart rate, lipolysis and the central nervous system.

In the presence of a dietary source of linoleic acid (along with Vitamin B_6) the body can synthesize *arachidonic* and *linolenic acids*, but no conversion of the other acids to linoleic acid occurs. *Linoleic acid* was shown to be a dietary essential for infants by Hansen, Wiese and associates,[9] who found that linoleic acid would prevent or cure a characteristic dermatitis (eczema) observed in infants fed a fat-free diet (Fig. 4–1). The only reported instances of essential fatty acid deficiency in adults are associated with long term fat-free intravenous feedings. See Chapter 12—Nutritional Deficiency Diseases.

EFA deficiency in animals produces not only poor growth and dermatitis but a poor reproductive capacity, lowered efficiency of energy utilization, decreased resistance to certain stresses such as x-ray and ultraviolet light, impairment of lipid transport and changes in the polyunsaturated fatty acid content of tissues. It is now theorized that some of the manifestations of EFAD may be due to resulting prostaglandin deficiency, since essential fatty acids are precursors of prostaglandins.[4]

The dietary requirement of linoleic acid for infants has been estimated to be between 1 and 3 per cent of the total calories. The requirement for the adult is relatively low. The minimum human requirement would appear to be near 2 per cent of the calorie intake.[7] The tissue storage of linoleic acid in the adult with the average dietary is high, so that an excess amount in the diet may be harmful. Excessive amounts of polyunsaturated fatty acids have been observed to reduce the vitamin E level in animal tissues to a dangerously low level, resulting in encephalomalacia and sterility in chicks and creatinuria in rats. Fortunately, vegetable oils supplying the linoleic content in a diet high in the EFA have a natural vitamin E content, which serves as a lipid antioxidant.

LIPIDS WITH SPECIAL FUNCTIONS

Phospholipids. Any lipid containing phosphorus is included in this classification. They

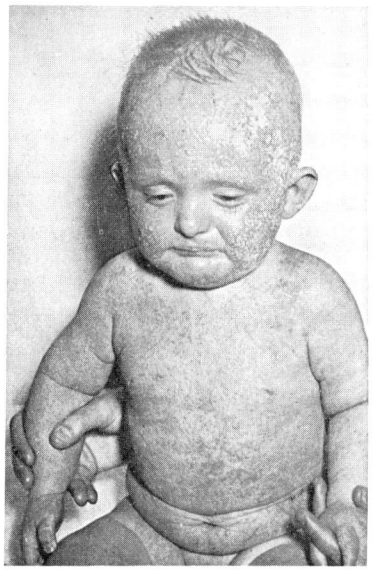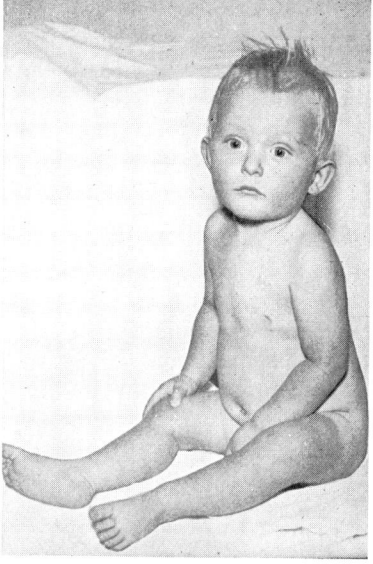

Figure 4–1   Certain fatty acids, found in fats of low melting point, must be furnished in the food. Skin troubles result when these essential fatty acids (linoleic and arachidonic acids) are lacking. Left, 6 month old infant with very resistant eczema since 2½ months of age. Right, same child six months later, after lard had been included in the diet. (Photos courtesy of Dr. A. E. Hansen.)

are the next largest lipid component of the body after the triglycerides. Phospholipids are formed in essentially all cells of the body, although a greater portion that enter the blood are formed in the liver cells and the intestinal mucosa. Because of their strong affinity for both water-soluble and fat-soluble substances in the molecule, large concentrations of phospholipids are found in combination with protein in cell membranes, where they facilitate the passage of fat in and out of the cell. The phospholipids function in maintaining the structural integrity of the cells rather than as fat stores. Despite the loss of body fat that occurs in extreme starvation the phospholipid content remains fairly constant, thus maintaining the integrity of tissue cells.

The *lecithins* contain glycerol and fatty acids as well as phosphoric acid and the nitrogen-containing base choline. They are the most widely distributed of the phospholipids; traces are present in liver and egg yolk and in unrefined vegetable oils such as corn oil. Lecithin is added to food products such as cheese, margarine and confections to aid in emulsification.

Phospholipids such as *cephalins* (which are similar in structure to lecithins), *lipontols* (which contain inositol, a compound with vitamin-like activity) and *sphingomyelins* (which contain no glycerol but a complex amino alcohol) are found in rather high concentrations in nerve tissue. A *cephalin* is needed to form thromboplastin for the blood clotting process. *Sphingomyelin* is found in the brain and other nerve tissue as a component of the myelin sheath. This substance acts as an insulator around the nerve fibers. Egg yolk and liver are good sources of these phospholipids.

As a rule, the invisible and not the visible fat of both plant and animal tissue contains appreciable amounts of phospholipids. The amount in oils, lard and butter is small owing to the processing which removes most of the phospholipids.

Glycolipids. The glycolipids include the *cerebrosides* and *gangliosides*. They contain the base sphingosine and fatty acids with 22 and 24 carbons. The carbohydrate component of the cerebrosides is galactose; the gangliosides contain, in addition, glucose and a complex compound containing an amino sugar. Structurally both the cerebrosides and gangliosides are components of nerve tissue and certain cell membranes, where they play a role in fat transport.

Lipoproteins. Lipoproteins are formed primarily in the liver and to a lesser degree in the intestine. They are found in cell and organelle membranes (mitochondria and lysosomes) and in the blood. Lipoproteins are combinations of triglycerides, phospholipids and cholesterol with protein which function to transport insoluble lipids in an aqueous medium. They are classified as (1) *chylomicrons* (formed in the chyle or lymph as lipids are absorbed), which consist of a core of triglyceride coated with phospholipid and protein; (2) *very low density lipoproteins (VLDL),* which contain mostly triglyceride and little protein; (3) *low density lipoproteins (LDL),* which contain less triglyceride and more cholesterol and protein; and (4) *high density lipoproteins (HDL),* which contain high concentrations of protein and low concentrations of triglycerides. *Non-esterified fatty acids* occur in combination with serum albumin.

Hydrocarbons. Mention should be made here of the term "oil," a confusing word that may refer to fats in a liquid state or to other substances which have the same properties but have no relation to fats. Examples are sulfuric acid, called oil of vitriol, and mineral oil, which is a hydrocarbon from petroleum. Motor oil is a hydrocarbon, and many hydrocarbon oils are physically like fats when cool (petroleum jelly, for example). Hydrocarbons have no nutritive value and are not metabolized or absorbed by the body. Some are used for specific purposes in medicine, such as mineral oil for its laxative and lubricating qualities in the bowel. Because the fat-soluble vitamins are readily carried in mineral oil and the latter is not absorbed, its administration in large amounts may reduce the absorption of the fat-soluble vitamins. Thus, it should not be used regularly and always with caution.

CHOLESTEROL

Cholesterol is a member of the large group of compounds called sterols. They all have the same complex ring structure. (See figure below.)

Cholesterol

The "-ol" ending indicates that cholesterol is an alcohol. *Cholesterol* is found only in animal tissues, but somewhat similar sterols are found in plants. *Ergosterol,* a yeast sterol, is converted to vitamin D_2 on exposure to ultraviolet light. Cholesterol is found not only as the free alcohol but also in combination with fatty acids as esters. It is an essential component of the structural membranes of all cells and is a major component of brain and nerve cells. It is the chief component of gallstones. Not only is cholesterol present in foods consumed (exogenous cholesterol), but it also can be synthesized in the cell (endogenous cholesterol).

Function. The structural function of cholesterol is not entirely understood. It is, however, a key intermediate in the biosynthesis of a number of other important *steroids*. These include the bile acids, adrenocortical hormones, estrogens, androgens and progesterone. The bile acids are compounds with a detergent-like action necessary for the proper absorption of fats from the intestines. The adrenocortical hormones help control the sodium-potassium stores of the body and the rates of metabolism of carbohydrate and nitrogen compounds. This group of steroids includes aldosterone, corticosterone and cortisone. The sex hormones (estrogens, androgens and progesterone) also participate in the development of typical secondary sex characteristics of the female and male. Cholesterol is converted by the intestinal mucosa to 7-dehydrocholesterol, the provitamin of vitamin D_3, cholecalciferol. This transformation is also effected by skin and other tissues. The provitamin, when irradiated with ultraviolet light, usually through exposure of the body to sunlight, is also transformed into active vitamin D_3. Cholesterol in the skin along with other lipids makes the skin resistant to the action of many chemical agents and to the absorption of water-soluble substances. Cholesterol and other lipids are highly inert to acids and certain solvents, which serve to prevent penetration into the body. Water evaporation from the skin is prevented by the presence of cholesterol and other lipids. Abnormal deposits of cholesterol in the tissues are associated with several conditions, including atherosclerosis, hypertension and diabetes mellitus.

Absorption and Excretion. Cholesterol esters are hydrolyzed in the intestinal tract but the cholesterol is largely re-esterified during the process of absorption. It is incorporated into the chylomicrons formed in the intestinal wall and transported via the lymphatic circulation to the liver. The absorption of cholesterol is dependent upon the absorption of fat and is stimulated by the presence of fatty acids. In the blood, cholesterol is present free or esterified with fatty acids as part of the lipoprotein complex.

The principal products of cholesterol breakdown are the bile acids, which are formed in the liver and are delivered into the small intestine in the bile secretions. About 80 per cent of the cholesterol metabolized is converted to bile acids. Both bile acids and cholesterol are continually reabsorbed from the terminal ileum and to a lesser extent from the large intestine, pass again into the liver, and are re-excreted in the bile. This is known as the *enterohepatic cycle*. The liver is also responsible for regulating the rate of loss of cholesterol from the body, which it does largely by converting it to cholic acid which is excreted in bile. Some cholesterol enters the intestinal tract by direct excretion across the intestinal mucosa as well as via the bile. In the lumen of the intestine a portion is hydrogenated to *coprosterol* by intestinal organisms. Coprosterol cannot be absorbed and is excreted in the feces. Very little cholesterol is excreted in the urine; some is lost by way of the skin.

Metabolism. The main sites of cholesterol synthesis are the liver cells and the intestinal cells, but it can also be synthesized in almost all other tissues. The liver is also a storage depot for cholesterol absorbed from the intestine. The rate of endogenous cholesterol synthesis is variable and is dependent upon the amount already present in the body and thus somewhat upon the amount in the diet. The enterohepatic cholesterol pool has been estimated to be about 2000 mg. (2 gm.).

The physiological and metabolic relationships among body fat, cholesterol, phospholipids, unsaturated fatty acids and atherosclerosis are complex and not completely understood, but are the object of much present-day medical research. (See Chapter 28 on cardiovascular diseases.)

Dietary Sources. Cholesterol occurs in largest amounts in egg yolk, liver, kidney, sweetbreads, brains and fish roe. Cholesterol is also present in smaller amount in the fat of meat, whole milk, cream, ice cream, cheese and butter. Foods that are low in cholesterol or contain no cholesterol are fruits, vegetables, cereals, breadstuffs, syrup, egg white, low-fat fish, very lean meats, soup stock made without fat and skim milk. (See Table 4–4 and Appendix Table 4 for a complete list of the cholesterol content of food.) However, it must be pointed

Table 4–4   CHOLESTEROL CONTENT OF SOME FOODS

	AMOUNT	MG. OF CHOLESTEROL
Kidneys	½ c. sliced pieces	562
Liver (beef, pork)	3 oz. slice (85 gm.)	372
Egg yolk	1 large yolk (17 gm.)	252
Custard, baked	½ c. (132 gm.)	139
Shrimp, canned	½ c. (64 gm.)	96
Crab, canned	½ c. (80 gm.)	80
Beef	3 oz. (85 gm.)	80
Halibut	1 fillet (125 gm.)	75
Pie, peach	⅛ of 9″ pie (114 gm.)	70
Chicken, breast	½ breast (80 gm.)	63
Lobster	½ c. of meat (72 gm.)	61
Oysters, canned	3 oz. (85 gm.)	38
Milk, whole	1 cup (244 gm.)	34
Cheese, cheddar	1 oz. (28 gm.)	28
Ice cream	½ c. (66 gm.)	26
Cheese, cottage, 1% fat	1 cup (267 gm.)	23

From Feeley, R. M., Criner, P. E., and Watt, B. K.: Cholesterol content of foods, J. Am. Diet. Assoc., *61*:134, 1972.

out that the amount synthesized and metabolized daily by the body itself is far greater than the amount usually consumed in the diet, of which only 50 per cent is absorbed. The level of cholesterol is influenced by the amount present in the diet and also by the amount of fat, especially saturated fat, in the diet. It is important that the nurse understand the limitations of diet in the lowering of blood cholesterol so that she can intelligently answer the numerous questions of her patients and prevent the omission of necessary nutrients such as vitamins A and D, protein and EFA.

REGULATION OF BLOOD LIPID LEVELS THROUGH DIETARY FAT AND CHOLESTEROL MANIPULATION

The dietary fat intake has been shown to have an effect on the serum cholesterol level of individuals. Populations (United States, Great Britain, Finland) consuming diets high in fat usually have relatively high serum cholesterol levels. Populations (Japan, Italy) with a low fat intake usually have relatively low serum cholesterol levels.

The total concentration of cholesterol in the blood plasma is highly variable, averaging about 200 mg. per 100 ml. (range between 150 and 250 mg. per 100 ml.) in the adult. The liver is primarily responsible for the maintenance of plasma cholesterol level. The blood cholesterol levels probably reflect the difference between the rate of synthesis and the rate of destruction. The dietary factors that affect the plasma con-

centration of cholesterol may be summarized as follows:

1. A high intake of *dietary cholesterol* normally increases the blood cholesterol level, a few milligrams per 100 ml. The liver normally compensates for the high exogenous intake of cholesterol by synthesizing smaller quantities of endogenous cholesterol and converting more cholesterol into bile acids. However, these control mechanisms vary from one person to another and possibly from one race to another. Intestinal cholesterol synthesis may also be involved.

2. A dietary containing only *saturated fat* (butter, coconut oil, fat of meat) increases the blood cholesterol level as much as 40 to 50 mg. per 100 ml. A high fat consumption increases blood cholesterol in two ways: (1) triglycerides in food enhance the absorption of cholesterol and (2) triglycerides presumably increase fat deposition in the liver which in turn increases the rate of fat metabolism and supplies increased amounts of acetyl-CoA in the liver cells for the manufacture of cholesterol. A decrease, therefore, in the amount of saturated fats rather than of cholesterol is indicated.

3. A dietary intake of the *polyunsaturated fats* such as corn oil, cottonseed oil and safflower oil effectively lowers serum cholesterol levels.

4. Evidence suggests that *dietary fiber* may lower serum cholesterol by binding with bile acids and preventing their reabsorption, or by favoring the growth of intestinal flora, which produce secondary bile acids that are not as well absorbed as primary bile acids.[5]

Other factors such as an excess secretion of the *thyroid hormone* decrease the blood cholesterol levels. *Estrogens* decrease serum cholesterol and *androgens* increase serum cholesterol. How this occurs is unknown. In *diabetes mellitus* the blood cholesterol level rises, probably because of the increase in the mobilization of lipids. The blood cholesterol level rises along with blood triglyceride and phospholipid levels in *renal retention diseases*, resulting from a diminished removal of lipoproteins from the blood owing to an inhibition of *lipoprotein lipase*.

Cholesterol is further discussed under diseases of the gallbladder and in relation to atherosclerosis. Diets with modified cholesterol and fat content appear on page 596. Also, see Appendix Tables 1 and 4 for cholesterol and fatty acid content of foods.

METABOLISM AND STORAGE OF FAT

Transport of Fat

Almost all the lipids of the diet are absorbed into the lymph from the intestinal mucosa. Only the medium chain fatty acids, absorbed directly into the portal blood, bypass the lymphatic system. The lipids are carried in the lymph as *chylomicrons*, droplets of fat with cholesterol and phospholipids with a small amount of protein adsorbed to their outer surface. The droplets are large enough to make the plasma appear milky after a meal containing fat. They empty into the venous blood at the thoracic duct and are carried to the liver or are removed from the blood by the adipose tissue.

Within a few hours after eating, chylomicrons have been removed from the blood by the action of *clearing-factor lipase* or *lipoprotein lipase* on the endothelial cells lining the capillaries in the adipose tissue. Lipoprotein lipase hydrolyzes the triglycerides and phospholipids into fatty acids and glycerol, which can pass into the adipose cell.

In the liver lipids may be metabolized, stored or converted to lipoproteins, in which form they are carried in the blood to the tissues for immediate use for energy or special functions. They may also then be carried to the adipose tissue for storage.

Metabolism of Fat

The first step in catabolism of triglyceride is hydrolysis to glycerol and fatty acid. The fatty acids are released as non-esterified fatty acid bound to serum albumin—it is not a component of lipoproteins. Although a great deal of fatty acid is transported in this form, its level in the plasma remains low, since it is picked up by the tissues very rapidly. Normal plasma has a fatty acid concentration of about 15 mg. per 100 ml. In the first stage of oxidation, fatty acids are broken down stepwise into two-carbon units complexed with coenzyme A (acetyl-CoA). This complex is also an intermediate metabolite in glucose metabolism and from this point fatty acids and glucose are oxidized by the same pathway. Glycerol also, after activation, may be converted to an intermediate of glucose oxidation. These steps will be discussed in detail in a later chapter. (See Chapter 6—Digestion, Absorption and Cell Metabolism.)

Almost all tissues can utilize fatty acids for energy. Contrary to earlier opinion they form a large portion of the energy for muscular tissue even when glucose is available. Glycerol can be oxidized in only a few tissues; most of it is carried to the liver, where it can be oxidized for energy or used in the synthesis of new triglycerides.

The liver is a major center of lipid metabolism and is largely responsible for regulation of lipid levels in the body. Among its important functions are (1) synthesis of triglycerides from carbohydrate and, to a smaller extent, from protein; (2) synthesis of other lipids such as phospholipids and cholesterol from triglycerides; (3) desaturation of fatty acids (oleic acid is the predominant acid in human adipose tissue); and (4) degradation of triglycerides for use as energy. Even under normal conditions the liver produces more acetyl-CoA than it can oxidize completely. Two molecules of acetyl-CoA condense to form acetoacetic acid.

$$2\ CH_3CO\ CoA + H_2O \underset{\text{Other Cells}}{\overset{\text{Liver Cells}}{\rightleftarrows}}$$

Acetyl-CoA

$$CH_3COCH_2COOH + 2\ H\ CoA$$

Acetoacetic Acid   Coenzyme A

The *acetoacetic acid* diffuses through the liver cell membranes and is carried to peripheral tissues where it is converted again to acetyl-CoA and oxidized. When the body is relying

almost entirely on fat for energy, as in diabetes mellitus or prolonged starvation, large quantities of triglyceride appear in the liver and the production of acetoacetic acid far outstrips the ability of the peripheral tissues to oxidize it and the level in the blood rises. Part of the acetoacetic acid is converted to beta-hydroxybutyric acid and acetone—the three compounds being known collectively as the *ketone bodies*. Acetoacidic acid and beta-hydroxybutyric acid are acids that must be carried in the blood and excreted in the urine in combination with base (sodium ion). This reduces the available base in the body and the condition, if unchecked, leads to a lowering of the pH of body fluids (*acidosis*) which may be fatal. In diabetic acidosis carbohydrate metabolism returns to normal when insulin and glucose are given and the breakdown of fat is slowed to a normal pace.

Hormonal Control of Fat Metabolism

The hormones secreted by the endocrine glands which have marked effects on carbohydrate metabolism also affect fat metabolism.

(1) *Insulin* in insufficient amount decreases fat synthesis and increases fat mobilization (lipolysis) and utilization. Excessive insulin inhibits fat utilization and increases fat synthesis. Insulin influences fat metabolism by activating clearing-factor lipase, or lipoprotein lipase, which results in triglyceride hydrolysis and uptake of the resulting fatty acids by adipose tissue.

(2) *Thyroxine* increases mobilization of fats indirectly by increasing the rate of energy metabolism of each cell.

(3) *Glucocorticoids* increase the rate of fat mobilization by increasing the fat cell membrane permeability.

(4) *Adrenocorticoids* (especially corticotropin) increase fat mobilization directly and by stimulating the secretion of glucocorticoids.

(5) *Epinephrine* and *norepinephrine* increase the rate of fat mobilization by releasing free fatty acids from fat cells for metabolism. Figure 4–2 shows in simple fashion the various excursions fat can take in the body.

Storage of Fat

In the human body there are two kinds of body fat—white fat and brown fat. The vast majority of this fat is *white fat* composed of white adipose cells which basically accumulate

in three places: (1) subcutaneous tissue—50 per cent, (2) abdominal cavity, around the internal organs—45 per cent, and (3) intramuscular tissue—5 per cent. These fat cells are modified fibroblasts which store up to 95 per cent of their volume as triglycerides in liquid form. Fat storage is not static; there is a constant turnover of fat even though the amount remains the same. Besides the presence of lipoprotein lipase activating the uptake of fatty acids, there is also a *cellular lipase* which causes the release of fatty acids from the cell during times of energy deficit.

Brown adipose tissue is much less abundant ·and occurs only in certain areas of the body, particularly the interscapular region and the back of the neck. The amount of this fat is higher in the neonate and decreases with age, but it can be increased somewhat with extended exposure to cold since it functions in *thermogenesis* in response to cold. Instead of releasing fatty acids into the blood, this fat cell has the ability to switch to oxidation of fatty acids for production of heat. The mitochondrial metabolism is changed so that oxidation and phosphorylation are uncoupled, and rather than the efficient entrapment of energy as ATP, the result is energy dissipated as heat, warming the body. As might be presumed, this *nonshivering thermogenesis* is especially active in the neonate.

CHANGES IN FAT CONSUMPTION

Fats supply roughly 42 per cent of the total calories available for consumption in the retail market in the United States. Total fat consumed from animal and vegetable sources has increased from 125 to 156 gm. per person per day from the period of 1909–1912 to 1972. (See Fig. 3–7.) This increase of 31 grams is equivalent to two and one-half additional tablespoons of butter or margarine. The consumption of vegetable fat during the same period has increased from 17 per cent of fat calories to 38 per cent, causing the animal fat component to fall from 83 to 62 per cent.[3] Figure 4–3 graphically illustrates the decreased consumption of animal fat. The most rapid increase in fat consumption, for the most part owing to an increased consumption of salad and cooking oils, has occurred within the last 15 years.

The amount of fat in the diet has increased, but the percentage of total calories from *saturated* fatty acids has remained about the same

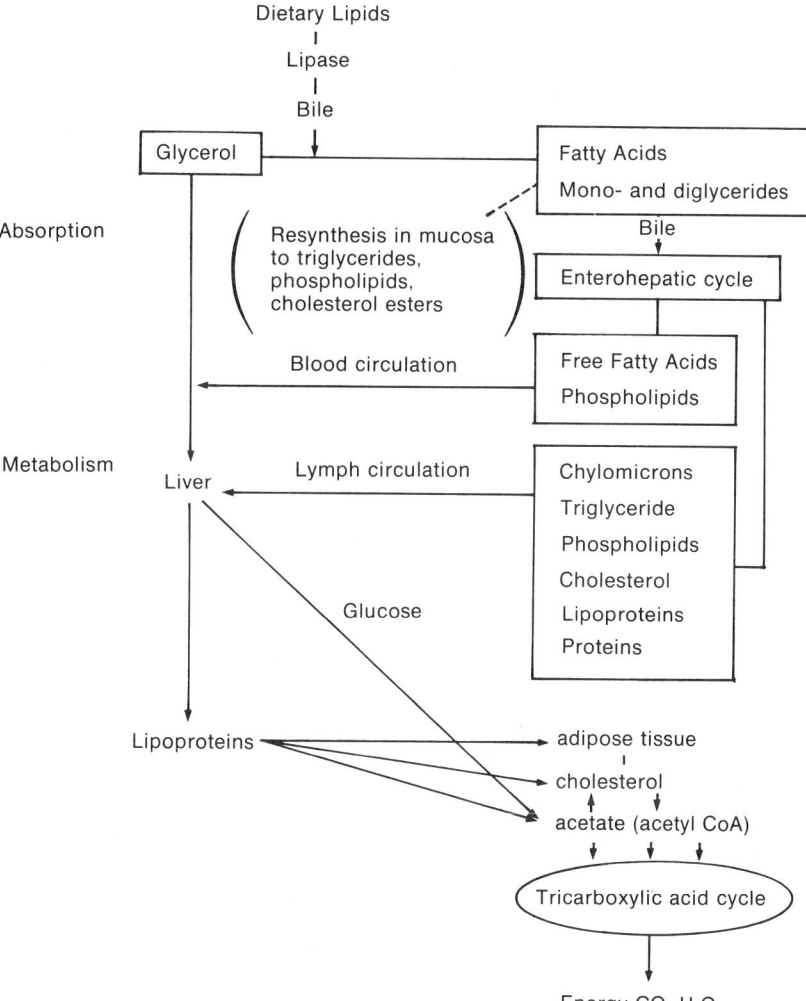

Figure 4–2   Brief summary of fat metabolism.

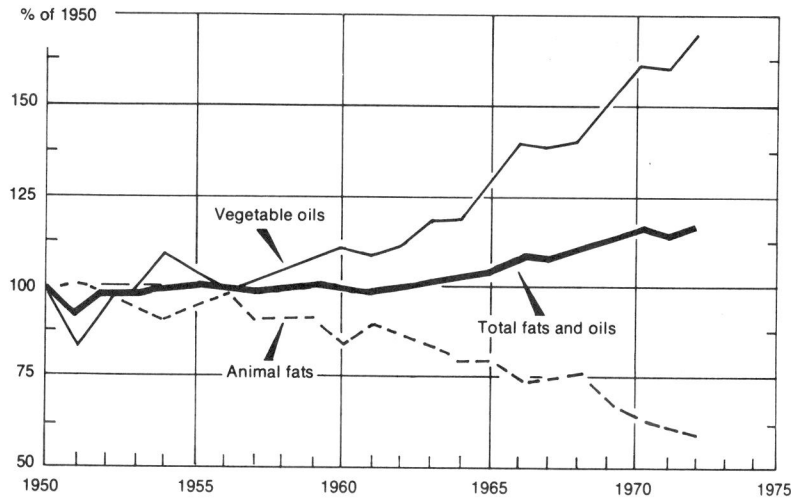

Figure 4–3   Consumption of fats and oils in the United States, 1950–1972. (From: Agricultural Research Service, U.S. Department of Agriculture.)

Table 4–5   FATTY ACIDS AVAILABLE, PER PERSON PER DAY, AND PER CENT OF TOTAL CALORIES

| YEAR | FATTY ACIDS | | | KCALORIES FURNISHED BY FATTY ACIDS | | | RATIO OF POLYUNSATURATED TO SATURATED FATTY ACIDS |
	Total Saturated, gm.	*Oleic Acid, gm.*	*Linoleic Acid, gm.*	*% Total Saturated*	*% Oleic Acid*	*% Linoleic Acid*	
1909–1913	50.3	51.5	10.7	12.9	13.3	2.7	0.20
1925–1929	53.3	55.2	12.5	13.7	14.2	3.2	0.23
1935–1939	52.9	54.5	12.7	14.4	14.8	3.5	0.24
1947–1949	54.4	58.0	14.8	15.0	16.0	4.1	0.27
1957–1959	54.7	58.2	16.6	15.6	16.6	4.7	0.30
1965	53.9	58.8	19.1	15.2	16.6	5.4	0.35
1972							0.41

(Adapted from Friend, B.: Nutrients in U.S. food supply. A review of trends 1909–1913 to 1965. Am. J. Clin. Nutr., *20*:911, 1967.)

at 13 to 15 per cent of total calories.[3] The ratio of polyunsaturated (linoleic acid) to saturated fatty acids progressively increased from 0.21 in 1909 to 0.27 in 1947 to 0.35 in 1965 and to 0.41 in 1972.[9] (See Table 4–5.) It should be pointed out that wastage, cooking and other losses are not considered in the statistics, so that the actual fat ingested is less than that available for consumption.

The trend toward a higher proportion of the calorie intake in the form of vegetable fat is due to several factors: consumption of corn, cottonseed and soybean oils in salad and cooking; the trend toward the substitution of margarines for butter; the increase in poultry consumption; and processing technology, which permits the manufacture of shortening entirely from vegetable oils. (See Fig. 4–4.)

Unfortunately the most current data on the actual *consumption* of nutrients by the U.S. population is 15 years old—that of the Household Food Consumption Survey of 1965–66. Some interesting data on fat consumption from

that survey are that 18–19-year-old males had the highest level of fat consumption—149 gm./person/day—and that among females the largest intake was by the 12–14-year-old group—100 gm./person/day.[2]

RECOMMENDED ALLOWANCE OF FATS IN THE DIET

The average American adult eats about 127 pounds of fat yearly, receiving perhaps 42 per cent of his total calories as fat. This includes both visible and invisible fats. Fats are popular because of their flavor and satiety value; however, their cost is greater than the cost of carbohydrates.

Americans consume more fat than is necessary and probably more than is good for them. The requirement of the human for the essential fatty acid has been estimated to be approximately 2 per cent of the calorie intake (infants, 1 to 3 per cent) of the diet. It is the consensus

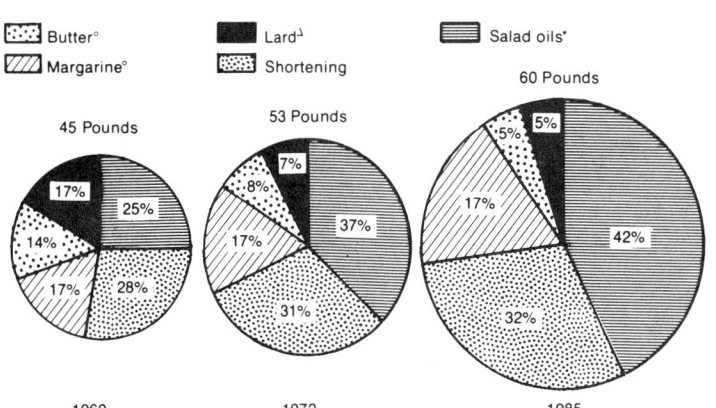

Butter°   Lard¹   Salad oils*
Margarine°   Shortening

Figure 4–4   Average amounts and percentages of saturated and unsaturated fats in the U.S. diet. (From White, P. L., Fletcher, D. C., and Ellis, M.: Nutrients in Processed Foods—Fats and Carbohydrates. Acton, Mass., Publishing Sciences Group, 1975.)

among nutritionists that the average diet should contain at least 25 per cent of its calories as fat. The precise amount of fat in the diets of the general public becomes less meaningful in the light of results published by several investigators which show that a decrease in dietary fat is usually accompanied by an increase in carbohydrate, which may correlate with a rise in blood triglycerides.

In the Report of the Inter-Society Commission for Heart Disease Resources the commission concluded that elevated serum cholesterol is a risk factor in the development of coronary heart disease and recommended dietary changes.[8] Furthermore, the Food and Nutrition Board, National Academy of Sciences, and the Council on Foods and Nutrition, AMA, state that the average level of plasma lipids of most American men and women is abnormally high and steps including dietary changes should be taken to alleviate this.[1] These changes, called by the American Heart Association the "Prudent Diet," are as follows:

    1. A caloric intake to achieve or maintain ideal body weight.

    2. A reduction in total fat calories from 40–45 per cent to 35 per cent of total calories.

    3. A reduction in dietary cholesterol to 300 mg. per day.

    4. An increase in complex dietary carbohydrate to replace calories from fat.

See Chapter 28 on cardiovascular disease for additional discussion of this topic.

Harm could result from severe reduction (0 to 15 per cent of total calories) of dietary fat, both in quantity and in proportion to other nutrients. Prolonged low fat regimens may lead to deficiencies of the essential polyunsaturated fatty acids. Since dietary fat is the carrier of the four fat-soluble vitamins (A, D, E, and K) and carotene, deficiencies in those nutrients may develop during prolonged periods of fat restriction.

Although the precise role of dietary fat in the pathogenesis of coronary atherosclerosis has not been determined, most authorities currently advocate some dietary restriction of total fat, saturated fatty acids, cholesterol and sucrose for the prevention of coronary artery disease. On the other hand, the increase in polyunsaturated fatty acid intake that is recommended can be overdone. More research is necessary to define the optimum level of PUFA intake in the light of vitamin E requirements, bile acid metabolism and the biological activities of of *trans*-fatty acids.

COOKING AND DIGESTIBILITY OF FATS

Cooking by the usual methods has no appreciable effect on the essential fatty acids. However, heating fat at very high temperatures burns the fat, resulting in the decomposition of the fat and the production of the substance *acrolein*. *Acrolein* may be very irritating to the nasal passages and to the gastrointestinal mucosa. Properly fried foods should have no adverse effect on normal digestion, but improperly fried foods do involve more effort on the part of the digestive system and therefore should never be served to the sick.

Digestibility of food fats varies to some degree and, of course, the hydrocarbon materials are not digestible or absorbable, as mentioned previously. Contrary to popular opinion, most fats are highly digestible; over 95 per cent of ingested fat is normally absorbed and utilized in the body. The absorption rate of fats varies, depending largely upon the melting point of the fat. Fats which are liquid at body temperature or more unsaturated are more rapidly absorbed than the solid fats. The rate of absorption is markedly enhanced by the presence of phospholipids and is also influenced by the quantity and type of mixture of fats eaten. In addition Ockner has discovered a *fatty acid binding protein (FABP)* in the mucosal cell which he feels may explain differences in rates of absorption of fatty acids. This protein exhibits an affinity for long chain unsaturated fatty acids.[6] The more rapidly absorbed fat is more quickly available to the tissues for energy. However, the more slowly absorbed fats remain in the intestines longer, thus extending the satiety period and producing much lower fluctuations in blood lipid levels following a meal.

PROBLEMS AND SUGGESTED TOPICS FOR DISCUSSION

1. List the amount of various fat foods you consume during a period of 24 hours. Calculate the percentage of total calories that were derived from fat.
2. Classify the fats in your diet for 1 day into "invisible" and "visible" fat foods; saturated and unsaturated.
3. What percentage of the daily dietary in the United States is consumed in the form of fat foods? What does this mean in terms of fat intake?
4. Why do you like to eat fat foods?
5. How do you obtain essential fatty acid in your diet?
6. Explain what is meant by saturated fat, unsaturated fat and hydrogenation. Explain their importance in nutrition and health.
7. Explain the metabolism and storage of fats in the body after absorption.

8. What is ketosis? Under what conditions does it occur?
9. Are fats a cheap or expensive source of energy? Explain.
10. What are the functions of fats in the body?
11. Survey the literature and report on the most recent research on human fat requirements in relation to cholesterol, saturated and unsaturated fats.
12. Evaluate the fats in your usual diet. How can your diet be improved?
13. What does the American Heart Association recommend for saturated fat, cholesterol and total fat intake?

CITED REFERENCES

1. Diet and coronary heart disease: a joint policy statement of the AMA Council on Foods and Nutrition and the Food and Nutrition Board of the NAS-NRC. JAMA, *222*:1647, 1972.
2. Food and nutrient intake of individuals in the United States, household food consumption survey 1965–66, Report No. 11. Washington, D.C., U.S.D.A., Agricultural Research Service, 1972.
3. Friend, B.: Nutrients in United States food supply—a review of trends, 1909–1913 to 1965. Am. J. Clin. Nutr., *20*:907, 1967.
4. Hansen, A. E., et al.: Role of linoleic acid in infant nutrition. Pediatrics, *31*:171, 1963.
5. Kritchevsky, D., and Story, J. A.: Binding of bile salts in vitro by nonnutritive fiber. J. Nutr., *104*:458, 1974.
6. Ockner, R. K., et al.: A binding protein for fatty acids in cytosol of intestinal mucosa, liver, myocardium, and other tissues. Science, *177*:56, 1972.
7. Recommended Dietary Allowances, 8th ed. Washington, D.C., Food and Nutrition Board, National Research Council, National Academy of Sciences, 1974.
8. Report of Inter-Society Commission for Heart Disease Resources, Primary prevention of the atherosclerotic diseases. Circulation, Vol. *42*, December 1970, revised April 1972.
9. Rizek, R. L., Friend, B., and Page, L.: Fat in today's food supply—level of use and sources. J. Am. Oil Chemists' Soc., *51*:244, 1974.
10. Van Dorp, D. A.: Essential fatty acid metabolism. Proc. Nutr. Soc., *34*:279, 1975.

ADDITIONAL REFERENCES

Babayan, V. K.: Tailoring fats for technical and nutritional needs. In White, P. L., Fletcher, D. C., and Ellis, M. (eds.): Nutrients in Processed Foods—Fats, Carbohydrates. Acton, Mass., Publishing Sciences Group, Inc., 1975.

Dairy Council Digest: Current research on dietary fatty acids. Chicago, National Dairy Council, *41*: No. 3, May–June, 1970.

Danon, A.: Prostaglandins and fat metabolism. In White, P. L., Fletcher, D. C., and Ellis, M. (eds.): Nutrients in Processed Foods—Fats, Carbohydrates. Acton, Mass., Publishing Sciences Group, Inc., 1975.

Feeley, R. M., Criner, P. E., and Watt, B. K.: Cholesterol content of foods. J. Am. Diet. Assoc., *61*:134, 1972.

Food Fats and Oils, 4th ed. Washington, D. C., Institute of Shortening and Edible Oils, Inc., 1974.

Goodhart, R. S., and Shils, M. E. (eds.): Modern Nutrition in Health and Disease, 5th ed. Philadelphia, Lea and Febiger, 1973, Chapter 4—Fats and other lipids.

Gorman, J. C., and Moore, M. E.: Fatty acids in vegetarian diets. J. Am. Diet. Assoc., *50*:372, 1967.

Guyton, A. C.: Textbook of Medical Physiology, 5th ed. Philadelphia, W. B. Saunders Company, 1976, Chapter 68—Lipid metabolism.

Latner, A. L.: Cantarow and Trumper Clinical Biochemistry, 7th ed. Philadelphia, W. B. Saunders Company, 1975, Chapter 2—Lipid metabolism.

Macdonald, I.: Interrelationships between the influences of dietary carbohydrates and fats on fasting serum lipids. Am. J. Clin. Nutr., *20*:345, 1967.

Myant, N. B.: The influence of some dietary factors on cholesterol metabolism. Proc. Nutr. Soc., *34*:271, 1975.

Sgoutas, D., and Kummerow, F. A.: Incorporation of trans-fatty acid into tissue lipids. Am. J. Clin. Nutr., *23*:1111, 1970.

Chapter 5

PROTEINS

DEFINITION AND IMPORTANCE

Protein derived its name more than a century ago from a Greek word meaning "of first importance." It was the first substance recognized as a vital part of living tissue. Proteins, the key components of all living organisms, are nitrogen-containing compounds which yield amino acids on hydrolysis. Proteins are the fundamental structural compounds of the cell, antibodies, enzymes and many of the hormones. They are essential constituents of the nucleus and protoplasm of every cell and they are almost the sole form in which man can replace nitrogen. Proteins are the most abundant of the organic compounds in the body. Most of the protein is found in muscle tissue; the remainder is distributed in soft tissues, bones, teeth, blood and other body fluids. Since proteins serve such important and essential functions in the body, and since certain indispensable protein components can be obtained solely through dietary intake, it is obvious that the quality and amounts of protein in the daily diet and a knowledge of protein sources and of protein metabolism are matters of considerable importance to those interested in dietetics and medical sciences.

THE COMPOSITION AND NATURE OF PROTEINS

Proteins, like fats and carbohydrates, contain carbon, hydrogen and oxygen but, in addition, they also contain about 16 per cent *nitrogen* along with sulfur and sometimes other elements such as phosphorus, iron and cobalt. The structural units of protein are the amino acids. They are united in long chains in various geometric structures and chemical combinations to form specific proteins, all of which are very large and complex molecules, each with its own physiological specificity. Despite their structural complexity, proteins can be hydrolyzed (broken down) into their amino acid constituents by enzymes or by boiling with acids and alkalis under certain conditions. Pure dry proteins are fairly stable, but under the conditions in which they are found in foods they tend to decompose at room temperatures, aided by bacterial action, and may form products that are toxic to the body; thus, the necessity for keeping protein foods such as eggs, fish, fowl, meat and milk refrigerated.

Plants obtain their nitrogen from the nitrates and ammonia in the soil, and from them synthesize their protein. Animals, in turn, obtain their nitrogen and protein from protein foods (plants and other animals). Animal metabolism, excretion and death finally return the nitrogen to the soil. This continuing process is known as the *nitrogen cycle*.

Amino Acids

Twenty two amino acids have been recognized as constituents of most protein. They are all alpha-amino carboxylic acids: that is, they have a basic amino group and an acid carboxylic group attached to the same carbon atom.

$$R-\underset{\underset{NH_2}{|}}{\overset{\overset{H}{|}}{C}}-COOH$$

They are differentiated by the remainder of the molecule (R), as illustrated above.

Amino acids, because they have both an acidic and basic group, have a buffer capacity. Depending on pH they can form salts with either acids or bases.

Structure of Proteins

Amino acids join together to form proteins by means of the *peptide link*: the carboxylic carbon of one acid attaches to the nitrogen of another acid with a molecule of water being

69

$$
\begin{array}{lll}
\text{O} & \text{H} \quad \text{COOH} \quad \text{H}_2\text{O} & \text{O} \quad\quad \text{COOH}\\
\| & \quad\quad | & \| \quad \text{H} \quad | \\
\text{C}-[\text{OH} \quad \text{H}]-\text{N}-\text{CH}\!\!<\!\! & & \text{C}-\text{N}-\text{CH}\\
| & \quad\quad | & | \quad\quad | \\
\text{H}_2\text{N}-\text{CH} & \quad\quad \text{CH}_2\text{OH} \quad \text{H}_2\text{N}-\text{CH} & \text{H}_2\text{N}-\text{CH} \quad \text{CH}_2\text{OH}\\
| & & | \\
\text{CH}_3 & & \text{CH}_3
\end{array}
$$

Alanine   Serine   Alanyl-serine

Formation of a Dipeptide

formed at the same time. The resulting compound has a free carboxyl group at one end and a free amino group at the other, so that the chain can continue to be built up from both ends.

Proteins vary in size from relatively small polypeptides such as ACTH with a molecular weight of 3200 (23 amino acid units) to very complex molecules with several hundred thousand amino acid units. The polypeptide chains take the form of a *helix*. Several chains may be linked together (usually through the S-S link of cystine). In addition, the entire chain may be wound upon itself into a globular or other form—the whole being held rigid by interatomic forces such as hydrogen bonds. The structure of a protein may thus be considered at three levels: the *primary structure* is the number, kind, and order of the amino acid chains; the *secondary structure* is the helical form; and the *tertiary structure* is the spatial arrangement. It is because of the almost infinite possibilities of variation offered by these structures that there are millions (or more) of different proteins with specific properties and biological functions.

Studies on the shape of protein molecules indicate that there are two general types: globular proteins, with a length:width ratio less than 10, and fibrous proteins with a ratio greater than 10. The *fibrous proteins* are used in the formation of structural elements. They may have several helical peptide chains twisted together to form a stiff rod. They are characterized by low solubility and high mechanical strength. Collagen of connective tissue, keratin of hair and myosin of muscle tissue are examples of fibrous proteins.

Globular proteins are found in the extracellular fluid of plants and animals, and in conjugated form constitute most intracellular enzymes. They are very soluble and are easily denatured.* Some globular proteins of interest in nutrition are casein in milk, egg albumin, the albumins and globulins of blood plasma, and hemoglobin.

Essential Amino Acids

There are eight amino acids which are classified as essential, since they must be supplied in the food. Body synthesis of these amino acids is lacking or so limited as to be unable to meet metabolic needs. These *essential amino acids* are valine, lysine, threonine, leucine, isoleucine, tryptophan, phenylalanine and methionine. One other amino acid, histidine, is required by infants, and recent work by Kopple and Swendseid suggests that it may also be essential for adults.[6] Without an adequate supply of the essential amino acids, protein cannot be synthesized or body tissue maintained. (See Figure 5–1.)

The other amino acids which can be synthesized by the body in adequate amounts for normal function are termed *non-essential:*

glycine	glutamic acid
alanine	proline
serine	hydroxyproline
cystine	citrulline
tyrosine	arginine
aspartic acid	norleucine
	hydroxyglutamic acid

This is not to suggest that these amino acids are not essential constituents of the proteins, but rather that the tissues can make their own supply from carbohydrate, fat and other amino

---

*Conditions that do not hydrolyze peptide bonds may still destroy the biological nature and activity of the protein. These are heat, air, ultraviolet radiation, alcohol, strong acids or bases, detergents, salts of heavy metals, alkaloidal reagents such as tannic acid and violent shaking. The protein usually coagulates after denaturation.

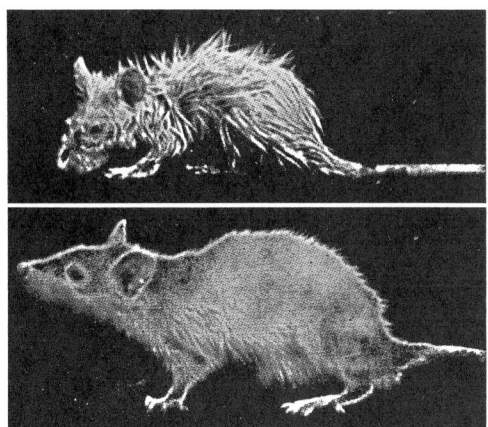

Figure 5–1 Effects of lack of one of the essential amino acids. The upper photograph shows a rat on the 28th day of valine deprivation. The lower photograph shows the same animal after valine had been administered for 25 days. (Photos courtesy of Rose and Eppstein and the Journal of Biological Chemistry.)

demonstrates that in this area of amino acid and protein requirements there are not clear-cut data and complete knowledge. Either of these patterns can be used to evaluate protein quality, which will be discussed later in this chapter.

Because of growth, infants and children require more protein per kilogram of body weight, and a greater percentage of their protein must be composed of essential amino acids—approximately 43 per cent for the infant and 36 per cent for the child, compared to 19 per cent for the adult. (See Figure 5–2.)

Special Functions of Amino Acids

Although virtually all the amino acids have certain unique functions in the body, a few are worth singling out. *Tryptophan* is a precursor of the vitamin niacin. Tryptophan is also a precursor of serotonin, a potent vasoconstrictor found in serum, and it is active in stimulating gastrointestinal activity. *Methionine* is a principal donor of methyl groups for the synthesis of various compounds such as choline and creatine. *Phenylalanine* is a precursor of tyrosine and together they lead to the formation of thyroxine and epinephrine. *Arginine*, *ornithine* and *citrulline*, all non-essential amino acids, are specifically involved in the synthesis of urea in the liver. *Glycine*, the simplest and perhaps most ubiquitous of the amino acids, combines with many toxic substances and converts them to harmless forms which are then

acids. The estimated requirements for the essential amino acids for the infant and the adult are listed in Table 5–1.

Having stated the estimated requirements, the Food and Nutrition Board went on to define the "ideal" protein or the protein with the amino acid pattern that would best fulfill the requirements. In 1973 a committee of FAO/WHO also defined the amino acid pattern for the ideal protein. (See Table 5–1.) You will note that they are somewhat different, which

Table 5–1 ESTIMATED AMINO ACID REQUIREMENTS OF MAN AND AMINO ACID PATTERNS FOR PROTEINS

AMINO ACID	REQUIREMENT (PER KG. OF BODY WT.), MG./DAY*			AMINO ACID PATTERN FOR HIGH QUALITY PROTEINS, MG./G. OF PROTEIN	FAO/WHO†† PROVISIONAL AMINO ACID SCORING PATTERN MG./G. PROTEIN
	Infant† (3–6 mo.)	*Child* (10–12 yr.)	*Adult*		
Histidine	33	?	?	17	—
Isoleucine	80	28	12	42	40
Leucine	128	42	16	70	70
Lysine	97	44	12	51	55
Total *S*-containing amino acids	45	22	10	26	35
Total aromatic amino acids	132	22	16	73	60
Threonine	63	28	8	35	40
Tryptophan	19	4	3	11	10
Valine	89	25	14	48	50

*FNB, Recommended Dietary Allowances, 8th ed., Washington, D.C., NRC, 1974.

†Two grams per kilogram of body weight per day of protein of the quality defined by the amino acid pattern would meet the amino acid needs of the infant.

††FAO/WHO, Energy and Protein Requirements, WHO Tech. Rep. No 522, 1973.

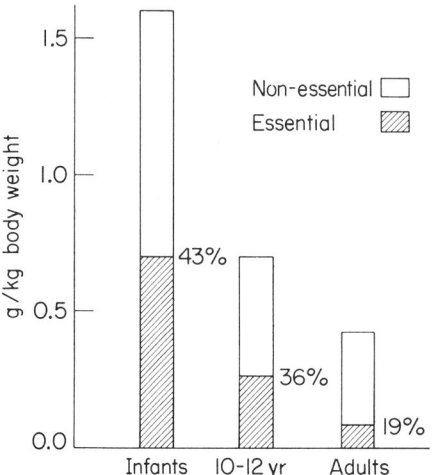

Figure 5–2 Proportion of total and essential amino acids required by various age groups as percentage of total nitrogen required. (From Scrimshaw, N. S.: Strengths and weaknesses of the committee approach: an analysis of past and present recommended dietary allowances for protein in health and disease. N. Engl. J. Med., 294:136, 1976.)

excreted. Glycine is also used in the synthesis of the porphyrin nucleus of hemoglobin and is a constituent of one of the bile acids (glycocholic acid). *Histidine* is essential for the synthesis of histamine which causes vasodilatation in the circulatory system. Epinephrine, synthesized from *tyrosine,* has a methyl group from methionine. Creatine, synthesized from *arginine, glycine* and *methionine,* combines with phosphate to form creatine phosphate. Creatine phosphate is an important reservoir of high energy phosphate in the cell. Glutamine, formed from *glutamic acid,* and asparagine, formed from *aspartic acid,* have important roles as reservoirs of amino groups throughout the body. In addition, hippuric acid, nicotinic acid, ornithine, pantothenic acid, purines and taurine are all derived from amino acids. These few examples illustrate some of the important intracellular substances synthesized from amino acids.

CLASSIFICATION OF PROTEINS

It is difficult to devise a consistent system for classification of the multitude of proteins. The following system is based partly on solubility and characteristic physical properties and partly on chemical composition. They are grouped as simple proteins, conjugated proteins and derived proteins.

Simple proteins are those which yield only

amino acids upon hydrolysis. They include the following, which exhibit various degrees of solubility: albumins, globulins, glutelins, prolamins, albuminoids, and histones and protamines (found in nuclei of cells). Those proteins such as albumins and globulins, which are soluble in water and dilute salt solution, are present in animal fluids, while less soluble ones such as myosin and muscle protein are present in tissues.

Conjugated proteins or proteids are combinations of simple proteins and some other non-protein substance, called a prosthetic group, attached to the molecule. They perform functions which neither constituent could properly perform by itself. These include

Nucleoproteins—combinations of simple proteins and nucleic acid. Deoxyribose nucleoproteins are the principal constituents of the genes, and ribose nucleoproteins are necessary for the synthesis of proteins in cytoplasm.

Mucoproteins and Glycoproteins—combinations of proteins and large quantities of complex polysaccharides. Example: mucin found in secretions from gastric mucous membranes.

Lipoproteins—compounds of proteins, triglycerides or other lipids. Example: phospholipid or cholesterol found in cell and organelle membranes.

Phosphoproteins—phosphoric acid joined by ester linkages to proteins. Example: casein of milk.

Chromoproteins—compounds of proteins and non-protein pigments. Example: flavoproteins, hemoglobin and cytochromes.

Metalloproteins—compounds of metals (copper, magnesium, zinc, iron) attached to proteins. Example: ferritin, hemosiderin, transferrin.

Derived proteins are products formed in the various stages of hydrolysis of the protein molecule. For example, proteoses are formed early in the hydrolysis process, while peptones, polypeptides and peptides are products that form near the final stages of protein breakdown.

NITROGEN BALANCE

To determine the extent of protein utilization, the nitrogen balance is studied. The amount of nitrogen is an accurate index of the amount of protein involved. Most proteins con-

Table 5–2   SUMMARY OF SIGNIFICANCE OF NITROGEN BALANCE DATA

CONDITION	MEASUREMENT	SIGNIFICANCE
Positive nitrogen balance	N intake > N excretion	Growth
Nitrogen equilibrium	N intake = N excretion	Maintenance and repair of tissue
Negative nitrogen balance	N intake < N excretion	Wasting of body; loss of weight

(From Guthrie, H. A.: Introductory Nutrition, 3rd ed. St. Louis, C.V. Mosby Co., 1975, p. 66.)

tain about 16 per cent nitrogen and this fact is utilized in determining the amount of protein in foods or body substances. The nitrogen content is determined chemically and this figure, multiplied by 6.25, gives the amount of protein present in the substance. Thus, if the amount of nitrogen that goes into the body in food and the amount that leaves the body in the excreta are determined, the portion used by the body can be calculated. If the nitrogen intake and the nitrogen output are equal, the individual is in *nitrogen balance* or *equilibrium*. Should the intake of nitrogen be greater than the amount in urine, feces and integumental loss, the individual is in a state of *positive balance;* that is, the build up (anabolism) or synthesis of tissue proteins is greater than the breakdown (catabolic) activities. There is a net gain of protein in the body. Should the excretion of nitrogen be more than that consumed, a state of *negative balance* exists; that is, the rate of protein breakdown is exceeding the rate of protein synthesis. (See Table 5–2.)

An adult may be maintained in nitrogen and protein equilibrium, or put into positive nitrogen balance (more intake of nitrogen than output in a given period of time) by feeding him

mixtures of pure essential amino acids. In other words, protein itself is dispensable, if necessary, so long as the essential amino acids are provided in correct amount and proportion. This fact is utilized medically in parenteral feeding with protein hydrolysate or amino acid mixtures if the patient cannot ingest food. It is necessary, however, to supply adequate calories, vitamins and minerals in these feedings for tissue synthesis to take place.

The Committee on Therapeutic Nutrition, Food and Nutrition Board, National Research Council compiled results to show that "when a mixture of only essential amino acids serves as the sole source of dietary nitrogen, it does not support growth at a rate commensurate with that of intact proteins in a diet of equicaloric and equal nitrogen content. The superiority of a diet containing all of the protein components may indicate that the synthesis of the nonessential amino acids, in addition to the formation of tissue structures, presents too great a burden upon the chemical resources of the cell. When tissue growth or tissue repletion is proceeding at a rapid pace, nonessential amino acids may become limiting factors in the anabolic processes."[13]

Figure 5–3   Stunting of growth owing to feeding an incomplete protein as sole source of protein in the diet. Contrast between two rats of same age kept on diets alike except for the protein, which was a complete protein (casein from milk) in the case of the rat pictured at top and an incomplete protein in the case of the rat pictured at bottom (gliadin from wheat). (From experiments by Osborne and Mendel, Connecticut Agricultural Experimental Station; pictures reproduced by courtesy of Yale University Press.)

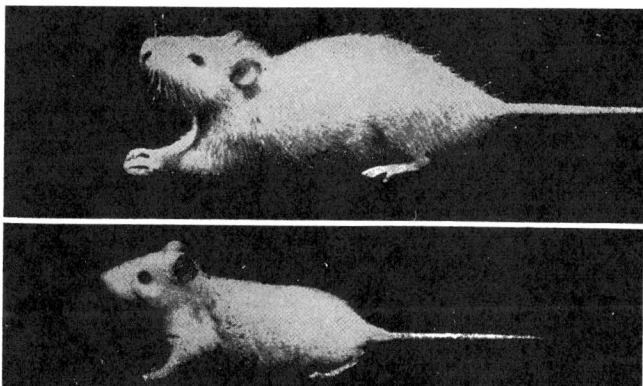

EVALUATION OF PROTEIN QUALITY

Complete and Incomplete Proteins

Proteins that contain all the essential amino acids in sufficient quantity and in the right ratio to maintain nitrogen equilibrium and permit growth of the young are known as *complete proteins.* Such proteins are ovalbumin, the main protein of egg, and casein, the principal protein in milk. Other complete proteins are those in meat, fish and poultry. Proteins that do not supply all the essential amino acids in appropriate amounts to maintain nitrogen equilibrium and growth are *incomplete proteins.* (See Fig. 5–3.) The proteins in vegetables and grains are classified as incomplete proteins. We also refer to the *biological value* of proteins. The biological value is high or low depending upon the completeness with which a protein supplies the essential amino acids. Foods of high biological value are largely of animal origin. Most grain and vegetable proteins are incomplete proteins and thus are of only fair or low biological value.

The incompleteness of proteins may be partial or total. *Partially incomplete proteins* will sustain life but, lacking sufficient amounts of amino acids, will not support normal growth. These are found in legumes (dried beans and peas, peanuts), nuts and grains. (See Fig. 5–4.) A food protein lacking an essential amino acid will not support life or growth. Zein, in corn, and gelatin, an animal protein, are examples of *totally incomplete proteins.* Plant foods generally contain an insufficient quantity of lysine, methionine, threonine and tryptophan. The amino acids which plant foods do contribute, however, are important and should be made use of by feeding simultaneously with small amounts of a complete protein food, or by providing a correct mixture of several plant foods which will give all the amino acids in appropriate amounts, or by adding synthetic amino acids to foods to make a complete protein.

Amino Acid Score

The distribution of the essential amino acids in eggs and human milk has been recommended

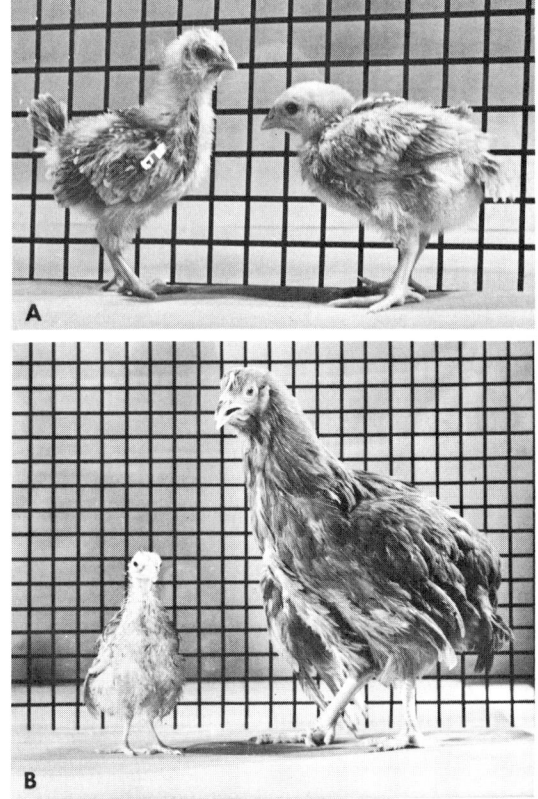

Figure 5–4 Effect of the amino acid tryptophan on growth and health. A, Week-old chicks. Chick at left to be fed a tryptophan-free diet. Chick at right will continue eating standard feed. B, Same chicks at nine weeks of age. The chick at left on tryptophan-free diet remains at approximately his week-old size. There are some changes in appearance, however, because most of the feathers, the beak and the eyes developed at normal rate. When tryptophan is restored to the diet, the chick will immediately begin to grow and mature, reaching maturation seemingly without ill effects. (Photos courtesy of Monsanto Chemical Company's Agricultural Experiment Farm, St. Louis, Missouri.)

by the Joint Committee of FAO/WHO for use as the ideal reference pattern. However, in 1973 a new provisional amino acid scoring pattern was devised based on additional data on amino acid requirements.[1] (See Table 5–3.) A protein is compared to this amino acid reference pattern and receives an *amino acid or chemical score* by the calculation shown below.

$$\text{Amino acid score} = \frac{\text{mg. of an amino acid in 1 gm. test protein}}{\text{mg. of that amino acid in 1 gm. reference pattern}} \times 100$$

Table 5–3 COMPARISON OF HUMAN MILK, COW'S MILK AND EGG PROTEIN TO FAO/WHO STANDARD AMINO ACID PATTERN

AMINO ACID	FAO/WHO 1973 PROVISIONAL AMINO ACID SCORING PATTERN MG. PER G. OF PROTEIN	REPORTED COMPOSITION			
		HUMAN MILK		COW'S MILK	EGG
		RANGE	MEAN		
Histidine	*	18–36	26	27	22
Isoleucine	40	41–53	46	47	54
Leucine	70	83–107	93	95	86
Lysine	55	53–76	66	78	70
Methionine + cystine	35	29–60	42	33	57
Phenylalanine + tyrosine	60	68–118	72	102	93
Threonine	40	40–45	43	44	47
Tryptophan	10	16–17	17	14	17
Valine	50	44–77	55	64	66
Total	360	390–552	434	477	490
+ histidine		408–588	460	504	512

*Did not define for histidine
(From Joint FAO/WHO Ad Hoc Expert Committee, Energy and Protein Requirements, WHO Tech. Rep. No. 522, Geneva, Switzerland, 1973.)

The amino acid for which a protein has the lowest score is the *limiting amino acid* and becomes the chemical score for the protein. Proteins such as whole egg, human milk and cow's milk with scores of 100 meet the reference pattern for all essential amino acids. (See Table 5–3.)

The amino acid score of a protein is a crude way to evaluate the quality of a protein because it does not take into account the digestibility of the protein, the availability of the amino acids, the utilization of those amino acids by the human body, or the ability of that protein to support cellular synthesis. Considering these biological factors, several measures of protein quality have been developed, but the most widely used is the net protein utilization (NPU).

Net Protein Utilization

Net protein utilization measures the biological value (BV) or percentage of absorbed nitrogen utilized by the body and the digestibility of the protein under standard conditions of total dietary protein, total energy intake and nutritional status of the individual. NPU quantifies food nitrogen utilization and in simplistic terms is equal to the N retained/N intake, which is equal to

$$\frac{\text{N intake} - \text{N output}}{\text{N intake}}$$

The NPU will usually be less than the chemical score of a protein. (See Table 5–4 for the NPU values and chemical scores of some common proteins.)

An observation of interest is that as the amount of protein in the diet reaches the amount needed to maintain N equilibrium, a smaller percentage is retained, and thus the NPU for a protein seems to decrease. Why this happens is not clear, but on lower intakes of protein, the body seems to be more efficient in its protein retention and utilization. Possibly, the body has a survival mechanism providing for greater utilization of protein when protein intakes are low; however, even this ability is limited.

Table 5–4 CHEMICAL SCORE AND NET PROTEIN UTILIZATION VALUES OF COMMON FOODS

PROTEIN	NEW PATTERN CHEMICAL SCORE	NPU MEASURED IN RATS
Whole egg	100	94
Human milk	100	87
Cow's milk	95	82
Soya bean	74	65
Sesame	50	54
Groundnut	65	47
Cottonseed	81	59
Maize	49	52
Millet	63	44
Rice, polished	67	59
Wheat, whole	53	48

(Adapted from Joint FAO/WHO Ad Hoc Expert Committee, Energy and Protein Requirements, WHO Tech. Rep. No. 522, Geneva, Switzerland, 1973, p. 67.)

FOOD SOURCES AND PROTEIN SUPPLEMENTATION

Most people tend to ingest a mixture of foods in a meal and the combination of proteins, complete and incomplete, in sufficient quality and quantity, are apt to complement or supplement one another to provide all the essential amino acids. The minimum requirement for the adult male, for example, is readily obtained in four slices of bread and one pint of milk (Table 5–5).

When the use of a complete protein is restricted, mixtures of a carbohydrate with a small amount of a complete protein will supply the essential amino acids. Examples of this *supplementation* are cereal with milk; macaroni and cheese; rice, beans and sofrito (meat or fish sauce). Small amounts of fish meal or skim milk may be added to vegetable or carbohydrate mixtures to provide the essential amino acids.

In areas where animal protein is scarce or unavailable, plant proteins may be combined according to the FAO reference pattern to form a complete protein. This mixture, referred to as mutual supplementation, supplies all the essential amino acids and has a higher biological value than either of the protein components used alone. (See Table 5–6 for the amino acid contributions of vegetable proteins. Also see Table 10–7 and Fig. 10–2.) One of the first of these products, Incaparina, was developed by the Institute of Nutrition in Central America and Panama (INCAP). It consists of a mixture of ground maize, sorghum, cottonseed flour, torula yeast and vitamin A. Suitable products have been developed in other countries to meet the protein needs, especially of infants and children.

Enrichment of grains and legumes with amino acids (lysine to bread; methionine to legumes) in which they are insufficiently supplied also has been done. However, if one amino acid is increased too greatly, the protein quality may be decreased, as evidenced by lower nitrogen retention. Supplementation with an amino acid other than the most limiting amino acid may be in excess and can possibly only depress food intake.[2]

Mutual supplementation of proteins is most effective when two principles are kept in mind:

1. The lower the quality of protein, the more protein is required to meet the minimum requirements for amino acids and total protein. In a vegetable protein diet, more total protein is required than in a mixed vegetable and animal protein diet.

2. For maximal utilization of amino acids for protein synthesis, all amino acids should be present in the blood stream after absorption from the gastrointestinal tract. This means that complementary proteins should be eaten at the same time or after a short interval.

The practical application of these principles with recipes is presented by Frances Moore Lappé in *Diet for a Small Planet*.

METABOLISM OF PROTEINS

The processes of digestion and absorption of proteins are discussed in Chapter 6. All proteins must be broken down into amino acids

Table 5–5   ESSENTIAL AMINO ACIDS SUPPLIED BY BREAD AND MILK (4 slices (100 gm.) of bread and 2 cups (480 gm.) of milk)

ESSENTIAL AMINO ACIDS	BREAD (White)-4 slices yield 8.5 gm. protein	MILK (Whole or skim)-2 cups yield 16.8 gm. protein	TOTAL	ADULT MINIMUM DAILY NEEDS (Male)
		Amounts in Grams		
Tryptophan	0.091	0.235	0.326	0.25
Threonine	0.282	0.773	1.055	0.50
Isoleucine	0.429	1.070	1.449	0.70
Leucine	0.668	1.651	2.319	1.10
Lysine	0.225	1.306	1.531	0.80
Methionine + cystine	0.342	0.562	0.904	1.10
Phenylalanine + tyrosine	0.708	1.670	2.378	1.10
Valine	0.435	1.152	1.587	0.80

See also Appendix Table 6, Amino Acid Content of Foods.

Table 5–6 AMINO ACID COMPOSITION OF SOME FOODS

ESSENTIAL AMINO ACIDS	CHEESE EGGS MILK MEAT	CORN	CEREAL	LE-GUMES	WHOLE GRAINS (WITH GERM)	NUTS SEED OILS SOYBEANS	SESAME & SUN-FLOWER SEEDS	PEANUT PROTEIN	GREEN LEAFY VEG. LEAF PROT.	GELA-TIN*	YEAST
Cystine**			—	—			x				
Methionine		x	x	—	x	—	x	—	—	—	x
Isoleucine	x										
Leucine	x										
Lysine	x	—	x	x	x	x	—	—		—	
Phenylalanine		—	—								
Threonine	x	—	—	x	—	x					x
Tryptophan		—		—	—		x			—	
Valine	x										

Symbols: X— High amount of amino acid present in that food.
 — Low amount of amino acid present in that food.
 Blank spaces indicate a general good balance of amino acids in the food.

* Gelatin is not a good source of all essential amino acids.
** Not essential but added because hard to get in a vegetarian diet. Methionine and cystine can be compared as one.

(From Erhard, D.: Nutrition education for the "now" generation. J. Nutr. Educ., 3: 135, 1971.)

and di- or tripeptides by digestion before absorption and use by the body. In the lumen are large amounts of endogenous protein from cell sloughing and cell secretions, which combine with exogenous protein to present a fairly constant amino acid pattern. Absorption through the intestinal lumen is an active process, not simple diffusion; it requires energy (ATP), pyridoxal phosphate (B₆) and manganese ion. There appear to be two systems, one for free amino acids and one for small peptides. The one for peptides appears to provide for intracellular hydrolysis of di- and tripeptides in the mucosal cell. As a group, the essential amino acids are better absorbed than nonessential amino acids. The amino acids are carried in the portal vein to the liver and then into the general circulation. Amino acids which are constantly being formed by breakdown of tissue proteins and non-essential amino acids synthesized in the body contribute to the circulating pool.

Protein Synthesis

The fundamental and most interesting use of the amino acid is as a building block for the body proteins, such as enzymes, hormones, vitamins and structural proteins. Each cell in the body has the capacity to synthesize an enormous number of specific proteins. For the synthesis of a protein all the essential amino acids must be available at the same time. Protein synthesis is not a step-wise process. Complete peptides are laid down in a short period of time and there is no provision for storage of incomplete sections. The non-essential amino acids must either be supplied as such or there must be suitable precursors, including amino groups from other amino acids, so that they can be synthesized. The synthesis of the characteristic proteins of each cell is controlled by the genetic material, *deoxyribose nucleic acid (DNA)* in the nucleus. DNA is used as a template for *transcription* or the synthesis of *ribose nucleic acid* (RNA), of which there are several forms. One form, *messenger* or *mRNA*, carries the information to the cytoplasm where the proteins are synthesized. DNA and RNA are composed of nucleotide units consisting of ribose (or deoxyribose), phosphoric acid and one of the four cyclic nitrogenous bases (a purine or pyrimidine). (See Fig. 5–5, Building Blocks of DNA.) They are strung together in long chains of pentose and phosphoric acid alternately with the purine and pyrimidine

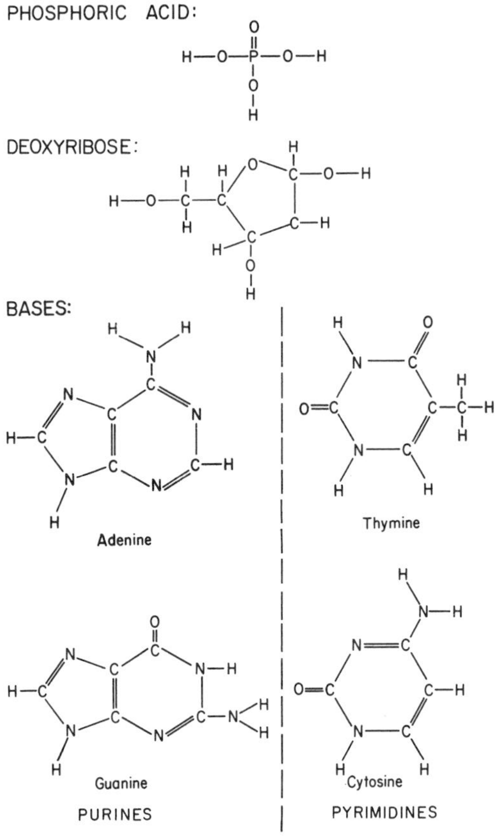

Figure 5–5 The basic building blocks of DNA. (From Guyton, A. C.: Textbook of Medical Physiology. 5th ed. W. B. Saunders Company, 1976.)

molecules as branches. DNA is a double-stranded molecule, the two chains in the form of a double helix held together by hydrogen bonds linking a purine and a pyrimidine. It may have a molecular weight of two billion, with a million or more bases arranged in a continuous line. RNA is a single strand. It is the sequence of the bases along the chain which specifies the arrangement of amino acids in the protein, each amino acid being defined by a set of three bases. In the cytoplasm are other RNA molecules, relatively small, one for each amino acid. These *t (transfer) RNA's* direct the amino acids to the appropriate position along the mRNA so that the peptide chain can be synthesized. In addition *r (ribosomal) RNA*, composed of a large and small RNA molecule, functions with the ribosome to bind tRNA to the ribosome and then provide enzymes that promote peptide linkage. Major steps in this intricate process are shown in Figure 5–6. Of course, among the proteins which must be synthesized are the enzymes needed to catalyze

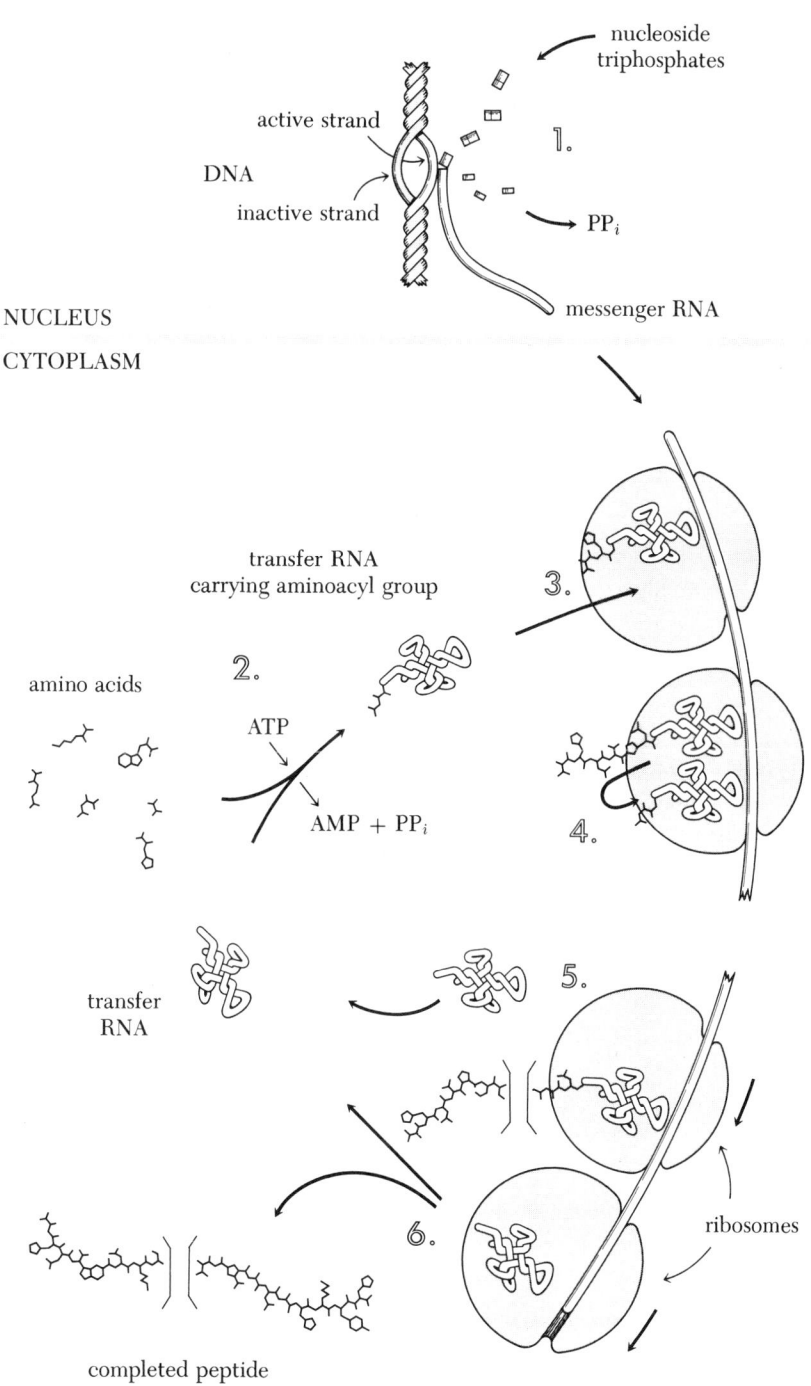

nucleoside triphosphates

active strand

DNA

inactive strand

1.

PP$_i$

NUCLEUS

CYTOPLASM

messenger RNA

transfer RNA
carrying aminoacyl group

3.

amino acids

2.

ATP

AMP + PP$_i$

4.

transfer
RNA

5.

6.

ribosomes

completed peptide

See legend on following page

the synthesis. Energy for synthesis is supplied by ATP, itself a nucleotide.

Protein Catabolism

There is no large reserve of free amino acids in the body and any amount above that needed for synthesis of tissue protein and the varied non-protein nitrogen-containing compounds is oxidized, providing high-energy phosphate molecules. The amino group is detached from the amino acid before oxidation of the remaining portion of the molecule. Most of the amino nitrogen is converted to urea in the liver and excreted in the urine. The liver is the main location for deamination and other early steps in amino acid metabolism (including synthesis of non-essential amino acids). The carbon skeletons are converted into some of the same intermediates formed during glucose and fatty acid catabolism. These can be carried to the peripheral tissues where they are needed for oxidation to produce high-energy phosphate. These fragments can also be used in synthetic processes to make glucose or fats. About 58 per cent of the protein consumed can be converted into glucose. The mechanisms of these reactions will be further discussed in Chapter 6.

Since most types of proteins of the body are regularly being built up and torn down, the amino acids used for protein synthesis also are eventually replaced and metabolized. The nitrogen from the protein must be excreted in the urine. Besides urea, the major excretory products are uric acid and creatinine. *Uric acid* is the end product of the metabolism of purines, important components of the nucleic acids. Disturbed metabolism of purines and uric acid is found in gout, discussed in Chapter 26. *Creatinine* is the excretion form of creatine, present in all muscle tissue and creatine phosphate, a store of high-energy phosphate. The amount of urea excreted is related to protein intake, while creatinine excretion is related to muscle mass and is relatively constant in any individual. In fact, it is so constant that it has been used to check the accuracy of 24-hour urine collections.

Metabolic Pool of Amino Acids

Metabolism of proteins is sometimes divided into two types: (1) *exogenous* metabolism, which includes the metabolism of all protein ingested in excess of essential body requirements and is obviously quite variable; and (2) *endogenous* metabolism, which includes all the necessary protein buildup and breakdown processes that are essential to life, growth and repair of the body. Creatinine excretion is regarded as a measure of the endogenous metabolism.

There is practically no storage of amino acids in the body. They are constantly being utilized to form other compounds and re-formed by breakdown and ingestion of protein, with the

---

Figure 5–6 Schematic summary of protein synthesis. *Top, step 1.* A molecule of DNA in the nucleus unfolds, and one of its strands is used as a template to direct the formation of messenger RNA (mRNA) from nucleoside triphosphates, which lose inorganic-pyrophosphate (PP_i) as they attach to the growing RNA chain. The completed mRNA moves to the cytoplasm *(bottom)*, where it binds ribosomes into a polysome, and acts as a template for protein synthesis.

The following steps are shown on separate ribosomes for clarity, but in fact they are repeated in sequence on each ribosome. The successive ribosomes grow longer and longer peptide chains as they move down the molecule of mRNA.

Step 2. Meanwhile, amino acids are combined with specific molecules of transfer RNA (tRNA) in the cytoplasm by a reaction that also involves the cleavage of adenosine triphosphate (ATP) into adenosine monophosphate (AMP) and PP_i.

Step 3. The tRNA molecules, carrying the amino acids in the form of aminoacyl groups, diffuse to the polysome, where the growing peptide chain is on another molecule of tRNA already attached. The incoming tRNA, which bears the next group required for the growing peptide (in this case leucyl residue), has the proper configuration to complex with mRNA on the ribosome.

Step 4. When the proper tRNA is in place, the peptide chain is transferred onto the amino group of the new residue brought in by tRNA, so that the chain is now one residue longer.

Step 5. When the transfer of the previous step is completed, the previously bound tRNA no longer carries a peptide chain and is free to dissociate from the ribosome, returning to the mixed pool of tRNA in the soluble cytoplasm, where it is available for transport of another molecule of its specific amino acid. The ribosome now moves along the mRNA molecule to the position where the placement of the next amino acid will be directed.

Step 6. Steps 3, 4 and 5 are repeated. As each amino acid residue adds to the peptide chain, the ribosome moves down the mRNA molecule. When a ribosome has reached the end of the molecule, the peptide is completed and is detached into the soluble cytoplasm. The ribosome itself can then move free of the mRNA and be available for attachment to the beginning of yet another molecule of mRNA (not shown). (From McGilvery, R. W.: Biochemistry—A Functional Approach. W. B. Saunders Company, 1970.)

excess being excreted as previously mentioned.

Any "storage" is in the form of cellular proteins themselves. There is an upper limit, however, after which excess amino acids are degraded and used for energy or stored as fat. As with fats and carbohydrates, there exists a state of dynamic equilibrium for amino acids, with constant buildup, breakdown, and interchange, and there exists a *metabolic pool* of amino acids in this state of dynamic equilibrium that at any given time may be called upon by the body for any appropriate need. The most active tissues for protein turnover are the plasma proteins, intestinal mucosa, pancreas, liver and kidney, while the muscle, skin and brain are much less active. Figure 5–7 summarizes the anabolic and catabolic reactions of amino acids. The direction taken depends on the supply of amino acids in the food and the needs of the body. Regulation is largely under hormonal control.

Hormonal Regulation

Hormones have anabolic and catabolic effects on protein metabolism. The *growth hormone* stimulates protein synthesis, thus increasing tissue concentration. *Insulin* also stimulates protein synthesis by accelerating amino acid transport across the cell membrane, and a lack of insulin reduces protein synthesis. Insulin and the gonad-stimulating hormones, especially *testosterone*, stimulate protein synthesis during growth periods. The *glucocorticoids* stimulate gluconeogenesis and ketogenesis from proteins and decrease protein in most tissues except for plasma and hepatic protein, which are increased. *Thyroxine* indirectly affects protein metabolism by increasing the rate of metabolism in all cells. As a result it increases the rate of normal anabolic and catabolic reactions of protein. In physiological doses with adequate calories and amino acids present, it will produce protein synthesis. With inadequate calories or in large doses (unphysiological), thyroxine will have a catabolic effect.

FUNCTIONS OF PROTEINS IN THE BODY

Dietary proteins furnish the amino acids for synthesis of tissue protein and other special metabolic functions. A concise summary of the

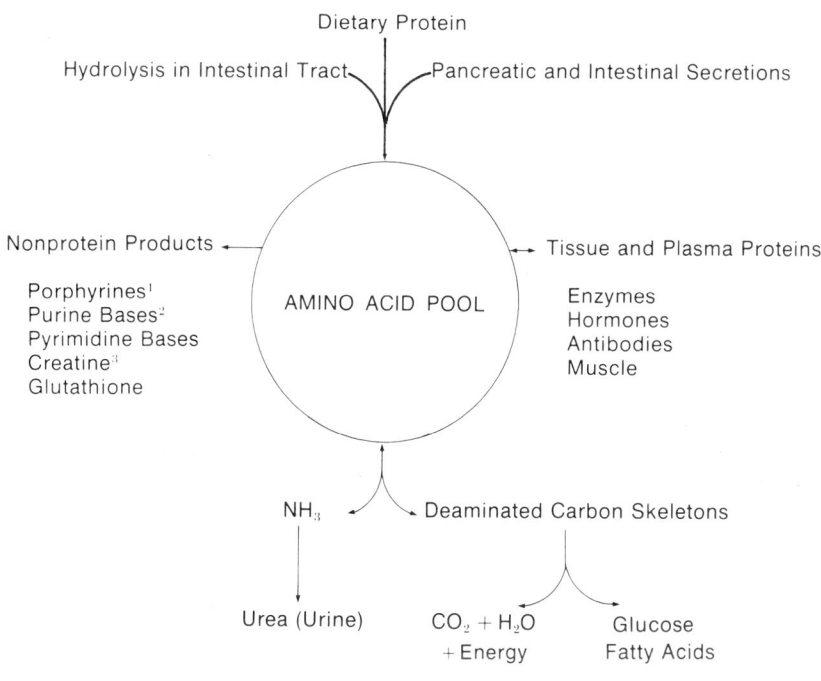

Figure 5–7 Amino acid pool.
[1]Excreted in bile as bilirubin.
[2]Excreted in urine as uric acid.
[3]Excreted in urine as creatinine.

numerous functions of proteins would be as follows:

1. Proteins are used *to repair worn-out body tissue proteins* (anabolism) resulting from the continued "wear and tear" (catabolism) going on in the body. This is a function provided only by protein. No other nutrients can do it because the amino acid building blocks of tissue are available only from protein.

2. Proteins are used *to build new tissue* (anabolism) by supplying the necessary amino acid building blocks. This is the reason for an increased protein need during periods of rapid growth, as in infancy, childhood, adolescence and pregnancy.

3. Proteins are a *source of heat and energy*. They supply 4 kcalories per gram, the same as does a carbohydrate, but in a more expensive fashion than a carbohydrate. Protein is not only a more expensive source of energy to buy and eat, but it will be remembered that protein has a greater specific dynamic action than carbohydrate, which adds to the total energy expended by the body (5 per cent of calories for carbohydrate and fat versus as much as 30 per cent for protein). However, in a mixed diet this difference is not significant. (See page 31 for definition of specific dynamic action.) Also, one of the end products of protein metabolism is nitrogen, which has to be excreted by the body, a function that involves a cost in work by the body. Carbohydrate, on the other hand, is cheap to obtain and burns completely to carbon dioxide and water.

4. Proteins *contribute to numerous essential body secretions and fluids*. Enzymes are proteins, and some hormones have protein or amino acid components. Mucus, milk and sperm are largely protein, as is the fluid in which sperm are contained. About the only protein-free body fluids are sweat, bile, and urine.

5. Plasma proteins of the blood, particularly albumin, are important in the *maintenance of normal osmotic relations* among the various body fluids. Indeed, one of the main signs of hypoproteinemia is the appearance of edema (excessive tissue fluid) as a result of a loss of osmotic balance.

6. Plasma proteins also function in the *transport of other substances*. Lipid-carrying proteins transport triglyceride, cholesterol, phospholipid and fat soluble vitamins. Transferrin transports iron, and calcium is transported bound to a protein. Albumin carries free fatty acids and bilirubin. In addition many drugs are carried in the blood bound to albumin.

7. Proteins in the form of *immunoglobulins (or antibodies) play a role in the resistance of the body* to disease.

8. Dietary proteins furnish the amino acids for a variety of metabolic functions. They are *components or precursors of many non-protein nitrogen-containing substances*. Some of these have been discussed (p. 73).

RECOMMENDED PROTEIN AND AMINO ACID ALLOWANCES

The daily recommended allowance (RDA) as defined by the Food and Nutrition Board, NRC, for the 70-kg. reference man and 58-kg. reference woman is approximately 0.8 gm. of protein per kg. of body weight per day.[15] This amounts to 56 gm. and 46 gm. per day for the reference man and woman, respectively (see Table 10–1), or approximately 8–9 per cent of the total daily calories. These recommendations are based on the amount of protein needed to compensate for the nitrogen lost in urine and feces by individuals adjusted to a protein-free diet; the amount to compensate for skin, sweat, hair and nail losses; and the amount necessary for the increase in body mass during normal growth.

Nitrogen losses are used to estimate the amount of ideal protein required. If the protein provides both the exact amount of nitrogen lost from the body and the precise mixture of amino acids needed, additional nitrogen will not be excreted. Nitrogen balance would be attained.

The minimum requirement of protein needed to maintain nitrogen balance has been determined to be about .47 gm. per kg. body weight daily, assuming adequate caloric intake. An increase of 30 per cent is made to account for individual variation (.47 × 1.30 = .61 gm./kg./day). This figure of .6 gm./kg./day is increased again to account for the fact that the mixed proteins in the U.S. diet have about 75 per cent efficiency of utilization. Thus the final recommended allowance for protein for the adult is .8 gm./kg./day.[15] For infants and children additional allowances are made for growth, and for the pregnant or lactating woman additional allowances are recommended for fetal development and milk production.

The Joint Committee of FAO/WHO has also defined protein allowances by defining the "safe level" of protein intake in terms of the highest quality protein (egg or milk) as .52–.57 gm./kg./day for the adult.[1] However, this amount must be increased, depending on the quality of the protein in the diet. (See Table 5–7.)

Meeting the RDA for Protein

The FNB recommended allowance of .8 gm. protein per kg. body weight allows for intake of some proteins of low biological value. It is good nutritional practice to include at least one-third of the protein intake from complete protein foods, although this is not absolutely necessary. Balanced and adequate protein intakes can be achieved by conscientious attention to the combination of incomplete proteins, but the protein requirement will be higher. (See Table 5–8 for the protein contents of various foods.)

Protein : Calorie Ratio

If the fat and carbohydrate in a diet are supplied in adequate amounts to meet energy requirements, there can be nitrogen equilibrium even when the intake of protein is very low. They will "spare" the proteins. Unless sufficient calories are available in the diet for energy needs, an increased amount of protein is metabolized to compensate for the dietary energy inadequacy. In this capacity of "protein sparing" carbohydrate seems to be more important than fat. Although the mechanism is not understood, it is supposed that because carbohydrate provides a major source of oxaloacetate for the citric acid cycle and the carbon skeletons for nonessential amino acids, in the absence of adequate carbohydrate, protein must perform these functions, which fat cannot do. This is why inadequate carbohydrate can cause a negative N balance.

In 1975 the Protein-Calorie Advisory Group of the UN published a report stating a recommended protein/calorie ratio of 1:20, i.e., 5–5.5 per cent of the calories, should come from protein.[12] This is the recommendation for a person with "moderate activity" who is consuming a high quality protein. "Light activity" with a lower calorie intake would require a higher concentration of protein in the diet and "heavy

Table 5–7 SAFE LEVEL OF PROTEIN IN TERMS OF DIETS OF PROTEIN QUALITIES OF 60%, 70% AND 80% RELATIVE TO MILK OR EGGS

AGE GROUP	BODY WEIGHT (KG.)	SAFE LEVEL OF PROTEIN INTAKE		ADJUSTED LEVEL FOR PROTEINS OF DIFFERENT QUALITY (GM. PER PERSON PER DAY)		
		(gm. protein per kg. per day)	*(gm. protein per person per day)*	*Score* [a] *80*	*Score 70*	*Score 60*
Infants						
6–11 months	9.0	1.53	14	17	20	23
Children						
1–3 years	13.4	1.19	16	20	23	27
4–6 years	20.2	1.01	20	26	29	34
7–9 years	28.1	0.88	25	31	35	41
Male adolescents						
10–12 years	36.9	0.81	30	37	43	50
13–15 years	51.3	0.72	37	46	53	62
16–19 years	62.9	0.60	38	47	54	63
Female adolescents						
10–12 years	38.0	0.76	29	36	41	48
13–15 years	49.9	0.63	31	39	45	52
16–19 years	54.4	0.55	30	37	43	50
Adult man	65.0	0.57	37	46 [b]	53 [b]	62 [b]
Adult woman	55.0	0.52	29	36 [b]	41 [b]	48 [b]
Pregnant woman, latter half of pregnancy			Add 9	Add 11	Add 13	Add 15
Lactating woman, first 6 months			Add 17	Add 21	Add 24	Add 28

[a] Scores are estimates of the quality of the protein usually consumed relative to that of egg or milk. The safe level of protein intake is adjusted by multiplying it by 100 divided by the score of the food protein. For example, 100/60 = 1.67, and for a child of 1–4 years the safe level of protein intake would be 16 × 1.67, or 27 gm. of protein having a relative quality of 60.

[b] The correction may overestimate adult protein requirements.

(From Joint FAO/WHO Ad Hoc Expert Committee, Energy and Protein Requirements, WHO Tech. Rep. No. 522, Geneva, Switzerland, 1973, p. 74.)

Table 5–8 PROTEINS AVAILABLE IN COMMON FOODS

FOOD	CHIEF PROTEINS PRESENT	COMPLEMENT OF ESSENTIAL AMINO ACIDS	AVERAGE SERVING		WEIGHT GRAMS
			Grams of Proteins	*Approximate Measure*	
Milk, whole	Casein and lact-albumin	Complete	9 gm.	1 glass (8 oz.)	244
Meat, lean	Albumin and myosin	Complete	22 gm.	2.5 oz.	72
Cheese, uncreamed cottage	Casein and lact-albumin	Complete	5 gm.	1 oz.	28
Egg	Ovalbumin and ovovitellin	Complete	6 gm.	1 egg	50
Navy beans	Phaesolin	Incomplete	7.5 gm.	½ cup	128
Peas, small, green	Legumin	Incomplete	4 gm.	½ cup	80
Corn, canned	Glutelin Zein	Incomplete Incomplete	2.5 gm.	½ cup	128
Bread	Gliadin	Incomplete	2 gm.	1 slice	23
Soy beans	Glycinin Legumelin	Complete Incomplete	3 gm.	½ cup	54
Dry, nonfat milk	Casein and lact-albumin	Complete	6 + gm.	¼ cup	17.5 gm.

activity" would require a lower concentration. The other variable is the quality of the protein. As the quality of the protein decreases, more is necessary to meet requirements, and thus protein must make up more of the calories. The 1973 FAO/WHO report states that populations of most countries, independent of income, select a diet containing approximately 11 per cent of the calories as protein.[1]

The practical implication is that proteins and amino acids should not be ingested by themselves. Protein is an expensive source of calories and during its catabolism yields nitrogen compounds which must be excreted by the kidney. The requirement for the essential amino acids is also "spared" by the dietary content of the non-essential amino acids, since they need not be deaminated to supply amino groups for non-essential amino acids.

Protein Requirements

The general belief has been that an inadequate protein intake compels the body to call upon "reserve" or body "store" of proteins in order to supply the necessary amino acids to meet situations of deprivation or stress. The depletion of the store is speeded up if the protein stores are also called upon to act as a source of energy. However, Holt et al.[5] have questioned the concept of a protein "store" or "reserve" ready to meet the needs of restriction and stress. After a critical examination of the literature and a review of some animal experiments, they conclude that there is

no virtue in feeding protein beyond the minimum adequate quantity. These authors believe there is no value in consuming extra proteins in anticipation of deprivation and stress but that the time for eating extra protein is during the untoward event and especially during convalescence, not before. The general trend at present is, however, toward a generous protein allowance for all ages.

Any condition of health or disease that imposes an increased nitrogen requirement upon the body (growth, pregnancy, lactation, burns, surgery, fever, hyperthyroidism and stress) must be met by increased protein intake if destruction of tissue and plasma proteins (negative nitrogen balance) is to be avoided.

Protein allowances should be based upon ideal body weight—what the person should weigh, not what he does weigh.

Refer to Table 10–1 for the allowances of protein recommended by the Food and Nutrition Board of the National Research Council.

Effect of Growth. During growth the need for protein is greater than at any other time in a person's life. Thus, infants and children need relatively more than the adult allowance because they accumulate new tissue of high protein content. Recommended allowances for children are 2.2 gm. per kg. of body weight for the infant of 0–6 months of age, 2.0 gm. per kg. for the infant of 6 months to 1 year, 1.7 gm. per kg. for 1–3 years, 1.2–1.5 gm. per kg. for older children and .9–1.0 gm. per kg. for adolescents. (See Chapters 14 and 15.)

Effect of Pregnancy and Lactation. Because pregnancy represents another form of rapid growth, the mother has an additional need for protein. The Food and Nutrition Board of the National Research Council (NRC) suggests that an additional 30 grams is needed daily over and above the normal allowance of .8 gm. per kg. of body weight. Lactation imposes an additional protein burden on the body inasmuch as 12 to 15 gm. of protein may be secreted daily in the breast milk. The NRC recommends an intake of an additional 20 gm. of protein above the normal allowance during lactation. (See Chapter 13.) In all these periods of growth requiring additional amounts of protein, additional calories are also necessary.

Effect of Age. The protein allowance of .8 gm. per kg. of body weight is maintained throughout adult life. However, a higher proportion of protein in the diet is required to achieve this level when the total calorie consumption is decreased with age. Proteins are essential in spite of the fact that the stomach secretes less acid and pepsin with age. Commonly we see older people who lose their zest for eating, or who, living alone, do not care to prepare well-balanced meals, or who have too little money for food. These people show the signs of dietary deficiencies, most commonly of proteins and vitamins. This is discussed in more detail in Chapter 16.

Effect of Exercise. The amount of physical work or exercise done is not of prime importance in determining protein allowance. Heavy work will require more expenditure of energy than light work will, but protein needs will not be increased, provided the calorie requirement is satisfied. During the period when a person is getting into "top physical condition," additional protein may be helpful during the period of muscle growth and increased muscle mass.[16] The actual protein needs of the athlete are similar to those of the non-athlete, provided the calorie requirements are satisfied.

Most people doing heavy work seem to prefer high protein intakes, perhaps because of the sense of well-being and vigor produced by high protein diets as well as the pleasant way of receiving the additional calories needed; however, it is not necessary.

Effect of Illness and Surgery. Any physical illness increases protein breakdown in the body. Indeed, merely staying in bed and decreasing food intake for several days will put a person into negative nitrogen balance. It is important therefore that these factors be considered in diet planning for the ill and convalescent person. Surgery is frequently preceded by a poor or precarious protein balance that should, when time permits, be corrected before surgical procedures are undertaken. Surgery itself contributes to establishing or continuing a negative nitrogen balance and such a balance retards wound healing and convalescence. (See Chapter 34.)

If the loss of protein is sudden, as occurs in hemorrhage following surgery or loss of blood plasma in burns, the patient will manifest shock. If the protein deficiency is gradual and prolonged, the following clinical signs of protein malnutrition may occur: loss of weight, skin changes (from soft, moist, pliable character to dry and scaly), reduced resistance to infection, impaired healing, hepatic insufficiency, nutritional edema, and changes in concentration of hemoglobin and plasma proteins.

Acute episodes of infection cause a negative N balance that depends on the severity and frequency of the infection and the response of the host. The negative N balance can be due to increased urinary N excretion owing to increased adrenocortical activity, decreased N absorption because of diarrhea, or anorexia. Protein supplementation during the infection does not prevent the negative balance, but it is important for replacing the nitrogen after the infection.

Protein malnutrition is best prevented through the consumption of sufficient protein foods of high biological value. In fact, the period of convalescence for the patient is shortened if protein deficiency does not develop, an important economic factor in the care of the sick. However, if the patient already has a protein deficiency, it should not be aggravated by inadequate dietary care. Instead, the backlog of poor nutrition needs to be improved along with the curing of the disease.

LOW AND HIGH PROTEIN INTAKE

The adult apparently can, if necessary, get along on protein intakes as low as 30 to 40 gm. daily, depending upon the quality of protein ingested. Concidentally, on such a low protein intake the urinary nitrogen output falls drastically, which indicates an adaptation process going on within the body to compensate for the low protein intake. If the protein in the diet is suddenly decreased, a negative nitrogen balance will exist for four to five days. Then, equi-

librium is reestablished at a lower level, unless the decreased intake of protein is below the critical point. Real protein deficiency is accompanied by edema, retardation of growth, wasting of body tissues, weakness, and loss of vigor. On the other side of the scale, people on very high intakes of protein have been studied and found to have no apparent harm. The normal kidney can handle large amounts of nitrogenous waste without difficulty. However, infants with normal immature kidneys do not tolerate excess protein intakes. One important condition in which a high protein intake is harmful is chronic kidney disease with nitrogen retention. The damaged kidney cannot excrete nitrogenous wastes, and giving excess protein only adds to the burden of a kidney that cannot do its normal work. Consequently, nitrogen retention is increased. However, in chronic kidney disease accompanied by low blood proteins (due to loss of protein through the injured kidney) and no excessive nitrogen retention, a high protein intake is indicated to make up for the urinary loss of protein. These conditions of disease and diet will be dealt with in more detail in Part Two.

MEETING PROTEIN AND ENERGY NEEDS FOR THE WORLD POPULATION

Intake of protein below the recommended allowance is found in many parts of the world and invariably it coincides with energy intakes below the recommended level. Protein malnutrition is a serious nutritional problem in the underdeveloped areas, particularly in its effect on infants and children who have a higher protein requirement on a per kg. or per kcal. basis than adults. Severe protein deficiency may lead to death. The chronic form leads more often to grossly retarded physical growth and development and increased susceptibility to acute and chronic infections. Mental development, learning and behavior may be impaired as well. Kwashiorkor was described by Cicely Williams as a disease in infants and children occurring when protein intake, especially animal protein, is severely restricted. (See Chapter 12.) This term has probably been overused in describing the malnutrition in the developing areas of the world. The situation of protein deficiency cannot be clearly separated from energy deficit, and a more accurate description of the problem is "protein-calorie" or "protein-energy malnutrition."[3, 8, 10] In 1974 McLaren stated:

Food consumption data and dietary surveys incriminate energy rather than protein deficit. Increasing the energy intake and not that of protein has produced catch-up growth in undernourished children. Lack of nutriment in general with an energy gap rather than a protein gap is the crux of the matter; but how to match the intake of the child with its requirements remains a problem of puzzling complexity.[8]

Only recently have we begun to realize that protein is not all of the problem, and that some of the efforts of the last 20 years which focused *only* on the problem of improvement of protein quality and quantity in the diet may not have reflected a broad enough approach to the problem. In 1973 the FAO/WHO committee stated: "When intakes of both energy and protein are grossly inadequate, the provision of protein-rich food of animal origin may be a costly and inefficient way of improving diets, since energy can generally be provided more cheaply than protein of good quality."[1]

One of the reasons for emphasis on protein is the observation that food sources of good protein are scarce in many parts of the world, and this is usually a result of inadequate total food production. In some countries there are possibilities for production of the desired protein, but the quality is not good, or information on food is lacking. The various divisions of the United Nations, particularly the Protein Advisory Group (PAG), have been attempting to advise on the suitability and safety of new protein foods for human consumption. Any new foods that are to find wide acceptance must be integrated into existing diets; they must be compatible with existing customs and food habits. A solution for one country may not be feasible in another country of different climate, geography, economic resources, social patterns and eating habits. Nutritional improvement of people or population groups takes place only if and when a better diet is actually consumed.

Sources of Protein

In a number of the technically underdeveloped areas and countries, efforts to develop vegetable sources of protein have been, to a great extent, stimulated and aided by WHO, FAO and UNICEF. In French West Africa and Zaire, peanut flour has been explored as a source of protein for child feeding. Soya and sunflower seed press cakes have been used in Uganda. In Japan, research is being conducted on soya products prepared by

traditional fermentation methods. Fish flour plants and ponds for raising fish have been set up to provide a low-cost source of animal protein in a number of countries (Fig. 1–2). Surplus skim milk has been made available in various countries through UNICEF for a number of years.

Worldwide endeavors have been made to develop protein-rich foods of low cost. In India, Zaire, and other parts of Africa and Central America, inexpensive mixtures of vegetable origin with a high protein content of good biological value have been contrived to be used as a dietary supplement, especially for children. Incaparina, already mentioned on page 77, is a good example.

In the United States, during World War II, a mixture providing 50 per cent protein known as MPF (Multi-Purpose Food) was compounded from toasted soy grits, calcium carbonate, vitamin C, niacin, riboflavin, vitamin B_6, thiamin, vitamin A and vitamin D, vitamin B_{12} and potassium iodide. It was precooked and could be sprinkled over ready-to-eat cereal or used in milk over cereal.

Development of New Sources of Protein

From the laboratory there is a new kind of food called Single Cell Protein (SCP). It is a tasteless, odorless mass of edible microorganisms (yeasts, bacteria and fungi) which are grown on the waste products of petroleum refinement and are then treated and dried. It is presently fed to animals, but it may become a food for humans. Other new high-protein foods called meat analogues also are on the market for consumer consumption. They include vegetable proteins such as spun soybean fiber and are called *textured vegetable protein* or TVP. These products contain 40 to 60 per cent protein of good biological value and are able to imitate, with varying degrees of acceptance, ground beef, diced chicken, ham, bacon, scallops and turkey.

In an attempt to salvage protein discarded after processing, new methods have been developed that enable the procurement of a protein from the cottonseed and groundnut after the oil has been extracted. *Whey,* a usually discarded by-product of cheese production, is now being processed for its protein and sugar content.

Leaf protein concentrates, processed from leaves that traditionally would not be harvested or because of fibrous material would have protein unavailable to humans, are now being extracted, processed and tested for utilization and acceptability. Antarctic krill, a plankton, is another potential source of protein if the supply is approached ecologically and correctly.

There is an increase in the use of synthetic essential amino acids to improve the quality of the proteins of cereals and other vegetable sources. For an example, lysine added to wheat flour dramatically improves the quality of wheat protein.

Attempts to grow more complete proteins have resulted in the development of a new strain of corn, *opaque-2*. It contains higher amounts of lysine and tryptophan (essential amino acids) than found in ordinary strains of corn. Its nutritive value approaches that of milk protein in feeding trials and there is much optimism concerning its potential impact in the corn-consuming countries of the world. Work is under way to develop soybean varieties containing larger amounts of methionine and wheat and sorghum containing more lysine.

Stature Related to Protein Intake

There is evidence that stature is influenced by the kind and amount of protein, as well as by heredity (Fig. 5–8). Orientals, who depend largely on a vegetable diet, are relatively short as contrasted with native New Zealanders, who are renowned meat-eaters and who are tall and have large physiques. Statistics[11] point out a remarkable increase in the stature of Japanese youth during the past decades, which is most marked in children born since the period of postwar shortages. Evidence, direct and indirect, indicates better nutrition has contributed to increased growth rate. From changes in average nutrient intake during the past decade, it is concluded that protein or nutrients associated with protein must have played a major role. Total protein consumption in Japan has increased 10 per cent in the past three decades with the intake of animal protein almost doubled.

TRENDS OF PROTEIN INTAKE IN THE AMERICAN DIET

According to the estimate of per capita consumption by Consumer and Food Economics Research Division, Agricultural Research Service, Department of Agriculture, protein decreased from 102 gm. in the 1909 to 1913 period to a low of 90 gm. per day in the 1935 to 1939 period. The figure for 1965 was 96 gm. and for

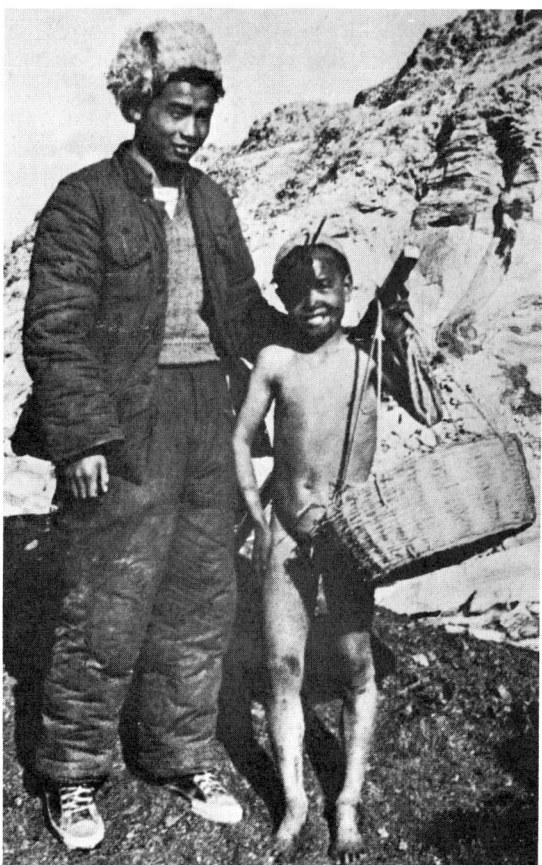

Figure 5–8 Two Asian boys of the same age. The boy on the right worked in a mine and received ordinary protein-poor local food. The other boy spent four years in a boarding school were he was well fed. (Photo courtesy of FAO.)

intake appeared to be adequate in all groups except possibly pregnant women.[4] The First Health and Nutrition Examination Survey (HANES, 1971–72) also showed that protein intake seemed to be adequate.[14] Protein deficiency does not appear to be a problem in the U.S., but rather our excess protein intake should be questioned.

Protein in Foods

The Home Economics Research Report No. 4, U.S. Department of Agriculture booklet entitled "Amino Acid Content of Foods," by M. L. Orr and B. K. Watt, contains data on 18 amino acids, both in terms of amino acids per gram of total nitrogen (202 food items) and in terms of amino acids in 100-gram foods (316 food items). Table 6 in the Appendix is taken from this pamphlet, which includes the average amount of amino acids per 100 grams of various foods for the essential amino acids necessary for growth; it can be used to calculate the essential amino acid content of foods.

Effect of Processing of Protein Foods. Processing of foods alters the nutritive value of protein.[9] Overheating, particularly in the absence of water (dry heat, frying), may either destroy certain essential amino acids such as lysine, which is heat labile, or alter them by tying them up in new chemical linkages so that the protein becomes resistant to digestive enzymes, or the release of individual amino acids in the intestinal tract is retarded. On the other hand, processing may have a favorable effect on protein foods by increasing the digestibility or increasing the liberation of individual amino acids. For example, cooking in the presence of water increases the nutritive value and digestibility of navy beans. High, dry heat exerts a deleterious effect on the nutritive value of wheat and oat protein. Similarly, toasting reduces the nutritive value of bread. Marked heat will decrease the availability of protein in soybeans, while mild heat is favorable. It appears that the nutritive value of meat proteins is not greatly diminished by ordinary cooking methods. However, severe heat treatment (such as autoclaving or pressure cooking) may lessen the nutritive value of meat proteins. Heat appears to reduce the nutritive value of milk used in cooking. On the other hand, the heat treatment involved in preparing evaporated or dried milk not only fails to decrease the nutritive value but enhances the digestibility and utilization of protein.

1974, 99 grams. The type of protein shifted from 56 per cent animal protein in the 1935 to 1939 period to 68 per cent in 1965, where it remained in 1974. Vegetable protein decreased from 47 per cent to about 30 per cent, where it had remained as of 1974. It is interesting to find that flour and cereal products contributed 36 per cent of the total protein available for consumption in the 1909 to 1913 period, but only 19 per cent in 1965 and 18 per cent in 1974. As these foods decreased in importance as sources of protein, dairy products, eggs, meat, poultry and fish increased in importance by contributing more of the total protein in the diet. In general, the North American diet provides protein in generous amounts, about two-thirds from animal source and one-third from plants. The Ten State Nutrition Survey (1968–70), which assessed the nutritional status of a large sample of poor families, revealed that protein

PROBLEMS AND SUGGESTED TOPICS FOR DISCUSSION

1. List the most popular protein foods. Classify them as to *complete* and *incomplete protein*.
2. What is meant by the term "essential amino acids"? Name them. What are the physiological functions of amino acids?
3. Give examples of specific functions of four of the amino acids.
4. List the amounts of various protein foods you consume during a period of 24 hours and a period of 3 days; calculate the protein content.
5. Evaluate the list of protein foods. Classify them into animal and vegetable-grain proteins. Which ones have high biological value? What percentage of your diet is protein? Was the total amount of protein consumed in 24 hours equally distributed between the three meals?
6. Give five reasons why you eat protein foods.
7. Design an adequate menu of complementary proteins for a vegetarian who does not eat eggs, milk products or animal flesh.
8. Plan a basic dietary pattern of protein foods you require daily. Divide into three meals, keeping in mind the recent findings as to quality and quantity.
9. How is the need for good protein being met throughout the world?
10. What is the trend in protein consumption in the United States? What changes should be made?
11. What is meant by a negative nitrogen balance? When might this occur? Describe two kinds of diets most likely to maintain nitrogen balance or equilibrium.
12. Using the ratio pattern for essential amino acids in Table 6 in the Appendix, determine the balance of amino acids in your food intake for one day. Is your diet properly balanced in essential amino acids? If not, show how it can be corrected.
13. Why are proteins considered to be a wasteful source of energy?
14. What effect does cooking have on protein foods? Explain and give examples.
15. Take a nutrition history of a patient on a normal diet. Plan a diet for the patient to follow when discharged from the hospital, keeping in mind the food budget, protein allowance, biological value of proteins, balance of essential amino acids, and any environmental factors involved.

CITED REFERENCES

1. Energy and Protein Requirements. Joint FAO/WHO Ad Hoc Expert Committee, World Health Organization, Tech. Report No. 522, Geneva, Switzerland, 1973.
2. Harper, A. E.: Amino acid excess. In White, P. L., and Fletcher, D. C. (eds.): Nutrients in Processed Foods—Proteins. Acton, Mass., Publishing Sciences Group, Inc., 1974.
3. Hegsted, D. M.: Protein needs and possible modifications of the American diet. J. Am. Diet. Assoc., 68: 317, 1976.
4. Highlights of the Ten-State Nutrition Survey, 1968–70. U.S. DHEW Pub. No. (HSM) 72–8134, 1972.
5. Holt, J. E., Jr., et al.: The concept of protein stores and its implication in diet. JAMA 181:699, 1962.
6. Kopple, J. D., and Swendseid, M. E.: Evidence that histidine is an essential amino acid in normal and chronically uremic men. J. Clin. Invest.,55:881, 1975.
7. Kuiken, K. A., and Lyman, C. L.: Availability of amino acids in some foods. J. Nutr., 36:359, 1948.
8. McLaren, D. S.: The great protein fiasco. Lancet, 2:93, 1974.
9. Melnick, D.: The influence of heat processing on the functional and nutritive properties of protein food. Food Tech., 3:57, 1949.
10. Miller, D. S.: Protein-energy interrelationships. In Porter, J. W., and Rolls, B. A. (eds.): Proteins in Human Nutrition. New York, Academic Press, 1973.
11. Mitchell, H. S.: Nutrition in relation to stature. J. Am. Diet Assoc., 40:521, 1962.
12. PAG Bulletin, 5 (3), September, 1975.
13. Pollack, H., and Halpern, S. L.: Therapeutic Nutrition. Washington, D.C., National Research Council, Pub. No. 234, 1952, p. 4.
14. Preliminary Findings of the First Health and Nutrition Examination Survey, U.S., 1971–72, Dietary Intake and Biochemical Findings. U.S. DHEW Pub. No. (HRA) 74–1219-1, 1974.
15. Recommended Dietary Allowances, 8th ed. Washington, D.C., Food and Nutrition Board, National Research Council, NAS, 1974.
16. Van Itallie, T.: If only we knew. Nutr. Today, 3(2):3, 1968.

ADDITIONAL REFERENCES

Adibi, S. A.: Intestinal phase of protein assimilation in man. Am. J. Clin. Nutr., 29:205, 1976.
Allison, J. B., and Wannemacher, R. W.: The concept and significance of labile and over-all protein reserves of the body. Am. J. Clin. Nutr., 16:445, 1965.
Guyton, A. C.: Textbook of Medical Physiology, 5th ed. Philadelphia, W. B. Saunders Company, 1976, Chapter 69—Protein Metabolism.
Harpstead, D. D.: High-lysine corn. Sci. Am., 225(2):34, 1971.
Howe, E. E., et al.: Amino acid supplementation of cereal grains as related to the world food supply. Am. J. Clin. Nutr., 16:315, 1965.
Irwin, M. I., and Hegsted, D. M.: A conspectus of research on protein requirements of man. J. Nutr., 101:385, 1971.
Lappé, F. M.: Diet for a Small Planet. New York, Ballantine Books, 1971.
Leverton, R. M.: Amino acid requirements of young adults. In Albanese, A. A. (ed.): Protein and Amino Acid Nutrition. New York, Academic Press, 1959, pp. 477–506.
Nasset, E. S.: Amino acid homeostasis in the gut lumen and its nutritional significance. World Rev. Nutr. Diet., 14:134, Basel, Karger, 1972.
Review: evaluation of the FAO amino acid reference pattern. Nutr. Rev., 21:101, 1963.
Rose, W. C., et al.: The amino acid requirements of man. J. Biol.Chem., 217:987, 1955.
Sanchez, A., et al.: Nutritive value of selected proteins and protein combinations. I. The biological value of proteins singly and in meal patterns with varying fat composition. II. Biological value predictability. Am. J. Clin. Nutr., 13:243, 1963.
Scrimshaw, N. S.: Strengths and weaknesses of the committee approach—an analysis of past and present recommended dietary allowances for protein in health and disease. N. Engl. J. Med., 294(3):136–142, (4):194–206, 1976.
Watson, I. D.: The Double Helix: A Personal Account of the Structure of DNA. New York, Academic Press, 1968.

Chapter 6

DIGESTION, ABSORPTION AND CELL METABOLISM

Most of the major nutrients in foods are bound in large molecules which cannot be absorbed from the intestine because of size or because they are not water-soluble. The reduction of these large molecules into smaller, readily absorbed units and conversion of the insoluble molecules into soluble forms is the work of the digestive tract.

The digestive system extends from the mouth to the anus. (See Figure 6–1.) It consists of the alimentary canal and the exocrine and endocrine functions of its appendage organs, e.g., the liver and biliary tree and the pancreas.

Functions. The functions of the digestive system include: (1) receipt, maceration and transport of ingested substances and waste

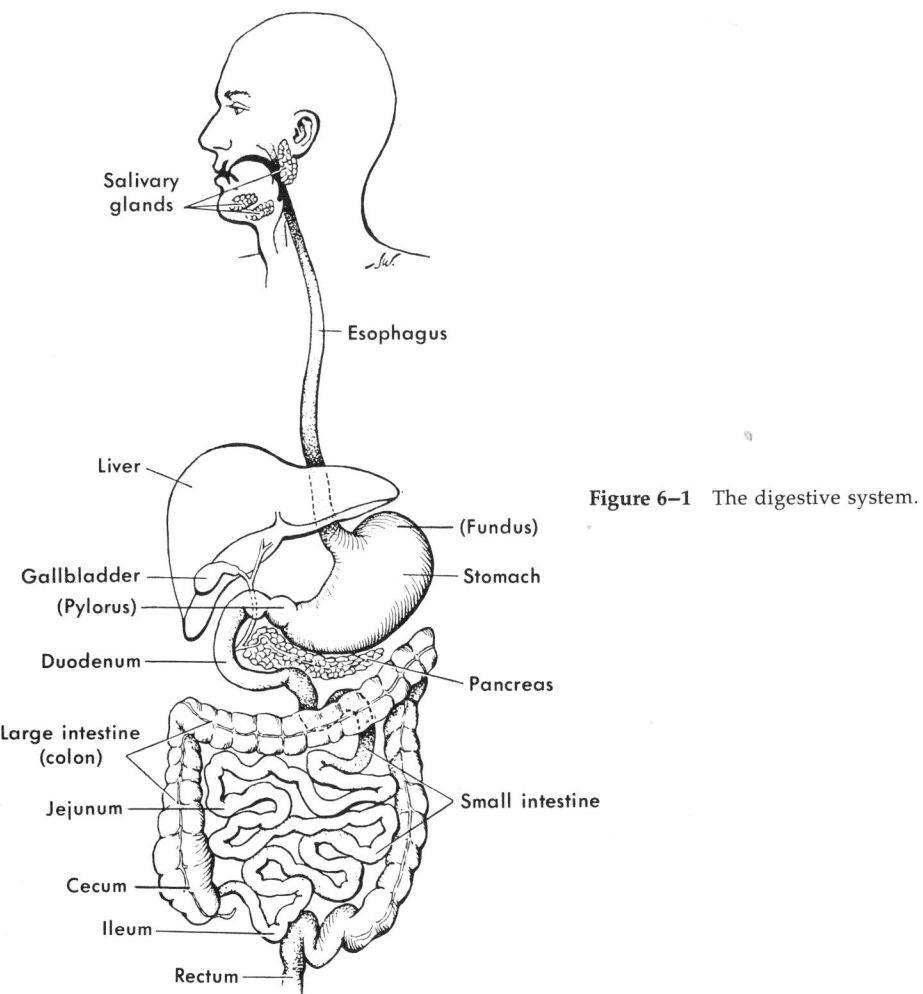

Salivary glands

Esophagus

Liver

(Fundus)

Gallbladder

Stomach

(Pylorus)

Duodenum

Pancreas

Large intestine (colon)

Jejunum

Small intestine

Cecum

Ileum

Rectum

Figure 6–1 The digestive system.

products; (2) secretion of acid, mucus, digestive enzymes, bile and other materials; (3) digestion of ingested foodstuffs; (4) absorption; (5) storage of waste products; (6) excretion; and (7) certain ancillary functions.

MOUTH   The mouth receives food into the oral cavity, reduces it in size by chewing and mixes it with saliva, mucus and the digestive enzyme ptyalin (salivary amylase).

ESOPHAGUS.   The esophagus functions to transport food and liquids from the oral cavity and pharynx to the stomach.

STOMACH.   The stomach and first portion of duodenum participate in the storage, digestion, and transport of ingested materials. The stomach secretes hydrochloric acid, intrinsic factor, the inactive protease pepsinogen, gastric lipase, mucus, and the gastrointestinal hormone gastrin. Only very lipid-soluble substances and weak acids such as alcohol and aspirin (acetylsalicylic acid) are absorbed from the stomach.

SMALL INTESTINE.   The small intestine functions to secrete and to participate in digestion, absorption, and transport of ingested materials. It consists of the duodenum, jejunum and ileum. Just past the pyloric sphincter are Brunner's glands, which secrete the much needed mucus to protect the duodenal mucosa from chyme acidity. The duodenum receives the secretions of the large accessory glands of digestion—the pancreas and the liver. The small intestine functions to continue digestion and to absorb the end products of digestion of carbohydrates, proteins and fats. It secretes the enzyme enterokinase, and its epithelial cells contain several peptidases, sucrase, lactase, α-dextrinase, maltase, amylase and small quantities of enteric lipase. The gastrointestinal hormones secretin and enterogastrone are formed in the wall of the duodenum.

LARGE INTESTINE AND RECTUM.   The large intestine and rectum absorb water, electrolytes and, in reduced amounts, some of the final products of digestion. They also provide a temporary storage for waste products which serve as a medium for bacterial synthesis of some nutritional factors.

ANUS.   The anus functions to control defecation. Power for this function is provided by the propulsive contractions of the colon and rectum which are normally coordinated with the involuntary and voluntary portions of the anal sphincter.

PANCREAS.   The pancreas functions to produce secretions required for the digestion and absorption of food. Enzymes excreted include pancreatic lipase, cholesterol esterase, pancreatic amylase, ribonuclease, deoxyribonuclease, carboxypolypeptidase, trypsin and chymotrypsin (in their respective inactive forms, e.g., procarboxypolypeptidase, trypsinogen and chymotrypsinogen). These are activated by trypsin only after they are in the intestinal lumen. Under the influence of secretin, the pancreas secretes fluid containing large amounts of the bicarbonate ion. Important endocrine secretions of the pancreas are insulin and glucagon.

LIVER AND BILIARY TRACT.   The major functions of the liver include the metabolism of protein, carbohydrate and lipid; the conjugation and detoxification of hormones, toxins and drugs; and the synthesis of proteins. In addition, the metabolism of bile pigments and bile salts takes place within the liver, and these products, important in the digestion and absorption of fats, are secreted into the duodenum through the biliary tract.

Each of these functions will be discussed in more detail.

DIGESTION AND ABSORPTION

Digestion and absorption do not take place one step at a time as isolated functions. They are continuous processes with many mechanical and chemical reactions taking place simultaneously; a defect in one phase hampers the other phase.

Normally, 92 to 97 per cent of the mixed American dietary is digested and absorbed. Foods are prepared for ingestion in a variety of ways and combinations; processing methods and cooking may begin a slight breakdown of complex compounds such as starch and collagen before they are eaten. Water, monosaccharides, alcohol and inorganic ions are usually absorbed in their original form. The di- and polysaccharides, lipids and proteins must be converted to their simple constituents before they are absorbed.

It is assumed that knowledge in this subject has been acquired elsewhere. However, a brief review is included for the purpose of integration. For additional details, it is recommended that the reader consult a textbook on physiology or biochemistry.

DIGESTION

Digestion is a series of physical and chemical changes by which food, taken into the body, undergoes hydrolysis (addition of water) and is

broken down in preparation for absorption from the intestinal tract into the blood stream.

The physical changes in food are brought about by grinding, crushing and mixing of the food with the digestive juices and propulsion of the mass through the digestive tract. The propulsive force of the gastrointestinal tract resides in the circular and longitudinal smooth muscles contained in its walls. These muscles churn and push the food mass (chyme) along the digestive tract in rhythmic waves (peristalsis) toward the anus. During the propulsion of the chyme through the gut, it is mixed at appropriate times with the digestive juices which begin their chemical changes of food. The active materials in the digestive juices which cause this chemical breakdown are enzymes, both endoenzymes and exoenzymes. The whole process is regulated through neural and hormonal mechanisms.

REGULATION OF GASTROINTESTINAL ACTIVITY

Neural Mechanisms. The neural control of gastrointestinal contractile and secretory activity is composed of two parts—a local system of internal plexuses and an external system of nerve fibers from the autonomic nervous system.

The local system consists of the *myenteric plexus* and the *submucosal plexus.* Located in the gut wall or mucosa are receptors sensitive to the composition of the chyme (acidity, for instance) and lumen stretch (fullness, for example). These receptors send impulses to the internal plexuses. From the plexuses impulses then go out on efferent fibers to muscle cells and secretory cells of the intestinal tract.

The autonomic innervation comes from the sympathetic postganglionic fibers, which run along blood vessels, and the parasympathetic preganglionic fibers in the vagus nerve. The *vagus nerve* has branches to the stomach, small intestine, and upper portion of the large intestine and carries impulses, either excitatory or inhibitory. This activity does not control but rather influences the local activity in the plexuses. An example of vagal activity is the stimulation of acid secretion from parietal cells which accompanies the sight or smell of food (the cephalic phase of digestion). Because of its ability to stimulate gastric acid secretion, the vagus nerve is frequently cut as a treatment for peptic ulcer disease when constant hyperacidity is present.

Hormonal Mechanisms. Our knowledge of the hormonal control of the gastrointestinal tract is mushrooming, as evidenced by the continual discovery of "candidate hormones" (a term coined by Grossman[1]). These candidate hormones are identified substances that could have definite physiological functions and thus be termed hormones after additional study. At present we believe that hormonal regulation of the gastrointestinal system is possibly controlled by many hormones, of which only three are fairly well defined local hormones: gastrin, secretin, and cholecystokinin.

Gastrin is released from G cells in the antral mucosa of the stomach, the duodenum and jejunum. Like all of the gastrointestinal hormones, gastrin is released into the blood stream, is carried in the venous system to the heart, and does not have its particular effect on gastrointestinal cells until it returns via the arterial blood flow. Thus a gastrointestinal hormone can affect any portion of the gastrointestinal (GI) system regardless of where it was produced. The release of gastrin from the antral mucosa of the stomach is initiated by (1) distention of the antrum (as after a meal), (2) impulses from the vagus nerve (as at the thought of food), and (3) the presence in the antrum of secretagogues, such as partially digested proteins, food extracts (e.g., bouillon), alcohol and caffeine. Unfortunately the intestinal release of gastrin is not as well understood.

The functions of gastrin are many, but the most important one is to increase gastric secretion through stimulation of parietal cell acid secretion, chief cell enzyme secretion and gastric antral motility. Some other effects are listed in Table 6–1. Through a feedback mechanism, gastrin release is inhibited when the lumen pH gets too low, and thus acid secretion is reduced.

Secretin, a hormone released from the duodenal wall into the blood stream, has several actions in opposition to gastrin and results in a lowering of acidity. Secreted in response to duodenal acidity, it stimulates the pancreas to secrete water and bicarbonate (HCO_3^-) into the duodenum. This bicarbonate neutralizes the acidity from the stomach, thus protecting the duodenal mucosa from prolonged exposure to acid and permitting the activity of duodenal enzymes, which require a neutral or slightly alkaline environment. Gastrin is inhibited by secretin, which leads to reduced acid secretion and a further lowering of lumen acidity. Table 6–1 lists some other activities of secretin.

Other cells of the duodenal mucosa secrete a

Table 6–1   IMPORTANT FUNCTIONS OF GASTROINTESTINAL HORMONES

HORMONE	SITE OF RELEASE	STIMULANT OF RELEASE	ORGAN AFFECTED	EFFECT ON ORGAN
gastrin	antral mucosa of stomach duodenum jejunum	polypeptides amino acids caffeine alcohol food extracts	esophagus	—increases resting pressure of lower esophageal sphincter
			stomach	—stimulates secretion of HCl and pepsinogen by parietal and chief cells, respectively —increases gastric antral motility
			gallbladder	—weakly stimulates contraction of gallbladder
			pancreas	—weakly stimulates pancreatic secretion of bicarbonate
secretin	duodenal mucosa	gut acidity (pH < 4–5)	esophagus	—reduces resting pressure of lower esophageal sphincter
			stomach	—reduces gastric and duodenal motility —stimulates pepsinogen secretion —inhibits gastrin stimulated secretion of acid
			duodenum	—decreases motility —increases mucous output of Brunner's glands
			pancreas	—increases output of H_2O and bicarbonate
			liver	—increases volume and electrolyte output of bile
Cholecystokinin-pancreozymin	duodenal mucosa	amino acids HCl fatty acids (< 9c.) food	stomach	—inhibits gastrin stimulated secretion of acid
			small bowel	—increases motility
			gallbladder	—causes contraction of gallbladder
			pancreas	—stimulates enzyme secretion —potentiates effect of secretin on pancreas

hormone *cholecystokinin-pancreozymin* or *CCK-PZ* whose release is stimulated by the presence in the duodenum of amino acids and fatty acids, the products of protein and fat digestion. The functions of this hormone are (1) stimulation of the pancreas to secrete enzymes and (2) stimulation of the gallbladder to contract.

The presence of a fourth hormone speculatively named *enterogastrone*, or gastric inhibitory polypeptide, has been postulated but has not been confirmed, since it has not been identified as a specific entity. The reason for suspecting an additional hormone is the fact that fatty foods in the duodenum, especially fatty acids, cause a slowing down of stomach emptying. It is thought that this is caused by this hormone (enterogastrone) released by the intestinal mucosa. However, secretin has a similar effect on stomach emptying and it may be the hormone in question.

Many other names appear in the gastrointestinal endocrinology literature—vasoactive intestinal polypeptide, enteroglucagon, somatostatin and others. Much more needs to be elucidated before these can be called true gastrointestinal hormones. See Rayford and associates[3] for a good review of the subject. In the healthy person, these hormonal and neural mechanisms, of which we understand so little, beautifully regulate and orchestrate the complex, interrelated and simultaneously occurring processes of digestion and absorption.

Digestion in the Mouth. In the mouth the teeth function to grind and crush the food into small particles. Simultaneously, the food mass is moistened and lubricated by saliva secreted by three pairs of glands: the parotid, submaxillary and sublingual glands.

These three pairs of glands produce about 1.5 liters of saliva daily. There are two types of saliva. One type is a serous secretion and contains α-amylase (ptyalin), which begins the digestion of starch; the other contains mucus, a protein that makes particles of food stick together and lubricates the mass for easier swallowing. The masticated food mass, now known as the bolus, passes back to the pharynx under voluntary control, but from there on and through the esophagus the process of swallowing is involuntary. Peristalsis then moves the food rapidly into the stomach.

Digestion in the Stomach. There is a mixing and propulsion of the food particles with gastric secretions in wave-like contractions. The churning and mixing waves are usually described as going from the fundus to the antrum of the pylorus. In the process of gastric digestion the food becomes semiliquid (chyme) and contains approximately 50 per cent water.

Active chemical digestion begins in the middle portion of the stomach. An average of 2000 to 2500 ml. of gastric juice is secreted daily and contains the enzymes, mucus and hydrochloric acid necessary for digestion. Foodstuffs, when taken alone, leave the stomach in the following order: carbohydrate first, protein next, then fat, which takes the longest. But when carbohydrate, protein and fat are mixed, they all take longer. The stomach normally is emptied in 1 to 4 hours, depending upon the amount and kinds of foods eaten.

Digestion in the Small Intestine. The small intestine, which has a total length of about 22 feet, is divided into three sections: the duodenum, the jejunum and the ileum. (See Fig. 6–1.) The acidic chyme slowly moves in spurts of a few milliliters through the exit valve (pylorus) at the junction of the stomach and duodenum into the duodenum, where it mixes with duodenal juices, bile (produced by the liver and stored in the gallbladder until needed), and the secretions from the pancreas.

The valves (sphincters) guarding the entrance to and the exit from the stomach prevent backflow of the mixture from the duodenum into the stomach and from the stomach into the pharynx. These structures open and close at the proper time; but because the nervous system influences their behavior, they often become too energetic during emotional upsets. When the exit pyloric valve tightens or goes into spasms, the pain is excruciating. Irritation from nearby ulcers also may alter the performance of this structure. Mild exercise is advantageous to the digestive process but violent exercise inhibits it. The chyme moves down the small intestine at a rate of 1 cm. per minute and takes from 3 to 10 hours to travel the entire length to the ileocecal valve. Most of the digestion process is completed in the duodenum, and the remainder of the small intestine (jejunum and ileum) functions principally in the absorption of nutrients.

ABSORPTION

Absorption from the Small Intestine. The remarkable structural feature of the small intestine is its tremendous absorptive area. The inner lining of the intestine, the mucosa, is in immediate contact with the products of digestion. The mucosa is folded to form *valvulae conniventes.* Covering these folds are finger-like projections called *villi.* The absorptive surface is further increased by the existence on each villus of *microvilli,* which make up the so-called *brush border.* The convolutions, villi and their microvilli give the small intestine an enormous absorptive surface of about 250 square meters, which rests on a supporting structure called the lamina propria. The lamina propria is composed of connective tissue in which are suspended the blood and lymph vessels. These vessels receive the absorbed nutrients from the mucosal cells. Figure 6–2 schematically represents the intestinal mucosa, and Figure 6–3 illustrates a villous absorptive or epithelial cell.

The Mechanism of Absorption. Absorption is an extremely complex process and all its ramifications are not completely understood. It is not simply a matter of diffusion of the nutrients through the mucosal cells into the blood stream for transport to other parts of the body. Diffusion does occur in certain instances in which the substance is lipid-soluble (e.g., fatty acids, alcohol) and is able to be dissolved in the lipid of the cell membrane and then diffused through the cell. Other more intricate processes are also involved and explain how large amounts of nutrients constantly enter and leave the cell. Physiologists and biochemists discuss current absorption theory in terms of pores, carriers, pumps and pinocytosis. (These mechanisms, though not proven fact, may apply equally to other tissues as well—liver, muscle, kidney, etc.) (See Fig. 6–4.)

PORES. The presence of a layer of lipoprotein in the wall of the microvilli makes the cell relatively impervious to water and water-soluble substances. It is postulated that these lipoprotein cell membranes are perforated by thousands of tiny pores which permit water, certain electrolytes and very small water-soluble molecules to enter the cell.

CARRIERS. Water molecules and other inorganic ions are sufficiently small to gain access to the inside of the epithelial cells through the pores. Amino acids, simple sugars and fats have molecules larger than water molecules and therefore cannot pass easily through small pores. It is proposed that these relatively large fat-insoluble substances are escorted across the cell membranes by a carrier, an agent that shuttles back and forth like a ferry. This carrier

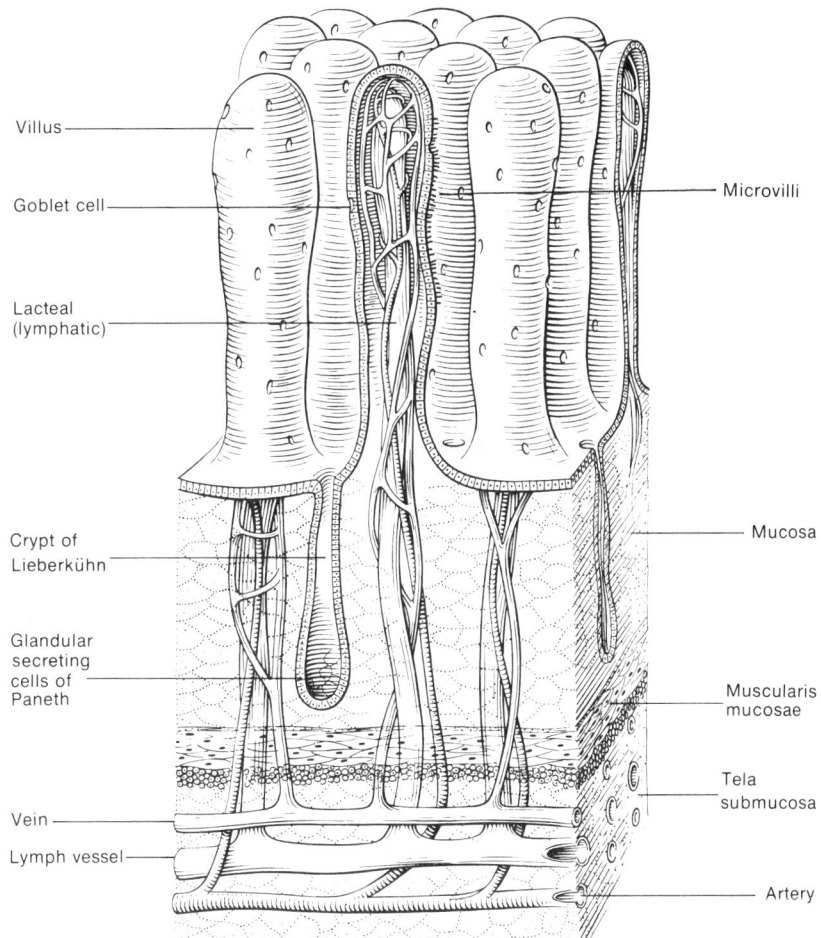

Villus

Goblet cell

Lacteal
(lymphatic)

Crypt of
Lieberkühn

Glandular
secreting
cells of
Paneth

Vein

Lymph vessel

Microvilli

Mucosa

Muscularis
mucosae

Tela
submucosa

Artery

Figure 6–2 Diagram of villi of human intestine showing their structure and blood and lymph vessels. (From: Villee, C. A., and Dethier, V. G.: Biological Principles and Processes, 2nd ed. Philadelphia, W. B. Saunders Co., 1976.)

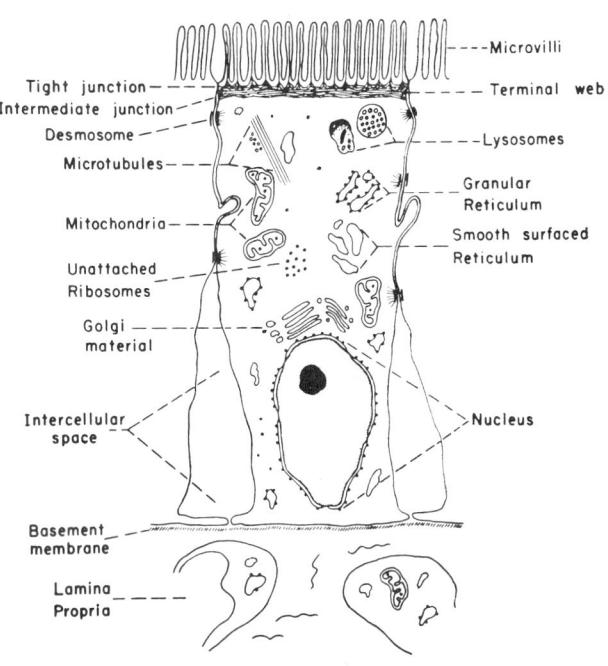

Tight junction
Intermediate junction
Desmosome
Microtubules

Mitochondria

Unattached
Ribosomes

Golgi
material

Intercellular
space

Basement
membrane

Lamina
Propria

Microvilli
Terminal web
Lysosomes
Granular
Reticulum
Smooth surfaced
Reticulum

Nucleus

Figure 6–3 Schematic diagram of a villous absorptive cell. (From: Trier, J. S.: Structure of the mucosa of the small intestine as it relates to intestinal function. Fed. Proc., 26:1392, 1967.)

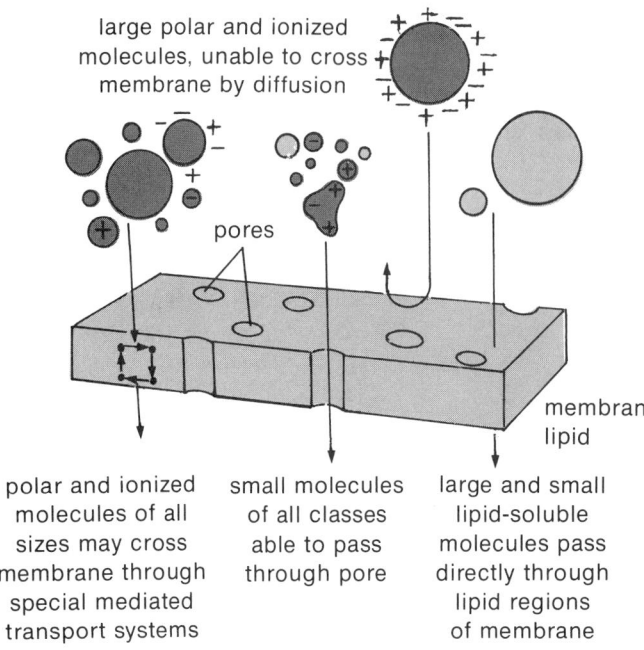

large polar and ionized
molecules, unable to cross
membrane by diffusion

pores

membrane
lipid

polar and ionized
molecules of all
sizes may cross
membrane through
special mediated
transport systems

small molecules
of all classes
able to pass
through pore

large and small
lipid-soluble
molecules pass
directly through
lipid regions
of membrane

Figure 6–4 Summary of the various pathways by which molecules can cross intestinal cell membranes. (From: Vander, A. J., Sherman, J. H., and Luciano, D. S.: Human Physiology: The Mechanisms of Body Function, 2nd ed. Copyright © 1975 by McGraw-Hill, Inc. Used by permission of McGraw-Hill Book Company.)

is thought to be a protein or lipoprotein. At one side of the membrane it combines with the material needing transport, shuttles it across the cell membrane and then releases it into the interior of the cell. In so doing, it is then free to return for another load. This system is also called *facilitated diffusion*—the carrier makes the molecule soluble in the lipid membrane and thus facilitates diffusion. It is apparent that there are specific carriers· for specific substances. Presumably, the transported substance sits in a "special chair" on the carrier similar to substrates which have specific sites of attachment on enzymes. Some nutrients may share the same carrier and thus may compete for absorption. Carrier systems can also become saturated and the absorption of the nutrient can be slowed. The best known carrier is that responsible for the absorption of vitamin B_{12}. A carrier protein called intrinsic factor is produced by the lining of the stomach. This specialized protein joins with vitamin B_{12} in the intestine and a carrier system provides for its absorption.

PUMPS. Some molecules require energy in order to move from the intestinal lumen into the mucosal cell, since the concentration within the cell is far greater than that in the lumen, and a pump is required. These pumps, which require cellular energy or ATP and a carrier, rapidly move certain nutrients into the cells and thence into the blood supply. The absorption of glu-

cose, sodium, galactose, potassium, magnesium, phosphate, iodide, calcium, iron and amino acids is thought to occur in this manner.

PINOCYTOSIS. Pinocytosis has been described by Ingelfinger[2] as a "drinking in" of a small drop of intestinal contents by the epithelial cell membrane. In this way, large particles such as whole proteins may be absorbed in small quantity. Even though it is doubtful that much nutrient is normally absorbed via pinocytosis, foreign proteins, which somehow find their way across the gastrointestinal tract into the blood stream and cause allergic reactions, probably result from pinocytosis.

Absorption from the Large Intestine. The large intestine is approximately five feet long and consists of the cecum, colon and rectum. (See Fig. 6–1.) It is the site of the absorption of water, salts and some of the vitamins leaving the mass in a semisolid state. Most of the water in the 500–1000 ml. of chyme that enters the colon each day is absorbed, leaving 100–200 ml. of fluid to be excreted in the feces. In the large intestine the sodium ion is actively absorbed by the mucosa, and because of the electrical potential thus created across the membrane, chloride and other negative ions as well as water move out of the colon into the intestinal mucosa. In addition, the large intestine serves to permit bacteria to reduce materials resistant to the previous digestive processes. Normally, as the contents of the colon move

forward at 5 cm. per hour, almost everything of nutritional value is utilized. The waste is composed mostly of cellulose, a number of other polysaccharides and related substances such as pectins and pentosans and other indigestible products. The feces contain some water, dead mucosal cells, bacteria, and some fat (2.5 to 5 per cent), which comes from the unabsorbed fatty acids from the diet, fat formed by bacterial action, and fat found in the sloughed epithelial cells. Passing of feces through the anus, or defecation, occurs with varying frequency, ranging from after every meal to once every 3 or more days.

Digestion and absorption do not always proceed in an orderly fashion. An irritant such as an infection may increase the rate of peristalsis, causing the intestinal contents to pass through the intestinal tract rapidly (diarrhea). If the condition becomes chronic, a considerable loss of body water and electrolytes may result, causing dehydration and electrolyte imbalance. When the contents pass through too slowly, so that a large amount of water is removed, the feces become excessively hard (constipation). Some of the diseases and disturbances will be discussed in Unit 6—Diseases of the Gastrointestinal System.

The Digestive Enzymes—Their Relation to Digestion and Absorption

The digestive enzymes are both exoenzymes and endoenzymes. Those enzymes concerned with metabolism of the cell are usually retained within the cell and are called endoenzymes. Those enzymes which are released by the cell and catalyze reactions in the environment of the cell are called exoenzymes. The latter are synthesized within specialized cells in the liver and pancreas, extruded and then delivered into the lumen of the intestine where they exert their catalytic action. After catalyzing necessary reactions, some of the enzymes from the pancreas may be partially reabsorbed and carried in the blood to the pancreas to be used again. The endoenzymes are localized in the lipoprotein membranes of the mucosal cells and attach their substrates as they enter the cell. Thus these cells have both a digestive and absorptive function. A discussion of the digestive enzymes is best considered in terms of the nutrient being digested and absorbed.

Carbohydrate Digestion and Absorption. In the mouth, the enzyme *salivary amylase (ptyalin),* which is neutral or slightly alkaline, starts the digestive action on starch, hydrolyz-

ing it to dextrins (or isomaltose) and maltose. Approximately 1500 ml. (3 pints) of saliva is secreted daily. The activity of amylase continues in the stomach until the hydrochloric acid destroys it. If the digestible carbohydrates remained in the stomach long enough, the acid hydrolysis could reduce much of it to the monosaccharide stage. However, the stomach usually empties itself before this can take place, and carbohydrate digestion takes place almost entirely in the small intestine, with the greatest activity in the duodenum. *Amylase* from the pancreas breaks the starches into dextrins and maltose, and maltase from the intestinal juice changes maltose to glucose. (See Fig. 6–5.) This breakdown occurs on the surfaces of the epithelial cells lining the intestines, the so-called *brush border* composed of microvilli. These outer cell membranes contain the endoenzymes *sucrase, lactase, maltase* and *isomaltase* (or *α-dextrinase*), which act on sucrose, lactose, maltose, and isomaltose respectively.

The resulting monosaccharides—glucose, galactose and fructose—pass through the

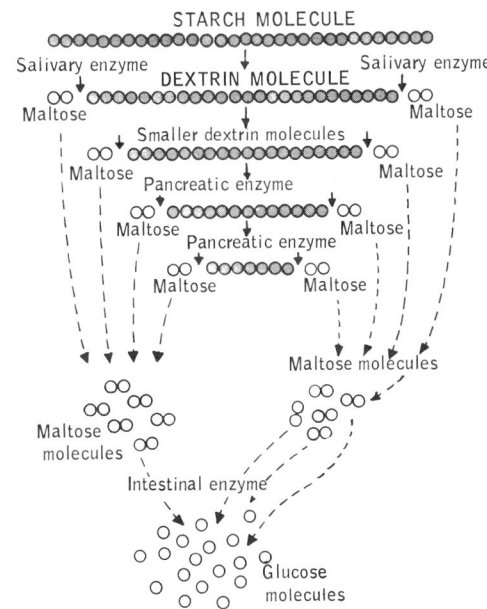

Figure 6–5 Breakdown of starch molecule to glucose. Gradual breaking down of large starch molecules by enzymes in digestion. The disaccharide maltose is split off by enzymes in the saliva and pancreatic juice, with smaller and smaller dextrin molecules formed as intermediate products, until the starch has been completely reduced to maltose. An intestinal enzyme then acts on the maltose molecules, splitting them into molecules of the monosaccharide, or simple sugar, glucose. (From: Bogert, L. J., et al.: Nutrition and Physical Fitness, 9th ed. Philadelphia, W. B. Saunders Co., 1973.)

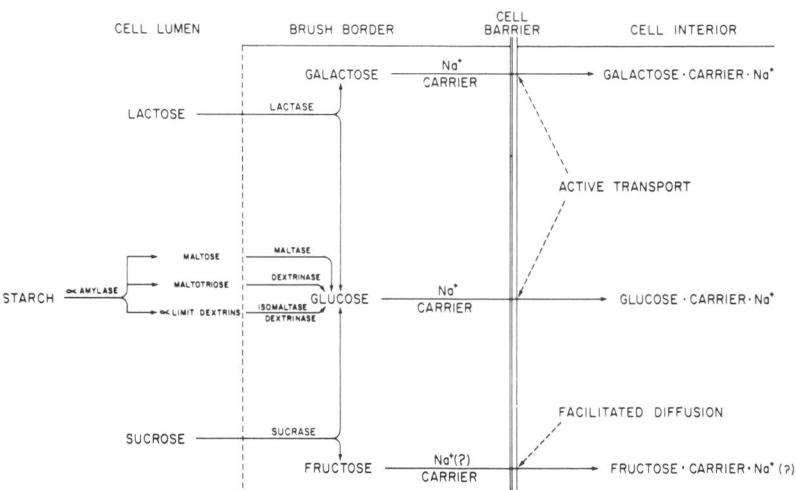

Figure 6–6 Digestion and absorption of carbohydrates. Sodium and either glucose or galactose combine with carrier. The sugar–carrier–sodium ion complex is transported across the cell membrane into the interior of the cell. Once inside the cell, the glucose diffuses passively across the serosal membrane, and the sodium is actively pumped back out of the cell. The driving force for glucose transport against a concentration gradient is the gradient of sodium ion across the membrane that contains the glucose carrier. (Modified from: Greene, H. L.: Developmental Nutrition: Carbohydrate Absorption. No. 12. Ross Laboratories, 1976.)

mucosal cell and are actively absorbed into the blood stream and delivered via the portal vein to the liver. In passing through the mucosal cell to the blood stream, specific carriers are used. (See Fig. 6–6.) In the case of glucose and galactose, there is one carrier system that is dependent upon the presence of sodium. Because it is the same active transport mechanism, glucose and galactose compete for absorption. Fructose is absorbed by a not fully understood facilitated diffusion mechanism that is less than half as rapid as the active absorption. Other sugars, such as mannose, xylose and arabinose, are absorbed even more slowly. (See Table 6–2.)

From the mucosal cell the glucose and galactose travel to the liver, and from the liver, glucose is transported to the tissues, although some glucose is stored in the liver and muscles

as glycogen until needed. A small amount of fructose may be converted to glucose before it passes from the intestinal cell into the blood stream, but most is transported as fructose to the liver where, like galactose, it is converted to glucose.

Glucose is the principle carbohydrate used by the body and is the sugar normally found in the blood. Within 1/2 to 1 hour after a meal, the blood glucose reaches its highest level of 130 mg. per 100 ml. Fructose and galactose are only found in the systemic circulation after very large ingestion of these sugars by normal people and in persons with liver damage. Lactose can be found in the blood of some normal lactating women, and fructose is commonly seen in seminal fluid. In some gastrointestinal disease conditions, disaccharides can be found in the urine, showing that they were absorbed from the GI tract. It is not understood how this happens.

Some forms of carbohydrate cannot be digested by man. Cellulose, hemicellulose, and lignin are excreted in the feces unchanged. Neither salivary amylase or pancreatic amylase has the ability to split the cellulose bond. The termite, cow and other lower animals, however, can digest cellulose with ease.

Fat Digestion and Absorption. Fat digestion starts in the stomach with the action of gastric lipase (tributyrinase), but it is only able to break naturally occurring short chain tri-

Table 6–2 RELATIVE RATES OF TRANSPORT OF SUGARS COMPARED TO GLUCOSE

galactose	1.1
glucose	1.0
fructose	.4
mannose	.2
xylose	.15
arabinose	.1

From Guyton, A. C.: Textbook of Medical Physiology, 5th ed. Philadelphia, W. B. Saunders Company, 1976, p. 889.

glycerides (found in butter) into fatty acids and glycerol. It is unable to attack the larger molecules of unemulsified fat; therefore, its digestive activity is minimal. The presence of fat in the diet causes food to be retained in the stomach for an extended period. As mentioned, fat eaten with a meal enters the small intestine and stimulates the release of enterogastrone, which inhibits gastric secretion and motility. Food may remain in the stomach as much as four hours or longer before being discharged to the small intestines, which gives a prolonged feeling of satiety. In the small intestine bile acts on the larger fat molecules to break them into smaller fat particles (emulsification).

Bile is a secretion of the liver composed of bile acids (glycocholic and taurocholic acids), bile pigments (which color the feces), inorganic salts, some protein, cholesterol, lecithin and many compounds metabolized and secreted by the liver, such as detoxified drugs. There are no enzymes in bile. From its storage place in the gallbladder, about 2 pints (1 liter) daily are secreted when it is called into the duodenum by the stimulus of food in the duodenum and stomach.

The emulsification by bile acids makes the fat globules more accessible to digestion by pancreatic and, to a lesser extent by enteric lipase, which usually splits off two of the three fatty acids from triglycerides. These resulting free fatty acids and monoglycerides along with bile salts form complexes called *micelles* which attach themselves to the surface of the microvilli, and the lipid part of the complex enters the cell presumably by simple diffusion. The bile salts are then released from their lipid components and re-enter the lumen of the gut. Most of the bile salts are actively reabsorbed in the terminal ileum and are recycled back to the liver to enter the gut via the liver and gallbladder. This efficient recycling is known as the *enterohepatic* circulation of bile acids. The pool of bile acids may circulate anywhere from 3 to 15 times per day, depending on the amount of food ingested.

The fatty acids and monoglycerides, now in the mucosal cell, are further digested into free fatty acids and glycerol. They are then reassembled to form triglycerides, which along with cholesterol and phospholipids are surrounded by a protein coat, betalipoprotein, forming *chylomicrons*. (See Fig. 6–7.) The chylomicrons pass into the lacteals of the villi and are transported by the lymph vessels to the thoracic duct, which empties at the junction of the left internal jugular and left subclavian veins. (See Fig. 6–8.) The triglycerides in the form of chylomicrons enter the blood stream and are carried to the liver and adipose tissue for metabolism and storage. Cholesterol is absorbed in a similar manner after being hydrolyzed from the ester form by pancreatic cholesterol esterase. The fat-soluble vitamins A, D, E, and K are also absorbed in a micellar fashion, although vitamin A and carotene can be absorbed without the presence of bile acids.

Under normal conditions about 60 to 70 per cent of ingested fat is absorbed via lymph vessels. The remaining medium and short chain fatty acids follow a different path of digestion and absorption. Because of shorter length and thus increased solubility, fatty acids of 10 carbons or less can be absorbed directly into the mucosal cell without the presence of bile and micelle formation. After entering the mucosal cell, they go directly (without esterification) into the portal vein by which they are carried to the liver. (See Table 6–3.)

The finding that shorter chain fatty acids (10 carbons or less) are absorbed quite differently than long chain fatty acids is of clinical usefulness. There are individuals who cannot efficiently absorb the usual types of dietary fat (long chain triglycerides) because they lack necessary bile salts for micellar formation or the means for transporting triglycerides out of the intestinal epithelial cells into the lymphatics (abetalipoproteinemia). In these cases *medium chain triglycerides*, C_8 and C_{10}, which bypass micellar formation and chylomicron formation, are used for the fat in the diet.

Increased motility, intestinal mucosa changes, and the absence of bile decrease absorption of fat, and undigested fat will appear in the feces—a condition known as *steatorrhea*. In the healthy adult only about 5 grams of fat should remain in the feces.

Protein Digestion and Absorption. Protein must be broken down into its constituents, the amino acids, to leave the cells in the lining of the intestine and pass through the capillary wall into the intracellular spaces and through the cell membrane into the cell. This involves breaking the peptide linkages that join the amino acids. Protein digestion begins in the stomach where the acid medium changes the pre-enzyme *pepsinogen* to *pepsin*, which hydrolyzes the protein into simpler molecules—polypeptides, proteoses and peptones. Unlike any of the other proteolytic enzymes, pepsin is able to digest collagen, the connective tissue of meat. However, in the total process of protein

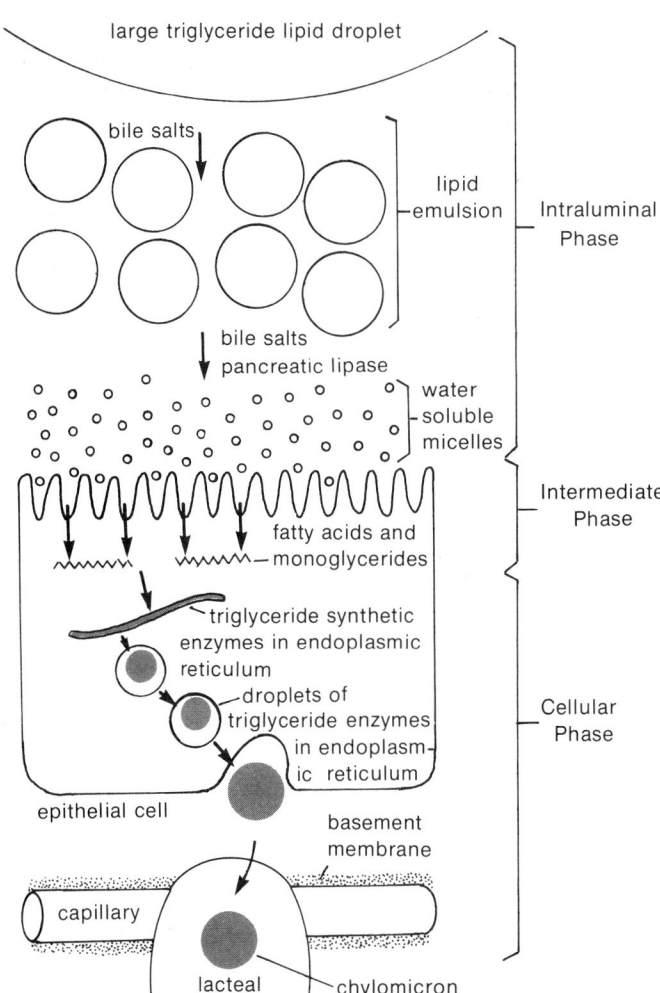

Figure 6–7 Summary of fat absorption across the walls of the small intestine. (Adapted from: Vander, A. J., Sherman, J. H., and Luciano, D. S.: Human Physiology: The Mechanisms of Body Function, 2nd ed. Copyright © 1975 by McGraw-Hill, Inc. Used by permission of McGraw-Hill Book Company.)

digestion the contribution of the stomach is small.

From the stomach, the partially digested protein moves into the duodenum. When the chyme reaches the intestinal mucosa, it causes the mucosa to release *enterokinase*, an enzyme that transforms inactive pancreatic *trypsinogen* into active trypsin. Trypsin in turn activates the other pancreatic proteolytic enzymes. Pancreatic *trypsin*, *chymotrypsin* and *carboxypolypeptidase* break down intact protein and continue the breakdown started in the stomach until simple peptides and amino acids are formed. *Proteolytic peptidases* thought to be located on the brush border also act on polypeptides and dipeptides, changing them to amino acids, which are absorbed. (See Table 6–4.) Possibly there is another distinct mechanism that involves the transport of some peptides across the membrane. Whole proteins may also be absorbed, presumably by pinocytosis. Fortunately this is very active in the newborn infant and accounts for the fact that the newborn breast-fed infant can absorb the protein antibodies in human colostrum and thus gain some of the immunity of the mother.

There are specific mechanisms for amino acid transport, and many of them are sodium dependent. Via these active transport systems, these amino acids are actively absorbed from the lumen of the small intestine into the mucosal cells, enter the blood stream and are then sent to the liver via the portal vein. There they are released into general circulation and carried to the various tissues and cells or built into new protein, as demanded by the body. Some amino acids may remain in the epithelial cell to be used in the synthesis of intestinal enzymes and new cells. Almost all of the protein has been absorbed by the time it reaches the end of the

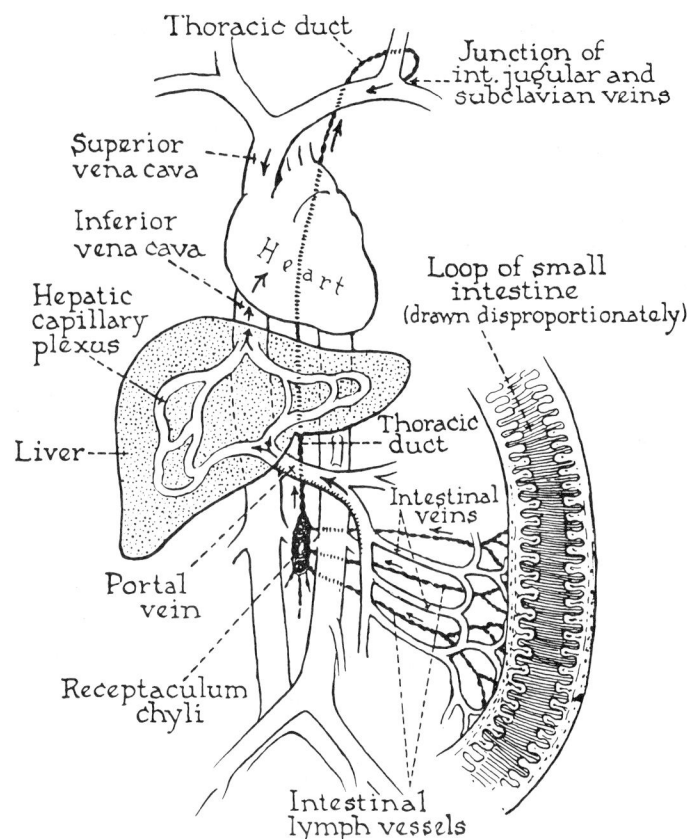

Figure 6–8 Routes by which the absorbed foods reach the blood of the general circulation. Intestinal veins converge to form, in part, the portal vein, which enters the liver and by repeated branchings assists in the formation of the hepatic capillary plexus; the hepatic veins carry blood from the liver and discharge it into the inferior vena cava; the intestinal lymph vessels converge to discharge their contents, chyle, into the receptaculum chyli, the lower expanded part of the thoracic duct; the thoracic duct discharges lymph and chyle into the blood at the junction of the internal jugular and subclavian veins. (Modified scheme after Bachman.)

Table 6–3   THREE PHASES OF FAT DIGESTION AND ABSORPTION (LONG CHAIN TRIGLYCERIDES, CHOLESTEROL AND PHOSPHOLIPIDS)

1. Intraluminal:	Emulsification—formation of smaller fat droplets to increase surface area of fat. Action of bile acids helps.
	Lipolysis—hydrolysis of triglycerides to glycerol, fatty acids and monoglycerides by lipases.
	*Micelle formation—grouping of fatty acids, monoglycerides, phospholipids, cholesterol and bile acids into lipid soluble molecules.
2. Intermediate:	Mucosal Uptake—release of fatty acids, monoglycerides and/or phospholipids and cholesterol into mucosal cells and return of bile acids to lumen.
3. Cellular:	*Esterification—resynthesis of triglycerides from glycerol and fatty acids.
	*Chylomicron formation—coating of cholesterol, triglyceride and phospholipid with single protein coat so that it is water soluble.
	*Lymphatic delivery—release of chylomicrons into lacteal of villus with subsequent travel through lymphatic system to be emptied into blood stream via left internal jugular or left subclavian vein for transport to liver.

*Denotes steps unnecessary in the digestion of medium and short chain triglycerides. Their transport is via the portal system, not the lymphatic system.

Table 6–4 SUMMARY OF ENZYMATIC DIGESTION AND ABSORPTION

SECRETION AND SOURCE OF SECRETION	ENZYME	SUBSTRATE	ACTION AND PRODUCTS OF ACTION	ABSORPTION
Saliva from salivary glands in mouth	Ptyalin (salivary amylase)	Starch	Hydrolysis to form disaccharides (dextrins and maltose) and branched oligosaccharides	
Gastric juice from gastric glands in stomach mucosa	Rennin	Casein (milk protein)	Curdles casein to prepare it for pepsin action (? presence in human infant)	
	Pepsin	Protein (presence of HCl)	Hydrolysis of peptide bonds to form polypeptides and amino acids	
	Lipase (tributyrinase)	Fat (tributyrin)	Hydrolysis to form free fatty acids	
Exocrine secretion from pancreas	Trypsin (activated trypsinogen)	Protein and polypeptides	Hydrolysis of interior peptide bonds to form polypeptides	
	Chymotrypsin (activated chymotrypsinogen)	Proteins and peptides	Hydrolysis of interior peptide bonds to form polypeptides	Pinocytosis of small peptides
	Carboxypolypeptidase	Polypeptides	Hydrolysis of terminal peptide bonds (carboxyl end) to form amino acids	Amino acids absorbed into blood
	Ribonuclease	Ribonucleic Acids-	Hydrolysis to form mononucleotides	
	Deoxyribonuclease	Deoxyribonucleic acids		
	Elastase	Fibrous protein	Hydrolyis to form peptides and amino acids	
	Lipase	Fat (presence of bile salts)	Hydrolysis to form simple glycerides, fatty acids and glycerol	
	Cholesterol esterase	Cholesterol	Hydrolysis to form esters of cholesterol and fatty acids	Micelles → mucosal cells → chylomicrons → lymph
	α-Amylase	Starch and dextrins	Hydrolysis to form dextrins and maltose	
Small intestine enzymes, most of which located in the "brush border"	Carboxypeptidase Aminopeptidase Dipeptidase	Polypeptides	Hydrolysis of peptide bonds to form amino acids	Amino acids absorbed into blood
	Nucleosidase	Nucleotides	Hydrolysis to form nucleosides and H_3PO_4	
	Nucleosidase	Nucleosides	Hydrolysis to form purines, pyrimidines and pentose	
	Enterokinase	Trypsinogen	Activates to trypsin	
	Lipase (enteric)	Monoglycerides	Hydrolysis to fatty acids and glycerol	Micelles → mucosal cell → chylomicrons → lymph
	Sucrase	Sucrose	Hydrolysis to glucose and fructose	glucose, galactose and fructose absorbed into blood
	α-dextrinase (isomaltase)	Dextrin (isomaltose)	Hydrolysis to glucose	
	Maltase	Maltose		
	Lactase	Lactose	Hydrolysis to glucose and galactose	

There are no digestive enzymes in the large intestine. Digestion and absorption are completed by the time the colon is reached. Only water, salt, vitamins and minerals are absorbed thereafter.

jejunum, and only 1 per cent of ingested protein will be found in the feces. Throughout the intestinal length not only is ingested protein absorbed, but also most of the endogenous protein from intestinal secretions and desquamated epithelial cells.

Most amino acids, especially alanine, stimulate the release of insulin, particularly in the presence of an elevated blood glucose concentration.

Other Nutrients. The vitamins, minerals and fluids are being absorbed simultaneously through the intestinal mucosa. Each day about 8 liters of fluid from the body pass back and forth across the membrane of the gut to keep the nutrients in solution. See Figure 6–9 for sites and routes of absorption of nutrients. Absorption of individual vitamins and minerals will be discussed in Chapters 7 and 8.

Factors Affecting Digestion

The term *digestibility* has several meanings. Atwater used the term to mean the proportion of food material actually digested. The most common interpretation, especially by laymen, is to refer to the rapidity rather than to the completeness of digestion. Who has not heard someone say, "I cannot digest that"? What he really means is that the food remains in the alimentary tract for a long period of time, yet in the end may be as completely digested and absorbed as food digested in much less time.

Atwater assembled results of many digestive experiments on men in which the apparent digestibility of a food was studied. It was found that over 90 per cent of the food in a mixed diet is utilized. The average coefficients of apparent digestibility (availability as Atwater used the term) for the nutrients in different food groups and for nutrients in a mixed diet are shown in Table 6–5.

Psychological Factors. Sight, smell and taste of food and even the thought of food increase secretions of saliva and the stomach juices and increase muscular activity of the gastrointestinal tract. The phrase "the sight of food makes my mouth water" applies to the psychic factor of digestion. Attractive food presentation in happy surroundings enhances digestion; unattractive food or unfamiliar tastes of food, served under emotional stress, retards digestion. Anger, fear, fright and worry have a depressing effect on the secretions and may delay digestion. Anger and fear produce an immediate effect in slowing down the process of digestion, and worry tends to produce a delayed effect. Emotions stimulate the

hypothalamus, which activates the autonomic nervous system to depress secretions, inhibit peristalsis and increase the tone of the sphincters. The propulsion of food through the gastrointestinal tract is slowed considerably. However, emotional stimuli may increase gastric secretion during the interdigestive period. The presence of this highly potent secretion when there is no food upon which to act is irritating to the intestinal mucosa and accounts for the play of emotional factors in the etiology of peptic ulcers. These are important points to remember when assisting individuals with dietary problems. The appearance of the food served, the combinations and the tastes of food along with the existing emotional stresses have an impact on the digestion of food.

Mechanical Factors. These are the physical changes brought about by the grinding, crushing and mixing of the food that occurs in the gastrointestinal tract. They facilitate the mixing of the food with the digestive juices and propel the mass through the digestive tract. Movements in the stomach are weak and shallow in the fundic wall and are strong and vigorous in the pyloric region. In the intestines the chyme is propelled caudally by waves of rhythmic contractions (peristalsis), mixed, and brought into contact with the intestinal mucosa containing layers of circular and longitudinal muscles which produce segmentation movements. Some of the reduction of food can be done before it enters the body. Foods prepared to have a fine consistency, such as mashed foods, purées and liquids, are frequently served patients who require easily swallowed and readily digested foods. Cellulose present in vegetables slows digestion and may increase putrefaction in the colon.

In general, properly cooked foods are more digestible than raw foods. Proper cooking of meat, for example, loosens the connective tissue, aids chewing and makes the meat more accessible to the digestive juices. Bolting of food has the result of introducing large chunks into the stomach, bypassing the benefit of mastication to break it down. It is an added tax on the digestive system. Small, frequent meals may be more easily tolerated than three large meals, an important factor to remember when feeding the sick.

Chemical Factors. These apply to the chemical reactions between food and the secretions of the digestive system. Fatty and improperly fried foods in which acrolein is produced will retard the flow of digestive juices, while meat extracts, for example, will stimulate digestion.

Some foods agree with many people and dis-

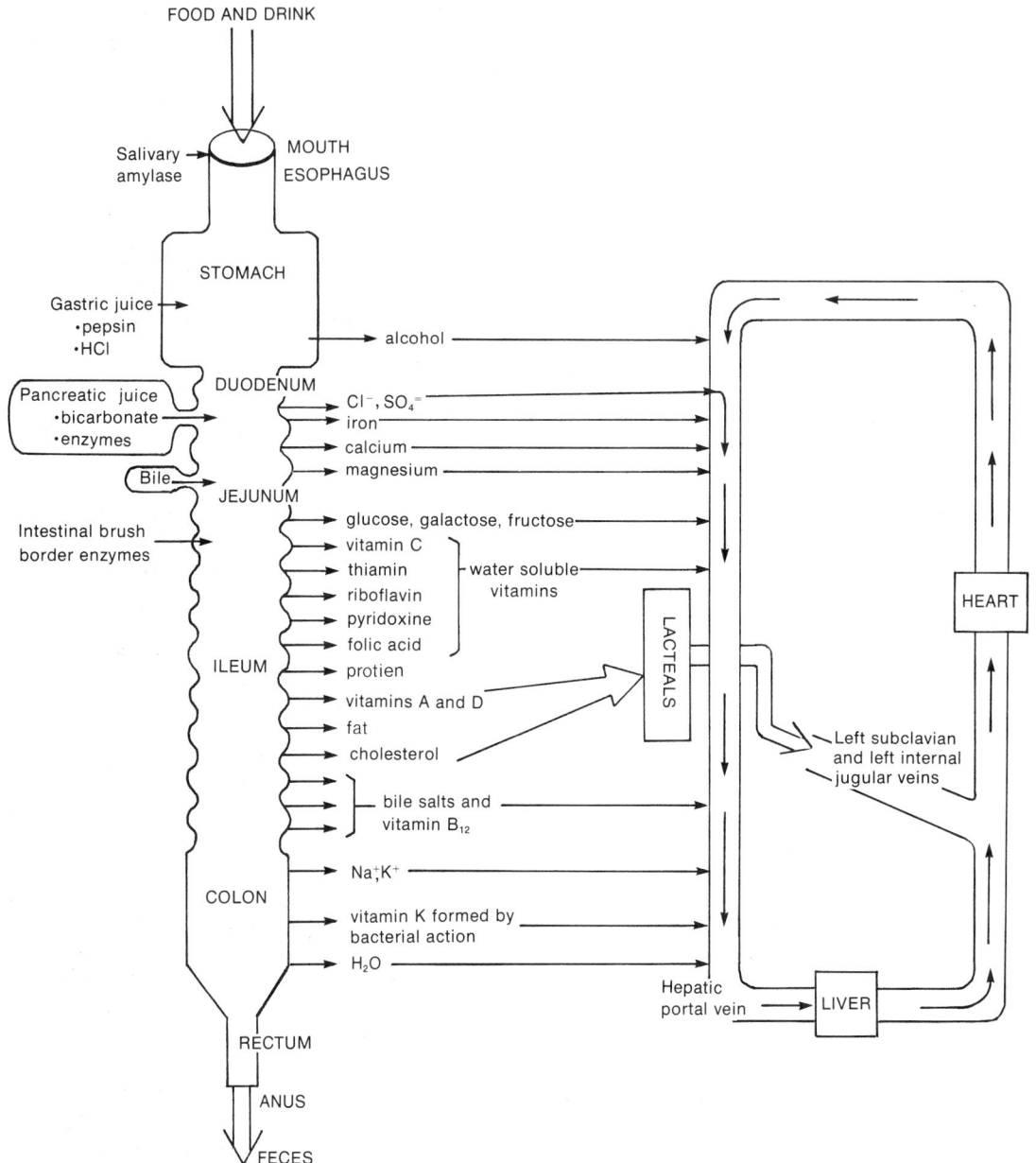

Figure 6–9 Sites of secretion and absorption in the gastrointestinal tract.

agree with others. Personal idiosyncrasy or an allergy may account for this. It has been suggested that there are people who are peculiarly sensitive to some chemical substances or to their physical states. For example, why do some people have distress from drinking orange juice? Although orange juice is considered a very easily digested food, there are those in good physical condition who claim it causes genuine distress, especially if ice cold and ingested when the stomach is empty.

There is evidence showing that digestive enzymes in the jejunum change in response to dietary substances. The change seems to take 2 to 5 days, the estimated turnover time of a human intestinal epithelial cell.[4] As these mechanisms of change become defined, some of the mystery surrounding individual intolerances of foods and indigestion will probably be dispelled.

Bacterial Action. The gut microflora make up a complex community in which about 100

Table 6–5   PER CENT DIGESTIBILITY OF
NUTRIENTS

FOOD GROUP	PROTEIN	FAT	CARBO-HYDRATE
	Per Cent	Per Cent	Per Cent
Animal Foods	97	95	98
Cereals	85	90	98
Legumes, dried	78	90	97
Sugars and starches			98
Vegetables	83	90	95
Fruits	85	90	90
Vegetable foods	84	90	97
Total food*	92	95	97

*Weighted by consumption statistics based on a survey of 185 dietaries.
From Merrill, A. L., and Watts, B. K.: Energy Value of Foods—Basis and Derivation. Washington, D.C., U.S. Department of Agriculture, Handbook No. 74, 1955.

species have been identified in the normal intestinal tract. At birth the gastrointestinal tract is essentially sterile, but implantation of various microorganisms soon takes place. *Lactobacillus* is the first organism to appear and is the chief component of the flora until the infant begins to eat solid foods. The *coli* become predominant in the distal ileum and the primary colonic flora appear to be *anaerobic,* with the *bacteroides* group most frequent. Lactobacilli are also present in the stools of most persons on an ordinary mixed diet.

Normally, there is very little bacterial action in the stomach, as the hydrochloric acid acts as a germicidal agent. However, in conditions in which there is decreased secretion of hydrochloric acid, resistance to bacterial action (both fermentative and putrefactive) is lowered. Occasionally gastritis, an inflammation of the gastric mucosa, may be due to bacterial inflammation.

Bacterial action is most intense in the large intestine with 10^{11} organisms per gm. feces, compared to 10^5 for the stomach, duodenum, jejunum and upper ileum and 10^8 per gm. for the distal ileum or transitional zone. Although dietary intake alters the fecal flora, the response varies markedly in degree from time to time and from individual to individual. Colonic bacteria contribute to the formation of (1) gases (hydrogen, carbon dioxide, oxygen, ammonia, methane), (2) acids (lactic, acetic, etc.), and (3) various toxic substances (indole, phenol, etc.). The ingestion of carbohydrate, in general, leads to increased fermentation in the large intestine; protein yields increased putrefaction. If large amounts of carbohydrate or protein reach the large intestine as a result of faulty absorption in the small intestine, bacterial action may give rise to the formation of excessive gas and also of certain toxic substances. Some of these toxic substances have been suspected in the etiology of colonic cancer. An example is cyclohexylamine, a potentially carcinogenic agent which is formed by intestinal bacterial action on cyclamate, a non-absorbed artificial sweetener. The colon also contains great numbers of bacteria which grow on the waste products and help generate compounds which account for the odor of the feces. The brown color of feces is caused by stercobilin and urobilin, derivatives of bilirubin.

Intestinal flora plays a much more important role in nutrition than was previously considered. Some of the intestinal organisms have the ability to synthesize a number of the vitamins of the B-complex (especially biotin and folic acid) and vitamin K. In addition, they contribute toward maintaining the intestines in a healthy condition. The organic acids produced help to check the growth of some of the less desirable bacteria. They also increase the solubility and therefore the absorption of calcium.

CELL METABOLISM

The absorbed nutrients including water and electrolytes are carried in the blood stream to the cells. The complex chemical changes for converting the nutrients in carbohydrate, fat and protein foods into energy (catabolism) and the synthesis of new molecules (anabolism) are continuous and proceed simultaneously. The metabolism of glucose, fats and amino acids is regulated and controlled by cellular enzymes, their coenzymes (many of which are the B vitamins), other co-factors (many of which are trace minerals) and hormones. The end products of glucose, fat and amino acids are the same, namely, carbon dioxide and water. In addition to carbon dioxide and water, the end products of amino acid metabolism are the nitrogenous wastes in the urine.

In earlier chapters the general metabolism of the carbohydrates, fats and proteins has been described. The present discussion will consider the nutrition of the individual cells, the intricate biochemical pathway by which the chemical energy of the foods is made available to the cells as needed, and the steps by which the three major nutrients enter this pathway. The same preliminary steps are needed

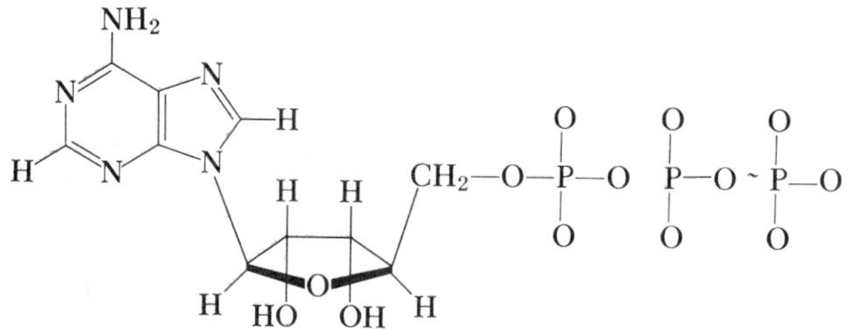

ATP
(adenosine triphosphate)

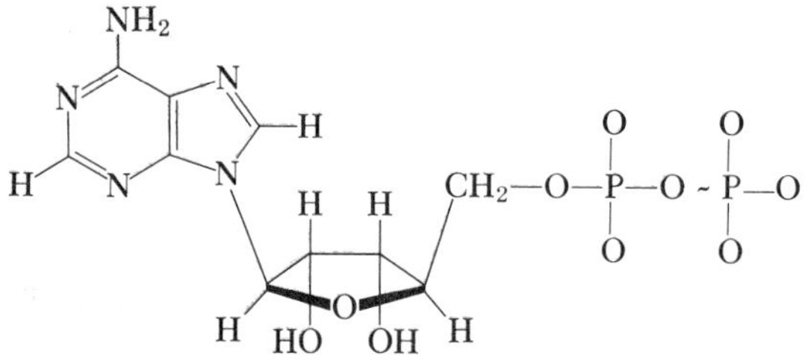

ADP
(adenosine diphosphate)

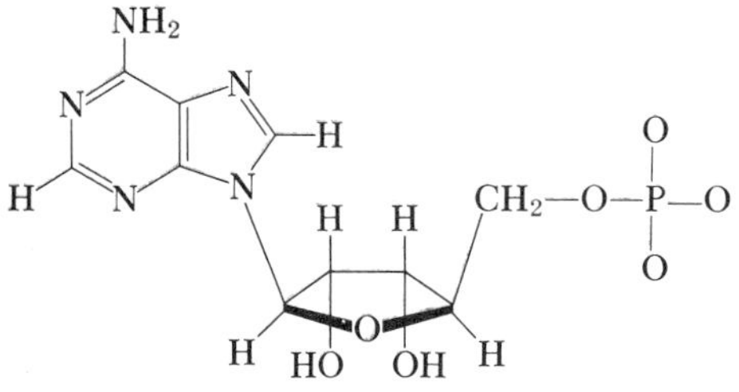

AMP
(adenosine monophosphate)

Figure 6–10 High-energy bonds of adenine nucleotides. (Adapted from: McGilvery, R. W.: Biochemistry: A Functional Approach. Philadelphia, W. B. Saunders Co., 1970.)

whether the nutrients are used immediately for energy or are transformed for other use or storage.

Adenine Nucleotides. The source of energy for the body is the oxidation of food. This energy must be in a utilizable form and for many processes, notably muscle contraction, it must be immediately available. The energy is trapped in certain organic phosphates and is released very rapidly when the compounds are hydrolyzed. The most important of these are the adenine nucleotides: tri-, di-, and monoadenosine phosphates, usually written ATP, ADP and AMP (Fig. 6–10). Hydrolysis of the terminal phosphate group of ATP or ADP releases a large amount of energy and the linkage is called a "high-energy phosphate bond" (~). When ATP is hydrolyzed, 12 kcalories are released per molecule. In the full oxidation of one molecule of glucose 38 high-energy phosphate bonds are formed, a total of 456 kcalories. Thus about 70 per cent of the total energy of the glucose (646 kcalories) is

made available for muscular work or other vital activity. This is very efficient transfer for any thermodynamic process.

A heavy demand for energy can outstrip the capacity of a muscle to regenerate ATP by complete oxidation of glucose or fatty acid. There are two mechanisms by which this need can be met. One is the use of another high-energy phosphate, *creatine phosphate*, to regenerate ATP. The other is by *glycolysis*, the conversion of glucose to lactic acid,* which will be discussed in the next section.

Glucose. The complete oxidation of glucose may be divided into two stages: anaerobic and aerobic. The first one, also called the *Embden-Meyerhof pathway*, takes place in the cell cytoplasm and converts one molecule of glucose into two molecules of pyruvic acid.

---

*It is convenient to use the term "lactic acid," but it must be remembered that at body pH the acids formed in metabolism do not exist as the free acid but as organic anions.

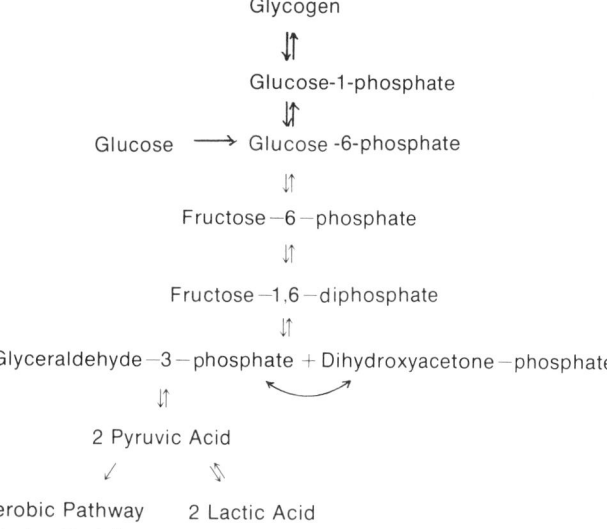

Glycogen

$\Updownarrow$

Glucose-1-phosphate

$\Updownarrow$

Glucose $\longrightarrow$ Glucose -6-phosphate

$\Updownarrow$

Fructose $-6-$ phosphate

$\Updownarrow$

Fructose $-1,6-$ diphosphate

$\Updownarrow$

Glyceraldehyde $-3-$ phosphate $+$ Dihydroxyacetone $-$ phosphate

$\Updownarrow$

2 Pyruvic Acid

Aerobic Pathway   2 Lactic Acid
(Krebs Cycle)

Figure 6–11 Simplification of Embden-Meyerhof anaerobic pathway.

This conversion requires 10 successive steps, each with its specific enzyme and its own requirements for cofactors. In the process 2 molecules of ATP are used and 4 are produced, a net gain of 2 molecules of ATP available for immediate use. Figure 6–11 gives an abbreviated outline of this pathway. There is no involvement of oxygen in the series of reactions. If there is heavy demand for muscular work and there is insufficient oxygen to continue with the aerobic pathway, the anaerobic reaction may go one step further with reduction of pyruvic acid to lactic acid (lactate). The lactic acid will diffuse out of the cells and its level in the blood stream will rise. This allows the concentration of pyruvic acid and H+ in the cell to remain low, and thus the anaerobic glycolysis can continue longer and provide energy to the cell. When O_2 is again present (as after completion of an exercise when "catching one's breath") the lactic acid can be converted to glucose in the liver and be used directly for energy or be converted into glycogen. This system in the muscle and liver whereby the following occurs—blood glucose → muscle glycogen → lactic acid → liver → glucose-6-phosphate → blood glucose—is called the *Cori cycle*. (See Fig. 6–12.) The steps indicated in the diagram can all occur in the reverse direction, but in a few steps the reverse reaction is catalyzed by a different enzyme.

Anaerobic glycolysis production of energy is inefficient, producing only two moles of ATP, compared to aerobic glycolysis with a production of eight moles of ATP. However, it is necessary and life-saving during muscular activity and periods of oxygen shortage. The heart muscle has the unique ability to utilize lactic acid and convert it to pyruvic acid, which is oxidized for energy production via the Krebs cycle.

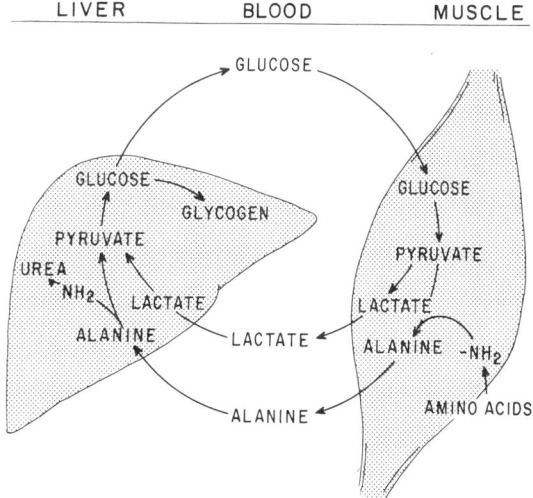

LIVER   BLOOD   MUSCLE

Figure 6–12 The relationship between the metabolism of muscle and liver during gluconeogenesis. Note the parallelism of the lactic acid (Cori) cycle and the alanine cycle. The latter represents the major pathway by which the amino groups from muscle amino acids are conveyed to the liver to conversion to urea. (From: Bondy, P. K., and Felig, P.: Disorders of carbohydrate metabolism. In: Bondy, P. K., and Rosenberg, L. E. (eds.): Duncan's Diseases of Metabolism, 7th ed. Philadelphia, W. B. Saunders Co., 1974.)

The second stage of carbohydrate metabolism, which cannot take place without the presence of molecular oxygen, is variously referred to as the *aerobic cycle, Krebs cycle* and the *tricarboxylic* or *citric acid cycle* (because of the formation of citric and several related 6-carbon acids). Pyruvic acid or pyruvate may be regarded as the starting point of the cycle, and it moves into the mitochondria for this oxidation. It was early recognized that the first step involved oxidative decarboxylation of pyruvic acid with formation of CO_2 and acetic acid. The acetic acid was in some active form; the nature of this acid form was elusive but was finally identified as a combination of acetic acid with a derivative of pantothenic acid. The coenzyme was called Coenzyme A and the active molecule *acetyl-CoA*. In another reaction, an adjunct to the Krebs cycle, pyruvic acid may combine with a molecule of CO_2 to form oxaloacetic acid. The significance of this reaction is that the body has the ability to assimilate CO_2 and synthesize the catalytic acid for the cycle—oxaloacetic acid. Figure 6–13 shows the cycle with oxaloacetic acid combining with acetyl-CoA to form citric acid (citrate). By a further series of steps, two atoms of carbon are oxidized to CO_2, and oxaloacetic acid is formed. The net result is the reformation of oxaloacetic acid, which can again combine with the activated acetyl unit (acetyl-CoA) and be metabolized through the cycle. The CO_2 is removed as a waste product.

Several steps in the cycle involve dehydrogenation. These steps cannot occur without simultaneous oxidation of hydrogen to water. This is brought about through what is called the *respiratory or electron transport chain*, a series of steps involving alternate oxidation and reduction of a sequence of coenzymes, culminating in the combination of hydrogen with molecular oxygen to form water.

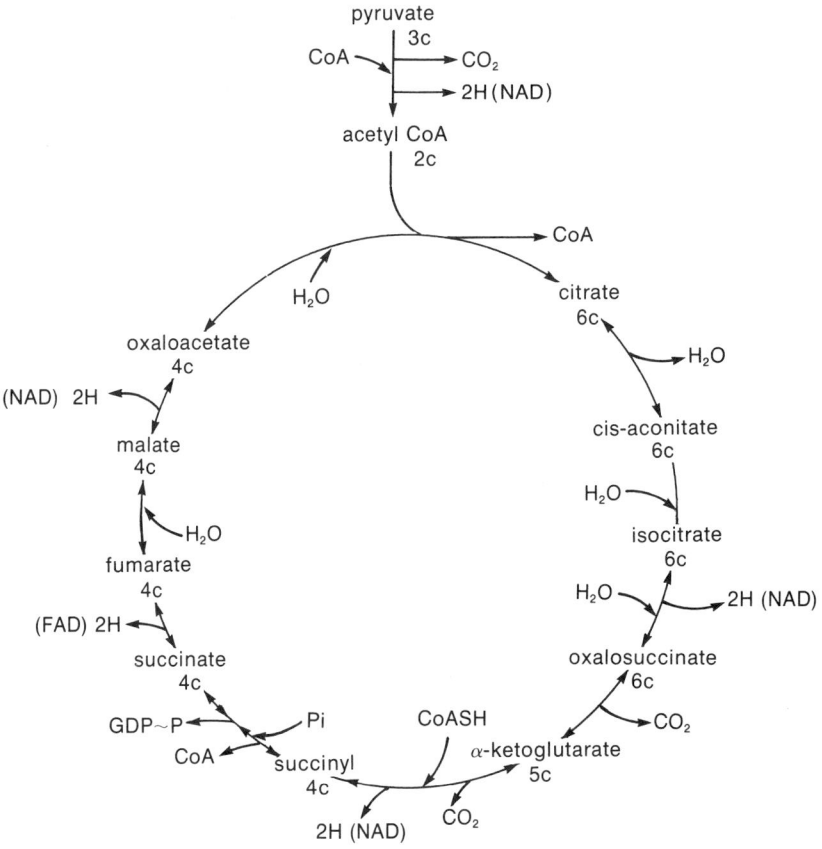

Net reaction per mole pyruvate: 1 Acetyl CoA + 3 H_2O + 1 Pi → 2 CO_2 + 8 H + 1 CoA + 1 GDP~P

Figure 6–13 The Krebs or citric acid cycle.

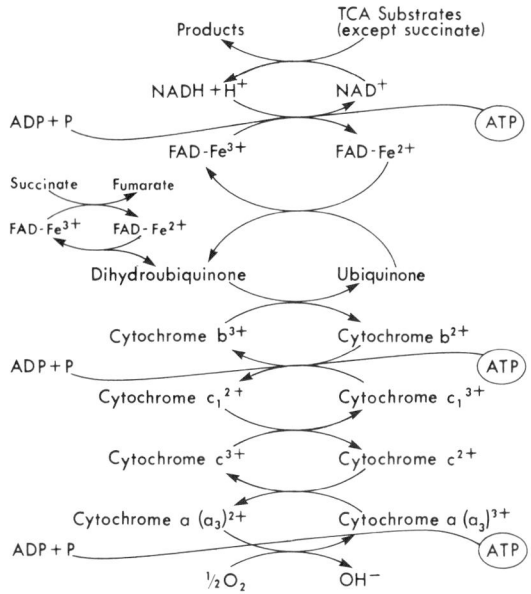

Figure 6–14 Electron transport and oxidative phosphorylation. (From: Pike, R. L., and Brown, M. L.: Nutrition: An Integrated Approach, 2nd ed. New York, John Wiley & Sons, 1975, p. 522.)

The whole process is called *oxidative phosphorylation*. If the hydrogen were combined with oxygen directly, much energy would be wasted as heat. Instead, the respiratory chain allows the capture of this energy by the formation of about 3 moles of ATP. See Figure 6–14 for the sites of the ATP formation in the transfer of electrons in the respiratory chain. Oxidation of hydrogen and phosphorylation are *coupled*. The two must occur together and ADP is essential for the operation of the respiratory chain. Recent studies of cell structure at the molecular level have shown that these enzyme systems are not randomly dispersed in the cell, but are arranged in an orderly fashion on the matrix and inside wall of the *mitochondrion* of the cell and carry out the reaction in production-line fashion. (See Fig. 2–3.) Because this is the site of ATP generation, the mitochondrion has been called the cellular "powerhouse." Other activities such as fatty acid and amino acid synthesis are carried out by the mitochondria, but the entrapment of energy is the most important.

An additional anaerobic pathway of glycolysis that is important to mention is the *pentose phosphate shunt* or *hexose monophosphate shunt*. This pathway is useful in at least three ways: (1) it does not require

ATP like the Embden-Meyerhof pathway; (2) it is one of the few reactions that produces reduced nicotinamide adenine dinucleotide phosphate (NADPH), a coenzyme involved in the transfer of hydrogens (or electrons) and which is required in some cellular reactions such as the synthesis of fatty acids; and (3) it provides a means for synthesis of ribose necessary for nucleic acids. This pathway is very active in mammary gland, testis, adipose, leukocyte, adrenal cortex, and liver tissue, but almost nonexistent in muscle tissue (striated muscle). (See Fig. 6–15 for an abbreviated diagram of the hexose monophosphate shunt.)

Sugars can be reduced to form alcohols such as sorbitol and myo-inositol or oxidized to form acids such as ascorbic acid (vitamin C). The reduction pathway or *polyol pathway* is important in galactosemia or diabetes mellitus, where the level of blood glucose or galactose is high. In these situations the reduction of these sugars in the cell is increased and there is a build-up of the alcohol sorbitol that is thought to account for many of the complications of diabetes, particularly cataracts.

It is of interest to note here some of the roles of the vitamins in tissue metabolism. All the vitamins of the B-complex are known to function as coenzymes in metabolic reactions. Thiamin pyrophosphate is the coenzyme for decarboxylation of α-ketoglutarate. Transamination requires vitamin B_6 coenzyme. Coenzyme-A is a derivative of pantothenic acid, and riboflavin and nicotinic acid are constituents of coenzymes of the respiratory chain. The role of vitamin E is less clear, but it also appears to be involved in electron transport in conjunction with the cytochromes.

Fats. The first step in utilization of fat in the body is hydrolysis to fatty acids and glycerol. This takes place largely in the adipose tissue by the enzyme *lipoprotein lipase*. This hormone-sensitive enzyme is located on the lumen surface of the capillary endothelial cell and is activated by insulin. Once activated, it hydrolyzes triglycerides and phospholipids into glycerol and fatty acids, which can diffuse into the fat cell. Glycerol diffuses back into the plasma since it can only be oxidized for energy in the liver and kidney cell. Fatty acids in the adipose tissue cells are resynthesized into triglycerides for storage, and the glycerol for this resynthesis comes from glucose, which also enters the adipose cell when insulin is present.

The activity of *lipoprotein lipase* varies with the state of the individual. In times of energy excess such as after a meal, the lipoprotein

lipase is active in adipose tissue when triglycerides are being taken out of the blood for storage. In energy-deficient situations such as fasting, the activity is high in muscle tissue when fatty acids need to be taken up for oxidation for energy.

Fatty acids are released from the adipose cells by the action of a *cellular lipase* in the adipose cell. They are carried in the blood bound to albumin as *free fatty acids* or *nones-terified fatty acids* (FFA or NEFA.) They travel to the liver, which can convert them to acetoacetic acid, β-hydroxybutyric acid, and acetone *(ketone bodies)*, which can be utilized by muscle tissue for energy. As early as 1905 Knoop proposed that fatty acids were metabolized by beta-oxidation (the beta carbon is the second from the carboxyl carbon). The chain was shortened by two carbons at a time, forming in each step acetic acid

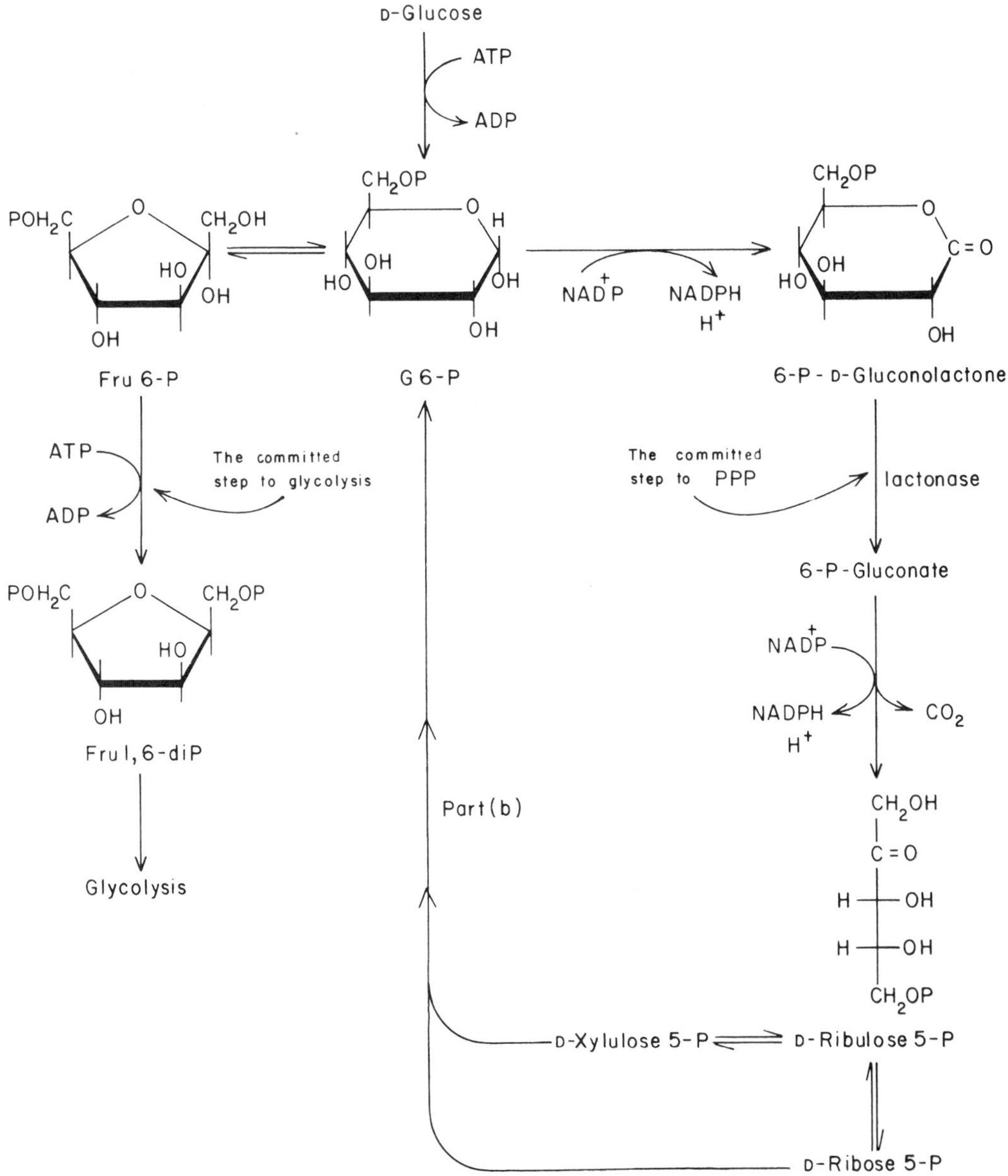

Figure 6–15 Pentose phosphate pathway or hexose monophosphate shunt. (From: Montgomery, R., et al.: Biochemistry: A Case-Oriented Approach. St. Louis, Mo., C. V. Mosby, 1974.)

R—CH$_2$—CH$_2$—CH$_2$—COOH

Fatty acid
(C$_n$)   (1)   ATP
                  CoASH

R—CH$_2$—CH$_2$—CH$_2$—C—SCoA
                         ‖
                         O
Fatty acid CoA ester

        (2)   —2H(FAD)

R—CH$_2$—CH=CH—C—SCoA
                    ‖
                    O
α-β-unsaturated acyl CoA

CH$_3$C—SCoA   (3)   H$_2$O
      ‖
      O
Acetyl CoA

C$_2$ C$_2$ C$_2$ C$_2$ C$_2$

R—CH$_2$—CHOH—CH$_2$—C—SCoA
                        ‖
                        O
β-hydroxyacyl CoA

        (4)   —2H(NAD)

R—CH$_2$—C—SCoA   (5)   R—CH$_2$—C—CH$_2$—C—SCoA
         ‖   ────   ‖   ‖
         O   CoASH   O   O
Fatty acid CoA ester   β-ketoacyl CoA
(C$_{n-2}$)

        +

CH$_3$C—SCoA   ⟶   Krebs Cycle
      ‖
      O
Acetyl CoA

Figure 6–16 Fatty acid oxidation. Enzymes are: (1) acyl CoA synthetase, (2) acyl CoA dehydrogenase, (3) enoyl CoA hydrase, (4) β-hydroxyacyl CoA dehydrogenase and (5) β-ketoacyl thiolase. (From: Pike, R. L., and Brown, M. L.: Nutrition: An Integrated Approach, 2nd ed. New York, John Wiley & Sons, 1975, p. 510.)

and a shorter fatty acid chain. This is still recognized as the major pathway of fatty acid oxidation. The mechanisms have been worked out as illustrated in Figure 6–16. The fatty acid forms an active complex with Coenzyme-A, this initial step being supplied with energy by ATP. As each acetyl-CoA molecule is formed it is oxidized via the citric acid cycle and energy results.

Amino Acids. It is impossible in a brief summary to show the catabolic pathways for all the amino acids. Important common steps may be illustrated. One of these steps is removal of the amino group. This occurs largely in the liver and usually involves oxidation with the formation of a *keto acid*. This may occur as oxidative *deamination* or, in many cases, as *transamination*, with exchange of an amino group and a keto group between two acids (Figure 6–17). The keto acids (particularly ketoglutaric and pyruvic acid) resulting from these reactions are members of the aerobic cycle (Krebs cycle). Either directly, as in these two cases, or after a longer series of preliminary reactions, the carbon skeleton of the amino acid can enter the citric acid cycle for complete oxidation. (See Fig. 6–13.)

TRANSAMINATION

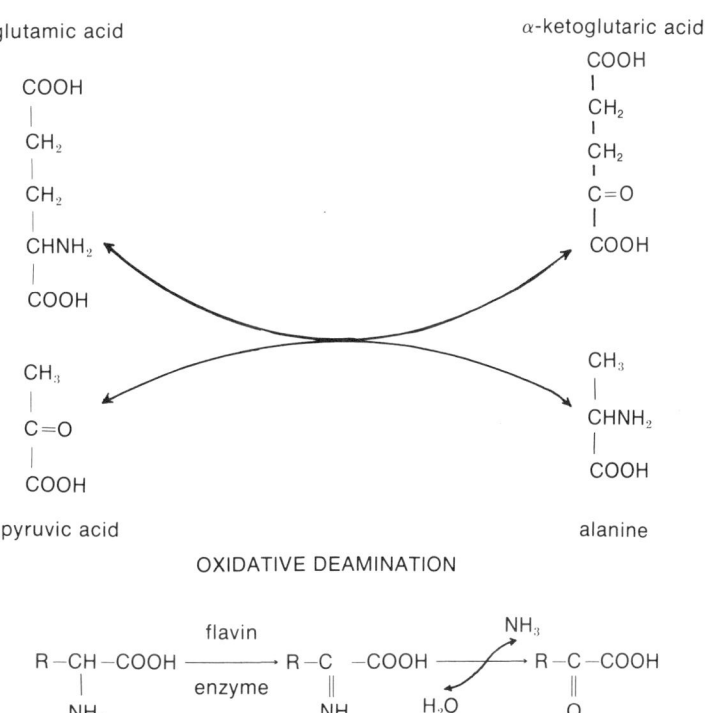

Figure 6–17 Transamination and deamination.

glutamic acid

COOH
|
CH$_2$
|
CH$_2$
|
CHNH$_2$
|
COOH

α-ketoglutaric acid

COOH
|
CH$_2$
|
CH$_2$
|
C=O
|
COOH

CH$_3$
|
C=O
|
COOH

pyruvic acid

CH$_3$
|
CHNH$_2$
|
COOH

alanine

OXIDATIVE DEAMINATION

                    flavin   NH$_3$
R—CH—COOH   ────────⟶   R—C —COOH   ──────⟶   R—C—COOH
      | enzyme   ‖   ‖
      NH$_2$ NH   H$_2$O   O

α-amino acid   α-amino acid   α-ketoacid

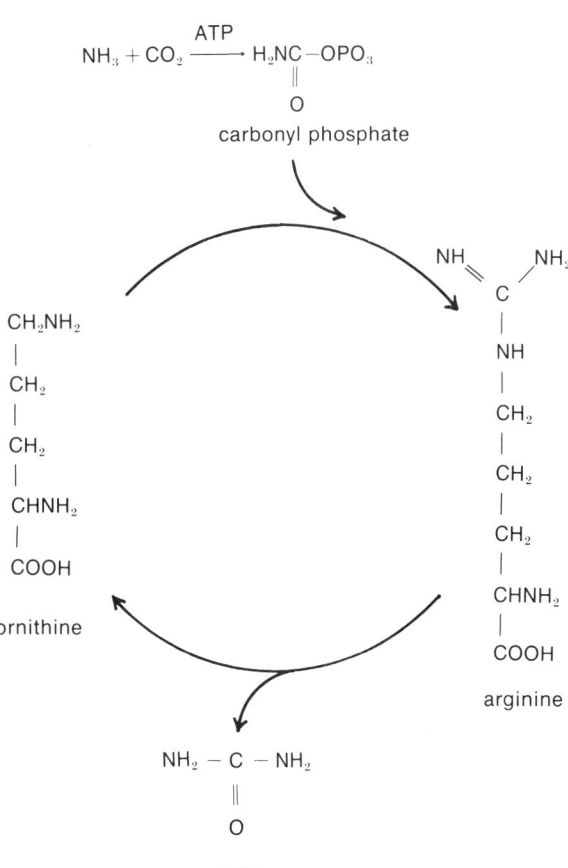

Figure 6–18 Urea formation.

Almost all amino acids are potentially glucogenic, but alanine is especially so. An alanine cycle has been identified, which, like the Cori cycle, is a glucose-yielding cycle between muscle and liver tissue. Pyruvate from glucose oxidation in muscle is transaminated to form alanine, which is transported to the liver where it is deaminated and the carbon skeleton is reconverted to glucose. This alanine cycle is significant as a source of glucose during periods of low exogenous glucose supply. It is also a way to move nitrogen from the muscle to the liver without the formation of ammonia.

The amino group of the amino acids is usually released as ammonia (chiefly as ammonium ion (NH_4^+ at body pH) and is used in synthetic processes or carried to the liver for conversion to urea, the form in which most of it is excreted. *Ammonia* is very toxic and so it is transported, in combination with glutamic acid, as glutamine. Most tissues are rich in the enzyme which catalyzes synthesis of glutamine. The liver and kidney, where ammonia will be used, have a large amount of the enzyme which catalyzes the hydrolysis of glutamine.

Synthesis of urea occurs through a process sometimes referred to as the *ornithine cycle* which is presented in condensed form in Figure 6–18. Carbon dioxide and NH_3 (with energy from ATP) combine with ornithine through a series of steps to form arginine. The arginine is hydrolyzed to yield urea and ornithine. Thus an ornithine molecule is used over and over in the formation of arginine and urea.

Common Metabolic Pathway.   Figure 6–19 is an integration of the metabolic pathways which have been described. It shows how carbohydrate, fat and protein may be utilized for energy by a common pathway; how carbohydrate may be converted to fat for storage or to cholesterol via acetyl-CoA; how some amino acids may be converted to glucose and some to fat and how some of the non-essential amino acids are synthesized. It should be noted that the step from pyruvic acid to acetyl-CoA is not reversible, so fatty acids cannot be used for net gain of

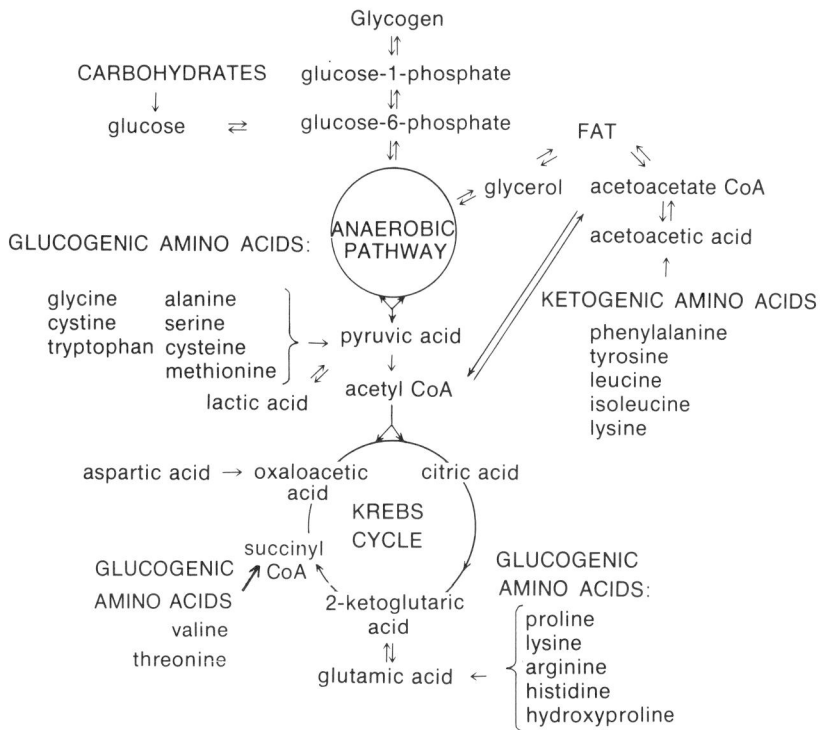

Figure 6–19 Metabolic integration of carbohydrate, fat and protein.

carbohydrate. It is by these interrelationships, and only a few of many have been shown, that the body can function smoothly under a variety of dietary and metabolic conditions.

Hormonal Control of Metabolism

In the presence of appropriate hormonal reaction, an enzyme in the plasma membrane, *adenyl cyclase,* forms *cyclic 3':5'-* AMP, cAMP from ATP. *cAMP* activates protein kinase which can then activate other necessary enzymes within the cell, resulting in a biochemical amplification. Cellular reactions are terminated by the conversion of cyclic AMP to 5'-AMP. Thus synthesis and catabolism of substances within the cell are controlled by enzymes activated by intracellular cAMP concentrations, and cAMP concentrations are controlled by adenyl cyclase, which is controlled hormonally. A second method for hormonal control of enzymatic activity is enzyme induction by direct effect of hormone on transcription of enzyme synthesis.

Adenyl cyclase in particular cells is only activated by certain hormones for which that cell has hormone-binding receptors. Receptors for both adrenalin and insulin have been identified on adipose cells. Lipolysis and glycogenolysis are two of the most important metabolic processes activated by this *hormone-cyclic AMP system.*

The processes of anabolism and catabolism are continuous and proceed simultaneously. Food intake in excess of body energy needs results in storage of glycogen and fat. When the food intake is inadequate to meet the energy needs of the body, body stores of glycogen and fat and, lastly, the tissue amino acids are oxidized. The composition of the body remains remarkably constant, but study with nutrients tagged with radioactive elements shows that there is constant exchange even in such tissues as bone or fat. Thus there is a state of dynamic equilibrium, constancy in the face of continuous change.

PROBLEMS AND SUGGESTED TOPICS FOR DISCUSSION

1. Describe what is meant by digestion; absorption. Describe the physical or mechanical factors of the alimentary canal; explain how they aid digestion and absorption.

2. Chart the digestive course of fruit juice, egg, toast, butter and milk.
3. What role does attractive food service play in digestion? Suggest some ways to make food service more attractive.
4. Describe the functions of the enzymes in digestion, mentioning the enzymes of the stomach, the small intestine and the pancreas; the material acted upon (substrate); and the products of the action.
5. Describe the function of bile.
6. Compare the rate of digestion and absorption of carbohydrate, protein and fat. Explain.
7. List all the factors that affect *your* food digestion in one day.

CITED REFERENCES

1. Grossman, M. I.: Candidate hormones of the gut, I. Introduction. Gastroenterology, *67*:730, 1974.
2. Ingelfinger, F. J.: Gastrointestinal absorption. Nutr. Today, *2*:2, 1967.
3. Rayford, P. L., Miller, T. A., and Thompson, J. C.: Secretin, cholecystokinin and newer gastrointestinal hormones. N. Engl. J. Med. Part 1, *294*(20):1093, 1976; Part 2, *294*(21):1157, 1976.
4. Rosenweig, N. S., and Herman, R. H.: Time response of jejunal sucrase and maltase activity to a high sucrose diet in normal man. Gastroenterology, *56*:500, 1969.

ADDITIONAL REFERENCES

Bogert, L. J., Briggs, G. M., and Calloway, D. H.: Nutrition and Physical Fitness. 9th ed. Philadelphia, W. B. Saunders Company, 1973.
Bondy, P. K., and Rosenberg, L. E.: Duncan's Diseases of Metabolism. 7th ed. Philadelphia, W. B. Saunders Company, 1974, Chapters 5, 6, 7, and 10.
Brown, J. C.: "Enterogastrone" and other new gut peptides. Med. Clin. N. Am., *58* (6):1374, 1974.
Davenport, H. W.: A Digest of Digestion. Chicago, Yearbook Medical Publishers, Inc., 1975.

Gangl, A., and Ockner, R. K.: Intestinal metabolism of lipids and lipoproteins. Gastroenterology, *68* (1):167, 1975.
Gorbach, S. L.: Intestinal microflora. Warren-Teed G. I. Tract, *5* (1):4, 1975.
Guyton, A. C.: Textbook of Medical Physiology. 5th ed. Philadelphia, W. B. Saunders Company, 1976, Part XI, pp. 850–901.
Latner, A. L.: Cantarow and Trumper Clinical Biochemistry. 7th ed. Philadelphia, W. B. Saunders Company, 1975.
Lehninger, A. L.: Biochemistry. 2nd ed. New York, Worth Publishers, Inc., 1975.
Levitt, M. D.: Intestinal Gas. Warren-Teed G. I. Tract, *4* (2):15, 1974.
Levitt, M. D., and Bond, J. H.: Volume, composition and source of intestinal gas. Gastroenterology, *59* (6):921, 1970.
Liebow, C.: Enteropancreatic circulation of digestive enzymes. Science, *189*:472, 1975.
Luckey, T. D.: Introduction: the villus in chemostat man. Am. J. Clin. Nutr., *27*:1266, 1974.
Mazur, A., and Harrow, B.: Textbook of Biochemistry. 10th ed. Philadelphia, W. B. Saunders Company, 1971.
McGilvery, R. W.: Biochemistry—A Functional Approach. Philadelphia, W. B. Saunders Company, 1970.
Montgomery, R., Dryer, R. L., Conway, T. W., and Spector, A. A.: Biochemistry—A Case Oriented Approach. St. Louis, C. V. Mosby Company, 1974.
Pike, R. L., and Brown, M. L.: Nutrition: An Integrated Approach. 2nd ed. New York, John Wiley & Sons, Inc., 1975.
Rosensweig, N. S.: Adaptive effects of dietary sugars on intestinal disaccharidase activity in man. In Sipple, H. L., and McNutt, K. W., (eds.): Sugars in Nutrition. New York, Nutrition Foundation, Inc., Academic Press, 1974.
Vander, A. J., Sherman, J. H., and Luciano, D. S.: Human Physiology: The Mechanisms of Body Function. 2nd ed. New York, McGraw-Hill Book Company, 1975, Chapter 12—Digestion and Absorption of Food.

Chapter 7

MINERALS

Revised by
DORICE M. CZAJKA-NARINS, Ph.D.*

Definition. By the term *"minerals"* we mean the elements in their simple inorganic form. In nutrition they are commonly referred to as *mineral elements* or, in the case of those present or required is small amounts, *trace elements* or *trace minerals*.

MINERAL COMPOSITION OF THE BODY

There are 21 mineral elements now known to be essential in nutrition. Analysis of mineral

*Associate Professor, Clinical Nutrition, Rush University.

ash shows the presence of more than 25. The minerals of the body are calcium, phosphorus, potassium, sulfur, sodium, chlorine, magnesium, iron, zinc, selenium, manganese, copper, iodine, molybdenum, cobalt, chromium, fluorine, vanadium, nickel, tin and silicon. There are also traces of barium, bromine, strontium, gold, silver, aluminum, bismuth, gallium, arsenic and others. Mineral elements exist in the body and in food in organic and inorganic combinations.

The human body contains relatively small amounts of individual minerals. Collectively, about 4 to 5 per cent of man's weight is in the form of minerals, compared with approximately 14 to 16 per cent protein and 12 to 20 per cent fat. For a man weighing 70 kg., there are approximately 2.8 kg. of minerals.

CLASSIFICATION

The minerals are found in the body and in food chiefly in their ionic form. Metals form positive ions (cations); non-metals form negative ions (anions). Sodium, potassium and calcium are cations. Non-metals forming anions include chlorine, sulfur (as sulfate) and phosphorus (as phosphate). Sodium chloride and calcium phosphate are typical salts. In bones and teeth the minerals are found as the fixed salts, primarily of calcium and phosphorus. In solution the salts dissociate and are found in body fluids as Na^+, K^+, Ca^{++}, Cl^- and $H_2PO_4^{--}$.

The minerals are also organic compounds such as phosphoproteins, phospholipids and hemoglobin. The hormone thyroxine contains four atoms of iodine. Phosphorus has been shown previously to occur in carbohydrates, fats and proteins; and sulfur has been shown to be an integral part of some amino acids and enzymes.

The essential minerals for nutrition are classified as *macronutrient elements* (>0.005 per cent body weight) and *micronutrient elements* (<0.005 per cent body weight). The minerals in these categories are listed in Table 7–1.

Table 7–1   MINERALS OF THE ADULT BODY

CLASSIFICATION	MINERAL	AMOUNT IN ADULT BODY (GRAMS)
Macronutrients essential at levels of 100 mg. or more per day for adult humans.	Calcium	1200
	Phosphorus	860
	Sulfur	300
	Potassium	180
	Chlorine	74
	Sodium	64
	Magnesium	25
Micronutrients essential at levels no higher than a few milligrams per day for adult humans.	Iron	4.5
	Fluorine	2.6
	Zinc	2
	Copper	0.1
	Iodine	0.025
	Chromium	0.006
	Cobalt	0.0015
Micronutrients essential, but amounts needed for humans can not be estimated at present.	Silicon	0.024
	Vanadium	0.018
	Tin	0.017
	Selenium	0.013
	Manganese	0.012
	Nickel	0.010
	Molybdenum	0.009
Minerals present in humans, function not known.	Strontium	T
	Bromine	R
	Gold	A
	Silver	C
	Aluminum	E
	Bismuth	
	Arsenic	
	Boron	

FUNCTION

Mineral elements have many essential roles, both in their ionic forms in solution in body fluids and as constituents of essential compounds. The balance of mineral ions in body fluids regulates the metabolism of many enzymes, maintains acid-base balance and osmotic pressure, facilitates membrane transfer of essential compounds, and maintains nerve and muscular irritability, and in some cases mineral ions are building constituents of body tissue. Indirectly many minerals are involved in the growth process. A few of the trace elements may be mere contaminants in the body.

Although the various minerals will be discussed individually, it must be remembered that their actions in the body occur in interrelated patterns and no one element can function, be deficient, or be overabundant in the body without affecting others.

REQUIREMENTS

The requirements for mineral elements vary greatly. Calcium, phosphorus, sulfur, potassium, chlorine, sodium and magnesium are required in amounts exceeding 100 mg./day. Iron, fluorine, zinc, copper, iodine, chromium and cobalt are required in amounts less than 20 mg./day.

The importance of many minerals has long been established and appreciated; however, the role of others is not clear, and since even the number of required minerals is not known, there is much need for additional work. Recent studies have established the essentiality of tin, silicon, nickel and vanadium in various species. These trace elements were earlier thought to be mere contaminants of the human body.

Of the minerals known to be needed by the human body, all must be supplied in the diet, particularly in high risk populations such as children under two years of age, and pregnant women, especially teenagers. The exact role of oral contraceptives in mineral metabolism has not been studied sufficiently to recommend that women using these drugs should take supplements; however, early work suggests that there are some effects on several micronutrients as well as on the metabolism of some vitamins.

The Food and Nutrition Board of the National Research Council has established recommended intakes of calcium, phosphorus, iodine, iron, magnesium and zinc. Specific allowances are not yet established for the other minerals because of the lack of sufficient information upon which to base the recommendation. With the increased realization of the importance of minerals in human nutrition, more and better information should provide a sound basis for making recommendations in the future. A varied or mixed diet of animal and vegetable products that meets energy and protein needs will also furnish adequate minerals. In those circumstances where oral intake is diminished or nil, such as during extended periods of total parenteral nutrition (see Chapter 35), there is great potential for mineral deficiency.

SOURCES

Most minerals are obtained from foods in which they exist as salts and organic compounds. The exception is sodium chloride (table salt), which is used as a condiment or a preservative. Highly processed foods and foods such as sugar contain few minerals. The mineral content of food is determined by first destroying the organic matter with heat and/or acid and analyzing the ash by flame photometry or atomic absorption spectroscopy.

MACRONUTRIENTS ESSENTIAL AT LEVELS OF 100 MG. OR MORE PER DAY FOR ADULT HUMANS

CALCIUM AND PHOSPHORUS

Calcium and phosphorus are frequently considered together because they are so closely related in the body. They are discussed here separately to emphasize their independent roles as well as their association in the way they function together in the body. The normal metabolism of calcium and phosphorus is maintained by a number of physiological mechanisms.

Calcium

The body needs calcium throughout life, but especially during periods of growth, pregnancy and lactation. Dietary intake is frequently low. According to the data obtained during the Ten-State Nutrition Survey, the median intake of people 60 years of age and over is approximately 400 mg. for females and approximately 500 mg. for males (RDA in both cases is 800 mg.).

Calcium is the most abundant mineral in the

body. It makes up about 1.5 to 2.0 per cent of the body weight and 39 per cent of the total minerals present; 99 per cent of it is in the hard tissues, bones and teeth. Thus an adult male has about 1200 grams of calcium and the adult female 1000 grams. The other 1 per cent is present in the blood, extracellular fluids and within the cells of soft tissues where it regulates many important metabolic functions.

In the bones, calcium occurs in the form of salts: *hydroxyapatite,* composed of calcium phosphate and calcium carbonate arranged in a characteristic crystal structure around a framework of softer protein material (organic matrix). The hydroxyapatite provides strength and rigidity to the soft matrix. Many other ions are also present in this crystal complex, including fluoride, hydroxyl, magnesium, zinc and sodium. Blood and lymph vessels, nerves and bone marrow pass through the matrix and between the crystal structures. The mineral ions diffuse into the extracellular fluid, bathing the crystals and permitting deposition of new mineral or its absorption from bones.

The same type of crystals are present in the enamel and dentin of teeth; however, the crystals are larger. There is little turnover of calcium in teeth, i.e., the calcium or phosphate is not readily available during periods of deprivation.

In the skeleton calcium exists in two chemically and physically distinct forms: a relatively *nonexchangeable* calcium component not available for short term regulation of calcium homeostasis and a rapidly *exchangeable* component used for metabolic activities. This calcium is part of the most recently deposited surface bone, which together with the calcium entering from the diet helps to maintain the serum levels within a defined range. The rapidly exchangeable component of the bone may be considered a reserve that may be built up when the dietary provides an adequate intake of calcium. This reserve is stored especially in the trabeculae, the ends of the long bones. It may be used to meet the body's increased need (growth, pregnancy, lactation) if calcium is not supplied in adequate amounts by the food intake. If there is no reserve, the calcium must be drawn from the more stable bone substance itself, which must be broken down before calcium is liberated. This results in a deficiency in the bone structure following prolonged inadequate intake. As it is with most components in the body, bone is constantly being synthesized and resorbed. Depending upon physiological state or age of the individual, one aspect of the process may predominate. In children, for example, bone synthesis is greater than the destruction of bone. In the normal adult these processes are in balance; approximately 600 to 700 mg. of calcium enter and leave the bones every day. In later adult life bone is lost as resorption predominates. Adult bone loss begins during the fifth decade in both sexes, but progresses more rapidly in the female (see osteomalacia and osteoporosis in Chapter 12—Nutritional Deficiency Diseases). Sixty per cent of serum calcium is ionized and physiologically active. Forty per cent is non-ionized and physiologically inert, thirty-five per cent bound to protein, and five per cent as the calcium salt of citrate, bicarbonate and phosphate. A significant increase in serum calcium can cause cardiac or respiratory failure. A decrease causes tetany.

Function. In addition to the major function of calcium to build and maintain bones and teeth, the remaining 1 per cent of the body's calcium is found in the body fluids and soft tissues. This calcium, present principally in ionic form has important metabolic functions. It is essential for the activity of certain enzymes, notably adenosine triphosphatase in the release of energy for muscular contraction and for the activity of cyclic AMP and monohydrogen phosphate as a "second messenger."

In the blood clotting process, calcium must be present to initiate the changes needed for the formation of the clot, fibrin. The ionized calcium stimulates the release of thromboplastin from the blood platelets, and it is also a necessary cofactor in the conversion of prothrombin to thrombin. Thrombin aids in the polymerization of fibrinogen to fibrin.

Calcium affects the transport function of cell membranes, possibly acting as a membrane stabilizer. Calcium also influences transmission of ions across membranes of cell organelles, the release of neurotransmitters at synaptic junctions, the synthesis, secretion and metabolic effects of protein hormones, and the release or activation of intracellular and extracellular enzymes. There are minute amounts of ionized calcium in the cytosol; it is found in the mitochondria and endoplasmic reticulum as a phosphate salt.

Calcium is required in nerve transmission and regulation of heart beat. The proper balance of calcium, sodium, potassium and magnesium ions maintains muscle tone and controls irritability.

Absorption and Utilization. Usually only 20

to 30 per cent of ingested calcium is absorbed and sometimes it is as low as 10 per cent. Calcium is absorbed in the duodenum in an acid medium, and its absorption ceases in the lower part of the intestinal tract when the food content becomes alkaline. Calcium is absorbed by active transport requiring energy and by passive diffusion. The amount absorbed depends largely upon the nature of the diet, for unless it is present in a water-soluble form in the intestine and is not precipitated by another dietary constituent, it will not be absorbed; unabsorbed calcium is excreted in the feces. Many factors influence the actual amount of calcium absorbed.

FACTORS WHICH INCREASE CALCIUM ABSORPTION. *Vitamin D.* Vitamin D in its active form $1,25-(OH)_2 D_3$ stimulates intestinal absorption of calcium through a complex series of steps including transfer of calcium across the mucosal brush border.

Acidity of Gastric Juices. The hydrochloric acid secreted in the stomach lowers the pH of the contents of the digestive tract in the small intestine and favors calcium absorption.

Lactose. In the presence of lactose, calcium absorption is improved. No definitive statement on the exact mode of action has been universally accepted. One hypothesis suggests that a relatively high ratio of lactose to calcium permits the formation of a sugar-calcium complex in the intestine that keeps the calcium in the form in which it can be transported to and across the intestinal mucosa.[1] It is also possible that the lactose-calcium complex prevents the precipitation of calcium in an insoluble complex as the contents of the intestinal tract change from acid to alkaline.

Fat. When fat is present in moderate amounts, transit time through the digestive tract increases, allowing more time for absorption.

Protein Intake. When the intake of protein is high, a greater percentage of calcium is absorbed than when the intake of protein is low. The action of certain amino acids upon intestinal pH and upon the formation of the soluble complex with calcium facilitates calcium absorption.

Physiological State. The body absorbs more effectively when in need. The greater the need and the smaller the dietary supply, the more efficient the absorption. During periods of growth, absorption is increased.

FACTORS WHICH DECREASE CALCIUM ABSORPTION. *Vitamin D Deficiency.* Lack of or insufficient amount of vitamin D in its active form $(1, 25-(OH)_2 D_3)$ decreases or prevents the absorption of calcium and thus it is not available to the body.

Fats. The excretion of large amounts of calcium in the feces of patients with steatorrhea suggested that diets high in fat might affect calcium absorption. Studies in humans and animals produced conflicting data. The effect may depend on the kind of fat in the diet.[28]

Oxalic Acid. The calcium availability from some fruits and vegetables depends upon the oxalic acid they contain. Oxalic acid combines in the digestive tract with calcium to form an insoluble compound, calcium oxalate. The calcium is not absorbed. Rhubarb, spinach, chard and beet greens contain oxalic acid in appreciable amounts.

Phytic Acid. Phytic acid, a phosphorus-containing compound found principally in the outer husks of cereal grains (especially oatmeal), combines with calcium to form calcium phytate which is insoluble and is not absorbed from the intestines.

Alkaline Medium. In an alkaline medium, calcium (and phosphorus) will form insoluble and non-absorbable calcium phosphate.

Gastrointestinal Motility. When the food passes through the intestinal tract too rapidly, calcium absorption is decreased.

Immobilization. Lack of exercise and lack of weight-bearing on the legs cause a decrease in the ability to absorb calcium.

Stress. Emotional instability may influence the efficiency of calcium absorption. Mental stress tends to decrease absorption and increase excretion of calcium. Under distress, emotional or physical, a higher intake of calcium is required to maintain calcium equilibrium. Whether increased calcium intake during time of stress will prevent losses has not been clearly shown.

Calcium-Phosphorus Ratio. The ratio of calcium to phosphorus in the diet has been stressed in the past. While excess phosphorus has an accelerating effect on resorption in animals, the importance in man has been overemphasized. In a recent study there was little effect of varying calcium and phosphorus intake on either calcium absorption or balance in adult subjects.[29]

Calcium is transported by the blood to the fluids bathing the tissues of the body and to the cells wherever needed. Most of the calcium is used in the bones. The calcium in the bone is in equilibrium with calcium in the blood. The parathyroid hormone, *parathormone,* and *cal-*

citonin, secreted chiefly by the thyroid gland, keep the serum calcium at a normal concentration of about 10 mg. per 100 ml. of blood serum. When it falls below this level, parathormone causes a transfer of exchangeable calcium from the bone into the blood. At the same time the parathyroid causes the kidney to reabsorb calcium which normally might be excreted in the urine and it stimulates more absorption of calcium from the intestines. When the blood calcium level is above normal, calcitonin acts to lower it by inhibiting further bone resorption, and since the processes of renal excretion and endogenous fecal secretion continue, the net effect is to lower serum calcium. Red blood cells are essentially calcium free.

Excretion. Normally most of the ingested calcium (65 to 75 per cent) is excreted in the feces and urine. Fecal calcium correlates with intake. Urinary calcium is relatively constant for a person over a wide range of intake, but varies among individuals. The amount of protein in the diet affects calcium metabolism. The urine of subjects taking 600 g. of protein contained eight times as much calcium as the urine of subjects on a protein-free diet.[16]

There are also some dermal losses: 1 to 2 per cent of tracer doses of which one-third was from body fluids and two-thirds from the skin itself. The loss of calcium in sweat is about 15 mg. per day. Strenuous physical activity will increase loss even in persons on low intake. In

cases of excessive urine excretion of calcium, calcium kidney stones may develop.

Dietary Sources. Calcium is assimilated better from some foods than from others. The calcium in milk is assimilated readily because of the lactose and vitamin D that are also present. Milk and milk products are the best sources of calcium. Dark green leafy vegetables such as kale, turnip greens, mustard greens and broccoli, and sardines, clams and oysters are good sources of calcium. It is difficult to meet the RDA for calcium without milk or milk products since 8 ounces of milk (whole or non-fat) daily would supply about 288 to 298 mg. of calcium. Along with foods from the bread-cereal, vegetable-fruit and meat groups in the amounts suggested (Table 10–4), approximately three-fourths of the recommended daily amounts of calcium would be provided for an adult.

Infants can easily meet the calcium intake because milk is their chief food. Children can best meet the requirement by including the amount of milk recommended for each age group (Table 10–4), or its equivalent, daily. Table 7–2 shows the calcium content of selected foods.

Recommended Dietary Allowance. Most of the data regarding calcium requirements for man have been obtained from calcium balance studies. (A controversy exists regarding the interpretation of the data and the use of the bal-

Table 7–2 CALCIUM AND PHOSPHORUS CONTENT OF FOODS

FOOD	AVERAGE SERVING		
	APPROXI-MATE MEASURE	MILLIGRAMS OF CALCIUM	MILLIGRAMS OF PHOS-PHORUS
Peanuts, roasted, with skins	⅔ cup	69	391
Turkey, roasted, flesh only	3 oz.	7	213
Fish (halibut, broiled with butter or margarine)	4.5 oz.	20	310
Pork loin, broiled, med. fat	2 oz.	7	181
Milk, nonfat (skim), fluid	1 glass (8 oz.)	296	233
Milk, whole, fluid	1 glass (8 oz.)	288	227
Chicken, roasted	3⅓ oz.	12	242
Loin lamb chop, broiled	3⅓ oz.	9	163
Beef, hamburger, cooked (reg. ground)	3 oz.	10	196
Oysters, raw	6 oysters	81	123
Cheese, cheddar	1 oz.	213	136
Peas, cooked	⅔ cup	25	105
Egg, poached	1 large	51	121
Wheat cereal, flakes	1 cup	12	83
Sweet corn, canned, vacuum packed	⅔ cup	4	102
Spinach, cooked	½ cup, packed	89	34
Bread, white, enriched	1 slice	21	24

From Agriculture Handbook Number 456. U.S. Dept. of Agriculture, Washington D.C., 1975.

ance studies as a basis for requirements.) These studies measure the intake and ouput of calcium over periods of time. To determine the minimum calcium requirement, the calcium intake is reduced until the person can no longer remain in balance (i.e., his excretion becomes greater than his intake). It is evident from these studies that man, if given time to adjust to changes in levels, can remain in calcium balance over a very wide range of calcium intakes. Man has been shown to adapt and maintain calcium balance on intakes as low as 200 to 400 mg./day. A higher proportion of calcium is utilized when intake is low.

The 1974 revision of Recommended Dietary Allowances of the National Research Council states that the normal adult male and female should receive 800 mg. of calcium daily. This amount covers basic needs and allows for a margin of safety. These allowances are greater than those recommended by the FAO/WHO Expert Group. This report concludes that intakes of 400 to 500 mg. per day would represent a suggested practical allowance for adults. The Committee felt that the usefulness of exceeding this has not been proven, and that this level can more readily be achieved by a larger segment of the world's population since sources of calcium are limited in the national food supply of many countries.

The Food and Nutrition Board, National Research Council justify the allowance of 800 mg. on the basis that calcium losses in metabolism amount to approximately 320 mg. per day. Since only 20–30 per cent of the dietary calcium is absorbed, 800 mg. would be required to maintain balance. Food sources of calcium are readily available to the population of the United States. Cognizance was also taken of the relatively high prevalence of osteoporosis in older persons and the possibility that minimal or moderate inadequacy in calcium intake over a period of years may contribute to the occurrence or accentuation of this disease. A preliminary recommendation has been made of 1000 mg. of calcium per day as an optimum for the prevention of osteoporosis.[15]

The need for calcium is increased during pregnancy and lactation. An increase in calcium is needed for the calcification of fetal bones and teeth and for the storage of calcium by the mother to meet the demands of lactation. The National Research Council has recommended an additional 400 mg. of calcium daily to meet the demands of the fetus and mother. Indications are that the pregnant woman may

absorb up to 40 per cent of dietary calcium, depending on the need.

The amount needed by the lactating mother is 400 mg. daily over normal requirements in order to provide adequate calcium in milk without causing depletion of the mother's calcium reserve or decrease in milk production. Since some women with a high production of milk may lose nearly 1 g./day of calcium directly via milk, calcium intakes must be adjusted on the basis of individual milk secretion.

During these periods of increased dietary needs for calcium the growing fetus or nursing child will satisfy his need for calcium at the mother's expense. If her dietary intake is deficient, presumably the mother will lose bone calcium.

The calcium requirement of the infant is not precisely known. A breast-fed infant receives about 60 mg. of calcium per kilogram body weight and retains about two-thirds of this amount. An infant fed a standard cow's milk formula receives about three times this amount of calcium per kilogram body weight, and retains 25 to 30 per cent. The National Research Council states that the recommended calcium intakes are 360 mg. for infants from birth to 6 months of age and 540 mg. for 6 months to a year of age. It is assumed that the calcium needs of the breast-fed infant have been met even though calcium intake is considerably less than that obtained on a cow's milk diet.

Children from ages 1 to 10 years need 800 mg. of calcium daily. From 11 to 18 years of age the recommendation for males and females is 1200 mg. daily.

Obviously an adequate intake of calcium is not enough. The conditions influencing the absorption and metabolism of calcium must be considered as well as the physiological state of the individual.

Calcium Deficiencies. These aspects will be considered in more detail in Chapter 12. Suffice it to state here that calcium deficiency in children may lead to *rickets* with retarded growth or, more likely, continued body growth, but with abnormal development of bones resulting in bowed legs and other bone deformities. (See Figs. 12–16 to 12–18.) Deficiency of calcium in adults may result in *osteomalacia* (sometimes referred to as adult rickets), a failure to mineralize the bone matrix, resulting in a reduction in the mineral content of the bone. Usually, rickets and osteomalacia are associated with a concurrent lack of vitamin D and imbalance in the calcium-phosphorus in-

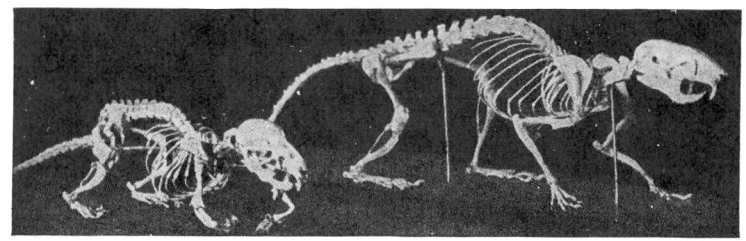

Figure 7–1 Skeletons of twin albino rats showing influence of calcium content of the diet on the growth and character of the bones. The rat fed a diet adequate in calcium (right) attained full growth and had strong bones; the one on the left received a diet deficient in calcium; its growth was stunted and bones were soft, brittle and more or less deformed. (Courtesy of Sherman and Macleod and the Journal of Biological Chemistry.)

take. In scurvy, the lack of ascorbic acid prevents the formation of bone matrix and normal mineralization does not occur.

Osteoporosis develops when the dietary intake of calcium is low over an extended period of time or when dietary needs are abnormally high because of poor absorption. Bone resorption occurs at an accelerated rate to maintain normal calcium blood levels. The bone is of normal composition but a reduced amount of bone is present. Patients with osteoporosis have generally been consuming diets lower in calcium than age-matched controls without bone demineralization and are in negative calcium balance. Since efficiency of absorption of calcium decreases with age, preventive therapy should be instituted early to obtain the best results.

Extremely low levels of calcium in the blood may increase the irritability of nerve fibers and nerve centers and result in muscle spasms such as leg cramps, a condition known as *tetany*. It sometimes occurs in pregnant women who have received too little calcium in their diets or who have received too much phosphorus. (The latter is responsible for hastening the excretion of calcium during pregnancy.) The rise in serum phosphorus causes a compensatory decrease in serum calcium. It sometimes occurs in newborn infants fed undiluted cow's milk, which contains more phosphorus than calcium. The kidneys of the infants cannot clear the phosphate.

A high intake of calcium and the presence of a high intake of vitamin D such as may occur in children is a potential source of *hypercalcemia* (elevated blood calcium levels). This may lead to widespread excessive calcification not only in bone but in the soft tissues such as kidneys.

Phosphorus

Phosphorus is one of the most essential elements, but it receives little attention by nu-

tritionists since it is a universal cell component available in all foods. Second to calcium in abundance, it comprises 22 per cent of the total minerals in the body. The bulk of phosphorus (about 80 per cent) is present as insoluble calcium phosphate (apatite) crystals in bones and teeth. One gram of phosphorus is required for every two grams of calcium retained. The other 20 per cent is very active metabolically and is distributed in every cell in the body and in the extracellular fluid in combination with carbohydrates, lipids and protein and a variety of other compounds.

The serum inorganic phosphorus is closely maintained at levels of 3 to 4 mg./100 ml. in adults. Levels in infants are somewhat higher. Usually, but not always, there is an adverse relationship to serum calcium.

Function.   In addition to its structural role, phosphorus has numerous functions, more than any other mineral element. A complete discussion would require consideration of every metabolic process in the body. Phosphorus is an essential component of nucleic acids, and phospholipids are key components in the structure of cell membranes. Glucose is phosphorylated as the first step in its utilization and at other steps. High energy phosphate compounds play a central role in many reactions, as does cyclic AMP. Phosphorus is part of some conjugated proteins, for example, casein from milk. Many of the B vitamins function as coenzymes only when in combination with phosphate. The phosphate buffer system is important particularly in intracellular fluid, where its concentration is much higher than in extracellular fluid, and in the tubular fluids of the kidney.

Absorption.   In older children and adults absorption from mixed diets varies between 50 and 70 per cent. Infants absorb more than 85 per cent from human milk and 65 to 75 per cent from cow's milk. Most favorable absorption of inorganic phosphate takes place when calcium

and phosphorus are ingested in approximately equal amounts. This makes milk a good source since calcium and phosphorus are present in equal amounts. (See Table 7–2.) As with calcium, the presence of vitamin D increases absorption. Simple phosphates such as calcium phosphate or potassium sodium phosphate are absorbed as such in the small intestine. In the digestion of complex compounds, phosphate is split off and absorbed. The factors that aid or deter the absorption of calcium act essentially in the same manner with regard to the absorption of phosphate. Phosphorus is present as phytic acid in some cereals and flours. If bread made from the flour is unleavened, the phytic acid can complex calcium and iron and depress their absorption. During the leavening process the phosphorus of phytic acid is converted to orthophosphate.

Dietary Sources. Meat, poultry, fish and eggs are excellent sources of phosphorus. Milk and milk products are good sources, as are nuts and legumes. Cereals and grains are good sources, but availability of the phosphorus as well as its effect on calcium absorption has been questioned because of the phytic acid, as explained previously. Table 7–2 shows the phosphorus content of average servings of various foods. Note that the good sources of protein are also good sources of phosphorus.

Recommended Dietary Allowance. The Food and Nutrition Board recommends that the daily intake of phosphorus at least equal that of calcium for all age groups except the young infant. The phosphorus allowances for young infants to one year of age are slightly less than those for calcium. (See Table 10–1.) Because phosphorus is so liberally distributed in foods, there is little possibility of a dietary inadequacy if the food intake contains adequate protein and calcium.

Deficiency. Phosphorus depletion has long been recognized in animals, but only recently has it been described in man in various disease states. The widespread, severe and ultimately fatal consequences of phosphorus depletion result from its widespread function, and are primarily the result of a decrease in ATP synthesis and other organic phosphate compounds. There are neuromuscular, skeletal, hematological and renal manifestations. Clinical phosphate depletion and hypophosphatemia are associated with administration of glucose or total parenteral nutrition without sufficient phosphate, excessive use of phosphate binding antacids, hyperparathyroidism, treatment of diabetic acidosis, alcoholism in patients with or without decompensated liver disease and other conditions.[14] Parenteral phosphate should be given for critically depleted patients; other patients can be given oral phosphate therapy.

SULFUR

Sulfur occurs principally as a constituent of the amino acids, cystine, cysteine and methionine. It is present in all proteins but is most prevalent in the keratin of skin and hair (4 to 6 per cent sulfur) and in insulin (3.2 per cent sulfur), the hormone which regulates carbohydrate metabolism. Glutathione, a tripeptide containing cysteine, is important in cellular reactions involving the sulfur amino acids in protein. Sulfur exists in a reduced form (—SH) in cysteine and in an oxidized form (—S—S—) as the double molecule, cystine. This is important in the specific configuration of some proteins and in the activity of some enzymes. Sulfur also occurs in carbohydrates such as heparin, an anticoagulant found in liver and some other tissues, and chondroitin sulfate in bone and cartilage. Two vitamins, thiamin and biotin, contain sulfur. The poisonous effects of arsenic are due to its ability to combine with sulfhydryl groups.

MAGNESIUM

The adult human contains approximately 20 to 28 grams of magnesium. Approximately 60 per cent is found in bone, 26 per cent in muscle, and the remainder in soft tissues and body fluids. Normal serum levels are usually in the range of 1.5 to 2.1 mEq. per liter. It is second to potassium as an intracellular cation. About half of the magnesium, including most in bone, is not exchangeable.

Absorption. The rate of absorption of magnesium ranges from 24 per cent to 85 per cent. The rest is excreted mainly in the feces. The kidney conserves magnesium efficiently. Renal reabsorption tends to vary inversely with that of calcium. The factors that increase the absorption of magnesium from the upper intestine are similar to those governing calcium absorption but vitamin D has no effect on magnesium absorption. The presence of fat, phytates, and calcium decreases magnesium absorption. As dietary calcium is reduced, magnesium absorption is increased.

Functions. This element is essential for the production and transfer of energy for protein synthesis, for contractility of muscle and excitability in nerves, and as an essential cofactor in numerous enzyme systems related to other

functions. Magnesium and calcium, having similar functions, may antagonize each other. An excess amount of magnesium will inhibit bone calcification. Calcium and magnesium also play antagonistic roles in normal muscle contraction, calcium acting as a stimulator and magnesium as a relaxer. An excessive amount of calcium may induce signs typical of magnesium deficiency.

A review of the role of magnesium in ischemic heart disease suggests that therapeutic use in the acute phase may be justified. Its usefulness is best explained by its metabolic effect within the cell, but the interrelationship with lipid metabolism and coagulation-fibrinolytic mechanisms may also be significant. The use of magnesium to inhibit atherogenesis or prevent ischemic heart disease or both requires further study.[27] It has also been shown that diets high in magnesium are partially effective in preventing the deposition of oxalate stones in the kidneys of rats deficient in vitamin B_6.

Deficiency. Magnesium deficiency is clinically manifested by anorexia, growth failure, ECG changes and neuromuscular changes. Low serum magnesium levels have been observed in various clinical conditions including alcoholism, diabetes, kwashiorkor, malabsorption syndromes, neuromuscular conditions in some cases associated with parathyroid diseases and in patients with extensive burns treated with daily saline baths and patients with vitamin D resistant rickets receiving massive doses of the vitamin.[3]

Recommended Dietary Allowance. Based on balance studies, the recommendation by the National Research Council (1974 revision) is 350 mg. per day for adult males and 300 mg. per day for adult females. For pregnant or lactating women the recommended allowance is 450 mg. per day. The recommended allowances for children have been estimated from the magnesium content of human milk (4 mg. per 100 ml.) and cow's milk (12 mg. per 100 ml.). Allowances for children and adolescents are only estimates, but they are intended to allow for increased needs during rapid bone growth. The allowances range from 60 to 250 mg. per day. (See Table 10–1.)

Food Sources. Magnesium intake varies widely. The average range for healthy adults in the United States and Western Europe is estimated to be 15 to 40 mEq. per day. The ordinary diet is generally believed to provide adequate amounts of magnesium, since it occurs abundantly in foods, particularly nuts, legumes, cereal grains, and dark green vegeta-

bles, where it is an essential constituent of chlorophyll. Other sources are seafood, cocoa and chocolate. High calcium, protein and vitamin D intakes, and alcohol all function to increase the requirement (particularly in those on low magnesium intake).

SODIUM, CHLORINE AND POTASSIUM

These three indispensable dietary constituents are so intimately related in the body that it is most convenient to discuss them together. Sodium constitutes 2 per cent, potassium 5 per cent, and chlorine 3 per cent of the total mineral content of the body. They are distributed ubiquitously throughout all body fluids and tissues, but sodium and chloride are primarily extracellular elements, while potassium is mainly an intracellular element. Sodium, potassium, and chloride are involved in at least four important physiological functions of the body:

1. Maintenance of normal water balance and distribution.
2. Maintenance of normal osmotic equilibrium.
3. Maintenance of normal acid-base balance.
4. Maintenance of normal muscular irritability.

All three elements are readily absorbed through the intestinal tract and are excreted through the urine, feces and sweat. These minerals are widely found in nature and in the ordinary diet. In a healthy person there is little chance of an occurrence of deficiency, but there is a chance of excess, particularly of sodium.

Hormonal control of sodium, potassium, and chloride is mediated through the adrenal cortex hormones and hormones of the anterior pituitary gland. An example of this important regulatory function is seen in Addison's disease, in which there is a decreased secretion of the adrenal cortex hormones with consequent sodium chloride loss and potassium retention by the body, causing weakness, muscle cramps, weight loss and other symptoms. The symptoms can be dramatically alleviated by giving sodium chloride alone or with adrenal cortex extract.

Sodium Chloride

Historically, the need for salt has been known ever since man and animals started living on this planet. The carnivora do not have an

urge for salt, because animal foods and milk contain sufficient salt, but the herbivorous animals and agricultural peoples demand salt because of the lack in cereals, grains, fruits and vegetables. The usual intake of sodium chloride is 6 to 18 gm. daily, much of which is added to foods. Present evidence indicates that 0.6 to 3.5 gm. is an adequate daily intake.[17] Salt is 40 per cent sodium and 60 per cent chloride. Several years ago the question was raised as to whether infants receiving much of their caloric intake from commercially prepared and processed foods may have a higher intake than that of an adult. The Committee of Nutrition of the American Academy of Pediatrics reviewed the available evidence and concluded that the intake was indeed larger than needed. Manufacturers complied with its recommendation and between 1969 and 1972 the sodium intake of infants decreased.

Low Salt Syndrome. Deficiency of sodium chloride occurs mainly during hot weather or as a result of heavy work in a hot climate when excessive sweating takes place. Water intoxication can occur if a large quantity of water is given either by mouth or intravenously without added salt. The simple provision of extra salt in food or in salt tablets will prevent or correct this condition for people working in a hot climate. Fifteen to 20 gm. daily, or even more, may be needed until acclimatization to heat is established.

Adrenal cortical insufficiency, or certain conditions such as marked vomiting and diarrhea, burns, surgical procedures with marked loss of blood, and long-term and overly vigorous treatment of heart failure or kidney disease with very low salt (sodium) diets, are some instances which may produce the "low salt syndrome." Clinical signs of salt depletion are anorexia, nausea, vomiting, headache, lassitude, muscular weakness developing into painful leg and abdominal cramps, alterations in appearance (sunken eyes, hollow cheeks, wrinkled skin) and, in severe cases, mental confusion. Resultant circulatory changes of low blood volume, low blood pressure and rapid pulse will manifest signs of "shock." (Low salt syndrome is also discussed in Chapter 28.)

Sodium

Sodium is readily absorbed in the intestine and carried by the blood to the kidneys, where it is filtered out and returned to the blood in the amounts needed to maintain blood levels re-

quired by the body. About 90 to 95 per cent of normal body sodium loss is via the urine and the rest is lost in perspiration and in the feces. Normally the quantity of sodium excreted daily equals the amount ingested, so that a state of sodium balance prevails. *Aldosterone,* a mineralocorticoid secreted by the adrenal cortex, controls the regulation of sodium balance. When blood sodium levels rise, the thirst receptors in the hypothalamus stimulate the thirst sensation. When blood levels are low, the excretion of sodium through the urine decreases. The levels of sodium in the urine reflect the dietary intake.

Daily requirements for sodium are not known. Deficiencies are rarely encountered under normal conditions and the body functions on a wide range of intakes through the mechanisms it has to conserve or excrete sodium. The sodium intake of Americans has been estimated to be 3 to 7 gm. per day (6 to 18 gm. of sodium chloride). Estimates of human requirements are as low as 200 mg. per day.

In addition to salt (sodium chloride) used in cooking, processing and as seasoning, sodium is present in most foods in varying amounts. (See Table 7–3 and Appendix Table 9.) Generally more sodium is present in the protein foods than in vegetables and grains. Fruits contain little or no sodium. The salt added to these foods in the preparation could be many times that found naturally in foods. The sodium content of the water supply varies considerably and in some areas of the country, the amount of sodium in water is of a sufficient quantity to be of significance in the total daily intake.

One of the problems of clinical medicine is the provision of palatable, diversified, sodium-restricted diets. It is frequently necessary to restrict sodium intake in order to control the over-retention of body water in various pathological states, particularly hypertension. The exact role of sodium in the etiology of hypertension is not clear cut. At the present time it appears that susceptibility to salt-induced hypertension is genetic. See Chapter 28, Nutritional Care for Patients with Cardiovascular Disease.

Chlorine

Chlorine is widely distributed throughout the body as chloride. It is the principal anion of the extracellular fluids. Together with sodium it helps to maintain water balance and osmotic pressure. The highest concentration is in the

cerebrospinal fluid and in the gastric and pancreatic juices of the gastrointestinal tract. In the gastric juice, chloride is secreted as hydrochloric acid which is necessary to maintain normal acidity of the stomach. Chloride is present in relatively small amounts in the alkaline pancreatic juice. Along with phosphate and sulfate, chloride helps to maintain acid-base balance in the body fluids. Chloride ions participate in the chloride-bicarbonate shift by having the ability to move in and out of the red blood cells and blood plasma, and to maintain osmotic equilibrium in face of the changing levels of carbon dioxide as bicarbonate in the plasma and red blood cells.

Chloride is almost completely absorbed in the intestine and excreted by the kidney. Most of the chloride ingested in the diet occurs as sodium chloride, and the amount in food and added table salt provides approximately 3 to 9 gm. daily. Whenever there are excessive losses of sodium, as in vomiting, diarrhea and in profuse sweating, there are losses of chloride ions.

Potassium

Potassium constitutes 5 per cent of the total mineral content of the body. It is the major cation of the intracellular fluid with a small amount in the extracellular fluid. Potassium with sodium is involved in the maintenance of normal water balance, osmotic equilibrium and acid-base balance. It is important with calcium in the regulation of neuromuscular activity. Any considerable increase or decrease of potassium in the extracellular fluid may be regarded as evidence of serious disturbances in muscle biochemistry, since the change in the extracellular fluid occurs late in the process.

Potassium is readily absorbed from the small intestine. It is excreted mainly in the urine. Very little is lost in the feces. The kidney maintains normal serum levels through its ability to filter, reabsorb, secrete and excrete potassium. The adrenal cortex hormone, *aldosterone,* influences potassium excretion. It conserves sodium, and ionized potassium is excreted in place of ionized sodium by means of the exchange mechanism in the renal tubule.

Potassium level in muscle is related to muscle mass; therefore if muscle is being formed, an adequate supply of potassium is essential. The same applies to glycogen storage.

A potassium deficiency from inadequate intake is not likely to happen in healthy individuals since potassium is widely distributed in foods. No requirement has been established.

The average intake is estimated to range from 0.8 to 1.5 gm. of potassium per 1000 kcalories (2 to 4 gm. for 2000 kcalorie dietary). An adequate intake of milk, meats, cereals, vegetables and fruits will provide ample potassium (see Table 9 in Appendix).

Excessive loss of extracellular fluid may result in potassium deficiency. The loss may be due to vomiting, diarrhea, excessive diuresis or prolonged malnutrition. These are conditions in which potassium from the intracellular fluid is transferred to the extracellular fluid. The serum potassium level is low and ionized potassium excretion is increased. The chief features of deficiency are muscular weakness and mental apathy. In hypokalemia cardiac failure can result from depletion of ionized potassium in heart muscle. Any condition giving rise to acidosis is liable to cause potassium loss. The acidotic patient has usually lost large quantities of water, potassium and sodium and accompanying anions, owing to osmotic diuresis. Diabetic acidosis requires replacement of potassium when insulin and glucose are given. Insulin is more effective if blood pH is normal and there is adequate renal blood flow to assure excretion of acid metabolites.

Intravenous feedings may lack sufficient potassium. Certain diuretics and adrenal cortical hormones may cause potassium depletion if efforts are not made to replace potassium in the diet.[17]

In hyperkalemia, the serum level is elevated resulting from kidney failure to clear ionized potassium. The symptoms are mental confusion, numbness of extremities, poor respiration and weakening of heart action.

MICRONUTRIENTS OR TRACE ELEMENTS

Certain elements, although present in minute amounts in the tissue, are as essential to optimal growth and development as those required in larger amounts. Inadequate intake may impair cellular and physiological function or cause illness. The recent development of instruments with increased sensitivity has enabled investigators to study the role of these micronutrients or trace elements more carefully.

To be considered essential, micronutrients must fulfill certain criteria. Cotzias postulated use of the following: (1) the element must be present in all healthy tissues; (2) its concentration in these tissues must be relatively constant; (3) withdrawal of the element from the

Table 7–3   MINERAL ELEMENTS IN HUMAN NUTRITION
(Known or Believed to Be Essential)

MINERAL	LOCATION IN BODY AND SOME BIOLOGICAL FUNCTIONS	RECOMMENDED DIETARY ALLOWANCE FOR ADULT MALE	FOOD SOURCES	COMMENTS ON LIKELIHOOD OF A DEFICIENCY
I. Macronutrients essential at levels of 100 mg. or more per day				
Calcium	99% in bones and teeth. Ionic calcium in body fluids essential for ion transport across cell membranes. Calcium is also bound to protein, citrate or inorganic acids.	800 mg.	Milk and milk products, sardines, clams, oysters, kale, turnip greens, mustard greens, broccoli.	Dietary surveys indicate that many diets do not meet recommended dietary allowances for calcium. Since bone serves as a homeostatic mechanism to maintain calcium level in blood, many essential functions are maintained, regardless of diet. Long-term dietary deficiency is probably one of the factors responsible for making osteoporosis (bone-thinning) a significant clinical problem.
Phosphorus	About 80% in inorganic phase of bones and teeth. Phosphorus is a component of every cell and of highly important metabolites, including DNA, RNA, ATP (high energy compound), and phospholipids. Important to pH regulation.	800 mg.	Cheese, egg yolk, milk, meat, fish, poultry, whole-grain cereals, legumes, nuts.	Dietary inadequacy not likely to occur if protein and calcium intake is adequate. However, increased need for phosphorus is postulated with diet leading to acid urine and during prolonged therapy with certain antacids.
Magnesium	About 50% in bone. Remaining 50% is almost entirely inside body cells with only about 1% in extracellular fluid. Ionic Mg functions as an activator of many enzymes and must influence almost all processes.	350 mg.	Whole-grain cereals, nuts, meat, milk, green vegetables, legumes.	Dietary inadequacy considered unlikely, but conditioned deficiency is often seen in clinical medicine, associated with surgery, alcoholism, malabsorption, loss of body fluids, certain hormone and renal diseases, etc. Magnesium deficiency has a profound effect on other animals.
Sodium	30 to 45% in bone. Major cation of extracellular fluid and only a small amount is inside cell. Regulates body fluid osmolarity, pH and body fluid volume.	2500 mg.	Common table salt, seafoods, animal foods, milk, eggs. Abundant in most foods except fruit.	Dietary inadequacy probably never occurs, although low blood sodium requires treatment in certain clinical disorders. Evidence is accumulating that requirements increase during pregnancy. Sodium restriction is practiced in certain cardiovascular disorders.

	Function and Metabolism	Amount	Sources	Comments
Chlorine	Major anion of extracellular fluid, functioning in combination with sodium; serves as a buffer, enzyme activator; component of gastric hydrochloric acid. Mostly present in extracellular fluid; less than 15% inside cells.	2000 mg.	Common table salt, seafoods, milk, meat, eggs.	In most cases dietary intake is of little significance except in presence of vomiting, diarrhea or profuse sweating, when a deficiency may develop.
Potassium	Major cation of intracellular fluid, with only small amounts in extracellular fluid. Functions in regulating pH and osmolarity, and cell membrane transfer. Ion is necessary for carbohydrate and protein metabolism.	2500 mg.	Fruits, milk, meat, cereals, vegetables, legumes.	Dietary inadequacy unlikely, but conditioned deficiency may be found in kidney disease, diabetic acidosis, excessive vomiting or diarrhea, hyperfunction of adrenal cortex, etc. Potassium excess may be a problem in renal failure and severe acidosis.
Sulfur	Bulk of dietary sulfur is present in sulfur-containing amino acids needed for synthesis of essential metabolites; functions in oxidation-reduction reactions. Sulfur also functions in thiamin and biotin, and as inorganic sulfur.	Need for sulfur is satisfied by essential sulfur-containing amino acids.	Protein foods (meat, fish, poultry, eggs, milk, cheese, legumes, nuts).	Dietary intake is chiefly from sulfur-containing amino acids and adequacy is related to protein intake.

II. Micronutrients essential at levels of a few milligrams

	Function and Metabolism	Amount	Sources	Comments
Iron	About 70% is in hemoglobin; about 26% stored in liver, spleen and bone. Iron is a component of hemoglobin and myoglobin, important in oxygen transfer; also present in serum transferrin and certain enzymes. Almost none in ionic form.	10 mg.	Liver, meat, egg yolk, legumes, whole or enriched grains, dark green vegetables, dark molasses, shrimp, oysters.	Iron-deficiency anemia occurs in women in reproductive years and in infants and preschool children. May be associated in some cases with unusual blood loss, parasites, and malabsorption.
Zinc	Present in most tissues, with higher amounts in liver, voluntary muscle and bone. Constituent of many enzymes and insulin; of importance in nucleic acid metabolism.	15 mg.	Milk, liver, shellfish, herring, wheat bran (widely distributed).	Extent of dietary inadequacy in this country not known. Conditioned deficiency may be seen in systemic childhood illnesses and in patients who are nutritionally depleted or have been subjected to severe stress, such as surgery.
Copper	Found in all body tissues; larger amounts in liver, brain, heart and kidney. Constituent of enzymes and of ceruloplasmin and erythrocuprein in blood. May be integral part of DNA or RNA molecule.	No R.D.A. Daily intake of 2 mg. appears to maintain balance; ordinary diets provide 2 to 5 mg./day.	Liver, shellfish, whole grains, cherries, legumes, kidney, poultry, oysters, chocolate, nuts.	No evidence that specific deficiencies of copper occur in the human.
Iodine	Constituent of thyroxine and related compounds synthesized by thyroid gland. Thyroxine functions in control of reactions involving cellular energy.	.14 mg.	Iodized table salt, seafoods, water and vegetables in non-goitrous regions.	Iodization of table salt is recommended especially in areas where food is low in iodine.

Table continued on the following page

Table 7–3   MINERAL ELEMENTS IN HUMAN NUTRITION (*Continued*)

(*Known or Believed to Be Essential*)

II. Micronutrients essential at levels of a few milligrams (*Continued*)

MINERAL	LOCATION IN BODY AND SOME BIOLOGICAL FUNCTIONS	RECOMMENDED DIETARY ALLOWANCE FOR ADULT MALE	FOOD SOURCES	COMMENTS ON LIKELIHOOD OF A DEFICIENCY
Manganese	Highest concentration is in bone; also relatively high concentrations in pituitary, liver, pancreas and gastrointestinal tissue. Constituent of essential enzyme systems; rich in mitochondria of liver cells.	Not established.	Beet greens, blueberries, whole grains, nuts, legumes, fruit, tea.	Unlikely that deficiency occurs in humans.
Fluorine	Present in bone. In optimal amounts in water and diet, reduces dental caries and may minimize bone loss.	Not established.	Drinking water (1 ppm. Fl), tea, coffee, rice, soybeans, spinach, gelatin, onions, lettuce.	In areas where fluorine content of water is low, fluoridation of water (1 ppm.) has been found beneficial in reducing incidence of dental caries.
Molybdenum	Constituent of an essential enzyme xanthine oxidase and of flavoproteins.	Not established.	Legumes, cereal grains, dark green leafy vegetables, organs.	No information.
Cobalt	Constituent of cyanocobalamin (vitamin B_{12}), occurring bound to protein in foods of animal origin. Essential to normal function of all cells, particularly cells of bone marrow, nervous system and gastrointestinal system.	3–5 μg. vitamin B_{12}	Liver, kidney, oysters, clams, poultry, milk; variable in vegetables and grains—depends upon selenium content of soil.	Primary dietary inadequacy is rare except when no animal products are consumed. Deficiency may be found in such conditions as lack of gastric intrinsic factor, gastrectomy and malabsorption syndromes.
Selenium	Associated with fat metabolism and vitamin E.	Not established.	Grains, onions, meats, milk, vegetables variable—depends upon selenium content of soil.	No known deficiency disease seen in man.
Chromium	Associated with glucose metabolism.	Not established.	Corn oil, clams, whole-grain cereals, meats, drinking water variable.	Deficiency found in severe malnutrition, diabetes and cardiovascular diseases.

diet must produce similar structural and physiological abnormalities in different species; and (4) these abnormalities must be prevented or reversed by addition of the element back into the diet.

Those elements fulfilling the requirements for essentiality are chromium, cobalt, copper, fluorine, iodine, iron, manganese, molybdenum, nickel, selenium, silicon, tin, vanadium and zinc. Six elements—fluorine, nickel, selenium, silicon, tin and vanadium—have been added only recently. Each element exhibits a spectrum of actions that depends on dosage and nutritional state of the recipient with respect to the element. Increasing amounts evoke an increasing biological response until a plateau is reached. Larger intakes may produce pharmacological actions, and still larger intakes may produce toxic effects. The toxic effects of fluorine and selenium were known before these elements were identified as essential nutrients.

FUNCTIONS OF MICRONUTRIENTS

Many enzymes contain a small amount of a trace metal that is required for full activity. Metals function in enzymes by: (1) direct participation in catalysis; (2) combination with substrate to form a complex upon which the enzyme acts; (3) formation of a metalloenzyme which binds substrates; (4) combination of metal with a reaction product; and (5) maintenance of quaternary structure.

ABSORPTION AND TRANSPORT

Absorption occurs in and is regulated at the mucosa of the small intestine. Except for chromium, excretion is predominantly through the gut. Ordinarily, urinary excretion of metals is negligible; however, it may increase markedly under conditions of stress, such as during prolonged starvation. The gastrointestinal tract is the site of important interactions between metals. Medication with iron may depress the absorption of copper. Copper in turn may lower iron and molybdenum absorption. Cobalt absorption is increased in patients with iron deficiency, but cobalt and iron compete and inhibit absorption of each other. These interactions probably reflect a lack of complete specificity of the mechanisms involved in absorption and transfer of the individual metals.

DIETARY SOURCES

For transport, metals are bound to a protein. Plasma concentrations of the micronutrients are regulated; concentration in plasma declines with low intake and increases with adequate intake.

In general, foods of animal origin are superior sources since concentrations tend to be higher and the metals are more available for absorption. Manganese is an exception, being readily available from plant sources. Trace elements are not evenly distributed in the wheat grain. Milling technology removes the germ and outer layers which contain the most minerals. While the mineral content of white flour is fairly low, those minerals left are more readily available since some of the metals in whole wheat flour are firmly complexed by phytate and fiber concentrations. Seafoods are usually rich in many micronutrients.

As the American diet changes to include more and more highly refined, processed and fabricated foods containing less and less micronutrients, there is increased concern that deficiencies may result. Added to this is the introduction of new varieties of plants and new processing techniques that may alter the mineral concentration in an as yet unknown fashion.

MICRONUTRIENTS ESSENTIAL AT LEVELS NO HIGHER THAN A FEW MILLIGRAMS PER DAY FOR ADULT HUMANS

IRON

Boussingault in the 1860's was the first to regard iron as an essential nutrient for animals. In the early 20th century there was great interest in iron absorption and excretion, even though the techniques used for analysis were tedious. By the 1920's, an animal model for the study of iron deficiency anemia was produced by feeding rats a milk diet. Interest in iron and iron deficiency anemia has continued to the present, and although there is more information on iron than on any of the other trace minerals, there are still unresolved questions and problems.

In a healthy adult there are 3 to 5 gm. of iron. An adult male has 40 to 50 mg. of iron per kilogram of body weight and the female 35 to 50 mg. per kilogram of body weight. In the new-

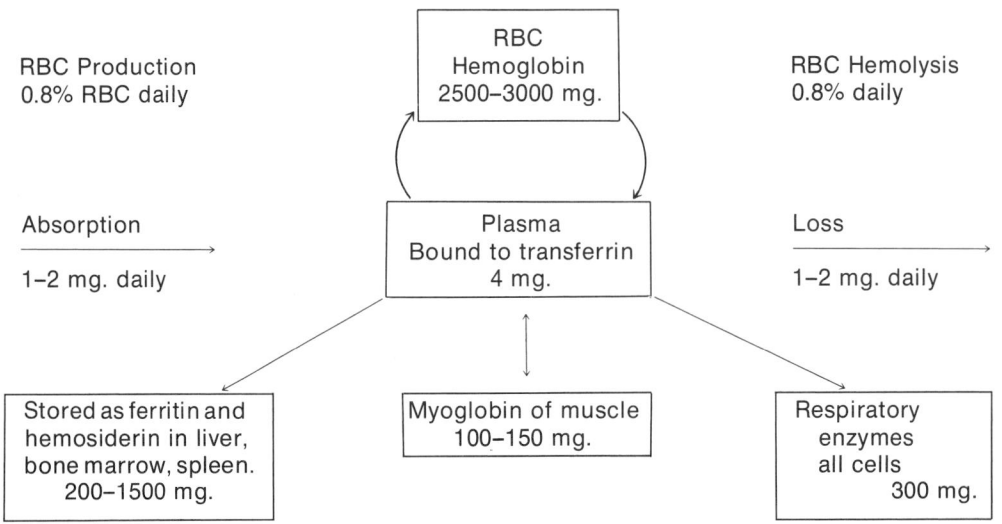

Figure 7–2 Distribution of iron in a 70 kg. man. Total body iron is about 4 gm. Although only 1–2 mg. must be absorbed to maintain equilibrium, the internal use is much greater.

born there are 70 mg. of iron per kilogram of body weight and a total of approximately 250 mg.

Sixty to seventy per cent of the iron in the body is classified as essential or functional iron, and thirty to forty per cent as storage or non-essential iron. The essential iron is incorporated into hemoglobin, myoglobin and certain respiratory enzymes which catalyze oxidation-reduction processes within the cell. If the total body contains approximately 4 gm. of iron, the distribution is as follows (Figure 7–2): 2.5 to 3.0 gm. is in the hemoglobin of erythrocytes (60 to 75 per cent); about 1 gm. is stored in the liver, bone marrow and spleen as ferritin and hemosiderin (25 per cent); 150 mg. is in the muscles as myoglobin (4 per cent); 3 to 4 mg. is in the plasma bound to the protein transferrin (1 per cent); and 300 mg. (6 per cent) is distributed among all of the cells as respiratory enzymes.

Functions. Iron plays a role in the transport of oxygen from the lungs to the tissues, in the transport of CO_2 away from the cells to the lungs, and in the process of cellular respiration.

The first two of these functions are accomplished by hemoglobin in the erythrocytes or red blood cells (RBC's). *Hemoglobin* is a metalloprotein with heme, an iron porphyrin, attached to the protein moiety. The iron combines with oxygen in the lungs, where the concentration is high, and releases the oxygen in the tissues where it is needed. *Myoglobin* within the muscle cell has a function similar to

that of hemoglobin. The *cytochromes*, present in all cells, do not combine with oxygen, but function in the respiratory chain in the transfer of electrons through alternate oxidation and reduction of iron ($Fe^{++} \leftrightarrow Fe^{+++}$). Catalase and peroxidase catalyze these oxidation-reduction processes within the cells.

In fetal life, the red blood cells are manufactured principally in the liver and the spleen. Fetal red blood cells contain a different form of hemoglobin, fetal hemoglobin, which has different association-disassociation characteristics. In the adult, RBC's are formed chiefly in the bone marrow. The erythrocytes begin as erythroblasts (immature cells). As they mature in the bone marrow, heme is synthesized from glycine and iron in the presence of pyridoxine and combined with the globin. Adequate amounts of amino acids must be available for the simultaneous synthesis of globin. The presence of copper and vitamin C are also essential for the synthesis of hemoglobin.

Since they are non-nucleated, red blood cells live only as long as the enzymes present at maturity remain functional. As cells age and approach the end of their life span (120 days), they become more fragile. Old cells are removed from circulation by the cells of the reticuloendothelial system. The iron is released from the porphyrin, taken up by the transferrin, and either returned to the bone marrow for the production of new blood cells or stored in the liver and spleen. Without this effective conservation it would be impossible to provide the

iron needed from dietary sources. The iron-free porphyrin is converted to bilirubin and carried to the liver for excretion in the bile. Deficiencies of ascorbic acid, vitamin E, folic acid, and vitamin B_{12} accelerate the rate of destruction of the RBC's.

The respiratory enzymes function in oxidation-reduction at the cellular level. There is evidence from animal studies that in a dietary deficiency the concentration of these enzymes may drop before the hemoglobin level in the blood drops. Although these enzymes represent only a small part of the total iron, a drop in the cellular concentration of these vital enzymes can still have a long-range effect.

There is considerable evidence that iron may also play a role in the conversion of beta-carotene to vitamin A, the synthesis of purines, the clearance of blood lipids and the detoxification of drugs in the liver. The answer to the question of whether iron status has an effect on immunocompetence and thereby on susceptibility to infection is not yet clear. Although iron is essential to the growth of microorganisms, it is also an integral part of enzymes and immune proteins needed to destroy the infectious organisms. *Lactoferrin* in breast milk is an iron-containing protein effective against *E. coli* of the gastrointestinal tract of infants.

Absorption. There are wide variations in the amount of iron that can be absorbed. The absorption of iron is affected by physiological factors and factors affecting the availability of iron from its source. Inorganic forms of iron ($FeSO_4$) are readily absorbed by the mucosa of the small intestine. The ferrous (Fe^{++}) salts appear to be more readily absorbed than are the ferric (Fe^{+++}) salts. The greatest absorption occurs in the upper duodenum because of the acidic environment. The rate of iron absorption seems to be controlled by the amount accepted by the intestinal mucosa in response to the body's requirement for iron, which is reflected by the amount available from the blood to meet the needs of newly formed cells (Fig. 7–3). There is no mechanism for excreting iron; therefore, the iron content of the body is regulated by the rate of absorption. Within the mucosal cell the iron may combine with *apoferritin* to form *ferritin,* the form in which iron is temporarily stored in the mucosal cells.

The rate at which the iron is released from the mucosal cells into general circulation may be regulated by the amount and saturation of *transferrin.* Transferrin is usually saturated to about one-third of its *total iron binding capacity* (TIBC). If iron is not needed, transferrin remains saturated, less is absorbed from the mucosal cells, and that remaining in the cells is sloughed with the cell at the end of their 2 to 3 day life. If iron is needed, the transferrin is less

Figure 7–3 Iron equilibrium in the intestinal mucosa. In normal subjects, mucosal cells contain iron supplied from body stores. The amount of iron which enters the cells is regulated, within limits, by the amount in the cells or the amount circulating bound to transferrin. In iron-deficient subjects, little iron is incorporated into the mucosal cells and less is present bound to transferrin. Therefore, iron absorption is increased and excretion is decreased. In iron-loaded subjects, both the mucosal cells and transferrin are saturated. This limits absorption and increases excretion.

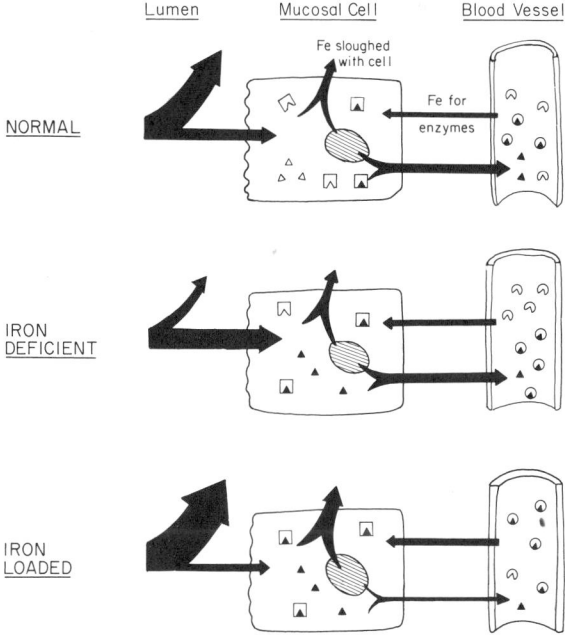

▲ IRON ▣ FERRITIN ⬚ APOFERRITIN ⊗ TRANSFERRITIN

saturated when it reaches the intestinal mucosal cells and more iron passes from the mucosal cell to the transferrin.

It is estimated that only 5 to 15 per cent of the iron in food is absorbed by adults with normal hemoglobin values, although it can be as high as 50 per cent in an iron-deficient person. From 2 to 10 per cent of iron in vegetables is absorbed, which may be due in part to the high fiber content. From 10 to 30 per cent of iron in animal protein can be absorbed. Heme iron is well absorbed and its availability is less influenced by other foods in the diet.

Factors That Enhance Absorption

1. *Ascorbic acid.* Bile contains ascorbate and other reducing substances which either chelate iron, reduce ferric to ferrous iron, or both. Dietary ascorbic acid improves the absorption of iron.
2. *Acid medium.* The degree of gastric acidity influences solubility and availability of iron in food.
3. *Calcium.* The presence of an adequate amount of calcium helps to remove phosphate, oxalate and phytate that would combine with iron and inhibit its absorption.
4. *Intrinsic factor.* Besides hydrochloric acid, gastric secretions include intrinsic factor and ascorbate. Intrinsic factor increases absorption of heme iron because of the structural similarity of heme and vitamin B_{12}.
5. *Physiological state.* During periods of increased rate of formation of blood, such as pregnancy and growth, absorption is increased. People with deficiency also absorb more iron.

Factors That Decrease Absorption

1. *Alkaline medium.* The lack of hydrochloric acid in the stomach or the administration of alkaline substances such as antacids interferes with iron absorption.
2. *Complexing agents.* Phytates, oxalates and phosphates form insoluble iron complexes, reducing absorption.
3. *Intestinal motility.* Increased motility decreases absorption by decreasing the contact time.
4. *Steatorrhea.* Decreases absorption.
5. *Chemical form of iron.* Studies have also indicated wide differences in the availability of iron from various compounds used for enrichment or supplementation. (See Fig. 7–4.) Ferrous, lactate, fumarate, glycine sulfate, succinate and glutamate are absorbed as well as ferrous sulfate. Ferrous citrate, tartrate and pyrophosphate are poorly absorbed.

When abnormally large amounts of iron are present as a result of long-term ingestion of extremely high amounts or excessive blood transfusions, the apoferritin in the liver becomes saturated and hemosiderin appears in large quantities. *Hemosiderin* is similar to ferritin but contains more iron and is very insoluble. Certain individuals with a genetic defect absorb more than an ordinary amount of iron and develop this iron storage condition which is called *hemosiderosis.* If the hemosiderosis is associated with tissue damage, it is called *hemochromatosis.*

Storage. Approximately 1000 mg. of iron are stored in the body as ferritin and hemosiderin; 30 per cent is in the liver, 30 per cent in the bone marrow and the rest in the spleen and muscles. Up to 50 mg. per day can be mobilized from storage iron. About 20 mg. of iron is used daily in hemoglobin synthesis. Iron is used very conservatively in the body. Approximately 90 per cent is conserved and used over and over again.

Excretion. Only very small amounts of iron are normally excreted from the body. The bulk of the iron lost in the feces consists of that not absorbed from food intake. The remainder is iron contained in exfoliated cells from the gastrointestinal epithelium, the excretion of bile, normal exfoliation of the cells of the skin and from bleeding. Virtually no iron is excreted in the urine and sweat.

The normal male loses about 1.0 mg. of iron daily. In the female, there is the additional loss of iron accompanying menstruation, which averages about 0.5 mg. per day—the amount of iron in the menstrual blood flow averaged over one month. Wide variations exist among individuals, and menstrual losses of over 1.4 mg. of iron per day have been reported in about 5 per cent of normal women.[5]

Metabolism. Figure 7–5 is a schematic outline of the essential steps in the metabolism of iron in adults.

Dietary Sources. By far the best source of dietary iron is liver, with oysters, shellfish, kidney, heart, lean meat and tongue as second choices. Dried beans and vegetables are the best plant sources. Some other foods that add iron are egg yolks, dried fruits, dark molasses, whole grain and enriched breads, wines and cereals. Milk and milk products are practically

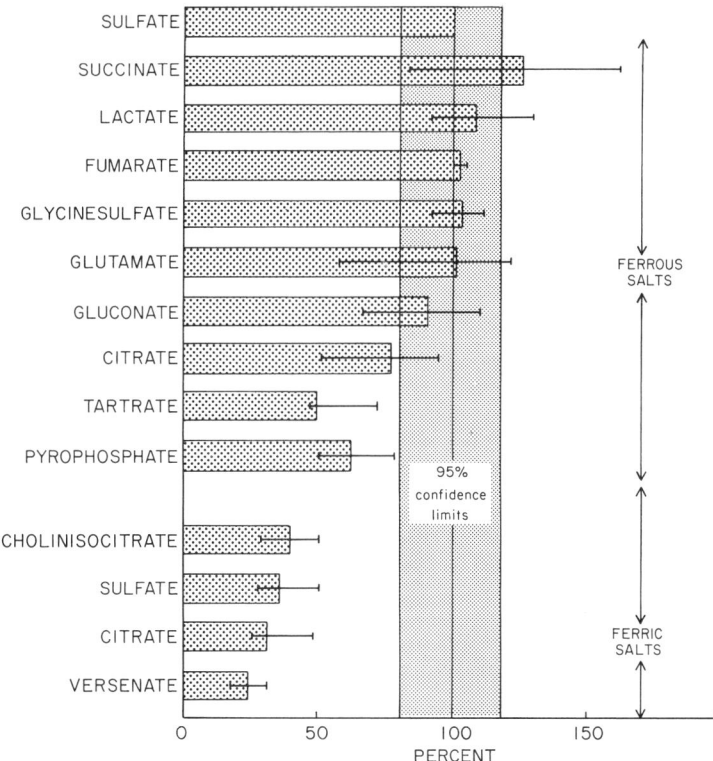

Figure 7–4 Absorption of iron from dose equivalent to 30 mg. elemental iron. Mean indicated by bar, range indicated by line.

devoid of iron. Foods high in iron content are shown in Figure 7–6. A more complete table is given in the Appendix Table 8.

The size of the average serving of food and the availability of the iron present in the foods must be taken into account when thinking of sources of dietary iron. For example, only half or less of the iron in whole grain cereals and some green leaves is available in utilizable form. Raisins, though popularly thought to be a good source of iron, really do not contribute a significant amount to the diet on a percentage basis because even though iron content may be good, the average serving is relatively small.

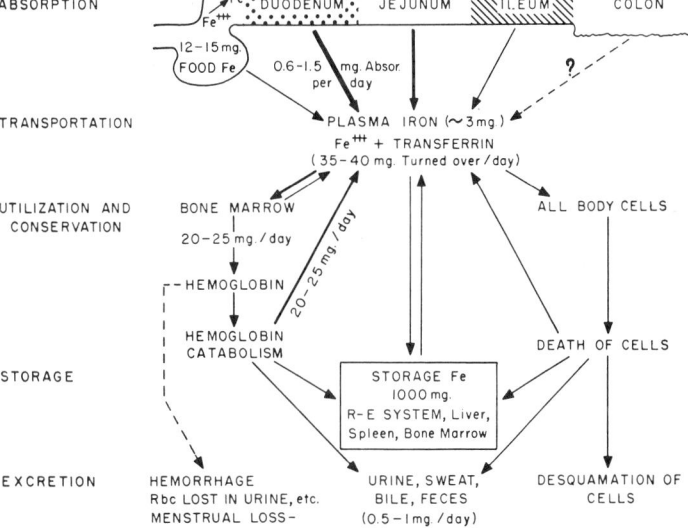

Figure 7–5 Schematic outline of iron metabolism in adults. (From Goodhart, R. S., and Shils, M. E. (eds.): Modern Nutrition in Health and Disease. 5th ed. Lea & Febiger, 1974.)

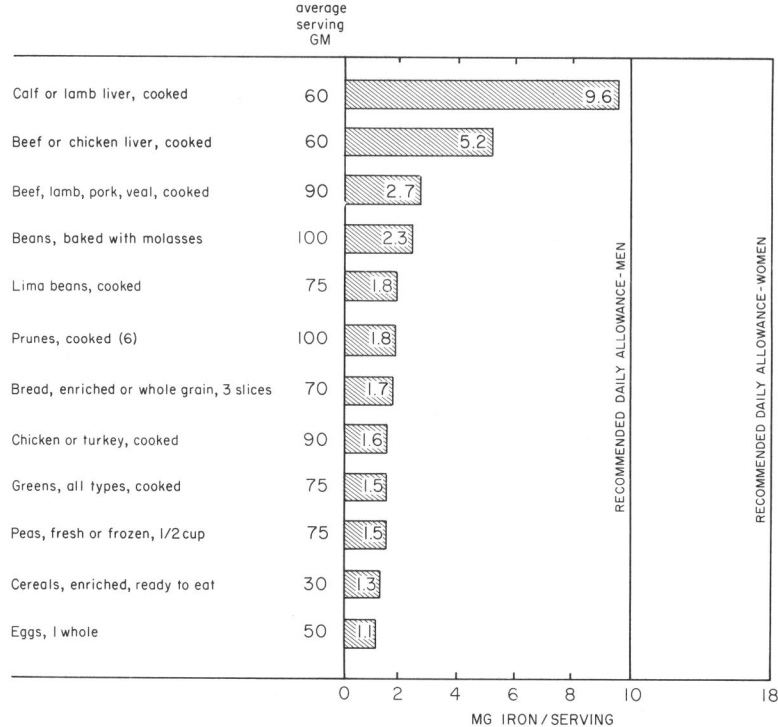

Figure 7–6   Iron in average servings of food compared to the RDA for men and women.

Iron fortification of cereals, flours and bread has added significantly to the total iron intake. Fortified infant cereal is a substantial source of iron for children up to 12 months of age.[23]

An otherwise adequate diet frequently contains no more than 6 mg. of iron per 1000 kilocalories. The average female, consuming 2300 kilocalories would only consume approximately 13.8 mg. of iron or approximately 75 per cent of the RDA. Since the RDA can be met by dietary intake only with difficulty and with good planning, there is a controversy as to whether it is set too high.

Another controversy surrounds iron fortification of foods. It has been suggested that iron fortification will cause more hemosiderosis in susceptible people. On the other hand, iron supplementation of more foods might prevent iron deficiency among the high risk population.

Recommended Dietary Allowance. A sufficient quantity of iron is needed in the diet to prevent the development of iron deficiency anemia. Iron requirements are determined by the demands for tissue growth and hemoglobin accretion and by replacement needs for iron lost in the urine, feces, and sweat and in the female in menstruation, pregnancy and lactation. Recommendations of the Food and Nutrition Board are for a daily intake of 10 mg. of iron for men and older women. An intake of 18

mg. per day is recommended for women during child-bearing years. This amount is required to cover menstrual losses and the demands of pregnancy lactation.

The infant is born with a reserve supply of iron and is apparently unable to utilize additional iron over and above that furnished by reduction of its hemoglobin mass shortly after birth. The recommended allowance for a normal term infant is based on an average need of 1.5 mg. per kg. of weight per day during the first year of life. Premature infants have limited stores since most of the iron is transferred during the last trimester of pregnancy, and premature infants are routinely given an iron supplemented formula. The need for iron to support rapid growth becomes apparent at approximately 3 months of age. The recommended allowance for the period from birth to 6 months is 10 mg.; for children 6 months to 3 years it is 15 mg.; for children ages 4 to 10 years it is 10 mg. The daily need for boys ages 11 to 18 years is 18 mg., dropping to 10 mg. for men 19 to 50 years and older. For girls ages 10 to 50, the RDA is 18 mg.; for women 50 years of age and older, it is 10 mg.

Iron Requirement in Relation to Age.   Figure 7–7 shows the absorbed requirement in relation to age. The requirement during infancy is the greatest in relation to food intake. The adoles-

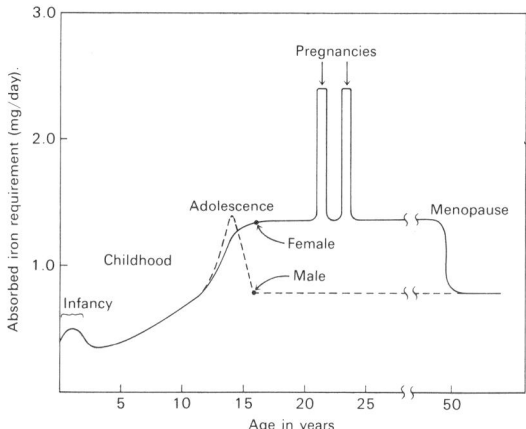

Figure 7–7 The absorbed iron requirement in males and females of various ages. The greatest requirements in relation to food intake occur during infancy. During childhood, requirements are the same for both sexes. During the adolescent growth spurt there is an increase in iron needs—more in the male than in the female. However, with the onset of menstruation, requirements for the female exceed those for the male. (From Wintrobe, M. S., et al.: Clinical Hematology. 7th ed. Lea and Febiger, 1974.)

cent growth spurt is another period of increased requirement, higher in the male than female; however, with the onset of menstruation the requirements of the female exceed the male.

Because of individual variation in absorptive capacity, the differences among foods in the availability of their iron for absorption, and the ability of the body to increase iron absorption during periods of deficiency, it is difficult to convert physiological requirements for iron into dietary allowances. The United States recommendations for iron set by the Food and Nutrition Board of the National Research Council and those set by the Joint FAO/WHO Expert Group differ, although they are based on the same considerations.

Iron Deficiency. A deficiency of iron has been cited as the commonest of all deficiency diseases in humans in both developing and developed countries. Iron deficiency manifests itself ultimately by the development of an anemia (hypochromic microcytic anemia), which is corrected by giving diets rich in iron and by providing iron supplements in the form of ferrous sulfate or ferrous gluconate. Iron deficiency anemia can be caused by blood loss through illness, injury or hemorrhage and is aggravated by a poorly balanced diet that is often deficient in dietary iron, protein and the vitamins folate, B_{12}, B_6, and C. Iron deficiency anemia may develop on a purely nutritional basis as a result of an inadequate diet or faulty

absorption of iron. The sequence of events in the development of iron deficiency anemia is: desaturation of tissue stores, diminished levels of certain enzymes, decreased serum iron levels, increased TIBC, and finally decreased hemoglobin and hematocrit. Clinical symptoms develop slowly and frequently are not perceived by the patient. In severe anemia, cardiac symptoms develop. During iron depletion, organs with rapid cell turnover become rapidly depleted of iron-dependent enzymes; in organs with slow turnover, enzymes may remain unaltered. (Also see discussions in Chapters 12 and 29.)

FLUORINE

Before 1972 fluorine was considered by some to be essential because of its beneficial effect on tooth enamel, conferring maximal resistance to dental caries. In 1972 studies from the laboratories of Schwarz[24] provided additional support for fluorine as an essential trace element by showing that animals fed purified diets supplemented with 250 μg. F/100 g. of diet gained 30.8 per cent more weight than did controls not receiving the supplement.

The skeleton of the average man contains 2.6 gm. of fluorine. The average daily intake of adults is approximately 4.4 mg. Of the greatest importance is the amount ingested in drinking water. The fluoride content of food varies according to the content of the soil in which it is grown. Table 7–4 lists the fluorine content of selected foods.

Table 7–4 FLUORINE CONTENT OF SELECTED FOODS

FOOD	FLUORINE CONTENT (PPM.)
Meats	
Beef liver	5.20–5.80
Chicken	1.40
Beef	2.00
Pork chops	1.0
Lamb	1.2
Veal	0.9
Fish	
Mackerel, fresh	26.89
Salmon, canned	4.5
Sardines, in olive oil	16.1
Eggs	
Whole	1.2
Yolk	0.6
Milk, whole	0.07–0.22
Cereals and cereal products	0.54
Vegetables	0.1–0.2
Fruits	0.1–0.2

(Adapted from Bell, M. E., et al.: The Supply of Fluorine to Man in Fluorides and Human Health, WHO Monograph No. 59, Geneva, Switzerland, WHO, 1970.)

Dental fluorosis may occur at fluoride concentrations of 2 to 7 ppm. and osteosclerosis at 8 to 20 ppm. To produce symptoms of chronic toxicity, daily intakes of 20 to 80 mg. or more must be consumed for years. In parts of the western United States the water sometimes contains 10 to 45 ppm. of fluoride and tooth mottling is endemic (Fig. 7–8). In other areas such as parts of Michigan and New York where fluorine is deficient, the incidence of dental decay is quite high. One mg. of fluorine per liter of drinking water for long periods produces a 60 to 70 per cent reduction in dental caries. For maximal effect, the fluoride must be used in the early years when teeth are forming. Approximately 10,000 communities in which the content is low have added this amount to water supplies serving over 100 million people. This practice is recognized as an important public health measure (see Dental Caries in Chapter 33). Studies have demonstrated that the hydroxyapatite crystals in bone are larger and more nearly perfect when the fluoride content of the diet is adequate. Bone containing fluoride is more stable and more resistant to degeneration. A further benefit may be a reduction in the incidence of osteoporosis and calcification of the aorta in areas where fluoride intake is adequate.

Although pills, drugs and fluoridated toothpaste are of some use, none combine the efficiency, effectiveness or the economy of water fluoridation.

ZINC

In 1934 Todd and associates[31] reported that zinc was necessary for life in animals and suggested that this included man. However, it was not until 1961 that Prasad and coworkers[21] described a group of zinc-deficient Iranian men who also had severe iron deficiency anemia,

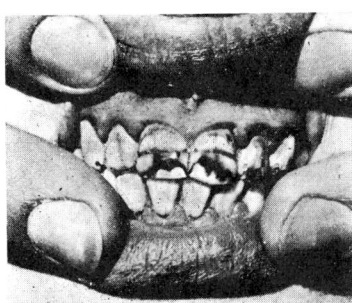

Figure 7–8 Mottled enamel caused by excess fluorine in water. (Fluorine and Dental Health Pub. No. 19. Am. Assoc. for the Advancement of Science, Washington, D.C., 1942.)

hepatosplenomegaly, short stature, marked hypogonadism and a history of geophagia (clay eating). There is now evidence that not only can zinc deficiency disease be found in malnourished populations, but also that disease and physical injury can alter zinc metabolism and excretion.

Zinc is ubiquitous in plants, microorganisms and animals. There are 1.4 to 2.3 grams of zinc in the body of an adult. The liver, pancreas, kidney, bone and voluntary muscles have the largest concentration. Other tissues with high concentrations include various parts of the eye, prostate gland and spermatozoa, skin, hair, fingernails and toenails. Plasma values range around 100 mg./dl. (S.D.±10 mg./dl.) Women have lower values than men and concentrations in children are lower than in adults. Red and white blood cells contain 6 to 8 times as much as the plasma. There is a slight *circadian periodicity* of plasma zinc, not more than 5 to 10 per cent from the baseline.

Studies using radioactive zinc as a tracer have shown that 5 to 15 per cent of the ingested zinc is absorbed primarily in the upper small intestine. The major route of excretion is via the gastrointestinal tract. Relatively little is known about the renal excreting mechanism. As much as 1 mg./liter may be lost as sweat. This may become significant in hot climates where the volume of sweat may be as much as 5 liters a day.

In rats the concentrations of zinc in newly grown hair correlate closely with zinc intake. In one study of human infants, the level of zinc in the plasma correlated well with the amount in the hair. However, in a group of Iranian children with low plasma zinc, the hair concentration was not correspondingly low.

Metabolic Functions. Many questions regarding the biological role of zinc in man are as yet unanswered; however, it is clear that zinc plays a role in a number of metabolic activities. There is a family of 70 or more metalloenzymes that require zinc to function. These include carbonic anhydrase, alkaline phosphatase, lactic dehydrogenase and carboxypeptidase. Zinc functions by maintaining spatial and configurational relationships necessary for enzymatic action. In this role it helps to bind enzymes to substrates and may modify the molecular shape of enzymes by simultaneously combining with amino acids at different places on the protein, thus affecting secondary, tertiary and quaternary protein structure. A number of zinc metalloenzymes are involved in the regulation of cellular growth.

In addition to its function in enzymes, zinc participates in the metabolism of nucleic acids and the synthesis of proteins. Although its role is not completely understood, zinc appears to be an integral part of the RNA molecule of a number of species and is thought to help maintain stable molecular configuration. Zinc may also have an important role in cell division since zinc deficiency causes adverse effects on the incorporation of thymidine into the DNA of rats. Zinc is required for DNA synthesis, and the DNA dependent RNA polymerase is a zinc dependent enzyme, as is thymidine kinase.

Absorption and Bioavailability. Zinc absorption is affected by body size, the level of zinc in the diet and the presence of interfering substances such as calcium, phytate, other chelating agents and vitamin D. Zinc is most available as zinc sulfate. Phytate (inositol hexaphosphate) present in cereal grains lowers zinc availability. When large quantities of unleavened bread are consumed as the main protein source, the phytate in the bread enhances the possibility of zinc deficiency. Leavening bread results in the destruction of phytate. The chelating properties of phytate may induce a wide variety of mineral deficiencies, depending on which element first becomes limiting. Rats treated with vitamin D were observed to absorb more dietary zinc; however, this effect may be the result of increased need secondary to increased skeletal growth, rather than improvement in absorption.

Excretion. Excretion is almost solely via the feces in normal individuals. Increased urinary excretion has been reported in patients with nephrosis, diabetes, alcoholism, hepatic cirrhosis and porphyria. Urinary excretion increased tenfold in individuals who were starving; however, plasma levels remained constant in spite of the increased excretion. In another study, urinary zinc in two patients reached a maximum about 10 days after surgery for total hip replacement and correlated well with urinary nitrogen. It was therefore suggested that urinary zinc may provide an index by which to monitor muscle catabolism. Further studies are needed to determine if this relationship is definite.

Deficiency. The clinical picture of zinc deficiency is most prominent in growing children. Symptoms include poor growth, loss of appetite, hypogonadism in males and loss of the senses of taste and smell. If the patient has had a surgical procedure, wound healing may be delayed. Hyperfunction of the adrenal cortex accompanies zinc deficiency, and corticosteroid therapy causes a rapid decline in serum zinc. (Also see Chapter 12—Nutritional Deficiency Diseases.)

Reexamination of the subjects of the early studies has raised some questions regarding the original observations. Selected subjects from the same area with normal growth and development also had low plasma zinc levels. While it appears that in some of the early Iranian and Egyptian studies other limiting nutritional factors may also have been involved, confirmatory studies have documented the zinc deficiency syndrome in females and a zinc responsive growth failure and sexual maturation in males.

The teratogenic effect of zinc deficiency in humans has not been demonstrated; however, there is a wealth of evidence demonstrating the effect in animals. Ingestion of a zinc deficient diet by rats during pregnancy results in a number of congenital anomalies, e.g., tail anomalies, clubfoot, syndactyly, hydrocephalus, scoliosis, and kyphosis.[8] There is sufficient circumstantial evidence suggesting a relationship between maternal zinc status and congenital anomalies to urge further careful study of this problem. One piece of circumstantial evidence involved a study of 8 children with multiple congenital anomalies born to alcoholic mothers. The anomalies are reminiscent of those seen in the progeny of zinc deficient rats. Low serum zinc and hyperzincuria may occur in alcoholics, and with the added stress of pregnancy and poor diet, these women may have been zinc deficient. Unfortunately, zinc status was not determined.[9]

Zinc therapy improves healing in patients with zinc deficiency. However, there is no conclusive evidence that zinc stimulates healing in the individual with an adequate zinc nutriture. Illnesses in which both serum and erythrocyte levels of zinc decrease include cirrhosis of the liver, hepatitis, nephrosis, malabsorption syndromes, chronic infectious diseases, myocardial infarction and hypothyroidism.

Deficiency of zinc has been associated with alterations in taste. Treatment with zinc, nickel or copper results in an improvement in taste perception. Children with low zinc content in the hair and poor growth, who also had loss of taste and smell, showed reversal of the abnormalities following zinc supplementation.

Acute zinc deficiency has recently been reported in patients receiving total parenteral alimentation. Urinary zinc losses can be very high in these patients because of the high rate of

catabolism; however, plasma zinc does not fall until there is sustained anabolism and weight gain. Four of thirty-seven adult patients followed by Key and colleagues[10] had low plasma zinc and a syndrome characterized by diarrhea, mental depression, paranoia, oral and peri-oral dermatitis and alopecia. Response to zinc therapy was rapid except for regrowth of hair, which took longer. A single case of acquired zinc deficiency of such severity as to cause the cutaneous manifestations of *acrodermatitis enteropathica* has been reported.

Based on the similarities between patients with sickle cell anemia and zinc deficiency, Prasad and associates[22] have suggested the possibility of a secondary zinc deficiency in people with sickle cell anemia. Zinc sulfate therapy produced some positive effects. Several subjects grew, all but one gained weight, and some of the males showed increased hair growth. More work is necessary before conclusions can be drawn. (See Chapter 29 for more discussion of sickle cell anemia.)

Excess. There are no known syndromes of dietary zinc excess. Accidental ingestion of excess zinc results in nausea, vomiting and diarrhea.

Recommended Dietary Allowance. An intake of 8 to 10 mg./day appears sufficient to achieve zinc equilibrium in healthy adults. Therefore, the RDA for 1974 was set at 15 mg./day for adolescents and adults, plus 15 mg. additional during pregnancy and 10 mg. during lactation. For preadolescents the requirement is estimated at 6 mg./day and the RDA has been set at 10 mg. There is limited information on the zinc requirements of infants. The RDA was, therefore, tentatively set at 3 mg./day. The American adult consuming a mixed diet has an average intake of 10 to 15 mg. For children 1 to 3 years of age, the intake has been estimated at 5 mg., increasing to 13 mg. for adolescents 10 to 13 years of age.

Dietary Sources. Zinc should come from a balanced diet that contains sufficient animal protein. Meat, liver, eggs and seafood (particularly oysters) are good sources of available zinc. Table 7–5 lists the actual zinc content of selected foods; a more complete list is included in the appendix. The content of most drinking water is negligible.

COPPER

An adult human body of 70 kg. contains 80 to 120 mg. of copper. Concentrations are highest in brain, liver, heart and kidney. Bone and

Table 7–5 ZINC CONTENT OF SELECTED FOODS

FOOD	ZINC MG./100 MG.
Meat	
Beef, separable lean, cooked	6.2
Liver, calf, cooked	6.1
Pork loin, separable lean, cooked	3.1
Sausages and cold cuts	
Bologna, beef	1.8
Braunschweiger	2.8
Beef and pork frankfurters	1.6
Turkey	
Light meat, cooked, dry heat	2.1
Dark meat, cooked, dry heat	4.4
Eggs, fresh, whole	1.0
Breads	
White	0.6
Whole wheat	1.8
Vegetables	
Dry beans, boiled, drained	1.0
Peas, canned, drained solids	0.8
Wheat cereals, ready-to-eat	
Bran flakes, 40%	3.6
Flakes	2.3
Germ, toasted	15.4
Shredded	2.8

(Adapted from Murphy, E. W., Willis, B. W., and Watt, B. K.: Provisional tables on the zinc content of foods. J. Am. Diet. Assoc., *66*:345, 1975.)

muscle have lower concentrations but contain one-half of the total because of their large mass.

The concentration of copper is greatest in the newborn, decreasing during the first year of life. Infants have an exceptional requirement of about .08 mg./kg. of body weight. Older children need only half this amount, and for adults .03 mg./kg. is sufficient.

Copper is a component of many enzymes and there are at least three functional areas of prime importance. It is involved in the development and maintenance of (1) cardiovascular and skeletal integrity, (2) central nervous system structure and function and (3) erythropoietic function.

Copper concentrations are higher in serum than in plasma, and values depend on copper intakes. Average plasma values for women range from 87 to 153 mg./dl. with a mean value of 120 mg./dl.; for men the range is 89 to 137 mg./dl. with a mean of 109 mg./dl. Approximately 90 per cent of the copper in the plasma is bound to *ceruloplasmin;* the rest is bound to albumin.

Absorption. Copper is absorbed from the stomach and upper gut by at least two mechanisms. One mechanism, facilitated by amino acids, is an energy dependent process and may

represent the absorption of copper complexes of amino acids. A smaller portion is absorbed by this mechanism. The bulk of the copper is absorbed by the second mechanism involving binding to two protein fractions of the small intestine. Transition elements such as cadmium or zinc, molybdenum and sulfate alter or interfere with copper absorption. Small amounts are present in urine, sweat and menstrual flow. Unabsorbed copper is found in the feces.

Metabolic Functions. The anemia of copper deficiency is probably due to a disruption of iron metabolism. Ceruloplasmin may aid the mobilization of iron from ferritin in the liver and other iron storage sites. There are numerous amine oxidases that are copper and pyridoxal phosphate dependent. Several cuproenzymes have well defined functions; however, a specific pathologic sign cannot be identified with each enzyme function. On the other hand, there are cuproenzymes associated with specific pathological signs. The bones of copper deficient chicks contain a higher than normal proportion of soluble collagen, and collagen crosslinking is impaired. Failure of the crosslink formation of collagen and elastin accounts for greater fragility and associated abnormalities. Cardiac failure, reported in animals raised on a copper deficient diet, may also result from failure of collagen and elastin crosslinking or from an as yet undefined muscular defect.[11]

Copper deficiency affects the developing central nervous system. The disease described in subprimate species is manifested by locomotion incoordination associated with a lack of myelination of the spinal cord. The amyelination is associated with the ataxia, but it is not known whether it is the cause.

In animals with pigmented hair, wool or feathers, copper deficiency results in a failure of melanin formation. Tyrosinase, a cuproenzyme, catalyzes the hydroxylation of tyrosine to DOPA (3, 4, dihydroxyphenylalanine) and the oxidation of DOPA to a quinone gives rise to melanin.

Deficiency. The signs of copper deficiency in order of appearance are: fall in serum copper and ceruloplasmin levels, failure of iron absorption, neutropenia, leukopenia, bone demineralization, failure of erythropoiesis and finally death. Neutropenia and leukopenia are the best early indications of copper deficiency in children.

Copper deficiency has not been reported in humans consuming a varied diet. Low serum copper values have been reported in patients receiving TPN solutions without copper supplementation. Low serum copper and ceruloplasmin provide supportive evidence of copper deficiency. With the resumption of oral feeding, serum copper rises rapidly.

Three deficiency syndromes have been recognized in infants. One is manifested by moderate to severe *anemia* in infants whose diet is based on cow's milk. For complete recovery, therapy with both copper and iron was required since serum levels of both were low. (See Chapter 29.)

The second syndrome is associated with *chronic malnutrition and diarrhea.* The use of modified cow's milk to alleviate the malnutrition contributed in some cases to the development of anemia.

The third syndrome, *Menke's kinky hair syndrome,* is a sex-linked recessive defect of copper absorption. The infants have retarded growth, defective keratinization and pigmentation of the hair, hypothermia, degenerative changes in aortic elastin, abnormalities of the metaphyses of long bone and progressive mental deterioration. Brain tissue is practically devoid of cytochrome c oxidase, a cuproenzyme, and there is a marked accumulation of copper in the intestinal mucosa. Parenteral administration of copper results in transient improvement.

Decreased plasma copper is seen in patients with several malabsorption diseases such as celiac, tropical and non-tropical sprue, protein-losing enteropathies and nephrotic syndrome. Decreased serum copper, as well as decreased zinc, may result in alterations of taste perception.

Klevay[13] has suggested that a metabolic imbalance produced by a high ratio of zinc to copper or an absolute deficiency of copper results in hypercholesterolemia. This hypercholesterolemia in turns leads to coronary heart disease. Additional studies are needed to provide evidence to confirm or deny this hypothesis. (See Chapter 28.)

Excess. HYPERCUPREMIA. Ceruloplasmin concentrations increase during pregnancy and in women taking oral contraceptives. Serum copper concentration is increased in some patients with acute and chronic infections, patients with liver disease and patients with pellagra. In the case of pellagra, ceruloplasmin does not increase, an exception to the usual close correlation between serum copper and ceruloplasmin concentrations.

WILSON'S DISEASE (HEPATO-LENTICULAR

DEGENERATION). At birth the child with Wilson's disease is indistinguishable from normal neonates. However, the physiologic increase in serum ceruloplasmin and decrease in hepatic copper do not occur. Hepatic copper continues to accumulate with age, producing fatty deposition, necrosis of cells, pigmentary changes and an excess of fibrous tissue. The central nervous system is also adversely affected. Copper deposits in the cornea, *Kaper-Fleischer rings,* do not interfere with vision and are of no pathologic significance. The clinical symptoms of Wilson's disease vary depending on which organs are most seriously affected. Patients are treated with a low-copper diet and with penicillamine, which chelates the copper and allows it to be excreted in the urine.

Food Sources. Copper is widely distributed and most diets provide about 2 mg./day. Foods high in copper are liver, kidney, oysters, chocolate, nuts, dried legumes, cereals, dried fruits, poultry, shellfish and animal tissues. Milk is as poor in copper as it is in iron, containing 0.015 to 0.18 mg./liter. Human milk content ranges from 0.15 to 1.05 mg./liter.

Recommended Dietary Allowances. While sufficient data are not available to set an RDA, copper intakes of 1.3 and 2 mg./day appear to maintain balance in adolescent girls and adults, respectively.

IODINE

The only known function of iodine is as an integral part of thyroid hormones. These hormones regulate a large number of activities which include (1) energy transformation through an effect on oxygen consumption and heat production; (2) growth; (3) reproduction; (4) neuromuscular function; (5) skin and hair growth; and (6) cellular metabolism.

The body normally contains 20 to 30 mg. of iodine. About 60 per cent of it is in the thyroid gland and the rest is diffused throughout all tissues, especially in the ovaries, muscles and blood.

Metabolic Function. Iodine metabolism and thyroid hormone production are under neuroendocrine control. *A thyrotropin releasing hormone* (TRH) secreted by the hypothalamus stimulates the secretion of *thyrotropin* by the adenohypophysis. This hormone acts on the thyroid, causing it to increase the entrapment of iodide and production of *triiodotyrosine (T_3)* and *thyroxine (T_4).* Increasing levels of circulating T_3 and T_4 inhibit the release of additional TRH and thyrotropin and so provide a negative feedback control on the concentration of the hormones in the circulation.

Iodides are readily absorbed from the intestinal tract and rapidly transported in the blood stream to the thyroid gland, where they are oxidized to iodine and utilized in the production of the hormones. About one-third of the absorbed iodine is utilized by the thyroid gland, while two-thirds are excreted in the urine. Iodine in the feces comes mainly from the bile.

Recommended Dietary Allowances. The National Research Council has suggested that an intake of 100 to 300 μg./day is sufficient for all adults. Growing children, especially girls and pregnant or lactating women, need more, and therefore the RDA for these groups is higher.

Dietary Sources. Iodine occurs in extremely variable amounts in food and drinking water. Seafoods, such as clams, lobsters, oysters, sardines and other fish, are rich sources of iodine. Salt water fish contain 300 to 3000 μg I/kg. of flesh; fresh water fish contain 20 to 40 μg. The iodine content of cow's milk and of eggs is determined by the iodides available in the diet of the animal, and the iodides in vegetables vary according to the amount in the soil in which they are grown. Increased iodide in cow's milk may result from the use of solutions containing iodine to clean milking machines.

The best way to obtain an adequate intake of iodine is to use iodized salt (76 μg. iodine per gram of salt) in the cooking of food. Only about 50 per cent of the table salt sold in the United States is iodized. Mandatory iodization has been adopted by many nations. In Europe 10 μg./gm. of salt is used. The importance of iodized salt should still be emphasized to prevent recurrence of goiter. Other methods of increasing iodine intake (adding iodine to water supply and to tablets) have been tried in the iodine deficient areas and were found to be impractical.

An active antithyroid substance, a *goitrogen,* found in cabbage, rutabagas, turnips and peanuts, interferes with iodine utilization and can produce thyroid enlargement. It is doubtful that humans consume enough to affect thyroid activity, except under highly unusual conditions. Cooking inactivates goitrogens.

Deficiency. Lack of iodine intake is associated with the development of a type of thyroid gland dysfunction known as *colloid, endemic* or *simple goiter.* This condition formerly was especially prevalent in the geographical areas of the United States known as the "goiter belt"; in these areas iodine was lacking in the water and soils. The goiter belt includes

the Great Lakes region, Nebraska, the Dakotas, Colorado, Montana, Utah, Oregon and Washington (See Fig. 12–21). Nowadays, with the rapid transportation of food, the regular use of iodized salt and iodized fertilizers, iodine deficiency is unlikely in the United States population generally. Goiter is one of the most prevalent nutritional diseases in the underdeveloped countries, particularly in those regions far from the sea. (See Chapter 12 and Chapter 26.)

With a deficient intake of iodine, thyroid cells increase in size and the gland becomes hypertrophied. The condition is known as *simple goiter*. Hyperfunction of the gland results in a *toxic goiter*. Administration of radioactive iodine is the most commonly used test of thyroid function. At present, radioactive technetium is sometimes used because the radiation is weaker and, therefore, produces less tissue damage. Plasma T_3 and T_4 concentrations can also be measured.

Excess. Data on 35,999 persons in the Ten-State Nutrition Survey revealed a 3.1 per cent prevalence of thyroid enlargement. However, urinary excretion of iodine was also high. Two other surveys confirm high levels of urinary iodine excretion by the U.S. population, thus reflecting high iodine intake. A study of dietary frequency histories from 754 children, ages 9 to 16 years, revealed that milk and bread made with iodine dough conditioners and iodized salt are significant dietary sources of iodine.[12] Accumulating evidence of increased iodine intake has caused sufficient concern to initiate study of possible untoward reactions. A review of the literature and opinions of experts indicates that at this point, adverse reaction to iodine in foods is not a significant clinical or public health problem in the United States.

CHROMIUM

In 1957 Schwarz and Mertz postulated the existence of a new dietary component, *glucose tolerance factor* (GTF), that contained chromium as an active component. Brewer's yeast is the richest source of this factor. As additional information became available, it appeared that there were two categories of chromium compounds: the *GTF type with insulin potentiating activity,* and *simple compounds.* Data from animal studies demonstrated that simple chromium salts did not meet the criteria for an essential element. Neither does GTF meet the description of a typical trace element.

Work on GTF suggests that it is a low molecular weight substance which is water soluble, heat stable in solution, and associated with chromium. Mertz[18] suggested the following hypothesis: "Man has varying ability to synthesize GTF from inorganic chromium, niacin and amino acids, with the result that different subjects depend on preformed GTF to different degrees. The site of synthesis may be the intestinal flora or the liver. In response to acute increase of insulin in the blood, GTF is released and exerts its action, the potentiation of insulin at the target organs." Clearly, additional studies are needed to clarify the relationship between GTF and chromium.

Chromium deficiency has been described in three animal species and man. In rats the first sign of mild chromium deficiency is an impairment of glucose tolerance. Under strictly controlled environmental conditions, the rats develop a syndrome consisting of impaired growth, fasting hyperglycemia, glycosuria and elevated serum cholesterol.

The chromium content of the blood of adults and children ranges from 4 to 18 µg./l. Chromium is transported in the plasma in combination with transferrin. Plasma chromium does not reflect chromium status. Unlike other metals, once chromium is absorbed it is almost entirely excreted in the urine. Therefore, urine chromium is a rough estimate of status.

Inorganic chromium is poorly absorbed. The average intake of 50 to 100 µg./day of inorganic chromium from food and water supplies only 0.25 to 0.5 µg. of the 7 to 10 µg. excreted in the urine each day. In contrast, 10 to 25 per cent of the chromium in yeast extracts is absorbed. Table 7–6 shows the chromium content of

Table 7–6   CHROMIUM IN FOODS

FOOD	µG./GM.	µG./100 KCAL.
Vegetable oils		
Margarine, corn oil	0.23	2.56
Corn oil	0.12	0.33
Cotton seed oil	0.05	1.0
Safflower oil	0.07	0.8
Butter, unsalted	0.21	2.3
Grains		
Buckwheat	0.38	11.0
Wheat	0.03	0.8
Cereal Products		
All bran	0.25	8.1
Puffed rice	0.71	18.2
Wheat germ	0.07	2.0
Molasses	0.22	10.0

(Schroeder, H. A., Nason, A. P., and Tipton, I. H.: Chromium deficiency as a factor in atherosclerosis. J. Chronic Dis. *23*:123, 1970.)

selected foods. At the present state of technology, it is not possible to distinguish biologically available GTF from chromium and inorganic chromium. Refining whole wheat removes most of the chromium, since it is largely contained in the germ and the bran. Refining sugar results in a fractionation of the chromium into the molasses. Brewer's yeast is an excellent source. Fruits and vegetables contain trace amounts. Drinking water supplies variable amounts. Expert committees of the National Academy of Science and WHO feel data are insufficient to estalish a chromium requirement for man.

COBALT

Cobalt is unique in that it must be supplied entirely in its physiologically active form, vitamin B_{12}. This is the only known biological function of cobalt. It has been suggested that cobalt and manganese are necessary for the synthesis of thyroid hormone in rats, but studies to confirm this relationship are very scant.[32] Vitamin B_{12} is essential for the maturation of red blood cells and normal functioning of all cells. Deficiency of the vitamin produces a macrocytic anemia or pernicious anemia. However, in the case of pernicious anemia, deficiency results from a genetic defect rather than a dietary inadequacy: failure of the gastric mucosa to form a mucoprotein necessary for absorption of the vitamin.

Although earlier it was thought to be poorly absorbed, cobalt is now known to be well absorbed. Cobalt absorption is increased in patients with iron deficiency, portal cirrhosis with iron overload, and idiopathic hemochromatosis. Cobalt may share at least part of the same intestinal transport mechanism with iron that causes increased absorption in the latter mineral. The major route of excretion is the urine, with small amounts excreted in the feces, sweat and hair. Most of the cobalt in the body is found in the liver, the main storage organ, with some found in the spleen, kidneys and pancreas. About $1 \mu g$. per 100 ml. is found in the blood plasma.

The dietary requirement of cobalt is $1 \mu g$. per day in the form of vitamin B_{12}. There is not sufficient information upon which to base the requirement for cobalt itself. Neither animals nor plants can synthesize vitamin B_{12}. Ruminants are dependent upon the symbiotic relationship with the microorganisms of their gastrointestinal tract, which synthesize vitamin B_{12}. The microor-

ganisms of monogastric species, such as man, have an extremely limited capacity for synthesis in areas where the vitamin can be absorbed; therefore, humans get their B_{12} from animal foods. Organ meats, such as liver and kidneys which contain 0.15 to 0.25 ppm. of cobalt on a dry weight basis, are excellent sources. Muscle meats contain approximately half that amount. Oysters and clams are also excellent sources. Fruits, vegetables and cereals contain none of their cobalt as vitamin B_{12}. Strict vegetarians, who avoid all animal products, are known to become deficient; however, it may take 3 to 6 years for the deficiency to develop.

Excess. A high intake of inorganic cobalt in animal diets has been shown to produce polycythemia (overproduction of red blood cells), hyperplasia of bone marrow, reticulocytosis and increased blood volume. In view of the levels of cobalt required, this should be regarded as a pharmacological rather than a physiological effect.

ESSENTIAL MICRONUTRIENTS—AMOUNTS NEEDED FOR HUMANS CANNOT BE ESTIMATED AT PRESENT

SILICON

Until recently silicon was thought to be an environmental contaminant of human tissue. In 1972, however, Schwarz[24] reported significant increases in the rate of growth of rats receiving silicon supplementation over deficient controls. The same year Carlisle reported that silicon deficient chicks also were growth retarded and had bone deformities. More recent studies indicate a role for silicon in connective tissue metabolism as a crosslinking agent contributing to the stability of mucopolysaccharides and/or other components. Hyaluronic acid and chondroitin sulfate from the human umbilical cord contain high concentrations of bound silicon (78–329 μg./gm. of tissue). Human cartilage contains large amounts of bound silicon as chondroitin sulfate and keratin sulfate. There is a trend toward decreasing concentrations with age in the human dermis and aorta. With the development of atherosclerosis, the concentration of silicon in the arterial wall decreases.[4] Animal foods, with the exception of chicken skin, are poor sources of silicon; plant foods, particularly unrefined grains, contain large amounts of silicon. The most concentrated source of silicon is beer, which contains 1200 μg./gm. [20]

VANADIUM

Data from four laboratories on studies of two different species have established vanadium as an essential nutrient. Vanadium deficiency in rats and chicks produced reduced growth, poor reproductive performance, changes in hematological parameters, bone defects and alterations of lipid metabolism.

Based on the effects seen in animals, Hopkins and Mohr[7] have suggested that the most important effect to humans may be the influence on lipid metabolism. Vanadium deficient chicks had high plasma cholesterol and triglyceride levels. It is most likely that vanadium functions as an oxidation-reduction catalyst. Human intake has been established to be 2 mg. daily in a "well balanced diet" for a person weighing 75 kg. Little information is available on either vanadium requirements or on the vanadium content of foods. However, if man continues to refine his diet, the intake of trace elements in general will drop. A diet could contain less than 100 ng. of vanadium per gram of diet if intake were exclusively milk, meat and certain vegetables.

TIN

Until recently, the presence of tin in tissues was attributed to environmental contamination. However, the accuracy of early quantitative data is questionable because of the considerable loss of the metal during analytical procedures—a loss which has been noted only recently. Careful work by Schwarz and colleagues[25] demonstrated that tin produced an acceleration of growth in rats and met the standards for essentiality. As a member of the fourth main chemical group of elements, tin has many chemical and physical properties similar to those of carbon, silicon, germanium and lead. Tin is similar to carbon in its tendency to form truly covalent linkages. A large proportion of tin is found in the lipid extractable portion of commercial fats. Recently, tin has been shown to exert a potent induction effect on heme oxygenase, enhancing heme breakdown in the kidney and impairing heme-dependent cellular functions, such as cytochrome P–450 mediated drug biotransformation.

SELENIUM

Although toxic in high doses, selenium is an essential nutrient for some species. Selenium prevents the development of exudative diathesis in chicks and muscular dystrophy in lambs and calves, as well as a number of other diseases. Some of the disorders also respond to vitamin E (tocopherol), thus establishing a relationship between it and selenium. Other disorders are not corrected by tocopherol, showing there is a separate need for selenium.

There is little information available on the concentration of selenium in various human tissues. Based on limited information, the highest concentration is in the kidney; the next highest is in the liver. Concentration in the blood depends on intake and varies widely. Selenium values in people living in selenious areas may be tenfold higher than those of people living in a region where the soil is low in selenium. Children with kwashiorkor have low blood concentrations of selenium.

Selenium is an important constituent of *glutathione peroxidase* in erythrocytes; this enzyme protects against accumulation of hydrogen peroxide. The antioxidant effects of selenium and vitamin E may reinforce each other by overlap of remedial action. Selenium functions with tocopherol to protect cell and organelle membranes from oxidative damage, to facilitate union between oxygen and hydrogen at the end of the metabolic chain, to transfer ions across cell membranes and to aid in immunoglobulin and ubiquinone synthesis.

Patients with cancer have lowered plasma selenium levels. Statistical analysis of data has shown lower cancer mortality in those states with higher levels of selenium in forage crops and grains. Another hypothesis suggests that human heart disease is due in part to dietary inadequacy of selenium and vitamin E.

The selenium content of foods is dependent on the amount in the soil. A study of four composite diets from three Canadian cities showed they contained 191, 220, 113 and 115 μg. of selenium.[30]

Cereals contain the most selenium, with meat, poultry and fish, and dairy products following in decreasing concentration. Selenium may be lost from foods by washing, cooking and storing.

MANGANESE

In 1972 the first report of manganese deficiency in man appeared.[6] Until that time there was doubt that manganese deficiency could occur in humans. The symptoms were weight loss, transient dermatitis, occasional nausea and vomiting, changes in hair and beard color and slow growth of hair and beard. Studies of manganese deficiency in animals revealed ef-

fects on reproductive capacity, pancreatic function and other aspects of carbohydrate metabolism which may relate to its role with pyruvate carboxylase. There are 10 to 20 μg. of manganese in the adult human body. It tends to be high in tissues rich in mitochondria. Serum concentration is reported to range from 1 to 200 μg./liter.

The manganese content of foods also varies greatly. The richest sources are blueberries, wheat bran, dried legumes, nuts, lettuce, beet tops and pineapple. Animal tissues, seafood and dairy products are poor sources. Instant coffee and tea have relatively high amounts. Human milk is relatively deficient in manganese.

Mechanisms of absorption from the gastrointestinal tract are unknown, but there is a specific manganese-carrying plasma protein, *transmanganin*. Absorbed manganese appears rapidly in the bile and is excreted in the feces. Selective excretion rather than selective absorption appears to regulate tissue levels.

The manganous ion is known to be an activator of many enzymes. However, it is not possible at this time to correlate effects on dependent enzymes with the deficiency state. Manganese appears to be essential for sulfomucopolysaccharide biosynthesis. Abnormalities of cellular ultrastructure include an increase in the vascular portion of the cell, abnormal mitochondria, enlargement of the Golgi apparatus and disorganization of the rough endoplasmic reticulum. Changes in the latter two organelles are particularly significant since they are felt to be the sites of mucopolysaccharide synthesis.[2] Information regarding the relationship between manganese and various hormones, nucleic acids and therapeutic applications is just beginning to be studied. Animal studies have established the essentiality of manganese for reproduction: deficiency results in sterility in both sexes. The most striking effects of manganese deficiency are the skeletal abnormalities and ataxia of the offspring of deficient mothers.

Manganese toxicity has been seen in miners as a result of absorption of manganese through the respiratory tract after prolonged exposure to dust. The excess accumulates in the liver and central nervous system. Symptoms resemble those found in Parkinson's and Wilson's diseases.

NICKEL

The physiological role of nickel has not been elucidated, but there is evidence that nickel is essential for some animals.[19] The most likely roles for nickel are in some aspect of hormonal action, membrane phenomenon or enzyme activation. Changes in the concentration of several metal ions are associated with increases or decreases in hormonal secretion; however, it is not known whether hypothalamic releasing factors influence trace element concentration. Excessive levels of nickel cause an increase in the release of prolactin-inhibiting factor, which in turn decreases the in vitro release of prolactin from bovine and rat pituitary glands. Increased and deficient intake of nickel are both associated with reduced litter size. Impaired reproduction in swine maintained on a nickel deficient diet has also been reported. Nickel deficiency results in changes in the livers of the animal species studied thus far. These changes include ultrastructural degeneration and reduced oxidative ability of the liver, as well as abnormalities of the polysome profile.

Nickel is present in human blood, lung, pancreas, adrenal glands, brain, teeth, bone, kidney, aorta and skin. Nickel has been shown to be consistently present in ribonucleic acids (RNA). Increased amounts of nickel are present in several pathological conditions. Patients with cancer, myocardial infarction or thyrotoxicosis have increased blood levels. Increased blood and skin levels are seen in patients with psoriasis, photodermatitis and several forms of eczema. There is a decrease in blood nickel in patients with vitamin B_{12} deficiency. The reasons for changes in the circulating level of nickel in these, as well as other conditions, are not known. Good sources of dietary nickel appear to be grains and vegetables; however, there is the possibility that some of the nickel may not be bioavailable. Foods of animal origin contain relatively little nickel. It would appear that diets high in foods of animal origin or fats might be low in nickel.

MOLYBDENUM

Molybdenum has been shown to be an integral part of xanthine oxidase and has been implicated in aldehyde oxidase and sulfite oxidase activities. Xanthine oxidase, which also contains iron, is involved in the formation of uric acid from the purine xanthine and is important in the mobilization of ferritin iron from liver reserves. An interrelationship between molybdenum, copper and sulfate absorption has been demonstrated in livestock. Copper and molybdenum each prevent the uptake of excessive amounts of the other, but these actions require the presence of inorganic sulfate. Seelig

suggests that the high copper intake of people in the United States lowers molybdenum and iron absorption.[26] Molybdenum is found in minute amounts in the body, is readily absorbed from the gastrointestinal tract and is excreted mainly in the urine. The daily requirement is not known. It is widely distributed in commonly used foods such as legumes, whole-grain cereals, dark green leafy vegetables, milk and liver.

ADDITIONAL TRACE ELEMENTS

In addition to the above, other minerals may have specific essential physiological functions. Research and interest is ever growing. Cadmium may play a role in control of blood pressure. High levels have been found in the kidneys of patients with hypertension. In contrast to other non-essential trace elements, cadmium has a specific pattern of distribution. The kidney has ten times the concentration of the liver, which has five times more than any other organ. There are no known functions or needs for *aluminum, arsenic, boron,* or *bromine,* although these elements are found in animal and plant tissues. They seem to be harmless for man in their naturally occurring concentrations.

PROBLEMS AND SUGGESTED TOPICS FOR DISCUSSION

1. Keep a record of your food intake for 24 hours and evaluate the intake for foods high in iron and calcium. Make suggestions for improvement in selection.
2. Plan a diet for yourself, omitting milk and milk products, and check for adequacy of calcium.
3. What is the importance to the body of (a) iodine, (b) zinc, (c) potassium, (d) sodium, (e) sulfur, (f) magnesium?
4. Which minerals are most important in maintaining the electrolyte balance of the body? How is this accomplished?
5. Which nutrients are involved in the synthesis of hemoglobin?
6. Survey the literature and report on a mineral now under investigation for its importance to human nutrition.

CITED REFERENCES

1. Alvioli, V.: Intestinal absorption of calcium. Arch. Intern. Med., *129*:345, 1972.
2. Burch, R. E., Hahn, H. K., and Sullivan, J. F.: Newer aspects of the roles of zinc, manganese, and copper in human nutrition. Clin. Chem., *21*:501, 1975.
3. Caddell, J. L.: Magnesium in the nutrition of the child. Clin. Pediatr., *13*:263, 1974.
4. Carlisle, E. M.: Silicon as an essential element. Fed. Proc., *33*:1758, 1976.
5. Cole, S. K., et al.: Haematological characteristics and menstrual blood losses. J. Obstet. Gynecol., *79*:994, 1972.
6. Henkin, R. I.: Trace metals in endocrinology. Med. Clin. North Am., *60*:779, 1976.
7. Hopkins, L. L., and Mohr, H. E.: Vanadium as an essential nutrient. Fed. Proc., *33*:1773, 1974.
8. Hurley, L. S.: Trace elements and teratogenesis. Med. Clin. North Am., *60*:771, 1976.
9. Jones, K. L., et al.: Pattern of malformation of offspring of chronic alcoholic mothers. Lancet, *1*:1267, 1973.
10. Kay, R. G., et al.: A syndrome of acute zinc deficiency during total parenteral alimentation in man. Ann. Surg., *183*:331, 1976.
11. Kelley, W. A., Kesterson, J. W., and Carleton, W. W.: Myocardial lesions in the offspring of female rats fed a copper deficient diet. Exp. Mol. Pathol., *20*:40, 1974.
12. Kidd, P. S., et al.: Sources of dietary iodine. J. Am. Diet. Assoc., *65*:420, 1974.
13. Klevay, L. J.: The ratio of zinc to copper of diets in the United States. Nutr. Reports Int., *11*:237, 1975.
14. Lee, D. B., and Kleeman, C. R.: Phosphorus in man. McGaw Clinical Digest 5, No. 3, 1976.
15. Lutwak, L.: Continuing need for dietary calcium throughout life. Geriatrics, *29*:171, 1974.
16. Margen, S., et al.: Studies in calcium metabolism: I. The calciuretic effect of dietary protein. Am. J. Clin. Nutr., *27*:584, 1974.
17. Meneely, G. R. and Battarbee, H. D.: Sodium and potassium. Nutr. Rev., *34*:225, 1976.
18. Mertz, W.: Effects and metabolism of glucose tolerance factor. Nutr. Rev., *33*:129, 1975.
19. Nielsen, F. H., and Ollerich, D. A.: A new essential trace element. Fed. Proc., *33*:1767, 1974.
20. Nielsen, F. H., and Sandstead, H. H.: Are nickel, vanadium, silicon, fluoride and tin essential for man? A review. Am. J. Clin. Nutr., *27*:515, 1974.
21. Prasad, A. S., Halsted, J. A., and Nadimi, M.: Syndrome of iron deficiency anemia, hepatosplenomegaly, dwarfism, hypogonadism and geophagia. Am. J. Med., *31*:532, 1961.
22. Prasad, A. S., et al.: Zinc deficiency in sickle cell disease. Clin. Chem., *21*:582, 1975.
23. Purvis, G. A.: What nutrients do our infants really get? Nutr. Today, *8*:29, 1973.
24. Schwarz, K.: Recent dietary trace element research exemplified by tin, fluorine and silicon. Fed. Proc., *33*:1748, 1974.
25. Schwarz, K., Milne, D. B., and Vinyard, E.: Growth effect of tin compounds in rats maintained in a trace element controlled environment. Biochem. Biophys. Res. Commun., *40*:22, 1970.
26. Seelig, M. S.: Review: relation of copper and molybdenum to iron metabolism. Am. J. Clin. Nutr., *25*:1022, 1972.
27. Seelig, M. S., and Heggtveit, H. A.: Magnesium interrelationships in ischemic heart disease: a review. Am. J. Clin. Nutr., *27*:59, 1974.
28. Speckman, E. W., and Brink, M. F.: Relationship between fat and mineral metabolism—a review. J. Am. Diet. Assoc., *51*:517, 1967.
29. Spencer, H., Kramer, L., and Norris, C.: Calcium absorption and balance during high phosphorus intake in man. Fed. Proc., *34*:888, 1975.
30. Thompson, J. M., Erdoby, P., and Smith, D. C.: Selenium content of food consumed by Canadians. J. Nutr., *105*:274, 1975.
31. Todd, W. R., Elvehjem, C. H., and Hart, E. G.: Zinc in the nutrition of the rat. Am. J. Physiol., *107*:146, 1934.
32. Underwood, E. J.: Cobalt. Nutr. Rev., *33*:65, 1975.

ADDITIONAL REFERENCES

GENERAL

Burch, R. E., and Sullivan, J. F., (eds.): Trace Elements. Med. Clin. North Am., *60*(4), 1976.

Davidson, S., et al.: Human Nutrition and Dietetics. 6th ed. Edinburgh, Churchill Livingstone, 1975.

Goodhart, R. E., and Shils, M. E. (eds.): Modern Nutrition in Health and Disease. 5th ed. Philadelphia, Lea & Febiger, 1974.

Mertz, W., and Cornatzer, W. E. (eds.): Newer Trace Elements in Nutrition. New York, Marcel Dekker, 1971.

Prasad, A. S., and Oberleas, D. (eds.): Trace Elements in Health and Disease. Vol. I and II, New York, Academic Press, 1976.

Present Knowledge of Nutrition. 4th ed. New York, The Nutrition Foundation, 1976.

The Ten-State Nutrition Survey 1968–70. U.S. Dept. of Health, Education and Welfare, US DHEW Publication No. HSM 72–8130–4.

Underwood, E. J.: Trace Elements in Human and Animal Nutrition. 3rd ed. New York, Academic Press, 1971.

CALCIUM, PHOSPHORUS AND MAGNESIUM

Agriculture Handbook Number 456. U.S. Dept. of Agriculture, Washington, D.C., 1975.

Gershoff, S. M., and Andrus, S. B.: Dietary magnesium, calcium and vitamin B_6 and experimental nephropathies in rats: calcium oxalate calculi, apatite nephrocalcinosis. J. Nutr., *73*:308, 1963.

Tsang, R. C., Donovan, E. F., and Steichen, J. J.: Calcium physiology and pathology in the neonate. Pediatr. Clin. North Am., *23*:611, 1976.

SODIUM, POTASSIUM AND CHLORIDE

Committee on Nutrition, American Academy of Pediatrics. Pediatr., *53*:115, 1974.

Dahl, L. K.: Salt intake and salt need. N. Engl. J. Med., *258*:1122, 1958.

Seftel, H. C.: Early and intensive potassium replacement in diabetic acidosis. Diabetes, *15*:694, 1966.

IRON

The dietary iron controversy. Nutr. Today, *7*:2, 1972.

Forth, W., and Rummel, W.: Iron absorption. Physiol. Rev., *53*:724, 1973.

Moore, C. V.: Iron. In Goodhart, R. S., and Shils, M. E. (eds.): Modern Nutrition in Health and Disease. 5th ed. Lea & Febiger, 1974.

Wintrobe, M. M., et al.: Clinical Hematology. 7th ed. Philadelphia, Lea & Febiger, 1974.

FLUORINE

Bell, M. E., et al.: The Supply of Fluorine to Man in Fluorides and Human Health. WHO Monograph, No. 59, Geneva, Switzerland, 1970.

Reinhold, J. G.: Trace elements—a selective survey. Clin. Chem., *21*:476, 1975.

ZINC

Coble, Y. D., et al.: Zinc levels and blood enzyme activities in Egyptian male subjects with retarded growth and sexual development. Am. J. Clin. Nutr., *19*:415, 1966.

Hambidge, K. M., et al.: Low levels of zinc in hair, anorexia, poor growth, and hypogeusia in children. Pediatr. Res., *6*:868, 1972.

Henkin, R. I., and Bradley, D. F.: Hypogeusia corrected by nickel and zinc. Life Sci., *14*:701, 1970.

Murphy, E. W., Willis, B. W., and Watt, B. K.: Provisional tables on the zinc content of foods. J. Am. Diet. Assoc., *66*:345, 1975.

Prasad, A. S., and Oberleas, D.: Thymidine kinase activity and incorporation of thymidine into DNA of zinc deficient tissue. J. Lab. Clin. Med., *83*:634, 1974.

Tucker, S. B., et al.: Acquired zinc deficiency. JAMA, *235*:2399, 1976.

COPPER

Everson, G. J., Shrader, R. E., and Wang, T.: Chemical and morphological changes in the brains of copper deficient guinea pigs. J. Nutr., *96*:145, 1968.

Schenker, J. G., et al.: Serum copper and zinc levels in patients taking oral contraceptives, Fertil. Steril. 22:229, 1971.

IODINE

Owen, G. M., et al.: A study of nutritional status of preschool children in the United States, 1968–70. Pediatrics, *53*, Part II Supplement, April, 1974.

CHROMIUM

Mertz, W., et al.: Current knowledge of the role of chromium. Fed. Proc., *33*:2275, 1974.

Schroeder, H. A., Nason, A. P., and Tipton, I. H.: Chromium deficiency as a factor in atherosclerosis. J. Chronic Dis., *23*:123, 1970.

Schwarz, K., and Mertz, W.: Chromium III and the glucose tolerance factor. Arch. Biochem. Biophys., *85*:292, 1959.

SILICON

Carlisle, E. M.: In vivo requirement for silicon in articular cartilage and connective tissue formation in the chick. J. Nutr., *106*:478, 1976.

Schwarz, K.: Recent dietary trace element research, exemplified by tin, fluorine and silicon. Fed. Proc., *33*:1748, 1974.

VANADIUM

Hafey, Y., and Kratzer, F. H.: The effect of dietary vanadium on fatty acid and cholesterol synthesis and turnover in the chick. J. Nutr., *106*:249, 1976.

Nielsen, F. H., and Ollerich, D. A.: Studies on vanadium deficiency in chicks. Fed. Proc., *32*:929, 1973.

Schwarz, K., and Milne, D. B.: Growth effects of vanadium in the rat. Science, *174*:426, 1971.

TIN

Kappas, A. and Maines, M. D.: Tin: a potent inducer of heme oxygenase in kidney. Science, *192*:60, 1976.

Shamberger, R. J., et al.: Antioxidants and cancer. I. Selenium in the blood of normal and cancer patients. J. Natl. Cancer Inst., *50*:863, 1973.

Webb, J., et al.: Analysis by pattern recognition techniques of changes in serum level of fourteen metals after acute myocardial infarction. Exp. Mol. Pathol., *25*:322, 1976.

MANGANESE

Doisy, E. A.: Micronutrient control of biosynthesis of clotting proteins and cholesterol. In Hemphill, D. D. (ed.): Proceedings of the University of Missouri's 6th Annual Conference on Trace Substances in Environmental Health. Columbia, MO, University of Missouri Press, 1973.

Mena, I.: The role of manganese in human disease. Ann. Clin. Lab. Sci., *4*:487, 1974.

NICKEL

Nielsen, F. H., and Sandstead, H. H.: Are nickel, vanadium, silicon, fluorine and tin essential for man? A review. Am. J. Clin. Nutr., *27*:515, 1974.

Sunderman, F. W., Decsy, M. I., and McNeely, M. D.: Nickel metabolism in health and disease. Ann. N.Y. Acad. Sci., *199*:300, 1972.

MOLYBDENUM

Schroeder, H.: Essential trace metals in man: molybdenum. J. Chronic Dis., *23*:481, 1970.

CADMIUM

Schroeder, H. A.: Cadmium as a factor in hypertension. J. Chronic Dis., *18*:647, 1965.

Chapter 8

VITAMINS

Definition. *Vitamins* are a group of unrelated organic compounds needed only in minute quantities in the diet but essential for specific metabolic reactions within the cell and necessary for normal growth and maintenance of health. Many act as coenzymes or a prosthetic group of enzymes responsible for promoting essential chemical reactions. They are often called "accessory food factors" in view of the fact that they do not supply calories nor contribute appreciably to body mass. Animals fed on pure mixtures of carbohydrate, fat, protein, water, and minerals fail to grow properly and thrive because, as is now known, they lack vitamins. Vitamins vary widely in chemical structure and in their body functions. Some are relatively simple while others are quite complex. With a few exceptions the body cannot synthesize vitamins; they must be supplied in the diet or in addition to the diet. Certain vitamins (K, thiamin, folacin and B_{12}) to some extent may be formed by microorganisms in the intestinal tract, and it is known that vitamins A, choline and niacin can be formed if their precursors are supplied. Vitamin D can be synthesized in the skin upon exposure to sunlight. Considering new evidence it is becoming increasingly difficult to differentiate between those vitamins that can be partially synthesized by the body and hormones. They are somewhat similar in their organic structure and modes of action.

Function. Vitamins have different functions in various animal species. For the most part, this discussion will be restricted to the functions known for man and to the effects of deficiencies in man. Vitamins regulate metabolism, help convert fat and carbohydrate into energy, and assist in forming bones and tissues. Although a great deal is known about the vitamins, investigations continue to determine their biochemical structures and functions.

History. Vitamin investigation began with

the search for the unknown accessory dietary factors which would prevent or cure the classic deficiency diseases. People have died or have lived miserable existences in poor health because of vitamin deficiencies, and the solutions of such medical riddles as pellagra, scurvy, rickets, night blindness, and hemorrhagic disease of the newborn, to name a few, through the elucidation of the etiologic role of vitamin deficiencies in these diseases, are among the brightest chapters in medical and nutritional history.

With the possible exception of scurvy, the classic deficiency diseases have largely disappeared in the United States. They do, however, exist in a number of developing countries, either through a scarcity of food or ignorance of the basic food principles. The reader is urged to consult treatises on the development of vitamin knowledge for stimulating and interesting reading on vitamin history.[15, 17, 25, 28]

While history cites evidence as far back as the Egyptians that indicates a knowledge of vitamins, the modern story dates back only to the close of the nineteenth century. Eijkman in 1897 described a disease in chickens and pigeons resembling beriberi in man. He induced this disease by feeding milled rice exclusively. The symptoms could be cured by feeding the rice polishings. This recognition of the importance of other factors, besides carbohydrate, fat and protein, to promote healthy nutrition stimulated investigations by many workers and led to the modern concept of vitamins. Today approximately 20 vitamins are known or believed to be important to human well-being, and the existence of several more has been postulated.

Nomenclature. The term "vitamine,"

meaning a vital amine, was introduced by Funk (a Polish chemist working at the Lister Institute in London) in 1912 to designate the accessory food factors necessary to life. The final "e" has been dropped, since the chemical nature of these various substances has been proved and most of them are not amines.

The vitamins were originally named by letter or by their function. For example, vitamin B was commonly called the antineuritic or antiberiberi vitamin because it was found to be definitely useful in preventing the onset of these conditions. When it was found that the semi-purified materials contained several active substances, additional letters or numerical subscripts were used to identify the newly discovered vitamins. This led to some confusion. As each vitamin was isolated in pure form and its chemical structure determined specific names were assigned. At present the names are generally related to the chemical structure. The original names of some of the vitamins are still in use. See Table 8–1 for the current nomenclature of the original vitamins.

Classification. It is convenient to divide the vitamins into two groups on the basis of solubility: (1) the fat-soluble vitamins A, D, E and K, which are found in foods in association with lipids, and (2) the water-soluble vitamins B-complex and C. As more is being learned about the vitamins it is becoming apparent that the differences between these two groups concern more than just solubility. Although the modes of action of the fat-soluble vitamins are not nearly as clear as those for the water-soluble vitamins, it is evident that their activities are different from the coenzyme activities of water-soluble vitamins.

Recommended Dietary Allowances (RDA).

Table 8–1　NOMENCLATURE OF THE VITAMINS*

ORIGINAL NAME	CURRENT NAME
Vitamin A (anti-infective)	Vitamin A (retinol)
Vitamin B₁ (antiberiberi, antineuritic)	Thiamin (vitamin B₁)
Vitamin G (B₂)	Riboflavin
Pellagra preventative factor	Niacin (nicotinic acid, niacinamide)
Vitamin B-complex	Vitamin B₆ (pyridoxine)
	Vitamin B₁₂ (cyanocobalamin)
	Folacin (folic acid, pteroylglutamic acid)
	Pantothenic acid
	Biotin
Vitamin C	Ascorbic acid
Vitamin D	Vitamin D (calciferol)
Vitamin E	Vitamin E (α-tocopherol)
Vitamin K	Vitamin K (menaquinone and phylloquinones)

*Only those vitamins proved to be essential to human nutrition are listed here.

Much work has been done to determine requirements of vitamins for the various age groups and in circumstances of additional needs such as pregnancy and lactation. The National Research Council's Food and Nutrition Board has established desirable levels, as revised in 1974, for those vitamins whose requirements are known to be essential to healthy man. These are intended to apply to persons whose physical activity is considered "normal" (neither sedentary nor heavy physical activity) and living in a temperate climate, and to provide a safety margin for each vitamin over the minimal level that will normally maintain health. (See Table 10–1, Chapter 10.)

THE U.S. RDA (U.S. RECOMMENDED DAILY ALLOWANCE). There is a difference between the RDA established by the Food and Nutrition Board and the U.S. RDA established in 1973 by the Food and Drug Administration for the purpose of nutrition labeling of foods. In essence, the U.S. RDA represents the highest allowance of each nutrient for persons from 4 years of age through adult life, with the exception of pregnant or lactating women. See Chapter 10 for a complete explanation of the U. S. RDA and its use.

The possibility of biochemical individuality is being intensively studied at present, and there is enough evidence to indicate that it might exist. Applied to human nutrition and particularly vitamin requirements, it may mean that individuals have very different requirements for various nutrients. However, much more research is needed on this subject before it can be put to clinical use.

With every innovation enthusiasm usually runs high, and in the vitamin era virtually all ailments have been blamed at some time on a shortage of vitamins. Under these circumstances it is not surprising that the vitamins should become imbued in the minds of many lay and professional people with far-reaching therapeutic qualities which they do not possess. However, it is important that sight should not be lost of the nature of these substances and their highly specific role in human nutrition.

Vitamins taken in excess of the finite amount utilized in the metabolic processes are valueless, since they will have no substrate upon which to act. Excessive water-soluble vitamins are excreted, mainly in the urine, and an excessive intake of fat-soluble vitamins will result in increased storage, having little or no beneficial effect, but rather, taken to extreme, producing actual toxicity.

Vitamin Supplementation. There is no reliable evidence that vitamin supplementation increases immunity in the otherwise well-nourished individual, nor will there be that extra surge of energy so confidently expected by some when taking a multivitamin capsule. While certain vitamin requirements may be increased by prolonged muscular exertion, the extra vitamins will be automatically provided if the exertion is counterbalanced calorically by the consumption of a reasonably mixed diet. The routine vitamin supplementation of the diet, as a prophylactic measure, is not justified, except in the case where the diet is known to be chronically poor, unbalanced or composed in large part of processed and unenriched and unfortified foods.

A vast amount of money is expended annually on vitamin concentrates that might better be used for providing health-building foods. Healthy persons who eat well-balanced meals rarely require vitamins as medication. Clinically manifested vitamin deficiencies are uncommon in this country except in alcoholics, the very poor or in persons with gastrointestinal or mental diseases. However, there possibly could be more subclinical vitamin deficiency than we realize because tests for blood and tissue levels of nutrients are not well defined or used much.

Synthetic vs. Natural. There is no evidence for the claim of the superiority of natural vitamins over synthetic vitamins. The structure of the vitamin is the same regardless of whether it was made in a laboratory or by a plant or animal, and it performs the same functions. Although his body cannot tell the difference, the consumer can tell by the price of natural vitamins, which often is twice that of the synthetic vitamins. (See food fads, fallacies and quackery in Chapter 1.)

Standardization. The early method of determining the vitamin potency of a food was of necessity based upon the direct measurement of its biological activity in preventing or curing certain specific pathological conditions in a predetermined experimental animal. This is known as the *bioassay* method and expresses measurement in terms of units. At present, three vitamins are still thought of in terms of "units," namely, A, D and E. The unitage of these will be discussed subsequently. The other vitamins are discussed in terms of actual weight of material as determined by chemical or microbiological assay.

Stability. In general, the fat-soluble vitamins are fairly stable to ordinary cooking methods and are not lost in the cooking water.

On the other hand, the water-soluble vitamins may be destroyed by overcooking and are easily dissolved in cooking water. A good rule to follow is to avoid long cooking at high temperature in the presence of air, under alkaline conditions, and to use as little water as is feasible. Steaming or pressure cooking of vegetables is a good vitamin retaining habit. Washing, dicing and failure to store under refrigeration are among other factors that cause loss of vitamins.

The potency of vitamins is directly related to their length of storage time.

Terminology. *Avitaminosis* means "without vitamins" and is a term applied to severe vitamin deficiency. For example, in cases of severe or complete deficiency of B-complex, we speak of "avitaminosis B." Less severe grades of deficiency would be "deficiency of B-complex." On the other hand, it is now known that excessive intake of certain vitamins can cause clinical abnormalities, characteristic of *"hypervitaminosis."* Vitamin deficiencies will be discussed in Chapter 12, Nutritional Deficiency Diseases.

FAT-SOLUBLE VITAMINS

These vitamins are absorbed along with dietary fats, and conditions not favorable to normal fat uptake will also interfere with their absorption. They can be stored in the body to some extent and are not normally excreted in the urine. *Mineral oil* interferes with absorption, and if used it should be taken on rising or long enough after a meal to prevent interference with the utilization of the fat-soluble vitamins. Antibiotics and certain other drugs and various disease states such as malabsorption syndromes decrease the absorption of vitamins, especially fat-soluble vitamins, from the intestinal tract. (See Chapter 21.)

VITAMIN A (Retinol)

History. Vitamin A was the first fat-soluble vitamin to be recognized. Two groups of research workers, McCollum and Davis at the University of Wisconsin, and Osborne and Mendel at Yale University, made the discovery almost simultaneously in 1913. They found that young animals became unhealthy and failed to grow on diets lacking natural fats. They also observed that, following a lack of growth, the eyes became inflamed and infected (see Fig. 8–1, *A*) but could be quickly relieved by the addition to the diet of a natural fat, such as butter fat or cod liver oil (see Fig. 8–1, *B*). In 1924, Bloch, working in Denmark, demonstrated that *xerophthalmia* in children could be prevented by feeding them butterfat or cod liver oil.

Vegetable foods also had vitamin A activity which was found to be related to their content of *carotenes* and *cryptoxanthin,* yellow pigments frequently found in association with chlorophyll and largely responsible for the color of red and yellow vegetables. By 1932 it was found that the carotenes were precursors

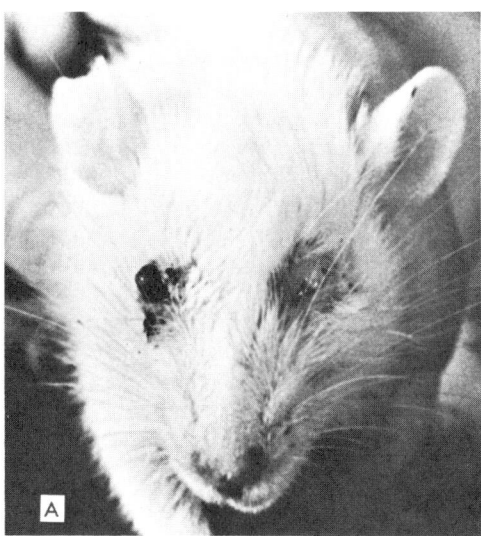
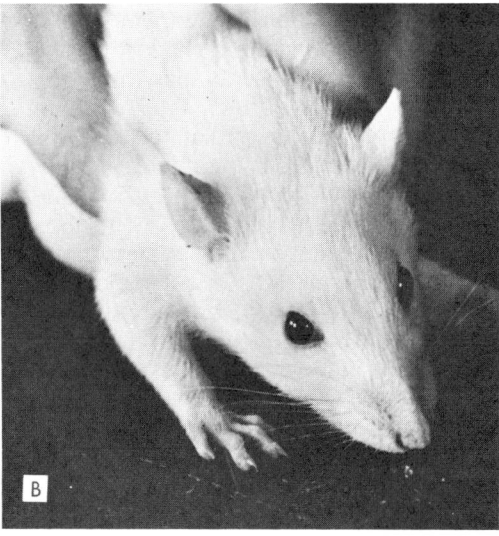

Figure 8–1 *A,* Typical eye condition produced by lack of vitamin A in the diet. *B,* Eyes restored to normal by feeding vitamin A. Three U.S.P. units (about 0.001 mg.) of vitamin A daily will cause resumption of growth and cure symptoms of vitamin deficiency in the white rat. (Courtesy of E. R. Squibb and Sons.)

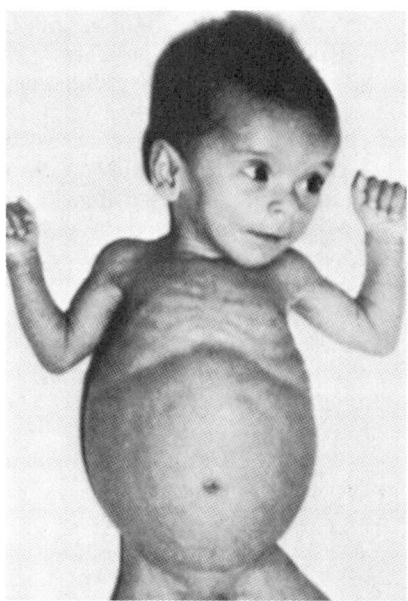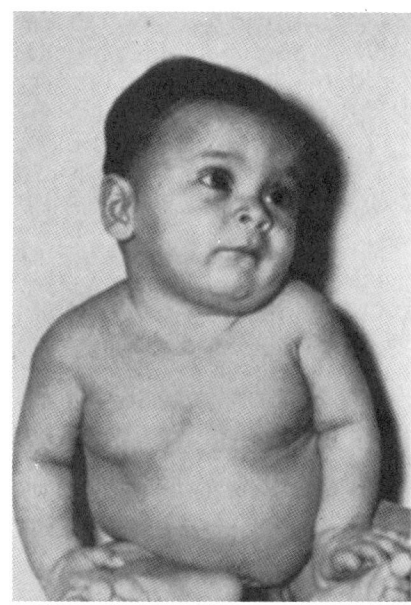

Figure 8–2 Malnutrition led to refractive errors in the eyes of this child from Bealback, Lebanon. Normal eye function returned when he was properly fed. (Courtesy of: Nutrition Today, March, 1968, p. 5.)

of vitamin A. *Beta carotene* was the most active, one molecule yielding two molecules of vitamin A; *alpha and gamma carotenes* yielded only one molecule of vitamin A, the other half of the carotene molecule being inactive. Carotene is referred to as a provitamin. Animals cannot synthesize it but can convert it to vitamin A. The human dietary includes not only the provitamin but the vitamin itself *preformed*, from animal foods and fish oils.

Chemistry and Utilization. Vitamin A has been isolated in pure form as pale yellow crystals which are fat-soluble and has been synthesized chemically. The condensed formula, $C_{20}H_{29}OH$ indicates that it is an alcohol. It has been named *retinol* because it has a specific function in the retina of the eye. Natural vitamin A usually is found esterified with a fatty acid (usually palmitic acid). Metabolically active forms of the vitamin include the corresponding aldehyde and acid *(retinoic acid).*

Absorption. The dietary vitamin A esters are hydrolyzed in the lumen of the small intestine to form retinol. Retinol passes across the mucosal cell wall where it is again esterified and is carried as retinyl ester to the liver where it is stored. Carotenoids are partially absorbed as such from the intestine and contribute to the yellow color of the blood serum. Most of the carotene is converted in the intestinal mucosa to *retinal* (vitamin A aldehyde). Both liver and intestinal mucosa have enzymes which catalyze reduction of the aldehyde to the alcohol.

Vitamin A and the carotenoids are fat-soluble. Therefore the factors which affect the absorption of the fat (bile salts, lipases, etc.) affect their absorption. In the blood stream vitamin A is transported with the lipids in the form of chylomicrons and lipoproteins in the lymph. It then enters the blood stream and is carried to the liver. Mobilization of retinol from the liver depends on adequate dietary protein since it has to be bound to retinol binding protein (RBP) to be carried in the blood.

Inadequate vitamin A and protein are probably two of the most common causes of malnutrition in the world today and the two deficiencies frequently occur together. It has been shown that protein deficient children afflicted with kwashiorkor have a vitamin A deficiency[5] also (Fig. 8–2).

Stability. Vitamin A is rather stable to light and heat, but prolonged heating in contact with air destroys it. It is easily destroyed by oxidation and ultraviolet light. A cool atmosphere and refrigeration tend to preserve it. Vitamin E may be used with vitamin A to prevent oxidation.

Measurement. The *international unit* (I.U.) of vitamin A activity was originally defined as the amount required per day to promote growth in a white rat receiving an otherwise vitamin A-free diet. This may now be expressed in chemical terms as 0.300 μg. of crystalline vitamin A alcohol. The unit for B-carotene is 0.6 μg. Thus dietary carotene has only about one-

half the activity of vitamin A. However, because of the poorer absorption of the provitamins as compared to retinol, the measurement of vitamin A activity in the diet as I.U. constantly had to be qualified as being from provitamins or retinol itself. In 1967 an FAO/WHO Expert Committee recommended that vitamin A activity be stated as an equivalent weight of retinol (retinol equivalents) and not as I.U., which is a measure of vitamin A activity regardless of its absorption. For example, 1 retinol equivalent is equal to 1 μg. of retinol, 6 μg. of β-carotene or 12 μg. of other provitamin carotenoids. (See Table 8–2). The Food and Nutrition Board of the NRC/NAS adopted this recommendation and the RDA for vitamin A is stated in I.U. and in R.E. until the change over to R.E. is complete.

Recommended Dietary Allowance. The requirement appears to be proportional to body weight. Levels of intake which provide 20 I.U. (6 μg.) of preformed vitamin A per kg. of body weight, or 40 I.U. (24 μg.) of beta carotene, have been demonstrated to meet minimal requirements. The male adult recommended allowance of 5000 I.U. daily assumes an intake evenly divided between preformed vitamin A (2500 I.U.) and vitamin A precursors (2500 I.U.). This translates into the new RDA of 1000 R.E. The RDA for women is lower (4000 I.U., 800 R.E.) to allow for smaller body size. Both are about twice that required to meet the minimal needs. During pregnancy 5000 I.U. (1000 R.E.) are recommended, and during lactation 6000 I.U. (1200 R.E.). Children need 1400 to 5000 I.U. (420 to 1000 R.E.) daily, the amount increasing with age from infancy to 14 years.

In the United States, according to the Food and Nutrition Board,[32] approximately 50 per cent of the vitamin A intake is in the form of the provitamin (carotene). Data on vitamin A status from the U.S. Ten-State Nutrition Survey, 1968–70, revealed that in the low income populations studied, there was a relatively high prevalence of low plasma vitamin A levels in children. This was most marked in the Spanish-American population.[37] Serum levels of vitamin A for healthy adults are about 30 to 65 μg. per 100 ml. (100 to 200 I.U. per 100 ml.), levels of 20 μg. per 100 ml. or less being indicative of marginal vitamin A status. Because vitamin A is stored, serum vitamin levels do not reflect recent vitamin A intake. Serum carotenoid level would more accurately reflect this. Serum carotenoid levels range from 80 μg. to 225 μg. per 100 ml.

Function. VISION. Vitamin A is essential to the integrity of night vision, being a constituent of the *visual purple (rhodopsin)* of the retina, which is necessary for normal dim light vision. The elucidation of the biochemical role of vitamin A in the visual system is a result largely of the investigations of Wald and his co-workers. *Retinal* is a prosthetic group of photosensitive pigment of both the rods (rhodopsin) and cones (iodopsin). The reaction involves the oxidation-reduction systems of retinol-retinal and stereochemical changes of the vitamin A molecule. When there is a deficiency of vitamin A the rods and cones cannot adjust to light changes, resulting in night blindness. An injection of vitamin A corrects this condition within a matter of minutes. Color blindness and other defects of vision cannot be cured by vitamin A.

GROWTH AND BONE DEVELOPMENT. Vitamin A is necessary for growth and development of skeletal and soft tissues through its effect upon protein synthesis and differentiation of the bone cells. It appears that the active metabolite in this capacity is retinoic acid and not retinol. A normal intake of vitamin A helps to provide for normal bone development. It also affects tooth formation in early life by being necessary for enamel-forming epithelial cells.

EPITHELIAL TISSUE DEVELOPMENT AND MAINTENANCE. Vitamin A also plays a role in the maintenance of normal epithelial structures. It is necessary in the differentiation of basal cells into mucous secreting epithelial cells. A deficiency of this vitamin is accompanied by keratinization of the mucous membranes which line the respiratory tract, the alimentary canal and the urinary tract, and by keratinization of the body skin and epithelium of the eye, which lowers the protective barrier role played by these membranes in protection of the body against infection. Thus, a ready entry for infections is provided. It is from this function that vitamin A has become known as the *anti-infective vitamin.* Actually, vitamin A

Table 8–2   RETINOL EQUIVALENTS

1 retinol equivalent = 1 μg. retinol
= 6 μg. β-carotene
= 12 μg. other provitamin A carotenoids
= 3.33 I.U. vitamin A activity from retinol
= 10 I.U. vitamin A activity from β-carotene

Table 8–3   VITAMIN A CONTENT OF
            SOME FOODS

FOOD	I.U.
Liver, beef, 100 gm.	43,900
Carrots, raw, 1	11,000
Sweet potato, baked, 1 sm.	8,100
Spinach, cooked, ½ cup	7,300
Apricots, dried, 8 lg. halves	5,500
Squash, winter, ½ cup	4,200
Cantaloupe, ¼ melon	3,400
Broccoli, 1 stalk	2,500
Crab, 100 gm.	2,170
Peach, 1 med.	1,330
Halibut, 125 gm.	850
Egg yolk, 1	580
Milk, whole, 1 cup	370
Cheese, cheddar, 1 oz.	370
Orange, 1 med.	300
Butter, 1 tsp.	165
Margarine, fortified, 1 tsp.	165
Apple, 1 med.	140
Peanuts, raw, 100 gm.	16

has nothing to do with an already present infection, but its lack sets up conditions whereby infection can more easily occur.

The keratinization related to the eye is known as *xerophthalmia*. If treatment is initiated early and is adequate (25,000 I.U. vitamin A daily) the pathological changes of xerophthalmia may be remedied. Otherwise, partial or complete blindness may result. Xerophthalmia is a major cause of blindness in developing countries.

REPRODUCTION. Animal studies have shown that vitamin A intake must be increased above that required for good growth in order to assure normal reproduction and lactation. Although the role of vitamin A in reproduction is not clear, it may be an involvement in steroid hormone synthesis or a more basic role in cellular differentiation.

The role of vitamin A in normal human metabolism continues to challenge clinicians and biochemists. It must be involved in some fundamental function in most tissues but the nature of this function still is not known. It is probably unrelated to the retinal-retinol interconversion of the visual pigments, since in some, but not all, tissues retinoic acid (which cannot be reduced to retinal) is active.

Storage.   The liver is considered the storage site of vitamin A, with small amounts in the fat depots, lungs, and kidneys. Through the years the liver accumulates a reserve supply which reaches its peak in adult life. Approximately 90 per cent of the vitamin A in the body is stored in the liver. This savings account of vitamin A in the system may be drawn upon if in any emergency the vitamin is wanting in the diet. This storage capacity allows for a less than daily intake of vitamin A.

Dietary Sources.   The dietary sources of *preformed vitamin A* are chiefly liver, kidney, butter and fortified margarine, egg yolk, whole milk and cream, cheese made with whole milk or cream and fortified skim milk. The *carotene* forms are found in dark green, leafy and yellow vegetables (collards, turnip greens, carrots, sweet potatoes, squash) and yellow fruit (apricots, peaches, cantaloupe). The deeper the green or the yellow of a vegetable, the more carotene (provitamin A) it contains. Cod and halibut fish oils are usually sources for therapeutic doses of vitamin A. (See Table 8–3.)

Deficiency.   If the diet is inadequate in vitamin A, a primary deficiency may occur. "Secondary" or "conditioned" deficiencies occur when (1) a bodily dysfunction interferes with the absorption or storage of vitamin A (as in ulcerative colitis, cirrhosis of the liver, obstruction of the bile duct); (2) a disorder interferes with the conversion of carotene to vitamin A (as in diabetes mellitus, hypothyroidism); and (3) any rapid bodily loss of vitamin A takes place (pneumonia, hyperthyroidism, scarlet fever and some respiratory infections in children). (See Chapter 12 for vitamin A deficiency disorders.)

Toxicity.   In normal doses no toxic effects are observed. *Hypervitaminosis A* has been observed in adults and children taking in excess of 50,000 I.U. per day for several years, or in the case of the synthetic water soluble form, 18,500 to 60,000 I.U. for a period of months. It has been noted to stunt growth or has left one leg two to three inches shorter than the other. The difference in leg length usually develops because the child tends to favor whichever leg becomes more painful. Transient hydrocephalus and vomiting are the prominent symptoms in children receiving overdoses of vitamin A. Bone fragility, thickening of long bones and deep bone pain, loss of appetite, coarsening and loss of hair, scaly skin eruptions, enlargement of the liver and spleen, irritability, double vision and skin rashes are among the symptoms of prolonged, excessive intake. (See Table 8–4.) Portal hypertension and ascites with cirrhotic-like changes have also been reported in two adults taking over 100,000 I.U. per day for eight years.[34] Toxicity can easily develop in an adolescent taking

Table 8–4　SIGNS OF VITAMIN A TOXICITY

Serum vitamin A of 250–6600 I.U./100 ml.
Bone pain and fragility
Hydrocephalus and vomiting (infants and children)
Dry, fissured skin
Brittle nails
Hair loss (alopecia)
Gingivitis
Cheilosis
Anorexia
Irritability
Fatigue
Hepatomegaly and abnormal liver function
Ascites and portal hypertension

25,000 to 50,000 I.U. per day for treatment of acne. If vitamin A toxicity is detected and stopped in time, the symptoms disappear in a few days after the vitamin is withdrawn, although this may take longer depending on the amount of vitamin A that has been ingested and the extent of the liver stores of vitamin A.

Hypercarotenemia from the ingestion of large amounts of foods containing carotene merely results in deposition of carotene in tissues, particularly the skin and eyes, and gives the person a disturbing yet harmless orange appearance.

VITAMIN D (Calciferol)

History.　The isolation of vitamin D was delayed because of its confusion for a time with vitamin A. Both of these vitamins are fat-soluble; hence, they occur together in nature. Since the Middle Ages cod liver oil has been used as a remedy for rickets, but not until the period of World War I was the cause of rickets and the scientific basis for its cure established. Mellanby produced bone development characteristic of rickets in dogs, and demonstrated that it was related to the anticalcifying effect of some cereals. It was next found that this abnormal development could be counteracted by a fat-soluble factor which McCollum separated from vitamin A in 1922. In 1924 Steenbock and Hess independently and simultaneously discovered that ultraviolet irradiation gave antirachitic properties to certain foods. In 1930 vitamin D was isolated in crystalline form and named *calciferol*. In 1936 Windaus demonstrated that the natural prehormone found in the skin which becomes calciferol on ultraviolet irradiation was 7-dehydrocholesterol. In 1968 Blunt, De Luca and Schnoes discovered that the metabolically active form of vitamin D was not calciferol but 25-hydroxycholecalciferol, which was synthesized in the body from calciferol. Since this time, more metabolites have been found and the metabolism of vitamin D has been clarified more every year.

Sources.　Vitamin D can be acquired either as *preformed vitamin D* by ingestion or by exposure to sunlight. It is found in only small and highly variable amounts in butter, cream, egg yolk and liver. The best food sources are the fish liver oils. In recent years approximately 98 per cent of all fluid milk[31] has been fortified with vitamin D, usually 400 I.U. per quart. Most dried whole milk and evaporated milk are fortified as well as some margarines, butter, certain cereals and infant formula products. (See Table 8–5.) Vitamin D_3 is formed in the body by the *action of sunlight* (ultraviolet rays) on 7-dehydrocholesterol in the skin. Since the provitamin can be synthesized in the body and needs only sunlight as an activator, classification of the active compound as a vitamin is not strictly accurate. In fact, now that we better understand its formation and functions it might more appropriately be called a prohormone; its active metabolite is a hormone.

Table 8–5　VITAMIN D CONTENT OF UNFORTIFIED FOODS (INTERNATIONAL UNITS/100 G. UNLESS OTHERWISE STATED)

Butter	35
Cheese	12–15
·Cream	50
Egg yolk	25 I.U./average yolk
Halibut	44
Herring	
Fresh, raw	315
Canned	330
Liver	
Beef, raw	9–42
Calves, raw	0–15
Lamb, raw	17–20
Pork, raw	44–45
Chicken, raw	50–67
Mackerel	
Fresh, raw	1100
Milk	
Cow's	0.3–4 I.U./100 ml.
Human	0–10 I.U./100 ml.
Oysters	5 I.U./3–4 medium-sized
Salmon	
Fresh, raw	154–550
Canned	220–440
Sardines	
Canned	1150–1570
Shrimp	150

(From Avioli, L. V. In Improved vitamin D bone therapy. *Med. World News*, October 19, 1973, p. 34.)

Stability. Vitamin D is remarkably stable, and preparations or foods containing it can be warmed or kept for long periods without its deterioration.

Chemical and Physical Properties. There are at least 11 sterols with vitamin D activity but only those called D_2 and D_3 are of practical importance. *Ergosterol,* a plant sterol closely related to cholesterol in structure is provitamin D_2 and *7-dehydrocholesterol* is provitamin D_3. They are converted to the active form by irradiation with ultraviolet light. *Ergocalciferol (D_2)* is prepared commercially for use as a vitamin supplement. *Cholecalciferol (D_3)* is the form synthesized in animal tissues. It is the chief form in the fish oils.

Measurement. The International Unit of vitamin D is the equivalent of $0.025 \mu g.$ of pure calciferol (D_2), produced by irradiation of ergosterol, and is based on certain biological activities in the rat. For all practical purposes, the U.S.P. unit and I.U. are identical.

Absorption and Storage. Ingested vitamin D is absorbed with the fats from the intestine with the aid of bile. Vitamin D from the skin is absorbed into the blood stream. Both are carried in the blood stream to the liver and transformed into the active form. Storage sites of vitamin D and its active forms are the liver, skin, brains, bones, and probably other tissues.

Function. Vitamin D is essential for normal growth and development and is important for the formation of normal bones and teeth. Vitamin D, along with parathormone and thyrocalcitonin, has an important role in the maintenance of the rather narrow range of serum calcium and phosphorus levels, in the growth and mineralization of the bones of children, and in the maintenance of mineralization of bones of the adult. In accordance with this overall purpose, vitamin D has the following functions:

1. It stimulates the active, energy-requiring intestinal absorption of calcium.
2. It stimulates the active phosphate-transport system in the intestine.
3. In conjunction with parathormone it acts to mobilize calcium from previously formed bone in order to maintain proper serum calcium levels.
4. It mobilizes phosphate from bone in order to maintain serum phosphate levels.
5. In a minor way, it acts to increase the reabsorption of calcium by the kidney. Ninety-nine per cent of calcium in renal filtrate is reabsorbed anyway, and vitamin D only affects the other one per cent.
6. It increases renal tubular reabsorption of phosphate.

Metabolism. Tracer studies indicate that vitamin D_3 is converted in the liver to the biologically active metabolite 25–hydroxycholecalciferol (25–OHD_3 or 25–HCC), which is five times as potent as vitamin D_3. It appears that the blood level of 25–OHD_3 is maintained at a constant level regardless of vitamin D intake, and as more is needed it is released by the liver. The most active form of vitamin D_3, though, is 1,25–$(OH)_2D_3$. It is produced by the kidneys, which convert 25–OH-D_3 to 1,25–dihydroxycholecalciferol (1,25–$(OH)_2D_3$). It is ten times as potent as vitamin D_3 and is the form which is presently thought to act on the intestine to increase calcium and phosphate absorption and on the bone to increase calcium and phosphate mobilization. (See Fig. 8–3.)

If 1,25–$(OH)_2D_3$ is produced by the kidney, then it could be termed a hormone, with the intestine and bone as the target organs. In fact, it has been shown that similar to a hormone, its synthesis is *feedback regulated* by the level of serum calcium and phosphorus. A low serum calcium results in increased production of

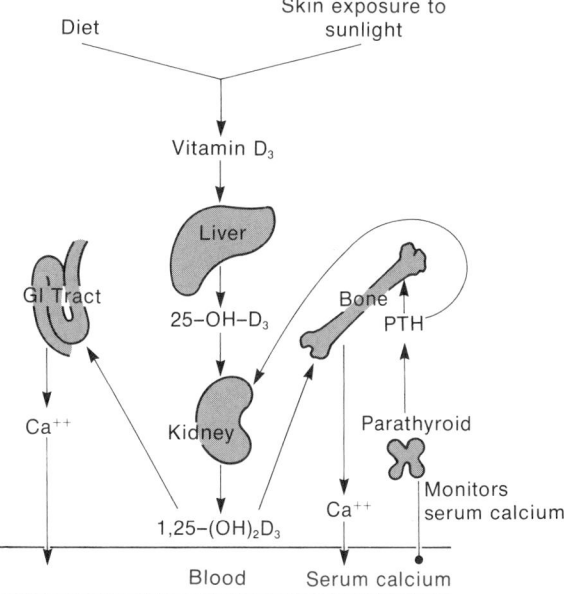

Figure 8–3 The metabolism and functions of vitamin D. Vitamin D_3 (cholecalciferol) is changed to its biologically active forms, 25-OHD$_3$ and 1,25-$(OH)_2D_3$. 1,25-$(OH)_2D_3$ acts on the intestine to increase calcium absorption and on the bones to increase calcium resorption.

1,25–$(OH)_2D_3$, a hypercalcemic effect and less synthesis of 24,25–$(OH)_2D_3$, another metabolite found in the blood. (The function of this metabolite is not clear at present.) When the serum calcium approaches normal, the synthesis of 1,25–$(OH)_2D_3$ is stopped and that of 24,25–$(OH)_2D_3$ stimulated. It appears that parathyroid hormone, which is released in response to low serum calcium, is the mediator that stimulates the production of 1,25–OH_2D_3 by the kidney in response to a low serum calcium level. Thus it is proposed that the level of calcium in the diet affects serum calcium, which in turn affects PTH secretion, and PTH controls kidney synthesis of 1,25–$(OH)_2D_3$. The intestine is then acted upon by 1,25–$(OH)_2D_3$, which increases absorption of calcium and acts on the bone to increase calcium mobilization. In fact, rats on low calcium diets produce large amounts of 1,25–$(OH)_2D_3$ and have a high efficiency of absorption of calcium, while rats on high-calcium diets have less 1,25–$(OH)_2D_3$ production and less calcium absorption efficiency. Dietary phosphate has a similar effect on 1,25–$(OH)_2D_3$ production, but does not require the intermediate action of parathyroid hormone. When dietary phosphate, and thus serum phosphate, are low, 1,25–$(OH)_2D_3$ production is stimulated and acts to stimulate the intestinal phosphate-transport system to be more efficient in absorption. It also acts to mobilize phosphate from bone.

In summary, for proper calcium and phosphorus homeostasis, functioning kidneys and intestine, parathormone, calcitonin, and adequate dietary calcium, phosphorous, and vitamin D are required.

Deficiency. Vitamin D is needed to prevent and to cure *rickets,* a disease formerly prevalent in infants and children, associated with malformation of bones due to deficient deposition of calcium phosphate (hydroxyapatite). In rickets the bones are not strong and rigid and cannot stand the ordinary stresses and strains expected of them, so that knock-knees, bowlegs, pigeon breast, and frontal bossing of the skull appear. When a deficiency of vitamin D occurs, and calcium is not well absorbed, the renal threshold for phosphate excretion is lowered and more phosphate than normal is excreted in order to maintain a balance between calcium and phosphorus in the blood. In the adult, the equivalent disease is *osteomalacia,* in which, however, there is a decalcification of the bone shafts and the tendency is for fractures rather than bending to occur.

With the discovery of the need for and function of vitamin D, the incidence of rickets and osteomalacia from vitamin D deficiency has dropped remarkably in the past generation. *Renal rickets,* caused by a certain type of kidney disease and altered calcium metabolism and *vitamin D resistant rickets* are not due to a deficient intake of vitamin D, but rather to an inability of the liver or kidney to synthesize the active metabolite. (See Chapter 12 for vitamin D deficiency disorders and Chapter 30 for a discussion of renal rickets.)

Toxicity. It is known that hypervitaminosis D can occur and cause pathological changes in the body when vitamin D is taken in excess. These changes consist of an exaggeration of the normal changes produced by the vitamin, namely excessive calcification of bone, and metastatic calcification (calcification elsewhere in the body). It encourages the formation of kidney stones. Headache, nausea and diarrhea may be the subjective findings. Infants given excessive amounts of vitamin D may suffer gastrointestinal upsets, calcification of soft tissues (kidney and lungs), bone fragility, retarded growth and mental retardation. However, these difficulties appear only with enormous doses given over an extended period of time, and the usual doses available in vitamin preparations are not likely to be harmful. (See Table 8–6.)

HYPERCALCEMIA. Excessive quantities of vitamin D (1000 to 3000 I.U. per kg. per day for children and adults) and hypersensitivity to vitamin D may lead to hypercalcemia (excess calcium in the blood). It can be cured if recognized in time, by medication and omitting vitamin D from the diet. A few infants who receive excessive amounts in association with a liberal calcium intake suffer this syndrome.

Because present intake of vitamin D seems to be more than adequate for the U.S. population, it has been recommended that fortification of foods other than those already standardly

Table 8–6   SIGNS OF VITAMIN D TOXICITY

Excessive calcification of bone
Kidney stones
Metastatic calcification of soft tissues
  (kidney and lung)
Hypercalcemia
  Headache
  Weakness
  Nausea and vomiting
  Constipation
  Polyuria
  Polydipsia

Table 8–7   VITAMIN D—AVERAGE DAILY
INTAKE AND CONTRIBUTING SOURCES

AGE OF SUBJECT (Yr.)	TOTAL (I.U.)	SOURCE		
		Vitamins (I.U.)	Milk (I.U.)	Foods* (I.U.)
0–1	462	201	257	4
2–5	660	283	309	68
6–8	532	146	280	106
9–11	578	151	276	151
12–14	579	92	308	179
15–17	477	0	367	110
All	547	145	300	102

*Other than milk.
(From Pale, A. E., and Lowenberg, M. E.: Consumption of vitamin D in fortified and natural foods and in vitamin preparations. J. Pediatr., 70:952, 1967.)

fortified (milk and margarine) be reduced or discontinued. (See Table 8–7.)

Recommended Dietary Allowance.   The normal adult is presumed to obtain sufficient vitamin D from exposure to sunlight and from the incidental ingestion of small amounts with food, such as fish and vitamin D fortified milk. The need for supplemental vitamin D by vigorous adults is believed unnecessary unless they are shielded from sunlight, as in the case of persons living in smoggy sunless areas; wearing clothes which cover the body; working at night and staying indoors as elderly persons may do. In these special cases a small daily supplement of vitamin D is believed desirable. The Food and Nutrition Board, National Research Council, sets the daily allowance of vitamin D at 400 international units as sufficient to meet the requirements of practically all healthy individuals who have no exposure to ultraviolet light. When the milk intake is one quart the 400 international units allowance for infants is provided. Because of more access to sunlight and various food sources of vitamin D, the requirement is more difficult to determine beyond infancy. For women during pregnancy and lactation, adequate vitamin D is needed to promote efficient use of the increased calcium and phosphorus in the diet. The optimum amount of vitamin D is not known, but on the basis of available evidence 400 units is recommended.

It must be emphasized that no good will come from the provision of adequate vitamin D unless the calcium and phosphorus requirements are met also. In cases of vitamin D deficiency, "therapeutic dosages" are needed, namely, 1500 to 2500 I.U. daily for several months.

VITAMIN E (Tocopherol)

History.   Vitamin E was first discovered by Evans and Bishop in 1922 when they found that rats reared on a basic diet failed to reproduce. In 1924 Sure gave it the name of vitamin E or antisterility vitamin. Evans, Emerson and Emerson isolated it from the unsaponifiable fraction of wheat germ oil in 1936, and it was chemically identified in 1938 and named tocopherol [*tokos* (Gr) = offspring].

Chemistry.   Four different tocopherols have been identified (alpha, beta, gamma, delta). They are oily yellow liquids, insoluble in water but soluble in fat solvents. They are stable to heat. Their most important chemical characteristic is their antioxidant property. Of the four tocopherols, alpha is the most active biologically. This may be related to better absorption from the intestine.

Function.   The function of vitamin E at the molecular level in the biological processes of the body is not fully determined.

ANTIOXIDANT FUNCTIONS.   That it acts *in vitro* as a lipid antioxidant is well documented. It serves to prevent the formation of peroxides from polyunsaturated fatty acids, thus preventing the oxidation of the unsaturated fats. Vitamin E also helps to enhance the activity of vitamin A by preventing its oxidation and loss of activity in the intestinal tract. Vitamin C in foods is similarly protected when vitamin E is present.

Vitamin E appears to protect the cell membranes from deterioration caused by lipid peroxidation. When insufficient vitamin E is present, the amount of unsaturated fats in the cells decreases. This causes abnormal structure and function of the mitochondria and the lysosomes. This ability of vitamin E to protect the membrane lipid has been related to aging, which is also characterized by cell membrane deterioration from lipid peroxidation. Vitamin E appears to control some of these processes. A theory relating vitamin E, selenium, glutathione peroxidase, cystine and polyunsaturated fats in the cell membrane has been proposed. While adequate levels of vitamin E appear to protect the organism from excessive oxidative damage, there is no evidence to say that increased amounts will prevent or delay the aging process.

It has also been postulated that the antioxidant properties of vitamin E may have a protective effect for lung tissue exposed to ozone, an oxidant in smog. At present, this has only been demonstrated in rats, and more information is

needed regarding its applicability to human populations.

While some authorities feel that the functions of vitamin E are only those of an antioxidant, there are others who feel that vitamin E has additional non-oxidant functions. Some of these specific functions will be discussed.

SPECIFIC FUNCTIONS. Increased hemolysis, megaloblastic anemia and creatinuria are found in some children with kwashiorkor and in vitamin E–deficient monkeys. The addition of vitamin E induced a reticulocyte response and urinary excretion of creatine decreased. Newborn infants have low tissue concentrations of vitamin E because of little transfer across the placenta. A hemolytic anemia has been noted in infants, especially premature infants who have serum α-tocopherol levels of less than 0.5 mg./100 ml. It appears to be due to a vitamin E deficiency. The amount of vitamin E in human milk is apparently sufficient to meet the infant's requirement. Cow's milk is relatively low in vitamin E content, having only 0.06 mg. vitamin E/100 ml., compared with 0.56 mg. vitamin E in the same amount of human milk.

A common instance of what appears to be a vitamin E deficiency is the muscle weakness, ceroid deposition in smooth muscle, creatinuria (resembling that in muscular dystrophy) and hemolysis in patients with severe fat malabsorption syndromes caused by celiac disease, cystic fibrosis, sprue and other diseases. These patients also have low levels of vitamin E in their serum.

It is well known that a deficiency of vitamin E causes a variety of symptoms in many species of animals. Some symptoms in animals attributed to vitamin E deficiency are listed.[33]

—in the female rat, the fetus dies and is reabsorbed, and in the male rat the testes atrophy usually resulting in sterility.

—in poultry, low hatchability and embryonic abnormalities and mortalities occur.

—in the dog, guinea pig, rabbit, chick, lamb and monkey, muscular dystrophy, anemia and various hematological symptoms are observed in deficient animals.

—in herbivorous animals, myocardial degeneration is found.

—in pigs, degeneration of skeletal and cardiac muscle and liver develops.

—in chicks, encephalomalacia with its neurological symptoms is manifested.

—in rats, a necrosis of the liver develops. The effect of vitamin E in prevention of this condition is augmented by small amounts of selenium.

The above brief mention of research reported in the literature suggests the possibilities for the role of tocopherols in human nutrition. However, the many previous enthusiastic claims for vitamin E in relieving or preventing rheumatic fever, muscular dystrophy, menstrual disorders, toxemias of pregnancy, spontaneous abortion, fibrositis, and sterility have not been substantiated for the human being, and the reader is cautioned against acceptance of claims for usefulness of this vitamin (and for so many other vitamins and drugs) until long term, controlled, and carefully studied results are forthcoming.

Absorption and Storage. Vitamin E is thought to be absorbed in the same way as the other fat-soluble vitamins in the presence of bile salts and fat. Vitamin E is stored primarily in the fatty tissues and not in the liver, unlike the other fat-soluble vitamins. The pituitary and adrenal glands have high concentrations of vitamin E.

Stability. Vitamin E is fairly stable to heat and acids and unstable to alkalies, ultraviolet light, and oxygen. It is also destroyed when in contact with rancid fats, lead, and iron. Since it is insoluble in water, there is no loss by extraction in cooking. Storage including deep freeze food processing and deep-fat frying destroy most of the tocopherol present. Esters of tocopherol such as tocopherol acetate are not appreciably destroyed. As in the intestine, the tocopherols protect vitamin A and carotene in foods from oxidative destruction. Exposure to oxygen, however, and development of rancidity result in the destruction of the tocopherols.

Measurement. One milligram of dl-alpha-tocopherol acetate is the international unit (1 mg. of dl-α-tocopherol, the naturally occurring form, is equal to 1.49 I.U.).

Recommended Dietary Allowance. The allowance for infants is 4 to 5 I.U. of vitamin E; for children and adolescents the range is 7 to 15 I.U.; for the adult male and female 15 I.U. and 12 I.U. respectively; in pregnancy and lactation 15 I.U. The RDA for infants with low birth weight is 4.5 I.U. per liter of formula. The requirement for vitamin E increases as the intake of polyunsaturated fatty acids (PUFA) in the diet is increased. The Food and Nutrition Board (FNB) recommends an α-tocopherol:PUFA ratio of 0.6 (mg./gm.). The average daily intakes of Americans have been estimated at between 7.4 mg. (11 I.U.) and 9.0 mg. (13.4 I.U.) of vitamin E and 21 gm. PUFA.[8, 10] This is equivalent to an α-tocopherol:PUFA ratio of approximately 0.4, somewhat lower than the guide. However, the ratio

of 0.6 is not proven and can only function as a guide. A great deal more information is needed about the dietary factors that influence vitamin E requirements.[7]

Toxicity. It has generally been assumed that there are no toxic effects from large doses of vitamin E.[16] This is fortunate considering the large amounts with which many people self-medicate themselves. However, recent evidence suggests that high levels of vitamin E may interfere with vitamin K activity in particular individuals.[11, 20, 23] There is an anticoagulant effect and prolonged blood clotting time. Large doses may be more toxic than we think.

Sources. Vitamin E is the most widely available of any of the vitamins in common foodstuffs. Wheat germ oil is the richest source of the vitamin, but other cereal germs, green plants, egg yolk, milk fat, butter, meat (especially liver), nuts, and vegetable oils (soybean, corn, cottonseed) also contain it. In the customary United States diet about 64 per cent of the vitamin E intake is supplied by salad oils, margarine and shortening; about 11 per cent by fruits and vegetables and about 7 per cent by grains and grain products.[32] It is produced synthetically, also.

Clinical Uses. α-Tocopherol use in treatment of hemolytic anemia of the newborn is effective and justified. Another use is in the treatment of intermittent claudication (tension and pain in the legs when walking).[18]

VITAMIN K

History. In 1935 Dam in Copenhagen discovered a severe hemorrhagic disease in newly hatched chickens on a ration adequate in all known vitamins and dietary essentials. By giving hog liver fat or alfalfa, normal clotting time was restored. It was suggested that the hemorrhage in chicks was due to a fall in prothrombin, a compound required for normal clotting of blood. Dam named the antihemorrhage factor vitamin K, or "Koagulationsvitamin." In 1939 vitamin K was isolated and only a few months later it was synthesized.

Chemical and Physical Properties. There are at least three forms of vitamin K all belonging to a group of chemical compounds known as *quinones*. The naturally occurring vitamins are K_1 *(phylloquinone)*, which occurs in green plants, and K_2 *(menaquinone)*, which is formed as the result of bacterial action in the intestinal tract. Vitamin K_1 was isolated from alfalfa and K_2 from putrefied fish meal. Water-soluble

forms of K_1 and K_2 are available for use by individuals unable to absorb the fat-soluble form. The fat-soluble synthetic compound, *menadione* (K_3), is about twice as potent biologically as the naturally occurring vitamins K_1 and K_2 on a weight basis because it lacks the long side chain of the natural vitamin. The body must add the side chain to the menadione before it can function as vitamin K. None of the forms of vitamin K are stored in appreciable amounts.

Stability. Vitamin K is fairly resistant to heat, but sunlight destroys the K_1. There is no destruction in ordinary cooking methods and, being fat-soluble, there is no loss in cooking water. All vitamin K compounds tend to be unstable to alkali.

Measurement. At present no specific unitage of vitamin K has been agreed upon. One of the most commonly used systems, however, states that 1 mg. of pure vitamin K_1 contains 1000 Thayer-Doisy units.

Function. Vitamin K is absorbed (with the aid of bile) in the upper intestinal tract and transported to the liver where it is essential for synthesis of *prothrombin* and several related proteins involved in the clotting of blood. The clotting mechanism, of which the final step is the conversion of *fibrinogen*, which is soluble, to *fibrin*, which is insoluble, and that forms the clot, is complex. It involves many factors. Those factors whose production is dependent upon vitamin K are II (prothrombin), VII, IX and X. (See Fig. 8–4.) It appears that a precursor protein to prothrombin is constantly being produced by the liver. The step whereby this precursor is converted to active prothrombin requires vitamin K.

Deficiency. A deficiency occurs when the diet lacks green vegetables and the growth of intestinal microorganisms is inhibited simultaneously by the administration of antibiotics or when the absorption of lipid is impaired.

Deficiencies of vitamin K usually occur from inadequate absorption from the intestinal tract or inability to utilize it in the liver. The latter occurs frequently in severe liver disease and is an instance in which large therapeutic doses of vitamin K are indicated.

Newborn infants are prone to have prothrombin deficiency during the first few days of life and are therefore susceptible to development of *"hemorrhagic disease of the newborn,"* a disease manifested by abnormal bleeding. This is due to poor placental transfer of vitamin K and failure to establish vitamin K–producing intestinal flora. Therefore, it is

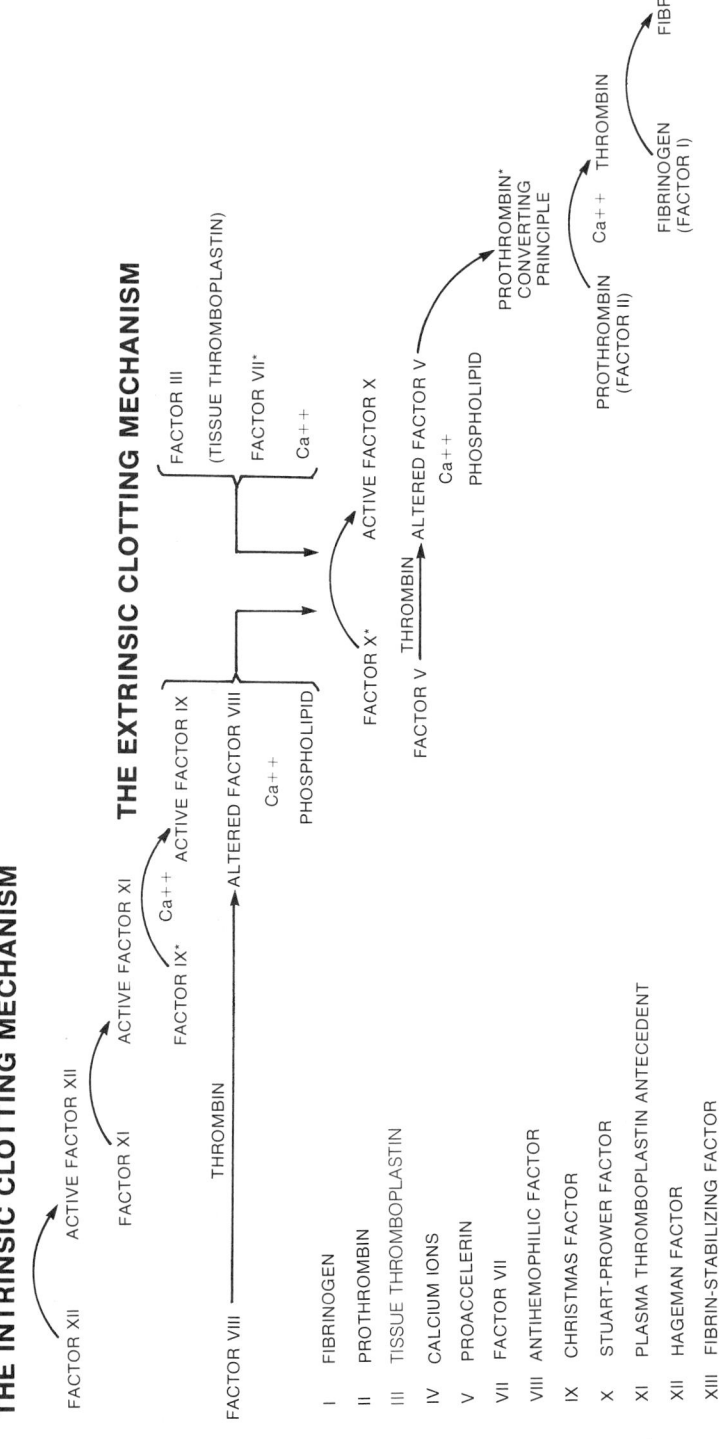

Figure 8–4 Cascade theory of blood coagulation. (Adapted from: Sauberlich, H. E., Skala, J. H., and Dowdy, R. P.: Laboratory Tests for the Assessment of Nutritional Status. Cleveland, Ohio, CRC Press, 1974, p. 85.)

*Vitamin K-dependent factors

necessary at times to administer vitamin K to the child upon delivery as a preventive measure against this disease. Furthermore, in the use of anticoagulants such as Dicumarol, bleeding occasionally occurs and this can be mitigated by the use of vitamin K. Frequently, it is given to patients before surgery to prevent abnormal bleeding. Excessive use of aspirin can prevent normal clotting of blood by interfering with platelet aggregation.

Toxicity. Excessive doses of synthetic vitamin K have produced hemolytic anemia in the rat and kernicterus in the infant. Because the toxicity of menadione causes an increase in breakdown of red blood cells and inhibits bilirubin glucuronide formation, menadione in over-the-counter supplements for pregnancy has been prohibited. The water miscible forms of vitamin K—Mephyton, Konakion and Mono-kay—have a much wider margin of safety.

Recommended Dietary Allowance. No quantitative estimate of vitamin K requirement has been made for human beings, but it is known that materials containing vitamin K activity in doses of 1 to 2 mg. will correct vitamin K deficiency in most cases. The Food and Nutrition Board, National Research Council, suggests that a single dose of 1 to 2 mg. of vitamin K_1 (0.5 to 1.0 mg. of the water miscible forms) immediately after birth is adequate to prevent hemorrhagic disease. Infants born to mothers receiving anticoagulant therapy should be given vitamin K_1 immediately after birth.

Vitamin K occurs in abundant quantities in the average diet, and is synthesized by intestinal bacteria, so that, with the exception of the newborn infant, there should be no dietary deficiency of it in the healthy person.

Sources. Vitamin K is found in green leafy vegetables, especially cabbage, spinach, kale and lettuce, cauliflower, tomatoes, wheat bran, soybeans and in oil, cheese, egg yolk and liver. It can be synthesized chemically. Vitamin K_2 has been shown to be formed by bacterial action of the flora of the human lower intestinal tract, so that an important supply of this vitamin may be available to the body even if it is not supplied in the diet. However, this source is only partially available for absorption.

WATER-SOLUBLE VITAMINS

These vitamins are not normally stored in the body in appreciable amounts; thus, a daily supply is desirable to avoid depletion and interruption of normal physiologic functions. Most of them are components of essential enzyme systems and are normally excreted in small quantities in the urine.

VITAMIN B-COMPLEX

History. Originally vitamin B was recognized as the preventive factor in the disease beriberi. Today more than a dozen separate B vitamins have been identified and found to play important roles in nutrition.

In 1897 Eijkman, a Dutch physician in Java, observed that chickens in the prison yard showed symptoms similar to those of his beriberi patients. The chickens ate the polished-rice table scraps discarded from the prisoners' meals, developed the malady and died. Eijkman found that addition of rice bran to the rice cured and prevented the beriberi in fowls. Although the findings were wrongly interpreted and shelved for years, the work of Eijkman laid the foundation for the conduct of future experiments. It was not until about 1911 that Funk and others described vitamin B.

Since later work showed that the original vitamin B actually consisted of several necessary accessory food factors, the anti-beriberi portion was christened B_1 or thiamin, and the other parts labeled B_2 and so forth as they were discovered. Today the members of the B-complex group are commonly referred to by their chemical names. Thiamin is B_1, riboflavin is B_2, pyridoxine is B_6, and we also have niacin (nicotinic acid), pantothenic acid, folacin, biotin, inositol, choline and cyanocobalamin (B_{12}).

The grouping of all these water-soluble compounds under the term "B-complex" is based upon their common source distribution, their close relationship in vegetable and animal tissues, and their intimate functional *interrelations*.

Function. One should think of the symptoms arising from avitaminosis B as a result of an attempt by the tissue cells to produce the energy needed for normal function in the absence of enough of the members of the B-complex group to accomplish the oxidation of food at the required rate. The B group, in general, plays an essential role in the metabolic processes of all living cells by serving as cofactors in the various enzyme systems involved in the oxidation of food and production of energy. They function as *co-enzymes* or as a prosthetic group bound to an apoenzyme, an enzyme protein. Coenzymes and prosthetic groups function similarly, since both contain

one of the active sites of the enzyme complex to which the substrate molecule is attached. The active site for most enzyme systems is a portion of the vitamin molecule. There exists such a close *interrelation* among the B vitamins that an inadequate intake of one may impair the utilization of others. Therefore, single discrete deficiencies of the B group are seldom seen clinically although the signs and symptoms of deficiency of a particular member of the group may predominate. Furthermore, the use of a single member of the group therapeutically may create a vitamin imbalance and precipitate deficiency of other members of the group. Thus, therapy with vitamin B should generally consist of therapy with all vitamin B-complex members rather than with any single substance of the group. Dry yeast is the richest natural source of the B-complex group.

Thiamin (Vitamin B₁)

History. Thiamin has been known as the antineuritic vitamin because it is needed for normal functioning of the nervous system. Deficiency of it in animals causes hindquarter paralysis. The symptom recognized by Eijkman in chickens and pigeons, and the beriberi described by workers in the Orient, was found to be concerned with the B_1 or thiamin fraction of the original B vitamin. In 1926 Jansen and Donath isolated thiamin in crystalline form, and in 1936 R. R. Williams accomplished the synthesis and determined the chemical formula. The vitamin was named thiamin to designate the presence of sulfur and an amino group in the complex molecule. For more of the history see Beriberi in Chapter 12.

Source. Thiamin is found in a large variety of animal and vegetable materials but in abundance in only a few foods. Lean pork, fresh and cured, and wheat germ are outstanding sources. Liver and all organ meats, liver sausage, lean meats, poultry, egg yolk, fish, dry beans and peas, soybeans, peanuts and whole grains are excellent sources. The whole grain and enriched grain products are the best sources of thiamin. The basic foods in the recommended amounts for an adult provide approximately 1 mg. of thiamin per day. Milk and milk products, fruit and vegetables are not good sources but when consumed in sufficient quantities they contribute materially to the day's total intake of thiamin.

Chemical Characteristics and Stability. Pure thiamin hydrochloride has been isolated and is a crystalline yellowish white powder with a salty, nutlike taste, and is water soluble. The dry vitamin is fairly stable, but solutions of it are unstable in the presence of heat or alkali. It is heat stable in acid solution. Loss of the vitamin in cooking is extremely variable, depending on the pH of the food, time, temperature, quantity of water used and discarded, and the use of sodium bicarbonate to enhance the green color of vegetables. Freezing has little or no effect on the thiamin content of foods.

Absorption, Synthesis and Storage. Thiamin is absorbed readily in the acid medium of the proximal duodenum and to some extent, in the lower duodenum. The maximum amount that can be absorbed is 5 mg. per day and any taken in excess of this will be excreted in the feces. When lumen concentration of the vitamin is low, an active, possibly Na^+ dependent process of absorption operates, and when lumen concentrations are high, a passive diffusion takes place. Thiamine is phosphorylated in the mucosal cell to thiamine phosphate, and in this form is carried to the liver by the portal circulation. It is not stored in any great quantity in the body and must, therefore, be supplied daily. The vitamin can be synthesized by microorganisms in the intestinal tract of animals and man, but the amount available to the human body to supplement the dietary supply seems to be small. Thiamin is excreted in the urine in amounts that reflect the intake and the amount stored. Fat and protein spare thiamin and a high intake of carbohydrate increases the need for thiamin. Thiaminase present in uncooked clams and fish destroys approximately 50 per cent of the thiamin.

Function. Thiamin is necessary throughout life for tissue respiration. Thiamin combines with phosphorus to form the coenzyme *thiamin pyrophosphate* (TPP), which functions as cocarboxylase. TPP is required for the oxidative decarboxylation of pyruvate to form active acetate and thence to acetyl Coenzyme A, the central compound of the Krebs metabolic pathway. TPP is required for the oxidative decarboxylation of other alpha-keto acids, alpha-ketoglutaric acid and the 2-ketocarboxylates derived from amino acids methionine, threonine, leucine, isoleucine and valine. TPP is also the coenzyme for the transketolase reaction which functions in the pentose phosphate shunt, an alternate pathway for glucose oxidation.

Thiamin is needed for the metabolism of carbohydrates, fats and proteins. However, all the evidence from the effects of thiamin deficiency link it with disturbance of carbohydrate

metabolism, especially in the brain. The thiamin requirement is linked to carbohydrate intake. This indicates that the decarboxylation of pyruvate, which is concerned only with carbohydrate metabolism, is the one which suffers first during thiamin inadequacy.

Thiamin Deficiency. As previously stated, severe thiamin deficiency of long duration causes beriberi, a disease formerly quite common in the Orient. Animals and humans with mild deficiencies may show fatigue, emotional instability, depression, irritability, retarded normal growth, loss of appetite, loss of interest in daily tasks, and general lethargy. (See Fig. 8–5.) Thiamin status of an individual is assessed by measuring the urinary excretion of thiamin since it decreases proportionately to thiamin intake. Erythrocyte transketolase may also be a useful measurement of thiamin nutriture.

EFFECT OF THIAMIN DEFICIENCY ON THE NERVOUS SYSTEM. Without thiamin the function of the central nervous system, which depends solely upon glucose for its energy, is greatly impaired. The neuronal cells show chromatolysis and swelling resulting in diminished reflex response. During thiamin de-

ficiency, degeneration of myelin sheaths of nerve fibers in the central nervous system and the peripheral nerves occurs. This causes the nerves to become irritable, which produces pain in the pathway of the peripheral nerves. Deep muscle pain in the calf is characteristic of thiamin deficiency. Progressive degeneration may cause paralysis and muscle atrophy.

EFFECT OF THIAMIN DEFICIENCY ON THE CARDIOVASCULAR SYSTEM. The heart muscle is weakened in thiamin deficiency and it may cause cardiac failure resulting in peripheral edema and ascites in the extremities. This is referred to as wet beriberi. A metabolic deficiency in smooth muscle of the vascular system causes peripheral vasodilatation.

EFFECT OF THIAMIN DEFICIENCY ON THE GASTROINTESTINAL TRACT. Gastrointestinal symptoms of thiamin deficiency are indigestion, severe constipation, anorexia, gastric atony and decreased hydrochloric acid secretion. This probably results from insufficient energy from carbohydrate metabolism for the smooth muscles and glands of the intestinal tract.

OTHER EFFECTS OF THIAMIN DEFICIENCY. Alcoholic polyneuropathy and amblyopia are

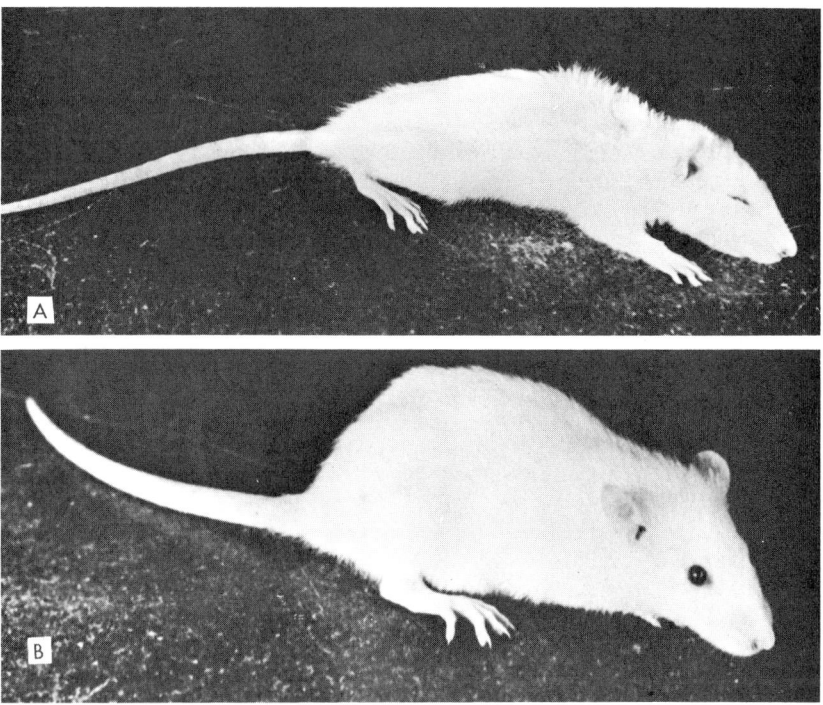

Figure 8–5   *A,* Prolonged deficiency of vitamin B₁ checks growth in young animals, causes loss of appetite and results in degenerative changes in the nervous system. *B,* Animal cured by administration of vitamin B₁ (thiamin chloride). A dose of from 0.006 to 0.009 mg. of thiamin chloride daily will cure symptoms of vitamin B₁ deficiency in these animals. (Courtesy of: E. R. Squibb and Sons.)

largely due to a thiamin deficiency. When treated early the symptoms of the Wernicke-Korsakoff syndrome respond to thiamin. Individuals whose intake of calories is markedly restricted are prone to development of thiamin deficiency symptoms. Exercise, fever, hyperthyroidism, major surgical operations and other stresses increase cellular energy requirements which increase the thiamin needs. Deficiency may be remedied by giving therapeutic doses of B-complex and thiamin plus an adequate diet.

Toxicity. There are no known toxic effects from thiamin.

Recommended Dietary Allowance. Many factors influence the thiamin needs of an individual. Among these are body weight, calorie intake, and the small amount synthesized in the intestinal tract. The amount of thiamin required is related to calorie needs, specifically to those obtained from carbohydrate. Liberal amounts of fat and protein in the diet exert a thiamin-sparing effect and will require less thiamin than will a high carbohydrate diet of the same caloric value. The Food and Nutrition Board recommends 0.5 mg. per 1000 kcalories for all ages. This allows for a margin of safety. A thiamin intake of 1.0 mg. per day is recommended for older adults even though they consume less than 2000 kcalories daily because it is believed that older persons use thiamin less efficiently. The allowance for pregnancy is 0.5 mg. per 1000 kcal. during the first two trimesters and 0.6 mg. per 1000 kcal. during the last trimester of pregnancy, which would make a total daily requirement of 1.3 to 1.5 mg. of thiamin per day during pregnancy. Recommended intake during lactation is 0.5 mg. thiamin per 1000 kcal. (See Table 10–1.)

Findings from the Ten-State Nutrition Survey, 1968–70, revealed adequate thiamin nutriture among the population studied.

Riboflavin (Vitamin B₂)

History. The existence of a yellow-green fluorescent pigment in milk whey was recognized in 1879. The biological significance of this pigment was not understood until 1932 when a group of German workers isolated "Warburg's yellow enzyme" from yeast and demonstrated that the material was necessary for activity of an intracellular respiratory enzyme. Almost simultaneously other investigators were studying a food factor that aided growth of laboratory animals. In 1933 Kuhn and his co-workers isolated the pigment from milk. They noted,

however, that it did not have all the activities ascribed to vitamin B₂. The compound was synthesized in 1935 by Kuhn and his co-workers and given the name *riboflavin*. Later investigations differentiated it from the pellagra-preventive factor with which it had first been confused.

Chemical Characteristics and Stability. Riboflavin belongs to a group of yellow fluorescent pigments called flavins. The flavin ring is attached to an alcohol related to ribose. It has been synthesized and in pure state appears as yellow crystals. It is stable to heat, oxidation, and acid; it is sparingly soluble in water but disintegrates in the presence of alkali or light, especially ultraviolet. Due to its heat stability and limited water solubility, very little is lost in the cooking and processing of foods. However, because it is sensitive to alkali, the addition of baking soda to soften dried peas or beans for faster cooking destroys much of their riboflavin content.

It has been demonstrated that bottled milk left outside the door in sunlight will lose a significant amount of riboflavin. Milk in paper containers is protected against such losses. Sun drying of fruits and vegetables as practiced in some countries can also cause considerable destruction of the riboflavin content.

Function. Riboflavin combines in the tissues with phosphoric acid to become part of the structure of two flavin coenzymes, *flavin mononucleotide (FMN)* and *flavin adenine dinucleotide (FAD)*. These coenzymes are the prosthetic group of the flavoprotein enzymes which catalyze oxidation-reduction reaction in the cells as hydrogen carriers in the mitochondrial electron transport system. They are coenzymes of the dehydrogenases which catalyze the first step in oxidation of several intermediates in glucose metabolism and of fatty acids. They are also active in oxidation deamination of amino acids. Riboflavin also is involved in the activation of vitamin B₆ and the conversion of folic acid to its coenzymes.

Riboflavin is essential for growth and is thought to have multiple functions in production of corticosteroids, formation of red blood cells, gluconeogenesis and thyroid enzyme regulating activity. (See Fig. 8–6.) Deficiency of riboflavin leads to cheilosis (cracking at the corners of the lips), glossitis (swollen and reddened tongue), seborrheic type of dermatitis, and ocular disorders such as itching, burning, lacrimation, sensitivity to light, and vascularization of the cornea. Other members of the B group are usually concur-

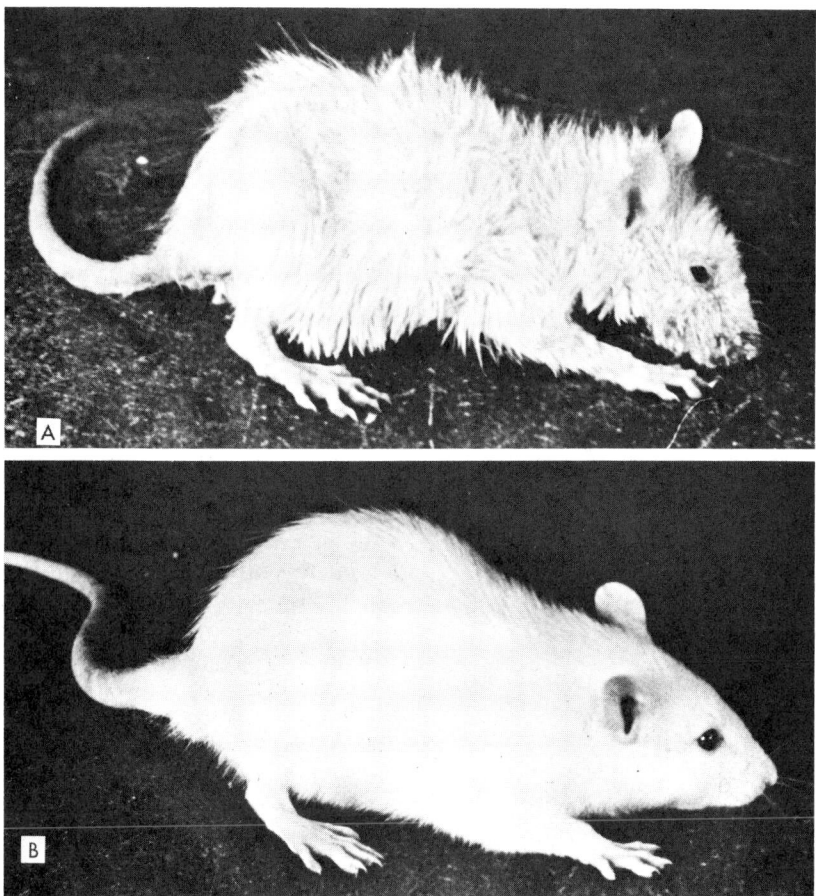

Figure 8–6 *A,* Deficiency of vitamin B₂ (riboflavin) affects growth and also induces certain changes in skin. *B,* Riboflavin deficiency symptoms cured. About 0.012 to 0.015 mg. daily is required. (Courtesy of: E. R. Squibb and Sons.)

rently deficient, and appropriate signs and symptoms of such deficiencies also appear. (See Chapter 12 for riboflavin deficiency disorders.)

Absorption and Storage. Riboflavin is easily absorbed through the walls of the proximal small intestine, where there is a specialized riboflavin transport process. It is phosphorylated to FMN before entering the blood stream. The absorption of riboflavin is increased by the presence of food in the gastrointestinal tract. Only 15 per cent of the vitamin is absorbed when taken alone, and 60 per cent of a 30 mg. dose when taken with food.[21] A decreased gastrointestinal transit time when food is present allows for greater absorption. It is carried by the blood to the tissues of the body and excreted in the urine. The amount excreted depends upon the intake and relative need of the tissues. Loss of riboflavin accompanies a loss of protein from the body. Although small

amounts of riboflavin are found in the liver and kidney, it is not stored to any great degree in the body and must therefore be supplied in the diet regularly.

Toxicity. There is no known toxicity to riboflavin.

Recommended Dietary Allowance. The riboflavin requirements of the human, according to the 1974 revision of the Food and Nutrition Board, are related to energy intake. The recommended amount for people of all ages is 0.6 mg./1000 kcal. During pregnancy an increase of 0.3 mg. per day and for lactation an additional daily intake of 0.5 mg. are recommended.

Adequacy of riboflavin is determined by urinary excretion of riboflavin. According to the Ten-State Nutrition Survey, 21.9 per cent of all blacks tested had riboflavin excretion levels suggestive of deficient or low riboflavin intake. Deficient or low intake was much less prevalent

in other groups. Perhaps these findings will direct more attention to possible riboflavin deficiency, which is usually ignored because it is rarely incapacitating.

Sources. Riboflavin is widely distributed in foods but in small amounts. The best daily sources in average servings are milk (fresh, canned or dried), cheddar cheese and cottage cheese. Although some of the riboflavin of cheese and cottage cheese is lost to the whey, they are good sources of riboflavin. Organ meats (liver, heart, kidney, liverwurst) contain appreciable amounts of riboflavin and other lean meats, eggs and green leafy vegetables are important sources in the amounts usually consumed. Breads and cereals enriched with riboflavin provide lesser amounts of riboflavin but contribute appreciably to the total daily intake.

Niacin (Nicotinic Acid)

History. It has been known for several centuries that pellagra occurred mainly where people used corn as a staple of the diet. It was described by Casál of Spain early in the 18th century and the disease was common in Italy at about the same time. Pellagra was described first in United States in the early 1900's. The United States Bureau of Public Health selected Dr. Joseph Goldberger to investigate the problem of pellagra that was rampant in the southern states. The condition based on evidence was related to a poor diet (high in cornmeal) as the cause. A diet of good quality protein foods prevented pellagra. Following the discovery in 1937 by Elvehjem that the disease blacktongue in dogs is due to a niacin deficiency, human pellagra was recognized by Spies and others as a niacin deficiency condition. In 1945 Krehl and his associates, in treating pellagra at the University of Wisconsin, found that tryptophan and niacin produce similar results. Since then it has been established that tryptophan is a precursor of niacin. However, recent findings indicate that pellagra is a mixed deficiency and that thiamin and riboflavin are also lacking.

In addition, the role of corn in the production of this disease has been recognized. Frequently those people who suffer from pellagra are on very inadequate diets in which corn is a mainstay. There is very little niacin in the diet and the tryptophan in the corn is unavailable and cannot be asorbed from the intestine. Subsequently, there is no tryptophan to be metabolized to niacin and a niacin deficiency

state results. In corn-based diets, such as that of Mexicans in which the corn is soaked in lye before use, the alkali makes the tryptophan available for absorption, and niacin deficiency is infrequent. Pellagra is further discussed in Chapter 12.

Source. Both niacin and its precursor, tryptophan, are included in determining the niacin in foods. Lean meats, poultry, fish and peanuts are rich daily sources of both. Organ meats, brewers' yeast, peanuts and peanut butter are the richest sources of niacin. Vegetables and fruits are poor sources. Milk and eggs contain small amounts of niacin but are excellent sources of tryptophan. To a lesser extent, beans, peas, other legumes, most nuts, and whole grains or enriched cereals also contain them. Of particular importance to the South is the niacin enrichment of corn products.

Most foods rich in animal protein are also rich in tryptophan. A dietary intake of 60 gm. predominantly complete protein provides 0.6 gm. (600 mg.) tryptophan. Since tryptophan is a niacin precursor, one niacin equivalent (1 mg.) is defined as 60 mg. of dietary tryptophan. A 60-gm. protein dietary would contribute 10 mg. of niacin equivalent* from tryptophan. Since nutrient composition tables give only the milligrams of preformed niacin in food, the total nicotinamide equivalent of the diet is underestimated.† To get an accurate intake it is necessary to also record the tryptophan in foods and divide it by 60.

Chemical Characteristics and Stability. Niacin, nicotinic acid, is a whitish crystalline material, stable when dry. It is easily converted to the active form *nicotinamide*. It is much more stable than thiamin and riboflavin, and is remarkably resistant to heat, light, air, acids and alkalies, although small amounts may be lost in discarded cooking water. It is frequently administered in the amide form, namely nicotinamide for therapeutic doses, since nicotinic acid acts as a vasodilator.

Absorption and Storage. Absorption takes place in the intestine. Little storage occurs in the body, and any excess is eliminated through the urine.

Function. Nicotinic acid functions in the body as a component of the coenzymes *nicotinamide adenine dinucleotide (NAD)* and *nicotinamide adenine dinucleotide phosphate*

---

*"Niacin equivalent" is used to express requirements for niacin.

†"Nicotinamide equivalent" is used to define the contribution to the diet of all nutritionally active forms of niacin, including tryptophan.

(NADP), known as the pyridine nucleotides. They were formerly known as coenzymes I and II and then DPN and TPN (diphosphopyridine nucleotide and triphosphopyridine nucleotide). These coenzymes are concerned with glycolysis, tissue respiration and fat synthesis. They serve as hydrogen acceptors capable of accepting and releasing hydrogen atoms as they are removed from food substrates by the many different types of dihydrogenases that are essential in the oxidation-reduction reactions in the release of energy from carbohydrates, fats and proteins. These coenzymes in their reduced forms (NADH and NADPH) deal with reduction of riboflavin-containing coenzymes and enzymes. Hydrogen is passed along from the reduced pyridine nucleotides to the riboflavin-containing coenzymes and then through mediation of the cytochromes finally to oxygen and the formation of metabolic water. Some niacin may be synthesized by the bacteria in the intestinal flora and some may be synthesized from tryptophan.

Deficiency. The symptoms of niacin deficiency are many. In the early stages muscular weakness, anorexia, indigestion and skin eruptions occur. Severe deficiency of niacin leads to pellagra which is characterized by dermatitis, dementia, diarrhea (the "3 D's" of pellagra) tremors, and sore tongue ("beef tongue"). The skin develops a cracked pigmented scaly dermatitis in the parts exposed to sun irradiations. Lesions appear in many parts of the central nervous system resulting in confusion, disorientation and neuritis. Many digestive abnormalities develop in niacin deficiency causing irritation and inflammation of the mucous membranes of the mouth and the gastrointestinal tract. Clinical symptoms of severe riboflavin deficiency appear. In fact many of the niacin deficiencies are similar, owing to the close interrelationships of riboflavin and niacin in cell metabolism. (See Chapter 12 for further discussion of pellagra.)

Clinical Uses. Niacin, but not nicotinamide, in massive doses of 3 gm. or more per day will lower serum cholesterol. The effect of niacin may be due to an interference of lipoprotein production or a stimulation of lipoprotein lipase which degrades lipoprotein. However, the use of niacin in reducing serum cholesterol is questionable because of evidence showing that it inhibits the use of free fatty acids for energy by the heart muscle. Consequently, the heart muscle must rely on glycogen and stored fat for energy, with the result that muscle glycogen is depleted.[14]

The use of massive doses of niacin (orthomolecular treatment) in the treatment of schizophrenia is also questionable.[2] See Chapter 32 for a discussion of orthomolecular psychiatry.

Toxicity. No real *toxic* effects are known, but large doses cause transient side effects such as tingling sensations, flushing of the skin and throbbing in the head due to its vasodilating action.

Recommended Dietary Allowance. The Food and Nutrition Board recommended allowances for niacin are expressed as niacin equivalents, and it is assumed that 60 mg. of tryptophan may be converted to 1 mg. of niacin. Requirement is based on caloric intake and the recommended allowance expressed in niacin equivalents is 6.6 mg. per 1000 kcalories and not less than 13 mg. at caloric intakes of less than 2000 kcalories. Daily requirement for niacin is influenced by the amount of tryptophan and thus by the amount and kind of protein available in the dietary. Excessive dietary leucine increases the requirement for niacin, as does the dietary sugar fructose.

Most diets consumed in the United States average 500 to 1000 mg. or more of tryptophan daily and 8 to 17 mg. of preformed niacin, for a total niacin equivalent of 16 to 33 mg. Thus, the daily allowance falls between 13 to 14 mg. for women and 14 to 18 for men, varying with the energy requirement. For pregnancy, the recommended allowance provides an increase of 2 mg. niacin per day based on the recommended increase in calorie intake. During lactation an additional daily allowance of 4 mg. niacin is recommended, based on the additional allowance of 500 kcal. See Table 10-1 for the niacin RDA, which includes dietary sources of niacin plus 1 mg. niacin equivalent for each 60 mg. of dietary tryptophan.

Vitamin B$_6$ (Pyridoxine, Pyridoxal and Pyridoxamine)

History. In 1938 pyridoxine was identified as another fraction of the vitamin B-complex, and synthesized in 1939. Later it was found that two derivatives of pyridoxine, namely *pyridoxamine* and *pyridoxal,* were also active. Therefore, vitamin B$_6$ is a complex of these three closely related chemical compounds of naturally occurring pyridines that are metabolically and functionally interrelated. Pyridoxine or B$_6$ is the term used to designate this group of vitamins.

Chemical Properties. Pyridoxine, a white,

crystalline, odorless compound, is soluble in water and alcohol. It is stable to heat in an acid medium and relatively unstable in alkaline solutions, but very unstable to light. It is absorbed in the upper small intestine and excreted from the body primarily as pyridoxic acid.

Function. This vitamin plays an essential role in many of the complex biochemical processes by which foods are metabolized in the body. Pyridoxine is found in cells in the active form, *pyridoxal phosphate (PLP),* a coenzyme that functions in protein, fat and carbohydrate metabolism. Its primary function as a coenzyme for many chemical reactions, however, is related to protein metabolism. Pyridoxal phosphate functions in the reactions involved in the non-oxidative degradation of amino acids, namely:

—transamination, the transfer of the amino group (NH_2) from one amino acid to form a different amino acid and the keto-analogue of the original amino acid. Transaminase activity in tissues is low in pyridoxine deficiency.

—deamination, the removal of amino groups from some amino acids not needed for growth, thus rendering the carbon residues available for energy.

—desulfuration, transfer of sulfhydryl group (HS) from one amino acid (methionine) to another (serine) to form cysteine.

—decarboxylation, the removal of the carboxyl group (COOH) from certain amino acids to form another compound. This decarboxylation is required for the synthesis of serotonin, norepinephrine and histamine from tryptophan, tyrosine and histidine respectively.

In addition, pyridoxal phosphate is necessary for the formation of a precursor of porphyrin compounds, which are an essential part of the hemoglobin molecule.

Vitamin B_6 is essential for the formation and metabolism of tryptophan and for the conversion of tryptophan to nicotinic acid (niacin). In this reaction pyridoxal phosphate plays a role in niacin supply. An individual with pyridoxine deficiency when given the tryptophan load test will accumulate xanthurenic acid (an intermediary product in the conversion of tryptophan to niacin). The amount can be measured in the urine and is used as an indication of the extent of available pyridoxine.

Pyridoxine as a part of the enzyme phosphorylase facilitates the release of glycogen from the liver and muscle as glucose-1-phosphate.

It is also involved in the conversion of the essential unsaturated fatty acid, linoleic acid, to the biologically important arachidonic acid. The formation of sphingolipids involved in the development of the myelin sheath surrounding nerve cells is also vitamin B_6 dependent.

Pyridoxine is involved in the maintenance of cellular immunity. Furthermore, it is involved in central nervous system metabolism, possibly by regulating the synthesis of brain enzymes that control central nervous system excitation.

Deficiency. Rats deficient in pyridoxine (B_6) develop a dermatitis, decreased rate of growth, fatty liver, anemia, decreased immune response, weakness and evidence of mental retardation. (See Figure 8–7.) The skin disturbance cannot be cured with niacin. Hamsters and monkeys given diets deficient in B_6 show an increase in dental caries.[39] Monkeys on a pyridoxine-deficient diet develop arteriosclerotic changes, indicating a possible role for pyridoxine in cholesterol metabolism.

Adults who were given a B_6 antagonist (deoxypyridoxine) developed depression, nausea, vomiting, seborrheic dermatitis, mucous membrane lesions and peripheral neuritis.[38]

Isoniazid (INH; isonicotinic acid hyrazide), used as a chemotherapeutic agent·for tubercular patients, is a potent antagonist of B_6. Patients develop peripheral neuritis and many of the symptoms of pyridoxine deficiency. The enzyme involved in decarboxylation of amino acids apparently is inactivated when isoniazid combines with pyridoxal phosphate. Urinary excretion of vitamin B_6 is greatly increased. The same is true with the medication penicillamine.

Spies found that certain symptoms in some pellagra and beriberi patients which were not relieved by niacin, thiamin or riboflavin responded to pyridoxine.

Vitamin B_6 deficiency has been shown to increase urinary oxalate excretion and has been implicated in renal calculi formation. This has been attributed to inability to convert glyoxalate to glycine and reflects the importance of this vitamin in metabolism of glycine and serine.

Pregnant women on "normal" diets have manifested pyridoxine deficiency when given the tryptophan load test and the abnormality was corrected by the administration of the vitamin. The placenta actively transports pyridoxine to attain a five-fold increase in fetal blood as compared with the mother. The vitamin has been used in the treatment of nausea

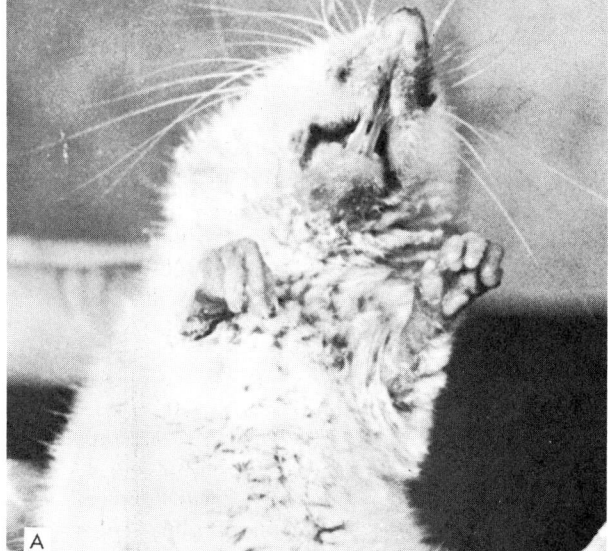

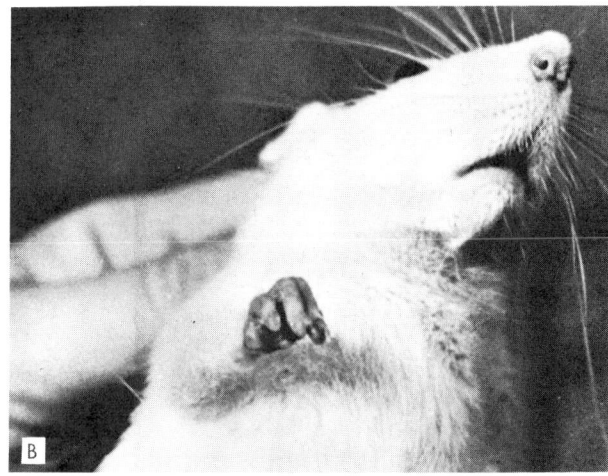

Figure 8–7 *A,* Typical dermatitis around the nose and paws caused by a lack of vitamin B$_6$. *B,* Animal cured of vitamin B$_6$ deficiency. A daily dose of 0.01 mg. of vitamin B$_6$ suffices to erase the symptoms of deficiency. (Courtesy of: E. R. Squibb and Sons.)

and vomiting of pregnancy and following radiation treatment with apparently good results. However, its efficiency in this use has not been proven.

Women taking oral steroid contraceptives have been shown to also have increased urinary excretion of tryptophan metabolites, suggestive of B$_6$ deficiency. This and accompanying states of malaise, depression, and glucose intolerance are relieved by vitamin B$_6$ supplementation. (See Chapter 21 on drug-nutrient interactions.)

Central nervous system abnormalities appear in extreme pyridoxine deficiency. Infants fed a liquid milk formula in which much of the vitamin was unknowingly destroyed in processing (autoclaving, high temperatures) developed irritability and convulsions. Urinary excretion of B$_6$ decreased and the trypto-

phan load test was positive with an increase in xanthurenic aciduria. Other infants fed a synthetic formula devoid of vitamin B$_6$ developed anemia and convulsions.[35] Infants recovered rapidly after an injection of the vitamin. It is apparent that enzyme systems of the central nervous system have a low order of binding capacity with coenzyme pyridoxal phosphate, making them susceptible to deficiency with resultant derangement of cellular metabolism and clinical abnormalities.

A deficiency syndrome has been identified in mentally retarded children with uncontrollable convulsions from birth due to inborn error of B$_6$ metabolism. Correction of the convulsions requires daily ingestion of large amounts of the vitamin and must be started in the neonatal period in order to prevent the development of irreversible mental

retardation. Another form in children with cryptogenic epilepsy which occurs at several years of age requires large doses of pyridoxine in order to correct the tryptophan load test and improve the EEG and seizure manifestations.

Source. The best sources of pyridoxine are yeast, wheat germ, pork, glandular meats (especially liver), whole grain cereals, legumes, potatoes, bananas, and oatmeal. Milk, eggs, vegetables and fruit contain small amounts. (See Table 8–8.) It is in most common foodstuffs and probably some can be synthesized by the intestinal flora.

Toxicity. Side effects, such as sleepiness, may follow injection of large doses (100 mg.).

Recommended Dietary Allowance. Results from a study by Baker et al.[6] with young adult male subjects indicate that the requirement is directly related to the protein intake. They conclude that the optimal daily vitamin B_6 requirement (as pyridoxine hydrochloride) for subjects on a high protein intake (100 gm.) appears to be 1.75 to 2.0 mg. per day; on a low protein intake (30 gm.) the requirement appears to be 1.25 to 1.5 mg. per day. In the 1974 revision, the Food and Nutrition Board provides for a margin of safety in recommending for adults a level of 2.0 mg. per day. (See Table 10–1.) The need increases in pregnancy and lactation (RDA of 2.5 mg. vitamin B_6 per day) and possibly with aging and in special situations such as radiation exposure, cardiac failure, use of oral contraceptives containing estrogen and in isoniazid therapy. The RDA is lower for infants and children. (See Table 10–1.)

Pantothenic Acid

History. The synthesis of pantothenic acid was completed in 1940. It is a part of Coenzyme A, which mediates acetylation and many other acylation reactions.

Source. Pantothenic acid is present in all plant and animal tissue, hence its name meaning "widespread." Egg, kidney, liver, salmon, and yeast are the best sources. Cauliflower, broccoli, beef (lean), potatoes (white and sweet), tomatoes, and molasses are good sources. It is also possibly synthesized by the intestinal flora. Approximately 33 per cent is lost in cooking meat and about 50 per cent is lost in the milling of flour.

Chemical Characteristics and Stability. Pantothenic acid is a white, crystalline compound (calcium pantothenate), bitter to the taste, more stable in solution than in dry form and easily decomposed by acid, alkali and dry heat. It is water-soluble and stable in moist heat in neutral solution.

Function. Pantothenic acid is known to be essential in the intermediary metabolism of carbohydrate, fat and protein. As part of Coenzyme A it has many metabolic roles in the cells. Because pantothenic acid is incorporated into CoA on which acetylation and other acylation reactions depend, it is involved in the release of energy from carbohydrate and in the degradation and metabolism of fatty acids. Besides functioning in the transfer of acetate groups to the Krebs cycle, CoA is involved as an acceptor acetate group for amino acids, vitamins

Table 8–8 PYRIDOXINE (B_6) CONTENT OF SELECTED FOODS
(MG./100 GM.)

Egg, white	.002	Prunes, dried	.24
Milk, human	.01	Egg, yolk	.30
Orange juice	.028	Chicken, dark meat	.325
Apple	.03	Peanut butter	.33
Bread, white	.04	Avocado	.42
Milk, whole	.04	Tuna, canned	.425
Yogurt	.046	Halibut	.43
Cornflakes	.065	Beef	.435
Apricots	.07	Pork	.45
Cheese, cheddar	.08	Banana, raw	.51
Potatoes, mashed	.091	Rice, brown	.55
Tomato, raw	.10	Chicken, light meat	.683
Frankfurter	.14	Salmon, fresh	.70
Oatmeal	.14	Walnuts	.73
Rice, white	.17	Soybeans, dry	.81
Brussels sprouts	.175	Liver, beef	.84
Bread, whole wheat	.18	Wheat germ, toasted	1.15
Corn, canned	.2	Sunflower seeds, kernels	1.25
Cauliflower	.21	Yeast, dry active	2.0

(From Orr, M. L.: Pantothenic Acid, Vitamin B_6 and Vitamin B_{12} in Foods. Home Econ. Res. Rep., No. 36, Agricultural Research Service, USDA, Washington, D.C., 1969.)

and sulfonamides. It is involved in the synthesis of cholesterol, steroid hormones, porphyrin for hemoglobin and phospholipids. It is known to be essential in the metabolism of man, chicks, dogs and rats, and prevents graying of the hair in certain animals.

It is so widely distributed in foods that a deficiency disease due to lack of the vitamin has not been observed in man on an adequate diet. Deficiency induced by administering an antagonist to volunteer subjects produced numerous physical and biochemical disturbances. Some of the subjects experienced pain and sensations in the arms and legs; others noted loss of appetite, nausea, and indigestion. Most became quarrelsome, sullen and depressed. Fainting attacks were common; the pulse tended to be rapid. An increase in susceptibility to infection seemed to follow. Pantothenic acid deficiency in both animals and man results in loss of antibody production. Pantothenic acid has been reported to improve the stress reactions of well-nourished subjects and to relieve the burning feet syndrome.

Toxicity. No toxic effects of this substance are known.

Recommended Dietary Allowance. According to the Food and Nutrition Board's 1974 revision the daily intake of 5 to 10 mg. is probably adequate for children and adults and there is no evidence for or against a greater requirement during pregnancy and lactation. However, there is not enough evidence to define a recommended allowance. Usual intake of pantothenic acid in the American dietary is about 10 to 15 mg. with a range of 6 to 20 mg. A deficiency is not likely.

Biotin

History. Biotin was first isolated in 1936 and synthesized in 1943. Previously the factor causing the syndrome manifested by eczema and characteristic alopecia around the eyes observed in rats and chicks fed large amounts of raw egg whites had been named vitamin H. A potent growth factor for yeast was called coenzyme R. These factors proved to be the same and the corrective factor found in egg yolk was called biotin.

Chemistry and Stability. Biotin is a monocarboxylic acid, stable to heat, soluble in water and alcohol, and susceptible to oxidation, to alkali and to strong acids.

Source. Biotin is found in a great many foods, and a considerable amount is synthesized by intestinal bacteria. It is known to occur in liver, milk, meat, egg yolk, most vegetables, mushrooms, a number of fruits (bananas, grapefruit, watermelon, strawberries), peanuts, and yeast in moderate abundance.

Function. Biotin is essential for the activity of many enzyme systems. It functions as the coenzyme for the process of carbon dioxide fixation (enzymatic reactions involving the addition or removal of carbon dioxide to or from active compounds). The synthesis and oxidation of fatty acids require biotin as a coenzyme. Biotin has a role in deamination as a coenzyme in the removal of NH_2 from certain amino acids (notably aspartic acid, threonine and serine). It is closely related metabolically to folic acid, pantothenic acid and vitamin B_{12}.

In animals its deficiency is associated with the characteristic dermatitis and can be produced only by adding egg white to a biotin-deficient diet. Thus, it has been known in animal research as the "egg-white-injury" factor. Avidin, a material in raw egg white, combines with biotin in the intestine, making it unavailable to the body. Biotin deficiency symptoms have also been induced in human beings by feeding raw egg whites, and the symptoms have been alleviated by giving a biotin concentrate. The experimental diet for man of 200 mg. dried egg white daily[36] induced the deficiency. This amount or its equivalent in raw egg white ingested daily in the American diet is unusual. The occasional raw egg whites would not precipitate a deficiency state. Avidin in raw egg whites is denatured upon cooking.

Biotin is frequently added to multiple vitamin preparations even though its need has not been definitely established.

Toxicity. There are no known toxic effects from this substance.

Recommended Dietary Allowance. In 1974 the Food and Nutrition Board, National Research Council, stated that 100 to 300 μg. of biotin per day is the probable daily intake by Americans; however, the minimum requirement and an RDA have not been established. In addition, biotin is furnished by bacterial synthesis in the intestinal tract and makes establishing an RDA very difficult. Cow's milk contains approximately 150 mcg. per liter and human milk contains from 1 to 8 mcg. with an average of 1.6 μg. biotin per liter.[32]

Folacin (Folic Acid or Pteroylmonoglutamate)

Folacin has been known under several names in the study of unidentified growth factors in bacteria and experimental animals and in the study and treatment of anemias. It was synthesized in 1946 and established as a dietary essential for man, many animals and microorganisms.

Chemical and Physical Properties. Folacin is a water-soluble, yellow, crystalline compound which belongs to a group of compounds known as "pterins," (Greek, "wing"; they were found in pigment of butterfly wings) and is also known chemically as pteroylglutamic acid, folate and *Lactobacillus casei* factor. Pteroylglutamic acid is formed by the linkage of three compounds; pterin and para-aminobenzoic acid (PABA) conjugated with one, three or seven molecules of glutamic acid. Some of the glutamic acid molecules must be split off to form an unconjugated folic acid molecule, pteroyl*mono*glutamic acid (PGA), which is the active form and is referred to as *folic acid*. This is done with the aid of specific enzymes and vitamin B_{12}. Folic acid in the presence of NAD (niacin-containing coenzyme) is reduced to *tetrahydrofolic acid* (THFA). THFA unites with a single carbon unit to form formyl-tetrahydrofolic acid or *citrovorum factor,* which is much more stable. Folic acid is an indispensable component of tissues, without which there is serious interference with cellular metabolism as shown by the use of folic acid antagonists or blocking agents that cause acute folic acid deficiency (for example, aminopterin). This antagonist, chemically related to folic acid, blocks the action of folacin by interrupting its conversion to tetrahydrofolic acid. Folacin, usually present in the polyglutamate form in food, is broken down to the monoglutamate form and then is readily absorbed by the gastrointestinal tract by active transport and diffusion and is stored primarily in the liver. It appears that folic acid absorption is decreased in an alkaline gastrointestinal tract.[26] Folate compounds are synthesized by intestinal microorganisms.

Source. It occurs widely in foods, and an adequate supply is easily obtained. It usually appears in the polyglutamate form. At this point we are not sure about the exact amount of food folate that is absorbed, but it is assumed that all of the free folic acid (PGA) and a good portion of the polyglutamates are absorbed.

Table 8–9 FOLACIN CONTENT OF SOME FOODS

	FOLACIN μG./GM.	
	Free	*Total*
Yeast		
brewer's	1.75	38.5
active, dry	1.40	40.9
Wheat germ	2.57	3.28
Wheat bran	1.34	2.58
Egg yolk	2.30	2.73
Romaine lettuce	.60	1.87
Cabbage	.43	.96
Whole wheat bread	.37	.62
Whole wheat flour	.59	.67
Fresh orange juice	.33	.66
Fresh orange	.35	.46
White bread	.22	.43
Banana	.36	.30
White flour, all purpose	.24	.28
Molasses, light	.07	.13
Milk, whole	.06	.15

(From Butterfield, S., and Calloway, D. H.: Folacin in wheat and selected foods. J. Am. Diet. Assoc., *60*:310, 1972.)

The best sources are liver, kidney beans, lima beans, fresh dark green leafy vegetables, especially spinach, asparagus and broccoli. Good sources are lean beef, potatoes, whole wheat bread and dried beans. Poor sources include most meats, milk, eggs, most fruits and root vegetables. (See Table 8–9.) Folacin is a potent substance, with 1 mg. causing certain physiological responses which will be discussed subsequently.

Stability. Folacin is unstable to heat in acid media, and stable to sunlight when in solution. There is considerable loss of folic acid in vegetables during storage at room temperature. Loss occurs in processing food at high temperatures. In dried milk, for example, folic acid activity is destroyed.

Function. Several coenzyme forms of folacin are known and their major role is the transfer of one-carbon units to appropriate metabolites in the synthesis of DNA, RNA, methionine and serine. The enzymes which utilize folacin coenzymes are known as pteroproteins.

Tetrahydrofolic acid is carrier for the single carbon groups (formyl, hydroxymethyl, or methyl groups) from one substance to another. It plays an important role in the synthesis of the purines guanine and adenine and of the pyrimidine thymine, compounds which are

utilized for the formation of nucleoproteins DNA (deoxyribonucleic acid) and RNA (ribonucleic acid) which are essential to cell division and the transmission of inherited traits.

Tetrahydrofolic acid participates in the interconversion of serine and glycine, the oxidation of glycine, methylation of homocysteine to methionine with B_{12} as co-factor, and the methylation of the precursor ethanolamine to the vitamin choline. The conversion of nicotinamide to N-methyl nicotinamide by addition of a single carbon (methyl group) and the oxidation of phenylalanine to tyrosine require folacin.

Folacin is required for one step in the conversion of histidine to glutamic acid. An impaired metabolism of histidine results in piling up of the intermediary product, formiminoglutamic acid (FIGLU), which is excreted in the urine.

Folacin is essential for the formation of both red and white blood cells in the bone marrow and for their maturation. It serves as a single carbon carrier in the formation of heme.

Deficiency. Deficiency of folacin results in poor growth, megaloblastic anemia, and other blood disorders, glossitis, and gastrointestinal tract disturbances arising from inadequate dietary intake, impaired absorption, excessive demands by tissues of the body and metabolic derangements. Folacin will control the macrocytic anemias of pregnancy and sprue and the megaloblastic anemia of infancy. Many patients with malabsorption syndrome have impaired absorption of folacin. Protein malnutrition may impair the utilization and function of folacin and conditions in which the demands for folacin are unusually great such as in hemolytic anemia, leukemia, Hodgkin's disease, certain drugs and carcinomatosis can cause a deficiency.

In pernicious anemia, folic acid will produce marked alleviation of the anemia, but the gastrointestinal symptoms and neurologic lesions progress. This is referred to as the "masking effect" of folacin in pernicious anemia. On the other hand, liver extract and vitamin B_{12} control all the aspects of pernicious anemia, namely, blood cell regeneration and the neurological condition.

Recommended Dietary Allowance. It has been estimated that daily intakes of healthy individuals range from 37 μg. to 297 μg. of free folacin.[32] Intestinal bacteria which synthesize folacin also provide some folacin. The daily recommendations are: 0.4 mg. for adults; 0.8

mg. in pregnancy and 0.6 mg. in lactation. Other stressful situations including disease states and the consumption of alcohol increase the requirement for folacin.

Vitamin B_{12} (Cobalamin)

In 1948 this compound was isolated from liver extract and shown to have high antipernicious anemia potency. It contains the heavy metal cobalt, chelated in a large tetrapyrrole ring very similar to the porphyrin ring of heme. The form of the vitamin originally isolated contained cyanide, which we ordinarily consider to be very toxic. Cobalamin is the generic name of vitamin B_{12} because of the presence of cobalt. Several of the different cobalamin compounds exhibit vitamin B_{12} activity. Of these compounds cyanocobalamin and hydroxycobalamin are the most active forms. The functional forms of the vitamin are called cobamide coenzymes.

Vitamin B_{12} is the extrinisic factor of food so necessary for treatment and prevention of pernicious anemia. It is considered to be identical with the antipernicious anemia factor and the erythrocyte maturation factor of Castle, as well as with the so-called animal protein factor.

Absorption. It is poorly absorbed from the intestinal tract unless the *intrinsic factor* (a mucoprotein enzyme called Castle's intrinsic factor) in the gastric secretion is present. The presence of hydrochloric acid is necessary to split vitamin B_{12} from its peptide bonds. The intrinsic factor combines with vitamin B_{12} in the food and in the bound form becomes adsorbed to a receptor in the membranes of the ileum through which it is transported into the cells in pinocytic vesicles. Calcium is necessary for the transfer.

After absorption, it is transported in the blood stream again bound to serum proteins (globulins), *transcobalamin I and II* (II being more important), and circulates to the various tissues. The tissues of normal persons contain vitamin B_{12} in varying amounts, with the highest concentration found in the liver and to some extent in the kidney. It is released as needed to the bone marrow and other tissues of the body. The body store of the vitamin (approximately 2000 μg.) is substantial. It may take five or six years for deficiency symptoms to appear after the body's supply from the natural sources has been restricted. An excess intake of the vitamin is excreted in the urine.

Absorption of B_{12} appears to decrease with

aging and with iron and B_6 deficiency and increases during pregnancy.

Function. Cobalamin has various physiological roles at the cellular level. It is essential for normal function in the metabolism of all cells, especially for those of the gastrointestinal tract, bone marrow, and nervous tissue, and for growth. It participates with folic acid, choline and methionine in the transfer of methyl groups in the synthesis of nucleic acids, purines and pyrimidine intermediates. Cobalamin coenzymes are necessary for reducing ribonucleotides to deoxyribonucleotides which function in the promotion of growth and the red blood cell maturation. Vitamin B_{12} affects myelin formation. It is involved in protein, fat and carbohydrate metabolism and associated with folic acid absorption and metabolism.

Deficiency. Failure to absorb vitamin B_{12} because of the absence of intrinsic factor in the gastric secretion results in a deficiency state of the vitamin. Surgical resection of the intrinsic-factor-secreting portions of the stomach (fundus and cardia) or the absorbing surfaces of the ileum may result in a deficiency of vitamin B_{12}. The anemia may not become apparent for several years after the surgery because of storage of the vitamin. Small bowel diverticula, intestinal infestations, sprue and other malabsorption syndromes may induce a vitamin B_{12} deficiency state. These conditions are complicated by deficiencies of folic acid as well as other essential nutrients. Vitamin B_{12} deficiency causes demyelination of the large nerve fibers of the spinal cord.

Vegetarians (persons living exclusively on vegetables) have a low dietary intake of vitamin B_{12}. They usually have low serum levels of this vitamin.

Chemical Characteristics and Stability. Vitamin B_{12} is slowly destroyed by dilute acid, alkali, light and oxidizing or reducing agents. It is water-soluble and forms red crystals. Red color is due to the presence of cobalt in the molecule. Its potency has been found to be amazingly high. One microgram of crystalline B_{12} equals 1 U.S.P. unit of purified liver extract. Approximately 70 per cent of the vitamin activity is retained during cooking.

Source. Vitamin B_{12} is present in animal protein foods. Liver and kidney are richest sources; fresh milk, eggs, fish, cheese and muscle meats are good sources. Pasteurized and evaporated milk have lost 40 to 90 per cent of the vitamin. (See Table 8–10.)

Toxicity. No toxic effects are known.

Recommended Dietary Allowance. Human

requirements for this factor are minute but essential. Doses of 0.5 to 1.0 μg., injected parenterally, have relieved pernicious anemia, and large doses have relieved or prevented progression of the neurologic complications of pernicious anemia.[19] It seems to act by allowing maturation of the red blood cells. Oral administration is ineffective unless administered in huge doses because IF is not present to allow its absorption. B_{12} also relieves nutritional anemia caused by folic acid deficiency (sprue, pregnancy) in many cases. Excesses are not absorbed. Limited bacterial synthesis in man occurs in the colon, past the terminal ileum, so it is not absorbed. Therefore, humans apparently do not derive sufficient vitamin B_{12} from endogenous bacterial synthesis and must rely on a supply of the preformed vitamin in the food intake. The usual American diet, adequate in proteins, provides minimum requirements. The 1974 revision of the Recommended Dietary Allowances suggests 3 μg. daily for adults, and 4 μg. during pregnancy and lactation. A diet containing 15 μg. daily will gradually replenish depleted stores.

ASCORBIC ACID (Vitamin C)

History. Vitamin C is the antiscorbutic vitamin, the preventive of and cure for scurvy. Many dramatic stories are in the scientific literature relating the use of citrus fruits for the cure of scurvy, the dreaded disease of explorers and voyagers. This disease was first described during the Crusades, and remained common among soldiers and sailors until the preventive value of lemon juice was discovered. The history of the relation between vitamin C and scurvy is further discussed in Chapter 12.

Although vitamin C was isolated in 1928 by Szent-Györgyi, who found it in adrenal tissue

Table 8–10   VITAMIN B_{12} CONTENT OF
SELECTED FOODS
μG./100 GM.

Milk, whole	.4
Chicken, fried	.42
Frankfurters, cooked	1.3
Egg	2.0
Beef, round	2.65
Oysters	18.0
Clams, canned	19.1
Liver, beef	80.0

(From Pennington, J. A.: Dietary Nutrient Guide. Westport, Connecticut, AVI Publishing Co., 1976.)

and in orange and cabbage and identified it as hexuronic acid, it was not until 1932 that C. Glenn King at the University of Pittsburgh re-isolated the compound from lemons and identified it as vitamin C, having the properties of preventing and curing scurvy in guinea pigs. Shortly thereafter its correct structural formula was established and synthesis was accomplished. It is known as L-ascorbic acid in the reduced form and as L-dehydroascorbic acid in the oxidized form. Ascorbic acid is the accepted name of the vitamin.

Source. Ascorbic acid is widely found in citrus fruits, raw leafy vegetables, and to-matoes. Canned or frozen citrus fruit, and to-matoes are good and inexpensive sources of ascorbic acid where fresh fruits are not abundant or not obtainable. Strawberries, cantaloupe, cabbage and green peppers are good sources. Potatoes are considered a good source when properly prepared because of the quantity eaten. An average serving of citrus fruit juices (½ cup) contains 45 to 60 mg. of ascorbic acid, cantaloupe (¼) 30 mg., strawberries (1 cup) 88 mg., sweet green pepper (1 raw) 94 mg., tomato (1 raw) 42 mg. and boiled potato (1 med.) 20 mg. The acerola tree, or Puerto Rican cherry, has an unusually high vitamin C concentration. Values obtained have averaged to 2000 mg. of ascorbic acid per 100 gm. of juice or fruit. A six-ounce glass of the juice contains as much as 8650 mg. of vitamin C—more than 85 times as much as an equal glass of orange juice. Other less common foods rich in ascorbic acid are black currants, and edible hips of the wild rose. Tropical foods high in the vitamin include the sapodilla, ceriman cherry, papaya, sour-sop, star apple, and guava. Turnip greens, broccoli, cabbage, spinach, Brussels sprouts, berries, and pineapples are good sources. Apples, peaches, pears and bananas are good sources when eaten in large amounts. Milk, eggs, meat and poultry contain little or no ascorbic acid.

Chemical Characteristics and Stability. Chemically, ascorbic acid is a white, water-soluble crystalline material that is stable in dry form. In solution it is easily oxidized, especially on exposure to heat. Oxidation can be accelerated by the presence of copper and by alkaline pH. Consequently, much ascorbic acid is lost in cooking or thrown out in the cooking water. Bruising, cutting, and allowing fruit and vegetables to be kept exposed to the air cause much loss of ascorbic acid. Less destruction and more retention of the vitamin occurs when the food is cooked quickly in small amounts of boiling water, and covered tightly. Quick freezing of foods preserves the vitamins. Refrigeration aids retention. Use of sodium bicarbonate in cooking vegetables to preserve and improve the color is very destructive of the vitamin. The ascorbic acid content of fruits and vegetables varies with the conditions under which they are grown, degree of ripeness when harvested, and conditions under which they are stored, and cooked.

Ascorbic acid is a hexose derivative and classified as a carbohydrate closely related to the monosaccharides. The reduced ($C_6H_8O_6$) form is the most active form and is readily oxidized to form dehydroascorbic acid ($C_6H_6O_6$). It may be reduced back to the original form (reversible oxidation-reduction). Both forms are antiscorbutic. Further oxidation of dehydroascorbic acid produces diketogulonic acid with no antiascorbic acid properties and cannot be reduced to form dehydroascorbic acid again. In plants several simple sugars are converted to ascorbic acid but in animals glucose and to some extent galactose are the precursors for the vitamin.

Absorption and Storage. Ascorbic acid is easily absorbed from the small intestine by an active mechanism and probably by diffusion and carried to the tissues by the blood. It readily passes into tissues of the adrenals, kidney, liver and spleen, most of which appear to be in equilibrium with serum level. It is stored in these tissues to some extent (1.5 gm.) through tissue saturation but should be supplied daily. Excess amounts ingested over the saturation level of various tissues are excreted in the urine as oxalic, threonic and dehydroascorbic acids and some is oxidized and exhaled as carbon dioxide. A very small amount is lost in the feces. It requires approximately 3 months for scurvy to develop in a person on a vitamin C deficient diet.

Function. Ascorbic acid has multiple functions in the body, either as a coenzyme or co-factor. Its function at the cellular level has not been resolved. It appears to be present and essential to the normal functioning of all cellular units including subcellular structures such as ribosomes and mitochondria. The ability of ascorbic acid to lose and take on hydrogen gives it an essential role in metabolism.

Ascorbic acid is required for production and maintenance of collagen, a protein substance found in all fibrous tissue (connective tissue, cartilage, bone matrix, tooth dentin, skin and tendon). The integrity of cellular structure de-

pends on it. Ascorbic acid is involved in the hydroxylation of proline to form *hydroxyproline* in the synthesis of collagen. Ascorbic acid maintains this intercellular cement substance with preservation of capillary integrity; promotes healing of wounds, fractures, bruises, pinpoint hemorrhages and bleeding gums; and reduces liability to infections. A high level of ascorbic acid is present during healing and in scar tissue.

It is essential for the oxidation of phenylalanine and tyrosine and for the conversion of folacin to tetrahydrofolic acid (THFA). It is also helpful in the reduction of ferric iron to ferrous iron in the intestinal tract to facilitate absorption, in the transfer of iron from plasma transferrin to liver and for the conversion of tryptophan to 5-hydroxytryptophan. Hydroxylation reactions appear specific for ascorbic acid. It also participates in the hydroxylation of certain steroids synthesized in adrenal tissue. Under stress, when adrenal cortical hormone activity is high, ascorbic acid concentration in the tissue is decreased. Injection of ACTH causes considerable loss of ascorbic acid from the adrenal cortex. During periods of emotional, psychological or physiological stress, the urinary excretion of ascorbic acid is increased.

Fevers and infections require additional amounts of ascorbic acid to maintain tissue levels. Adequate tissue concentration of ascorbic acid helps the body to maintain resistance to infection. The value of large amounts of ascorbic acid to prevent and cure the common cold has been reported, but these findings are still controversial.

Vitamin C and the Common Cold.   Interest in the use of vitamin C for treatment of the common cold dates from the 1940s, but it was not really popularized until Linus Pauling, a Nobel laureate, wrote his book that made claims for vitamin C as a protective agent against the common cold.[29] Sales of the vitamin skyrocketed in the presence of a great deal of controversy among nutrition authorities regarding this new information. In subsequent years several studies have been performed that tend to modify the original hypothesis:

1. Anderson and colleagues conducted a double blind, large scale trial on 818 individuals. One group consumed a placebo, and a second group took 1 gm. vitamin C daily and 4 gm. daily during the first 3 days of a cold. Anderson found that those taking vitamin C did experience less illness, but the differences were smaller than those claimed and statistically were not significant. However, when those taking vitamin C did contract a cold, it was less severe and resulted in 30 per cent fewer days of disability.[3, 4]

2. In a study involving 641 children taking a placebo or 1 to 2 gm. vitamin C, Coulehan and colleagues found a decrease of 28 to 34 per cent in the number of days of sickness in those children contracting a cold who were also taking vitamin C. Coulehan did not find that vitamin C prevented getting a cold.[13] However, a more recent study by the same investigator could not confirm the effectiveness of 1 gm. daily doses in reducing the severity of cold symptoms.[12] At this point it appears that large daily doses of vitamin C (no one is sure about how large) will possibly reduce the severity and duration of symptoms of a cold.

3. Wilson and colleagues have found that prophylactic doses of 200 to 500 mg. daily resulted in reduced cold symptoms in girls, but had no effect in boys.[40]

One investigator concluded that ascorbic acid had an antihistamine effect.[9]

Deficiency.   The earliest signs of ascorbic deficiency may begin during the first month of deprivation, depending on the rate of catabolism. Deficiency appears after the serum level has fallen below 0.2 mg. per 100 ml. Severe deficiency of ascorbic acid causes scurvy. It is characterized by decreased urinary excretion, plasma concentration, tissue and leukocyte concentration. Other symptoms include weakness, poor appetite and growth, anemia, tenderness to touch, swollen and inflamed gums, loosened teeth, swollen wrist and ankle joints, shortness of breath, petechial hemorrhages from the venules, beading or fracture of ribs at costochondral junctions, fracture of epiphysis, multiple subcutaneous and subperiosteal hemorrhages with pain on motion of the body. Secondary infections develop easily in the bleeding areas. All these characteristics can be attributed primarily to collagen defects.

Neurotic disturbances consisting of hypochondriasis, hysteria and depression followed by decreased psychomotor performance have been reported in ascorbic acid deficiency.[22] The symptoms of scurvy clear rapidly with therapeutic doses of ascorbic acid. (See Fig. 8–8 *A* and *B*.) Although scurvy is rare today, dietary surveys indicate that many Americans receive insufficient amounts of this vitamin for optimum health.

Apparently cigarette smoking adversely affects the body's ability to utilize ascorbic acid. Less ascorbic acid is available in smokers for

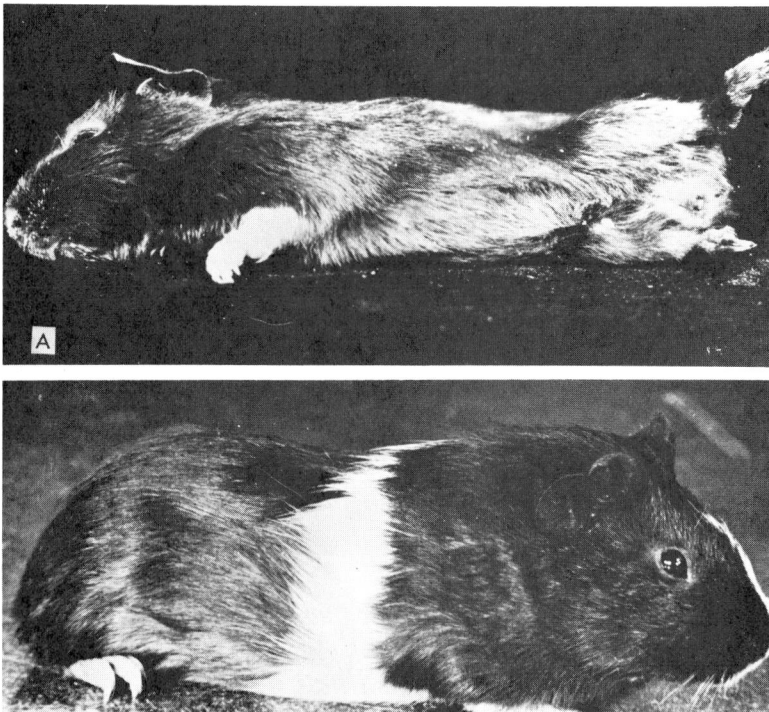

Figure 8–8 *A,* The guinea pig is very susceptible to vitamin C deficiency and rapidly develops scurvy, one evidence of which is seen in the enlarged joints. If completely deprived of vitamin C, the animals generally die in about three weeks. Untreated scurvy is also fatal in man. *B,* Guinea pig cured of scurvy by treatment with crystalline vitamin C (ascorbic acid). (Courtesy of: E. R. Squibb and Sons.)

utilization and storage, indicating the lower amount absorbed. Smokers appear to oxidize more ascorbic acid to dehydroascorbic acid which isomerizes to diketogulonic acid in the gastrointestinal tract due to the secretion of an oxidative enzyme, ceruloplasmin, involved in the oxidation of serotonin. Serotinin is known to be released by nicotine. The average smoker probably needs twice as much ascorbic acid as the non-smoker to have a comparable blood level.[30]

Toxicity. Excess ascorbic acid excreted in the urine gives a false positive test for sugar. It could cause formation of urate, cystine or oxalate stones.[24]

It has also been reported that those on massive intakes of vitamin C have a "rebound" scurvy when they stop taking the massive doses. This is possibly due to a high rate of vitamin C catabolism as an adaptation to hypersaturation. This catabolism does not return to a normal level immediately upon reducing vitamin C intake, and a vitamin C deficiency state results.[27]

Recommended Dietary Allowance. According to the Food and Nutrition Board, National Research Council the minimal daily intake of ascorbic acid needed to prevent scurvy is approximately 10 mg. The revised recommended allowances (1974) are 45 mg. daily for an adult female or male. Infants need 35 mg. daily the first year. A daily allowance of 60 mg. is recommended in pregnancy and 80 mg. during lactation. (See Table 10–1.)

Table 8–11 summarizes the information on vitamins.

OTHER VITAMIN-LIKE FACTORS

This chapter might be summarized by stating that, to date, the metabolic function in man of the following vitamins has been clearly demonstrated: vitamins A, D, E, K, ascorbic acid, thiamin, riboflavin, niacin, folic acid, B_{12}, B_6, pantothenic acid and biotin.

Exact minimal quantitative requirements for vitamins are difficult to state. The standards set by the Food and Nutrition Board of the National Research Council are aimed toward generous and safe margins of intake in the light

Table 8–11   SUMMARY OF INFORMATION ON VITAMINS

FAT-SOLUBLE VITAMINS

Name	Daily Recommended Allowances for Adults	Rich Food Sources	Pharmaceutical Sources	Stability	Biological Role
Vitamin A (retinol; provitamin A; α, β, γ carotene)	4000–5000 I.U. or 800–1000 R.E.	Liver, kidney, milk fat, fortified margarine, egg yolk, yellow and dark green leafy vegetables, apricots, cantaloupe, peaches.	Fish liver oils.	Stable to light, heat and usual cooking methods. Destroyed by oxidation, drying, very high temperature, ultraviolet light.	Essential for normal growth, development and maintenance of epithelial tissue. Essential to the integrity of night vision. Essential for health of the eyes. Helps provide for normal bone development and influences normal tooth formation. Toxic in large quantities.
Vitamin D (calciferol)	Sunlight and normal diet are adequate. (400 I.U. in children, pregnancy and lactation.)	Vitamin D milk, irradiated foods, some in milk fat, liver, egg yolk, salmon, tuna fish, sardines.	Fish liver oils, concentrates.	Stable to heat and oxidation.	Essential for normal growth and development; important for formation of normal bones and teeth. Influences absorption and metabolism of phosphorus and calcium. Prevents and cures rickets and osteomalacia. Toxic in large quantities.
Vitamin E (tocopherols)	12–15 I.U.	Wheat germ, vegetable oils, green leafy vegetables, milk fat, egg yolk, nuts.	Wheat germ oil, synthetic.	Stable to heat and acids. Destroyed by rancid fats, alkali, oxygen, lead, and iron salts, and ultraviolet irradiation.	Is a strong antioxidant. As such may help prevent oxidation of unsaturated fatty acids and vitamin A in intestinal tract and body tissues. Protects red blood cells from hemolysis. Role in reproduction (in animals).
Vitamin K (menadione)	Not established. Oral dose of 1–2 mg. considered adequate for healthy persons.	Liver, soybean oil, other vegetable oils, green leafy vegetables, tomatoes, cauliflower, wheat bran. (Synthesized in intestinal tract.)	Synthetic.	Resistant to heat, oxygen, and moisture. Destroyed by alkali and ultraviolet light.	Aids in production of prothrombin, a compound required for normal clotting of blood. Toxic in large amounts.

WATER-SOLUBLE VITAMINS

Name	Daily Recommended Allowances for Adults	Rich Food Sources	Pharmaceutical Sources	Stability	Biological Role
Thiamin (vitamin B_1)	0.5 mg. per 1000 kcalories; older person 1.0 mg. per day.	Pork, liver, organ meats, legumes, whole grain and enriched cereals and breads, wheat germ, potatoes. (Synthesized in intestinal tract.)	Yeast, wheat germ, synthetic.	Unstable in presence of heat or alkali or oxygen. Heat stable in acid solution.	Prevents beriberi. As part of cocarboxylase, aids in removal of CO_2 from alpha-keto acids during oxidation of carbohydrates. Essential for growth, normal appetite, digestion and healthy nerves.
Riboflavin (vitamin B_2)	0.6 mg. per 1000 kcalories.	Milk and dairy foods, organ meats, green leafy vegetables, enriched cereals and breads, eggs.	Yeast, liver concentrates, synthetic.	Stable to heat, oxygen, and acid. Unstable to light (especially ultraviolet) or alkali.	Essential for growth. Essential for health of the eyes. Plays enzymatic role in tissue reproduction, and acts as a transporter of hydrogen ions. Coenzyme forms FMN and FAD. Prevents fissures at corners of mouth, around nose and ears, eye irritation, photophobia.

Table 8–11 SUMMARY OF INFORMATION ON VITAMINS (*Continued*)

WATER-SOLUBLE VITAMINS

Name	Daily Recommended Allowances for Adults	Rich Food Sources	Pharma-ceutical Sources	Stability	Biological Role
Niacin (nicotinic acid)	13–18 mg. niacin equivalent or 6.6 mg. per 1000 kcalories.	Fish, liver, meat, poultry, many grains, eggs, peanuts, milk, legumes, enriched grains.	Yeast, liver concentrates, synthetic.	Stable to heat, light, oxidation, acid and alkali. ι	As part of enzyme system, aids in transfer of hydrogen, acts in metabolism of carbohydrates and amino acids. Prevents pellagra, nervous depression, neuritis. Involved in glycolysis, fat synthesis and tissue respiration.
Vitamin B₆ (pyridox-ine, pyridoxal and pyridoxamine)	2.0 mg.	Pork, glandular meats, cereal bran and germ, milk, egg yolk, oatmeal, and legumes.	Yeast, wheat germ, liver concentrates.	Stable to heat, light and oxidation.	As a coenzyme, aids in the synthesis and breakdown of amino acids and in the synthesis of unsaturated fatty acids from essential fatty acids. Essential for conversion of tryptophan to niacin. Prevents hypochromic anemia, seborrheic dermatitis, mucous membrane lesions and peripheral neuritis. Essential for normal growth.
Pantothenic acid	Level not yet determined but believe 5–10 mg. adequate. Supplied in normal diet.	Present in all plant and animal foods. Eggs, kidney, liver, salmon and yeast are best sources.	Yeast, wheat germ, liver concentrates.	Unstable to acid, alkali, heat and certain salts.	As part of coenzyme A, functions in the synthesis and breakdown of many vital body compounds. Essential in the intermediary metabolism of carbohydrate, fat, and protein.
Biotin	Not known but 100 to 300 μg. will provide daily needs.	Liver, mushrooms, peanuts, yeast, milk, meat, egg yolk, most vegetables, banana, grapefruit, tomato, watermelon, and strawberries. (Synthesized in intestinal tract.)	Yeast, liver concentrates.	Stable.	Probably an essential component of a coenzyme. Appears to be involved in synthesis and breakdown of fatty acids and amino acids through aiding the addition and removal of CO_2 to or from active compounds, and the removal of NH_3 from amino acids. It is closely related metabolically to folic acid and pantothenic acid.
Folacin (folic acid)	0.4 mg.	Green leafy vegetables, organ meats (liver), lean beef, wheat, eggs, fish, dry beans, lentils, cowpeas, asparagus, broccoli, collards, yeast. (Synthesized in intestinal tract.)	Yeast, concentrates.	Stable to sunlight when in solution; unstable to heat in acid media.	Appears essential for biosynthesis of nucleic acids and probably for normal fat metabolism. Appears essential for normal maturation of red blood cells. Functions as a coenzyme: tetrahydrofolic acid.
Vitamin B₁₂ (cyanocobalamin)	3 μg.	Liver, kidney, milk and dairy foods, meat, eggs. Complete vegetarians require supplement.	Concentrates, synthetic.	Slowly destroyed by acid, alkali, light and oxidation.	Involved in the metabolism of single-carbon fragments. Essential for biosynthesis of nucleic acids and nucleoproteins, and thereby in normal red blood cell formation; role in metabolism of nervous tissue; probably essential for normal fat metabolism. Related to certain anemias, especially pernicious anemia. Related to growth.

Table continued on the following page

Table 8–11   SUMMARY OF INFORMATION ON VITAMINS (*Continued*)

WATER-SOLUBLE VITAMINS

Name	Daily Recommended Allowances for Adults	Rich Food Sources	Pharmaceutical Sources	Stability	Biological Role
Ascorbic acid (vitamin C)	45 mg.	Puerto Rican cherry, citrus fruits, tomatoes, melons, peppers, greens, raw cabbage, guava, strawberries, pineapple, potatoes.	Synthetic.	Unstable to heat, alkali, and oxidation, except in acids. Destroyed by storage.	Essential for growth. Possibly functions as coenzyme in the metabolism of amino acids, particularly phenylalanine and tyrosine; facilitates conversion of folic acid to folinic acid and is essential for many hydroxylation reactions. Role in tooth and bone formation. Maintains intracellular cement substance with preservation of capillary integrity. Promotes healing of wounds and fractures; and reduces liability to infections. Enhances absorption of iron. Essential for production of collagen, the basic substance of connective tissue. Related in some way to biosynthesis of steroid hormones. Prevents scurvy.

of present knowledge and continued revisions of these figures in the future are to be expected.

There are many other food factors, some of which have no known specific functions, and others which have functions known for certain animal species. A brief presentation of a few with vitamin-like properties follows.

CHOLINE

Choline has been known for over a century as an essential component of animal tissues and it is classified as having vitamin-like activity in experimental animals. Man, however, can synthesize choline from methionine. Choline is widely distributed in animal and plant tissues, and in an average diet no inadequacy of it will occur. The body can synthesize choline from the amino acid, serine, providing methionine is present to supply methyl groups and with vitamin B_{12} and folacin to act as coenzymes. However, the rate at which it is synthesized is insufficient to meet the need of most higher animals. For this reason choline is considered an essential nutrient. Choline is a source in the body for labile methyl groups. These are used for various synthetic processes and for detoxification of many toxic compounds. Choline is an integral part of phospholipids, lecithin (important in the metabolism of fat in the liver)

and sphingomyelin in brain and nerve tissue. Choline serves also as a precursor of acetylcholine.

Function. Its function in man is in the metabolism of and in the transport of fat from the liver, preventing the development of fatty liver. As a component of several phospholipids, it functions in triglyceride transport and cell membrane structure. In the liver choline forms *lecithin,* and during the process fatty acids are removed from the glycerides of the liver, resulting in the decrease of triglyceride content in that organ. As a constituent of *acetylcholine,* choline plays a role in the transmission of nerve impulses. As a dietary source of labile methyl groups it is essential for synthesis of methionine. Betaine, methionine and choline function as donors of methyl groups. Each serves to partially make up for a shortage of one of the others. This process is known as a transmethylation. The action of these substances serves to prevent the development of fatty liver.

Deficiency is associated with fatty deposition in the liver. Fatty infiltration of the liver is observed in chronic alcoholics and in kwashiorkor, but cannot be related to a methionine deficiency and thus a choline deficiency. Choline deficiency in man has not been demonstrated.

Choline deficiency in animals leads to many

abnormal findings, including hemorrhagic lesions in the kidney and fatty liver.

Source. The richest known dietary source is egg yolk. Other food sources are liver, brain, kidney, heart, lean meat, yeast, soy beans, peanuts, beans, peas and wheat germ. Fruit, fruit juices, milk and vegetables generally are not sources of choline. Neutral fats are essentially devoid of choline.

Recommended Dietary Allowance. Daily requirements are not known and no toxic effects have been observed. The average diet has been estimated to contain 400 to 900 mg. per day of choline, including its natural precursor betaine, according to the 1974 revision of the Recommended Dietary Allowances.

INOSITOL

Inositol has long been known as a chemical compound, but only since 1940 has it been considered a vitamin. It is found in fruits, grains, vegetables, nuts, legumes, and organ meats (liver, heart). It occurs abundantly in the average diet. Chemically, inositol is a colorless, water-soluble crystalline material. It is a cyclic 6-carbon compound with 6-hydroxyl groups and so is related to glucose. *Myoinositol,* known as "muscle sugar," occurs in animal tissues as a component of phospholipids. In plants it is found as *phytic acid* (hexaphosphate ester of inositol). Phytic acid interferes with the absorption of calcium and iron. It binds both to form an insoluble complex. Inositol is concentrated in the brain and occurs in skeletal and heart muscles and other tissues.

Inositol's physiological role is related to its presence in phosphoinositols and thus to the function of phospholipids. It is considered to have lipotrophic activity. It is thought to be metabolized to glucose through glucuronic acid and this may be the reason for its increased excretion in diabetics.[1] There is no evidence that inositol is a vitamin for man.

LIPOIC ACID

Lipoic acid, a fat-soluble, sulfur-containing fatty acid, is not a true vitamin, since it can be synthesized in the body. It functions as a coenzyme and is essential together with the thiamin-containing enzyme, pyrophosphatase (TPP), for reactions in carbohydrate metabolism which convert pyruvic acid to acetylcoenzyme A. Lipoic acid with two sulfur bonds combines with the TPP to reduce pyruvate to active acetate. It joins the intermediary products of protein and fat metabolism in the Krebs cycle in the reactions involved in producing energy from these nutrients. A metal ion (magnesium or calcium) is involved in this oxidative decarboxylation along with vitamins, thiamin, pantothenic acid, niacin, riboflavin and lipoic acid.

No dietary requirement for lipoic acid for humans is known. The amounts needed to participate in the reactions in the tissues may be synthesized in the body. It is found in liver and yeast.

UBIQUINONE (Coenzyme Q)

A lipid-like substance similar to vitamin K, ubiquinone belongs to a group of compounds known as ubiquinones. Ubiquinones are a group of coenzymes. Attached to the basic quinone ring structure are 30 or more carbon atoms in a side chain. Coenzyme Q is present in all cell nuclei and microsomes. It is concentrated in the mitochondria and functions in the respiratory chain in which energy is released from the energy-yielding nutrients as ATP. The ubiquinones appear to be synthesized in the body and cannot be classified as vitamins.

ANTIVITAMINS
(Vitamin Antagonists or Antimetabolites)

There are a growing number of instances of antivitamin activity of special interest in nutrition. An antivitamin or antagonist may be defined as a substance or condition that interferes with the synthesis or metabolism of vitamins. Many vitamin antagonists are compounds similar in structure to the active vitamin molecule. They can prevent incorporation of the vitamin units in the coenzyme structure by attaching themselves to the enzyme. They block the action of the coenzyme, which results in a true vitamin deficiency. Experimental vitamin deficiencies have been produced by using vitamin antagonists. An established example of another type of antivitamin is avidin, found in raw egg white, which combines with biotin and forms a compound which cannot be absorbed from the intestinal tract. A biotin deficiency can be produced in experimental animals and humans who are fed extremely large quantities of raw egg white. Antibiotics used in medical and surgical treatment may destroy the bacteria in the intestinal tract which are necessary to synthesize certain vitamins (K and several members of the B-complex group).

Isonicotinic acid hydrazide (INH), which is used as a chemotherapeutic agent in the treatment of tuberculosis, is an antagonist for pyridoxine. Aminopterin, an antagonist of folacin, has reduced the number of leukocytes in leukemia. Dicumarol, which is an anticoagulant, acts as an antagonist to vitamin K. (See Chapter 21 on drug-nutrient interactions.)

PROBLEMS AND SUGGESTED TOPICS FOR DISCUSSION

1. Evaluate your dietary pattern for the foods high in vitamins A, D, thiamin, riboflavin, niacin, and ascorbic acid. Make suggestions for improvement.
2. Select references from the suggested reading list pertaining to vitamins and vision, thiamin and mentality, folic acid and anemia, vitamin B_6 and depression, and the relationship of enzymes and vitamins, for either an oral or written report.
3. What are the functions of vitamins A, D, E and K?
4. List the fractions of the vitamin B-complex that are recognized as necessary for humans. What is the function of each?
5. What effects may handling, storage, and cooking of foods have on vitamins A, thiamine, riboflavin, niacin, folic acid, B_{12} and ascorbic acid?
6. Does the normal healthy person on an adequate well-rounded diet need vitamin supplements? Explain.
7. Search the literature and make a list of drugs with antivitamin activity that are of special interest in nutrition.
8. List the vitamins that should be supplied daily. List the vitamins stored in the body. List the vitamins that are known to be synthesized in the body.

CITED REFERENCES

1. Alam, S. Q.: Inositols, IX. Biochemical Systems. In Sebrell, W. H., and Harris, R. S. (eds.): The Vitamins. Vol. III, New York, Academic Press, 1971, pp. 380–394.
2. American Psychiatric Association Task Force on Vitamin Therapy in Psychiatry: Megavitamin and Orthomolecular Therapy in Psychiatry. Washington, D.C. Publications Services Division, Am. Psychiatric Assoc., 1973.
3. Anderson, T. W.: Large scale trials of vitamin C. Ann. N.Y. Acad. Sci., 258:498, 1975.
4. Anderson, T. W., Reid, D. B., and Beaton, G. H.: Vitamin C and the common cold: a double-blind trial. Can. Med. Assoc. J., 107:503, 1972.
5. Arroyave, G., et. al.: Alterations in serum concentration of vitamin A associated with the hypoproteinemia of severe protein malnutrition. J. Pediatr., 62:920, 1963.
6. Baker, E. M., et al.: Vitamin B_6 requirement for adult men. Am. J. Clin. Nutr., 15:59, 1964.
7. Bieri, J. G.: Vitamin E. Nutr. Rev., 33:161, 1975.
8. Bieri, J. G., and Evarts, R. P.: Tocopherols and fatty acids in American diets. J. Am. Diet. Assoc., 62:147, 1973.
9. Bouhuys, A.: Colds and antihistamine effects of vitamin C. N. Engl. J. Med., 290:633, 1974.
10. Bunnell, R. H., et al.: Alpha-tocopherol content of foods. Am. J. Clin. Nutr., 17:1, 1965.
11. Corrigan, J. J., and Marcus, F. I.: Coagulopathy associated with vitamin E ingestion, JAMA, 230:1300, 1974.
12. Coulehan, J. L., et al.: Vitamin C and upper respiratory illness in Navaho children: preliminary observations (1974). Ann. N.Y. Acad. Sci., 258:513, 1975.
13. Coulehan, J. L., et al.: Vitamin C prophylaxis in a boarding school. N. Engl. J. Med., 290:6, 1974.
14. Darby, W. J., McNutt, K. W., and Todhunter, E. N.: Niacin. Nutr. Rev., 33:289, 1975.
15. Essays on the History of Nutrition and Dietetics. Chicago, American Dietetic Association, 1967.
16. Farrell, P. M., and Bieri, J. G.: Megavitamin E supplementation in man. Am. J. Clin. Nutr., 28:1381, 1975.
17. Food: The Yearbook of Agriculture. Washington, D.C., USDA, 1959, pp. 1–23.
18. Haeger, K.: Long-time treatment of intermittent claudication with vitamin E. Am. J. Clin. Nutr., 27:1179, 1974.
19. Herbert, V.: Nutritional requirements for B_{12} and folic acid. Am. J. Clin. Nutr., 21:743, 1968.
20. Hypervitaminosis E and coagulation. Nutr. Rev., 33:269, 1975.
21. Jusko, W. J., and Levy, G.: Absorption, protein binding, and elimination of riboflavin. In Rivlin, R. S. (ed.): Riboflavin. New York, Plenum Press, 1975.
22. Kinsman, R. A., and Hood, J.: Some behavioral effects of ascorbic acid deficiency. Am. J. Clin. Nutr., 24:455, 1971.
23. Korsan-Bengsten, K., Elmfeldt, D., and Holm, T.: Prolonged plasma clotting time and decreased fibrinolysis after long-term treatment with α-tocopherol. Thromb. Diath. Haemorrh., 31:505, 1974.
24. Lamden, N.: Dangers of massive vitamin C intake. N. Engl. J. Med., 284:336, 1971.
25. Lowenberg, M. E., et al.: Food and Man. 2nd ed. New York, John Wiley & Sons, Inc., 1972.
26. MacKenzie, J. F., and Russell, R. I.: The effect of pH on folic acid absorption in man. Clin. Sci. Mol. Med., 51:363, 1976.
27. Mašek, J.: Contribution to the problem of vitamin C requirement in adults. Rev. Czech. Med., 12:54, 1966.
28. McCollum, E.V.: A History of Nutrition. Boston, Houghton-Mifflin Company, 1957.
29. Pauling, L.: Vitamin C and the Common Cold. San Francisco, W. H. Freeman & Co., 1970.
30. Pelletier, O.: Cigarette smoking and vitamin C. Nutr. Today, 5:12, 1970.
31. Recent Developments in Vitamin D. Chicago, National Dairy Council, Dairy Council Digest, 47(3), 1976.
32. Recommended Dietary Allowances. 8th ed. Washington, D.C., Food and Nutrition Board, National Research Council, NAS, 1974.
33. Roels, O. A.: Present knowledge of vitamin E. In Present Knowledge of Nutrition, 3rd ed. New York, The Nutrition Foundation, 1967.
34. Russell, R. M., and Boyer, J. L.: Hepatic injury from chronic hypervitaminosis A resulting in portal hypertension and ascites. N. Engl. J. Med., 291:435, 1974.
35. Snyderman, S. E., Carreterro, R., and Holt, L. E.: Pyridoxine deficiency in the human being. Fed. Proc., 9:371, 1950.
36. Sydenstricker, V. P., et al.: "Egg-white injury" in man and its cure with a biotin concentrate. JAMA, 118:1199, 1942.

37. Ten-State Nutrition Survey, 1968–70. DHEW Publ. No. (HSM) 72–8134, 1972.
38. Vilter, R. W., et al.: The effect of vitamin B_6 deficiency induced by desoxypyridoxine in human beings. J. Lab. Clin. Med., 42:335, 1953.
39. Williams, M. A.: Present knowledge of vitamin B_6. In Present Knowledge in Nutrition. 3rd ed. New York, The Nutrition Foundation, Inc., 1967, pp. 67 and 70.
40. Wilson, C. W., and Loh, H. S.: Common cold and vitamin C. Lancet, 1:638, 1973.

ADDITIONAL REFERENCES

GENERAL

Nutrients in Processed Foods, Vitamins and Minerals. American Medical Association, Acton, Mass., Publishing Sciences Group, Inc., 1974.
Carter, J.: The Ten-State Nutrition Survey: An Analysis. Atlanta, Georgia, Southern Regional Council, Inc., 1974.
Guthrie, H. A.: Introductory Nutrition. 3rd ed. St. Louis, Missouri, C. V. Mosby Co., 1975.
Hardinge, M. G., and Crooks, H.: Lesser known vitamins in foods. J. Am. Diet. Assoc., 38:240, 1961.
Jolliffe, N.: Clinical Nutrition. 2nd ed. New York, Harper and Brothers, 1962, Chapters 13 through 22.
Levitan, R., and Wilson, D. E.: Absorption of water soluble substances. In Jacobson, E. D., and Shanour, L. (eds.): Gastrointestinal Physiology. Baltimore, University Park Press, 1974.
Mangay Chung, A. S., et al.: Folic acid, vitamin B_6, pantothenic acid and vitamin B_{12} in human dietaries. Am. J. Clin. Nutr., 9:573, 1961.
Orr, M. L.: Pantothenic Acid, Vitamin B_6 and Vitamin B_{12} in Foods. Home Economics Research Report No. 36, Washington, D.C., Agricultural Research Service, USDA, 1969.
Preliminary Findings of the First Health and Nutrition Examination Survey, United States, 1971–72, Dietary Intake and Biochemical Findings. Washington, D.C., DHEW Publ. No. (HRA) 74–1219–1, 1974.
Sauberlich, H. E., Skala, J. H. and Dowdy, R. P.: Laboratory Tests for the Assessment of Nutritional Status. Cleveland, Ohio, CRC Press, 1974.
Watt, B. K., and Merrill, A. L.: Composition of Foods. Agriculture Handbook No. 8, Washington, D.C., Agriculture Research Service, USDA, 1963.

VITAMIN A

Ames, S. R.: Factors affecting absorption, transport, and storage of vitamin A. Am. J. Clin. Nutr., 22:934, 1969.
Bergen, S. S., and Roels, O. A.: Hypervitaminosis A, report of a case. Am. J. Clin. Nutr., 16:265, 1965.
Chopra, J. G., and Kevany, J.: Hypovitaminosis A in the Americas. Am. J. Clin. Nutr., 23:231, 1970.
Interrelationships between vitamins A and E. Nutr. Rev., 23:82, 1965.
Mori, S.: Primary changes in eyes of rats that result from deficiency of fat soluble A. JAMA, 79:197, 1922.
Pereira, S. M., et al.: Vitamin A therapy in children with kwashiorkor. Am. J. Clin. Nutr., 20:297, 1967.
The therapeutic use of vitamin A acid. Acta Derm. Venereol. [Suppl.], 55:74, 1976.
Wald, G., and Hubbard, R.: The synthesis of rhodopsin from vitamin A. Proc. Natl. Acad. Sci. USA, 36:92, 1950.

VITAMIN D

Blunt, J. W., De Luca, H. F., and Schnoes, H. K.: 25-hydroxycholecalciferol: a biologically active metabolite of vitamin D_3. Biochem., 7:3317, 1968.
De Luca, H. F.: New forms of vitamin D and their potential applications. Nutr. News, 36(4), 1973.
De Luca, H. F.: Vitamin D endocrinology. Ann. Int. Med., 85:367, 1976.
Food and Nutrition Board, NRC/NAS: Hazards of overdose of vitamin D. Am. J. Clin. Nutr., 28:512, 1975.
Fraser, D. R., and Kodicek, E.: Unique biosynthesis by kidney of a biologically active vitamin D metabolite. Nature, 228:764, 1970.
Holick, M. F., et al.: Isolation and identification of 1,25-dihydroxycholeciferol. A metabolite of vitamin D active in intestine. Biochem., 10:2799, 1971.
Lawson, D. E., et al.: Identification of 1,25-dihydroxycholeciferol, a new kidney hormone controlling calcium metabolism. Nature, 230:228, 1971.
MacIntyre, I.: Vitamin D metabolism (Letter), N. Engl. J. Med., 288:471, 1973.

VITAMIN E

Dicks-Bushnell, M. W., and Davis, K. C.: Vitamin E content of infant formulas and cereals. Am. J. Clin. Nutr., 20:262, 1967.
Horwitt, M. K.: Vitamin E: a reexamination. Am. J. Clin. Nutr., 29:569, 1976.
Horwitt, M. K., et al.: Polyunsaturated lipids and tocopherol requirements. J. Am. Diet. Assoc., 38:231, 1961.
Oski, F. A., and Barnes, L. A.: Vitamin E deficiency: a previously unrecognized cause of hemolytic anemia in the premature infant. J. Pediatr., 70:211, 1967.
Tapple, A. L.: Reactions of vitamin E, ubiquinol, and selenoamino acids and protection of oxidant-labile enzymes. In De Luca, H. F., and Suttie, J. W. (eds.): The Fat Soluble Vitamins. Madison, Wisconsin, University of Wisconsin Press, 1970.

VITAMIN K

Crosse, V. M., et al.: Kernicterus and Prematurity. Arch. Dis. Child., 30:501, 1955.
Nutrition and blood clotting. Dairy Council Digest, 43(3), 1972.
Olson, R. E.: Vitamin K. In Goodhart, R. S., and Shils, M.E. (eds.): Modern Nutrition in Health and Disease. 5th ed. Philadelphia, Lea & Febiger, 1973.
Suttie, J. W.: Vitamin K and prothrombin synthesis. Nutr. Rev., 31:105, 1973.
Udall, J. A.: Human sources and absorption of vitamin K in relation to anticoagulation stability. JAMA, 194:127, 1965.
Vietti, T. J., Stephens, J. C., and Bennett, K. R.: Vitamin K_1 prophylaxis in the newborn. JAMA, 176:791, 1961.

THIAMIN

Brin, M.: Erythrocyte as a biopsy tissue for functional evaluation of thiamine adequacy. JAMA, 187:762, 1964.
Rindi, G., and Ventura, U.: Thiamine intestinal transport. Physiol. Rev., 52:821, 1972.

RIBOFLAVIN

Rivlin, R. S. (ed.): Riboflavin. New York, Plenum Press, 1975.

NIACIN

Roe, D. A.: A Plague of Corn: The Social History of Pellagra. Ithaca, New York, Cornell University Press, 1973.

VITAMIN B₆

Coursin, D. B.: Vitamin B₆ requirements. JAMA, *189*:27, 1964.

Jacobs, F. A.: Role of vitamin B₆ in intestinal absorption of amino acids in situ. JAMA, *179*:523, 1962.

Miller, L. T., and Linkswiler, H. M.: Effect of protein intake on the development of abnormal tryptophan metabolism by men during vitamin B₆ depletion. J. Nutr., *93*:53, 1967.

Polansky, M. M., and Murphy, E. W.: Vitamin B₆ in fruits and nuts. J. Am. Diet. Assoc., *48*:109, 1966.

Vitamin B₆ components in various foods. Nutr. Rev., *23*:78, 1965.

Vitamin B₆ deficiency and immune responses. Nutr. Rev., *34*:188, 1976.

PANTOTHENIC ACID

Further studies of pantothenic acid deficiency in man. Nutr. Rev., *17*:200, 1959.

Wirtschafter, Z. T., and Walsh, J. R.: Hepatocellular lipoid changes in pantothenic acid deficiency. Am. J. Clin. Nutr., *10*:525, 1962.

FOLACIN

Butterfield, S., and Calloway, D. H.: Folacin in wheat and selected foods. J. Am. Diet. Assoc., *60*:310, 1972.

Streiff, R. R.: Folate levels in citrus and other juices. Am. J. Clin. Nutr., *24*:1390, 1971.

Streiff, R. R., and Little, A. B.: Folic acid deficiency in pregnancy. N. Engl. J. Med., *276*:776, 1967.

Thenen, S. W.: Food folate values (letter). Am. J. Clin. Nutr., *28*:1341, 1975.

VITAMIN B₁₂

Drapanas, T., et al.: Role of the ileum in the absorption of vitamin B₁₂ and intrinsic factor (IF). JAMA, *184*:337, 1963.

Herbert, V.: Folic acid and vitamin B₁₂. In Goodhart, R. S., and Shils, M. E. (eds.): Modern Nutrition in Health and Disease. 5th ed. Lea & Febiger, 1973.

Hines, J. D.: Megaloblastic anemia in adult vegan. Am. J. Clin. Nutr., *19*:260, 1966.

Hsu, J. M.: Effect of deficiencies of certain B vitamins and ascorbic acid on absorption of vitamin B₁₂. Am. J. Clin. Nutr., *12*:170, 1963.

Wilson, T. H.: Intrinsic factor and B₁₂ absorption—a problem in cell physiology. Nutr. Rev., *23*:33, 1965.

VITAMIN C

Hodges, R. E.: The effect of stress on ascorbic acid metabolism in man. Nutr. Today, *5*:11, 1970.

Hodges, R. E. et al.: Experimental scurvy in man. Am. J. Clin. Nutr., *22*:535, 1969.

King, C. G., and Burns, J. J. (eds.): Second conference on vitamin C. Ann. N.Y. Acad. Sci., vol. 258, 1975.

Schwartz, F. W.: Ascorbic acid in wound healing—a review. J. Am. Diet. Assoc., *56*:497, 1970.

Shaffer, C. F.: Ascorbic acid and atherosclerosis. Am. J. Clin. Nutr., *23*:27, 1970.

Sherlock, P., and Rothchild, E. O.: Zen diets and scurvy. JAMA, *199*:794, 1967.

Stevenson, N. R.: Active transport of l-ascorbic acid in the human ileum. Gastroenterology, *67*:952, 1974.

Vitamin C toxicity. Nutr. Rev., *34*:236, 1976.

Chapter 9

WATER AND ELECTROLYTES

DISTRIBUTION OF WATER WITHIN THE BODY

Water constitutes about two-thirds of the total body weight and is the body's principal component from the anatomical as well as the physiological point of view. Next to oxygen, it is the most important constituent for maintenance of life. A person can live for several weeks without food but only a few days without water. Dehydration (water loss) will kill far quicker than starvation.

A man can lose most of his fat and glycogen and half his protein (40 per cent loss of body

weight) and survive, but a 20 per cent loss of body water may cause death, and a loss of only 10 per cent of water causes severe disorders.

Life goes on in a milieu of water. Water is an essential component of all protoplasm and plays a major role in cellular metabolism. Structurally 70 per cent of the mass of fat-free body weight consists of water. It is classified as intracellular and extracellular water. *Intracellular* water is within the cells of the body. *Extracellular* water includes the water in the blood, lymph, spinal fluid and secretions, and the *intercellular* or *interstitial* water that is found between and around the cells (Fig. 9–1).

The water in the blood constitutes about 5 per cent and the interstitial water about 15 per cent of body weight. The intracellular water will approximate 50 per cent of the body weight. The distribution of body water is not fixed but can vary under differing circum-

stances, but the total amount in the body remains relatively constant.

FUNCTIONS OF WATER IN THE BODY

Water is the solvent in which all of the metabolic changes take place. It is not only a solvent but acts catalytically as well.

Water functions in digestion, absorption, circulation and excretion. It leaves the body through the skin, lungs, kidneys and feces. Water helps to maintain the electrolytic balance of the body. Only so long as the osmotic pressure exerted by solutes remains in equilibrium is it possible to have good health.

Water plays a role in the maintenance of body temperature. Perspiration during warm weather and in fevers keeps the skin moist; by evaporation of perspiration the body is cooled.

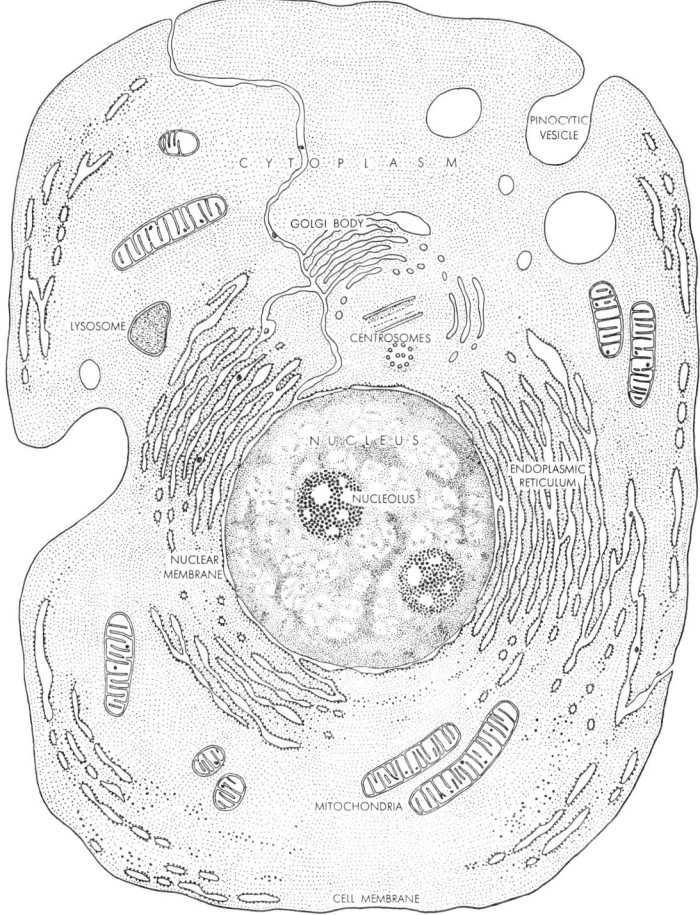

Figure 9–1   Diagram of a typical cell based on what is seen in electron micrographs. (From: Brachet, J.: The living cell. Sci. Am., *205*:50, 1961. © 1961 by Scientific American, Inc. All rights reserved.)

Water acts as a transporting medium for nutrients and all body substances.

Metabolic waste products generated in the cells of the body are transported in the water solution via the blood to the kidneys where the wastes are excreted in urine.

Water substances in the body act as lubricants. Special water-soluble substances are in saliva to make foodstuffs slippery and around bones to lubricate the joints.

Water serves as a building material for growth and repair of the body. It is a part of all body tissues and fluids.

Water in the intestinal tract aids elimination.

WATER BALANCE

Because the water content of the fat-free body weight remains fairly constant, it is evident that balance must exist. That is, the amount of water taken in daily is approximately equivalent to the amount of water lost.

Water Intake. In health water intake is controlled largely by thirst sensations. The thirst control center located in the hypothalamus is apparently activated when osmotic pressure of the body fluids increases or there is a lower extracellular volume. The sensation of thirst occurs and serves as a signal to seek fluids.

Water is ingested as such and as part of ingested food. Most adults in the United States consume 1.5 to 2.0 liters of fluids daily. Almost all foods contain some water. They may be composed of from 4 to 98 per cent water. Table 9-1 shows the percentage of water in some common foods.

In addition to the water contained in ingested foods, the oxidation of these foods in the body also produces water as an end-product. The oxidation of 100 gm. of fat, carbohydrate or protein yields 107, 55 and 41 gm. of water, respectively. Such water is known as "metabolic water" and must be considered in the calculations of water balance. The amount of water as a result of the oxidation of food is 10 to 14 grams per 100 kcalories or approximately 300 to 350 ml. per day.

In addition to water taken into the digestive tract by mouth, a large amount of extracellular fluid is transferred daily into the stomach and intestines. This may amount to 8200 ml. daily. The sources of this fluid are shown in Table 9-2. These fluids function in digestion and absorption and then pass on into the ileum and colon. Here the water is almost entirely reabsorbed except for a small amount, about 100 ml., which is excreted in the feces. Because this

Table 9–1 PERCENTAGES OF WATER IN SOME COMMON FOODS

Lettuce (iceberg)	96
Snapbeans, radishes, celery	94
Watermelon	93
Cabbage (raw)	92
Broccoli, carrots, beets, collards	91
Orange	88
Milk	87
Cereals (cooked)	87
Apples	85
Potatoes (boiled)	80
Bananas	76
Eggs	74
Corn	74
Chicken (boiled)	71
Fish (baked)	68
Prunes (cooked)	66
Beef (lean)	60
Cheese	40
Bread	36
Cake (sponge)	32
Butter	16
Nuts	5
Soda crackers, dry cereals	4
Sugar (white)	trace
Oils	0

From Nutritive Value of Foods, U.S. Department of Agriculture. Home Garden Bull. No. 72, revised 1964. Appendix Table 1.

volume of reabsorbed fluid is about twice that of the blood plasma (3500 ml.) the loss of large amounts from the gastrointestinal tract (diarrhea) may be of serious consequence to the individual.

When water cannot be taken orally, it may be given intravenously, subcutaneously or rectally in the form of salt (saline) solutions which resemble closely the fluids of the body. Water also may be given intravenously as glucose solutions or as blood, plasma or protein hydrolysate mixtures.

Water is absorbed rapidly from the digestive tract into blood and lymph because it moves freely by diffusion through membranes. The

Table 9–2 SOURCES OF WATER IN THE DIGESTIVE JUICES*

Saliva	1500 ml.
Gastric secretions	2500 ml.
Bile	500 ml.
Pancreatic secretions	700 ml.
Intestinal mucosa secretions	3000 ml.
Total	8200 ml.

*Gamble, J. L.: Chemical Anatomy, Physiology and Pathology of Extracellular Fluids. Cambridge, Harvard University Press, 1954.

movement of water is controlled mostly by osmotic forces generated by the inorganic ions found in solution in the body.

Water Elimination. Water is lost from the body through the kidneys as urine, through the bowel in feces, through the lungs with expired air, and through the skin as perspiration. The kidney is by far the main regulator of water loss.

Insensible water loss is that which goes on constantly and usually unconsciously, namely through the skin and lungs, and amounts to 800 to 1000 ml. daily in normal conditions. Sensible water loss is that excreted through the bowel and kidneys.

Lung water goes out of the body as tiny droplets in the expired air. Water loss through the kidneys, perspiration and feces carries out waste products and minerals with it, thus accounting for the need to replace minerals daily by the diet, as discussed in Chapter 7.

Abnormal losses of water occur through vomiting, diarrhea, hemorrhages, draining fistulas, exuding of burns, nasogastric tubes, draining surgical tubes and from the ingestion of diuretics. When water intake is insufficient or water loss occurs, the kidney attempts to compensate by conserving water and thereby excretes a more concentrated urine. Concentration of urine is measured by *specific gravity,* which is normally between 1.010 and 1.030. During dehydration the specific gravity is increased. This action of the kidney is controlled by the pituitary antidiuretic hormone (ADH), which stimulates the renal tubules to increase the reabsorption of water. When water is lost, changes in electrolyte balance occur. When the water losses are excessive (dehydration), the extracellular fluid becomes concentrated and osmotic pressure increases and causes a drain of water from the cells into the extracellular fluid to compensate for the loss. Usually the individual becomes extremely thirsty and nauseated. There are many recognized specific imbalances of body fluids.

Water Balance. Water balance is directly related to the homeostatic functioning of the internal environment: hydrogen ion concentration, water and electrolyte concentration, osmotic pressure, temperature, and other balances of the interstitial fluids.

For a person to be in metabolic equilibrium, water intake must equal water output. The typical daily water intake and output is shown in Table 9–3.

This table could be changed markedly by varying environmental conditions. For exam-

Table 9–3 WATER BALANCE

WATER INTAKE	
Fluids	1250 ml.
Water in food	900 ml.
Water from oxidation of food in the body	350 ml.
Total	2500 ml.

WATER OUTPUT	
Urine	1400 ml.
Water in feces	100 ml.
Skin (perspiration)	700 ml.
Lungs (expired air)	300 ml.
Total	2500 ml.

ple, in cold weather, less water would be lost through the skin and more would then be passed as urine. In very hot weather, both skin and lung water output would be much greater, urine output would be less, and intake of drinking water would be greater.

The body has no place to store water. Water held in the bladder is of no metabolic use. Therefore, the amount lost every 24 hours must be replaced to maintain health and efficiency.

WATER IN FOODS

Vegetables and fruits contain approximately 90 per cent water (Table 9–1). Milk is 87 per cent water, meat 60 to 75 per cent water. Even dried foods such as figs and raisins contain about 20 per cent water. Only truly dried foods, the commercially dehydrated foods, do not contain water. In addition to the actual water present in foods is the water that becomes available as an end product of food metabolism, as previously stated.

Recommended Allowance of Water. The water requirement depends upon the losses through the various routes—sensible and insensible. The Food and Nutrition Board in 1974 states that under the most favorable conditions (low solute diet), minimal physical activity and absence of sweating, the total water supplied from food, beverages and metabolic water should be at least 1.5 liters per day. A reasonable allowance based on recommended caloric intake is suggested to be 1 ml./kcal. for adults and 1.5 ml./kcal. for infants. A suitable daily allowance for adults in most instances is 2½ liters or approximately 2½ to 3 quarts. A large percentage of this is contained in pre-

pared foods. Diets such as the Zen macrobiotic diet, which recommends severely restricted intakes of water and/or fluid, can be extremely dangerous.

Thirst is usually an adequate guide for water intake except for infants and the sick. In cases of extreme heat or excessive sweating thirst may not keep pace with the actual water requirement. Special attention to water needs should be given to infants on high protein formulas; to comatose patients; to those individuals with fever, excessive urine loss or diarrhea or who are consuming high protein diets; and to all persons in hot environments.[1]

WATER AND ELECTROLYTES

When a salt, acid or base is dissolved in water it dissociates into its constituent ions. Because these charged particles can conduct an electric current they are known as electrolytes. Glucose, alcohols, urea, protein and many other substances involved in metabolism which do not separate into charged particles are called nonelectrolytes because these molecules do not ionize.

There are some major differences in the electrolyte composition of extracellular and intracellular fluids. The composition of the extracellular fluid is well known because blood, the main extracellular fluid, is readily available for study. Obtaining representative samples of intracellular fluids for analysis is no easy task. Thus the data on their composition is less reliable than that of extracellular fluids. The substances present in the fluid between the cells (interstitial fluid) closely resemble those found in blood plasma except that the concentration of proteins is lower.

Electrolytes are of importance in relation to their concentration (number of particles per unit volume) and because of their number of charges. Electrolyte concentrations are conventionally expressed in terms of *milliequivalents* (mEq.) When the concentrations of each ionic constituent of extracellular or intracellular fluids are expressed in terms of milliequivalents per liter, the sum of all the positively charged ions *(cations)* exactly equals the sum of all the negatively charged ions *(anions)*. Thus, every positively charged ion is exactly balanced by a negatively charged ion. This concept will be evident from perusal of the values in Table 9–4. The average sum of the concentration of all the cations in serum is about 150 mEq. per liter. This is balanced by

Table 9–4   NORMAL ELECTROLYTE CONCENTRATIONS OF THE EXTRACELLULAR AND INTRACELLULAR FLUIDS (in mEq./liter)

	IN EXTRA-CELLULAR FLUID	IN INTRA-CELLULAR FLUID
Cations		
Sodium	135 to 147	10
Potassium	3.5 to 5.5	150
Calcium	4.5 to 5.5	1 to 2
Magnesium	1.5 to 3.0	40
Anions		
Chloride	98 to 106	4
Bicarbonate	26 to 30	10
Phosphate	2 to 5	140
Sulfate	2 to 5	10
Organic Acids (lactic, pyruvic)	3 to 6	
Proteins	15 to 19	40

Adapted from Gamble, J. L.: Chemical Anatomy, Physiology and Pathology of Extracellular Fluids. Cambridge, Harvard University Press, 1954.

150 mEq. per liter of anions to make a total serum osmolarity of about 300 mEq. per liter.

Osmotic Pressure. The body seeks to equalize the total salt concentrations (in milliequivalents) of the intracellular and extracellular fluids. Reference is being made to total cation and anion concentrations and not the concentrations of individual ions because it has already been noted that sodium and potassium, for example, are normally distributed in quite a different manner between intracellular and extracellular fluid.

In an effort to maintain these equal concentrations, small shifts of water may take place. These shifts are due to a force called osmotic pressure which is directly proportional to the number of particles in solution. If the salt content of the tissues (intracellular fluid) gets too high, water passes from the surrounding fluid (extracellular fluid) into the cell and thus reduces the salt concentration in the cell and also increases the concentration of salt in the extracellular fluid. If, on the other hand, the salt concentration in the intracellular fluid is too low, water passes out of the cells into the extracellular fluid. It is convenient (although not entirely accurate) to consider that the osmotic pressure of the intracellular fluid is largely a function of its content of potassium because this cation predominates, whereas the osmotic pressure of the extracellular fluid may be conveniently considered to relate to its content of

sodium—this being the major cation present. Shifts in the distribution of these ions are the principal cause of shifts of water between the various fluid compartments, although chloride and PO_4 can also influence H_2O balance.

Proteins, non-diffusible because of their size, also play an important part in maintaining osmotic equilibrium. Their presence in the plasma exerts a colloidal osmotic pressure which helps to retain water within the blood vessel lumen and thereby prevents the leakage of water from the plasma into the interstitial fluid. In some disease states, such as protein calorie (energy) malnutrition, when the protein content of plasma is exceptionally low, water does leak into the interstitial fluids, resulting in edema.

Electrolyte Control of Body Hydration. An important difference in the distribution of sodium and potassium has been noted (i.e., sodium is largely confined to extracellular fluids, whereas potassium occurs largely within the cells). Also it has been noted that phosphate anions predominate within cells and chloride anions (Cl^-) predominate in the extracellular fluids.

Sodium and potassium concentrations are of major influence in directing the movement of water from one body compartment to another (i.e., from extracellular fluid into cells and vice versa). These two cations are in control of total hydration of the body (i.e., control over the amount of water to be retained in any given compartment). The shifts in water from one compartment to another are due to changes occurring in the extracellular concentrations of electrolytes. When water loss exceeds electrolyte loss, the extracellular fluid becomes *hypertonic* to the intracellular fluid (i.e., the osmotic pressure of the extracellular fluid is higher than the osmotic pressure of the intracellular fluid) and water shifts from the cells to the extracellular space to compensate. When water enters the extracellular fluid with the electrolytes in amounts insufficient to maintain normal density of the solutions, the extracellular fluid becomes *hypotonic* to the intracellular fluid (i.e., the osmotic pressure of the extracellular fluid is lower than the osmotic pressure of the intracellular fluid) and water shifts from the extracellular space into the cell. The reduction of the extracellular fluid continues until osmotic equilibrium between intracellular and extracellular fluids is reestablished. When the body is unable to maintain osmotic equilibrium, dehydration or edema may result. Causes of dehydration or edema are discussed later in the text.

ACID-BASE REGULATION

Acid-Base Balance. The reaction of the body fluids is slightly basic (pH 7.35 to 7.4). The body normally maintains this narrow range of pH with remarkable precision even though large amounts of acid are produced during metabolism and various amounts of acids are ingested in foodstuffs. The reason that pH is maintained in the face of these threats is that the food and metabolic acids are rapidly neutralized by buffers present in the blood. The main buffers operating in this regulatory system are the bicarbonate-carbonic acid system, the phosphate system, and the protein systems.

When acids are ingested or formed in metabolism the hydrogen ion combines with bicarbonate ion in the blood plasma to form carbonic acid which is only slightly ionized and traps the hydrogen ion in non-ionized form. In the lungs the carbonic acid is decomposed to form carbon dioxide and water. The carbon dioxide is excreted. The organic anion is excreted in the urine along with a cation (usually sodium). This process, if allowed to continue, would deplete the amount of sodium ion in the body. There are two main mechanisms in the kidney for saving cation. The urine is usually more acid than blood, with a pH of 6.0 to 7.0 and may be as low as 4.7. This is accomplished through the phosphate buffer system. In the plasma most of the phosphate is present as Na_2HPO_4, with smaller amounts of NaH_2PO_4. In the urine the ratio may be reversed. Hydrogen ion is exchanged for sodium ion in the kidney, and the sodium returned to the plasma. Also ammonium ion (NH_4^+) may be formed in the kidney chiefly by hydrolysis of the amino acid glutamine. The ammonium ion is excreted and a sodium ion saved.

Acids and Bases. An acid is defined as a substance (ion, molecule) that yields hydrogen ions (protons) in solution. Conversely, a base is anything that combines with hydrogen ions. Accordingly, when the common acids dissociate into their respective cations and anions, the anionic component may be considered to be a base. Bases are weak or strong depending on their affinity for the hydrogen ion. HCO_3^-, $HPO_4^=$, $H_2PO_4^-$, and protein are relatively strong because they have a strong affinity for hydrogen ion. On the other hand, HCl is almost completely ionized, thus Cl^- is an extremely poor base because it has little ability to bind hydrogen ions. Clinically the term base is frequently applied to the cations (Na^+, K^+, Mg^{++}, Ca^{++}) of the body fluids and the term acid is commonly applied to the anions (Cl^-,

HCO_3^-, $SO_4^=$, $HPO_4^=$). The term "total base" is frequently used in reference to the sum of the cations.

The term *alkali reserve* is frequently used by clinicians to refer to plasma bicarbonate concentration. This anion is available to neutralize acids that might enter the plasma. The term alkali reserve should really refer to all the relatively strong buffer bases of the body fluids, i.e., HCO_3^-, $H_2PO_4^-$, $HPO_4^=$, protein, etc., but under ordinary conditions the bicarbonate levels will reflect the condition of the entire buffer complex. It must be remembered that carbon dioxide is constantly being formed in metabolism and though carbonic acid is a much weaker acid (HCO_3^- a much stronger base) than those we have been discussing and serves as a buffer for them, the amount formed would cause an appreciable change in the pH of the blood if it were not buffered. Hemoglobin is in large measure responsible for the buffering of the metabolic CO_2. Conditions in which respiration is depressed (pneumonia, emphysema, etc.) cause retention of carbon dioxide and a condition referred to as respiratory acidosis.

Potential Acid-Base Reaction of Foods. Foodstuffs, when burned in the body, yield mineral residues which are acidic or basic in reaction. If approximately equal quantities of cations and anions are left in the residue, then the residue will be essentially neutral and the body will not have to make any particular adjustment in the pH of its fluids. If, on the other hand, there is an excess of cations (Na^+, K^+, Ca^{++}, Mg^{++}), the body must draw on its anion reserve to restore pH of blood. The cations will be excreted in the urine largely as dicationic phosphate (Na_2HPO_4, K_2HPO_4) and the urine will be more alkaline in reaction. If there is an excess of anions ($SO_4^=$, $PO_4^=$), the urine will be acid, as described in the previous section, and ammonium ion may be formed.

In general, meats and cereals produce acidic residues such as phosphates and sulfates which result in an acid urine. Conversely, vegetables and fruits produce basic residues which tend to produce alkaline urine. It would seem a curious anomaly that the consumption of citrus fruits and tomatoes results in an alkaline urine. This is because the cations in fruits (chiefly Na^+, K^+) are associated with weak organic anions such as malate or citrate which can be oxidized in the body leaving a cationic residue. A typical mixed diet contains a reasonable balance of acidic and basic substances. Thus the body often does not have to draw strenuously upon its buffering systems to take care of these ingested compounds. The principal threat to the buffer systems of the body are the many acidic products of metabolism. Fortunately, its buffer defenses are quite biased toward the excretion of excess acid and the usual pH of the body fluids is maintained. For this reason, the usual pH of urine is on the acid side of neutral.

Occasionally, foods that will produce acid, basic or neutral ashes are used to produce acidic or basic urine for various therapeutic purposes. For example, the daily ingestion of cranberry juice, which produces an acid residue and acidic urine, is often recommended as a preventive measure to avoid urinary tract infections. Table 9–5 contains a list of foods and indicates their potential acid-base reaction.

Functions of Electrolytes of Body Fluids. The most important cations and anions of body fluids have been listed in Table 9–4 and other

Table 9–5   POTENTIAL ACID-BASE REACTION OF CERTAIN FOODS

ACID ASH FOODS	BASIC ASH FOODS	NEUTRAL ASH FOODS
Breads and crackers	Fruits (except prunes,	Butter and margarine
Cakes and cookies, plain	plums, cranberries)	Cooking fat and oils
Cereals and cereal products	Jams, jellies, honey	Cream
(macaroni, spaghetti, noodles)	Milk	Starch
Cheese	Nuts (Coconut)	Sugars and syrups
Eggs	(Almond)	
Fish	(Chestnut)	
Meats	Vegetables (except corn	
Peanuts, walnuts	and lentils)	
Poultry		
Prunes		
Plums		
Cranberries		
Corn		
Lentils, dried		

mineral elements essential for many vital processes in human metabolism are listed in Table 7–3. They are delivered to the body in the food ingested daily.

The functions of sodium, potassium and chloride, the electrolytes which are the major constituents in extracellular and intracellular fluids, along with the other mineral elements essential in nutrition are presented in Chapter 7, Minerals.

PROBLEMS AND SUGGESTED TOPICS FOR DISCUSSION

1. Keep a record of your water and fluid intake for a period of 24 hours. Evaluate it.
2. Select references from the suggested list pertaining to water and salt relationship for either an oral or written report.
3. What are the routes of water elimination from the body?
4. What is insensible water loss? What is the usual amount? When would it be increased? Decreased?
5. List the functions of water in the body.
6. List the conditions that affect water balance in the body.
7. What is meant by the acid-base regulation of the body? Evaluate your food intake as to whether it is predominately acid or alkaline.

CITED REFERENCE

1. Food and Nutrition Board, Recommended Dietary Allowances. 8th ed. Washington, D.C., National Research Council/NAS, 1974, p. 24.

ADDITIONAL REFERENCES

Baker, E. M., Plough, I. C., and Allen, T. H.: Water requirement of men as related to the salt intake. Am. J. Clin. Nutr., 12:394, 1963.

Bland, J. H.: Clinical Metabolism of Body Water and Electrolytes. Philadelphia, W. B. Saunders Company, 1963.

Brooke, C. E.: Oral fluid and electrolytes. J.A.M.A., 179:792, 1962.

Burton, B. T. (ed.): Human Nutrition. 3rd ed. New York, McGraw-Hill Book Company, Inc., 1976. Chapter 3, Fluid Electrolyte and Acid-Base Balance.

Camien, M. N., et al.: A critical reappraisal of acid-base balance. Am. J. Clin. Nutr., 22:786, 1969.

Chow, B. F., et al.: Diet and urinary output of water. Am. J. Clin. Nutr., 12:333, 1963.

Gamble, J. L.: Chemical Anatomy, Physiology and Pathology of Extracellular Fluid. 6th ed. Cambridge, Harvard University Press, 1954.

Goldberger, E.: A Primer of Water Electrolyte and Acid-Base Syndromes. 2nd ed. Philadelphia, Lea & Febiger, 1962.

Goodhart, R. S., and Shils, M. E. (eds.): Modern Nutrition in Health and Disease. 5th ed. Philadelphia, Lea & Febiger, 1973, Chapter 7, Water, electrolytes and acid-base balance.

Jolliffe, N. (ed.): Clinical Nutrition. 2nd ed. New York, Harper & Bros., 1962. Chapter 12, Sodium, Potassium and Chloride Malnutrition, including Water Balance and Shock.

Metheny, N. M., and Snively, W. D.: Nurses' Handbook of Fluid Balance. 2nd ed. Philadelphia, J. B. Lippincott Co., 1974.

Statland, H.: Fluids and Electrolytes in Practice, 3rd ed. Philadelphia, J. B. Lippincott Company, 1963.

Weisberg, H. E.: Water Electrolytes and Acid-Base Balance, Normal and Pathological. Baltimore, Williams & Wilkins, 1962.

UNIT TWO

NUTRITIONAL STATUS

Chapter 10

RECOMMENDED DIETARY ALLOWANCES AND THE ADEQUATE DIET

INTERPRETATION OF AN ADEQUATE DIET

An adequate diet is composed of the various nutrients which the body needs for maintenance, repair, the living processes and growth or development. It is a diet which meets in full all the nutritional needs of the person. There is no *ideal* diet, since such a diet is a matter of individual requirement. It is the purpose of the daily meals to supply the essential elements. Regional availability of foods, socioeconomic conditions, taste preferences, food habits, age of the family members, storage and preparation facilities, and cooking skills are factors to consider when nutritious meals are planned.

In the preceding chapters the various nutrients needed by the body have been discussed. In this chapter, application of the information gained will be made by translating the nutrients into a daily diet. This chapter is important in that it is the translation of principles of nutrition into the selection of an adequate diet and the foundation of therapeutic nutrition.

DIETARY INTERRELATIONSHIPS

All studies of the interaction of nutrients indicate the need for a balanced diet. Clinical reports show that often when an individual is found deficient in one nutrient, such as a vitamin, deficiencies in others are also found. For example, a deficiency of vitamin A may result also in symptoms and damage associated with deficiency of ascorbic acid. Scurvy has been produced in animals by depriving them of vitamin A. Today it is an established fact that the presence or absence of one essential nutrient may affect the availability, absorption, metabolism, or dietary need for others.

Interrelationships exist not only among the vitamins but among the minerals. Vitamins interact with minerals just as both vitamins and minerals are related to fat, protein and carbohydrate functions and requirements. Numerous experiments have extended understanding of the broad nutritional import of interrelationships or "balance" among nutrients. While certain interrelationships have long been known, the recognition of the large number of them re-emphasizes the basic soundness of the principle of maintaining variety in foods in order to provide the most complete diet. Much current research is being devoted to dietary interrelationships.

PROGRESS IN DETERMINING HUMAN DIETARY NEEDS

The history of the development of the science of nutrition and dietary standards is outlined in Chapter 1. The dietary standards set up by the Food and Nutrition Board of the National Academy of Sciences–National Research Council (Table 10–1) are universally accepted as the guide or yardstick for planning and evaluating diets and food supplies for population groups and individuals in the United

States. FAO/WHO has established standards for people in developing countries and several other countries have their own standards for human nutrient requirements. These standards represent years of research by many workers on both animals and human beings. The U.S. standards, revised in 1974 (eighth revision; original edition published in 1943), represent the latest U.S. interpretation of human nutritional needs by a large number of nutrition authorities.

RECOMMENDED DAILY DIETARY ALLOWANCES (RDA)

The purposes and the applicability of the recommended dietary allowances can best be explained by quoting from the 1974 revised publication.[11]

1. "The Recommended Dietary Allowances are the levels of intake of essential nutrients considered in the judgement of the Food and Nutrition Board on the basis of available scientific knowledge, to be adequate to meet the known nutritional needs of practically all healthy persons."
2. ". . . we are well aware that present knowledge of nutritional needs is incomplete. Requirements for many nutrients have not been established. Therefore, to ensure that possibly unrecognized nutritional needs are met, RDA should be provided from as varied a selection of food as possible."
3. "RDA should not be confused with requirements. Differences in the nutrient requirements of individuals that derive from differences in their genetic makeup are ordinarily unknown. Therefore, as there is no way of predicting whose needs are high and whose are low, RDA (except for energy) are estimated to exceed the requirements of most individuals and thereby ensure that the needs of nearly all are met."
4. "RDA . . . meet the needs of healthy people and do not take into account special needs arising from infections, metabolic disorders, chronic diseases or other abnormalities that require special dietary treatment."
5. "In addition to being a source of nutrients, food has psychological and social values that are difficult to quantify . . . however, as food has no nutritional value unless and until it is eaten, RDA should be provided from a selection of foods that are acceptable and palatable."

The RDA are stated as the amounts of nutrients to be consumed by individuals. They do not take into account the nutrient losses that occur during processing and preparation of food.

The RDA have been used as guides in planning nutritionally adequate diets for groups. They are used in the interpretation of the adequacy of nutrient intakes of individuals in dietary surveys. They are to be used as a reference. Any deviations of the individual intakes from the recommended nutrient allowances should be regarded as significant only in terms of the individual's total health status. The nutritional status is the sum total of the food consumption: present and past nutrient intake, clinical signs and symptoms, growth and development, biochemical data and excretory levels of nutrients. (See Chapter 11–Assessment of Nutritional Status.)

Individuals whose diets do not meet the RDA standards are not necessarily suffering from malnutrition. Equally invalid are statements to the effect that "the average intake of a population meets the RDA; therefore there is no problem of nutritional inadequacy as applied to individuals." The RDA allow for a margin of safety for individual variations. The recommended allowances are designed for the population of the United States and are revised periodically in order to include new research findings. Nutritional surveys are also needed periodically to determine the nature, causes and location of malnutrition in the United States.

In the 1968 revision recommended allowances were added for vitamins E, B_6, B_{12} and folacin and for minerals iodine, magnesium and phosphorus. The 1974 revision added allowances for zinc. (See Table 10–2.) The fact that recommendations for four vitamins and four minerals have been made within the last 10 to 15 years gives an idea of how new and rapidly expanding the knowledge of human nutrition really is. The age and sex groupings include two periods of infancy up to one year, three age groupings for children and seven age groups of males and females from 11 years to 51 years of age and beyond. The "reference" man (wt: 154 lb. or 70 kg., ht: 69 in. or 172 cm.) and "reference" woman (wt: 128 lb. or 58 kg., ht: 65 in. or 162 cm.), with two age groups—23 to 50 years of age and 51+ years of age—are used. They are presumed to live in an environment with a mean temperature of 20°C. (70°F.). Their physical activity is considered "light" (neither sedentary nor heavy physical activity).

Certain of the 1974 RDA require comments:

Calories. This is the one "nutrient" for which the RDA does not include a margin of safety. Because of the concern over the fact that a considerable segment of the American

Table 10–1 FOOD AND NUTRITION BOARD, NATIONAL ACADEMY OF SCIENCES–NATIONAL RESEARCH COUNCIL RECOMMENDED DAILY DIETARY ALLOWANCES,[a] Revised 1974

Designed for the maintenance of good nutrition of practically all healthy people in the U.S.A.

| | AGE | WEIGHT | | HEIGHT | | ENERGY | PROTEIN | FAT-SOLUBLE VITAMINS | | | |
| | | | | | | | | Vitamin A Activity | | Vitamin D | Vitamin E Activity[e] |
	(years)	(kg.)	(lb.)	(cm.)	(in.)	(kcal.)[b]	(g.)	(R.E.)[c]	(I.U.)	(I.U.)	(I.U.)
Infants	0.0–0.5	6	14	60	24	kg × 117	kg × 2.2	420[d]	1,400	400	4
	0.5–1.0	9	20	71	28	kg × 108	kg × 2.0	400	2,000	400	5
Children	1–3	13	28	86	34	1,300	23	400	2,000	400	7
	4–6	20	44	110	44	1,800	30	500	2,500	400	9
	7–10	30	66	135	54	2,400	36	700	3,300	400	10
Males	11–14	44	97	158	63	2,800	44	1,000	5,000	400	12
	15–18	61	134	172	69	3,000	54	1,000	5,000	400	15
	19–22	67	147	172	69	3,000	54	1,000	5,000	400	15
	23–50	70	154	172	69	2,700	56	1,000	5,000		15
	51+	70	154	172	69	2,400	56	1,000	5,000		15
Females	11–14	44	97	155	62	2,400	44	800	4,000	400	12
	15–18	54	119	162	65	2,100	48	800	4,000	400	12
	19–22	58	128	162	65	2,100	46	800	4,000	400	12
	23–50	58	128	162	65	2,000	46	800	4,000		12
	51+	58	128	162	65	1,800	46	800	4,000		12
Pregnant						+300	+30	1,000	5,000	400	15
Lactating						+500	+20	1,200	6,000	400	15

[a] The allowances are intended to provide for individual variations among most normal persons as they live in the United States under usual environmental stresses. Diets should be based on a variety of common foods in order to provide other nutrients for which human requirements have been less well defined.

[b] Kilojoules (kJ) = 4.2 × kcal.

[c] Retinol equivalents.

[d] Assumed to be all as retinol in milk during the first six months of life. All subsequent intakes are assumed to be half as retinol and half as β-carotene when calculated from international units. As retinol equivalents, three fourths are as retinol and one fourth as β-carotene.

[e] Total vitamin E activity, estimated to be 80 per cent as α-tocopherol and 20 per cent as other tocopherols.

population is overweight, and the belief that the average adult exerts much less energy than was allowed in the 1958 and 1964 RDA, the 1968 and 1974 calorie allowances are lower and reflect the lowest energy intake thought to be compatible with health for males and females in certain age groups. The RDA for men and women are 2700 and 2000 kcal., respectively. The factor of 4.2 kjoules/kcalorie has been included for conversion of kcalories to kjoules.

Energy intake should be adjusted for variations in age, physical activity or climate so that an individual maintains ideal weight. Since the RDA for the reference man and woman are set for persons of "light" activity, those with moderate activity should add 300 kcal./day, and those who are very active may need to add 600 to 900 kcal./day. The same numbers do not apply to individuals in other age categories, but their energy intake may also need to be modified to allow for activity, proper growth, development and weight maintenance. Varia-

tions in body size from the reference figures also influence energy requirements. (See Chapter 2—Energy.)

Children or adults who gain excessive weight while habitually consuming the number of kcalories recommended for their age and sex category should be encouraged to increase their activity to achieve the desired weight, rather than decrease their caloric intake below the RDA. It is difficult to obtain adequate intakes of all the other nutrients when the caloric intake is much below the RDA, unless sugar, alcohol and fats are greatly restricted, which is not the habit in most American families. These foods are of extremely low nutrient density (the ratio of nutrient content to caloric value) and contribute many kcalories to the daily intake, yet contribute few nutrients.

Protein. Knowledge regarding human protein requirements is not complete. This is evident by the fact that in the last two revisions of the RDA, adult protein requirements have

Table 10–1 FOOD AND NUTRITION BOARD, NATIONAL ACADEMY OF SCIENCES–NATIONAL RESEARCH COUNCIL RECOMMENDED DAILY DIETARY ALLOWANCES, Revised 1974 (*Continued*)

Designed for the maintenance of good nutrition of practically all healthy people in the U.S.A.

		WATER-SOLUBLE VITAMINS							MINERALS				
Ascorbic Acid (mg.)	Folacin[f] (μg.)	Niacin[g] (mg.)	Ribo-flavin (mg.)	Thiamin (mg.)	Vitamin B_6 (mg.)	Vitamin B_{12} (μg.)	Calcium (mg.)	Phosphorus (mg.)	Iodine (μg.)	Iron (mg.)	Magnesium (mg.)	Zinc (mg.)
35	50	5	0.4	0.3	0.3	0.3	360	240	35	10	60	3
35	50	8	0.6	0.5	0.4	0.3	540	400	45	15	70	5
40	100	9	0.8	0.7	0.6	1.0	800	800	60	15	150	10
40	200	12	1.1	0.9	0.9	1.5	800	800	80	10	200	10
40	300	16	1.2	1.2	1.2	2.0	800	800	110	10	250	10
45	400	18	1.5	1.4	1.6	3.0	1,200	1,200	130	18	350	15
45	400	20	1.8	1.5	2.0	3.0	1,200	1,200	150	18	400	15
45	400	20	1.8	1.5	2.0	3.0	800	800	140	10	350	15
45	400	18	1.6	1.4	2.0	3.0	800	800	130	10	350	15
45	400	16	1.5	1.2	2.0	3.0	800	800	110	10	350	15
45	400	16	1.3	1.2	1.6	3.0	1,200	1,200	115	18	300	15
45	400	14	1.4	1.1	2.0	3.0	1,200	1,200	115	18	300	15
45	400	14	1.4	1.1	2.0	3.0	800	800	100	18	300	15
45	400	13	1.2	1.0	2.0	3.0	800	800	100	18	300	15
45	400	12	1.1	1.0	2.0	3.0	800	800	80	10	300	15
60	800	+2	+0.3	+0.3	2.5	4.0	1,200	1,200	125	18+[h]	450	20
80	600	+4	+0.5	+0.3	2.5	4.0	1,200	1,200	150	18	450	25

[f]The folacin allowances refer to dietary sources as determined by *Lactobacillus casei* assay. Pure forms of folacin may be effective in doses less than one fourth of the recommended dietary allowance.

[g]Although allowances are expressed as niacin, it is recognized that on the average 1 mg. of niacin is derived from each 60 mg. of dietary tryptophan.

[h]This increased requirement cannot be met by ordinary diets; therefore, the use of supplemental iron is recommended.

been decreased from 1.0 gm./kg./day in 1963 to 0.9 gm./kg./day in 1968 to 0.8 gm./kg./day in 1974. These allowances are established to cover the needs of most people in the age and sex categories who encounter the stresses of normal living. Allowances are increased for pregnancy, lactation and growth and may also need to be increased during stress. (See Chapter 5—Protein.)

Since high protein foods also are good sources of vitamins B_6, B_{12} and trace elements not included in the RDA but still essential, there has been some concern that the intake of these nutrients will be inadequate on the low protein intake being recommended. The protein intakes of Americans, however, are generally larger than those recommended by the FNB.

Vitamin E. It is interesting to note that the 1974 RDA for vitamin E, 15 I.U. for the reference male and 12 I.U. for the female, are about half that stated in 1968. They reflect the incomplete knowledge regarding the functions of vitamin E in the human and the level of optimal tissue saturation and intake. (See Chapter 8—Vitamins.)

Ascorbic Acid. This vitamin is another good example of the controversy that exists about the optimal level of intake of a nutrient. The optimal amount can be assessed as the daily intake required to prevent scurvy (10 mg./day), on the one extreme, or the amount required to maintain maximum tissue concentration and body stores (80 mg./day)[7] at the other extreme. Which is optimal? The 1974 RDA place the allowance for vitamin C for adults at 45 mg./day. Compare this to the Canadian and British recommendations of 30 mg./day.

Calcium. The calcium allowance illustrates how the interaction between a mineral and protein must be considered when setting the RDA. The FNB set the RDA for calcium at 800 mg. per day, considerably above the FAO/WHO allowance of 400 to 500 mg. per day.[1] This is based on evidence that calcium excretion is increased by a high protein intake and that Americans have a known high protein intake.[8]

Iron. Because of the wide individual variability in its absorption and availability in various foods, iron is the most problematic nutrient. Absorbability is assumed to be about 10 per cent of the food intake of iron. For males

Table 10–2   NUTRIENTS KNOWN TO BE ESSENTIAL FOR THE HUMAN BEING

Protein Vitamin A Vitamin D Vitamin C Thiamin Riboflavin Niacin Calcium Iron		RDA first established in 1963 or earlier
	Vitamin E Folacin Vitamin B$_6$ Vitamin B$_{12}$ Phosphorus Magnesium Iodine	RDA first established in 1968
	Zinc	RDA first established in 1974
		Essential fatty acids Carbohydrate Vitamin K Choline Pantothenic acid Biotin Sodium Potassium No RDA yet established Chloride Copper Fluorine Chromium Manganese Molybdenum Other trace minerals?

the 10 mg. per day recommended may be attained readily from the average American diet, but the RDA of 18 mg. per day for females on 2000 kcal. per day may be difficult to obtain from the dietary sources. Fortification of foods is indicated.

Zinc. A recommended allowance for this nutrient was first established in 1974 after accumulation of enough data to give an estimate of human requirements. The RDA for adults have been set at 15 mg./day. This recommendation will probably undergo many refinements in the ensuing revisions of the RDA.

See Table 10–2 for nutrients known to be essential, but for which there is not enough data to define an average human requirement. Since the recommended allowance is derived from the average human requirement, there are no RDA for these nutrients, although they are discussed in *Recommended Dietary Allowances.*

The RDA for a 70 kg. man are summarized in Figure 10–1. About 9 gm. of nitrogen is present in the 56 gm. of protein required. Leucine and tryptophan are shown in the figures to represent the extremes of essential amino acid need.

Dietary standards have been formulated for other countries, which differ in philosophy and purpose from those of the American standards, and thus specific recommendations differ. The allowances proposed in the Canadian standard[3] are considered to be adequate for the maintenance of health among the majority of people (Table 10–3); values recommended in the British standard are for maintenance of good nutrition in the average person; allowances recommended in the United States standards are for the maintenance of good nutrition in substantially all normal persons. Comparative dietary standards of selected countries and UN agencies may be found in the Appendix of the 1968 edition of the RDA.

Although the recommended daily dietary allowances are designed for *groups* of people, with proper interpretation and use, they can serve as a helpful criterion to judge, evaluate and plan the nutritional status of an *individual* and are referred to repeatedly throughout this

text. When new research findings alter the previous recommendations new standards are issued.

The scientific bases for the Recommended Dietary Allowances are described in full in the publication, and for proper and intelligent use of this table, it is strongly recommended that the report be read in its entirety.

ESSENTIALS OF AN ADEQUATE DIET

The task of planning nutritious meals centers on the inclusion of the essential nutrients in optimal amounts and adequate calories. Because some of the essential nutrients do not have established RDA, and others may not even be known, we must continue to rely on the principle of consumption of a wide variety of foods to provide for these unknowns. Provision of the financial ability to buy food and the

education to choose the proper foods must be provided simultaneously. The Expanded Food and Nutrition Education Program (EFNEP) of the USDA is an example of an effective nutrition education program.

Proteins, carbohydrates, fats, vitamins, minerals, cellulose and water need to be provided through the daily meals in sufficient quantity to meet the needs of the body.

Protein. Animal proteins are furnished through meats (muscle and organs), fish, fowl, eggs, milk and products made from milk, such as cheese. Vegetable proteins are furnished through nuts, legumes, grains, and some of the vegetables and fruits. A blend of the two types of proteins is needed to provide the essential amino acids.

Carbohydrate. Carbohydrates are supplied through grains, fruits, vegetables, starches and sugars.

Fat. Fats are furnished through the "invisible" fat content of meats, eggs, cheese, and nuts, and the "visible" fats, such as butter,

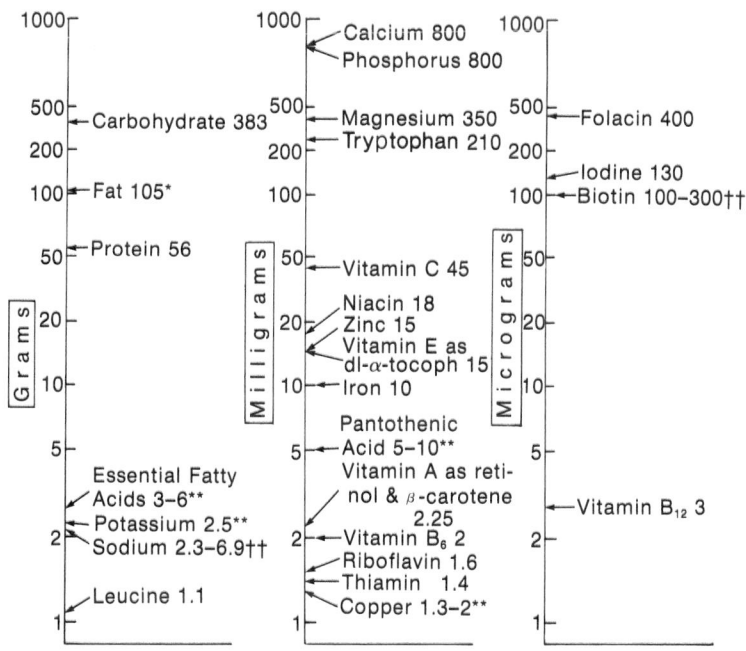

*Based on Am. Heart Assoc. recommendation of 35% of kcals from fat.

†Based on best estimates that 1–2% of kcals should be from EFA.

**Based on best estimates of adequate intake.

††Based on reports of present daily intake.

Figure 10–1 Summary of the 1974 Recommended Dietary Allowances for a 70-kg., 172-cm. reference man consuming 2700 kcal. daily.

Table 10–3 DIETARY STANDARD FOR CANADA—RECOMMENDED DAILY NUTRIENT INTAKE—REVISED 1975

Age	Sex	Weight (kg.)	Height (cm.)	Energy[a] (kcal.)	Energy[a] (M.J.)[b]	Protein (g.)	Thiamin (mg.)	Niacin (NE.)	Ribo-flavin (mg.)	Vita-min B$_6$[g] (mg.)	Folate[h] (µg.)
0–6 mo	Both	6	—	kg × 117	kg × 0.49	kg × 2.2(2.0)[e]	0.3	5	0.4	0.3	40
7–11 mo	Both	9	—	kg × 108	kg × 0.45	kg × 1.4	0.5	6	0.6	0.4	60
1–3 yrs	Both	13	90	1400	5.9	22	0.7	9	0.8	0.8	100
4–6 yrs	Both	19	110	1800	7.5	27	0.9	12	1.1	1.3	100
7–9 yrs	M	27	129	2200	9.2	33	1.1	14	1.3	1.6	100
	F	27	128	2000	8.4	33	1.0	13	1.2	1.4	100
10–12 yrs	M	36	144	2500	10.5	41	1.2	17	1.5	1.8	100
	F	38	145	2300	9.6	40	1.1	15	1.4	1.5	100
13–15 yrs	M	51	162	2800	11.7	52	1.4	19	1.7	2.0	200
	F	49	159	2200	9.2	43	1.1	15	1.4	1.5	200
16–18 yrs	M	64	172	3200	13.4	54	1.6	21	2.0	2.0	200
	F	54	161	2100	8.8	43	1.1	14	1.3	1.5	200
19–35 yrs	M	70	176	3000	12.6	56	1.5	20	1.8	2.0	200
	F	56	161	2100	8.8	41	1.1	14	1.3	1.5	200
36–50 yrs	M	70	176	2700	11.3	56	1.4	18	1.7	2.0	200
	F	56	161	1900	7.9	41	1.0	13	1.2	1.5	200
51+ yrs	M	70	176	2300[c]	9.6[c]	56	1.4	18	1.7	2.0	200
	F	56	161	1800[c]	7.5[c]	41	1.0	13	1.2	1.5	200
Pregnancy				+300[d]	1.3[d]	+20	+0.2	+2	+0.3	+0.5	+50
Lactation				+500	2.1	+24	+0.4	+7	+0.6	+0.6	+50

[a] Recommendations assume characteristic activity pattern for each age group.

[b] Megajoules (10^6 joules). Calculated from the relation 1 kilocalorie = 4.184 kilojoules and rounded to 1 decimal place.

[c] Recommended energy intake for age 66+ years reduced to 2000 kcal. (8.4 M.J.) for men and 1500 kcal. (6.3 M.J.) for women.

[d] Increased energy intake recommended during 2nd and 3rd trimesters. An increase of 100 kcal. (418.4 kJ.) per day is recommended during the 1st trimester.

[e] Recommended protein intake of 2.2 gm./kg. body wt. for infants age 0–2 mo. and 2.0 gm./kg. body wt. for those age 3–5 mo. Protein recommendation for infants 0–11 mo. assumes consumption of breast milk or protein of equivalent quality.

[f] 1 N.E. (niacin equivalent) is equal to 1 mg. of niacin or 60 mg. of tryptophan.

[g] Recommendations are based on estimated average daily protein intake of Canadians.

[h] Recommendation given in terms of free folate.

fortified margarine, oil, cream, and products made from cream. Saturated fats are found in animal products and rare vegetable oils such as coconut oil, while unsaturated fats are found in vegetables and vegetable products.

Vitamins and Minerals. Vitamins and minerals are supplied through meats, fish, fowl, eggs, milk and products made from milk, and through nuts, legumes, grains, and some of the fruits and vegetables. Some foods have higher vitamin and mineral content than others. It is important to know the best sources in relation to the availability in the region and the socio-economic status. The tables of food values are used as guides. (See Appendix Tables 1 and 2.)

Fiber. Cellulose or fiber is furnished through the skins, peelings and pulp of fruits and vegetables, and the hulls of grains.

Water. Water is supplied as such, and through the water content of foods and liquids.

Table 10–3 DIETARY STANDARD FOR CANADA—RECOMMENDED DAILY NUTRIENT INTAKE—REVISED 1975 *(Continued)*

WATER-SOLUBLE VITAMINS *(Continued)*		FAT-SOLUBLE VITAMINS			MINERALS					
Vitamin B_{12} (µg.)	Vitamin C (mg.)	Vitamin A (R.E.)[j]	Vitamin D (µg. cholecalciferol)[k]	Vitamin E (mg. d-α-tocopherol)	Calcium (mg.)	Phosphorus (mg.)	Magnesium (mg.)	Iodine (µg.)	Iron (mg.)	Zinc (mg.)
0.3	20[i]	400	10	3	500[m]	250[m]	50[m]	35[m]	7[m]	4[m]
0.3	20	400	10	3	500	400	50	50	7	5
0.9	20	400	10	4	500	500	75	70	8	5
1.5	20	500	5	5	500	500	100	90	9	6
1.5	30	700	2.5[l]	6	700	700	150	110	10	7
1.5	30	700	2.5[l]	6	700	700	150	100	10	7
3.0	30	800	2.5[l]	7	900	900	175	130	11	8
3.0	30	800	2.5[l]	7	1000	1000	200	120	11	9
3.0	30	1000	2.5[l]	9	1200	1200	250	140	13	10
3.0	30	800	2.5[l]	7	800	800	250	110	14	10
3.0	30	1000	2.5[l]	10	1000	1000	300	160	14	12
3.0	30	800	2.5[l]	6	700	700	250	110	14	11
3.0	30	1000	2.5[l]	9	800	800	300	150	10	10
3.0	30	800	2.5[l]	6	700	700	250	110	14	9
3.0	30	1000	2.5[l]	8	800	800	300	140	10	10
3.0	30	800	2.5[l]	6	700	700	250	100	14	9
3.0	30	1000	2.5[l]	8	800	800	300	140	10	10
3.0	30	800	2.5[l]	6	700	700	250	100	9	9
+1.0	+20	+100	+2.5[l]	+1	+500	+500	+25	+15	+1[n]	+3
+0.5	+30	+400	+2.5[l]	+2	+500	+500	+75	+25	+1[n]	+7

[i] Considerably higher levels may be prudent for infants during the first week of life to guard against neonatal tyrosinemia.

[j] R.E. (retinol equivalent) corresponds to a biological activity in humans equal to 1 µg. retinol (3.33 I.U.) or 6 µg. β-carotene (10 I.U.).

[k] One µg. cholecalciferol is equivalent to 1 µg. ergocalciferol (40 I.U. vitamin D activity).

[l] Most older children and adults receive vitamin D from irradiation but 2.5 µg. daily is recommended. This intake should be increased to 5.0 µg. daily during pregnancy and lactation and for those confined indoors or otherwise deprived of sunlight for extended periods.

[m] The intake of breast-fed infants may be less than the recommendation but is considered to be adequate.

[n] A recommended total intake of 15 mg. daily during pregnancy and lactation assumes the presence of adequate stores of iron. If stores are suspected of being inadequate, additional iron as a supplement is recommended.

APPLICATION OF DIETARY ALLOWANCES

In the previous discussion and chapters the physiological necessities for specific nutrients have been presented. These nutrition facts can be arranged now into a basic pattern to assist in the planning of meals.

The various quantities of nutrients recommended as allowances may generally be obtained from usual portions of commonly available foods in the United States. As previously pointed out, variety in foods is of considerable advantage in the selection of an adequate diet, since it offers the potential of affording many essential nutrients in natural proportions. Some foods are unique because of their important contributions to the diet. For example, milk is an important source of calcium, protein, and riboflavin; citrus fruits and tomatoes provide relatively large amounts of ascorbic acid.

These foods known to be high in necessary nutrients are called "protective" foods, because when they are included regularly as the basis for a diet, they protect against certain vitamin and mineral deficiencies. Table 10–12 lists foods especially high in various nutrients. Table 10–4 offers a guide to the foods that should be included daily in meals. Table 10–5 presents a daily food guide for an ovo-lacto vegetarian.

This basic pattern forms a *foundation* for a good diet providing the essential nutrients. It will supply the adult with approximately one half the caloric allowance, all the protein, vitamin A, riboflavin, ascorbic acid and calcium needed. Almost all the thiamin and niacin al-

lowances are provided but the iron supply is about half that needed by the female adult. Other foods are added, as necessary, to meet the caloric requirement, to meet unknown requirements, and to add palatability. These may be more of the same foods listed above, or others. Since butter, margarine, other fats, oils, sugars, and refined cereal foods are usually combined with other specified foods, they are not included in the food plan. See Table 10–6 for an evaluation of the foundation of an adequate diet for an adult.

Using the basic four food groups is not the only way to obtain a good diet. For example, a vegetarian can avoid meat and all foods in the milk group and still obtain an adequate diet if

Table 10–4 FOUNDATION OF AN ADEQUATE DIET—DAILY FOOD GUIDE

SERVINGS RECOMMENDED	WHAT COUNTS AS A SERVING
MEAT GROUP 2 or more	2 to 3 ounces of lean cooked meat, poultry or fish. As alternates: 1 egg, ½ cup cooked dry beans or peas, or 2 tablespoons of peanut butter may replace ½ serving of meat.

MILK GROUP
  CHILD, under 9 . . . . 2 to 3
  CHILD, 9 to 12 . . . . 3 or more
  TEENAGER . . . . 4 or more
  ADULT . . . . 2 or more
  PREGNANT WOMAN . . . . 3 or more
  NURSING WOMAN . . . . 4 or more
	One 8-ounce cup of fluid milk: whole, skim, buttermilk or evaporated or dry milk, reconstituted. As alternates: 1⅓ ounces cheddar-type cheese, or 1⅓ cups cottage cheese, 1⅔ cups ice cream, 1 cup yogurt.

VEGETABLE–FRUIT GROUP 4 or more, including:	½ cup of vegetable or fruit; or a portion, for example, 1 medium apple, banana, or potato, half a medium grapefruit or cantaloupe.
   1 good or 2 fair sources of vitamin C	Good sources: Grapefruit or grapefruit juice, orange or orange juice, cantaloupe, guava, mango, papaya, raw strawberries, broccoli, Brussels sprouts, green pepper, sweet red pepper.
	Fair sources: Honeydew melon, lemon, tangerine or tangerine juice, watermelon, asparagus, cabbage, cauliflower, collards, garden cress, kale, kohlrabi, mustard greens, potatoes and sweet potatoes cooked in the jacket, rutabagas, spinach, tomatoes or tomato juice, turnip greens.

  1 good source of vitamin A—at least every
    other day
	Good sources: Dark-green and deep-yellow vegetables and a few fruits, namely: apricots, broccoli, cantaloupe, carrots, chard, collards, cress, kale, mango, persimmon, pumpkin, spinach, sweet potatoes, turnip greens and other dark green leaves, winter squash.

BREAD–CEREAL GROUP 4 or more	COUNT ONLY IF WHOLE-GRAIN OR ENRICHED. 1 slice of bread or similar serving of baked goods made with whole-grain or enriched flour, 1 ounce ready-to-eat cereal, ½ to ¾ cup cooked cereal, cornmeal, grits, spaghetti, macaroni, noodles or rice.

OTHER WHOLESOME FOODS AS NEEDED
  To round out meals and meet energy requirements.

Table 10–5 FOOD GUIDE FOR AN OVO-LACTO VEGETARIAN

FOOD GROUPS (servings per day)	SIZE OF SERVING	FOOD SOURCES OR EXCHANGES
I. Milk Group (2 or more servings)	1 c. milk	½ c. evaporated milk 1 c. yogurt 1 c. skim milk 1 oz. cheese ¼ c. cottage cheese 1 c. soymilk 4 T. powdered soymilk
II. Vegetable Protein Foods (2 or more servings)	1 c. legumes (beans, garbanzos, lentils, peas) 2–3 oz. meat analogs	4 T. peanut butter 20–30 gm. dry textured vegetable proteins 4 oz. soy "cheese" or curd 1½ T. nuts or oil seeds
III. Fruits and Vegetables (4 or more servings)	½ c. cooked vegetables and/or fruits 1 c. raw vegetables ½ c. juice	1 serving vitamin C rich foods: citrus, cabbage and tomatoes, melon, green pepper, strawberries 1–2 servings of green leafy vegetables and yellow vegetables and fruits (carotene-rich)
IV. Bread and Cereals (4 or more servings)	1 slice of whole wheat or enriched bread ½–¾ c. cooked cereal, whole grain ¾–1 c. dry cereal	½–¾ c. enriched or whole rice ½–¾ c. enriched noodles, macaroni, or spaghetti ½ c. granola ½ hamburger bun Crackers: graham (2) saltines (5) wheat thins (8)
V. Other Foods Eggs (3–4 per week) Fats (1 T. per day)	1 egg 1 t. oil 1 t. soft margarine	

(From Vyhmeister, I.B., Register, U.D., and Sonnenberg, L.M.: Safe vegetarian diets for children. Pediatr. Clin. North Am., *24*:203, 1977.)

vegetables high in iron and calcium (such as kale) are included regularly. A person can avoid all fruits and still obtain adequate amounts of vitamin C if vegetables known to be good vitamin C sources such as cabbage and broccoli are included frequently.

On the other hand, an individual can follow the basic four food pattern and still have an inadequate intake of iron, folic acid, zinc and possibly fiber, depending on the foods selected in each group. It is important to look at the individual diet. The Basic Four Food Groups, however, can still serve as a practical guide in planning meals.

The Milk Group is counted on to provide most of the calcium requirement. In addition, it provides riboflavin, high quality protein, other vitamins and minerals, carbohydrate, and fat. The milk allowance is used in the form of fluid whole or skim milk, buttermilk, evaporated milk, dry milk, and cheese. A portion may be used in cooking. Approximate equivalents of 1 cup of fluid milk, according to calcium content, are given on page 807.

The Meat Group provides generous amounts of protein of high quality. In addition, iron, thiamin, riboflavin, niacin, phosphorus and zinc are supplied. At least once a week, liver, kidney and salt water fish such as salmon, oysters and mackerel are included in the animal protein allowance. See Chapter 40.

There are several non-meat alternatives that provide the same nutrients as animal flesh. In addition, the complete vegetarian can combine

Table 10-6 EVALUATION OF THE FOUNDATION OF AN ADEQUATE DIET FOR AN ADULT

FOOD	AVERAGE SERVING Household Measure	AVERAGE SERVING Weight Gm.	KILO-CALORIES	PRO-TEIN Gm.	FAT Gm.	CAR-BOHY-DRATE Gm.	MINERALS Calcium Mg.	MINERALS Iron Mg.	MINERALS A. (I.U.)	VITAMINS Ascorbic Acid Mg.	VITAMINS Thiamin Mg.	VITAMINS Ribo-flavin Mg.	VITAMINS Niacin Mg.
Milk, whole (or equivalent)	1 pt.	488	320	18.0	18	24	576	.2	700	4	.16	.84	.2
Meat group													
Eggs	1	50	80	6.0	6	tr.	27	1.1	590	—	.05	.15	tr.
Meat, poultry, fish[1]	3 oz. (cooked)	85	237	23.0	15	0	10	2.4	10	—	.09	.21	4.7
Vegetable—fruit group													
Vegetables:													
Deep green or yellow[2]	1 salad or cooked	50 raw or 75 cooked	27	1.4	tr.	6	36.7	.6	3016	20.5	.046	.08	.4
Other, cooked[3]	½ cup	80	41	2.5	tr.	7.7	15	.93	225	11	.12	.06	1.5
Potato, peeled, boiled	1 medium	122	80	2.0	tr.	18	7	.6	tr.	20	.11	.04	1.4
Fruits:													
Citrus[4]	1 serving	125	57	.8	tr.	14	28	.35	302	58	.09	.03	.36
Other (fresh and canned)[5]	1 serving	150	92	.5	tr.	24	8	.5	164	5	.03	.04	.4
Bread-cereal group													
Cereal (whole grain and enriched)[6]	½ cup cooked	28 (dry)	88	2.2	1	17.7	7.7	.6	—	—	.11	.02	.3
Bread (whole grain and enriched)	3 slices	69	180	6.0	3	36	57	1.8	tr.	tr.	.18	.15	1.8
Totals[7]			1202 (5000 kJ.)	62.4	43	147.4	772.4	9.1[8]	5007[8]	118.5	.986[9]	1.62	11.6[10]
Recommended Daily Dietary Allowances*													
Man (age 23–50, wt., 70 kg., ht., 172 cm.)			2700	56			800	10	5000	45	1.4	1.6	18[11]
Woman (age 23–50, wt., 58 kg., ht., 162 cm.)			2000	46			800	18	4000	45	1.0	1.2	13[11]

Evaluation based on Table 1 in the Appendix.

[1] Evaluation based on figures for cooked (lean and fat) beef, lamb, and veal.

[2] Evaluation based on lettuce, cooked carrots, green beans, winter squash and broccoli.

[3] Evaluation based on average for cooked peas and beets.

[4] Evaluation based on Florida orange and white and pink grapefruit: whole and juice.

[5] Evaluation based on canned peaches, applesauce, raw pears, apples and bananas.

[6] Evaluation based on oatmeal and cornflakes.

[7] With the addition of more of the same foods, or other foods, to meet calorie requirement, the totals will be increased.

[8] With the use of liver this figure will be markedly increased.

[9] With the use of pork, legumes and liver this figure will be markedly increased.

[10] The average diet in the United States, which contains a generous amount of protein, provides enough tryptophan to increase the niacin value by about a third.

[11] These figures are expressed as niacin equivalents, which include dietary sources of the preformed vitamin and the precursor, tryptophan.

* Recommended Dietary Allowances. Washington, D.C., National Research Council, 1974.

Table 10–7 EXAMPLES OF COMPLEMENTARY PROTEINS

COMBINATIONS	SUGGESTED RECIPE EXAMPLES
1. Rice + Legumes	a) Hopping John
	b) Roman Rice and Beans
	c) Crusty Soybean Casserole
2. Rice + Wheat + Soy	a) Mexican Grains
3. Rice + Sesame Seed	a) Sesame Vegetable Rice
4. Rice + Milk	a) Con Queso Rice
	b) Spinach Casserole
	c) Spinach Rice Loaf
5. Wheat Products + Milk	a) Lasagna
	b) French Fondue
	c) Macaroni and Cheese Puff
6. Wheat + Beans	a) Tabouili
7. Cornmeal + Beans	a) Mexican Pan Bread
8. Beans + Milk	a) Bean Chowder
9. Peanuts + Milk	a) Peanut Butter Sandwich and Milk

(From Goodwin, M. T.: Better Living Through Better Eating. 2nd ed. Montgomery County Health Department, Maryland. 1974. p. 19.)

incomplete proteins to meet the complete or high quality protein requirement. See Table 10–7 and Fig. 10–2.

The Bread and Cereal Group furnishes thiamin, protein, iron, niacin, carbohydrate and cellulose at a relatively low cost. The enrichment of breads and cereals with iron, thiamin, riboflavin, and niacin substantially contributes additional amounts of these nutrients to the diet. See Table 40–4.

The Vegetable and Fruit Group is an important supplier of fiber, vitamins and minerals, particularly vitamins A and C. Dark green and deep yellow vegetables are especially valuable for carotene, a precursor of vitamin A, and citrus fruits for vitamin C. Folic acid is found in the dark leafy vegetables and other fresh vegetables. See Chapter 40.

Salt pork, fatback and bacon are considered fat, not meat. Molasses, syrups, honey, jellies, jams, sugars, and candies are considered sweets.

When the daily food guide was designed, certain nutrients, such as phosphorus, zinc,

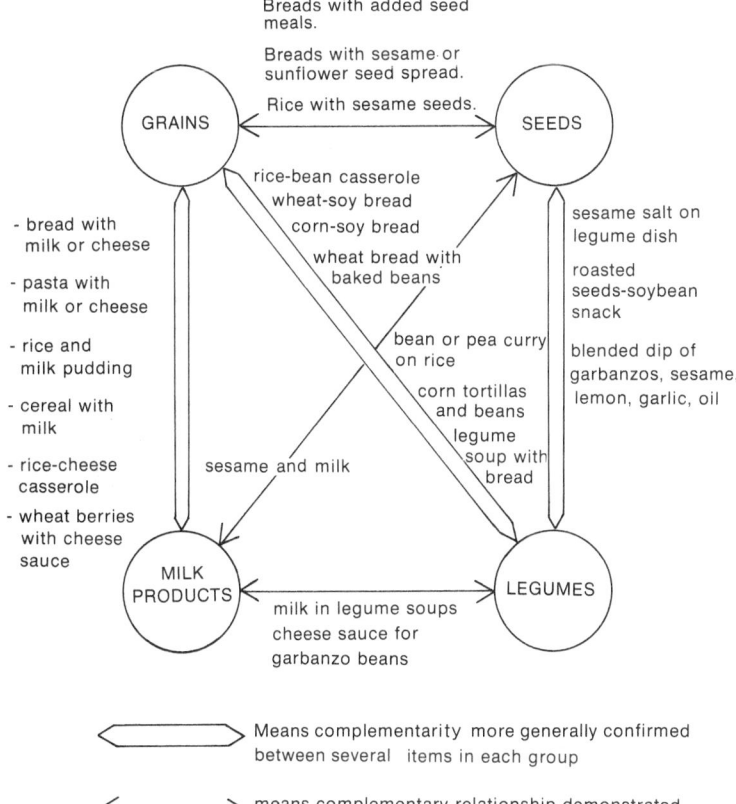

Figure 10–2 Summary of complementary protein relationships. (From: Lappé, F. M.: Diet for a Small Planet. New York, Ballantine Books, 1971.)

iodine, vitamins B_6, B_{12}, E and K, folacin, pantothenic acid, biotin, and trace minerals were not considered in the calculations. However, since most of these nutrients are found in many foods, the intake of a variety of foods within the four food groups will probably provide the needed amounts.

Presently there is a great deal of criticism of the use of the Four Food Groups as a basis for nutrition education for the public. The main arguments against its use are:

1. An individual can eat the proper number of servings from the four food groups and still not be getting an adequate intake of some vitamins and minerals, iron in particular.

2. Following the food guide can result in a high saturated fat and cholesterol, low fiber intake that many authorities feel does not constitute the optimal diet for health.

3. The additional assumption by educators using the guide that persons eating a wide variety of foods will meet other unknown requirements is fallacious since "a wide variety of foods" is ill defined in our society.

This last point is especially frustrating for the person trying to apply nutrition principles and select and prepare an adequate diet. The "wide variety" could be a variety of snack foods and drinks that add calories and no nutrients, or a variety of vegetables and fruits that add large amounts of nutrients and few calories.

Nutrient Density

The problem of selecting an adequate diet becomes especially difficult when in the presence of tremendous variety and abundance there are the constraints of calories and money. In situations of limited calories (owing to concern regarding overweight) and limited financial resources, the food selections must have a high nutrient/energy (calorie) ratio. The protective foods such as milk, liver, dark green and yellow vegetables, high vitamin C fruits and whole grain or enriched breads and cereals have high nutrient/calorie ratios, while most snack foods, such as cola drinks, cookies, cakes, candy and other heavily processed foods, have low ratios and less nutrient density. Because these low nutrient density foods add cost and calories to a diet, it is important to counsel people regarding their use. Hansen and associates [5, 13] have designed an index of food quality based on nutrient density. Although the concept is not new, it may be more practical now that there is nutritional labeling of most U.S. foods.

Nutritional Labeling

To aid in the translation of nutritional requirements into foods and meals, the FDA in 1973 developed a system of nutritional labeling of foods to replace the old system using MDR—minimum daily requirements. A standard was defined to be used in nutritional labeling—the *U.S. RDA* This is not to be confused with the NRC-RDA discussed earlier in this chapter, although the U.S. RDA is derived from the 1968 RDA.

In general the U.S. RDA is the highest value recommended for the nutrient in any age category in the RDA. Unlike the RDA, the U.S. RDA has only three age categories constituting three U.S. RDA standards: (1) adults and children over 4 years of age (the standard used in most nutrition labeling of foods), (2) infants and children under 4 years of age (the standard used on baby foods and vitamin-mineral supplements for infants and small children), and (3) pregnant or lactating women (the standard used on vitamin-mineral supplements for this group of women). See Table 10–8 for the U.S. RDA. You may want to compare this to the 1974 RDA in Table 10–1.

How Nutritional Labeling Can Help in Food Selection and Meal Planning. Nutritional labels express the nutrient composition of the food in terms of the U.S. RDA. The label must state (1) the serving size, (2) the percentage of the U.S. RDA that the serving meets for protein, five vitamins, iron and calcium (see Table 10–9), (3) the amount of protein, carbohydrate and fat in grams, and (4) the calories from protein, carbohydrate and fat. Listing of the percentage of the U.S. RDA for 12 other vitamins and minerals is optional. Cholesterol, polyunsaturated and saturated fat and sodium content may also be given. See Fig. 10–3 for a nutrition label.

Since the nutrient contribution of each food serving is stated on the label, except in the case of unpackaged fresh produce, meat and some other products, it is possible to compose an adequate daily intake by adding the percentages for the nutrients contributed by the servings of food throughout the day. A booklet and educational tool have been devised by the USDA to explain and teach the nutritional label.[9, 10] Table 10–10 shows how a typical day's intake for a 25-year-old woman is expressed as a percentage of the U.S. RDA. The contributions from all foods are totaled and the day's intake is compared to the U.S. RDA.

The U.S. RDA provides for a margin of

Table 10–8 U.S. RECOMMENDED DAILY ALLOWANCES (U.S. RDA)

VITAMINS AND MINERALS	UNIT OF MEASUREMENT	ADULTS AND CHILDREN 4 OR MORE YEARS OF AGE*	INFANTS AND CHILDREN UNDER 4 YEARS OF AGE	PREGNANT OR LACTATING WOMEN
Protein	Grams	65[a]	28	[b]
Vitamin A	International Units	5,000	2,500	8,000
Vitamin D	"	400	400	400
Vitamin E	"	30	10	30
Vitamin C	Milligrams	60	40	60
Folic Acid	"	0.4	0.2	0.8
Thiamin	"	1.5	0.7	1.7
Riboflavin	"	1.7	0.8	2.0
Niacin	"	20	9.0	20
Vitamin B_6	"	2.0	0.7	2.5
Vitamin B_{12}	Micrograms	6	3	8
Biotin	Milligrams	0.3	0.15	0.3
Pantothenic Acid	"	10	5.0	10
Calcium	Grams	1.0	0.8	1.3
Phosphorus	"	1.0	0.8	1.3
Iodine	Micrograms	150	70	150
Iron	Milligrams	18	10	18
Magnesium	"	400	200	450
Copper	"	2.0	1.0	2.0
Zinc	"	15	8.0	15

*These U.S. RDA values are on most nutrition labels

[a] If protein efficiency ratio of protein is equal to or better than that of casein, U.S. RDA is 45 gm. for adults and 20 gm. for infants.

[b] Not specified because this U.S. RDA used only in vitamin and mineral supplements for pregnant or lactating females.

[c] Presence optional for adults and children 4 or more years of age in vitamin and mineral supplements.

safety sometimes even higher than that of the RDA; so the fact that the diet does not meet the U.S. RDA does not necessarily mean that it is

Table 10–9 U.S. RECOMMENDED DAILY ALLOWANCE (U.S. RDA)*

NUTRIENT	U.S. RDA
Vitamin A	5,000 I.U.
Vitamin C (ascorbic acid)	60.0 mg.
Thiamin (vitamin B_1)	1.5 mg.
Riboflavin (vitamin B_2)	1.7 mg.
Niacin	20.0 mg.
Calcium	1.0 g.
Iron	18.0 mg.
Vitamin D	400 I.U.
Vitamin E	30 I.U.
Vitamin B_6	2.0 mg.
Folacin (folic acid)	0.4 mg.
Vitamin B_{12}	6.0 mcg.
Phosphorus	1.0 g
Iodine	150 mcg.
Magnesium	400 mg.
Zinc	15 mg.
Copper	2.0 mg.
Biotin	0.3 mg.
Pantothenic acid	10.0 mg.

*First seven nutrients listed require label listing or disclaimer. Others may be included.

inadequate. Table 10–11 shows the 1974 RDA interpreted in terms of U.S. RDA percentages necessary to meet allowances for each age group. Table 10–12 gives the percentage of U.S. RDA for eight nutrients for selected foods. From examination of caloric content and nutrient contribution as percentage of U.S. RDA, one can easily recognize nutrient rich foods.

Family Meal Planning and Sample Menu

The suggested basic pattern for meals applies to the entire family group. Serving size and number can be changed to meet the requirements of children, adolescents, pregnant women, lactating mothers or elderly people in the family. Changes can also be made for activity, disease, or food preferences. For example, a lactating mother can have 4 cups of milk instead of 2 and fulfill her increased requirements for calcium, phosphorus, riboflavin and protein.

If the working members of the family and schoolchildren carry lunch, then some of the vegetable and meat allowances may be made into a sandwich filling. There are also dessert

Text continued on page 214

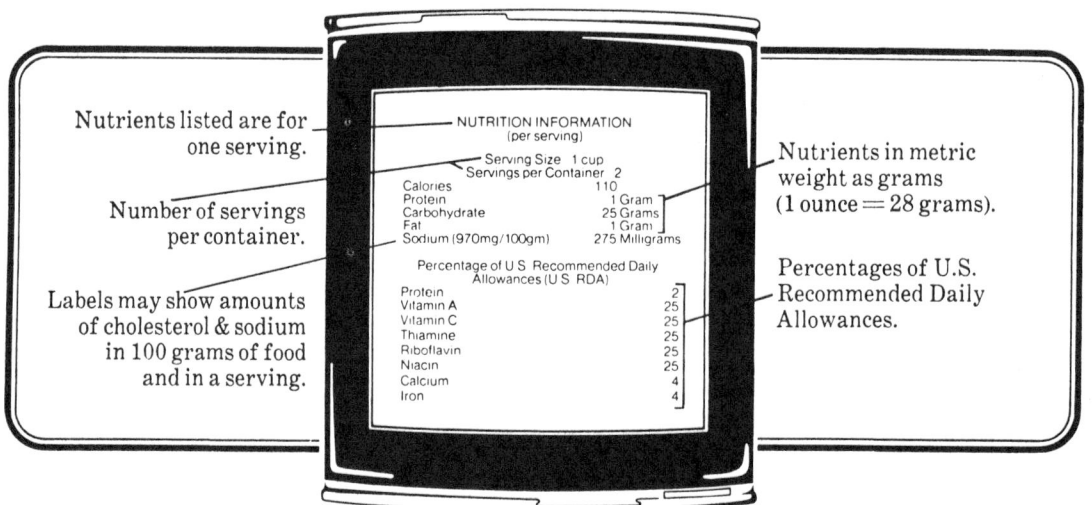

Figure 10–3   Example and explanation of a nutrition label.

Table 10–10   EVALUATION OF DIET USING THE U.S. RDA

FOOD FOR A DAY, WOMAN, 25 YEARS OLD

| | | | | | | Percentage of U.S. RDA | | | | |
Food	Amount eaten	Calories	Protein	Vita-min A	Vita-min C	Thia-min	Ribo-flavin	Niacin	Cal-cium	Iron
Ready-to-eat cereal	1 ounce	110	4	20	20	25	25	20	—	20
Milk	½ cup	80	10	3	2	2	12	—	15	—
Orange juice	½ cup	60	1	5	100	8	1	2	1	1
Peanut butter	2 tbsp.	180	16	—	—	4	1	2	1	1
Bread	2 slices	160	8	—	—	8	8	8	4	8
Jelly	1 tbsp.	50	—	—	2	—	—	—	—	2
Margarine	1 pat	35	—	4	—	—	—	—	—	—
Banana	1	100	2	4	20	4	4	4	—	4
Milk	1 cup	160	20	6	4	4	25	—	30	—
Ham	1 ounce	180	60	—	—	35	15	25	2	20
Mashed potatoes	¾ cup	150	4	6	22	9	4	8	3	3
Spinach	½ cup	20	4	145	40	4	8	2	8	10
Applesauce	½ cup	115	—	1	2	2	1	—	—	4
Brownie	1	100	2	—	—	2	2	—	—	2
Iced tea	1 glass	—	—	—	—	—	—	—	—	—
Ice cream	½ cup	130	8	6	1	2	8	—	10	—
Total:		1630	139	200	213	109	114	71	74	75
Goal for a 25-year-old woman		2000	75	80	75	70	75	30	80	100

Evaluation: The day's food provided less calcium and iron than recommended for a 25-year-old woman. The food provided fewer calories than many women need to maintain their weight, but may have provided enough for this woman.

Table 10-11 ALLOWANCES FOR FOOD ENERGY AND PERCENTAGES OF THE U.S. RECOMMENDED DAILY ALLOWANCES NEEDED TO MEET THE RECOMMENDED DIETARY ALLOWANCES FOR CHILDREN, MEN, AND WOMEN OF DIFFERENT AGES

AGE	FOOD ENERGY[a]	PRO-TEIN[b]	VITA-MIN A	VITA-MIN C	THIA-MIN	RIBO-FLAVIN	NIACIN[c]	CAL-CIUM	IRON
Years	Calories	.... Percent of U.S. Recommended Daily Allowance							
Child:									
1–3	1300	35	40	70	50	50	30	80	85
4–6	1800	50	50	70	60	65	35	80	60
7–10	2400	55	70	70	80	75	50	80	60
Male:									
11–14	2800	70	100	75	95	90	55	120	100
15–18	3000	85	100	75	100	110	55	120	100
19–22	3000	85	100	75	100	110	60	80	60
23–50	2700	90	100	75	95	95	45	80	60
51+	2400	90	100	75	80	90	35	80	60
Female:									
11–14	2400	70	80	75	80	80	45	120	100
15–18	2100	75	80	75	75	85	30	120	100
19–22	2100	75	80	75	75	85	35	80	100
23–50	2000	75	80	75	70	75	30	80	100
51+	1800	75	80	75	70	65	25	80	60
Pregnant	+300 kcal.[d]	+50[d]	100	100	+20[d]	+20[d]	35	120	100+
Nursing	+500 kcal.[d]	+35[d]	120	135	+20[d]	+30[d]	35	120	100

[a] Calorie needs differ depending on body composition and size, age, and activity of the person.

[b] U.S. RDA of 65 grams is used for this table. In labeling, a U.S. RDA of 45 grams is used for foods providing high-quality protein, such as milk, meat and eggs.

[c] The percentage of the U.S. RDA shown for niacin will provide the RDA for niacin if the RDA for protein is met. Some niacin is derived in the body from tryptophan, an amino acid present in protein.

[d] To be added to the percentage for the girl or woman of the appropriate age.

(From U.S. Recommended Daily Allowance, "Food Labeling," Federal Register, vol. 38, no. 49, part II, March 14, 1973. Recommended Dietary Allowances, 8th ed. 1974, National Academy of Sciences, National Research Council.)

Table 10-12 LIST OF FOODS THAT ARE IMPORTANT SOURCES OF NUTRIENTS*

VITAMIN A		
Food	Percentage of U.S. RDA	Amount of food
MEAT AND MEAT ALTERNATES:		
Liver, beef	910	3 ounces
Liver, calf	560	3 ounces
Liver, hog	250	3 ounces
Liver, chicken	60	1 ounce
Chicken or turkey potpie, home recipe.	60	⅓ of 9-inch pie
Beef and vegetable stew	50	1 cup
VEGETABLES AND FRUIT:		
Carrots, canned	470	1 cup
Sweetpotatoes, mashed	400	1 cup
Carrots, cooked	330	1 cup
Spinach, canned	330	1 cup
Pumpkin, canned	310	1 cup
Sweetpotatoes, pieces, canned.	310	1 cup
Collards, cooked	300	1 cup
Peas and carrots, cooked	300	1 cup
Spinach, cooked	290	1 cup
Dandelion greens, cooked.	250	1 cup
Carrots, raw, grated	240	1 cup
Sweetpotatoes, boiled in skin.	240	Medium potato
Turnip greens, canned, solids and liquid.	220	1 cup
Cress, garden, cooked	210	1 cup

*The foods that are the best sources of each nutrient are shown. Foods are listed in descending order for each nutrient according to the percentage of the U.S. RDA they provide. Consider the amount of food specified.

Percentages have been rounded off to the nearest percentage that would be shown on labels.

Consider a food superior to another food as the source of a nutrient only if it provides a substantially higher percentage of the U.S. RDA. Labeling regulations allow a manufacturer to claim that his food is superior to another food only if it contains at least 10 per cent more of the U.S. RDA per serving specified on the label. (From Nutrition Labeling. Tools for Its Use. Agricultural Information Bull. No. 382, Agric. Res. Serv., USDA, Washington, D.C., 1975)

Table continued on the following page

Table 10–12   LIST OF FOODS THAT ARE IMPORTANT SOURCES OF NUTRIENTS *(Continued)*

Food	Amount	Measure
Chard, Swiss, cooked	190	1 cup
Mango, raw	190	1 fruit (⅔ pound)
Cantaloupe, raw	180	½ of 5-inch-diameter melon
Kale, cooked	180	1 cup
Mustard greens, cooked from frozen.	180	1 cup
Sweetpotatoes, baked in skin.	180	Medium potato
Turnip greens, cooked	180	1 cup
Vegetables, mixed, cooked.	180	1 cup
Squash, winter, baked	170	1 cup
Mustard greens, cooked	160	1 cup
Apricots, dried, cooked	150	1 cup
Beet greens, cooked	150	1 cup
Cabbage, spoon, cooked	110	1 cup
Sweetpotatoes, candied	110	3-ounce piece
Broccoli, chopped, cooked from frozen.	100	1 cup
Apricots, canned	90	1 cup
Broccoli, cooked	90	Medium stalk
Spinach, raw, chopped	90	1 cup
Apricots, dried, uncooked.	80	10 medium halves
Broccoli, cut, cooked	80	1 cup
Melon balls, frozen, in syrup	70	1 cup
Pepper, red	70	1 pod
Apricots, raw	60	3 fruits
Peaches, dried, cooked	60	1 cup
Plums, canned	60	1 cup
Carrots, strips, raw	60	6–8 strips (2½–3 inches long)
Papaya, raw, cubed	50	1 cup
Tomatoes, cooked	50	1 cup
Watermelon, raw	50	4 × 8-inch wedge (2 pounds)

CEREAL AND BAKERY PRODUCTS:

Food	Amount	Measure
Pie, pumpkin	80	4¾-inch sector
Pie, sweetpotato	70	4¾-inch sector

MISCELLANEOUS:
Soup:

Food	Amount	Measure
Vegetable, with beef broth.	60	1 cup
Vegetable, vegetarian	60	1 cup
Vegetable beef	60	1 cup
Apricot nectar	50	1 cup

	VITAMIN C	
Food	*Percentage of U.S. RDA*	*Amount of food*

MEAT AND MEAT ALTERNATES:

Food	Percentage	Amount
Peppers, stuffed	120	1 pepper (6.5 ounces)
Lobster salad	80	A salad
Chop suey, with beef and pork, home recipe.	60	1 cup
Liver, calf	50	3 ounces

VEGETABLES AND FRUIT:

Food	Percentage	Amount
Broccoli, cooked	270	Medium stalk
Pepper, red, raw	250	1 pod
Collards, cooked	240	1 cup
Broccoli, cut, cooked	230	1 cup
Brussels sprouts, cooked	230	1 cup
Strawberries, frozen, sweetened.	230	1 cup
Pepper, green, cooked	220	1 cup
Orange juice, fresh	210	1 cup
Orange juice, from frozen or canned concentrate.	200	1 cup
Broccoli, chopped, cooked from frozen.	180	1 cup
Kale, cooked	170	1 cup
Turnip greens, cooked	170	1 cup
Orange juice, canned	170	1 cup
Peaches, frozen	170	1 cup
Pepper, green, raw	160	1 pod
Grapefruit juice, fresh or from frozen unsweetened concentrate.	160	1 cup
Cantaloupe, raw	150	½ of 5-inch-diameter melon
Orange sections, raw	150	1 cup
Strawberries, raw	150	1 cup
Grapefruit sections, raw, white or pink.	140	1 cup
Grapefruit juice, canned, unsweetened.	140	1 cup
Grapefruit juice, from frozen sweetened concentrate.	140	1 cup
Grapefruit sections, canned, syrup pack.	130	1 cup
Grapefruit juice, canned, sweetened.	130	1 cup
Papaya, raw, cubed	130	1 cup
Grapefruit sections, canned, water pack.	120	1 cup
Mango, raw	120	1 fruit (⅔ pound)
Cauliflower, cooked	120	1 cup
Cauliflower, raw	110	1 cup
Mustard greens, cooked	110	1 cup
Orange, raw	110	2⅝-inch-diameter orange
Tangerine juice, from frozen concentrate.	110	1 cup
Tomatoes, cooked	100	1 cup
Raspberries, red, frozen	90	1 cup
Tangerine juice, canned	90	1 cup
Cabbage, cooked	80	1 cup
Cress, garden, cooked	80	1 cup
Spinach, cooked	80	1 cup
Strawberries, canned	80	1 cup
Cabbage, raw, finely shredded.	70	1 cup
Cabbage, red, raw, shredded.	70	1 cup

Table 10–12 LIST OF FOODS THAT ARE IMPORTANT SOURCES OF NUTRIENTS *(Continued)*

Rutabagas, cooked	70	1 cup
Tomatoes, raw	70	3-inch-diameter tomato
Turnips greens, canned, solids and liquid.	70	1 cup
Tomato juice, canned or bottled.	70	1 cup
Sauerkraut juice	70	1 cup
Grapefruit, white or pink, raw.	70	½ medium fruit
Lemons, raw	70	1 lemon
Asparagus, pieces, cooked or canned.	60	1 cup
Cabbage, common or savoy, raw, coarsely shredded.	60	1 cup
Okra, sliced, cooked	60	1 cup
Peas, green, cooked	60	1 cup
Sauerkraut, canned	60	1 cup
Sweetpotatoes, canned, mashed.	60	1 cup
Turnips, cooked	60	1 cup
Coleslaw	60	1 cup
Honeydew melon, raw	60	2 × 7-inch wedge (½ pound)
Loganberries, raw	60	1 cup
Melon balls, frozen, syrup pack.	60	1 cup
Beans, lima, Fordhook, cooked from frozen.	50	1 cup
Beans, lima, immature seeds, cooked.	50	1 cup
Mustard greens, cooked from frozen.	50	1 cup
Potato, baked in skin	50	Medium potato
Spinach, canned	50	1 cup
Blackberries, raw	50	1 cup
Raspberries, red, raw	50	1 cup
Watermelon, raw	50	4 × 8-inch wedge (2 pounds)
Pineapple juice, from frozen concentrate.	50	1 cup
CEREAL AND BAKERY PRODUCTS:		
Spanish rice	60	1 cup
Pie, strawberry	50	4¾-inch sector
MISCELLANEOUS:		
Orange juice, from dehydrated crystals.	180	1 cup
Grapefruit juice, from dehydrated crystals.	150	1 cup
Cranberry juice cocktail	70	1 cup
Grape juice drink, canned.	70	1 cup
Orange-apricot juice drink.	70	1 cup
Pineapple-orange juice drink.	70	1 cup
Pineapple-grapefruit juice drink.	70	1 cup

THIAMIN

Food	*Percentage of U.S. RDA*	*Amount of food*
MEAT AND MEAT ALTERNATES:		
Sunflower seeds	190	1 cup
Pork, loin, chopped, lean	100	1 cup
Brazilnuts, shelled	90	1 cup
Pork, fresh or cured, ham or shoulder, chopped, lean.	60	1 cup
Pork, loin, sliced, lean only.	60	3 ounces
Pecans, halves	60	1 cup
Pork, loin, sliced, lean and fat.	50	3 ounces
Pork, loin chop, lean and fat.	50	2.7 ounces
Pork, fresh or cured, ham or shoulder, ground, lean.	45	1 cup
Pork, loin chop, lean	40	2 ounces
Cashew nuts, whole kernels, roasted.	40	1 cup
Filberts, whole kernels, shelled.	40	1 cup
Pork, fresh or cured, ham or shoulder, sliced, lean.	35	3 ounces
Pork, cured, shoulder, sliced, lean and fat.	30	3 ounces
Pork, fresh, ham or shoulder, sliced, lean and fat.	30	3 ounces
Kidney, beef	30	3 ounces
Peanuts	30	1 cup
Pork, cured, ham, sliced, lean and fat.	25	3 ounces
Spareribs	25	3 ounces
Spaghetti (enriched) with cheese, canned.	25	1 cup
Cowpeas, dry, cooked	25	1 cup
Soybeans, dry, cooked	25	1 cup
Almonds, whole, shelled	25	1 cup
Chestnuts, shelled	25	1 cup
Pumpkin kernels	25	1 cup
Walnuts, English, chopped.	25	1 cup
Liver, hog	20	3 ounces
Beef potpie, home-prepared from enriched flour.	20	1/3 of 9-inch pie
Chicken or turkey potpie, home-prepared from enriched flour.	20	1/3 of 9-inch pie
Chop suey, with beef and pork, home recipe.	20	1 cup
Beans, navy (pea), dry, cooked.	20	1 cup
Peas, split, dry, cooked	20	1 cup
Walnuts, black, chopped	20	1 cup
Bacon, Canadian	15	1 slice
Lamb, leg or shoulder, chopped, lean.	15	1 cup
Heart, beef, sliced	15	3 ounces

Table continued on the following page

Table 10–12   LIST OF FOODS THAT ARE IMPORTANT SOURCES OF NUTRIENTS (*Continued*)

Liver, calf or beef	15	3 ounces
Polish sausage	15	2.4-ounce link
Pork sausage	15	1-ounce pattie or 2 links
Crab, deviled	15	1 cup
Lobster salad	15	A salad
Macaroni (enriched) and cheese, home recipe.	15	1 cup
Spaghetti (enriched) with cheese, home recipe.	15	1 cup
Spaghetti (enriched) with meatballs, home recipe.	15	1 cup
Beans, canned, with pork and tomato sauce.	15	1 cup
Beans, lima, Great Northern, or kidney, dry, cooked.	15	1 cup

VEGETABLES AND FRUIT:

Cowpeas, cooked	35	1 cup
Peas, green, cooked	30	1 cup
Peas and carrots, cooked	20	1 cup
Beans, lima, fresh, cooked.	20	1 cup
Asparagus, pieces, cooked.	15	1 cup
Collards, cooked	15	1 cup
Cowpeas, canned, solids and liquid.	15	1 cup
Okra, sliced, cooked	15	1 cup
Soybeans, sprouted seeds, raw or cooked.	15	1 cup
Turnip greens, cooked	15	1 cup
Vegetables, mixed, cooked.	15	1 cup
Potato salad, with cooked salad dressing.	15	1 cup
Orange juice, fresh or from unsweetened frozen or canned concentrate.	15	1 cup
Pineapple, canned, water or syrup pack.	15	1 cup
Pineapple, frozen, sweetened.	15	1 cup

CEREAL AND BAKERY PRODUCTS:

Hoagie roll, enriched	35	11½-inch-long roll
Cereal, ready-to-eat (check label).	25	1 ounce
Hard roll, enriched	15	1 roll (1.8 ounces)
Spoonbread	15	1 cup
Oatmeal, cooked	15	1 cup
Oat and wheat cereal, cooked.	15	1 cup
Macaroni, enriched, cooked.	15	1 cup
Noodles, enriched, cooked.	15	1 cup
Spaghetti, enriched, cooked.	15	1 cup
Rice, white, enriched, cooked.	15	1 cup
Gingerbread, with enriched flour.	15	1/9 of 9-inch-square cake
Pie, pecan	15	4¾-inch sector

MISCELLANEOUS:

Orange juice, from dehydrated crystals.	15	1 cup
Soup, split pea	15	1 cup
Bread pudding, with enriched bread.	15	1 cup

RIBOFLAVIN

Food	Percentage of U.S. RDA	Amount of food

MILK AND MILK PRODUCTS:

Food	Percentage of U.S. RDA	Amount of food
Cheese, cottage	35	1 cup
Milk, partially skimmed	30	1 cup
Malted beverage	30	1 cup
Custard, baked	30	1 cup
Milk, whole or skim	25	1 cup
Milk, nonfat dry, reconstituted.	25	1 cup
Buttermilk	25	1 cup
Chocolate drink	25	1 cup
Cocoa	25	1 cup
Ice milk, soft-serve	25	1 cup
Pudding, from mixes, with milk.	25	1 cup
Pudding, vanilla, home recipe.	25	1 cup
Rennin desserts	25	1 cup
Yogurt	25	1 cup
Ice cream, soft-serve	20	1 cup
Pudding, chocolate, home recipe.	20	1 cup
Tapioca cream	20	1 cup

MEAT AND MEAT ALTERNATES:

Food	Percentage of U.S. RDA	Amount of food
Kidney, beef	240	3 ounces
Liver, hog	220	3 ounces
Liver, beef or calf	210	3 ounces
Almonds, whole	80	1 cup
Fish loaf	60	4⅛ × 2½ × 1-inch slice
Heart, beef, sliced	60	3 ounces
Almonds, sliced	50	1 cup
Liver, chicken	40	1 ounce
Beef, dried, chipped, creamed.	30	1 cup
Welsh rarebit	30	1 cup
Lamb, leg or shoulder, chopped, lean.	25	1 cup
Pork, fresh, ham or loin, chopped, lean.	25	1 cup
Veal, stewed or roasted, chopped.	25	1 cup
Braunschweiger	25	1 ounce
Chicken a la king, home recipe.	25	1 cup
Macaroni (enriched) and cheese, home recipe.	25	1 cup
Beef, chuck or rump, chopped, lean.	20	1 cup
Lamb, leg or shoulder, chopped, lean and fat.	20	1 cup

Table 10-12 LIST OF FOODS THAT ARE IMPORTANT SOURCES OF NUTRIENTS (*Continued*)

Pork, cured, ham or shoulder, chopped, lean.	20	1 cup	Tuna, canned in oil, drained.	50	3 ounces
Pork, fresh shoulder, chopped.	20	1 cup	Tuna salad	50	1 cup
Pork, fresh, ham or shoulder, ground, lean.	20	1 cup	Lamb, leg, chopped, lean	45	1 cup
			Kidney, beef	45	3 ounces
Veal, loin, chopped	20	1 cup	Pork, loin, chopped, lean	45	1 cup
Veal, rib, ground	20	1 cup	Veal, stewed, chopped	45	1 cup
Turkey, dark meat, chopped.	20	1 cup	Veal, rib, ground	45	1 cup
			Chicken, canned	45	1 cup
Chicken or turkey potpie, home-prepared from enriched flour.	30	⅓ of 9-inch pie	Chicken, stewed, light meat, sliced.	45	3 ounces
			Turkey, light meat, sliced.	45	3 ounces
Chop suey with beef and pork, home recipe.	20	1 cup	Swordfish, broiled	45	3 ounces
Pepper, stuffed	20	1 pepper (6.5 ounces)	Chicken, broiled	40	3 ounces
			Goose	40	3 ounces
			Lamb, shoulder, chopped, lean.	40	1 cup
Spaghetti (enriched) with meatballs, home recipe.	20	1 cup	Pork, fresh, ham, chopped, lean.	40	1 cup
			Veal, loin, chopped	40	1 cup
VEGETABLES AND FRUIT:			Turkey potpie, home-prepared from enriched flour.	40	⅓ of 9-inch pie
Broccoli, cooked	20	Medium stalk			
			Salmon steak, broiled or baked.	40	3 ounces
Broccoli, cut, cooked	20	1 cup			
Corn pudding	20	1 cup	Sunflower seeds	40	1 cup
Collards, cooked	20	1 cup	Beef, rump, chopped, lean.	35	1 cup
Turnip greens, cooked	20	1 cup			
Avocado, Florida, raw	20	½ fruit	Pork, fresh or cured, shoulder, chopped, lean.	35	1 cup
Avocado, Florida or California, raw, cubed.	20	1 cup	Veal, rib, sliced	35	3 ounces
			Heart, beef, sliced	35	3 ounces
CEREAL AND BAKERY PRODUCTS:			Chicken, stewed, dark meat, sliced.	35	3 ounces
Cereals, ready-to-eat (check label).	25	1 ounce	Chicken, roasted, dark meat, chopped.	35	1 cup
Spoonbread	25	1 cup	Halibut, broiled	35	3 ounces
Hoagie roll, enriched	20	11½-inch-long roll	Mackerel, broiled	35	3 ounces
			Rockfish, oven-steamed	35	3 ounces
MISCELLANEOUS:			Shad, baked	35	3 ounces
Bread pudding, with enriched bread.	35	1 cup	Beef, chuck, chopped	30	1 cup
			Beef, rump, ground, lean	30	1 cup
Oyster stew, home recipe	25	1 cup	Pork, cured, ham, chopped, lean.	30	1 cup
Rice pudding	20	1 cup			
Soup, cream of mushroom, with milk.	20	1 cup	Pork, cured, shoulder, ground, lean.	30	1 cup
			Pork, loin, sliced, lean	30	3 ounces

	NIACIN	
Food	*Percentage of U.S.RDA*	*Amount of food*

MEAT AND MEAT ALTERNATES:		
Peanuts	120	1 cup
Liver, hog	100	3 ounces
Chicken, light meat, chopped.	80	1 cup
Turkey, light meat, chopped.	80	1 cup
Liver, calf or beef	70	3 ounces
Chicken, breast	60	½ breast (3.3 ounces)
Chicken, stewed, dark meat, chopped.	60	1 cup
Veal rib, chopped	60	1 cup
Tuna, canned in water	60	3 ounces
Chicken, roasted, light meat, sliced.	50	3 ounces
Turkey, canned	50	1 cup
Rabbit, domesticated	50	3 ounces

Chicken fricassee, home recipe.	30	1 cup
Turkey, dark meat, chopped.	30	1 cup
Salmon, pink, canned	30	3 ounces
Beef potpie, home-prepared from enriched flour.	30	⅓ of 9-inch pie
Beef, chuck, ground, lean	25	1 cup
Beef, steak (club, porterhouse, T-bone, or sirloin), lean.	25	3 ounces
Beef, steak (round)	25	3 ounces
Ground beef	25	3 ounces
Lamb, leg, sliced	25	3 ounces
Lamb, loin chop, lean and fat.	25	3.5 ounces
Lamb, shoulder, sliced, lean.	25	3 ounces

Table continued on the following page

Table 10–12 LIST OF FOODS THAT ARE IMPORTANT SOURCES OF NUTRIENTS *(Continued)*

Pork, cured, ham, ground, lean	25	3 ounces
Pork, fresh, ham, sliced, lean.	25	3 ounces
Pork, loin chop, lean and fat.	25	2.7 ounces
Pork, loin, sliced, lean and fat.	25	3 ounces
Veal, stewed, sliced	25	3 ounces
Veal, loin or cutlet	25	3 ounces
Chicken, roasted, dark meat, sliced.	25	3 ounces
Chicken a la king, home recipe.	25	1 cup
Chicken potpie, home-prepared from enriched flour.	25	⅓ of 9-inch pie
Salmon, red, canned	25	3 ounces
Salmon rice loaf	25	6-ounce piece
Sardines, canned, drained.	25	3 ounces
Beef and vegetable stew, home recipe.	25	1 cup
Chop suey, with beef and pork, home recipe.	25	1 cup
Corned beef hash, canned.	25	1 cup
Peppers, stuffed	25	1 pepper (6.5 ounces)
Spaghetti (enriched) with cheese, canned.	25	1 cup
Beef, chuck, sliced	20	3 ounces
Beef, rump, sliced	20	3 ounces
Beef, rib, sliced, lean and fat.	20	3 ounces
Beef, flank steak	20	3 ounces
Beef, plate, lean	20	3 ounces
Beef, steak (club, porterhouse, T-bone, or sirloin), lean and fat.	20	3 ounces
Lamb, rib chop, lean and fat.	20	3.2 ounces
Lamb, loin chop, lean	20	2.3 ounces
Lamb, shoulder, sliced, lean and fat.	20	3 ounces
Pork, cured, ham, sliced, lean.	20	3 ounces
Pork, fresh, ham, sliced, lean and fat.	20	3 ounces
Pork, fresh or cured, shoulder, sliced.	20	3 ounces
Pork, loin chop, lean	20	2 ounces
Chicken, thigh	20	2.3-ounce piece
Turkey, dark meat, sliced.	20	3 ounces
Chicken and noodles, home recipe.	20	1 cup
Chow mein, home recipe	20	1 cup
Spaghetti (enriched) with meatballs, home recipe.	20	1 cup
Lobster salad	20	A salad
Lobster Newburg	20	1 cup
Crab, deviled	20	1 cup

VEGETABLES AND FRUITS:

Dates, pitted, chopped	20	1 cup
Peaches, dried, cooked, unsweetened.	20	1 cup
Peas, green, cooked	20	1 cup

CEREAL AND BAKERY PRODUCTS:

Hoagie roll, enriched	25	11½-inch-long roll
Cereals, ready-to-eat (check label).	20	1 ounce

CALCIUM

Food	Percentage of U.S. RDA	Amount of food
MILK AND MILK PRODUCTS:		
Cheese, Parmesan, grated.	40	1 ounce
Milk, partially skimmed	35	1 cup
Pudding, uncooked, from mix.	35	1 cup
Milk, whole or skim	30	1 cup
Milk, nonfat dry, reconstituted.	30	1 cup
Buttermilk	30	1 cup
Chocolate drink, made from whole milk.	30	1 cup
Cocoa	30	1 cup
Malted beverage	30	1 cup
Custard, baked	30	1 cup
Pudding, vanilla, home recipe.	30	1 cup
Rennin desserts	30	1 cup
Yogurt, made from partially skimmed milk.	30	1 cup
Chocolate drink, made from skim milk.	25	1 cup
Cheese, cottage, creamed	25	1 cup
Cheese, Swiss	25	1 ounce
Yogurt, made from whole milk.	25	1 cup
Ice cream or ice milk, soft-serve.	25	1 cup
Pudding, cooked, from mix, with milk.	25	1 cup
Pudding, chocolate, home recipe.	25	1 cup
Cheese, American, process.	20	1 ounce
Cheese, Cheddar, natural	20	1 ounce
Cheese, cottage, uncreamed.	20	1 cup
Ice cream or ice milk, hardened.	20	1 cup
MEAT AND MEAT ALTERNATES:		
Welsh rarebit	60	1 cup
Sardines, canned, drained.	35	3 ounces
Macaroni (enriched) and cheese, home recipe.	35	1 cup
Potatoes au gratin	30	1 cup
Beef, dried, chipped, creamed.	25	1 cup
Cheese souffle	20	1 cup
Lobster Newburg	20	1 cup

Table 10–12　LIST OF FOODS THAT ARE IMPORTANT SOURCES OF NUTRIENTS *(Continued)*

Macaroni (enriched) and cheese, canned.	20	1 cup
VEGETABLES AND FRUIT:		
Collards, cooked	35	1 cup
Cabbage, spoon, cooked	25	1 cup
Spinach, canned	25	1 cup
Turnip greens	25	1 cup
Kale, cooked	20	1 cup
Mustard greens, cooked	20	1 cup
Rhubarb, cooked	20	1 cup
CEREAL AND BAKERY PRODUCTS:		
Spoonbread	25	1 cup
Farina, enriched, instant	20	1 cup
MISCELLANEOUS:		
Bread pudding	30	1 cup
Oyster stew, home recipe	30	1 cup
Rice pudding	25	1 cup
Soup, with milk:		
Green pea	20	1 cup
Cream of celery	20	1 cup
Cream of mushroom	20	1 cup
Cream of asparagus	20	1 cup

IRON

Food	Percentage of U.S. RDA	Amount of food
MEAT AND MEAT ALTERNATES:		
Liver, hog	140	3 ounces
Pumpkin kernels	90	1 cup
Liver, calf	70	3 ounces
Kidney, beef	60	3 ounces
Sunflower seeds	60	1 cup
Liver, beef	40	3 ounces
Walnuts, black, chopped	40	1 cup
Clams, canned, drained, chopped.	35	1 cup
Beans, lima, dry, cooked	35	1 cup
Beans, with pork and sweet sauce, canned.	35	1 cup
Almonds, whole, shelled	35	1 cup
Beef, chuck or rump, chopped, lean.	30	1 cup
Pork, cured, shoulder, chopped, lean.	30	1 cup
Pork, fresh, ham or loin, chopped, lean.	30	1 cup
Heart, beef, sliced	30	3 ounces
Clams, raw	30	4 or 5 clams
Beef potpie, home-prepared from enriched flour.	30	⅓ of 9-inch pie
Beans, navy (pea), dry, cooked.	30	1 cup
Beans, white, dry, canned, solids and liquid.	30	1 cup
Cashew nuts, whole kernels, roasted.	30	1 cup
Beef, chuck or rump, ground, lean.	25	1 cup
Pork, cured, ham, chopped, lean.	25	1 cup
Pork, fresh, shoulder, chopped.	25	1 cup
Pork, fresh, ham, ground, lean.	25	1 cup
Veal, chopped	25	1 cup
Chicken or turkey potpie, home-prepared from enriched flour.	25	⅓ of 9-inch pie
Chile con carne with beans, canned.	25	1 cup
Chop suey, with beef and pork, home recipe.	25	1 cup
Corned beef hash, canned.	25	1 cup
Beans, Great Northern or red kidney, dry, cooked.	25	1 cup
Beans, red kidney, dry, canned, solids and liquid.	25	1 cup
Lentils, dry, cooked	25	1 cup
Soybeans, dry, cooked	25	1 cup
Beans, with frankfurters, canned.	25	1 cup
Beans, with pork and tomato sauce, canned.	25	1 cup
Beef, chuck, sliced, lean	20	3 ounces
Beef, flank steak	20	3 ounces
Beef, plate, lean	20	3 ounces
Beef, steak, sirloin, lean	20	3 ounces
Pork, cured, ham or shoulder, ground, lean.	20	1 cup
Pork, fresh, shoulder, ground, lean.	20	1 cup
Pork, fresh, ham, sliced, lean.	20	3 ounces
Pork, loin, sliced, lean	20	3 ounces
Turkey, dark meat, chopped.	20	1 cup
Veal, rib, ground	20	1 cup
Peppers, stuffed	20	1 pepper (6.5 ounces)
Spaghetti (enriched) in tomato sauce, with meatballs; canned or home-prepared.	20	1 cup
Cowpeas, dry, cooked	20	1 cup
Peas, split, dry, cooked	20	1 cup
Beef, chuck, lean and fat, sliced.	15	3 ounces
Beef, corned	15	3 ounces
Beef, plate, lean and fat	15	3 ounces
Beef, rump, sliced	15	3 ounces
Beef, rib, sliced, lean	15	3 ounces
Beef, steak (round)	15	3 ounces
Beef, steak (club, porterhouse, or T-bone), lean.	15	3 ounces
Beef, steak (sirloin), lean and fat.	15	3 ounces
Ground beef	15	3 ounces
Lamb, shoulder, chopped, lean.	15	1 cup
Lamb, leg, chopped	15	1 cup
Pork, cured, shoulder, sliced.	15	3 ounces
Pork, cured, ham, sliced, lean.	15	3 ounces
Pork, fresh, loin or ham, sliced, lean and fat.	15	3 ounces
Pork, loin chop, lean and fat.	15	2.7 ounces

Table continued on the following page

Table 10-12 LIST OF FOODS THAT ARE IMPORTANT SOURCES OF NUTRIENTS (*Continued*)

Pork, fresh, shoulder, sliced.	15	3 ounces	Mustard greens, fresh or frozen, cooked.	15	1 cup
Veal, sliced	15	3 ounces	Peas, green, cooked	15	1 cup
Veal, cutlet or loin	15	3 ounces	Sauerkraut juice	15	1 cup
Beef and vegetable stew, home recipe.	15	1 cup	Vegetables, mixed, cooked.	15	1 cup
Chicken, dark meat, chopped.	15	1 cup	Boysenberries, canned	15	1 cup
Chicken, canned	15	1 cup	Plums, canned, water or syrup pack.	15	1 cup
Spaghetti (enriched) with tomato sauce and cheese, canned.	15	1 cup	Prunes, dried, uncooked.	15	10 prunes
			CEREAL AND BAKERY PRODUCTS:		
Turkey, canned	15	1 cup	Farina, instant, enriched, cooked.	90	1 cup
Chow mein, chicken, home recipe.	15	1 cup	Farina, regular and quick-cooking, enriched, cooked.	70	1 cup
Chicken a la king, home recipe.	15	1 cup	Hoagie roll, enriched	40	11½-inch-long roll
Crab, deviled	15	1 cup			
Sardines, canned	15	3 ounces	Cereals, ready-to-eat (check label).	20	1 ounce
Shrimp, canned	15	3 ounces	Cottage pudding with enriched flour and chocolate sauce.	20	1/6 of 8-inch-square cake
Lobster salad	15	A salad			
Tuna salad	15	1 cup			
VEGETABLES AND FRUIT:			Gingerbread, with enriched flour.	20	1/9 of 9-inch-square cake
Peaches, dried, uncooked	60	1 cup			
Prune juice, canned	60	1 cup			
Dates, pitted, chopped	30	1 cup	Pie, pecan	20	4¾-inch sector
Raisins, seedless	30	1 cup			
Spinach, canned	30	1 cup	Coffeecake, with enriched flour.	15	2.5-ounce piece
Asparagus, pieces, canned.	25	1 cup			
Beans, lima, canned	25	1 cup	Cottage pudding, with enriched flour and strawberry sauce.	15	1/6 of 8-inch square cake
Beans, lima, fresh or frozen, baby, cooked.	25	1 cup			
Apricots, dried, cooked	25	1 cup	Hard roll, enriched	15	1 roll (1.8 ounces)
Peaches, dried, cooked	25	1 cup			
Cowpeas, cooked	20	1 cup	Spoonbread	15	1 cup
Cowpeas, canned, solids and liquid.	20	1 cup	MISCELLANEOUS:		
Peas, green, canned	20	1 cup	Bread pudding, with raisins and enriched bread.	20	1 cup
Spinach, cooked	20	1 cup			
Turnip greens, canned, solids and liquid.	20	1 cup	Oyster stew, home recipe	20	1 cup
			Molasses, blackstrap	20	1 tablespoon
Prunes, dried, cooked	20	1 cup			
Beans, lima, Fordhook, cooked.	15	1 cup	Apple brown betty, with enriched bread.	15	1 cup
Beet greens, cooked	15	1 cup			
Chard, Swiss, cooked	15	1 cup	Syrup, sorghum	15	1 tablespoon

types of sandwiches which have fillings of chopped raisins and peanuts, sliced banana and peanut butter, orange marmalade or jam with cottage cheese, and chopped prunes and peanut butter.

The art of planning nutritious meals incorporates the knowledge of nutrition facts, the regional availability of foods, and cookery skills. Thought should be given to texture and color for "eye appeal," which is important for both the well and the sick. If meals are planned in advance there is less chance of guesswork or the omission of essential nutrients. A shopping list is made from the menus; however, the shopping list should be sufficiently flexible to take advantage of good buys or sales on foods that the family regularly eats.

There are many choices of food around the world which will provide adequate meals for the day. From the nutrition point of view, a meal should contain a complete protein or two or more complementary proteins, sufficient calories for energy needs and a good percentage of the vitamin and mineral requirements.

An adequate diet pattern for the daily meals for a family is suggested below.

BREAKFAST

Fruit or fruit juice
Egg and/or ham, sausage, fish, cheese or complementary protein dish
Whole grain or enriched toast; griddle cakes; or rolls; or cereal with milk
Butter or fortified margarine
Milk or milk drink for children
Coffee or tea for adults

DINNER

Main dish of meat, fish, fowl, cheese, eggs or other protein-rich food combination
Potato or other starch food (rice, grits, spaghetti, macaroni, noodles)
Cooked green or yellow vegetable
Raw vegetable salad
Whole grain or enriched bread, biscuits or roll and butter or fortified margarine
Dessert
Milk or milk drink for children
Coffee or tea for adults

SUPPER OR LUNCH

Casserole, stew or soup
Sandwich with filling of meat or peanut butter or cheese and chopped vegetable, tuna or egg salad
Cooked or raw fruit
Milk or milk drink

SNACK

(during day or evening)
Milk for children and teenagers
Cereal, graham cracker, roll, cookies, pizza or hamburger (for children or adults requiring extra calories)

Omitting a Meal. If any meal is omitted or neglected, there is too much nutritional load put on the remaining meals in a day's intake. For example, if breakfast is omitted, the intake of nutrients for the day is inadequate, or one's food intake is concentrated later in the day instead of divided throughout the twenty-four hours. Many times poor snacks, which are mainly "empty" calorie foods and drinks, comprise the entire day's food intake for teenagers.

The neglect of breakfast is more common in cities than in rural areas and does not seem to be related to income. Eating breakfast has been found essential for maximum efficiency—both physical and mental—during the morning hours. Skipping or slighting breakfast results in decreased output and decreased mental alertness. Four separate studies conducted at the University of Iowa Medical School showed the basic or medium breakfast, providing 25 per cent of the day's calories, permits, in most cases, a greater work output than a breakfast supplying 40 per cent of the day's calories. Unfortunately, one may not recognize the damage being done to the body through poor food habits until it is too late.

Sometimes five or six small meals are preferable to the usual three meals, in which case the milk and/or fruit allowance could be taken between meals. Some authors report this increases efficiency. It is important to prepare the foods tastily, and serve them attractively to favorably influence the appetite. Contrast in textures and color are other influential factors.

When planning meals, some nutritionists classify foods into (1) the essential protective foods or foods with high nutrient/calorie ratios and (2) the energy foods. The essential protective foods form the framework of the meal plans and the calorie requirements are completed by the energy foods.

Cost Comparison. To determine the economy of a choice of food, it is helpful to make a cost comparison. For example, to decide the form of milk which is most economical for the family food budget, the following cost analysis for the equivalent of 7 quarts of fluid milk could be made:

Whole milk: 7 quarts at . . . cents a quart would cost . . .

Evaporated milk: 7 tall (14½ oz.) cans at . . . cents a can would cost . . .

Skim milk: 7 quarts at . . . cents a quart would cost . . .

Dry whole milk: 23 ounces at . . . cents an ounce would cost . . .

Dry skim milk: 23 ounces at . . . cents an ounce would cost . . .

For food values, Tables 1 and 2 in the Appendix should be consulted.

The same procedure may be followed to determine the most economical source of the other foods and nutrients, as for example, vitamin C, to fit the family food budget: orange juice, canned or frozen grapefruit juice, canned tomatoes, fresh strawberries, raw cabbage, raw turnips or rutabagas.

The Daily Food Guide (Table 10–4) and Table 10–12 have been devised to assist with meal planning in order to include all the nutrients in the daily diet.

NUTRITION IN THE MIDDLE-AGE PERIOD

Leaders in the field of nutrition point to these years (ages 30 to 60) as the most promising period for discovery and prevention of advancing and preventable illness and disability. It can be called the last chance for effective prevention of unnecessary aging. The middle-age period is frequently referred to as the active, productive period of life. Wise eating habits can play a profound role in prolonging these years and in maintaining vitality and general well-being. It is during these years that the body is most generally neglected and abused. The stress and nervous strain of business and work are greatest and the amount of relaxing and conditioning is the lowest. Hurried meals, frequently skipped meals, irregular eating times and improper selection of foods take their toll in gastrointestinal problems, diabetes mellitus and coronary heart disease.

Overweight and underweight are also problems, but the former is much more common and serious from the standpoint of longevity. It is during middle age that metabolism and activity are slowing down, and adequate modifications in food intake should be taken to extend the productive years of life. Obese individuals are prone to develop the common chronic diseases, such as diabetes, hypertension, osteoarthritis, and the degenerative cardiovascular diseases. (See Chapter 27.)

Recommended Daily Dietary Allow-

ances. The Food and Nutrition Board lists the recommended daily dietary allowances for ages 23–51 and over 51 years of age (see Table 10–1), which can be attained with a great variety of common foods, as previously described in this chapter.

THE OPTIMAL DIET FOR HEALTH

The optimal diet for the best health is an individual practice that is tempered by the genetic makeup and the environment of the individual. Because it is so complex, and because much of nutrition is not completely understood, authorities do not agree on the optimal diet, although they would agree on the foundations of an adequate diet as already described. The optimal diet would be the one that allowed the development of an individual to his or her fullest potential, promoted the best mental and physical performance, afforded the greatest resistance to infection and disease, and did not accelerate the aging process. Many feel that this means saturated fat and cholesterol should be limited, sodium reduced, sugar omitted or protein limited. Others would say food additives and colorings should be reduced, or fiber and vitamin C increased. At this point we do not have enough information to design the optimal diet for each person's biological individuality, but we can say which basics should be included in the adequate diet for most people.

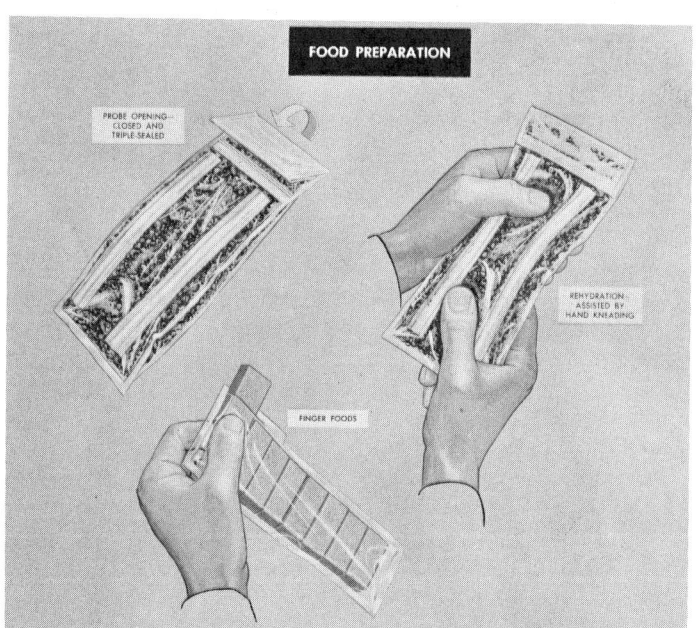

Figure 10–4 Food package that serves as storage vessel, food preparation utensil and eating device. (Courtesy of Beatrice Finkelstein and J. Am. Diet. Assoc.)

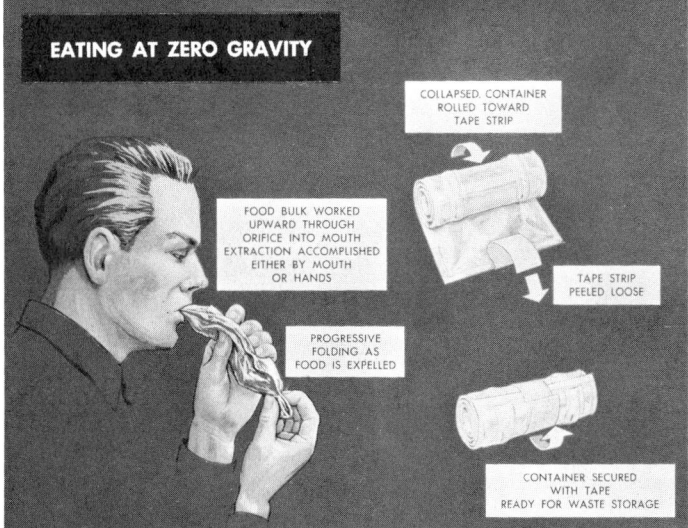

Figure 10–5 Eating at zero gravity by expelling food from food package. (Courtesy of Beatrice Finkelstein and J. Am. Diet. Assoc.)

ADEQUATE NUTRITION FOR ASTRONAUTS IN SPACE

Adequate nutrition for man in space offers many problems, and with the anticipation that more people will be traveling in space, the problems increase. The astronaut is a particularly healthy man by virtue of selection, but he still requires all the nutritional factors required by earth man. The calorie intake must not increase body mass or lose body weight. Lack of knowledge concerning the influence of the space conditions on man—weightlessness, lack of sunlight, confinement—makes it difficult to predict the energy required for activity. The main tasks in flight are classified as

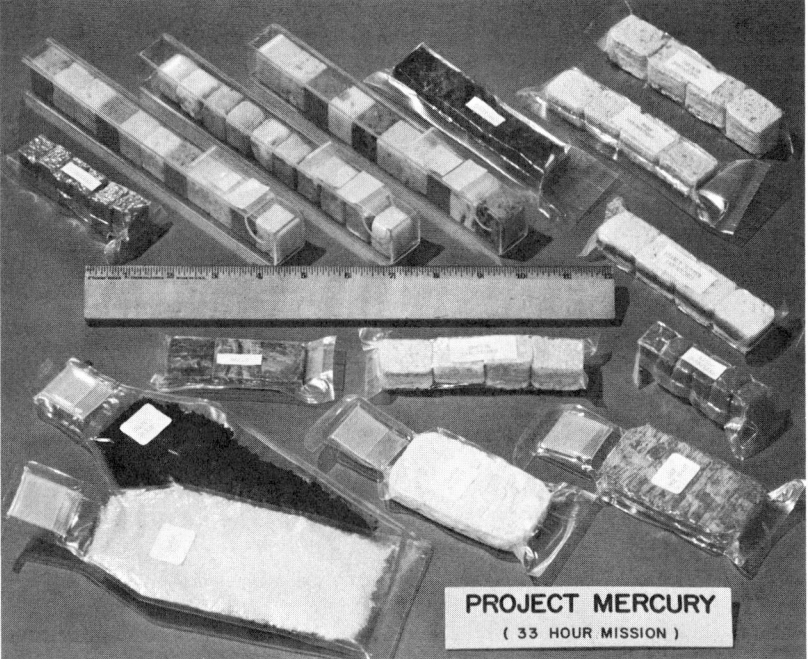

Figure 10–6 Bite-size foods available for astronauts' selection in Project Mercury. Top, left to right: cornflake cubes; three dispensers containing nine varieties of bite-size dessert-type cubes; fruit cake; beef sandwiches and chicken sandwiches. At the end of the ruler: peanut butter sandwiches. Below the ruler: orange juice, grape juice, bacon squares, cheese sandwiches, chicken and gravy, and rice-cornflakes cubes. (U.S. Army photo.)

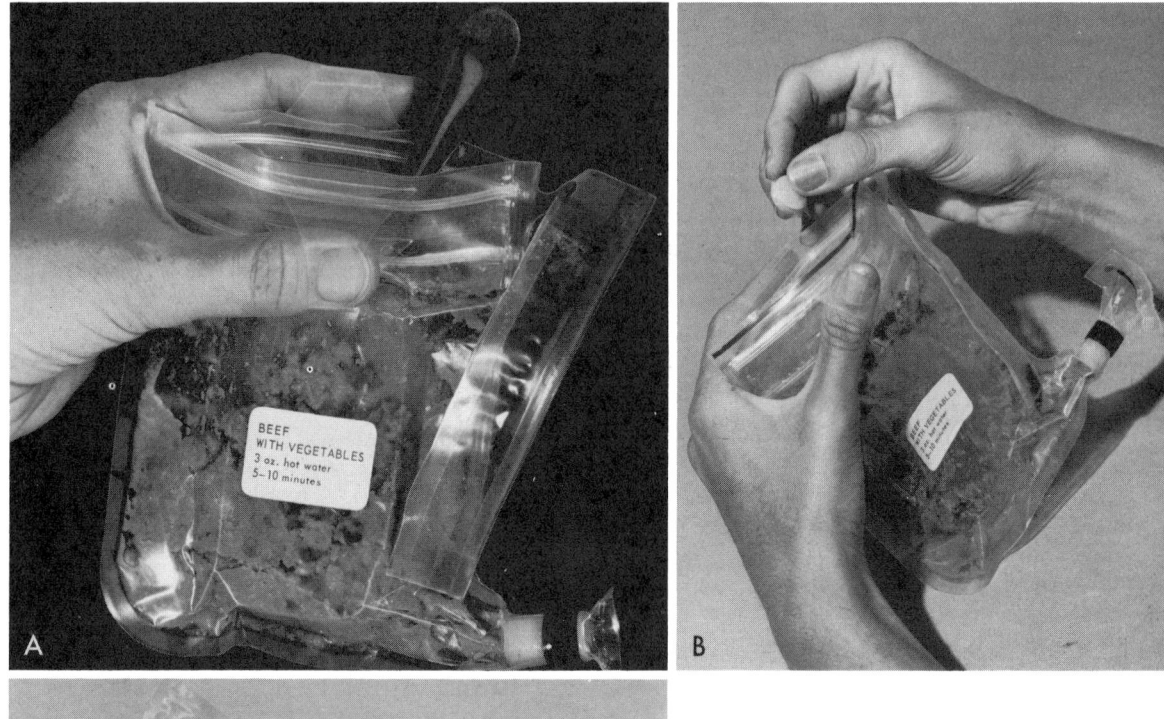

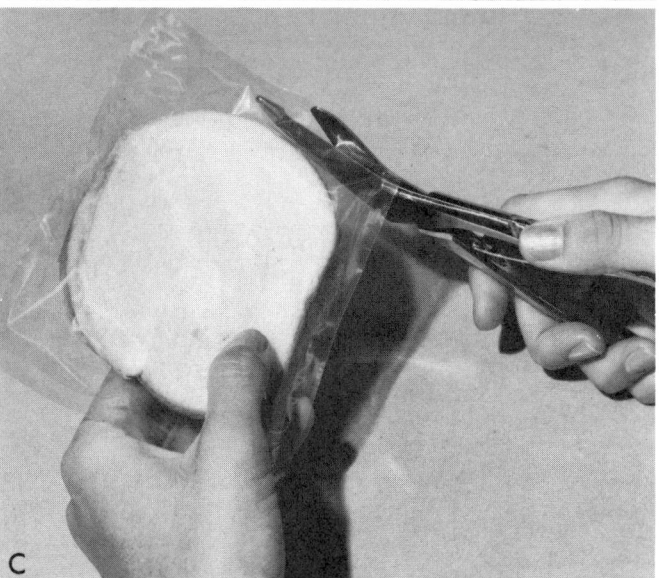

Figure 10–7 Familiar and tasty foods and using utensils in space missions. (Photos courtesy NASA.)

largely sedentary. The precise estimation of energy requirements are critical and based on the need for oxygen. Calloway[2] estimates a 2800 calorie diet as a safe allowance for routine space missions. Consideration of calorie density suggests that 50 per cent of the diet, or approximately 150 gm. should be derived from fat. On the basis of present knowledge, 0.9 gm. protein/kg. of body weight, or approximately 75 gm./day is allowed. Therefore, a total of approximately 285 gm. of carbohydrate is needed to make up the balance of calories. The minerals calcium, sodium, potassium and magnesium are provided in amounts 10 per cent above normal requirements to meet needs of anticipated stress. All other minerals are supplied by a mixed diet of processed foods. Animal research indicates that increased levels of ascorbic acid, vitamin E, and possibly thiamin are beneficial at high altitude. Liberal allowances of all vitamins are recommended, particularly ascorbic acid and vitamin E.

Foods. Foods must be compact, conveniently prepared and easily eaten in space. (See Figs. 10–4 and 10–5). Conditions dictate the predominant use of precooked, dehydrated, spray- or drum-dried foods. Some can be obtained from commercial sources and some will need to be custom produced. It is emphasized that "gas-producing" foods must be avoided in space diets on the basis that the gases produced are noxious and flammable. In addition, at reduced atmospheric pressure, expansion of gas volume can cause incapacitating pain due to distention.

Food preparation in the first missions consisted of the addition of water (hot or cold) in specified amounts. Food packaging and eating devices were designed and developed by the Food and Container Division of the U.S. Army Natick Laboratories, Natick, Massachusetts[6] working with the National Aeronautics and Space Administration (NASA) (See Fig. 10–6). Twenty-three bite-size foods and 37 dehydrated foods were included in the early missions. An average of 45 ounces (1330 ml.) water was required to reconstitute one day's menu. Approximately 2500 ml. water (5.5 lb.) was required per man per day for drinking and for the reconstitution of foods and beverages. A feeding system for one man per day contained 1.5 lb. of food which when packaged weighed approximately 1.67 lb. and occupied 225 cu. in. of space.[4]

In the voyage to the moon the astronauts Armstrong, Aldrin and Collins enjoyed a variety of food, enough to satisfy their hunger and to enable them to maintain performance. The first meal on the moon consisted of a light meal of fortified candy sticks, intermediate-moisture fruit, ham salad sandwich and rehydratable beverage. The food consumption on this mission (Apollo XI) was estimated to average 1800 to 2000 kcal. a day. In this mission the food supply came closer to meeting all the engineering, physiological and psychological requirements than in any previous flight. The problem of acceptability of foods in space is present. Eating habits are not easily changed or ignored. The food presented to man in the manner to which he is accustomed provides good nutrition. Astronauts now help plan the menus. The reader will recall the comments made when Borman, Lovell and Anders opened a surprise food package on Christmas Day and found natural chunks of turkey and brown gravy, bright red cranberry applesauce and an honest-to-goodness spoon. That meal proved it was possible to have familiar and tasty foods and be able to eat them with utensils, too (Fig. 10–7). The moon flight recorded considerable information about energy requirements. Every food program is influenced by the health of the people for which it is planned and the astronauts are no exception. Engineers, biologists, physicians and nutritionists have a challenge to design a feeding program for the space food system that will stimulate the appetite, allay hunger, be easy to prepare, be familiar in texture and flavor, provide pleasure and impart a sense of security.[12]

PROBLEMS AND SUGGESTED TOPICS FOR DISCUSSION

1. List your food intake for a week and compare with the basic food pattern on page 200. List any necessary adjustments for improvement.
2. Compare the daily nutritional allowances suggested for each member of the following family as determined from Table 10–1: Mother, age 35, overweight 30 pounds, who does own housework; father, age 40, who works as a mason and carries his lunch; girls, ages 3 and 6; active boy, age 12, 10 pounds underweight, who goes to school and comes home for lunch.
3. Compare costs of different available sources of milk to meet the daily calcium allowance. Follow the same procedure to compare costs of foods containing ascorbic acid; iron.
4. Define what you think your optimal diet should be. What improvements would you need to make to achieve it? Why is this your optimal diet?
5. Keep a record of your intake for two days in terms of percentage of U.S. RDA from the labels of foods you eat. What are some difficulties in this method? How does your total day's intake compare to the U.S. RDA and to the RDA?
6. How many different foods, with the exclusion of spices and condiments, do you eat in a week? Compare this intake with others. Count the *major* ingredients in such mixed items as stews and casseroles.

CITED REFERENCES

1. Calcium Requirements. FAO/WHO Expert Committee on Calcium Requirements, WHO Tech. Rep. Series 230, Rome, FAO, 1962.
2. Calloway, D. H.: Nutritional aspects of gastronautics. J. Am. Diet. Assoc., *44*:347, 1964.
3. Dietary Standard for Canada. Bureau of Nutritional Sciences, Food Directorate, Information Canada, 171 Slater St., Ottawa, 1975.
4. Finkelstein, B., and Symons, J.: Feeding concepts for manned space stations. J. Am. Diet. Assoc., *44*:353, 1964.
5. Hansen, R. G.: An index of food quality. Nutr. Rev., *31*:1, 1973.
6. Klicka, M. V.: Development of space foods. J. Am. Diet. Assoc., *44*:358, 1964.
7. Lowry, O. H., et al.: The interrelationship of dietary serum white blood cell and total ascorbic acid. J. Biol. Chem., *166*:111, 1946.
8. Margen, S., et al.: Studies in calcium metabolism. I. The calciuretic effect of dietary protein. Am. J. Clin. Nutr., *27*:584, 1974.

9. Nutrimeter. Student's Guide and Teacher's Guide. USDA, Agric. Res. Serv., Consumer and Food Economics Instit., Washington, D.C., May, 1975.

10. Nutrition Labeling. Tools for Its Use. USDA Agricultural Information Bulletin No. 382, U.S. Government Printing Office, Washington, D.C., 1975.

11. The Recommended Dietary Allowances. 8th ed. Food and Nutrition Board, Washington, D.C., National Research Council, NAS, 1974.

12. Smith, M., and Berry, C. A.: Dinner on the moon. Nutr. Today, *4*:37, 1969.

13. Sorensen, A. W., and Hansen, R. G.: Index of food quality. J. Nutr. Educ., *7*:53, 1975.

ADDITIONAL REFERENCES

Adams, C. F.: Nutritive Value of American Foods in Common Units. Washington, D.C., Agricultural Handbook No. 456, Agric., Res. Serv., USDA, 1975.

Bulletin. Conserving the Nutritive Values in Foods. Washington, D.C., U.S. Department of Agriculture, Home and Garden Bulletin Number 90, 1963.

Bulletin. Family Fare: A Guide to Good Nutrition. Washington, D.C., U.S. Department of Agriculture. Home and Garden Bulletin Number 1, Revised, 1970.

Bulletin. Food for the Young Couple. Washington, D.C., U.S. Department of Agriculture, Home and Garden Bulletin No. 85, 1967.

Bulletin. Food for Fitness—A Daily Food Guide. Washington, D.C., U.S. Department of Agriculture, Leaflet 424.

Burton, B. T.: Human Nutrition, 3rd ed. New York, McGraw-Hill Book Company, 1976, Chapter 13—Human Nutritional Requirements and Chapter 15—The Normal Adult Diet.

Church, C. F., and Church, H. N.: Food Values of Por-

tions Commonly Used. 12th ed. Philadelphia, J. B. Lippincott Company, 1976.

Dairy Council Digest: Recommended Dietary Allowances. Revised 1974, Chicago, National Dairy Council, *45*(3), May-June, 1974.

Deutsch, R.: Nutrition Labeling—How It Can Work for You. Chicago, The Nutrition Consortium, American Dietetic Association, 1976.

Goodwin, M. T.: Better Living Through Better Eating. 2nd ed. Rockville, Maryland, Montgomery County Health Department, 1974.

Harper, A. E.: Recommended dietary allowances: are they what we think they are? J. Am. Diet. Assoc., *64*:151, 1974.

Hayes, J. (ed.): Food for Us All. Yearbook of Agriculture, 1969. U.S. Government Printing Office, Washington, D.C.

Leverton, R. M.: Basic nutrition concepts. J. Home Econ., *59*:346, 1967.

Leverton, R. M.: The RDAs are not for amateurs. J. Am. Diet. Assoc., *66*:9, 1975.

Ohlson, M. A., and Hart, B. P.: Influence of breakfast on total day's food intake. J. Am. Dietet. A., *47*:282, 1965.

Recommended dietary allowances up to date—a symposium. J. Am. Diet. Assoc., *64*:149, 1974.

Turner, D.: Handbook of Diet Therapy. 5th ed. Chicago, University of Chicago Press, 1970, Chapters 1 and 2.

Walker, A. R. P.: Optimal intake of nutrients. Nutr. Rev. *23*:231, 1965.

Watt, B. K., and Merrill, A. L.: Composition of Foods. Agricultural Handbook No. 8, Agric. Res. Serv., USDA, Washington, D.C., 1963.

Wilson, E. D., Fisher, K. H., and Fuqua, M. E.: Principles of Nutrition. 3rd ed. New York, John Wiley & Sons, 1975, Chapter 16—Selecting an adequate diet.

Williams, R. J.: We abnormal normals. Nutrition Today, *2*:19, 1967.

Chapter 11

THE ASSESSMENT OF NUTRITIONAL STATUS

Even though the U.S. is the largest producer of food in the world, and even though for most citizens the food supply is adequate, we cannot assume that Americans will or can eat the food optimal for their well being, performance and growth. The method for measuring the influence of the nutrition factor on the health of the individual is through assessment of nutritional status.

Nutritional status or nutriture is the degree to which the individual's physiological need for nutrients is being met by the food he or she is eating. It is the state of balance in the individual between the nutrient intake and the nutrient expenditure or need. See Fig. 11–1. Evaluation of nutritional status involves examination of the individual's physical condition, growth and development, behavior, the urinary, blood or

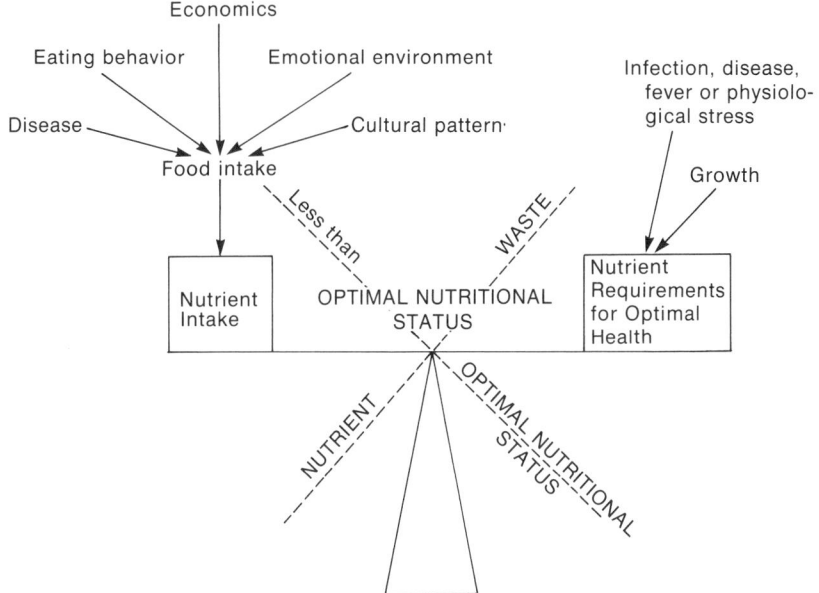

Figure 11–1 Optimal nutritional status as a balance between nutrient intake and nutrient requirements.

tissue levels of nutrients, and the quality and quantity of the nutrient intake. Information on present medication, stress or chronic illness, economic situation, nutrition knowledge, cultural patterns and living conditions is also useful because these factors influence nutritional intake and sometimes nutritional requirements, and thus nutritional status. In a thorough *nutritional status assessment,* all of the following aspects are considered:

1. Dietary history and intake data
2. Biochemical data
3. Clinical examination
   —pertinent medical history
4. Anthropometric data
5. Psychosocial data

Besides adding to the assessment of health, this information will give the health professional information for *anticipating* problems and preventing poor nutrition before it develops.

In situations of limited time, money, or professional staff, less information can be gathered, and of necessity the assessment must be abbreviated, although it is still useful. For an example, see Appendix Tables 22 and 23, which can form the basis for minimal assessment of nutritional status.

With regard to all the aspects of nutritional status assessment—the dietary intake, psychosocial information, biochemical data and anthropometric measurements—a finding below the standard only means that the individual is likely to have a subclinical deficiency. He is "at

risk" of developing a clinical nutritional deficiency, which is verified by a clinical examination.

ASSESSMENT OF THE COMMUNITY

Although this chapter will emphasize the nutritional status of the individual, an individual's nutritional status reflects the nutritional well-being of his community. For this reason an assessment of the community is important for any health worker concerned with the nutritional status of the community's individuals. Table 11–1 outlines those aspects of a community that should be evaluated. The factors affecting nutritional status are many and varied, and the assessment of the community will involve considerable exposure to the people and collection of information from many different records, agencies, and workers in the community.

ASSESSMENT OF THE INDIVIDUAL

DIETARY INTAKE

The accurate recording and evaluation of the dietary intake of an individual is the most difficult and frustrating aspect of nutritional assessment. First, it is difficult to record a person's food intake without influencing it. When

Table 11–1 INFORMATION FOR COMMUNITY ASSESSMENT

Demographic Information
  —age
  —ethnicity
  —sex
  —population density
Socioeconomic Stratification
Health Statistics: Morbidity and Mortality
  —birth rate
  —number of births weighing <2500 gm.
  —births to mothers <18 yr. of age
  —deaths and causes of death
  —prevalence or incidence of various diseases
Local Health Resources
Dental Health and Dental Health Resources
Cultural Factors
Community Political Organization
Housing
Food Supply
  —cost
  —enrichment or fortification
  —stores
School Nutrition or Elderly Feeding Programs
Social Welfare Programs
  —programs available
  —population receiving programs
Transportation
Education
  —language spoken
Occupational Data
Geography and Environment

(Adapted from Christakis, G. (ed.): Nutritional Assessment in Health Programs. Washington, D.C., Am. Pub. Health Assoc., Inc., 1973.)

people are watched, questioned about what they eat, or asked to write down what they eat, eating patterns tend to change. The extent of change depends on how well the person understands the dietary history, or to what extent he or she is influenced by what he or she thinks the nurse, nutritionist or physician wants to see or hear. Secondly, many people simply cannot remember the types or amounts of food they ate. Third, it is impossible to *accurately* evaluate the nutrient composition of the food eaten unless the intake is tightly controlled, as in a metabolic ward. Food composition tables are neither complete nor necessarily accurate for foods Americans are eating today. Many of the new processed foods are not listed in present tables and the information must be obtained from food manufacturers. Methods of cooking vary and can greatly affect nutrient values. The area in which a fruit or vegetable is grown can affect its nutrient content. Fortunately, as the U.S. Nutrient Data Center gets underway, food composition data should become more complete.[6, 10]

Methods for Assessing Dietary Intake

24-Hour Recall. The most popular and easiest method for obtaining an idea of a person's dietary intake is the *24-hour recall*. The individual completes a questionnaire or is interviewed by a dietitian/nutritionist or nurse experienced in dietary interviewing and is asked to recall everything that he or she ate within the last 24 hours, or the previous day. In surveys of population groups this has been found to be a fairly good tool. However, there are significant sources of error: (1) the person may not be able to accurately recall the amounts of food eaten; (2) the previous day's intake may be atypical of the usual intake; and (3) the person may not be telling the truth for a variety of reasons, one of which may be embarrassment. For instance, in one study Young found that there was a tendency to underestimate portion size as the portion size increased and overestimate portion size as the portion size decreased.[12] Foods least accurately reported are sauces, gravies, fruits and snack items.

Food Frequency Questionnaire. To help overcome some of the weaknesses inherent in the 24-hour recall method, a *food frequency questionnaire* may also be completed. Using this tool, the health professional can collect information on how many times per day, week or month the individual eats particular foods. This information can aid in validating the accuracy of the 24-hour recall data and clarify the picture of the person's real food consumption pattern. The food frequency questionnaire may be selective, with questions about foods suspected of being deficient or excessive in the diet, or general, with questions concerning all foods likely to be eaten. See Table 11–2 for a typical 24-hour recall questionnaire. Table 11–3 is a general food frequency questionnaire. Table 11–4 is a selective food frequency questionnaire.

Dietary History. The dietary history is more complete than either the 24-hour recall or food frequency questionnaire, although it usually includes both of these sources. The dietary history (see Table 11–5) contains additional information about the following:

  1. Economics
    a. income—frequency of paycheck
    b. amount of money for food each week or month and individual's perception of its adequacy for meeting food needs

c. eligibility for food stamps and cost of stamps

d. public aid recipient?

2. Physical activity
   a. occupation—type, hours/week, shift, energy expenditure
   b. exercise—type, amount, frequency (seasonal?)
   c. sleep—hours/day, (uninterrupted?)
   d. handicaps

3. Ethnic or cultural background
   a. influence on eating habits
   b. religion
   c. education

4. Homelife and meal patterns
   a. number in household (eat together?)
   b. person who does shopping
   c. person who does cooking, and relationship
   d. food storage and cooking facilities (stove, refrigerator)
   e. type of housing (home, apartment, room, etc.)
   f. ability to shop and prepare food

5. Appetite
   a. good, poor, any changes
   b. factors that affect appetite
   c. taste and smell perception

6. Allergies, intolerances or food avoidances
   a. foods avoided and reason
   b. length of time of avoidance

7. Dental and oral health
   a. problems with eating
   b. foods that cannot be eaten
   c. problems with swallowing, salivation, food sticking

8. Gastrointestinal
   a. problems with heartburn, bloating, gas, diarrhea, constipation, distention
   b. frequency of problems
   c. home remedies
   d. antacid, laxative or other drug use

9. Chronic disease
   a. treatment
   b. length of time of treatment
   c. dietary modification—physician prescription?, date of modification, education, compliance with diet

10. Medication
    a. vitamin and/or mineral supplements—frequency, type, amount
    b. medications—type, amount, frequency, length of time on medication

Text continued on page 228

Table 11–2 24-HOUR RECALL FORM AND FOOD GROUP EVALUATION

The following question pattern may be used for conducting the 24-hour recall. The information should then be recorded in the chart at the end.

"In order to get a more complete picture of your family's health, I need to know more about your eating habits. Would you please tell me everything you ate or drank, all day yesterday. Let's begin with:"

1. What time did you go to bed the night before last? _____ (typical versus atypical day)
   Was this the usual time? _____
2. What time did you get up yesterday? _____
   Was this the usual time? _____
3. When was the first time you had anything to eat or drink? _____ What did you have and how much?

_____

4. When did you eat again? _____ Where? _____ What and how much?_____

_____

5. When did you eat next? _____ What did you eat and how much?_____

_____

6. Did you eat or drink anything else? _____
   a. Anything from 1st to 2nd "meal?" _____
   b. Anything from 2nd to 3rd "meal?" _____
   c. Anything from 3rd "meal" to bedtime? _____
7. Was this day's food intake different from usual? _____ If so, how? _____
8. Is weekend eating different? _____ If so, how?_____

Table continued on the following page

Table 11–2   24-HOUR RECALL FORM AND FOOD GROUP EVALUATION *(Continued)*

FOOD AND FLUID INTAKE FROM TIME OF AWAKENING UNTIL
THE NEXT MORNING—24-HOUR RECALL

TIME	FOOD AND DRINK CONSUMED		NUMBER OF SERVINGS IN THE FOOD GROUPS							
	Name and Type	*Amount*	*Milk Grp.*	*Meat Grp.*	*Vit A Grp.*	*Vit C Grp.*	*Other F & V*	*Bread & Cereal*	*Butter, Fat, Oil*	*Miscellaneous (Candy, etc.)*
TOTALS										
		Amount	*Milk Grp.*	*Meat Grp.*	*Vit A Grp.*	*Vit C Grp.*	*Other F & V*	*Bread & Cereal*	*Butter Fat, Oil*	*Miscellaneous (Candy, etc.)*
Recommended No. of Servings Daily										
Children 6 or under			2–3 c.	2	3/wk	1	2	4	2 TBSP.*	†
Adolescent			4 c.	2	3/wk	1	2	4	2TBSP.	
Adult			2 c.	2	3/wk	1	2	4	2 TBSP.	
Pregnant or Lactating			4 c.	2	3/wk	1	2	4	2 TBSP.	
			Milk Grp.	Meat Grp.	Vit A Grp.	Vit C Grp.	Other F&V	Bread & Cereal	Butter, Fat, Oil	Miscellaneous (Candy, etc.)
Evaluation L = Low A = Adequate E = Excessive										

*2 Tbsp./day recommended to meet calorie and essential fatty acid needs. Excessive amounts in this group usually mean excessive caloric intake.

†Servings of high calorie, low nutrient items such as sugar, candy, soda pop. Excessive amounts in this group usually mean excessive caloric intake and possibly dental caries.

Table 11–3   A GENERAL FOOD FREQUENCY QUESTIONNAIRE

For the frequency of food use, the following pattern of questions may be useful. However, you may have to modify questions after learning some information from the 24-hour recall. For instance, if the patient has said he had a glass of milk yesterday, you wouldn't ask "Do you drink milk?", but rather "How much milk do you drink?" Record answers as 1/day, 1/wk., 3/mo., for example, or as accurately as possible. It may just have to be noted as "occasionally" or "rarely."

1. Do you drink milk? If so, how much? _____ What kind? Whole _____ Skim _____
2. Do you use fat? If so, what kind? _____ How much? _____
3. How many times do you eat meat? _____ eggs _____ cheese _____ beans _____
4. Do you eat snack foods? If so, which ones? _____ How often? _____ How much? _____
5. What vegetables do you eat? (in each group) How often?
   a. Broccoli _____ greenpeppers _____ cooked greens _____ carrots _____
      sweet potato _____
   b. Tomatoes _____ raw cabbage _____
   c. Asparagus _____ beets _____ cauliflower _____ corn _____
      cooked cabbage _____ celery _____ peas _____ lettuce _____
6. What fruits and how often?
   a. Apples or applesauce _____ apricots _____ banana _____ berries _____
      cherries _____ grapes or grape juice _____ peaches _____ pears _____
      pineapple _____ plums _____ prunes _____ raisins _____
   b. Oranges _____ orange juice _____ grapefruit _____ grapefruit juice _____
7. Bread and cereal products
   a. How much bread do you usually eat with each meal? _____ between meals _____
   b. Do you eat cereal (daily, weekly) cooked _____ dry _____
   c. How often do you eat foods such as macaroni, spaghetti, noodles, etc. _____
8. Do you use salt? _____ Do you salt your food before tasting it? _____
   Do you cook with salt? _____ Do you "crave" salt or salty foods? _____
9. How many tsp. of sugar do you use/day (1 packet = 1 tsp.)? _____
   (Be sure and ask patient about sugar on cereal, fruit, toast and in coffee, tea, etc.)
10. Do you drink water? _____ How often during the day? _____
    How much each time? _____ How much would you say you drink each day? _____
11. Do you drink alcohol? _____ How often? _____ How much? _____
    Beer, wine, liquor? _____

Table 11–4   SELECTIVE FOOD FREQUENCY QUESTIONNAIRE FOR INQUIRING ABOUT CHOLESTEROL, FAT, SODIUM, IRON OR SUGAR INTAKE

FREQUENCY OF FOOD USE: RECORD AS TIMES/WK. OR DAY OR N = NEVER, R = RARE

High or Moderately High in:	Use of		High or Moderately High in:		
CHOLESTEROL:	Eggs	_____	UNSATURATED FAT:	Soft margarine	_____
	Liver	_____		Vegetable oils	_____
	Shellfish	_____			
	Beef	_____	SODIUM:	Prepared frozen foods	_____
	Pork	_____		Sausages or franks	_____
				Snack foods, e.g.,	
SATURATED FAT:	Beef	_____		pretzels, potato chips,	
	Pork	_____		salted peanuts	_____
	Butter	_____		Softened water	_____
	Whole milk	_____		Olives, pickles	_____
	Cream	_____		Smoked fish; canned fish	_____
	Pastries	_____		Ham & other canned	
	Gravies	_____		meat	_____
	Ice cream	_____			
			IRON:	Iron supplements	_____
SUGAR:	Cakes	_____		Dark green leafy veg.	_____
	Pastries	_____		Enriched cereals	_____
	Cookies	_____		Dried beans	_____
	Coke	_____		Meat, fish, or poultry	_____
	Soda pop	_____		Eggs	_____
	Candy	_____			

Table 11–5 DIETARY HISTORY INFORMATION

The information in this section most likely can be obtained from the patient's past medical record or hospital chart. Any interview should be prefaced by a review of this record, because the purpose of the dietary history is to add to and complete the data base on a patient.

DATE	PATIENT'S NAME & HOSPITAL OR CLINIC NUMBER	INTERVIEWER

| MARITAL STATUS | ADDRESS | PREGNANT? _____ |
| | | LACTATING? _____ |

| AGE | SEX | ETHNIC AND/OR RELIGIOUS BACKGROUND AS RELATED TO DIET | PROBLEMS |
| | | | 1. _____ |

RECENT ILLNESS OR SURGERY?	FEVER?	PRIMARY DIAGNOSIS	2. _____
			3. _____
			4. _____

The information in this section can be obtained either from the patient's record or by asking the patient directly. For instance "What do you do?" or "Are you employed?" or "Do you exercise?", "What type of exercise?", or "How often."

| PRESENT MEDICATIONS | SLEEP _____ hr./24 hr. | HEIGHT _____ | ANY RECENT WEIGHT CHANGES |
| | | WEIGHT _____ | |

OCCUPATION

HOURS/WEEK AND SHIFT

FACTORS OR PHYSICAL HANDICAPS THAT PREVENT ACTIVITY OR EXERCISE

PHYSICAL EXERCISE—TYPE & AMOUNT & FREQUENCY

ASSESSMENT OF PATIENT'S ACTIVITIES

sedentary   mod. active   very active

DIET ORDERED PRIOR TO HOSPITALIZATION OR OUTPATIENT VISIT

Type _____   Followed most of time _____ Yes _____ No _____ How Long? _____

RECENT CHANGES IN EATING HABITS AND REASONS FOR CHANGES

FOOD ALLERGIES OR FOOD IDIOSYNCRACIES (i.e., Foods Disliked, Avoided, etc.)

DENTAL PROBLEMS

OTHER FACTORS INTERFERING WITH CONSUMPTION, DIGESTION OR ASSIMILATION OF FOOD

AMOUNT OF MONEY SPENT ON FOOD

FOOD STAMPS

OTHER PERTINENT ECONOMIC FACTORS

11. Dietary or nutritional problems (as perceived by patient)

Remember that dietary habits are personal and an individual may be unwilling to talk about them, especially if he or she perceives the interviewer as being judgemental. It is necessary to be as objective as possible when interviewing in order to gain a complete and accurate insight into a person's eating patterns. The reader is also referred to one of the many good books on interviewing. Interviewing regarding dietary patterns is discussed further in Chapter 19.

Food Diary or Record. This method involves more time, understanding, and motivation on the part of the patient or client. The subject is asked to write down everything he or she eats or drinks for a certain time period. Three days, particularly two week days and one weekend day, have been found to be a representative time period for most people. The length of time that the food diary must be kept in order to accurately reflect usual nutrient intake depends on whether the person has a regular food pattern. A daily food pattern requires fewer days of recording than a random, haphazard eating style. The nutrient contribution for each food is calculated; the total day's intake for each nutrient is totalled and then divided by the number of days to give an average daily intake. The health practitioner can gain information about lifestyle, companions, and meal eating atmosphere by asking the person to also note the time, place and people with whom he or she eats. See Fig. 11–2 for a typical page in a food diary. Recall can be combined with the food diary method when the nutrition counselor goes over the food record with the patient and asks the patient to supply additional information regarding amounts and types of preparation of the food. This is a very good way to get to know a person's lifestyle, since food habits are an intimate part of that lifestyle. A food diary is most complete and accurate if the patient is instructed to record it immediately after eating.

Observation of Food Intake. Observation of food intake is the most accurate method of dietary intake assessment, but also the most time consuming, expensive and difficult. Observation must be non-intrusive and is most easily done when the person's meals are provided for him, as in the case of a hospitalized person, nursing home resident or child at a boarding school. It requires knowing the amount and kind of food presented to the person and a record of the amount actually eaten.

The ultimate in a controlled situation is that in a metabolic unit when a weighed amount of food is presented, the amount of uneaten food is re-weighed, and the difference is recorded as the amount eaten.

Household Food Consumption. This method involves visiting a household periodically and recording the amounts and types of food purchased for that household and the disappearance of that food. The food unaccounted for is assumed to be that consumed by the family. It is most commonly used in large population surveys and is not a good evaluation of individual intake, because of food wastage and lack of a record of the individual household members' consumption. However, in attempting to gain insight into the nutrition situation in the community, this information can be very valuable. It can be traced backward from the food in the household to the income of the household to the food available in the market, and so on. See Fig. 11–3. This flow chart would apply more to a rural or less developed economy where climate and food transportation have more effect on the food available in the market than in a developed country. However, the "food available in the market" could be significant in the case of the inner city dweller, such as an elderly person who is trapped into shopping at the corner market that might not carry certain needed items such as bran flakes, diet soda, salt-free crackers or good fresh fruits. Depending on the situation, different factors in the food chain should be scrutinized.

Evaluation of Food Intake Data

The intakes of vitamins A and C and folic acid are the most variable intakes in the majority of U.S. diets. Because they are not widely present in foods, except for particular fruits and vegetables that are concentrated sources, the intake of these vitamins is greatly influenced by specific food choices during a day. Secondly, the intake of these nutrients frequently is seasonal, with a higher intake in the summer and fall when abundant amounts of fresh fruits and vegetables are more available either because they are cheaper or because the family has a fruit and vegetable garden. Riboflavin, calcium and vitamin D intakes are largely dependent on the intake of milk and milk products. The dietary intake of thiamin, niacin, protein, phosphorus, calories, vitamin E, iron, and B_{12}, which are present in a wide variety of foods, is more consistent each day.

Evaluation by Food Group Methods. The

DAY_____

DATE_____

Time	Place	With Whom	Situation	Amount	Name and Type of Food

Figure 11–2   Food diary.

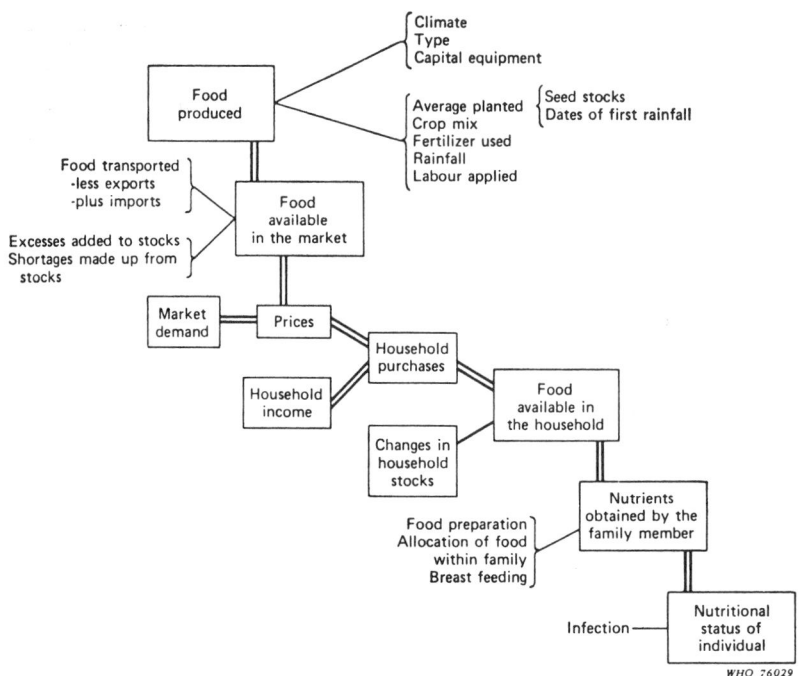

Figure 11–3   Flow chart for household food consumption: a food chain. (Adapted from: Methodology of Nutritional Surveillance. Joint FAO/UNICEF/WHO Expert Committee. Geneva, WHO, 1976.)

simplest, fastest, yet crudest way to evaluate food intake data is to determine how many servings from each of the four food groups were consumed during the recorded day. The number of servings from each group is then compared with the number of servings suggested in the Basic Four or Seven Food Group Plans. See Table 11–2 and Table 10–4. Gross deficiencies of protein, iron, calcium, riboflavin, vitamin A and vitamin C in the diet can be detected in this way. It becomes more difficult to use this method if the diet has many food mixtures or unusual cultural foods that do not fit into one of the food groups.

A more accurate assessment of the calories, protein and fat in the diet can be derived by quantifying the food intake in terms of diabetic exchanges. See Table 25–4. These figures can then be compared with the individual's recommended daily allowances (RDA, Table 10–1) for calories and protein and the American Heart Association recommendation that 35 per cent of the calories in the diet come from fat.

Evaluation by Nutrient Composition. The dietary intake can be evaluated more accurately by calculating the amounts of each nutrient in each food consumed, which can be done by hand or with the use of a computer.

The nutrient values for foods can be obtained from several sources: USDA Handbook No. 8 *Composition of Foods,*[11] Handbook No. 456, *Nutritive Values of American Foods,*[1] *Food Value of Portions Commonly Used,*[2] and nutrition labels and food manufacturers' information on the nutrient composition of the food (see Chapter 10).

After recording the nutrient composition for the various foods in the diet, the nutrient composition of the total diet can be determined.

A more accurate, yet far more difficult and expensive method is to prepare a total day's food intake identical to that taken by the patient and have it chemically analyzed for its nutrient content. Again, this is usually done in a metabolic unit where extreme accuracy is essential.

The intakes of most nutrients are interdependent. Guthrie postulates that for U.S. preschool children, the intakes of iron and energy are as indicative of the adequacy of the dietary intake as a more complete evaluation.[5] In other words, only the caloric and iron content of the diet would need to be calculated. If these were adequate, one could assume that the diet would be adequate for the rest of the nutrients needed by healthy children 12 to 72 months of age.

Standard for Evaluation of Nutrient Intake—the RDA

The standards usually used for evaluating the intake of specific nutrients are the Recommended Dietary Allowances (RDA). See page 193, Chapter 10 for a complete discussion of the meaning of these allowances. Although the RDA are frequently used to evaluate an *individual's* diet, this is theoretically an *improper* use of them. The RDA are set at a level above the requirement in order to include all those individuals within the population who might have an increased need for a particular vitamin or mineral above the mean requirement of the population. Because the RDA include this "safety factor," they are probably higher than a typical individual's requirement. Nutrition professionals frequently use two-thirds of the RDA as a satisfactory or adequate intake when evaluating an individual's intake of a nutrient. The exception is the RDA for calories, which does not include a safety factor. Calorie and protein intake should be evaluated on a per kilogram body weight basis. With these limitations in mind regarding the evaluation of the dietary intake of an individual, the RDA can be used to evaluate in a general manner the dietary intake of an individual.

It is impossible to judge the adequacy of a person's intake of a nutrient by looking at dietary intake alone. The practitioner must also evaluate serum and tissue levels of the nutrient, examine the person for clinical signs of a deficiency and take a thorough history. For example, one cannot assume that if the vitamin A intake of Joyce, age 20, is only 1000 I.U. per day, she is deficient in vitamin A. The serum levels of carotene, vitamin A, liver stores of vitamin A and examination for clinical signs such as follicular hyperkeratosis, Bitot's spots and night blindness would complete the assessment.

DEVELOPMENT OF NUTRITIONAL DEFICIENCY

Nutritional deficiency is a progressive phenomenon and different techniques of assessment detect different stages of nutritional adequacy or deficiency. Obviously, the ideal methods are those which detect nutritional deficiency in its early stages of development so that dietary intake can be improved through therapy and nutritional counseling before the more severe deficiency lesion appears.

The early stage of a nutritional deficiency is characterized by body adaptation to the decreased intake and less than optimal amounts of the nutrient present in the blood and tissues. For example, plasma vitamin A will be less, or urinary riboflavin excretion will fall. A more severe or prolonged nutritional deficiency would result in a biochemical "lesion" or a tissue enzyme deficiency or malfunction. By using biochemical tests, the clinician attempts to detect a nutritional deficiency in these early stages. The most severe nutritional deficiency states are reflected in changes in the functions of organs (e.g., dark maladaptation in vitamin A deficiency) and changes in tissue structure (e.g., histopathology of xerophthalmia). These stages are detected by clinical examination.

Somewhere between the initial stage of deficiency development and the biochemical lesion is the effect of nutritional deficiency on growth and anthropometric measurements, hence the reason for these measurements, especially in children.

BIOCHEMICAL MEASUREMENTS

There is considerable controversy over what constitutes optimal nutritional status, and the discussion is more heated for some nutrients than for others. For example, are the lower hemoglobin levels routinely seen in black people when compared with whites of all ages indicative of iron deficiency, or do they reflect a genetic difference?[4]

There are, however, some principles of biochemical evaluation upon which authorities agree.

First, heredity probably does influence the biochemical nutritional profile, but we do not know to what extent or how it is separate from dietary and other environmental influences.

Second, the level of a nutrient in the body is affected by the sex and age of the person. Therefore, in establishing the standards for nutritional biochemical data, separate values are given for some nutrients. In others, our knowledge is not complete enough to be able to give sex and age specific standards.

Third, there is not a definite value for a biochemical test that clearly delineates the deficient person from the non-deficient person. For this reason, standards are somewhat arbitrary and are usually given as ranges. Being deficient implies less than optimal growth, health or performance, and this must be defined by clinical examination.

Fourth, some biochemical values reflect

immediate nutrient intake, while others reflect past or long-term intake. For example, vitamin C, plasma carotene and plasma triglycerides reflect immediate intake.

Lastly, a biochemical value for one nutrient can be influenced by the intake or body level of another nutrient. For example, serum folate is influenced by the individual's vitamin B_{12} status.

Biochemical data regarding nutritional status can be obtained from examination of plasma, red blood cells, white blood cells, urine, or tissues such as liver, bone, hair and fingernails. Obviously, the latter two tissues are much easier to obtain and ideally we would like more information on the biochemical data of these tissues as reflections of nutrient intake. Clinicians and researchers are beginning to analyze hair root samples in order to evaluate protein, energy and zinc status.[9] Fingernails may possibly reflect protein nutriture, and knowledge in this area is developing rapidly.

Biochemical data indicative of immunologic function are also valuable. Cellular defense mechanisms are suppressed in protein-calorie malnutrition. Total white blood cell count, lymphocyte count, and cellular immunity skin testing (e.g., PPD and DNCB) indicate the status of the immunocompetence and thus protein nutriture. The level of serum transferrin (not percentage saturation) is indicative of the body's ability to make serum proteins as well as withstand bacterial invasion. See Chapter 35.

The accepted test for biochemical evaluation for each nutrient is given in Table 11–6. Most likely the test and the accepted values will change just as the RDA change as more information becomes available on the functions of the nutrients. The standard by which to judge the biochemical measurement and nutritional status is given in Appendix Table 18.

CLINICAL EXAMINATION

Clinical examination includes a complete physical examination and a medical history. In the clinical examination special attention should be given to the skin, hair, teeth, gums, lips, tongue, and eyes, and in men the genitalia, since these are areas which evidence signs of nutritional deficiencies. Hair, skin and mouth are susceptible because of the rapid cell turnover of epithelial and mucosal tissue. Early ramifications may also be reflected in the gastrointestinal tract such as diarrhea because of GI mucosal changes.

The medical history should include questions about mastication and swallowing. Are the teeth painful? Are teeth missing? Does the patient wear dentures, and if so, do they fit well? Any dryness of mouth or throat owing to decreased salivation? Does this prevent eating certain foods? Appetite, food avoidances or preferences, and digestion problems should be delved into thoroughly. These habits or problems all affect food intake, and thus nutritional status.

Through the history one can also learn of any behavioral or functional *changes* in gastrointestinal, neuromuscular or cardiovascular systems that may not be apparent to the clinician but remarkable to the patient or the patient's family.

Table 11–7 gives the clinical signs of possible nutritional significance in the examination of the patient.[8] A description of the clinical terms in this table is included in Appendix 30. Very few of these signs are diagnostic for specific nutritional deficiencies (although some are more reliable than others), which means that other causes such as environmental factors or underlying disease must be ruled out. Clinical signs of nutritional deficiency should always be confirmed with biochemical and dietary data. A clinical symptom can and usually does reflect the presence of more than one nutritional deficiency.

ANTHROPOMETRIC MEASUREMENTS

An important part of the clinical examination, especially in infants, children, adolescents and pregnant women, is measurement and evaluation of growth and development. The lack of proper growth is usually an early sign noticed by the clinician and should immediately arouse suspicion that nutrition may be at fault. This information is most valuable when obtained over a *period of time* with regular, accurate and consistent recording of anthropometric measurements and development. Physical measurements reflect the total nutritional status over a lifetime. Some measurements, such as height and head circumference, reflect past nutrition or chronic nutritional status. Others such as mid-arm circumference, weight and skinfold thickness reflect present nutritional status. See Table 11–8.

Height and weight are the most common measurements made, but because their significance and importance are not appreciated, they are frequently measured sloppily, incor-

Table 11–6 BIOCHEMICAL MEASUREMENTS OF NUTRITIONAL STATUS

NUTRIENT	MORE SENSITIVE	LESS SENSITIVE
Protein	Plasma amino acids Hair root morphology Serum albumin Urinary creatinine/height Urinary hydroxyproline	Total serum protein
Lipids	Serum cholesterol Serum triglycerides Lipoproteins	
Vitamin A	Serum vitamin A Serum carotene	
Vitamin D	Serum 25–OH–vitamin D_3 Serum alkaline phosphatase	Serum calcium Serum phosphorus
Vitamin E	Hydrogen peroxide erythrocyte hemolysis test Serum or plasma tocopherol	
Vitamin K		Prothrombin time
Thiamin	Urinary thiamin Erythrocyte transketolase activity	Blood pyruvate
Riboflavin	Urinary riboflavin Erythrocyte glutathione reductase	
Nicotinic Acid	N^1 methyl nicotinamide	Urinary pyridone
Vitamin B_6	Tryptophan load test (mg. xanthurenic acid excreted in urine)	Urinary pyridoxine excretion (mcg./gm. creatinine) Blood transaminase
Folic Acid	Red cell folate	Serum folate Bone marrow film Thin blood film Urinary FIGLU excretion
Vitamin B_{12}	Serum B_{12} Serum thimidylate synthetase Urine methylmalonic acid	Bone marrow film Thin blood film Schilling test
Vitamin C	Serum ascorbic acid	Urinary ascorbic acid
Iron	Iron deposits in bone marrow Serum iron % saturation of transferrin	Hemoglobin Hematocrit Thin blood film
Iodine		Urinary iodine Tests for thyroid function
Zinc	Serum and plasma zinc	Hair zinc
Magnesium	Serum magnesium	

Table 11–7 PHYSICAL SIGNS INDICATIVE OR SUGGESTIVE OF MALNUTRITION

	NORMAL APPEARANCE	SIGNS ASSOCIATED WITH MALNUTRITION	POSSIBLE DIS-ORDER OR NUTRIENT DEFICIENCY	POSSIBLE NON-NUTRITIONAL PROBLEM
Hair	Shiny; firm; not easily plucked	Lack of natural shine; dull and dry Thin and sparse Silky and straight; fine Dyspigmented Flag sign Easily plucked (no pain)	Kwashiorkor and, less commonly, maras-mus	Excessive bleaching of hair Alopecia
Face	Skin color uniform; smooth, pink, healthy appearance; not swollen	Nasolabial seborrhea (scaling of skin around nostrils) Swollen face (moon face) Paleness	Riboflavin Iron Kwashiorkor	Acne vulgaris
Eyes	Bright, clear, shiny; no sores at corners of eye-lids; membranes a healthy pink and moist; no prominent blood vessels or mound of tissue or sclera	Pale conjunctiva Red membranes Bitot's spots Conjunctival xerosis (dryness) Corneal xerosis (dullness) Keratomalacia (soften-ing of cornea) Redness and fissuring of eyelid corners Corneal arcus (white ring around eye) Xanthelasma (small yellowish lumps around eyes)	Anemia (e.g., iron) Vitamin A Riboflavin, pyridoxine Hyperlipidemia	Bloodshot eyes from exposure to weather, lack of sleep, smoke or alcohol
Lips	Smooth, not chapped or swollen	Angular stomatitis (white or pink lesions at corners of mouth) Angular scars Cheilosis (redness or swelling of lips and mouth)	Riboflavin	Excessive salivation from improper fitting dentures
Tongue	Deep red in appearance; not swollen or smooth	Scarlet and raw tongue Magenta tongue (purplish) Swollen tongue Filiform papillae atrophy or hyper-trophy	Nicotinic acid Riboflavin Niacin Folic acid Vitamin B_{12}	Leucoplakia
Teeth	No cavities; no pain; bright	Mottled enamel Caries (cavities) Missing teeth	Fluorosis Excessive sugar	Malocclusion Periodontal disease Health habits
Gums	Healthy; red; do not bleed; not swollen	Spongy, bleeding Receding gums	Vitamin C	Periodontal disease
Glands	Face not swollen	Thyroid enlargement (front of neck swollen) Parotid enlargement (cheeks become swollen)	Iodine Starvation	Allergic or inflam-matory enlarge-ment of thyroid

Table 11–7   PHYSICAL SIGNS INDICATIVE OR SUGGESTIVE OF MALNUTRITION (*Continued*)

	NORMAL APPEARANCE	SIGNS ASSOCIATED WITH MALNUTRITION	POSSIBLE DISORDER OR NUTRIENT DEFICIENCY	POSSIBLE NON-NUTRITIONAL PROBLEM
Skin	No signs of rashes, swellings, dark or light spots	Xerosis (dryness)	Vitamin A	Environmental exposure
		Follicular hyperkeratosis (sandpaper feel to skin)		
		Petechiae (small skin hemorrhages)	Vitamin C	
		Pellagrous dermatosis (red swollen pigmentation of areas exposed to sunlight)	Nicotinic acid	
		Excessive bruising	Vitamin K	Physical abuse
		Flaky paint dermatosis	Kwashiorkor	
		Scrotal and vulval dermatosis	Riboflavin	
		Xanthomas (fat deposits under skin around joints)	Hyperlipidemia	
Nails	Firm; pink	Koilonychia (spoon-shaped)	Iron	
		Brittle; ridged		
Subcutaneous tissue	Normal amount of fat	Edema	Kwashiorkor	
		Fat below standard	Starvation; marasmus	
		Fat above standard	Obesity	
Muscular and skeletal systems	Good muscle tone; some fat under skin; can walk or run without pain	Muscle wasting	Starvation, marasmus, Kwashiorkor	
		Craniotabes (thin, soft skull bones in infant)		
		Frontal and parietal bossing (round swelling of front and side of head)	Vitamin D	
		Epiphyseal enlargement (swelling of ends of bones)		
		Persistently open anterior fontanelle (soft area on head closes late)		
		Knock knees or bow legs		
		Musculoskeletal hemorrhages	Vitamin C	
		Calf muscle tenderness	Thiamin	
		Thoracic rosary	Vitamin D; Vitamin C	
		Fractures in elderly	Osteoporosis	
Cardiovascular system	Normal heart rate and rhythm; no murmurs or abnormal rhythms; normal blood pressure for age	Cardiac enlargement	Thiamin	
		Tachycardia		
		Elevated blood pressure	Sodium?	
Gastrointestinal system	No palpable organs or masses (in children, however, liver edge may be palpable)	Hepato-splenomegaly	Kwashiorkor	

Table continued on the following page

Table 11–7   PHYSICAL SIGNS INDICATIVE OR SUGGESTIVE OF MALNUTRITION (*Continued*)

	NORMAL APPEARANCE	SIGNS ASSOCIATED WITH MALNUTRITION	POSSIBLE DIS-ORDER OR NUTRIENT DEFICIENCY	POSSIBLE NON-NUTRITIONAL PROBLEM
Nervous system	Psychological stability; normal reflexes	Psychomotor changes	Kwashiorkor	
		Mental confusion	Nicotinic acid; thiamin	
		Depression	Pyridoxine;	
		Sensory loss	vitamin B_{12}	
		Motor weakness		
		Loss of position sense		
		Loss of vibration	Thiamin	
		Loss of ankle and knee jerks		
		Burning and tingling of hands and feet (paresthesia)		

(Adapted from Jelliffe, D. B.: The Assessment of the Nutritional Status of the Community. WHO Monograph No. 53, Geneva, 1966.

McLaren, D. S.: Nutritional assessment. In McLaren, D. S., and Burman, D.: Textbook of Pediatric Nutrition. Edinburgh, Churchill Livingstone, 1976, pp. 91–102.

Christakis, G. (ed.): Nutritional Assessment in Health Programs, Washington, D.C., Am. Pub. Health Assoc., Inc., 1973.)

rectly or inconsistently. Height is a measure of chronic nutrition or undernutrition and should be measured as accurately as possible. Children less than 36 months should be measured in the recumbent position (crown-heel length) and the length plotted on the chart for children 1 to 36 months of age. For young children the recumbent length is generally greater than stature by about 2 cm. or almost 1 inch. After 4 or 5 years the difference is closer to 1 cm. or about 1/2 inch. In any case, when the child can stand, the measurements should be *consistent*. Figure 11–4 shows a child being measured and gives guidelines for proper measurement of crown-heel length. Measuring the child by holding a tape measure at the child's head and stretching it to the heel does not give an accurate measurement of length.

Weight in children is a sensitive measure of growth and can be an early clue to growth problems and nutritional inadequacy. It reflects more recent nutrition of the child or adult than does length or height. In adults regular weight measurements are particularly important when there is chronic illness. By documenting weight loss in a previously normal-weight individual, one verifies the inability of that individual to meet nutritional requirements.

Height and weight are properly measured in the following manner:

Height
1. The person should be barefoot or wearing only socks or stockings.

2. The person's feet should be together with the heels against the upright bar of the scale.
3. The person should be standing erect, neither slumped nor stretching, looking straight ahead, without tipping the head up or down.
4. The horizontal bar then should be lowered to rest flat on the top of the head.
5. Read the height to the nearest 1/4 in. or .5 cm.

Weight
1. Use a beam balance scale, not a spring scale, whenever possible.
2. Periodically calibrate the scale for accuracy, using known weights.
3. The person should be weighed in light clothing without shoes.
4. Record weight to the nearest 1/2 lb. or .2 kg. for adults, and 1/4 lb. or .1 kg. for infants.

The height and weight measurements are evaluated by comparing them to various standards. See Appendix Tables 16, 17, and 24 to 27 for the NCHS growth curves for children, Appendix Tables 14 and 15 for desirable weights for men and women, Figure 13–2 for the standard weight gain curve for pregnant women and Figure 37–1 for the intrauterine growth curve of a fetus. Curves for early growth of premature infants have also been developed and are given in Fig. 37–3. In general, premature infants

Table 11–8   SOME ANTHROPOMETRIC MEASUREMENTS APPLIED IN NUTRITIONAL ASSESSMENT

MEASURE-MENTS	AGE GROUPS	NUTRITIONAL INDICATION	ADVAN-TAGES	DISAD-VANTAGES	INTERPRETATION
1. Weight	All groups	Present nutr. status; under and over	Common in use	Difficult in field; can't tell body composition; need accurate age; need proper scales	Adults—compare with Metropolitan Life Tables, Appendices 14 & 15. Children—compare with NCHS growth charts, Appendices 16, 17, 24–27. Height and weight should be at approximately the same percentile on the growth grids.
2. Height	All groups	Chronic nutr. status (under) Chronic under nutr. in early childhood	Common in use Simple to do in field	Differs by time of day Other factors play a role	Children—compare with NCHS growth charts, Appendices 16, 17, 24–27.
3. Head circumference	0–4 yr.	Intrauterine & childhood nutr. (chronic undernutrition; mental abilities)	Simple	Other factors play a role	Compare with NCHS growth charts, Appendices 25 and 27.
4. Mid-arm circumference	All groups	Present under- and overnutrition	Simple, age independent; child need not be denuded; suitable for rapid survey	No limits for over-nutrition; no standard for adult	Compare with standards in Appendix Table 20. <75% severe; 75–80% moderate; 80–85% mild malnutrition; >85% normal
5. Skin-fold thickness	All groups	Present under- and over nutrition	Measure body composition; detect obesity in adults	Need expensive callipers Difficult with child and in the field	Children and adults—compare with standards in Appendix Table 19.
6. Weight/height ratio	All ages	Present under- and over nutrition	Index of body build; age independent; 1–4 yr. and adults	Need proper scales; need trained personnel	<75% severe; 75–85% moderate; 85–90% mild malnutrition; 90–110% normal; 110–120% over; >120% obese
7. Mid-arm/head ratio	3 mo. to 48 mo.	Present undernutrition	Simple; age independent; sex independent; any person can do it for field	No standard for adults	<0.25 severe; 0.25–0.28 moderate; 0.28–0.31 mild malnutrition; 0.31–0.35 normal; >0.35 obese
8. Chest/head circs. ratio	1–5 yr.	Present undernutrition	Simple; age independent	For limited age; no classification method	<1 malnourished; >1 normal
9. Mid-arm/ height ratio	0–10 yr.	Present over and undernutrition	Simple; age and sex independent; only tape measure needed		<85–90% malnourished

(Adapted from Bengoa, J. M.: Nutrition, National Development and Planning. Massachusetts, MIT Press, 1972, p. 110.)

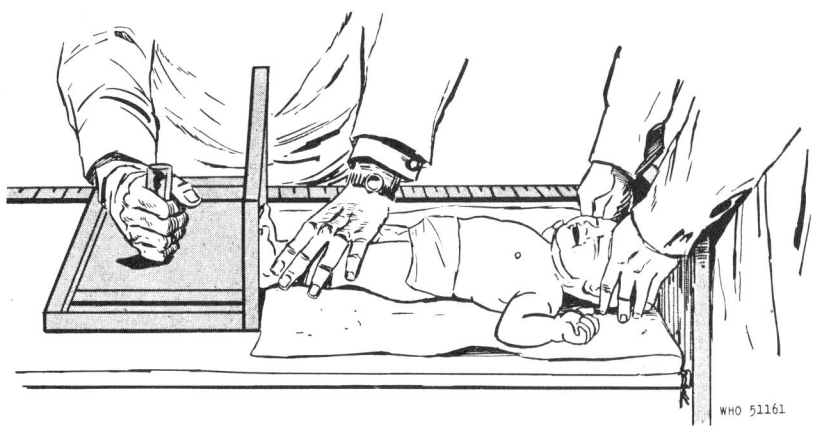

Figure 11–4   Measurement of length of an infant. Crown-heel length should be measured in children 36 months and younger in the following manner: (1) The child is laid on a ruled board that has an attached piece of wood at one end and a movable piece at the other. (2) Make sure that the child is stretched out on the board to give the most accurate measurement. This may require two people. The top of the child's head is placed against the immovable end. (3) The movable end is placed so that it is flat against the bottom of the child's foot, and the length is read from the side of the board. (4) Without a measuring board, the child can be stretched out on a piece of paper on a table and marks made at his heel and the crown of his head. (5) After the child is removed, the distance between the marks is measured to the nearest ¼″ or 0.5 cm. and recorded. (From Jelliffe, D. B.: The Assessment of the Nutritional Status of the Community. WHO Monograph No. 53. Geneva, WHO, 1966.)

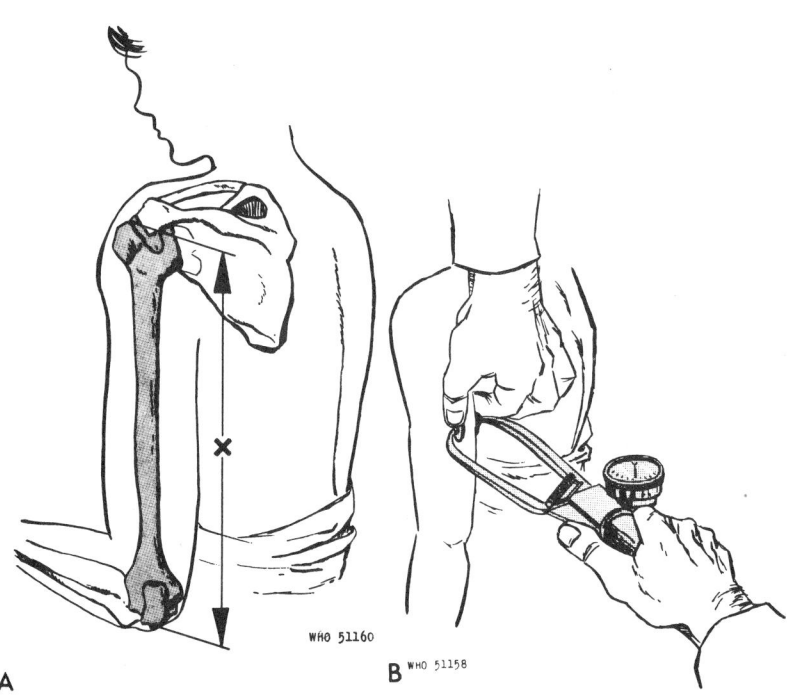

Figure 11–5   *A*, Determining midpoint of arm. *B*, Measuring the triceps skinfold with calipers. The following procedure is used to measure the triceps skinfold thickness of the left arm: (a) Ask the person to let the arm rest relaxed in the lap. With a tape measure, measure the length between the acromial process of the scapula and the tip of the elbow and mark this point *(A)*. (3) About an inch above this point, pinch the skin over the triceps between the thumb and forefinger. (4) Pull the skin slightly away from the muscle. (5) Gently pinch the skin and fat between the prongs of the calipers at the point marked, which is just below the pinch. (6) Read the measurement on the caliper in mm. (From: Jelliffe, D. B.: The Assessment of Nutritional Status of the Community. WHO Monograph No. 53. Geneva, WHO, 1966.)

would be somewhat smaller than term infants until the age of 4 years, when they will have caught up to term infants. See Chapter 37. The child's weight or height are recorded as a percentage of the total population of children having that height or weight at that age, and the child's growth at each age or growth "curve" can be followed. Weight and height can be compared with each other in an evaluation of growth by using the weight for length standard curve. This has an advantage in that one does not need to know the child's exact age.

The NCHS growth charts presented in the Appendix are new and more acceptable than the previous charts based on data from too small a population of white middle class children in Boston and Iowa. These new charts are based on data from children of all ethnic backgrounds from all over the U.S. Additional data suggest that children of different races may grow at different rates, particularly in the first 2 years of life, and a growth chart may be required for each race of children. Present evidence suggests that black children grow more rapidly than white children who grow more rapidly than Oriental children.

The measurement of head circumference is somewhat useful in children, especially in those under the age of 3, because it reflects brain growth, which is so rapid in the first 2 years of life. Presumably, severely malnourished children would have fewer brain cells, smaller brains and thus a small head circumference. However, head circumference must always be related to body size. Head circumference grossly inappropriate to the body which contains it is more significant.

The measurement of chest circumference is most valuable during the second and third years of life. Up until 6 months of age, the head and chest circumference are about the same, but after this the chest grows more rapidly. Between 6 months and 5 years of age, if the chest circumference is less than the head circumference (chest circumference:head circumference ratio less than 1), there possibly is a failure to develop or a wasting of muscle and fat from the chest wall, which is indicative of protein-calorie malnutrition. See Table 11–8.

Skinfold thickness is an anthropometric measurement that is coming into greater use as health practitioners become more concerned with preventing obesity. Skinfold thickness measures the amount of subcutaneous fat over either the triceps, biceps, scapula or several other sites, although it is generally agreed that

the triceps and scapular measurements are the best ones to use. See Figure 11–5 A and B for a description of the triceps skinfold measurement. The amount of body fatness and the presence of excess body fat can be determined since the volume of subcutaneous fat is related to the volume of body fat. Since women of normal weight have a greater percentage of body weight as fat, 24 per cent as compared to 17 per cent in the normal-weight male, their skinfold measurements will be larger by about 55 per cent.[3] Figure 27–6 shows how the subcutaneous fat looks when it is being measured by the skinfold calipers. The standards for triceps skinfold thickness are given in Appendix Table 19.

Mid upper arm circumference has been shown to be closely correlated with clinical and other anthropometric parameters of nutritional status.[7] It is an indication of protein-calorie nutriture. Standards for arm circumference are given in Appendix Table 20. See Figure 11–6.

When the mid upper arm circumference is combined with the skinfold thickness measurements, an even better assessment of protein and calorie nutriture can be made. It becomes possible to indirectly determine the arm *muscle* circumference, which, of course, would be im-

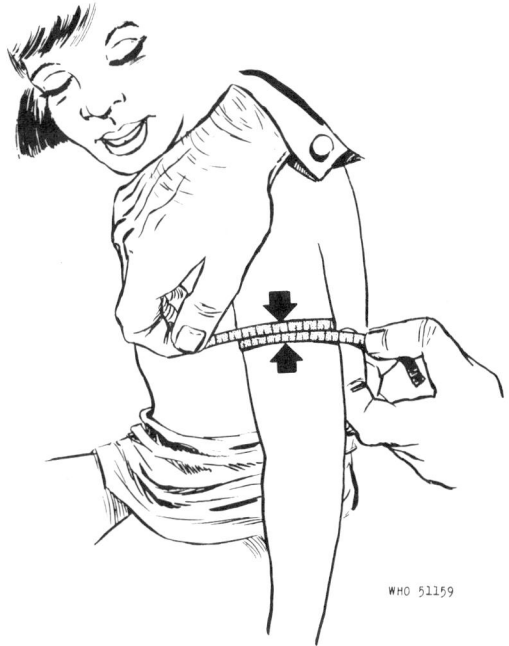

WHO 51159

Figure 11–6   Measurement of mid upper arm circumference. (From: Jelliffe, D. B.: The Assessment of Nutritional Status of the Community. WHO Monograph No. 53. Geneva, WHO, 1966.)

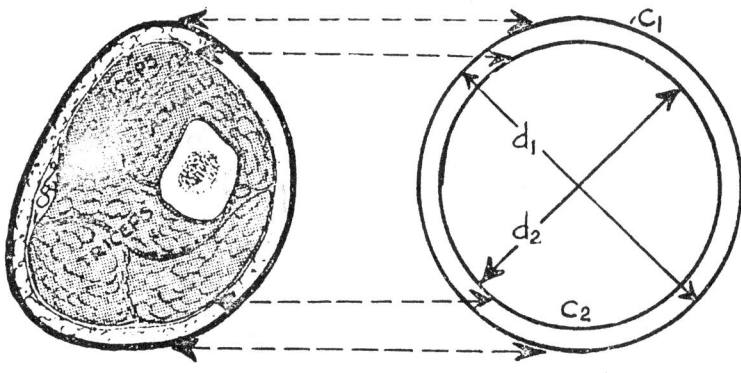

Figure 11–7 Calculation of arm muscle circumference. (1) Measure the mid upper arm circumference in cm. (C_1) and convert it to mm. (2) Measure the triceps skinfold in mm. (S). $S = 2x$ subcutaneous fat. (3) Let d_1 = arm diameter. $C_1 = \pi d_1$. Let d_2 = muscle diameter. $C_2 = \pi d_2$. (4) $S = d_1 - d_2$. (5) Let muscle circumference = $C_2 = \pi d_1 - \pi S$. (6) $C_2 = C_1 - \pi S$.

To avoid calculation of the arm muscle circumference, see nomograms in Appendices 28 and 29.

possible to measure directly. See Figure 11–7 for the method of calculating the muscle circumference. The muscle circumference is a good indication of the lean body mass and thus the skeletal protein reserves. This is important in growing children and is especially valuable in evaluating the person who may be protein-calorie malnourished from chronic illness, stress or multiple surgeries. Nomograms for adults and children appear in the Appendix, p. 931; they allow muscle mass to be determined without lengthy calculations. Standards for arm muscle circumference are given in Appendix Table 21.

BEHAVIOR EVALUATION

Behavior and changes in behavior are an elusive, hard to quantify aspect of the clinical examination. It is difficult to separate nutritional influence from the social and psychological environment. Unfortunately, there are no standards for this area, but the overall appearance of an adult or child can give an impression of nutritional status. Listlessness is very apparent in severe protein-calorie malnutrition of early childhood. The child is apathetic, withdrawn and uninterested in his surroundings.

NUTRITIONAL ASSESSMENT FOR VARIOUS AGE GROUPS

Assessments can be carried out at various levels. Nutritional assessment can also be tailored for each age group. In the Appendix Tables 22 and 23 guidelines are given for the assessments of nutrition at various levels. These guidelines are given for infants, children and adults and can be modified for adolescents.

USE OF THE NUTRITIONAL STATUS ASSESSMENT

An assessment of nutritional status should be done routinely for all persons in a health care system, although it is usually done in greater depth for those people in which a nutritional problem is suspected. The information in the nutritional assessment is usually used as the basis for designing the nutritional care plan and nutritional education. See Chapter 20. A thorough nutritional assessment makes the planning of effective nutrition education or counseling much easier. Through thorough interviewing, a good rapport is established with the patient, making necessary education and behavioral change much more possible. The patient has a better idea of the goal of the nutritional care and the importance of nutrition to his overall health.

PROBLEMS AND SUGGESTED TOPICS FOR DISCUSSION

1. Is it accurate to say, based solely on dietary data, that a person is deficient in a nutrient? Explain.
2. Perform a complete nutritional status assessment on a patient in your care.
   a. What problems did you have in collecting data?
   b. Are you missing necessary data?
   c. Were clinical findings confirmed by biochemical and dietary data?
   d. From the nutritional assessment, state the nutritional problems of your patient.
3. Evaluate a patient with a below normal nutritional biochemical finding. What does this indicate about his or her nutritional status? What additional information would be helpful?
4. Which anthropometric measurements are helpful in assessing the nutritional status of an individual? Explain. What are the inherent weaknesses in the use of these measurements?

CITED REFERENCES

1. Adams, C. F.: Nutritive Value of American Foods, Agricultural Handbook No. 456, Agricultural Research Service, Washington, D.C., U. S. Government Printing Office, 1975.
2. Church, C. F., and Church, H. N.: Food Values of Portions Commonly Used. 12th ed. Philadelphia, J. B. Lippincott Company, 1975.
3. Edwards, D. A.: Differences in the distribution of subcutaneous fat with sex and maturity. Clin. Sci., *10:*305, 1951.
4. Garn, S. M., Smith, N. J., and Clark, D. C.: The magnitude and the implication of apparent race differences in hemoglobin values. Am. J. Clin. Nutr., *28:*563, 1975.
5. Guthrie, H. A., Owen, G. M., and Guthrie, G. M.: Factor analysis of measures of nutritional status of preschool children. Am. J. Clin. Nutr., *26:*497, 1973.
6. Hertzler, A. A., and Hoover, L. W.: Development of food tables and use with computers. J. Am. Diet. Assoc., *70:*20, 1977.
7. Lowenstein, M. F., and Phillips, J. F.: Evaluation of arm circumference measurement for determining nutritional status of children and its use in an acute epidemic of malnutrition: Owerri, Nigeria following the Nigerian war. Am. J. Clin. Nutr., *26:*226, 1973.
8. Manual for Nutrition Surveys. Interdepartmental Committee on Nutrition for National Defense, National Institute of Health, Bethesda, Maryland, U.S. Government Printing Office, 1963, pp. 53–72.
9. McKigney, J. L., and Munro, H. N.: Nutrient Requirements in Adolescence. Cambridge, Mass., MIT Press, 1976, pp. 304–6.
10. Murphy, E. W., Watt, B. K., and Rizek, R. L.: Tables of food composition: availability, uses, and limitations. Food Technology, *27:*40, 1973.
11. Watt, B. K., and Merrill, A. L.: Composition of Foods. Agricultural Handbook No. 8, Agricultural Research Service, Washington, D.C., U.S. Government Printing Office, 1963.
12. Young, C. M.: Subjects' estimation of food intake and calculated nutritive value of the diet. J. Am. Diet. Assoc., *29:*1216, 1953.

ADDITIONAL REFERENCES

Beal, V. A.: The nutritional history in longitudinal research. J. Am. Diet. Assoc., *51:*426, 1967.
Burk, M. C., and Pao, E. M.: Methodology for Large-Scale Surveys of Household and Individual Diets. Home Economics Research Report No. 40, Agriculture Research Service, Washington, D.C., U.S. Government Printing Office, 1976.
Burke, B. S.: The dietary history as a tool in research. J. Am. Diet. Assoc., *23:*1041, 1947.
Christakis, G. (ed.): Nutritional Assessment in Health Programs. Washington, D.C., Am. Pub. Health Assoc., 1973.
Hamill, P. V., and Moore, W. M.: Contemporary growth charts: needs, construction and application. Dietetic Currents, *3*(5), 1976.
Jelliffe, D. B.: The Assessment of the Nutritional Status of the Community. WHO Monograph No. 53, Geneva, WHO, 1966.
Jelliffe, E. F., and Jelliffe, D. B.: The arm circumference as a public health index of protein-calorie malnutrition of early childhood. J. Trop. Pediatr., *15:*177, 1969.
McLaren, D. S. (ed.): Nutritional in the Community. New York, John Wiley & Sons, 1976.
McLaren, D. S.: Nutritional assessment. In McLaren, D. S., and Burman, D.: Textbook of Paediatric Nutrition. Edinburgh, Churchill Livingstone, 1976.
Methodology of Nutritional Surveillance. Joint FAO/UNICEF WHO Expert Committee, WHO Tech. Rep. No. 593, WHO, 1976.
Sauberlich, H. E., Skala, J. H., and Dowdy, R. P.: Laboratory Tests for the Assessment of Nutritional Status, Cleveland, Ohio, CRC Press, Inc., 1974.
Ten-State Nutrition Survey, 1968–70. U.S. Department of HEW, DHEW Publ. No. (HSM) 72–8130–33, Washington, D.C., U.S. Government Printing Office, 1972.

Chapter 12

NUTRITIONAL DEFICIENCY DISEASES

GENERAL DISCUSSION

Scientific progress in research, plus improved economic status, has reduced frank fully developed deficiency diseases in the United States from endemic proportions to a comparative few. However, there are still and probably always will be patients with the traditional forms of nutritional deficiency diseases, and it is important that the medical team be familiar with the manifestations. They are seen among the poor, the uneducated, the ne-

glected, the chronically or severely ill, persons on long-term or permanent medication, chronic alcoholics, psychiatric patients or persons consuming bizarre diets. Youmans[37] points out, "There is likelihood of their being missed because of a low index of suspicion, due to unfamiliarity and lack of experience with them.... Cases of common nutritional-deficiency disease are being missed because it is assumed that they no longer occur and because their diagnostic features have been forgotten."

Definition. A nutritional deficiency disease is usually defined as a pathologic condition caused by a diet which lacks one or more of the essential elements. However, this is not always the case. Actually, nutritional deficiency signifies a tissue deficiency of an essential nutrient, not necessarily a dietary inadequacy. Jolliffe[16] classifies nutritional deficiency diseases into two groups: primary (dietary) and secondary (conditioned) in origin. In *primary nutritional inadequacy,* the deficiency state results from an inadequate intake of nutrients either in amount or kind, or there is an imbalance of nutrients. In *secondary or conditioned nutritional inadequacy,* the deficiency state is produced by factors other than inadequate food intake, such as interference with the ingestion, absorption or utilization of nutrients consumed due to a disease. Other secondary factors which may cause malnutrition are: metabolic or functional conditions that increase the requirement for, or cause unusual destruction, or abnormal excretion of nutrients. For example, an increase in the dietary requirement, which occurs in certain diseases such as fever and hyperthyroidism and in pregnancy, can cause a secondary malnutrition. Rapid elimination and failure to absorb, which may occur in diarrhea as a result of too rapid transit of ingested foods through the intestinal tract, is another example of secondary malnutrition. A last example is liver failure, which can result in a defective utilization of nutrients.

Multiple deficiencies are present in most individuals who have deficiency conditions. Seldom is an isolated or single deficiency observed in clinical practice. This is apparent when one considers the fact that neither primary dietary failure nor conditioning factors are selective for any particular nutrient.

While classical deficiency diseases, such as rickets, scurvy and pellagra, have long been recognized to be of dietary origin, little was known about the relation of nutrition to other pathological conditions. There are indications that the answer to many medical problems may be found in the field of nutrition. As far back as 1939, Kruse wrote: "Every disease, sooner or later, involves nutrition."

Assessment of Nutritional Status. There are several stages of deficiency disease. Each specific deficiency requires recognition of its pathogenesis, severity and rate of development. The rate of development is interpreted as acute, subacute or chronic in duration. Severity is described as being mild, moderate or severe, and the pathogenesis can be either primary or conditioned. With the present methods and equipment for early diagnosis, the "subclinical" or "marginal" state of nutritional deficiency can be detected.

Many clinicians assert that they do not see deficiency disease among their patients. This may be attributed to a number of reasons. It is probable that many cases pass unrecognized because deficiency diseases can be present in other forms besides the clearly defined classic picture. It is also possible that the "subclinical" state may exist without clinical symptoms and would only be detected by a biochemical test. Individuals may go along for years in a mild deficiency state during which they are neither acutely ill nor at their most effective and efficient state of nutrition. These are the cases requiring closer, focused attention.

The medical history, dietary history, and physical examination of the patient are the most important tools of the physician in his provision of medical care in assessing nutritional status. The information thus acquired will often indicate the need for certain laboratory procedures to confirm the diagnosis. The sequence of events leading to a clinical nutritional deficiency is expressed diagrammatically by Pearson in Figure 12–1.

Many deficiency diseases, particularly in the beginning, show that the levels of essential substances in some of the tissues are lowered or decreased at the expense of others. This parasitic action is typical and most noticeable with vitamin deficiency symptoms.

Vitamin deficiencies immediately come to mind when nutritional deficiency diseases are discussed; however, protein-calorie malnutrition, nutritional anemia, simple goiter and osteoporosis are a few other equally prevalent deficiency diseases. See Chapter 11— Assessment of Nutritional Status.

Malnutrition Problems in the U.S. Overt classic nutritional deficiency diseases are uncommon in the United States today, but a significant amount of nutritional deficiency dis-

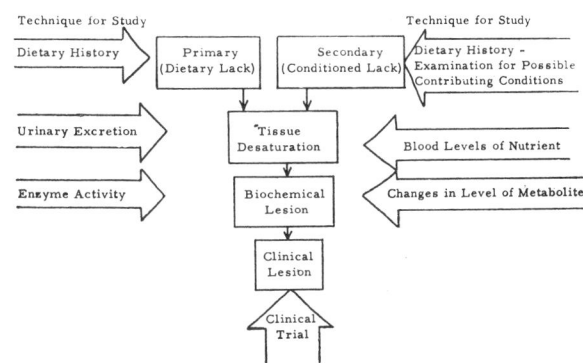

Figure 12–1 Sequence of events leading to clinical nutrition lesion. (From: Pearson, W. N.: Biochemical appraisal of the vitamin nutritional status in man. JAMA, *180*:49–55, 1962.)

ease still remains. Marginal or mild cases are present in a significant segment of the population, particularly growing children who are not well fed either because of insufficient funds, lack of knowledge or poor dietary habits. There is continued need for better nutritional education and improved living standards, especially for the poor.

America has been alerted to the extent of malnutrition within its boundaries by the Citizens' Board of Inquiry report, "Hunger U.S.A." and by the television program, "Hunger in America." The Senate Select Committee on Nutrition and Related Human Needs held hearings for several years, copies of which are available upon request. Malnutrition, more prevalent than hunger per se, is manifested in this country by widespread incidence of iron deficiency anemia, growth impairment and obesity, while the incidence of classical deficiency diseases such as scurvy, beriberi and pellagra is small.

During the period from 1968 to 1970 the Ten-State Nutrition Survey, the first and most extensive survey of the poor in this country, was conducted. The findings confirmed what had been suspected: that there is a good deal of malnutrition right here in a country as rich as this one. For example, 90 per cent of the poor who were evaluated had at least one out of six biochemical nutritional measurements in the low or deficient range.[5, 6]

Malnutrition in the Developing Countries. In evaluating the populations in developing countries, joint FAO/WHO Expert Committees on Nutrition report a number of nutritional problems of major importance.[8] Figure 12–2 illustrates areas and countries (22) in the world where ICNND nutrition surveys have been conducted. In the countries studied, ariboflavinosis and goiter were the most prevalent nutritional diseases encountered. However, preventable blindness (vitamin A deficiency), nu-

tritional anemias, beriberi, kwashiorkor, protein and calorie malnutrition, and pellagra occur widely throughout the world. Those who seem to suffer the greatest degree of malnutrition are infants, and pregnant or lactating women.

VITAMIN DEFICIENCY DISEASES

The list of vitamin deficiency conditions becomes longer each year. Research is constantly bringing to light new or old diseases attributed to vitamin deficiency. Only those diseases definitely established as being due to vitamin deficiency in human beings will be discussed. Although animal research has indicated there are many others, the evidence still needs to be applied to human nutrition.

An optimal mental and emotional status is dependent upon an adequate supply of all vitamins. The actions of vitamins are closely interrelated, and the lack of any one vitamin may affect the metabolism of the others.

Vitamin deficiency, except in severe injury or illness, is most frequently due to the lack of water-soluble vitamins. Secondary deficiencies are common in alcoholics or in persons with gastrointestinal or mental disease. Occasionally, vitamin deficiencies arise as a result of drug or medical therapy that alters metabolism of, increases the requirements for, or prevents the absorption of one or several nutrients. When such deficiencies develop, they are usually multiple. See Chapter 21—The Interactions Between Drugs, Nutrients and Nutritional Status.

Requirements in Disease. It is believed that the accepted standards of the Recommended Dietary Allowances for normal healthy persons (Table 10–1) are not always adequate for the sick and injured. As previously stated, it is common practice to administer up to ten times

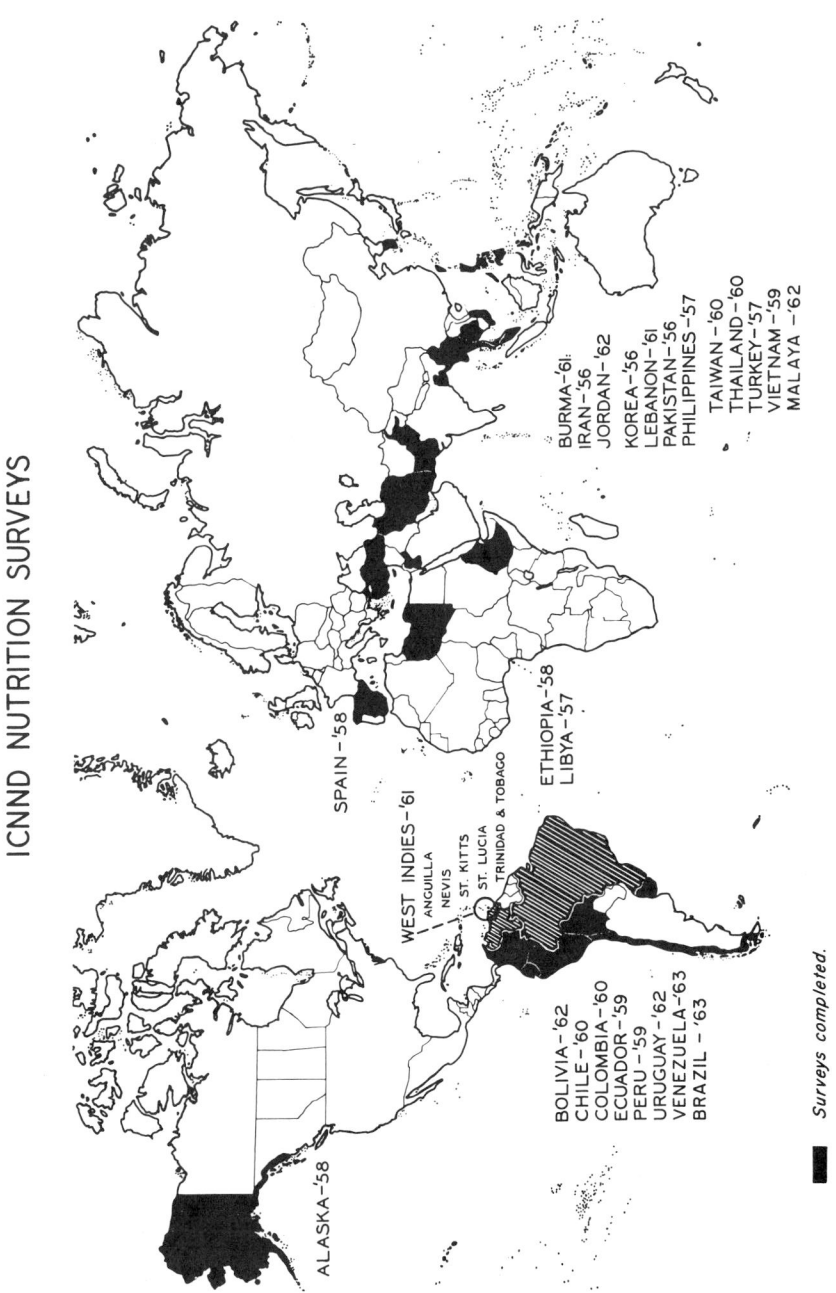

ICNND NUTRITION SURVEYS

ALASKA-'58

WEST INDIES-'61
ANGUILLA
NEVIS
ST. KITTS
ST. LUCIA
TRINIDAD & TOBAGO

SPAIN-'58

ETHIOPIA-'58
LIBYA-'57

BOLIVIA-'62
CHILE-'60
COLOMBIA-'60
ECUADOR-'59
PERU-'59
URUGUAY-'62
VENEZUELA-'63
BRAZIL-'63

BURMA-'61
IRAN-'56
JORDAN-'62

KOREA-'56
LEBANON-'61
PAKISTAN-'56
PHILIPPINES-'57

TAIWAN-'60
THAILAND-'60
TURKEY-'57
VIETNAM-'59
MALAYA-'62

■ Surveys completed.
▨ Surveys requested and planned.

Figure 12-2 World map showing areas and countries in which ICNND nutrition surveys have been conducted. (Courtesy of Interdepartmental Committee on Nutrition for National Defense (ICNND), National Institutes of Health, Bethesda, Maryland, and J. Am. Diet. Assoc. 42:296, 1963.)

the recommended normal daily allowances under stress situations.

Chapter 8, devoted to a discussion of vitamins, should be reviewed for the chemistry, function and sources of the vitamins.

VITAMIN A DEFICIENCY DISORDERS

Prolonged deficiency of vitamin A may produce skin changes, night blindness and corneal ulcerations. In extreme deficiency states, the mucous membrane of the respiratory, gastrointestinal, and genitourinary tracts may be affected. The relation of vitamin A deficiency to the common cold is controversial, although recent research demonstrates that the vitamin A content of the blood may be decreased in severe acute illness. It is suggested that this may be due to some increased utilization of the vitamin, to interference with conversion of the precursor carotene into vitamin A, or to failure of liberation of vitamin A from the liver.

More likely is the role of vitamin A in maintaining the cilia and mucous membranes of the trachea and bronchi. When vitamin A nutriture is deficient, the membranes do not function optimally and are less of a defense against infecting organisms.

Night Blindness (Nyctalopia)

History. Over one hundred years ago Lewis and Clark, on their exploration of the Northwest, observed a condition of night blindness among the Idaho Indians. Later, in 1865, Gamo Lobo described a similar condition of the eyes of Brazilian natives. For the next fifty years observations of definite symptoms were reported which were unexplainable by the medical knowledge of the time. Then scientists suggested there must be some unrecognized constituent in food. In 1913 the factor was found and named vitamin A.

Etiology. Night blindness is attributed to functional failure of the retina in the proper regeneration of *visual purple*. Vitamin A, by uniting with a protein in the retina to form visual purple, is the precursor of visual purple as well as the product of its decomposition. This formation of visual purple is a continuous process and depends upon a sufficient supply of vitamin A.

The ability to perceive details at low levels of illumination is related to tiny nerve endings called rods. These rods are found in the retina, which is made up of rods and cones. The latter are more numerous in the center and are concerned primarily with day sight and the perception of color. The rods are more profuse about the edges and control night vision. Individuals afflicted with night blindness (nyctalopia) cannot see in a dim light or at twilight. Impairment of dark adaptation, the ability to adapt from a bright light or glare to darkness (encountered in night driving or on entering a dark room from a brightly lighted one), is symptomatic of vitamin A deficiency.

Diagnosis. Special photometric instruments are used in the dark adaptation test to measure vitamin A deficiency. The dependability of the tests has been a provocative topic for discussions.

Xerophthalmia or Xerosis Conjunctivae

Xerophthalmia, one of the serious eye conditions caused by vitamin A deficiency, occurs rarely in the United States and is usually associated with malabsorption, chronic cachexia and weight loss from a debilitating disease such as cancer. It is more commonly found throughout much of the Far East and in parts of India, the Near East, Africa and Latin America. It is associated with atrophy of the periocular glands, hyperkeratosis of the conjunctiva and, finally, involvement of the cornea, leading to softening or *keratomalacia* and blindness. Table 12–1 describes the progression of eye disease caused by vitamin A deficiency. Unfortunately it proceeds more rapidly and is most severe in very young children. It also may progress quickly to keratomalacia without the presence of *Bitot's spots* (Fig. 12–3). Avitaminosis A is reported to be the leading cause of preventable blindness in India and in Southeast Asia today. It appeared in epidemic form in Denmark during World War I, when dairy products were replaced in the diets by fats lacking vitamin A. Although most common in infants and young children, it may appear at any age.

Cutaneous Changes

Characteristic changes in the skin texture as a result of vitamin A deficiency are the "goose flesh" or "toad skin" (*follicular hyperkeratosis*) appearance as shown in Figure 12–4, or the "fish skin" or "alligator skin," known as *xeroderma,* shown in Figure 12–5. In follicular hyperkeratosis, the hair follicles are blocked with plugs of keratin from their epithelial lining. It is not only seen with vitamin A deficiency,

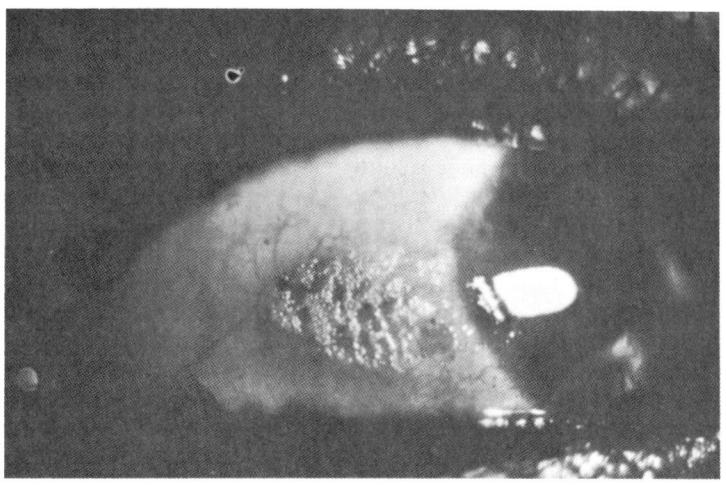

Figure 12–3 Bitot's spot. (From: McLaren, D. S., and Burman, D. (eds.): Textbook of Paediatric Nutrition. New York, Longman. © 1976 by Longman Group Ltd.)

but may also be caused by essential fatty acid deficiency, a vitamin B deficiency, exposure to sunlight or lack of cleanliness. The skin becomes dry, scaly and rough. At first the forearms and thighs are affected, but in advanced stages, the entire body may be involved. "Xeroderma" means dryness of the skin, and often a layer of fine, dry dandruff is seen over the skin, particularly the legs.

Prevention and Treatment of Avitaminosis A

Evidence exists to substantiate the fact that mild avitaminosis A, manifested by low serum vitamin A levels, does exist among the poor in this country. However, the Ten-State Nutrition Survey, which reported these findings, did not include clinical examination for night blindness. No xerosis, Bitot's spots or keratomalacia was noted.

Avitaminosis A has been reported in countries where skim milk powder was provided as

Table 12–1   XEROPHTHALMIA OF VITAMIN A DEFICIENCY

Stage I   *Xerosis of conjunctiva* — dryness with "lack luster" appearance, thickening, wrinkling, and diffuse pigmentation of conjunctiva.

Stage II   *Bitot's Spots* — usually triangular-shaped collections of desquamated keratinized epithelial cells and mucous.

Stage III   *Xerosis of cornea* — dryness of cornea leading to keratinization and a hazy or milky appearance.

Stage IV   *Keratomalacia* — ulceration, distortion and softening of the cornea with eventual perforation and iris prolapse and infection.

a relief food for infant feeding without supplementary vitamin A. For a number of years, UNICEF has been including vitamin A supplementation as part of programs in which skim milk is distributed to children whose diets are inadequate in vitamin A activity. FAO and UNICEF have, in addition, encouraged and supported school and home gardens in a number of developing countries as a means of supplying vegetable sources of vitamin A activity.

Although diet alone cannot ordinarily be depended upon to supply the needed vitamin in corrective dosage, a liberal, well-balanced diet is an essential element in the therapy. In any primary deficiency there can be no favorable prognosis unless the patient improves his diet permanently. In the long run, the increased consumption of various green leafy vegetables and yellow fruits and vegetables will correct existing vitamin A deficiencies, unless there is a disturbance of the process of conversion of the precursor, carotene, to vitamin A because of gastrointestinal or liver disease. The administration of a commercial vitamin A preparation such as a fish liver oil concentrate, which is packaged in 5000 and 10,000 I.U. to the capsule, is used when a more potent source is indicated (30,000 I.U. or 10 mg. of retinol— vitamin A— is a usual daily dose). Protein should also be given to assure the presence of enough prealbumin and retinol binding protein (RBP) to transport vitamin A.

The various symptoms of vitamin A deficiency respond to diet and supplementation in about the same order as they appear. For example, night blindness, an early manifestation of vitamin A deficiency, responds very quickly. On the other hand, the skin abnor-

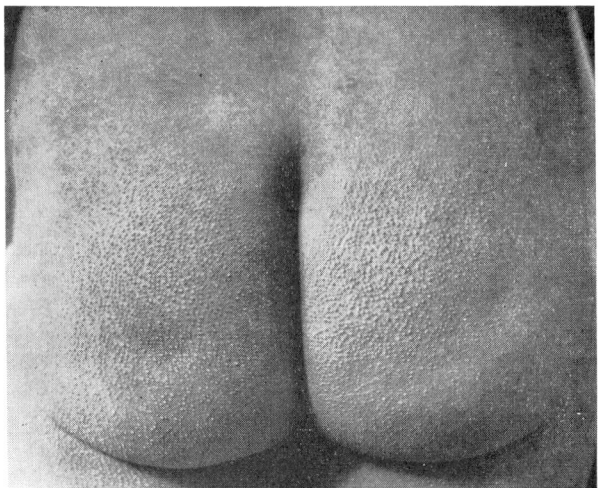

Figure 12–4 Vitamin A deficiency showing early follicular hyperkeratosis resembling "goose flesh." (Reproduced by courtesy of Section of Dermatology and Syphilology, Mayo Clinic, Rochester, Minn.)

malities may take several weeks to disappear. Members of vitamin B-complex (riboflavin, thiamin, and niacin) have been reported to be effective in alleviating night blindness and other vitamin deficiency signs when vitamin A failed to bring response.

The production and consumption of carotene food sources must be increased in the developing countries of the world through agricultural and educational guidance. Whenever economically feasible, enrichment with vitamin A of popular fatty foods should be considered.

India and Guatemala are considering fortifying tea and sugar, respectively, with a water-miscible form of vitamin A. In India and Bangladesh large prophylactic doses (200,000 I.U.) of retinol are being given to children every six months in an attempt to avoid vitamin A deficiency and blindness. This therapy shows much promise for reducing blindness,

although there are some transient toxic reactions. Since the most severe forms affect the infant and young child, special attention should be focused on adequate infant and child feeding. (Consult Table 10–12 for food sources of vitamin A. Also consult Chapter 8, Vitamins.)

VITAMIN B-COMPLEX DEFICIENCY DISORDERS

Thiamin Deficiency Disorders

Beriberi and its Cause. From the results of the experimental production of beriberi by diet in 1897, the conception of deficiency disease was formulated. Beriberi is a metabolic disease caused by an extended period of continuous lack or deficiency of vitamin B_1 (thiamin), resulting from faulty diet, faulty utilization, or poor absorption of food. It has been known to the Chinese since 2600 B.C. It occurs during food shortages, famine or war, when the diet is very restricted, or when the staple food is polished rice. In 1880 the Japanese navy suffered a siege of beriberi. When whole barley was substituted for part of the rice rations the disease was controlled. Thus it became known that the lack of a certain food substance caused beriberi. In 1912 the vitamin theory was proposed, and in 1916 vitamin B was isolated. Not until 1926 was it discovered that vitamin B was composed of several vitamins.

CLASSIFICATION. Beriberi is classified into several types. The *acute, mixed type* of beriberi is characterized by nervous and cardiac symptoms producing neuritis and heart failure. It has been shown that myocardial metabolism is largely dependent upon aerobic glycolysis and that drastic reduction in cardiac pyruvate

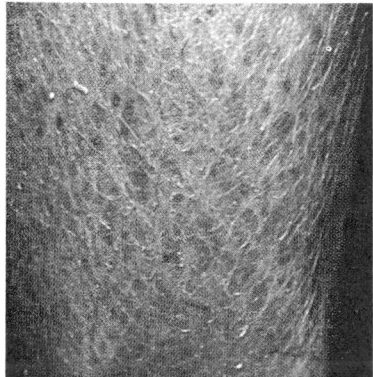

Figure 12–5 Vitamin A deficiency showing advanced xerosis, usually called ichthyosis, resembling "fish skin." (From: Jolliffe, N. (ed.): Clinical Nutrition, 2nd ed. New York, Harper & Bros., 1962.)

Figure 12–6

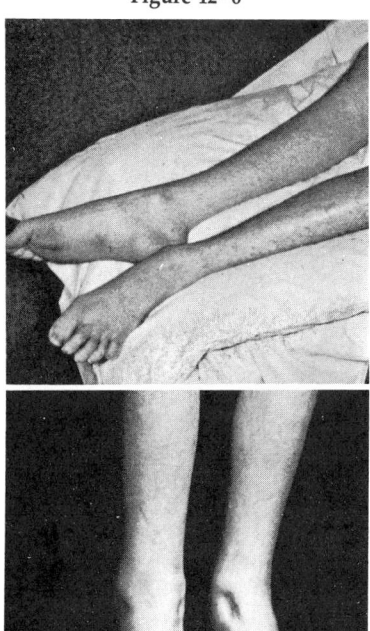

Figure 12–7

Figure 12–6 Advanced polyneuropathy with muscle atrophy and foot and toe drop in a patient with dry beriberi. (From: Jolliffe, N.(ed.): Clinical Nutrition, 2nd ed. New York, Harper & Bros., 1962.)

Figure 12–7 Edema in a patient with wet beriberi. (From: Jolliffe, N. (ed.): Clinical Nutrition, 2nd ed. New York, Harper & Bros., 1962.)

utilization is caused by thiamin deficiency. There are two other types, namely, the "dry" and the "wet" beriberi. In the *"dry" type* of the disease the nervous manifestations, with loss of function or paralysis of the lower extremities, are predominant; hence the term *polyneuritis* is synonymous (Fig. 12–6). In the *"wet" type* the edema of heart failure is the most striking sign (Fig 12–7). The edema is due to high blood pyruvate levels, the result of incomplete carbohydrate metabolism, which is thiamin dependent. Indefinite digestive disorders and emaciation are additional symptoms. See Table 12–2 for the clinical features of beriberi. A large number of diseases may have symptoms resembling those of beriberi, so that the diagnosis of beriberi should be confirmed by the RBC transketolase test and TPP effect and a dietary history.

INCIDENCE. This nutritional disease occurs primarily among population groups which subsist on a diet of highly polished rice. The neuri-

tic form is seen most frequently in the United States, particularly among alcoholics. Infantile beriberi occurs in breast-fed infants of mothers who have the disease. The disease is widespread geographically, occurring endemically or sporadically in all parts of the world. However, since foods, especially rice, have been enriched with thiamin, and milling practices have been used that remove less of the bran, the incidence of beriberi has fallen dramatically. In Thailand, Burma, and Vietnam it is a cause of death among infants 2 to 5 months of age. Although the most serious form of vitamin B_1 (thiamin) deficiency (beriberi) is rare in the United States, mild and borderline cases are not uncommon.

RELATION TO ALCOHOLISM. The neuritis of alcoholics is similar if not identical to the polyneuritis of beriberi. Also the encephalopathy of alcoholism, the *Wernicke-*

Table 12–2 CLINICAL FEATURES OF THIAMIN DEFICIENCY

Early stage of both wet and dry beriberi:	Anorexia
	Malaise
	Heaviness and weakness of legs
	Calf muscle tenderness
	"Pins and needles" and numbness in legs
	Anesthesia of skin, particularly at the tibia
	Increased pulse rate and palpitations
Wet beriberi:	Edema of legs, face, trunk and serous cavities
	Tense calf muscles
	Fast pulse
	Distended neck veins
	High blood pressure
	Decreased urine volume
Dry beriberi:	Worsening of polyneuritis of early stage
	Difficulty walking
	Wernicke-Korsakoff syndrome: encephalopathy may occur
	—loss of immediate memory
	—disorientation
	—nystagmus (jerky movements of eyes)
	—ataxia (staggering gait)
Infantile beriberi (2–5 months of age):	Acute
	—decreased urine output
	—excessive crying; thin and plaintive whining
	—cardiac failure
	Chronic
	—constipation and vomiting
	—fretfulness
	—soft, toneless muscles
	—pallor of skin with cyanosis

Korsakoff syndrome, has been attributed to a thiamin deficiency.[34] (See Chapter 32, p. 656.) Research studies reveal that it is due in part, if not entirely, to a deficiency of thiamin, and in some cases this is conditioned by a damaged gastrointestinal tract. It can be treated with improved diet habits emphasizing an adequate diet supplemented with vitamin B-complex, especially thiamin.

RELATION TO OTHER CONDITIONS. Since thiamin requirements are proportional to body weight, metabolism and calorie intake, the allowance should be increased under certain conditions, such as hyperthyroidism, infections, unusual exercise, and during pregnancy. The polyneuritis of pregnancy, resulting from increased metabolic demands, can be treated successfully with a diet abundant in thiamin and, when indicated, administration of thiamin concentrate.

TREATMENT. Thiamin treatment, 25 mg. two times a day for three days, is started immediately. The effect of treatment in wet beriberi is rapid, with easier breathing, slower pulse rate and diuresis within a few hours of thiamin administration. A daily oral dose of 10 mg. should be continued until return to complete health. The recovery in dry beriberi is not as rapid. Infantile beriberi is treated by giving thiamin to the lactating mother and the infant.

The diet for beriberi and other thiamin deficiencies should be well balanced nutritionally. Foods high in thiamin content, such as whole and enriched grains, vegetables (especially legumes); lean pork, eggs, liver, and milk should be included in abundance. Since most patients suffer from multiple deficiencies, frequently the B-complex concentrate is prescribed. If the damage to the nervous system is not too great, the response to treatment is usually good. In cases where acute heart failure has developed, the outlook is grave.

PREVENTION OF THIAMIN DEFICIENCY. Education to prevent deficiencies is of primary importance. People need to learn about the composition of foods and how to prepare foods to preserve the nutrients. In Burma, Thailand and Vietnam, beriberi was prevalent because the rice was processed with gasoline-driven mills. Formerly, the grain was hulled by pounding it at home. Thus, it still contained an appreciable amount of thiamin in the bran left on the kernel of rice. Rice is still being highly polished by the machines, but more thiamin is being consumed in other foods as these countries become more developed. In addition, manufacturers of cereals and millers of flour are restoring vitamins to their products, thereby enriching cereals and flours to normal potency. In Japan and the Philippines beriberi has practically disappeared as a result of the prophylactic use of thiamin and the enrichment of rice. The daily thiamin intake of predominantly rice eating populations can be increased to adequacy through consumption of under-milled or enriched rice. The extension of health services has also increased the use of medicinal thiamin, especially in maternal and child health centers.

Riboflavin Deficiency Disorders

Ariboflavinosis. Ariboflavinosis is a disease caused by riboflavin (vitamin B_2) deficiency, and is usually found in individuals who consume a marginal diet devoid of animal protein sources and leafy vegetables. The intake of riboflavin must be low for several months before the signs of deficiency develop. It is characterized by the development of *angular stomatitis* (Fig. 12–8), cracks in the skin at the corners of the mouth *(cheilosis),* a greasy eruption of the skin (Fig. 12–9), a purplish tongue and by capillary overgrowth around the cornea of the eye. See Table 12–3.

The angular stomatitis of ariboflavinosis can easily be mistaken for the effects of ill-fitting dentures, and poor hygiene may cause the dyssebacea of the nasolabial folds. Since riboflavin deficiency rarely appears alone, but is usually in the presence of multiple nutritional deficiencies, and because its symptoms are not specific for riboflavin deficiency alone, its diagnosis is difficult. Similar symptoms are characteristic of niacin, iron and pyridoxine deficiencies. A history of a dietary intake of less than .6 mg. of riboflavin per day for several months also helps to confirm the diagnosis of ariboflavinosis. A urinary excretion of less than 27 μg. riboflavin per gm. creatinine is also suggestive of deficiency. Other tests of riboflavin dependent enzymes in the red blood cell can also be used. See Chapter 11, Assessment of Nutritional Status.

TREATMENT. The diet for ariboflavinosis should include liberal amounts of foods rich in riboflavin. Riboflavin is distributed widely in foods of plant and animal origin, and liver, milk, milk products, eggs, meat, green leaves and buds may be considered the best and most reliable sources for the human dietary. Seeds or whole grain cereals, which are an important source of thiamin, are poor sources of riboflavin unless enriched.

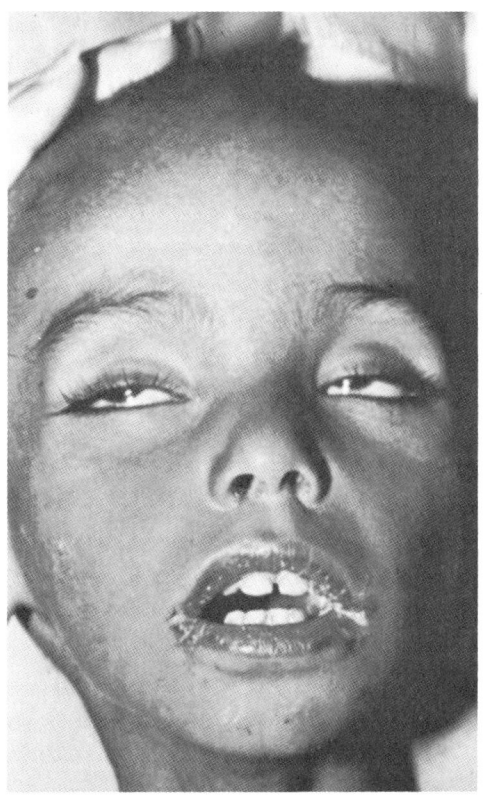

Figure 12–8 Angular stomatitis and cheilosis. (From: McLaren, D. S., et al.: Vitamin deficiency, toxicity and dependency. In: McLaren, D. S., and Burman, D.: Textbook of Paediatric Nutrition. New York, Longman.© 1976 by Longman Group Ltd.)

Supplements of the crystalline riboflavin in oral doses of 5 mg. two or three times per day, as well as other B-complex factors, are often prescribed, especially if the underlying cause of the deficiency is faulty utilization or poor absorption of the vitamin. The lesions respond rapidly and heal within a few days or weeks.

Prevention of Ariboflavinosis. In many developing countries, conditions do not permit use of dairy products and meat. For such areas, an effective remedial step for increasing the riboflavin intake is the enrichment of the basic grain of the country—rice, wheat, or corn.

Niacin Deficiency Disorders

Pellagra. Pellagra is a disease caused by a deficiency of the niacin fraction of the vitamin B-complex or the amino acid tryptophan. Tryptophan is a precursor of niacin, and it has been shown that pellagra can be cured by the administration of tryptophan alone, although the disease is manifested by multiple deficien-

cies. Pellagra was described originally as occurring in individuals who subsisted on a diet of maize. It was also noted among those people who consumed bad whiskey or had intestinal disturbances of such severity that absorption of food was hindered.

INCIDENCE. Pellagra occurs most commonly among the people of poor socioeconomic status and is usually associated with a diet composed primarily of corn. In the United States most cases become obvious in the Southeastern states during spring and early summer because of the characteristic skin lesions that appear upon exposure to the sun. During the winter, the patient has usually subsisted on cornmeal, salt pork and molasses. Cornmeal has an unusually low tryptophan content. Secondly, the niacin that is present in corn is bound as *niacytin* and is unavailable for absorption unless the corn has been soaked in lye—as it is in the Central American preparation of the tortilla—or roasted, as practiced by the Hopi Indians in Arizona.

LEUCINE AND VITAMIN B_6 RELATIONSHIP. An excess of leucine in the diet, as in the case of the sorghum or millet eaters in central India, also seems to be associated with

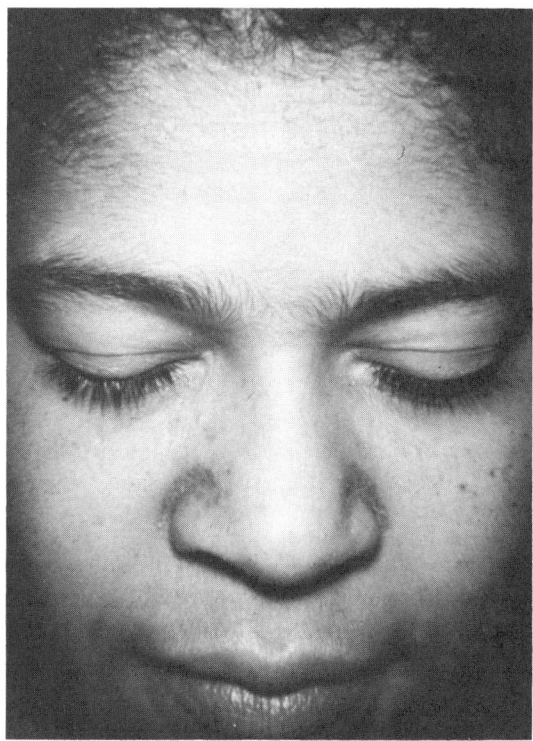

Figure 12–9 Riboflavin deficiency. Seborrheic dermatitis of nasolabial folds. (From: Rivlin, R. S. (ed.): Riboflavin. New York, Plenum Press, 1975.)

Table 12–3 SIGNS OF POSSIBLE RIBOFLAVIN DEFICIENCY

Soreness and burning of lips, mouth and tongue*
Cheilosis*
Angular stomatitis*
Glossitis*
Seborrheic dermatitis of nasolabial folds, vestibule
    of nose, and sometimes the ears and eyelids,
    scrotum and vulva
Ocular pathology (sometimes)
    —inflammation of conjunctiva
    —superficial vascularization of cornea
    —ulcerations of cornea
    —photophobia
Anemia—normocytic and normochromic
Neuropathy
Purplish or magenta tongue*
Hypertrophy or atrophy of tongue papillae*

*Tongue and mouth changes are difficult to differentiate from those in niacin, folic acid, thiamin, vitamin B_6 or vitamin B_{12} deficiency.

(Adapted from Goldsmith, G. A.: Riboflavin deficiency. In Rivlin, R. S. (ed.): Riboflavin. New York, Plenum Press, 1975.)

the occurrence of pellagra. It appears that excess leucine in the diet results in increased requirements for vitamin B_6. Since B_6 in the diet may already be low, this precipitates a B_6 deficiency. Several of the enzymes in the tryptophan-niacin pathway are B_6 dependent. In the presence of a deficiency of this vitamin, there are disturbances in this pathway and deficient niacin production, which can eventually result in pellagra.[19]

PREVENTION OF PELLAGRA. Enrichment of corn with niacin is one solution to the pellagra problem. Goldberger, working among the pellagrins of the South, was the first to demonstrate that the disease was due to a vitamin deficiency. The vitamin was called P-P or pellagra-preventive and later named vitamin B_2 or G. Still later this vitamin proved to have several fractions, one of which was found to be nicotinic acid.

Pellagra is endemic in several countries, particularly Turkey, Yugoslavia, Egypt, Syria, South Africa and Southern Rhodesia. Vitamin enrichment of the maize and redistribution of cereals within a country are being suggested as aids by FAO in preventing the disease. When the person learns to select enriched corn (and corn products) and other whole or enriched grains along with the food groups (meat-milk-vegetable-fruit) an adequate diet will be obtained. Another measure is the use of opaque-2 corn, a hybrid which contains three times as much tryptophan as normal corn.

SYMPTOMS. The early symptoms of pellagra are weakness, lassitude, anorexia, and indigestion, followed by a sore ulcerated mouth and tongue (Fig. 12–10) and diarrhea. The typical dermatitis of skin eruptions and scaly skin usually simplifies the diagnosis (Fig. 12–11). Neurological symptoms and mental changes occur in the more advanced cases. The various symptoms, especially the skin lesions, are aggravated by exposure to sunlight (e.g., Casal's necklace). The typical "sore tongue" has suggested to various investigators that the condition is analogous to the disease in dogs called "blacktongue." Both conditions are treated successfully with niacin.

Laboratory evidence of pellagra includes diminished urinary excretion of the major niacin metabolites. Plasma tryptophan is also very low. Biochemical data are necessary to differentiate niacin deficiency from kwashiorkor since many of the skin, mouth and gastrointestinal changes are similar. Pellagra could easily occur simultaneously with kwashiorkor.

DIETARY TREATMENT. Niacin and/or tryptophan is now used widely in the treatment of pellagra, but it is most effective when used in conjunction with other vitamins, especially thiamin and riboflavin, because pellagrins suffer usually from multiple deficiencies.

In severe cases of pellagra, oral administration of 150–600 mg. nicotinic acid or nicotinamide per day in several doses is effective. Nicotinamide is preferred because it does not cause the unpleasant flushing and burning sensations that accompany nicotinic acid therapy. Within 24 hours there is a response to nicotinamide, with cessation of diarrhea and less redness of the tongue. Unfortunately, some of the mental problems do not ever respond, probably because of the previous prolonged state of malnutrition.

A well-balanced diet containing foods high in niacin and tryptophan content is recommended. Liver, whole grains, yeast, lean meats, poultry and canned salmon are rich sources. Vegetables, fruits, milk and nuts are good sources. Because of the sore tongue symptom, it may be necessary to start patients with a liquid diet and progress gradually to a normal diet.

**Vitamin Deficiencies Producing
Anemia–Deficiencies of Vitamins B_6,
B_{12} and Folate**

Deficiencies of these vitamins are only briefly mentioned here. They are more fully

discussed in Chapter 29—Nutritional Care for Patients with Diseases of the Blood and Blood Forming Organs, because anemia is one of the prominent signs. Deficiency of vitamin B_6 is associated with a microcytic, hypochromic anemia that responds to pyridoxine therapy. Other non-specific signs of pyridoxine deficiency are dermatitis, peripheral neuropathy and depression. Folate and vitamin B_{12} deficient states are characterized by a megaloblastic anemia and neurological pathology.

ASCORBIC ACID DEFICIENCY DISORDERS AND SCURVY

History. Scurvy is a metabolic disease resulting from a deficiency of ascorbic acid. For hundreds of years the malady was known as "the plague of the seas." Men journeying on long voyages, military or exploring expeditions, settlers in new countries, or people in famine areas were afflicted with scurvy. Nothing was known about vitamins, but somehow the Dutch authorities discovered that the feeding of oranges, lemons or limes prevented the dreaded disease. English sailors are called by the nickname "limey," actually a misnomer, since early rations included not limes but lemons as a scurvy preventive. The specific relationship between scurvy, citrus foods and ascorbic acid was not established until the twentieth century. In the 1930's, ascorbic acid was discovered, isolated and synthesized as cevitamic acid. In 1939 the name cevitamic acid was changed officially to ascorbic acid.

Incidence. Few cases of severe ascorbic acid deficiency are seen today. A deficiency may be found among people who consume a diet devoid of fruits and vegetables such as the indigent, the mentally ill, food faddists, alcoholics, patients on restricted therapeutic diets consisting chiefly of milk and cereals (diet for gastric ulcer), and patients severely and chronically ill who are under a great deal of physiological stress. Infants who have been taken off breast milk (4–7 mg. vit. C/100 ml.) and put on whole milk (2 mg. vit. C/100 ml.) without solid foods containing vitamin C can manifest symptoms of ascorbic acid deficiency. Since the introduction of the potato, a source of ascorbic acid, the epidemics of scurvy, which formerly occurred at the end of every winter in Western Europe, have disappeared.

Determinations. Ascorbic acid content of the white blood cells is the most useful measurement of vitamin C nutriture. A value of 20 μg per 10^8 leukocytes is indicative of adequate vitamin status. Although low blood levels of

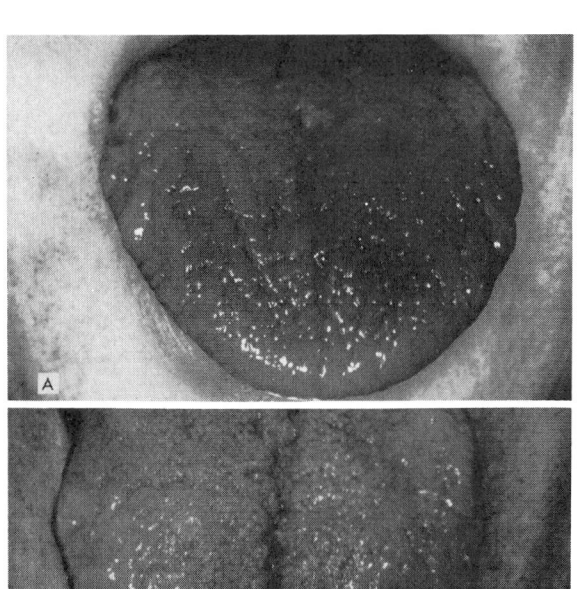

Figure 12–10 Chronic diseases, such as pellagra, may be caused by severe malnutrition. *A,* Glossitis is an early sign of this disease. *B,* Same patient after dietary treatment. (From: S. L. Halpern: Nutrition and Chronic Disease; reprinted from Health News, New York State Department of Health, September 1955.)

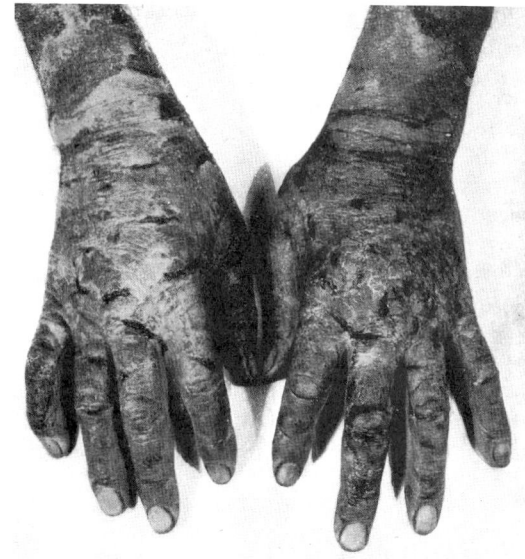

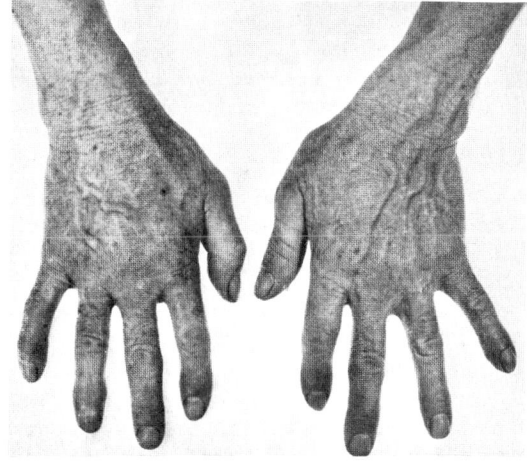

Figure 12–11 *Top,* Lesions on the backs of the hands are typical of pellagra. *Bottom,* The same patient after two weeks of nicotinamide therapy. (From: Spies: Rehabilitation through Better Nutrition.)

tracellular substance that binds together cells in capillaries, bone, teeth and connective tissue. (See Fig. 12–12.) In infants, periosteal hemorrhages occurring around the bones of the lower extremities, skeletal changes and failure to grow are manifestations of the deficiency. Bleeding in the muscle tissue (Fig. 12–13) and bloody diarrhea are not uncommon signs. Black and blue areas often appear on the surface of the skin because of the hemorrhages. These individuals are classified as bruising easily. Anemia may occur if there is significant blood loss, although there may also be increased hemolysis.

Wounds fail to heal in scurvy and scars of previous wounds may break down, leaving open sores, although this may only appear in very severe scorbutic states.

Many of the symptoms are seen every day in mild cases of ascorbic acid deficiency and are frequently overlooked or ignored.

Dietary Treatment. The treatment for deficiency is the administration of ascorbic acid. In severe cases, ascorbic acid is given in massive doses orally or parenterally. In addition, a well-balanced diet with foods rich in ascorbic acid is recommended. In many mild deficiency cases, the corrective diet is sufficient. Citrus fruits (lemons, limes, oranges, and grapefruit) are excellent sources. Tomatoes, spinach, cabbage, cauliflower, broccoli, berries, and fresh greens are likewise excellent sources, while most of the fresh vegetables and fruits are good sources. Because ascorbic acid is destroyed easily by heat and oxidation, fresh or raw foods are recommended. Fruit juices and tomato juice should be covered when

vitamin C do occur without evident manifestations of scurvy, the result of the determination indicates an intake of ascorbic acid below the amount necessary to maintain the individual's body reserve at the highest level.

Symptoms. Scurvy is characterized by general debility, pallor, poor appetite, sensitivity to touch, pains in the limbs and joints, especially the knee joints, sensitive and swollen gums, with bleeding and loosening of the teeth. With present knowledge these scorbutic changes can be explained on the basis of the physiologic function of vitamin C in the formation of *hydroxyproline*. Hydroxyproline is a necessary constituent of collagen, the in-

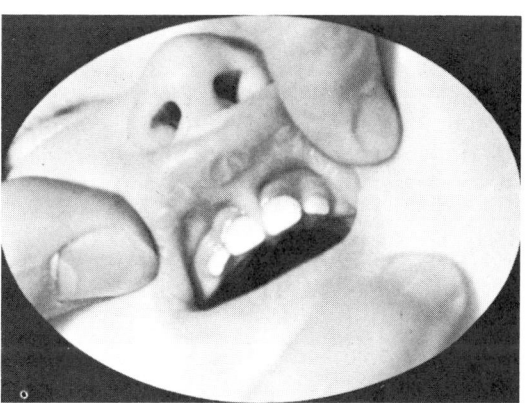

Figure 12–12 Scurvy. Note the bleeding swollen gums. (Courtesy of University of Rochester, Rochester, New York.)

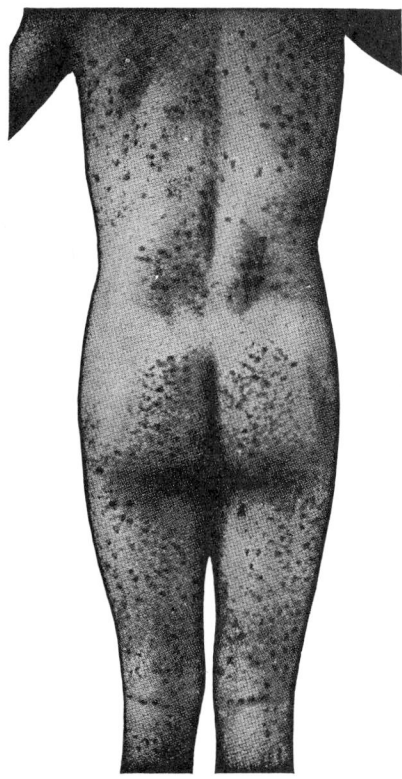

Figure 12–13 A typical case of adult scurvy, showing the numerous petechiae—spots where blood has effused to the skin. (From: L. J. Harris: Vitamins in Theory and Practice. New York, Macmillan Co.)

stored in the refrigerator to avoid loss of ascorbic acid through oxidation.

Because of sore gums and tongue, the diet may at first be composed of liquids and advanced gradually to solid foods. The administration of the indicated foodstuffs plus ascorbic acid is followed by miraculous improvement, which is most encouraging, both to the patient and the nurse.

Prevention of Ascorbic Acid Deficiency. In areas where there is evidence of widespread deficiency of ascorbic acid, efforts must be made to increase the production, distribution and availability of fresh fruits and vegetables. Educational efforts should be directed toward helping people make proper selection of foods to supply ascorbic acid.

VITAMIN D DEFICIENCY DISORDERS

Rickets

Rickets is a nutritional and metabolic disease of infancy and early childhood, in which cal-

cification of the bones does not take place normally. It is usually caused by deficiency of vitamin D, with accompanying metabolic disturbances in the calcium-phosphorus ratio. An inadequate, unbalanced diet lacking in sufficient calcium and/or phosphorus may result in rickets. So may poor absorption of these substances. Parathyroid activity results from the fall in serum calcium and rise in serum phosphate, and it is postulated that this activity may account for some of the biochemical and skeletal abnormalities in the disease.

Vitamin D is known at the antirachitic vitamin. It controls the utilization of calcium and phosphorus which are important in the formation and proper development of bones. Vitamin D is concerned with the intestinal absorption of calcium and phosphorus and the reabsorption of calcium and phosphorus from bone that is already formed. It has been reported that one of the first signs of deficiency of vitamin D is the decrease in the amount of calcium in the urine, followed by an increase of calcium in the stool, which progresses until a negative calcium balance exists. The changes in the metabolism of phosphorus differ only in the fact that the urinary excretion of phosphorus is increased. These changes may be reversed with very small doses of vitamin D.

Incidence. The existence of rickets has been noted throughout the world, its frequency and severity varying in different localities. Scientific advances in nutrition and an improved standard of living have almost eliminated the disease as a pediatric problem in North America. However, children with rickets still appear. Rickets in breast-fed infants not receiving a vitamin D supplement and infants receiving non-fortified fluid milk can be seen in the United States, especially in large cities where poor housing, inadequate diets, and limited exposure to sunshine prevail. It occurs particularly in children who grow very rapidly or who have a malabsorptive disease that deters the absorption of vitamin D and calcium. It also can occur in children receiving long-term anticonvulsant therapy for epilepsy. Speaking in general, the disease has been reported to be more prevalent in the north temperate zone and less frequent in the tropical and subtropical areas, where infants and children have more opportunity to be exposed to the sun.

Particularly vulnerable are Indian children whose families are living in northern countries such as England or Scotland. In addition to little exposure to sun, their diet contains little natural vitamin D, since their mothers do not

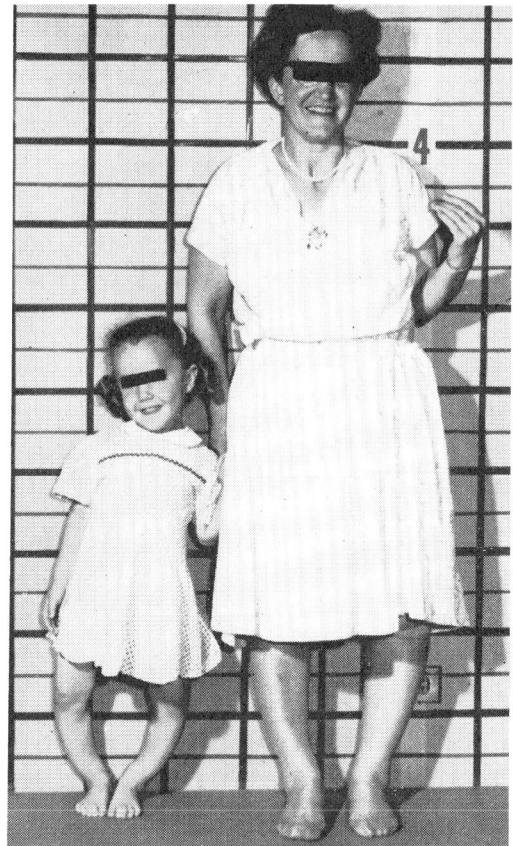

Figure 12–14 Illustration of hypophosphatemic vitamin D–refractory rickets of simple type. Mother and 4 year old daughter show typical deformities. (Courtesy of Fraser, D., and JAMA, *176*:281, 1961.)

use typical vitamin D fortified products, such as margarine or milk in cooking. These children respond well to vitamin D supplementation.[9]

On the other hand, there are a group of cases which belong to a heterogeneous class of patients in whom active rickets persists despite the administration of conventional doses of vitamin D. *Hypophosphatemic vitamin D refractory rickets* of the simple type, resulting from renal tubular dysfunction, is the most common. It may be classified as an inborn error of metabolism and is genetically determined. However, not all examples of vitamin D refractory rickets have an inherited background established. This form of rickets may develop in infancy but not infrequently appears in late childhood, or it may not appear until adult life. Currently, oral administration of massive doses of vitamin D_2 (50,000 to 500,000 I.U. per day) are used, but the treatment of choice is use of one of the active metabolites of vitamin

D_3—25-OHD_3 or 1,25 $(OH)_2D_3$ (25-hydroxy-cholecalciferol and 1,25-dihydroxycholecalciferol, respectively)—or a synthetic analogue. Use of these forms will bypass the metabolic defect that is causing the vitamin D deficient state and rickets. See Chapter 8 on vitamins for a discussion of the metabolism of vitamin D and its hormonal functions. The rickets is rarely completely cured and the stature remains short. (See Fig. 12–14.)

Symptoms. The first adequate description of rickets occurred in 1650. The disease usually develops during the first two years of life. It has the chief characteristic of failure to appropriate or retain calcium in the bones. The softened and deformed bones cause deformities such as pigeon chest, enlarged wrists and ankles (Figs. 12–15 and 12–16), and bowed legs or knock knees. (See Fig. 12–17.) The severity of the condition may be determined chemically through studies of the calcium and phosphorus content of the blood and clinically with roentgenograms of the bones. There may be an increase in the serum concentration of alkaline phosphatase, an enzyme released by the osteoblasts, because it cannot be used in growth owing to deficiency of calcium. Radiological evidence is a loss of metaphyseal definition.

Because teeth are made up of material similar to bone, it is believed by many authorities that vitamin D has a related effect on the development of teeth. Delayed tooth development may be a sign of subclinical rickets.

The beginning visible symptoms of rickets in infants are profuse sweating, restlessness, and the sleeping infant moving his head from side to

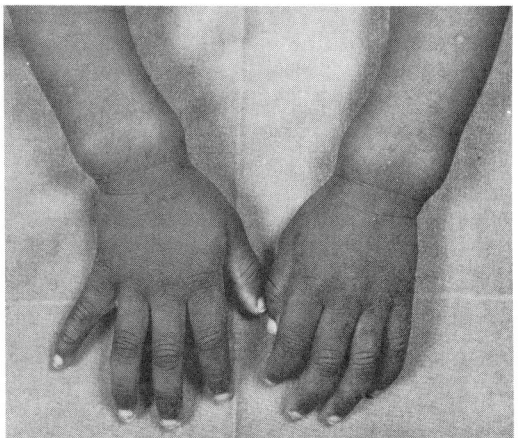

Figure 12–15 Rickets. Note the marked enlargement of wrists. (Courtesy of University of Rochester, Rochester, New York.)

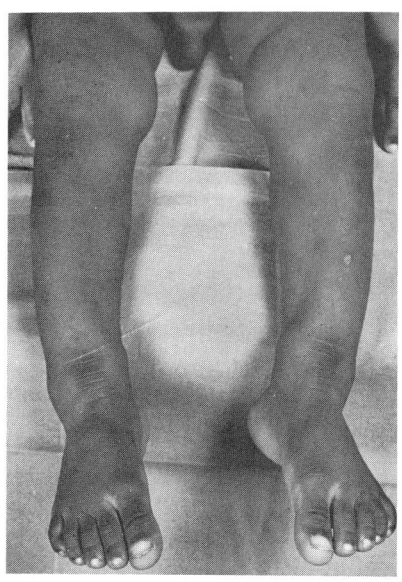

Figure 12–16 Rickets. Note the bowing and increase in width at epiphyses. (Courtesy of University of Rochester, Rochester, New York.)

side and rubbing off his hair. Contrary to the usual deficiency disease symptoms, the patient does not become thin or emaciated. Often parents will not recognize the symptoms of rickets until the child starts to walk. The legs will bow because the bones are soft and not strong enough to support the child's weight. A pot belly and beading of the ribs (the rachitic rosary) may pass unobserved in a plump, yet malnourished baby. (See Fig. 12–18.) If the deficiency appears during the third or fourth month of life, when the skull is growing rapidly, the structure of the head will be larger than normal. The shape is inclined to be square, with bulging on the sides and front. Lesser defects sometimes ensue when the ailment is mild.

Prevention and Dietary Treatment. Vitamin D, when it is converted to the active metabolite, acts to stimulate intestinal absorption of calcium and mobilization of calcium from bone. To prevent rickets in the newborn baby, the importance of starting the administration of vitamin D in appropriate amounts early and continuing throughout the growth period cannot be emphasized too much. If rickets is present, massive doses of vitamin D are given. Vitamin D concentrates of the fish liver oils, such as cod liver oil and viosterol, are often prescribed. One teaspoon (4 ml.) of cod liver oil contains 360 I.U. of vitamin D. Irradiated

ergosterol is also an excellent source. However, mothers should be warned against the simultaneous use of several preparations, since it is possible to give too much.

The therapeutic dose of vitamin D is 1000–5000 I.U./day, depending on the severity of the rickets. Calcium supplements should also be given in severe cases. In addition, the mother should be encouraged to allow the child to play in the sunshine if possible.

Many foods are being fortified with vitamin D and milk is an example (400 I.U./qt.). Since milk contains calcium and phosphorus, it becomes a good antirachitic food when vitamin D is added. A child drinking one quart of milk per day, which provides the RDA, would not need a vitamin D supplement.

Osteomalacia

Etiology and Symptoms. Osteomalacia is a disease of adulthood similar to rickets in infants and children. It is a nutritional disease usually attributed to (1) a defect in renal tubular reabsorption, or (2) a failure to respond to vitamin D, or (3) a deficiency of vitamin D or (4) an inadequate intake of calcium or (5) a loss of excessive amounts of calcium in the feces. In most cases seen in the United States, this condition is associated with steatorrhea. It is characterized by pronounced softening of the bones, which leads to deformities, especially of the limbs, spine, thorax, and pelvis. Radiographic findings in the bones are translucent bands (Looser's zones), which are diagnostic of osteomalacia. Typical symptoms are a rheumatic type of pain and general weakness. There may also be a waddling gait and tetany manifested by facial twitching. Although it is seen occasionally in men, it is most often ob-

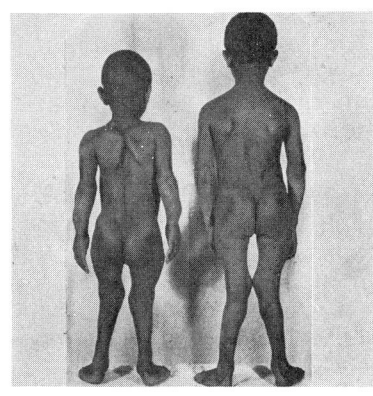

Figure 12–17 Rachitic deformities. Note knock knees and enlarged joints. (From: Jolliffe, N. (ed.): Clinical Nutrition, 2nd ed. New York, Harper & Brothers, 1962.)

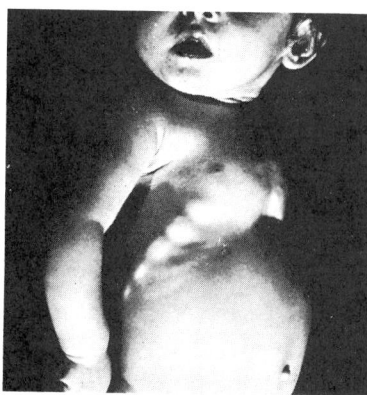

Figure 12–18 Child suffering from rickets. Note rachitic rosary and pot belly. (From: Jolliffe, N. (ed.): Clinical Nutrition, 2nd ed. New York, Harper & Brothers, 1962.)

served in women of child-bearing age who have become depleted of calcium because of multiple pregnancies and inadequate diet.

Secondary hyperparathyroidism may accompany cases of osteomalacia. This is due to the constant hypocalcemia that induces parathyroid activity. If hyperparathyroidism is also present, the bones will also exhibit lesions of osteitis fibrosa cystica.[29] (See Chapter 30—Nutritional Care for Patients with Diseases of the Kidney.)

Incidence. Although clinical osteomalacia is seldom seen among the people in developed countries, there are areas where it is a medical problem. It is distributed widely in India, most frequently among the women of the upper and middle classes who practice seclusion or purdah after marriage. It is also prevalent in the Orient, especially among the women, whose diets are extremely low in calcium, who get little sunshine, and who have frequent pregnancies and nurse their infants over extended periods.

In the United States, osteomalacia is sometimes encountered among elderly persons living alone, consuming an inadequate diet, and getting inadequate sunshine or other source of vitamin D. It is seldom encountered among the lower classes who wear less clothing and who work outdoors in the sun, or among people who have an abundant diet. It can also develop as a consequence of malabsorption of vitamin D from chronic digestive disease or as a result of anticonvulsant therapy. (See Chapter 21.)

Osteomalacia is frequently confused with a disease having similar symptoms, osteoporosis, discussed in this chapter under Mineral (Calcium and Phosphorus) Deficien-

cies. They frequently occur together, with osteomalacia developing after osteoporosis.

Prevention and Treatment. Because the average diet furnishes little vitamin D, it seems reasonable to assume that either the requirement of vitamin D for man is extremely low or his needs are usually provided by exposure to sunlight. Most authorities agree that the normal adult requires only a small amount of vitamin D. For osteomalacia the recommendations are an adequate diet liberal in protein of high biologic value, with an abundance of milk and milk products plus a supplement of vitamin D. The doses of vitamin D are usually 1000–5000 I.U. per day unless there is evidence of malabsorption, in which case the dose should be 50,000 I.U. daily. Calcium supplements may also be necessary. The pain and weakness will usually disappear within 1 to 2 months after starting treatment.

Prevention of rickets and osteomalacia is possible through the supply of adequate and correct proportions of calcium and phosphorus in the diet. Milk or its equivalent is necessary in the diet to provide calcium. In addition vitamin D must be assured from either sunshine, ultraviolet lamp, natural food source, fortified food source, or a concentrated supplement. Prevention is paramount since once the deformities of rickets or osteomalacia develop they are irreversible and can only be corrected by orthopedic surgery.

MINERAL DEFICIENCIES

Chapter 7, devoted to the subject of minerals, should be reviewed before reading this section.

CALCIUM AND PHOSPHORUS

The relationship and necessity for calcium and phosphorus in the prevention and treatment of rickets, tetany and osteomalacia have been discussed. It has been demonstrated that these diseases can develop when an imbalance or longstanding lack occurs of either or both calcium and phosphorus.

A moderate degree of calcium deficiency is believed to be quite prevalent during pregnancy, and also in childhood; it is usually much worse during adolescence. During the adolescent period the requirement is increased while in contrast too often the intake of calcium-rich foods is decreased. The desire to remain slim is a factor, especially among girls. It is during the

Table 12–4   THE DIFFERENTIAL DIAGNOSIS OF OSTEOMALACIA AND OSTEOPOROSIS

	OSTEOMALACIA	OSTEOPOROSIS
Clinical features		
Skeletal pain	A major complaint and usually persistent	Episodic and usually associated with a fracture
Muscle weakness	Usually present and producing disability and, when severe, a characteristic gait	Absent
Fractures	Relatively uncommon; healing delayed	The usual presenting feature; heals normally
Skeletal deformity	Common, especially kyphosis	Only occurs where there is a fracture
Radiographic features		
Loss of density of bone	Widespread	Irregular and often most marked in the spine
Loss of bone detail	Characteristic	Not a feature
Looser's zones	Diagnostic	Absent
Biopsy		
Histological changes	Excess osteoid tissue with bone present in normal quantity	Bone reduced in quantity but fully mineralized
Biochemical changes		
Plasma Ca and P	Often low	Normal
Plasma alkaline phosphatase	Often high	Normal
Urinary calcium	Often low	Normal or high
Response to treatment		
Vitamin D	Dramatic	None

(From Davidson, S., et al.: Human Nutrition and Dietetics. 6th ed. Edinburgh, Churchill Livingstone, 1975. p. 326.)

adolescent period that dental caries tend to become prevalent, a condition believed to depend on nutritional status and calcium metabolism. Milk and milk products are the best food sources. Calcium salts are considered useful under special circumstances.

Osteoporosis. Osteoporosis is a metabolic disorder which may be defined as a reduction in the *amount* of bone without any changes in its chemical composition. That is, the absolute amount has been diminished, but the bone remaining is normal in chemical composition. With bone loss, skeletal strength cannot be maintained and fractures occur with just minimal stress. Osteoporosis (deossification) is frequently confused with osteomalacia (demineralization). See Table 12–4.

INCIDENCE AND ETIOLOGY. Osteoporosis is encountered in persons after age 50 and especially in women after the menopause. Practically all people begin to lose bone at about age 55. Although the reasons are unclear, it seems to be physiologically normal. It is more common in women by a ratio of about four to one. It can be shown by measuring the cortical thickness of the long bones, particularly the femur, by x-ray. The disease is either *idiopathic* (unknown etiology) or secondary to some known disorders. There are four types of idiopathic osteoporosis: (1) juvenile, (2) presenile, (3)

postmenopausal and (4) senile, depending upon the age and sex of the patient. *Secondary osteoporosis* is usually endocrine, gastrointestinal, or renal induced. The majority of osteoporosis is the idiopathic type. See Table 12–5 for causes of osteoporosis. The most common type is osteoporosis of aging (senile) in females (postmenopausal). It is believed that

Table 12–5   SUSPECTED CAUSES OF OSTEOPOROSIS

PRIMARY DISEASE	SECONDARY DISEASE
Common causes	
Estrogen deficiency	Hyperparathyroidism
Inactivity	Hypercortisolism
High phosphate intake	Renal osteodystrophy
	Multiple myeloma
Uncommon causes	
Calcium deficiency	Hyperthyroidism
Vitamin D deficiency	Acromegaly
Immobilization	Heparin therapy
	Gastrectomy
	Anticonvulsant therapy
	Celiac disease
	Cirrhosis
	Scurvy
	Steatorrhea

(Adapted from Jowsey, J.: Osteoporosis. It's Nature and Role of Diet. Postgrad. Med., *60*:75, 1976.)

Figure 12–19 *A* illustrates a case of secondary osteoporosis in which, upon treatment of the underlying cause, the person either regains normal bone mineralization or *B*, proceeds with normal physiological demineralization of bone at a lower level. *C* illustrates active deteriorating osteoporosis. (Adapted from: Kuhlencordt, F.: Osteoporosis: A clinical review. *In:* Nielsen, S. P., and Kruse, H. (eds.): Calcified Tissue, 1975. Copenhagen, Fadl Publishing Co., 1976.)

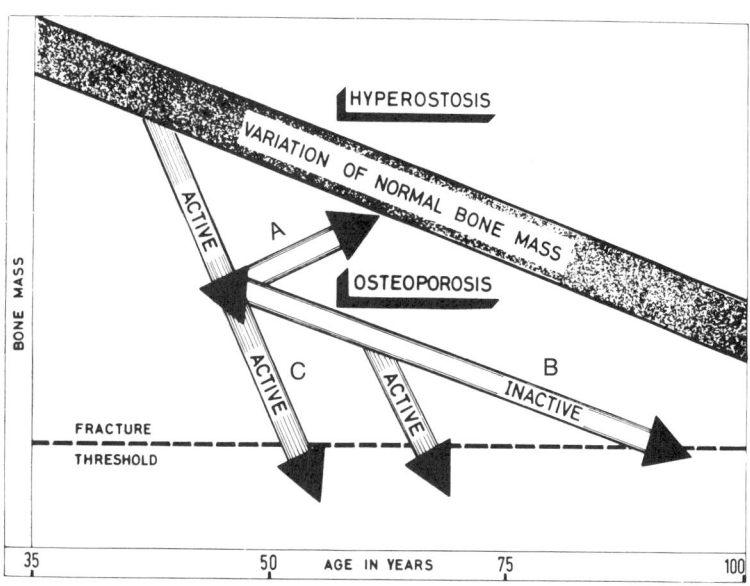

in these women and men the estrogen that is present is not effective, and the consequent lack of estrogen activity leads to the pathogenesis of the bone. Probably, osteoporosis is the result of a variety of factors, of which hormonal change is one. It is also the general consensus that osteoporosis does not come on suddenly in old age, but develops over a lifetime. (See Fig. 12–19.)

Calcium. It is not clear whether deficient calcium intake is a factor in the etiology of osteoporosis. It has been shown that persons with osteoporosis are in negative calcium balance and that the daily calcium loss may be as high as 90 mg. per day.[24] Over a lifetime this could result in a significant loss of skeleton. Also, calcium absorption from the intestine decreases with age, as does the usual dietary intake of calcium. Nordin postulates that this decreased absorption could be due to inadequate vitamin D or to a vitamin D "resistance." This vitamin D resistance could result from an increased sensitivity of bone to parathyroid hormone. This would elevate serum calcium and lead to less g.i. absorption of calcium. Another cause may be impaired renal function, which accompanies aging. Decreased renal function results in a decreased intestinal absorption of calcium. These suppositions have support in the fact that the elderly require large doses of vitamin D_2 but will respond to small doses of 1α-OH-D_3, the analogue of 1-OH D_3, the active vitamin D hormone.[25]

Phosphate. Serum inorganic phosphorus level increases after phosphate ingestion. Unlike calcium, whose absorption is only minimally dependent on dietary intake, phosphate absorption is dependent on the amount ingested. The increased serum phosphate results in a fall in serum calcium, which stimulates parathyroid hormone excretion. PTH causes an increase in serum calcium by mobilizing calcium from the bone.

Calcium: Phosphorus Ratio. The ratio of the calcium to the phosphorus in the diet appears to be a factor in osteoporosis development. The Ca:P ratio should be 1 in the adult diet and more than 1 in the diet of a growing child. However, the average American in 1960 had a dietary intake with a Ca:P ratio of 1:2.8, and today it is probably at least 1:4.[20] The ratio usually remains the same, regardless of whether the person drinks milk or not, because milk and milk products are good sources of both calcium and phosphorus in equal proportions.

The phosphate intake is so high because many popular foods—bread, cereal, meat and potatoes—contain phosphate and almost no calcium. See Table 7–2. Foods that contain considerable calcium and no phosphorus are few and little used, e.g., sesame seeds, maple syrup and seaweed. From her extensive research in this area, Jowsey recommends calcium supplements for people beginning at the age of 25.

Protein. A high protein intake has been found to result in increased calcium excretion, and a negative calcium balance could occur

since calcium absorption is not increased. It is postulated that the calcium excretion is due to a change in acid-base balance that necessitates the use of bone calcium as a buffering agent.[15, 35]

Parathyroid Hormone. Berlyne and associates show that in senile osteoporosis, serum PTH levels are increased and are related to the degree of osteoporosis. He explains the increased PTH by the fact that normal aging produces nephron death and decreased glomerular filtration rate. BUN rises and the decreased renal function causes an increase in parathyroid hormone and mineral resorption from the bone. The normal aging process then stimulates PTH excretion, and the low postmenopausal level of estrogen makes the bone sensitive to the action of PTH, which contributes to the osteoporotic process along with dietary factors.[1]

Exercise. Lack of exercise of many aging persons may be a factor; there is lack of stimulation to maintain calcium in the bony areas of stress and wear. This is especially evident during immobilization.

SYMPTOMS. Osteoporosis is acquired slowly, and many years may elapse before the individual is aware of the change. See Fig. 12–19, which shows progression of osteoporosis. Weakness is the initial manifestation, along with loss of appetite and pain in the back and hips associated with fractures. Fractures often occur easily; for example, individuals may break a hip from tripping over a rug or stepping down a low curb. Involvement of leg bones is followed by pain, tenderness and muscle cramps. Bowing occurs when bone tissue becomes too soft to support the weight of the body. Deformity such as stooped posture is frequently marked, along with decrease in height due to shrinkage of the spine. Hypercalciuria may occur in the beginning stage, and renal stones frequently develop.

TREATMENT AND PREVENTION. Androgens and estrogens have been shown to be slightly protective against osteoporosis and have been used in therapy. Calcium infusions have been used also to improve calcium retention, enhance bone formation and reduce bone resorption. An increase in vitamin D and calcium intake is indicated, as well as exercise to prevent atrophy of bone. The diet should be adequate in all respects to assure normal, or increased, calcium availability. Sufficient vitamin D must be present to permit utilization of the calcium taken into the body. Vitamin D intake may have to be 10,000–20,000 I.U. in order to achieve a response if there is any "vitamin D resistance." An adequate protein intake and positive nitrogen balance are important, as is a positive calcium balance.

Beneficial effects of fluoride have been reported but are controversial. Some feel that the bone formation stimulated is of inferior quality. Others such as Jowsey have produced good bone formation when the fluoride treatment (15–45 mg./day) is combined with calcium (1000 mg./day) and vitamin D (50,000 I.U. twice weekly).[17] It is believed that the effect in bone is similar to that which helps prevent dental caries. These studies also showed that calcified aortas occurred much less often with optimal fluoride intake. If these findings are confirmed, fluoride in some way helps to keep the calcium in the bone and to prevent its deposition in the blood vessel.[13]

IRON

The relationship and necessity for iron in the prevention and treatment of anemias is discussed in detail in Chapter 29.

Anemias. Iron deficiency is the most prevalent type of nutritional anemia and in the adult person is recognized generally by the presence of microcytic hypochromic anemia. Iron deficiency anemia is an important nutritional problem among infants and women of childbearing age throughout the world, including the United States. However, the Ten-State Nutrition Survey, 1968–70 unexpectedly revealed significant iron deficiency anemia among black male adolescents.[32] Although lack of dietary iron is the basic cause of this disorder, in the United States and the rest of the world other concurrent endemic diseases which contribute to blood loss (hookworm) or interfere with absorption (gastrointestinal diseases) are important contributing factors. Nutrition surveys, such as those made in the United States and by ICNND and the WHO, have disclosed iron deficiency anemia as a major impairment of health and working capacity and, as a consequence, a cause of economic loss. As high as 30 to 50 per cent or more of the underdeveloped countries have been found to be affected. See Chapter 29, Diseases of the Blood and Blood-Forming Organs, page 606 for discussion of Nutritional and Iron Deficiency Anemias; Chapter 13 for anemia in pregnancy; and Chapter 38 for anemia in infancy and childhood.

Prevention of Iron Deficiency Anemia. Careful selection of iron-rich foods in the daily dietary is necessary for all persons. In areas where

iron deficiency anemia results from parasitic infections, eradication of the parasites plus the introduction of adequate iron into the diet is the objective for prevention. In acute areas, iron may be supplied in the form of ferrous sulfate through the health center distribution program. Iron fortification of other foods besides bread and cereal products is contemplated.

IODINE

Although iodine is distributed extensively throughout the products of nature, the chief storehouse is in the surface soil. Since the amount varies with the local geologic conditions of the soil and water, there is an uneven distribution.

The thyroid gland is the storehouse for iodine in the human body. Iodine is an essential component of thyroxine, the active constituent of the thyroid gland.

Simple or Endemic Goiter. Simple goiter is a state of enlargement of the thyroid gland which develops through a deficiency of ingested iodine. The deficiency may be absolute, especially in areas of subnormal iodine intake, or relative, subsequent to various demands of the body which increase the need for thyroid secretion in the female during adolescence, pregnancy, and lactation. See Chapter 26 for a discussion of iodine deficiency and goiter.

INCIDENCE. The highest incidence in goitrous areas usually occurs in females 12 to 18 years of age and males 9 to 13 years. The incidence of goiter can be correlated with the iodine intake from the water and food of a specific region. In the regions known as the "goiter belt" in the United States the soil is iodine poor, producing iodine-poor food. This inadequacy is reflected in a prevalence of goiter among the population. The WHO has estimated that there are approximately 200 million goitrous individuals in the world today, and few countries are exempt.

The food iodine is an important factor determining the goiter incidence in a region. Nutritional iodine is derived essentially from the food and to a lesser degree from supplemented salt or water. The amount of iodine in the local drinking water may be regarded as a measure of the iodine content of the soil and, consequently, of the iodine content of the fruits, grasses, and vegetables grown in the region. However, the iodine content of water is not important as a souce of nutritional iodine except in unusual circumstances.

Goitrogens in food can also cause goiter. These are natural inhibitors of the thyroid gland. Some foods containing goitrogen are cabbage, turnips, rapeseeds, mustard seeds, groundnuts, cassava, soya beans and Brassica seeds (rarely eaten by humans).

Other studies suggest that local water may contain goitrogen substances from geologic origin or possibly from *Escherichia coli* in the water.[7] This may explain the prevalence of goiter in some areas where it does not seem dependent on iodine deficiency alone.

PREVENTION AND TREATMENT. Simple goiter can be prevented and frequently cured by the administration of iodine. To supply the needed iodine, the use of iodized salt is advised. People residing along the seacoast may obtain iodine from fresh shellfish (rich in iodine) and foods grown in iodine-rich soil. However, even the regional differences in iodine consumption have become less pronounced with the increase in interstate transportation of foods, beverages, vegetables, fruits, and fertilizers. People living in the goiter belt who consume local produce especially should be urged to use iodized salt.

Endemic goiter is still widespread in the underdeveloped areas and a significant number of cases have been found in the United States. (See Figures 12–20 and 12–21). The international agencies, particularly WHO and ICNND, have addressed a great deal of attention toward effective salt iodization.

MAGNESIUM

Magnesium deficiency may develop under conditions of stress and in the course of disease process. A deficiency may precipitate from any condition in which there is a decreased intake or increased loss of magnesium or a shift in electrolyte balance.

The hypomagnesemic tetany syndrome deficiency is reported to be almost identical to hypocalcemic tetany (p. 548) and can be differentiated chemically. Prominent signs are depression, muscular weakness, vertigo and tendency to convulsions. Administration of magnesium promptly relieves the symptoms. Patients observed with the deficiency all have a dietary inadequacy. In addition, one or more of the following factors are present: (1) excessive loss of magnesium from persistent vomiting or from removal of intestinal contents by mechanical suction, (2) intestinal malabsorption, or (3) administration of large amounts of magnesium-free parenteral fluids to postsurgical patients. Treatment with intramuscular

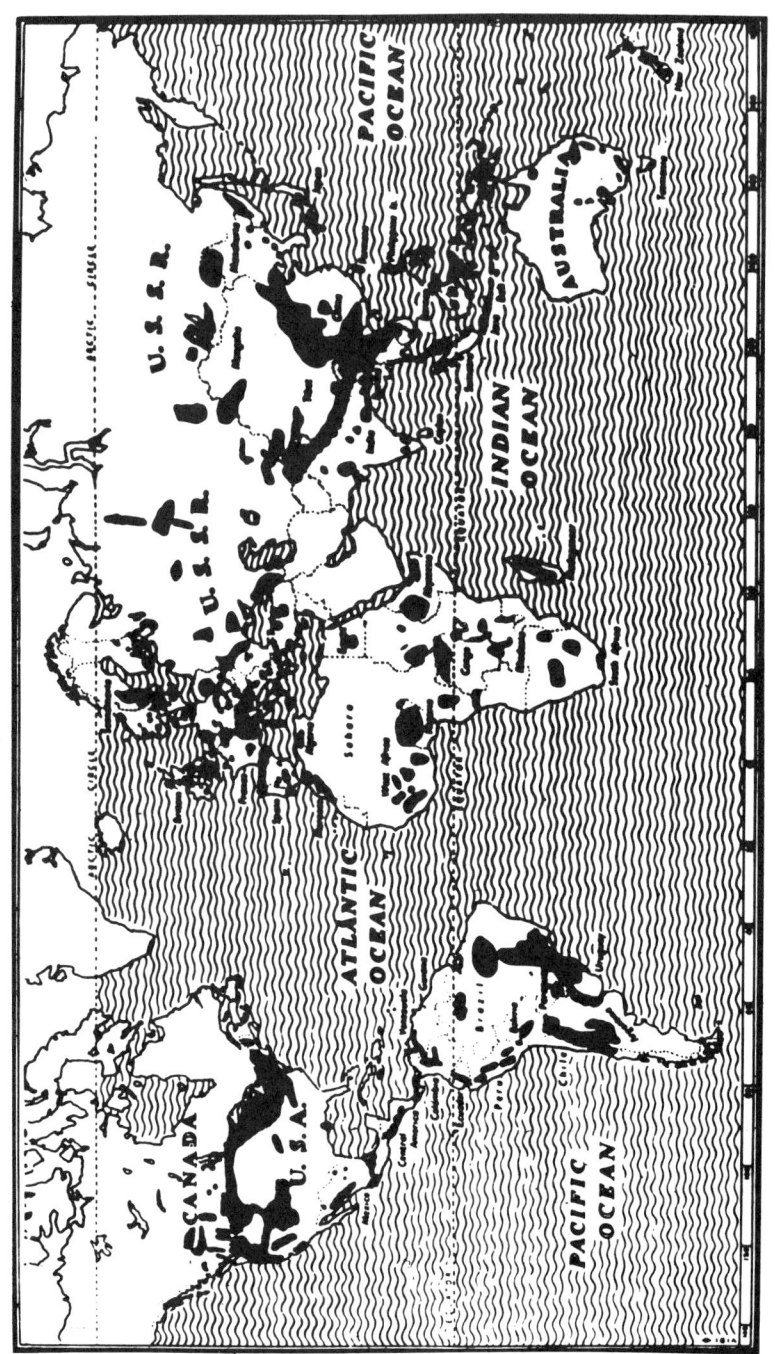

Figure 12–20   Goiter areas of the world. (From: Volume III, Agriculture. Science, Technology, and Development. U.S. papers prepared for the United Nations Conference on the application of Science and Technology for the Benefit of the Less Developed Areas, 1962.)

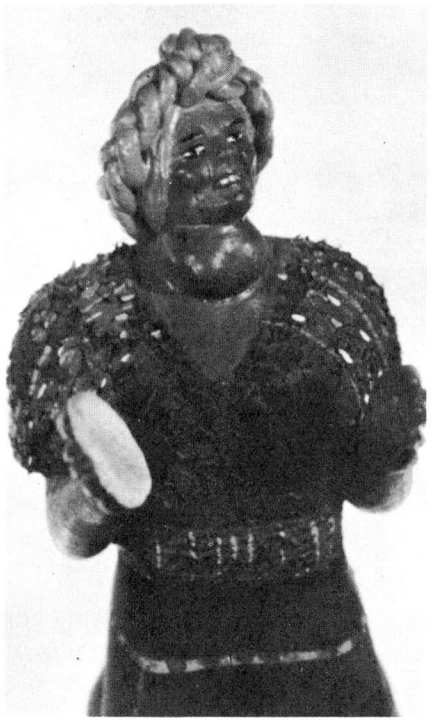

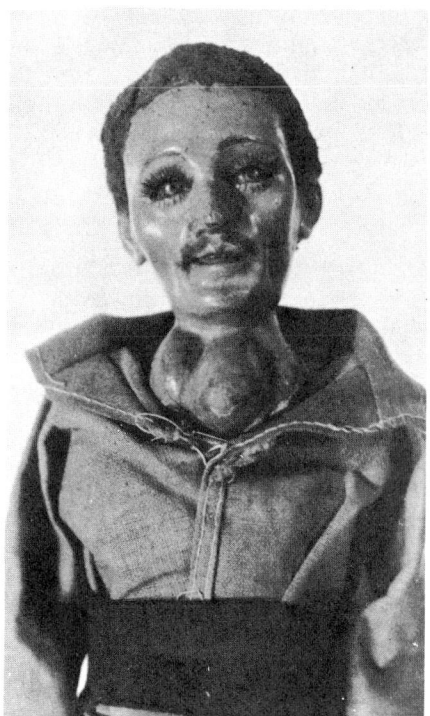

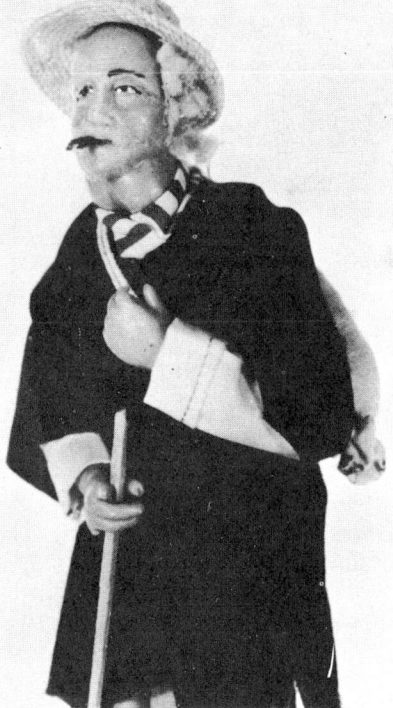

Figure 12–21 Dolls with goiter from the goitrous belt of Middle America. *Above,* figure of village woman making tortillas, made in local village and purchased in Guatemala City market; *lower left,* old religious statue from Antigua, Guatemala; *lower right,* doll of recent data manufactured in village in Colombia. All illustrate the acceptance of goiter as a normal physical feature. (From Volume III, Agriculture. Science, Technology, and Development. U.S. papers prepared for the United Nations Conference on the application of Science and Technology for the Benefit of the Less Developed Areas, 1962.)

magnesium sulfate promptly reverses the condition. Magnesium is present in a large number of foods, especially those of vegetable origin, since it is an essential component of chlorophyll.

Conditions in which acute deficiencies may develop are renal disease, diuretic therapy, malabsorption, hyperthyroidism, acute alcoholism, kwashiorkor, diabetes, parathyroid gland disorders, and post-surgical stress.

ZINC

The zinc deficient state, although previously known in animals, was fist described in man a little over 15 year ago. Prasad and others described the syndrome in adolescents in poor peasant communities in Egypt and Iran.[11, 26] See Fig. 12–22.

Symptoms. The clinical entity first described in young males was characterized by short stature, hypogonadism, mild anemia and low plasma zinc levels. After supplementation with zinc sulfate the boys began to grow and pubertal changes occurred. The anemia may have been due to a coexisting protein and/or iron deficiency. Additional symptoms such as *hypogeusia* (decreased taste acuity), delayed wound healing, alopecia, and a dermatitis called *acrodermatitis enteropathica* have also

been found to be part of the zinc deficiency syndrome.

Etiology and Incidence. The deficiency described in young males in Iran and Egypt was caused by the high phytate or fiber content of the diet from unrefined cereal and unleavened bread. The phytate or fiber in the intestine chelates with zinc and prevents its absorption, which results in a conditional deficiency.

In the United States Hambidge performed zinc analyses on hair in 338 middle and upper class children and adults in Denver, Colorado. He found ten children with very low hair zinc levels (less than 70 ppm.). Most of these children also had a history of poor appetite, were below the tenth percentile for height and had hypogeusia. All of these conditions improved upon administration of zinc sulfate. The diets of these children had consisted of very little meat and a great deal of milk, a poor source of zinc.[12]

In 1974 Moynahan described *acrodermatitis enteropathica,* a lethal inherited zinc deficiency which results in eczematoid skin lesions, alopecia, diarrhea, low plasma zinc levels, poor growth and development, malnutrition, intercurrent bacterial and yeast infections and eventually death if left untreated.[22] It usually shows up in infancy upon changing from breast milk to cow's milk. It has been

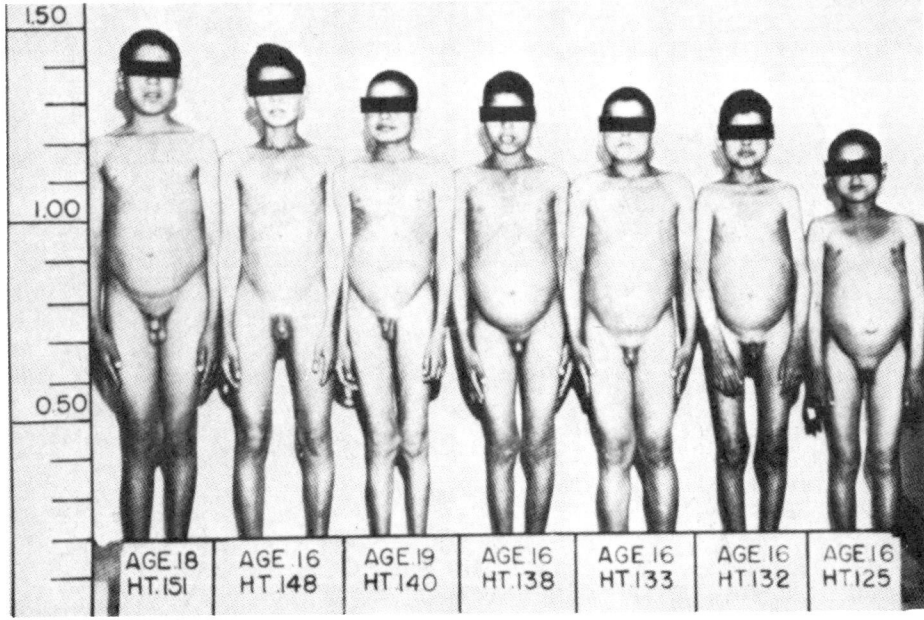

Figure 12–22 Zinc deficiency in dwarfs. (From: Prasad, A. S., et al.: Zinc metabolism in patients with the syndrome of iron deficiency anemia, hepatosplenomegaly, dwarfism and hypogonadism. J. Lab. Clin. Med., *61*:537, 1963.)

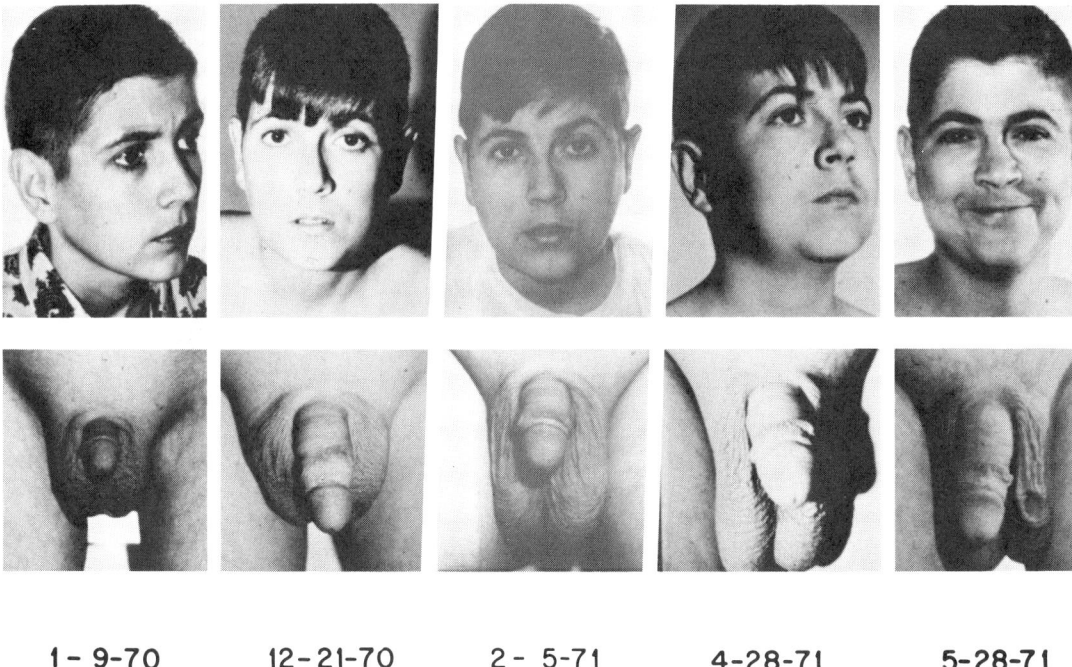

1-9-70   12-21-70   2-5-71   4-28-71   5-28-71

Figure 12–23   Zinc deficiency from malabsorption and after treatment with zinc sulfate. Note the physical maturation and growth that result from zinc supplementation. (From: Sandstead, H. H.: Zinc as an unrecognized limiting nutrient. Am. J. Clin. Nutr., 26:790, 1973.)

postulated that cow's milk contains a peptide that these children cannot digest and that chelates with zinc and prevents its absorption. The treatment is to provide zinc sulfate in amounts large enough to overcome this chelation effect and allow zinc absorption. Neldner and Hambidge found that zinc supplementation at a level of 22 mg. of elemental zinc was enough to cause remission of the disease in an adult.[23]

Other cases of low serum zinc levels as a result of chronic illness, malabsorption or long term zinc-free parenteral feedings have also been reported. See Fig. 12–23. In addition several investigators have demonstrated an accelerated healing of wounds in patients receiving zinc sulfate.

Treatment and Prevention.   Treatment is alleviation of the situation causing the reduced zinc absorption and supplementation with zinc sulfate. The patient should eat a diet high in foods containing zinc, such as meat, liver, wheat germ and nuts. Particularly good sources are oysters. See Appendix Table 13 for the zinc content of various foods.

After studying human zinc requirements and the level of zinc in the U.S. diet, Sandstead feels that a significant portion of the population, particularly those subsisting on low-income diets, may have a marginal zinc intake.[30] These people may be adversely affected by this marginal zinc intake, especially if they are subjected to stress or trauma.[33]

PROTEIN-CALORIE MALNUTRITION

An inadequate dietary intake of calories and proteins of good quality is the most widespread, serious nutritional problem in technically underdeveloped areas, and is particularly devastating in its effect on children.

In the United States, serious protein-calorie malnutrition (protein-energy malnutrition), including typical kwashiorkor and marasmus, is observed occasionally in neglected infants brought to large city hospitals and in low income families. The general improvement in the clinical or physical symptoms is usually satisfactory but in many instances there is evident lack of improvement in the functional capacities of the developing brain. Studies to solve the relationship of nutrition to central nervous system activity are of immense practical and theoretical importance. Findings regarding the profound effects of semi-starvation

Table 12–6 "WELLCOME" CLASSIFICATION OF PEM

	BODY WEIGHT AS % OF STANDARD*	EDEMA	DEFICIT IN WEIGHT FOR HEIGHT†
Underweight child	80–60	0	Minimal
Nutritional dwarfing	<60	0	Minimal
Marasmus	<60	0	+ +
Kwashiorkor	80–60	+	+ +
Marasmic kwashiorkor	<60	+	+ +

*Standard taken as 50th percentile of the Harvard values.

†Weight for height = $\dfrac{\text{weight of patient}}{\text{weight of normal subject of same height}} \times 100$

(From FAO/WHO Expert Committee on Nutrition. Eighth Report. WHO Technical Report Series, No. 477, Geneva. WHO, 1971.)

on the behavior patterns of man are equally important.[18]

Protein-calorie inadequacy problems that are secondary to other diseases are many. Serious caloric undernutrition occurs in association with chronic fevers such as tuberculosis, with malignancy, in diseases of the gastrointestinal tract that interfere with intake or absorption of food and in patients with psychiatric problems. Protein deficiency is a complication of numerous pathologic states. Protein may be lost in diarrheas and malabsorption syndromes, or in the urine in certain diseases of the kidney.

Trauma of all kinds, including surgery, can result in a negative nitrogen balance; cirrhosis of the liver is commonly associated with protein deficiency. In addition to physiological stress, psychological or emotional stress can result in a negative nitrogen balance.

Iatrogenic protein-calorie malnutrition can result from many modern medical treatments. Radiation therapy and chemotherapy for cancer can result in malabsorption, increased requirements and a consequent protein-calorie deficient state.

Definition. The phrase *protein energy malnutrition* (PEM) refers to a spectrum of clinical disorders caused by various degrees of deficiency and additional physiological insults and stresses. *Marasmus* commonly refers to a condition in which there is a deprivation of both calories and protein, a starvation condition, to which the child has adjusted by reduced growth. *Kwashiorkor* is a condition with a different clinical picture. It is characterized by more metabolic derangements and is more severe. This extreme protein deficiency is usually in the presence of calorie deficiency. The two diseases are at the extreme end of protein-energy malnutrition.

Several clinicians have attempted to provide means of classifying the severity of protein-energy malnutrition. One system devised by the FAO/WHO Expert Committee on Nutrition is shown in Table 12–6. Other systems, such as that of McLaren, include a scoring system. See Table 12–7.

It has been postulated that kwashiorkor and marasmus are two facets of the same disease process. No differences have been found between the diets that produce kwashiorkor or marasmus in children.[10] Therefore, the growth retardation of marasmus may be an "adaptation" to the stress of inadequate calories and protein, and metabolic processes, including liver function, are able to be well preserved. Kwashiorkor is a "dysadaptation" to the protein and calorie deficiency that is characterized by the edema and metabolic changes.[28] This "dysadaptation" is frequently caused by an infection such as malaria, measles or gastroenteritis. See Table 12–8.

Table 12–7 SCORING SYSTEM FOR SEVERE FORMS OF PEM

SIGNS PRESENT		POINTS
Edema		3
Dermatosis		2
Edema plus dermatosis		6
Hair change		1
Hepatomegaly		1
Serum albumin (or serum total protein)	(gm./100 ml.)	
<1.00	(<3.25)	7
1.00–1.49	(3.25–3.99)	6
1.50–1.99	(4.00–4.74)	5
2.00–2.49	(4.75–5.49)	4
2.50–2.99	(5.50–6.24)	3
3.00–3.49	(6.25–6.99)	2
3.50–3.99	(7.00–7.74)	1
≥4.00	(≥7.75)	0

Score = sum of points; 0–3 = marasmus (67.5 per cent or less expected weight by Harvard standard); 4–8 = marasmic kwashiorkor, 9–15 = kwashiorkor.

(From McLaren, D. S., and Burman, D.: Textbook of Pediatric Nutrition. Edinburgh, Churchill Livingstone, 1976, p. 109.)

Table 12–8 SOME CHARACTERISTICS OF MARASMUS AND KWASHIORKOR

	MARASMUS	KWASHIORKOR
General features		
Occurrence	World-wide	Limited
Usual age	Infancy	Second and third years
Adaptation to stress	Good	Poor
Response to treatment		
immediate	Poor	Good (occasional sudden death)
ultimate	Fair	Good
Long-term effects		
mental	Severe	Nil
physical	Severe	Mild
liver damage	Nil	Nil
Clinical signs		
Edema	Absent	Present
Dermatosis	Rare	Common
Hair changes	Common	Very common
Hepatomegaly	Common	Very common
Mental changes	Uncommon	Very common
Wasting of fat	Severe	Mild
of muscles	Severe	Mild
Anemia	Common and severe	Mild
Vitamin deficiencies	Uncommon	Common
Laboratory findings		
General		
Total body water	High	High
Extra-cellular water	Some increase	More increase
Body potassium	Some depletion	Much depletion
Malabsorption	Some	More
Fatty infiltration of liver	Absent	Severe
X-ray bone loss	Mild	Mild
Renal function	Impaired	Impaired
I.V. glucose tolerance	Normal	Impaired
Response to adrenaline	Exaggerated	Lowered
Serum		
Albumin	Slightly low	Very low
Enzymes (in general)	Normal	Low
Copper, zinc, sodium	Normal	Low
Non-essential/essential amino-acids	Normal	High
Triglycerides	Normal	Normal
Cholesterol	Normal	Low
Non-esterified fatty acids	Normal	High
β-Lipoprotein	High	Low
Insulin	Low	Low
Growth hormone	Low or normal	High
Glucose	Low	Very Low
Urine		
Urea/total N	Above 65 per cent	Below 50 per cent
Imidazole acrylic acid	Nil	Present
Hydroxyproline index	Low	Low
Liver		
Urea cycle enzymes	Low	Low
Amino-acid-synthesizing enzymes	High	High

(From McLaren, D. S.: Nutrition and Its Disorders. Baltimore, Williams & Wilkins Co., 1972, p. 107. © 1972 by The Williams & Wilkins Company.)

PROTEIN DEFICIENCY

The simplest, most obvious, common cause of protein deficiency is the lack of adequate protein in the food consumed and inadequate calorie intake. This may be due to one or more of these reasons: inadequate knowledge about sufficient protein intake, ingestion of poor quality protein, poor economic status, unavailability of good quality protein, misinformation, or the existence of some local or generalized disease which results in anorexia and dietary inadequacy. Other causes resulting in a *conditioned or secondary protein deficiency* are:

1. Impaired digestion or absorption of protein foods—chronic diarrhea, fistula and so on.

2. Inadequate synthesis of plasma protein—liver disease.

3. Increased breakdown of body protein stores: febrile states, elevated basal metabolic rate and the like.

4. Excessive loss of protein, such as nephrotic syndrome, ascites or hemorrhage.

Hypoproteinemia and Nutritional Edema

Nutritional edema invariably accompanies periods of famine following war and rapidly disappears when the afflicted are given sufficient food of good quality. Along with the general malnutrition, an inadequacy of proteins appears to be the most important factor in the production of the syndrome. The severe restriction of protein and calories in the diet may lead to the use of body proteins for fuel. If prolonged, a large protein deficit may occur in the body with *hypoproteinemia* and *edema*.

In mild cases the edema is usually confined to the lower limbs but when the condition is severe it extends to all parts of the body.

The edema, although in reality a late stage in protein deficiency, is almost the first clinical sign of the deficiency, according to present knowledge. The readiness with which it appears and its clinical picture depend to some extent upon the amount of ingested salt and water. One of the characteristics of the edema is the lack of association with symptoms which suggest other causes of edema, notably heart and kidney disease. Actual loss of weight is usually masked by the edema. In fact, there may be sudden increase in weight, accompanied by weakness and lassitude because of the holding of fluids in the tissues. Subclinical or marginal forms of the hypoproteinemia without edema may occur in debilitating disorders, such as following surgery, severe burns, severe wounds, kidney disease, and in disease with prolonged temperature rise. The most significant and most useful clinical test for protein deficiency is a laboratory test—the measurement of the concentration of the plasma or serum protein.

Dietary History. The dietary history of the patient is of great importance. (See p. 222.) The inquiry into diet should be made with care because small deficits existing over a long period can cause a deficiency. It is advisable to obtain a record of the kinds and amounts of food eaten during a period of one week or more. From the history a dietary intake can be calculated and an estimate made of the probable intake over a longer period. The calculated intake should be compared with the known standard requirements. Consideration should also be given to the possible deficiency of protein and one or more of the essential amino acids. Thus, the significance of the protein content, quality and utilization, as well as other factors of the diet, such as calorie intake, minerals and vitamins, should be evaluated.

Nutritional Care. In addition to a well-balanced diet, adequate in all the nutritional essentials, proteins of good quality must be provided in abundance. Calories must be adequate to maintain normal weight and to spare body protein. Not only must enough food be available to meet the usual optimal daily requirements, but the body weight and protein deficits produced through years of semistarvation must be replaced.

The return to normal serum protein concentration is slow. Approximately 30 gm. of protein must be deposited in the tissues before 1 gm. is retained in the circulation.

PROTEIN CONCENTRATES. Food by mouth is the choice route for the administration of protein and calories. However, for some patients with considerable body protein deficiency, especially if associated with anorexia, it may not be possible to supply sufficient protein orally. Other routes of administration must be used and concentrated protein given by hyperalimentation or stomach tube or parenterally in the form of human plasma, human albumin, gelatin, various hydrolysates of casein, or whole blood.

Supplementary nourishments prepared with protein concentrates are an effective method of increasing the protein intake with limited effort exerted by the patient. The various preparations of hydrolyzed protein rich foods, especially prepared for oral administration, like

soybean flours (45 per cent protein), casein (85 per cent protein), dry skim milk (35 per cent protein), wheat germ (35 per cent protein), and "Pro-Mix" (80 per cent protein), can be incorporated into such dishes as puddings, hot cereals, breads, soups, sandwich spreads, and also stirred into milk, fruit juice or tomato juice. They are, however, unpalatable and disturb digestion in some patients. (See also p. 703.) In situations of poor protein digestion, a predigested protein consisting of peptides and/or amino acids should be given orally. Examples are Vivonex (elemental amino acids, Eaton Labs) and Flexical (peptides, Mead Johnson, Evansville, Indiana).

When rehabilitating the protein malnourished adult or child it is important that all the other required nutrients be supplied also. For instance, protein rehabilitation without vitamin A can result in a vitamin A deficiency, as the protein vitamin A carrier, now available, depletes the liver of the small vitamin A stores that were present. Magnesium and potassium must also be given at the same time. Depletion of these electrolytes accompanies protein deficiency and may account for some of the neurological symptoms of the disease. Their repletion and balance are as important as the protein and calorie intake.

Kwashiorkor

Incidence. The term "kwashiorkor" was given to native children of a certain section of Africa, in whose dialect it means "the disease of the deposed baby when the next one is born." It is a comparatively new disease, being first mentioned in literature in 1933 by C. D. Williams, a Jamaican pediatrician working in the African Gold Coast. The disease appears among infants and young children in the late breast feeding, weaning and postweaning phases (usually between the ages of 1 and 4 years) wherever children are fed on high carbohydrate, low or poor quality protein diets and, if untreated, has a high mortality. Even among children receiving medical and hospital care, mortality still may be as high as 10 to 30 per cent.

Etiology. This disease is caused by insufficient good quality protein, associated with a deficiency of calories. It is often aggravated by one or other infectious processes and accompanied by severe vitamin A deficiency and may result in permanent blindness. In most of the dietary patterns in areas where kwashiorkor is endemic, the intake of animal protein foods is extremely low. The diets are also high in starchy foods and unbalanced in minerals and vitamins. That this disease is, in fact, primarily the result of lack of protein in the diet is supported by the findings of Brock and coworkers.[3, 4] These show that administration of a mixture of amino acids, without supplementary vitamins or other nutrients, is capable of initiating cure.

Symptoms. Infants and children afflicted with the disease have a feverish, generally ill condition, accompanied by universal edema, reddish pigmentation of the skin and hair, fatty liver, and loss of the enzymes from the pancreas and intestinal secretions. Additional clinical symptoms are retardation of growth and maturation, weight loss (often masked by edema), diarrhea and a variety of dermatoses. They also have a reduced number of T-cell lymphocytes and diminished cell-mediated immune response.[31] Consequently they frequently suffer from secondary infections. (See Figs. 12–24, 12–25 and 12–26.)

Treatment and Prevention. Clinical symptoms of kwashiorkor can usually be cured in four to six weeks with a diet adequate in

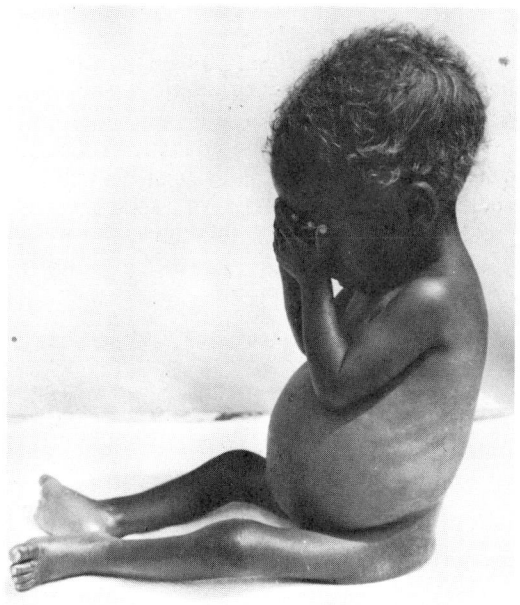

Figure 12–24 An African child suffering from kwashiorkor, the regional name for protein malnutrition. Note uncurled, graying hair, edema and skin lesions. The condition is common in areas where diets are high in starchy foods and low in protein and can be cured by protein-rich foods or by skim milk. (Courtesy Food and Agriculture Organization of the United Nations. Photo by M. Autret).

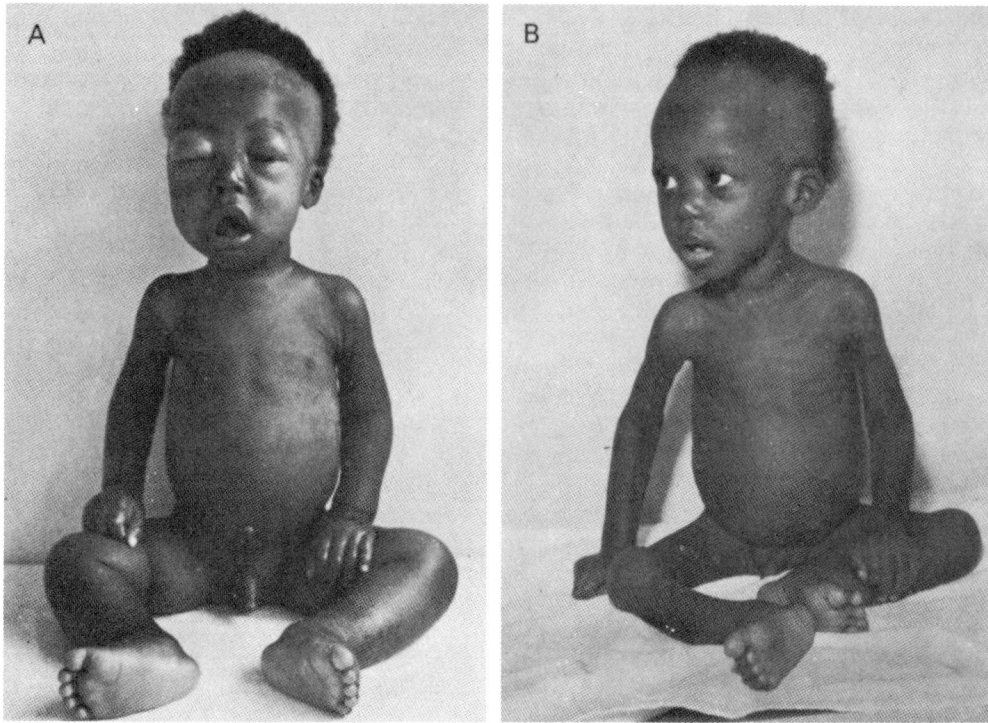

Figure 12–25   Child with kwashiorkor *(A)* on admission and *(B)* after the loss of his edema. (From: McLaren, D. S., and Burman, D.: Textbook of Paediatric Nutrition. New York, Longman, 1976, p. 122, © 1976 by Longman Group Ltd.)

nutrients and high quality protein; however, the affected mental development seems to remain throughout life.

The more difficult problem is the prevention of kwashiorkor. In areas of high prevalence, where economic factors and racial customs limit the variability and availability of proteins, including those of animal origin, prevention is difficult. Treatment and prevention of kwashiorkor lie in education and adoption of infant and preschool child feeding patterns which supply more proteins of relatively high biologic quality when infants are weaned.

A good protein supplement is dry skim milk

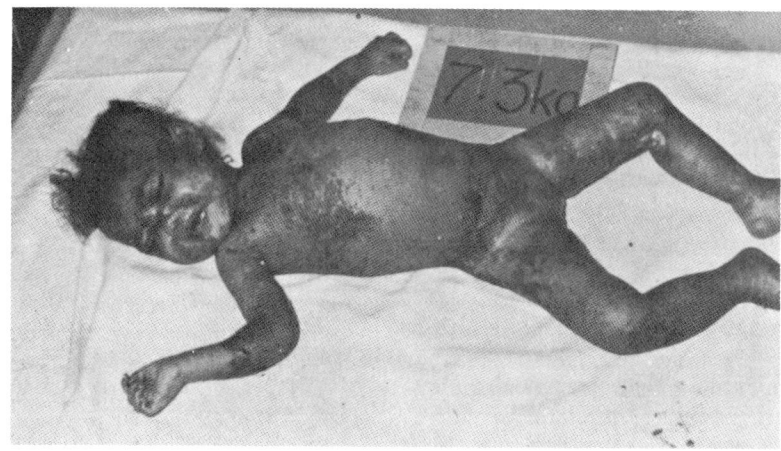

Figure 12–26   Dermatosis of kwashiorkor. (From: McLaren, D. S., and Burman, D.: Textbook of Paediatric Nutrition. New York, Longman, 1976, p. 123. © 1976 by Longman Group Ltd.)

fortified with vitamin A. However, milk is often too costly and/or unavailable where kwashiorkor is prevalent. Thus, the sources of protein must be sought and developed such as a properly selected mixture from available plant or animal sources (mutual supplementation). When economically feasible, powdered dried milk may be included, and this can be extended by judicious mixing with cheaper, locally available concentrates.

A large program for study, evaluation and improvement of children's diets has been carried out in cooperation with the government departments of Africa, sponsored jointly by UNICEF, FAO, WHO, and other agencies, particularly the United States Food and Nutrition Board. This program has culminated in the appearance of low cost nutrition foods such as Incaparina evolved by INCAP. This food mixture consists of 29 per cent ground whole maize, 29 per cent ground whole sorghum grain, 38 per cent cottonseed flour, 3 per cent Torula yeast, 1 per cent calcium carbonate, and 4500 units of added vitamin A per 100 gm. The nutritional value of this mixture in infant feeding has been established on practical as well as theoretical grounds.

FAO fostered a survey by Brock and Autret[2] in central and tropical Africa. In their report they suggest long-term measures of prevention of kwashiorkor which include (1) encouragement of an increase in the production of protective foods, especially fish, to supplement the present low protein of cereals, cassava and potatoes, (2) storage of food throughout the year to lessen the effect of the hungry months, (3) education, particularly of mothers, in better dietary practices, and (4) the development of a demonstration area, where preventive measures may be introduced, such as the use of more digestible foods and the mixing of proteins. Currently, FAO is encouraging increased protein production for human consumption. It appointed a Protein Advisory Group, which works in close liaison with the staffs of WHO, FAO and UNICEF, and is giving special attention to suitability of such low cost nutritious protein foods as oil seed presscakes, fish meal and soya products for human use. Better utilization of available food supplies is an important part of this program. Also, provision of cleaner water, removal of wastes and education in child care are needed since infections and parasitic diseases contribute to the development and appearance of kwashiorkor and malnutrition.

In India where protein-calorie malnutrition is prevalent, protein blends containing peanut protein isolate combined with either casein, lysine and methionine or dry skim milk were scientifically tried on groups of children afflicted with the disease. All groups showed satisfactory clinical responses.[36] In Mexico, Peru and Africa fish flour of *high quality* was found to be of considerable value in treatment of convalescent kwashiorkor as a supplement to maize meal diets.[27] Fish flour has a high protein content. In addition, it is a rich source of calcium and phosphorus, and contains considerable magnesium.

Amino acid supplementation of cereal grains and of protein concentrate is of benefit to the people in the cereal-consuming developing countries.[14]

Just supplying protein-rich foods is not enough to prevent protein-energy malnutrition. The entire scope of the problem, including housing, water, infections, digestibility of food and mother-child interaction must be appreciated and changed or improved. In the words of McLaren: "The malnourished child is deprived in many ways other than its nutrition and is a sick member of a sick community. The whole society is the patient."[21]

MALNUTRITION

Malnutrition adversely affects the life, development, and health of more people throughout the world than any disease. In certain areas of the United States and in the underdeveloped areas of other parts of the world, malnutrition results from the intake of too few calories, too little high quality protein, and multiple deficiencies of minerals and vitamins. It is complicated further by parasitic, bacterial, and viral infections. See Fig. 12–27.

The numerous dietary surveys which have been conducted during the past 10 years show, without exception, that malnutrition is widespread in this country. Although there are relatively few cases of severe malnutrition, there are many mild, chronic cases.

As previously pointed out, malnutrition signifies not a dietary inadequacy but a tissue deficiency of an essential nutrient. (See Chapter 11.)

Etiology. Probably the most important cause of the tissue deficiency is the failure to eat an adequate diet because of poor food habits, lack of knowledge, or economic status. An adequate diet does not only mean eating enough food to satisfy the appetite but eating the right kinds of food to provide the nutrients

SOME CAUSES OF MALNUTRITION

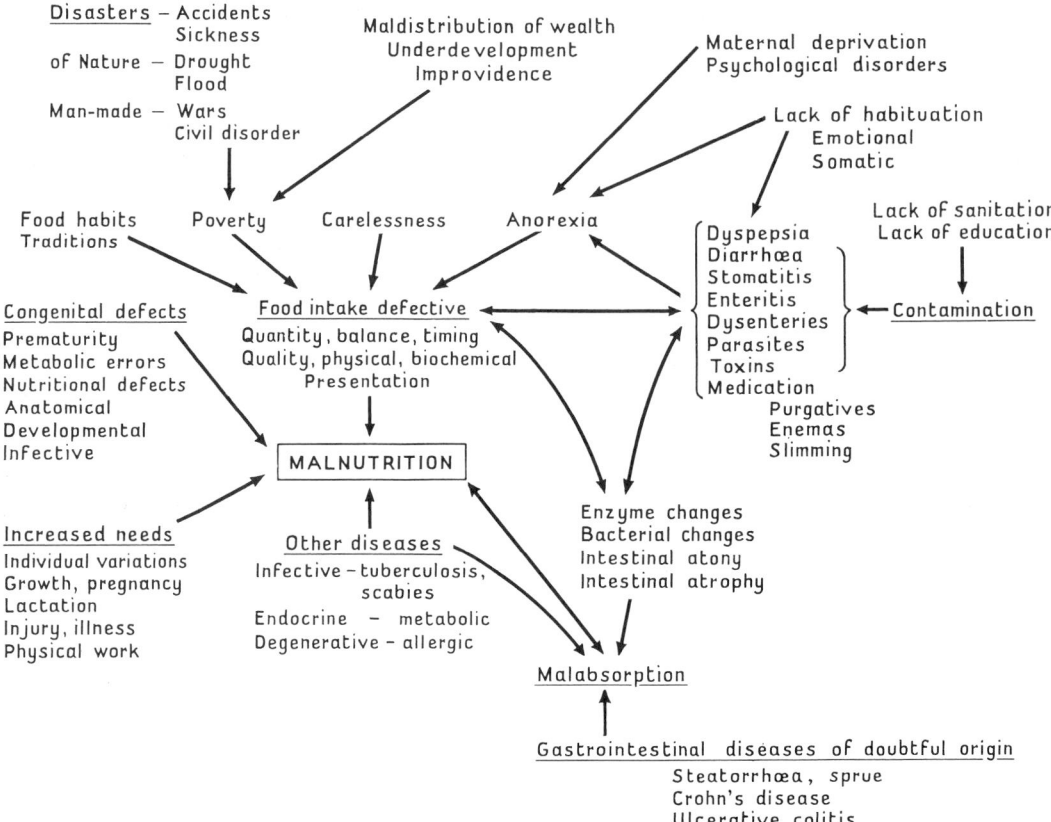

Figure 12–27 Some causes of malnutrition. (From: Williams, C. D.: Malnutrition. Lancet, 2:342, 1962.)

that are needed to build, repair, and regulate the body processes.

Sometimes a normal adequate diet is inadequate because factors either interfere with the absorption or utilization of the essential nutrients or increase the destruction, excretion, or requirements for minerals and vitamins. Many people do not eat an adequate diet every day, yet they show no apparent ill effects. This is because their diet is generally good or their requirements are less during the short period of inadequacy. If their diets were faulty for numerous or protracted periods, their bodies would show eventually that they are not getting the proper food.

Formerly, malnutrition was thought of as synonymous with underweight. It has since been demonstrated that weight is an inaccurate yardstick if used as the sole measure to judge the state of nutrition. An overweight person may be malnourished. Judging the nutritional status is not limited to one method of evalua-

tion. Individualization is of utmost importance to the successful diagnosis and treatment of malnutrition. Malnutrition is frequently associated with several other deficiency diseases that are discussed in this chapter. And, as already mentioned, malnutrition is frequently associated with chronic illness and aggressive and long-term medical and surgical treatment. See Chapters 11, 34 and 35.

PROBLEMS AND SUGGESTED TOPICS FOR DISCUSSION

1. List the predominating nutrients which are lacking in each of the following deficiency diseases: (1) night blindness, (2) beriberi, (3) ariboflavinosis, (4) pellagra, (5) scurvy, (6) rickets, and (7) simple goiter. How can a dietary history contribute to the diagnosis?
2. Find a child on the pediatric ward who is suffering from either primary or secondary malnutrition. What are his height and weight compared with the standards? Evaluate a dietary history for nutritional composition. What is being done for the malnutrition?
3. In what areas and countries is kwashiorkor prevalent?

Why is it found in these areas, and at what age is it most likely to occur? Why? Outline the dietary treatment.
4. Read and prepare a report on recent progress in early recognition and treatment of malnutrition.
5. Discuss the similarities and differences of osteoporosis and osteomalacia. What is a possible cause of each? What segment of the population is usually afflicted? What is the prevention and treatment for each?
6. What adult nutrition deficiency diseases are found in the United States today? What ages and conditions favor deficiency diseases?
7. What is being done in the developing countries to eliminate deficiency diseases?
8. Make a survey of the patients in the hospital for gastrointestinal surgery. Are any of them malnourished? What do their dietary histories reveal regarding their intake prior to the surgery?

CITED REFERENCES

1. Berlyne, G. M., et al.: The etiology of osteoporosis. The role of parathyroid hormone. JAMA, 229:1904, 1974.
2. Brock, J. F., and Autret, M.: Kwashiorkor in Africa. FAO Publ. No. 8, 1950.
3. Brock, J. F., and Hansen, J. D. L.: The role of amino acids in kwashiorkor. Am. J. Clin. Nutr., 4:286, 1956.
4. Brock, J. F., et al.: Kwashiorkor and protein malnutrition. Lancet, 2:355, 1955.
5. Carter, J.: The Ten-State Nutrition Survey: An Analysis. Atlanta, Georgia, Southern Regional Council, Inc., 1974, p. 21.
6. Council on Foods and Nutrition: Malnutrition and Hunger in the United States. JAMA, 213:272, 1970.
7. Endemic goiter and antithyroid agents. Nutr. Rev., 33:171, 1975.
8. FAO/WHO Expert Committee on Nutrition, Report VI, WHO Technical Report Series No. 245 and FAO Nutrition Report Series No. 32.
9. Geol, K. M., et al.: Florid and subclinical rickets among immigrant children in Glasgow. Lancet, 1:1141, 1976.
10. Gopalan, C., and Narasinga Rao, B. S.: Nutritional constraints on growth and development in current Indian dietaries. Indian J. Med. Res. (suppl.), 59:143, 1971.
11. Halsted, J. A., et al.: Zinc deficiency in man—the Shivaz experiment. Am. J. Med., 53:277, 1972.
12. Hambidge, K. M., et al.: Low levels of zinc in hair, anorexia, poor growth, and hypogeusia in children. Pediatr. Res., 6:868, 1972.
13. Hegsted, D. M.: Nutrition, bone and calcification. J. Am. Diet. Assoc., 50:107, 1967.
14. Howe, E. E., et al.: Amino acid supplementation of cereal grains as related to the world food supply. Am. J. Clin. Nutr., 16:315 and 321, 1965.
15. Johnson, N. E., Alcantara, E. N., and Linkswiler, H.: Effect of level of protein intake on urinary and fecal calcium and calcium retention of young adult males. J. Nutr., 100:1425, 1970.
16. Jolliffe, N. (ed.): Clinical Nutrition. 2nd ed. New York, Harper and Brothers, 1962.
17. Jowsey, J., Riggs, B. L., and Kelly, P. J.: Long term experience with fluoride and fluoride combination treatment of osteoporosis. In Kuhlencordt, F., and Kruse, H. (eds.): Calcium Metabolism, Bone and Metabolic Bone Disease. New York, Springer-Verlag, 1973.
18. Keys, A., et al.: The Biology of Human Starvation. Vol. II, Minneapolis, The University of Minnesota Press, 1950, pp. 1213–1215.
19. Krishnaswamy, K., et al.: Effect of vitamin B_6 on leucine induced changes in human subjects. Am. J. Clin. Nutr., 29:177, 1976.
20. Lutwak, L.: Dietary calcium and reversal of bone demineralization. Nutrition News, 37(1), 1974.
21. McLaren, D. S.: Nutrition and Its Disorders. Baltimore, Williams & Wilkins Company, 1972.
22. Moynahan, E. J.: Acrodermatitis enteropathica: a lethal inherited human zinc deficiency. Lancet, 2:399, 1974.
23. Neldner, K. H., and Hambidge, K. M.: Zinc therapy of acrodermatitis enteropathica. N. Engl. J. Med., 292:879, 1975.
24. Nordin, B. E. C.: Metabolic Bone and Stone Disease. Baltimore, Williams & Wilkins Co., 1973.
25. Nordin, B. E. C., et al.: Calcium absorption in the elderly. In Nielsen, S. P., and Hjörting-Hansen, E. (eds.): Calcified Tissues, 1975. Copenhagen, Fadl Publishing Co., 1976.
26. Prasad, A. S., et al.: Zinc metabolism in patients with the syndrome of iron deficiency anemia, hepatosplenomegaly, dwarfism, and hypogonadism. J. Lab. Clin. Med., 61:537, 1963.
27. Pretorius, P. J., and Wehmeyer, A. S.: An assessment of nutritive value of fish flour in the treatment of convalescent kwashiorkor patients. Am. J. Clin. Nutr., 14:147, 1964.
28. Rao, K. S.: Evolution of kwashiorkor and marasmus. Lancet, 1:709, 1974.
29. Rizvi, S. N. A., and Vaishnava, H.: Secondary hyperparathyroidism in nutritional osteomalacia. J. Indian Med. Assoc., 64:199, 1975.
30. Sandstead, H.: Zinc nutrition in the United States. Am. J. Clin. Nutr., 26:1251, 1973.
31. Schopfer, K., and Douglas, D. S.: In vitro studies of lymphocytes from children with kwashiorkor. Clin. Immunol. Immunopath., 5:21, 1976.
32. Ten-State Nutrition Survey, 1968–1970, DHEW Publ. No. (HSM) 72–8134. Health Services and Mental Health Administration, Washington, D.C., 1972.
33. Tucker, S. B., et al.: Acquired zinc deficiency. Cutaneous manifestations typical of acrodermatitis enteropathica. JAMA, 235:2399, 1976.
34. Victor, M., Adams, R. D., and Collins, G. H.: The Wernicke-Korsakoff Syndrome. Philadelphia, F. A. Davis Co., 1971.
35. Walker, R. M., and Linkswiler, H.: Calcium retention in the adult human male as affected by protein intake. J. Nutr., 102:1297, 1972.
36. Webb, J. K., et al.: Peanut protein and milk protein blends in the treatment of kwashiorkor. Am. J. Clin. Nutr., 14:331, 1964.
37. Youmans, J. B.: The changing face of nutritional disease in America. JAMA, 189:672, 1964.

ADDITIONAL REFERENCES

Acrodermatitis Enteropathica-Hereditary Zinc Deficiency. Nutr. Rev., 33:327, 1975.
Autret, M. A., and Behar, M.: Sindrome Policarencial Infantil (Kwashiorkor) and Its Prevention in Central America. Rome, Italy, Food and Agricultural Organization of the United Nations, October, 1954.
Baum, J. L., and Rao. G.: Keratomalacia in the cachetic hospitalized patient. Am. J. Opthamol., 82:435, 1976.

Bhagavan, R. K., et al.: Use of isolated vegetable proteins in the treatment of protein malnutrition (kwashiorkor). Am J. Clin. Nutr., *11*:127, 1962.

Bloom, W. L., and Flinchum, D.: Osteomalacia with pseudofractures caused by the ingestion of aluminum hydroxide. J.A.M.A., *174*:1327, 1960.

Butterworth, C. E., and Blackburn, G. L.: Hospital malnutrition. Nutr. Today, *10*:8, 1975.

Cartwright, G. E., and Deiss, A.: Sideroblasts, siderocytes and sideroblastic anemia. N. Engl. J. Med., *292*:185, 1975.

Coursin, D. B.: Effects of undernutrition on central nervous system function. Nutr. Rev., *23*:65, 1965.

Davidson, S., et al.: Human Nutrition and Dietetics. 6th ed. Edinburgh, Churchill Livingstone, 1975.

Downs, E. F.: Nutritional dwarfing: A syndrome of early protein-calorie malnutrition. Am. J. Clin. Nutr., *15*:275, 1965.

Gershoff, S. N.: Who is well nourished? Nutr. Rev., *19*:321, 1961.

Human pantothenic acid deficiency. Nutr. Rev., *14*:37, 1956.

Ingelfinger, F. J.: For want of an enzyme. Nutrition Today, *3*:2, 1968.

John, T. J., et al.: Kwashiorkor not associated with poverty. J. Pediatr., *90*:730, 1977.

Jolliffe, N.: Clinical Nutrition, 2nd ed. New York, Harper & Brothers, 1962.

Lozoff, B., and Fanaroff, A. A.: Kwashiorkor in Cleveland. Am. J. Dis. Child., *129*:710, 1975.

Lymphocyte number and function in protein malnutrition. Nutr. Rev., *34*:208, 1976.

McLaren, D. S., and Burman, D.: Textbook of Pediatric Nutrition. Edinburgh, Churchill Livingstone, 1976, Chapter 8—Vitamin deficiency, toxicity and dependency.

McLaren, D. S.: Xerophthalmia: A neglected problem. Nutr. Rev., *22*:289, 1964.

Nizel, A. E., and Shulman, J. S.: Interaction of dietetics and nutrition with dentistry. Recent advances and needs. J. Am. Dietet. A., *55*:470, 1969.

Nutrition in oral health: research and practice. Dairy Council Digest, *40*(6), 1969.

Pak, C. Y. C., et al.: The treatment of osteoporosis with calcium infusions. Am. J. Med., *47*:7, 1969.

Pereira, S. M., and Begum, A.: Prevention of vitamin A deficiency. Am. J. Clin. Nutr., *22*:858, 1969.

Review. Gluten enteropathy. Nutr. Rev., *21*:300, 1963.

Review. Goiter and iodine deficiency. Nutr. Rev., *22*:169, 1964.

Review. Intestinal calcium and bone formation. Nutr. Rev., *23*:6, 1965.

Roe, D. A.: Plague of Corn. A Social History of Pellagra. Ithaca, New York, Cornell University Press, 1973.

Schaefer, A. E.: Nutritional deficiencies in developing countries. J. Am. Dietet. A., *42*:295, 1963.

Schwartz, M. K., et al.: The effect of a gluten-free diet on fat, nitrogen and mineral metabolism in patients with sprue. Gastroenterology, *32*:232, 1957.

Scrimshaw, N. S.: Synergism of malnutrition and infection. J.A.M.A., *212*:1685, 1970.

Scrimshaw, N. S., et al.: Kwashiorkor in children and its response to protein therapy. J.A.M.A., *164*:555, 1957.

Sherlock, P., and Rothchild, E. O.: Scurvy produced by a zen macrobiotic diet. J.A.M.A., *199*:130, 1967.

Shils, M. E.: Experimental human magnesium depletion. I. Clinical observations and blood chemistry alterations. Am. J. Clin. Nutr., *15*:133, 1964.

Sunderman, F. W.: Current status of zinc deficiency in the pathogenesis of neurological, dermatological and musculoskeletal disorders. Ann. Clin. Lab. Sci., *5*:132, 1975.

Swaminathan, M. C.: Prevention of vitamin deficiency by administration of massive doses of vitamin A. Proc. First Asian Congress Nutr., Hyderabad, 1972, p. 695.

Tandon, M. I., et al.: Small intestine in protein malnutrition. Am. J. Clin. Nutr., *21*:813, 1968.

Webb, J. K., et al.: Peanut protein and milk protein blends in the treatment of kwashiorkor. Am. J. Clin. Nutr., *14*:331, 1964.

Whitehead, R. G., and Dean, R. F. A.: Serum amino acids in kwashiorkor. I. Relationship to clinical condition. Am. J. Clin. Nutr., *14*:313, 1964.

Williams, C. D.: Kwashiorkor. A nutritional disease of children associated with a maize diet. Lancet, *2*:1151, 1935.

Chapter 13

NUTRITION FOR PREGNANCY AND LACTATION

NUTRITION AND FETAL GROWTH

It is not known completely how nutrition or malnutrition affects growth, but knowledge in this area is rapidly expanding. With new techniques for measuring cell number and cell size, it is now possible to measure cellular growth and to gain new insights into the way organisms grow.

Each cell contains the specific amount of deoxyribonucleic acid (DNA) in its nucleus that is peculiar to its species; the human cell contains 6.0 picograms (pg.) of DNA. By determining the total amount of DNA in an organ and dividing this by the standard amount of DNA per cell, it is possible to calculate the number of cells in the organ. By weighing the organ to establish the total amount of protein, then dividing this by the number of cells, the amount of protein in each cell may be computed. This is a measure of cell size. The ribonucleic acid (RNA) of a cell, contained only in the cytoplasm, is an indication of the extent of cellular differentiation. These techniques have helped to determine three stages of growth:

1. *Hyperplasia.* In this stage the DNA content and the cell protein content increase at equal rates. Cell number is increasing.

2. *Hyperplasia and hypertrophy.* In this stage DNA synthesis slows and protein synthesis continues at the previous rate. Cell number continues to increase, but cell size increases at a faster rate.

3. *Hypertrophy.* In this stage DNA synthesis stops and protein synthesis continues. Cell size increases, while cell number stays the same.

All these phases of growth depend on the presence of the proper amount of nutrients for enzyme and cellular construction. The effect of a lack of the proper nutrients depends on the timing, severity and duration of the deficiency.

Laboratory rats malnourished from birth to weaning, were small and did not achieve normal size, even though there was some "catch-up" growth after termination of malnutrition and subsequent nutritional rehabilitation. Rats malnourished later in life were smaller than normal at the end of the period of malnutrition, but after rehabilitation, they achieved normal size. For these rats the "catch up" growth was complete. This time factor probably explains why nutritional rehabilitation after childhood malnutrition results in the attainment of normal size in some children and not in others. Malnutrition at some periods in development is more detrimental than at other times, and the fetal period seems to be a most vulnerable one.

How malnutrition during fetal or infant growth affects the development of the brain has attracted a great deal of attention, and well it should, considering its importance for human-

ity, particularly in developing countries where childhood malnutrition is rampant. In the human brain, cell division (hyperplasia) stops shortly after the age of 12 to 18 months. Malnutrition severe enough to cause death within the first year of life can also result in a brain with fewer cells. However, we cannot assume that a smaller brain in a smaller body (as most of these children have) is necessarily detrimental. Women usually have smaller bodies and smaller brains than men do. Evidence of reduction in dendritic growth, myelinization or in neurochemical development is probably more important as a determinant of retarded brain growth.

Different parts of the brain grow at different rates throughout the fetal period and the first year of postnatal life. The effect that retarded growth of areas at various stages of development has on later intellectual performance and behavior is still unclear. It is difficult to separate malnutrition-induced growth retardation from that caused by the social, physical or cultural environment surrounding the growing infant. However, the majority of children with fetal malnutrition have behavioral difficulties and an impaired capacity for learning.[11, 14]

The extent of the "catch-up" growth following nutritional rehabilitation (if it is provided) depends on the timing of the nutritional care. Early nutritional rehabilitation, when cells are still dividing, can result in an increase in cell number and in the capacity for attainment of normal size. Later rehabilitation, when cells have stopped dividing, results in cell growth only, and there is no potential for achieving maximal organ or organism size.

PREGNANCY

The nutritional status and nutritional intake of the mother during pregnancy is one of the most important parts of the "matroenvironment."* Many studies, nutrition surveys,[5, 12, 17, 38] observations in Holland of the effect of war starvation on pregnancy[34] and food supplementation programs for pregnant women[18, 29] affirm this fact. It is important to identify malnourished women (see Chapter 11, Assessment of Nutritional Status) and rehabilitate them prior to conception or as soon as possible after conception, through the provision of food, nutritional counseling and good prenatal care.

During pregnancy, the body requirements for food differ from those of a normal nonpregnant woman. Immediately following fertilization, the maternal organism begins a readjustment to provide the environment it needs to support life and the normal growth of the fetus and to support lactation after the birth of the infant. The metabolic and physiological changes involving all organs and systems of the mother's body take place during pregnancy. For the child, nine months old at birth, the intrauterine months represent the period of most rapid growth and development of the entire life cycle. All dietary essentials are increased proportionately to supply the additional demands of the mother and the growing fetus (Fig. 13–1).

Although the adage that the pregnant woman must "eat for two" is not accurate quantitatively, it does denote the increased nutritional demands of the woman during pregnancy. Although the fetus is parasitic on the mother to a degree that depends on her nutritional state and her diet during pregnancy, if the mother is sufficiently depleted nutritionally, the fetus may suffer to spare her. The diet of the mother during pregnancy affects the condition of her infant at birth and during the first two weeks of life; the better diet produces babies in better physical condition. Stillborn, low birth weight, premature and congenitally defective infants are more frequently born to mothers who have had an inadequate diet prior to and during pregnancy. It appears that the mother also benefits from being in good nutritional condition during pregnancy. Burke and colleagues[6, 8] found a greater incidence of complications, owing largely to a higher percentage of toxemia, among women with poor diets.

Most authorities agree that the nutritional status of the mother prior to conception is important. Baird concluded that the nutritional status of the mother, the result of her lifetime dietary habits, had a greater influence on the outcome of pregnancy than her diet during pregnancy.[1]

It may even be that the nutritional status of her own mother will influence the outcome of her pregnancy.[26, 39] Foundations are laid down during prenatal life and early childhood. Many other factors—genetic, biological, socioeconomic and psychological—are involved. An understanding of the role of nutrition in reproduction is based on the concept that pregnancy is a normal state and not a pathological one.

---

*Word coined by John E. Gordon to describe the physiological, biological and sociocultural environment that a mother provides for her infant.

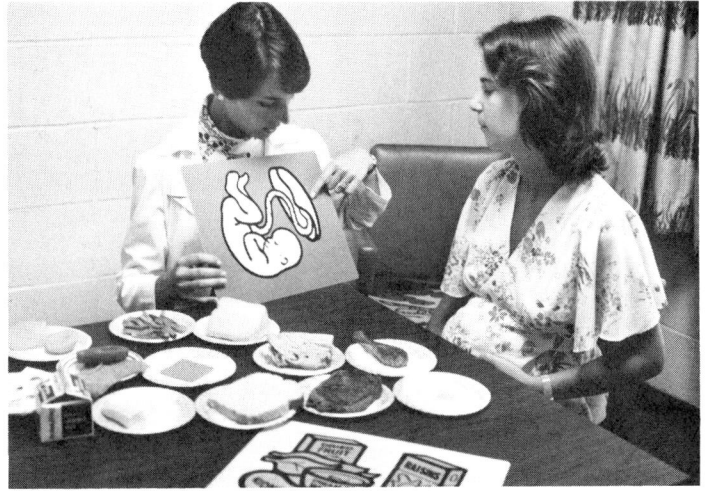

Figure 13–1 A pregnant woman learning about food in relation to her pregnancy. (Photograph courtesy of Nutrition Department, Lutheran General Hospital, Park Ridge, Illinois.)

PHYSICAL AND BIOCHEMICAL CHANGES

Many physical and biochemical changes occur in normal pregnancy. As the blood volume increases, concentration of hemoglobin is reduced. Plasma albumin falls. Amino acids may be excreted in the urine. Edema is sometimes present. Changes occur in cardiac and pulmonary functions. Serum alkaline phosphatase may rise markedly and other enzymes increase in amount. Most plasma lipid fractions rise during pregnancy. The thyroid gland often enlarges because of the loss of inorganic iodine in the urine. A renal loss of folate occurs in some individuals. During late pregnancy, the ability to excrete a water load is below normal and the water may pool in the lower limbs. This fluid retention is normal. The stomach shows signs of depressed function. (Histamine is depressed and pepsin production is reduced.) A reduced secretion of hydrochloric acid could have a depressing effect on calcium and iron absorption. Reduced motility of the gastrointestinal tract can result in constipation. A relaxed cardiac sphincter may produce regurgitation into the esophagus and "heartburn." Appetite and thirst increase during the first trimester. Once the early morning nausea subsides the ravenous appetite often returns. Cravings for or aversions to certain foods are common. *Pica*, the desire to eat non-food substances such as clay, laundry starch or cigarette ashes, develops in some women. Digestion and assimilation of foods are generally efficient. Clinical standards considered "normal" for the non-pregnant woman cannot be used as standards for the pregnant woman.

Weight gain reflects the physiological effects of pregnancy. The recommended weight gain during pregnancy is 24 pounds (12.5 kg.). However, this varies considerably. Young women tend to gain more weight than older women, primigravidas more than multigravidas and thin women more than fat women.

The height of the woman appears to be an important factor in the course and outcome of her pregnancy. In 1952, Baird showed that the incidence of stillbirths and difficult labor was higher among short women. Short stature may reflect the mother's poor nutrition from childhood, which pevented her from achieving her full genetic potential. Her poor nutritional status could result in a less than optimal environment for the fetus.

The incidence of low birth weight infants and closely related neonatal mortality rates are affected by the socioeconomic status of the mother. Other factors such as biological immaturity (under 17 years of age), low prepregnancy weight for height, small weight gain during pregnancy, short stature, poor nutritional status, smoking, infectious agents, chronic disease, history of unsuccessful pregnancies and complications of pregnancy are affected by the socioeconomic status of the mother. The most vulnerable individuals are those born and brought up in poor homes and in large families, where access to food, education and medical care is inadequate. However, women who have had sufficient income may also arrive at childbearing age with poor nutritional status and poor health habits.

Investigations into the psychological factors associated with fetal and infant mortality and morbidity are inconclusive. Anxiety has been

shown to be a predictor of poor outcome of pregnancy when it occurs late in pregnancy. In addition, anxiety usually affects an adequate intake of the protective foods and thus leads to poor nutrition. The pregnant woman may overeat or may suffer deprivation.

THE FETUS AND THE PLACENTA

How the placenta controls the supply of nutrients to the fetus is unclear. The placenta is responsible from early gestation for the transfer of sufficient amounts of all substances needed for growth and development to the fetus and for the return of nutrient excesses and waste products to the maternal circulation. Transfer of the nutrients takes place in several stages. Diffusion may be at one stage and active transport at another. Conversions and syntheses probably take place within the substances as they pass through.

Most of the nitrogen reaches the fetus as amino acids. Concentrations of amino acids, calcium and phosphorus are higher in fetal than in maternal blood. Active transport apparently takes place at the stage of their passage through the placenta. Glucose is transported to the fetus. From glucose the fetus receives energy and makes its own glycogen and fat. Essential fatty acids are transferred. Other fats are synthesized from glucose. The level of blood glucose apparently influences the rate of fetal growth. If the blood sugar is low near term, the fetus fails to store glycogen in its liver.

Periods of fasting even as short as 12 hours in the pregnant woman result in lower serum glucose levels, greater ketosis and less glyconeogenesis than in non-pregnant women. Although the serum ketones and glucose in the fetus cannot be measured, concentration of glucose in the amniotic fluid falls and ketone concentration rises. This probably reflects the resulting hyperketonemia and increased use of ketones by the developing fetal brain. What this means for the development of brain and other fetal tissue is unknown, but the practice of restricting weight gain with a low carbohydrate diet and periods of fasting should be condemned.[13] The data suggest that the human placenta is better able to buffer protein deficiencies by maintaining higher amino acid levels in the fetal circulation than it is able to buffer caloric deficiencies.

Sufficient amounts of iron, ascorbic acid, pyridoxine, folacin and cobalamin are transported to meet the demands of the fetus even at the expense of maternal reserves. The fetus and maternal tissue compete for riboflavin, thiamin and vitamin D. More vitamins A and E are present in maternal circulation than in the fetus.

The DNA increases linearly to about 35 weeks' gestation and then diminishes. Protein and RNA increase linearly to term. In infants with intrauterine growth retardation, placentas have a reduced DNA concentration, a markedly elevated RNA–DNA ratio and a decrease in total cell number. The high RNA–DNA ratio in the placenta may be a useful tool for studying malnutrition in the fetus.

It is suspected that some circulatory changes brought about by smoking may interfere with normal transport of nutrients to the placenta. More research is needed to determine the maternal factors that influence the supply line to the fetus.

ADOLESCENCE

Currently, the number of women under the age of 17 who become pregnant and have their babies is increasing. If the prospective mother is an adolescent, her diet requires individual attention to include the needs for her own growth as well as that of the developing fetus. Many of these girls enter into pregnancy with inadequate nutritional stores and are poorly equipped to meet the demands of motherhood. (See Chapter 15, Nutrition in Childhood and Adolescence.)

Girls who become pregnant before they are 17 years of age are at great risk both biologically and psychologically. Mortality rates are high among infants born to very young mothers. The psychological aspects of adolescence superimposed on those inherent in pregnancy add to the emotional burden carried by the adolescent. There is a great deal of risk for a teenager's first baby, but it appears that the second and third babies present bigger problems—the infant death rate is even higher.

The increase in the nutritional requirements for the adolescent and the woman during pregnancy in relation to those of the normally active and healthy non-pregnant woman is shown in the recommendations of the Food and Nutritional Board of the National Research Council. These requirements are given in Table 13–1 (from Table 10–1, Chapter 10). The increased allowances are only guides and must be carefully adjusted to the needs of the individual; they will vary with the age, the weight and the activity of the mother. The increased amounts recommended are based on the assumption

Table 13–1   RECOMMENDED DIETARY ALLOWANCES*

	NON-PREGNANT FEMALES				Pregnancy	Lactation
	11–14 yr.[a]	15–18 yr.[b]	19–22 yr.[c]	23–50 yr.[c]		
Energy (kcal.)	2400	2100	2100	2000	+300	+500
Protein (g.)	44	48	46	46	+30	+20
Vitamin A (I.U.)	4000	4000	4000	4000	5000	6000
Vitamin D (I.U.)	400	400	400		400	400
Vitamin E (I.U.)	12	12	12	12	15	15
Ascorbic acid (mg.)	45	45	45	45	60	80
Folacin (mcg.)	400	400	400	400	800	600
Niacin (mg.)	16	14	14	13	+2	+4
Riboflavin (mg.)	1.3	1.4	1.4	1.2	+0.3	+0.5
Thiamin (mg.)	1.2	1.1	1.1	1.0	+0.3	+0.3
Vitamin B_6 (mg.)	1.6	2.0	2.0	2.0	2.5	2.5
Vitamin B_{12} (mcg.)	3	3	3	3	4	4
Calcium (mg.)	1200	1200	800	800	1200	1200
Phosphorus (mg.)	1200	1200	800	800	1200	1200
Iodine (mcg.)	115	115	100	100	125	150
Iron (mg.)	18	18	18	18	†	18
Magnesium (mg.)	300	300	300	300	450	450
Zinc (mg.)	15	15	15	15	20	25

*From: Food and Nutrition Board, National Academy of Sciences–National Research Council, 8th ed., 1974.
[a]Weight 44 kg. (97 lb.), height 155 cm. (62 in.)
[b]Weight 54 kg. (119 lb.), height 162 cm. (65 in.)
[c]Weight 58 kg. (128 lb.), height 162 cm. (65 in.)
†The increased requirements of pregnancy cannot usually be met by ordinary diets; therefore, the use of supplemental iron is recommended.

that the woman is in sound nutritional condition at conception.

NUTRITION IN PREGNANCY

Calories

During the course of pregnancy, the total energy cost of storage plus maintenance (additional work of the maternal heart and uterus and the steady rise in basal metabolism) amounts to approximately 80,000 kcal. The energy cost of pregnancy then is about 300 kcalories a day. Energy intake should be 36 kcal. per kg. of pregnant weight per day. (One kg. equals approximately 2.2 pounds.) Present evidence suggests that in a population such as ours where women are sedentary, there is no reduction of activity during the last trimester of pregnancy and therefore no saving of calories.[4]

Weight Gain

The components of the maternal weight gain are shown in Table 13–2 and in Figure 13–2. The weight of the blood volume and the enlargement of the reproductive organs are fairly constant. If the weight gain is less than the weight of the maternal components in pregnancy the growth of the fetus calls on the reserves of the mother. Although weight gain

varies, general agreement is found in the literature that the normal curve of weight gain is sigmoid in shape. During the first trimester there is a small gain, a more rapid gain the second trimester and a slower rate of gain in weight during the third trimester (Fig. 13–3).

The Committee on Maternal Nutrition and the Course of Pregnancy recommended an average gain in weight during pregnancy of 24 pounds (range 20 to 27 lb). This amount is commensurate with a better than average course and outcome of pregnancy. The curve of weight gain would be that shown in Figure 13–3. A gain of 1.5 to 3.0 lb. (0.7 to 1.3 kg.) during the first trimester and a gain of 0.8 lb.

Table 13–2   MATERNAL WEIGHT GAIN

TISSUE	WEIGHT (Pounds)
Fetus	7.5
Uterus	2.0
Placenta	1.5
Amniotic fluid	2.0
Blood volume	3.0
Extracellular fluid accretion	2.0
Breast tissue	1.0
Fat	9.0
Total	28.0

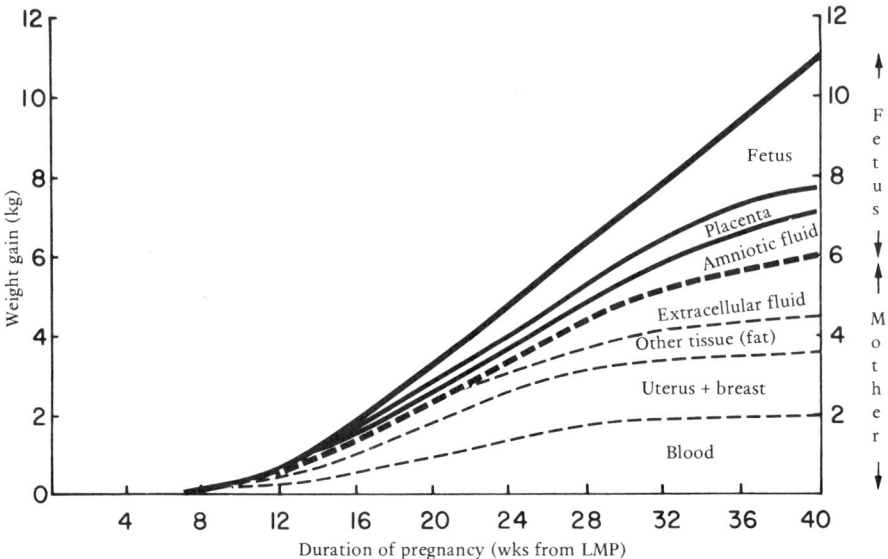

Figure 13–2 Average pattern and components of maternal weight gain during pregnancy. (From: Schneider, H. S.: Nutritional Support of Medical Practice. New York, Harper & Row, 1978.)

(0.35 kg.) per week during the remainder of pregnancy is a guideline. The pattern of weight gain is more important than the total amount gained. A sudden gain in weight after the twentieth week of pregnancy may indicate water retention and the possible onset of pre-eclampsia.

The energy stored as fat in the maternal tissue is found in fat deposits primarily, with a small deposit in the mammary glands. Fat serves as energy reserve and prevents catabolism of the mother's tissues, especially during lactation. After delivery of the baby the added fat is usually lost in a short time, particularly if the infant is breast-fed.

Approximately 1800 to 2800 kcalories of foods carefully selected for their nutritive value are necessary to meet essential requirements. Any regimen below this would be inadequate in nutrients. Severe calorie restriction limits the nutrients essential for the growth and development of the fetus and those essential to the mother. Weight control should be based on an adequate dietary program and not on the restriction of water and salt. An overweight woman should not correct her weight problem during pregnancy. It is better to increase exercise than to restrict caloric intake to less than the Recommended Daily Allowance (RDA). An adolescent under 17 years old should not be restricted in calories below energy needs for her own growth and that of the fetus, about 2400 to 2700 kcalories. If obese, the young

adolescent should still be expected to gain weight. The standardized diets used in most prenatal clinics are unsuited to the nutritional needs of the adolescent. Each adolescent requires special individual counseling.

Protein

The Food and Nutrition Board of the National Research Council suggests adding 30 gm. of protein daily in addition to the usual 0.8 gm. per kg. body weight. Adjusted for body size, this is 1.3 gm. per kg. pregnant weight for mature women 19 years or older, 1.5 gm. per kg. pregnant weight for the 15 to 18 year old teenager and 1.7 gm. per kg. pregnant weight for the younger girl. The additional protein provides for the increase in maternal tissue and for the growth of the fetus. Two thirds of the proteins should be of animal origin of the highest biological values (meat, milk, eggs, cheese, poultry and fish), since they furnish all the essential amino acids.

If protein needs are met, all other nutrients except ascorbic acid, vitamin A and vitamin D will probably be provided because of their association with protein in food. If protein is inadequate in the pregnant woman's diet, calcium, phosphorus, iron and B vitamins will usually also be inadequate.

The additional protein, calorie and calcium needs can be met by drinking one quart of skim

Prenatal Gain In Weight

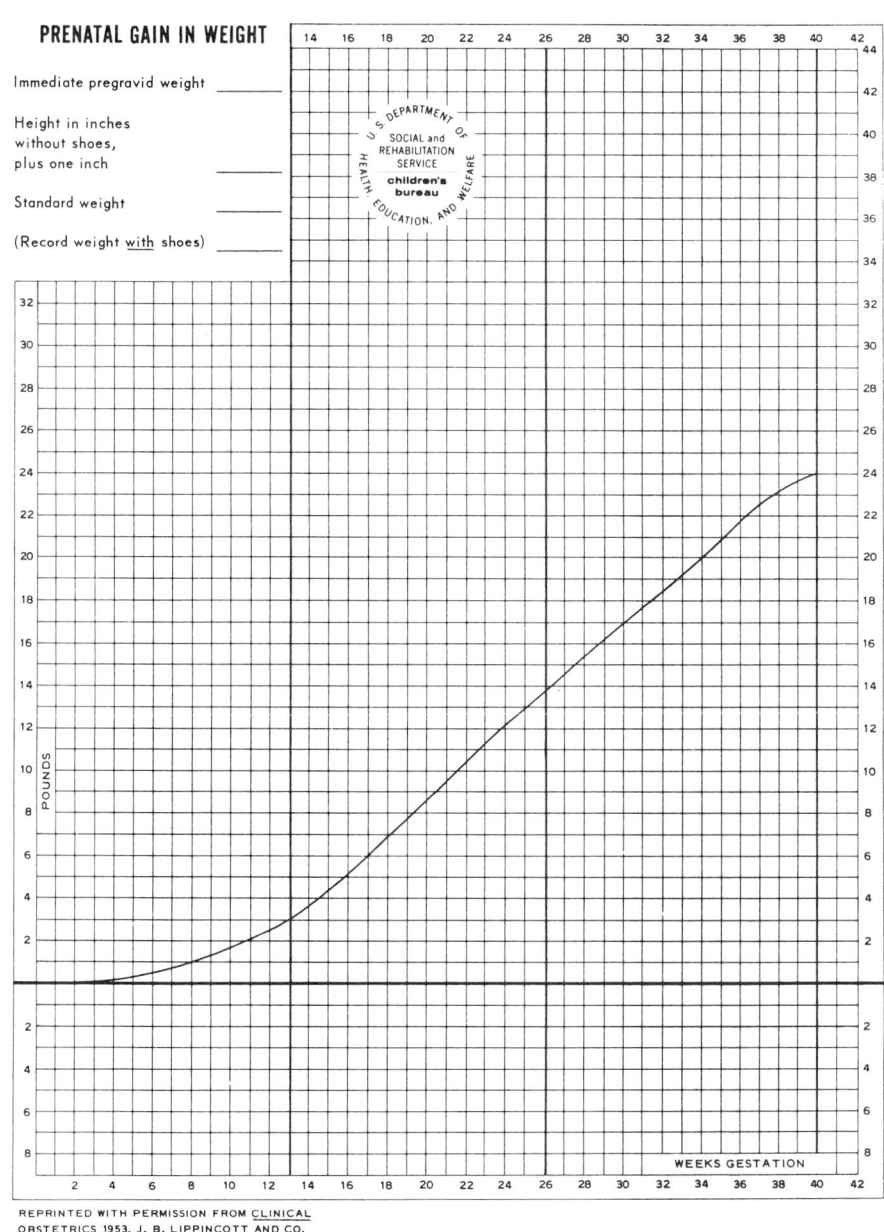

PRENATAL GAIN IN WEIGHT

Immediate pregravid weight _____

Height in inches
without shoes,
plus one inch _____

Standard weight _____

(Record weight <u>with</u> shoes) _____

POUNDS

WEEKS GESTATION

REPRINTED WITH PERMISSION FROM <u>CLINICAL</u>
<u>OBSTETRICS</u> 1953, J. B. LIPPINCOTT AND CO.

Figure 13–3 Curve of normal weight gain during pregnancy.

milk a day, which is why milk drinking is usually recommended for the pregnant woman.

Inadequacies in the protein content of the diet of the pregnant woman may lead to nutritional edema. Some research workers believe that a diet low in proteins may be a cause of toxemia of pregnancy. Other disorders of pregnancy that may result from a low protein intake are anemia, poor muscle tone of the uterus, abortion, lowered resistance to infection and insufficient lactation. The studies of Burke and co-workers[7] show that the weight, length and general condition of the infant at birth are related to the amount of protein con-

sumed by the mother. Consequently, the investigators suggest that "less than 75 gm. of protein daily during the latter part of pregnancy result in an infant who will tend to be short, light in weight, and most likely receive a low pediatric rating in other respects."[7]

An extensive study by Dieckmann and coworkers[10] revealed that women who increased their protein consumption throughout pregnancy had less anemia, no miscarriages and healthier babies, as compared with women who did not receive extra protein foods. No correlation was found, however, between the weight and length of the infants and the protein intake of the mother, although an increase in caloric intake is positively correlated with an increase in birth weight.[22]

Furthermore, protein increases the absorption of calcium. In the presence of a high protein intake, 15 per cent of the calcium was absorbed, while in the low protein diet only 5 per cent of the calcium was absorbed.[23] Amino acids probably facilitate calcium absorption. This could be significant in cases in which calcium intake is low and absorption is poor. A high protein diet may convert a calcium deficiency into sufficiency.

Calcium, Phosphorus and Vitamin D

Calcium is one of the most important elements of the diet for the pregnant woman. Since phosphorus and vitamin D are linked so closely with calcium metabolism, they are considered here at the same time. An adequate supply of vitamin D is essential for utilization of the calcium and phosphorus necessary for the calcification of the fetal bones and teeth, as well as for the gravid woman's own needs. If a pregnant woman's diet is inadequate in calcium she will have to sacrifice calcium from her bones in the interests of the developing fetus. Approximately 30 gm. of calcium is needed by the infant before birth, two thirds of it during the last trimester of pregnancy. The need for approximately 16 gm. of phosphorus by the fetus follows a similar pattern. Despite evidence showing that calcium absorption is increased during pregnancy and lactation, the daily intake of calcium must be increased from 0.8 gm., the standard non-pregnant adult daily allowance, to 1.2 gm. to satisfy these additional needs. Calcium intake recommendations for the pregnant young adolescent are the same: 1.2 gm. per day. Meeting the requirement for phosphorus is less of a problem, since it is present in many processed foods, in meat and

in many calcium-rich foods. If the woman drinks vitamin-fortified milk or is exposed to the sun, her vitamin D requirements will be met. If protein and calcium requirements are fulfilled, the need for phosphorus likely will be met as well.

Iron

During pregnancy there is an increased need for iron to supply the growing fetus. Iron is stored in the liver of the fetus for use during the first three to six months of life. During the second half of pregnancy the mother requires 6 mg. of iron daily to increase her own blood volume and transfer necessary iron to the placenta and fetus. To this must be added 0.5 to 1 mg. of iron to replace that lost through the intestine, urinary tract and integument. Thus the daily requirement for iron in the second half of pregnancy is about 7 mg. This 7 mg. comes from the maternal stores, from her diet and from supplementary iron. Iron stores are very often insufficient to meet the requirements of pregnancy. Dietary intake does not provide all the necessary iron. American women usually ingest 9 to 12 mg. of iron daily or only 1.5 to 1.8 mg. of absorbed iron. That is why the RDA is set at 18 mg. throughout pregnancy, so that stores will be increased. Fortunately, the rate of absorption of iron is increased in pregnancy. However, the Food and Nutrition Board in its 1974 revision of Daily Dietary Allowances also recommended iron supplementation of the diet to meet the demands for iron during pregnancy. Because an otherwise adequate diet contains approximately 6 mg. of iron per 1000 kcalories and because women often enter pregnancy with suboptimal stores and low hemoglobin values, a daily supplement of 30 to 60 mg. of iron in the form of ferrous salt daily during the second and third trimesters is recommended. From 120 to 240 mg. of iron per day is recommended for women who do not have iron stores, as would be reflected in a low serum iron level and a high total iron binding capacity (TIBC). If the additional demands for iron are not met, hypochromic anemia usually results (see Chapter 29).

Hemoglobin production also requires an adequate supply of protein to furnish essential amino acids, sufficient calories to protect the protein from catabolic degradation and iron and other minerals such as copper, zinc, folic acid, vitamin B_{12} and other co-factors involved in the synthesis of heme and globin.

Iodine

This mineral is of special importance in pregnancy to meet the added demands placed upon the metabolism by the thyroid gland, to meet the needs for fetal development and to provide for the deficiency of iodine due to urinary loss during pregnancy. The RDA for iodine for the pregnant woman is 125 μg, as compared to 100 μg for the non-gravid woman. An inadequate intake of iodine may result in goiter in the mother, especially the adolescent. The child may have a goiter also or, in the case of severe iodine deficiency, the child may develop cretinism. The regular use of iodized salt is recommended. Provisions for iodine supplementation are indicated when salt in the diet is severely restricted.

Other Minerals

Routine sodium restriction in pregnancy is not recommended. Evidence of increased need of sodium in pregnancy has been demonstrated and a severe restriction is hazardous. During pregnancy there is a normal gradual retention of sodium, which is distributed between the fetus and the mother. The glomerular filtration rate increases 50 per cent during pregnancy, but this is accompanied by increased reabsorption of sodium to prevent sodium depletion and circulatory collapse. Because the natural physiological mechanisms of pregnancy retain sodium and maintain a unique sodium balance, sodium restriction during pregnancy is not indicated.

Undesirable changes in the fetus have been associated with the intake of very low or excessive amounts of zinc, magnesium and manganese.

Vitamins

The RDA for most vitamins are higher during pregnancy (see Table 13–1). Increased needs for the B vitamins will be met when the food intake becomes greater to meet the additional need for calories, protein and calcium.

Folic Acid. Folic acid requirements are markedly increased during pregnancy because it is a period of rapid cell multiplication and of DNA synthesis. Evidence of folate depletion, including megaloblastic anemia, is common. Thus, the RDA for folic acid is an additional 400 μg per day, bringing the total requirement to 800 μg per day. This normally cannot be met by diet alone. A daily folic acid supplement of 400 to 800 μg is recommended.

Vitamin D. In most climates supplementary amounts of vitamin D should be given. Vitamin D-fortified milk contains 400 I.U. per quart, the amount required daily for maximum calcium retention. On the other hand, there is evidence that excessive vitamin D intake during pregnancy may cause abnormal calcium deposition in the fetus, producing increased density of the bones, especially the base of the skull, chalky deposits in the aorta, nephrocalcinosis and mental retardation.

Vitamin E. Considerable experimental research has been carried on to show the relationship between vitamin E and reproduction. No conclusive results have been demonstrated. However, experimental and clinical data suggest that vitamin E is necessary for the normal development of the fetus and the completion of pregnancy.

Vegetable oils that supply the essential polyunsaturated fatty acid (linoleic acid) also supply vitamin E.

Vitamin A. In animals, congenital malformations during early stages of gestation and poor reproductive performance result when they have a deficiency of vitamin A.

Vitamin K. When the vitamin K status of the mother has been unsatisfactory or is unknown at the time of labor, it is advisable to give the infant 1 to 2 mg. of vitamin K soon after birth to prevent hemorrhagic disease of the newborn. It is recommended that infants born to mothers receiving anticoagulant therapy be given 2 to 4 mg. of vitamin K.

Ascorbic Acid. A one-third increase in the RDA for the non-pregnant female is recommended for pregnant women. This brings the RDA during pregnancy to 60 mg. Ascorbic acid is essential in the formation of intercellular cement substance in connective tissue and in the vascular system of the fetus.

FOOD ALLOWANCES FOR THE NORMAL PREGNANT WOMAN

To meet the increased requirements of pregnancy, the adequate diet pattern (Chapter 10) is used plus a few important changes and additions (see Table 13–3).

Four cups of milk per day are recommended. This will provide the additional 30 gm. of high quality protein needed, will increase the calcium intake to 1.2 gm. and will provide an additional 320 kcalories from skim milk or 640 kcalories from whole milk. A number of choices are available: whole milk, skim milk, fluid and non-fat powdered milk, buttermilk,

Table 13–3 DAILY FOOD PATTERN TO ENSURE OPTIMAL NUTRITION DURING PREGNANCY

FOOD	AMOUNT	PROTEIN (gm.)
Milk, whole	3 or 4 8-oz. glasses.	24 to 32
Meat (lean), poultry, fish, liver is desirable at least once each week, cheese	2 servings/day, in all at least 4 oz. or equivalent in grams of protein.	28
Egg	One	7
Fruit	At least 2 servings. Two servings of citrus fruit or equivalent should be eaten. (1 serving equals 4 oz. of orange juice, 1 med. orange, 8 oz. of tomato juice, or ½ med. grapefruit.)	1
Potato	1 med. (150 gm.), preferably cooked in skin.	3
Other vegetables cooked and/or raw	2 or more servings. (1 serving equals ½ cup.) Dark green leafy or deep yellow vegetables often.	4
Bread and cereal	3 to 4 servings. (1 serving equals 1 slice of bread or ½ cup of cereal.) Whole grain or enriched.	6 to 8
Vegetable oil or special margarine, butter or fortified margarine	1 tablespoon	
Vitamin D	An amount to supply 400 I.U. such as vitamin D–fortified milk (1 qt.)	0
Total		73 to 83

evaporated milk, yogurt and cheese. Those who find drinking milk disagreeable may utilize the required amount in soups, custards, puddings, ice cream or flavored beverages. Also, milk products such as evaporated, homogenized or the powdered variety may be incorporated into the meal plan. The use of non-fat skim powder is an inconspicuous and acceptable way to add milk to the diet. Approximately 1½ ounces (5 tablespoons) of dried skim milk will equal 1 cup of fluid milk. Milk can be made richer in calcium, protein and calories by adding 2 tablespoons of dried nonfat milk to a glass of fluid milk. Dried non-fat milk may be used as a dry ingredient in the preparation of meatloaf, soups, mashed and scalloped potatoes, sandwich spreads, cooked cereals, homemade breads, cookies, pastries or puddings with little difficulty. The non-fat milk powder may be added also as a dry ingredient to cottage cheese, scrambled eggs, macaroni or spaghetti and cake. For women who have lactose intolerance, present in a large percentage of the black, Oriental and Mexican American populations, cheese, which contains very minute quantities of lactose, may be used. A small amount of milk may be beneficial in preventing or treating constipation. Commercial calcium preparations such as calcium lactate or carbonate may have to be prescribed.

The daily consumption of whole-grain or enriched bread and cereals, leafy green and yellow vegetables and fresh and dried fruits should be encouraged to provide additional minerals,

vitamins and fiber. Careful attention to the selection of foods that are good sources of iron and folic acid (see Table 8–9) within the food groups is stressed to provide as much dietary iron and folic acid as possible. Liver should be included in the diet at least once a week.

Three to four cups of milk fortified with vitamin D provide 300 to 400 I.U. of that vitamin. If milk is used in limited amounts, a vitamin D supplement may be necessary, especially if the woman has very little or no exposure to sunlight. See Table 13–4, Sample Menu for Pregnancy.

Total Fluids. The drinking of six to eight glasses (two liters) of water daily is encouraged. Intestinal stasis is often encountered as a result of the necessary restrictions of activities and the pressure of the enlarging uterus. However, for most individuals the bulky content of the protective diet plus the suggested amount of water will counteract any difficulty. Mineral oil is discouraged, since it may interfere with the absorption of the fat-soluble vitamins.

NUTRITION EDUCATION

Usually the prospective mother is anxious to have a normal, healthy baby and seeks obstetric care early. Nutrition advice, well presented at this time, is more apt to be accepted than at any other stage or period in life. However, unless such advice is based on previous food habits, customs and food budget, it may not be followed. Any improvement in food pattern

Table 13–4   SAMPLE MENU FOR PREGNANCY*

BREAKFAST
    Orange juice, 4 oz.
    Oatmeal, ½ cup
    Soft cooked egg
    Whole grain or enriched toast, 1 slice
    Butter or fortified margarine, 1 pat
    Coffee or tea

MID-MORNING
    Orange juice, 4 oz.
    Wheaties, ¾ cup
    Milk, 4 to 8 oz.

LUNCH
    Meat or cheese sandwich with rye or whole bread
        and 1 pat butter
    Lettuce and tomato salad
    Grapefruit, half
    Milk, 8 oz.

MIDAFTERNOON
    Milk, 8 oz.

DINNER
    Broiled beef liver, 4 oz.
    Baked potato with 1 pat butter or fortified margarine
    Peas and carrots
    Crisp celery
    Baked custard

BEDTIME
    Hot or cold milk, or cocoa, 8 oz.

*Kcalories are adjusted for desired weight. If the gravid individual is an adolescent, additional milk, fresh fruits or vegetables, whole-grain bread and butter or margarine are suggested.

depends upon how the person perceives the task of change. With few exceptions, a woman whose diet is poor during pregnancy can be considered as having been on a poor diet prior to conception. The average gravid adolescent girl especially requires individualized counseling on the basis of her specific needs. A printed diet list is of little or no value. Full discussion of individual needs with involvement of the person in planning for the necessary changes is the only effective approach. Even then the results may be disappointing, since many women do not take their nutritional supplements or do not change their eating habits after intensive counseling. (See Food Habits, Chapter 1; Teaching Nutrition, Chapter 19.)

To gain cooperation for diet improvement from the prospective mother, a discussion of the dietary habits of the prospective father and any other members of the family is also necessary. A prospective father, convinced that it is an essential part of his duties as a parent, will join in improving their food pattern and food habits. The counselor utilizes this interest and helps them to move in the direction of changes needed to provide an adequate diet. If each parent tends to watch the other's diet, both will improve their food habits. Thus, if both parents adopt an adequate diet, another family is started with good nutritional habits.

COMPLICATIONS OF PREGNANCY IN WHICH DIET IS A FACTOR

OBESITY

An obese woman at conception or one who gains an excessive amount of weight during pregnancy is in jeopardy. Complications develop that affect the course and outcome of pregnancy. Quite apart from the dangers to both mother and child during the pregnancy, another hazard of excessive antepartum weight gain is the development of permanent obesity and its resultant complications, some of which may not appear until later in life. While many patients who gain excessive weight during pregnancy lose it again spontaneously after delivery, too many women do not return to normal weight unless they make positive attempts to do so, either alone or with help. An adequate diet with sufficient calories to provide the energy required for the fetus and activity of the woman is an essential approach to weight control in the preventive concept of medicine.

The obese pregnant woman can control her rate of weight gain so that it follows the curve in Figure 13–2 without compromising the basic dietary requirements simply by decreasing the total calorie content through restriction of fats and carbohydrates. However, *she should not lose weight* but should gain 20 to 27 pounds as recommended.

Skim milk (320 kcalories per quart) may be substituted for whole milk (640 kcalories per quart). Sugar and ''empty'' calorie foods can be restricted or omitted. Protein intake is maintained at the prescribed level, and the diet should meet requirements for minerals and vitamins. In other words, the nurse or nutritionist counseling the obese pregnant woman should not be concerned with calories, but with changing the woman's eating habits so that she omits extraneous, non-nutritious calories and improves the calorie-nutrient ratio of her diet. She should eat the recommended number of servings from all of the food groups.

In a study of 12,847 cases of teenage gestation, excess weight gain was the most frequent

complication, occurring in over 30 per cent of the patients.[33] The incidence of pre-eclampsia and eclampsia is correlated with increasing weight gain, and perinatal mortality increases with the severity of the disease. As pointed out, it is the rate of gain during pregnancy that is important. Any sharp or sudden gain is indicative of the possible onset of complications.

ANEMIA

During pregnancy there is a high incidence of various types and degrees of anemia. In the second and third trimesters, physiological hemodilution lowers the red blood cell count, hematocrit and hemoglobin readings, so that normochromic normocytic anemia (hydremia) must be distinguished from *true* anemia.

True anemias of mild degree are managed with appropriate medications. Hypochromic anemia, the most common variety, is treated with iron preparations. Megaloblastic anemia is relatively common in pregnancy and most frequently is caused by a deficiency of folic acid. It has been estimated that one third of the pregnant women in the world suffer from this nutritional deficiency. Folic acid supplementation is necessary (see Chapter 29). Pernicious anemia is treated with vitamin B_{12}.

Hypochromic microcytic anemia is most commonly the result of iron deficiency, impaired utilization of iron, acute loss of blood, or low maternal stores of iron. In pregnancy, the maternal and fetal hemoglobin synthesis requires considerable iron. Maternal iron is lost to the fetus during the gestation period, and maternal blood is lost from bleeding at delivery. A diet inadequate in animal protein of high biological value is another significant cause of anemia.

Iron stored in the body in sufficient amount prior to pregnancy, plus an adequate diet, will usually provide the necessary iron during pregnancy. Unfortunately, the amount required for pregnancy is more than most women have stored. If the diet or absorption has been faulty and the iron stores are insufficient, iron must be provided through the food intake or through medication if iron deficiency anemia is to be avoided. It is well known that once anemia becomes established, it is impossible to raise the iron level by diet, regardless of the amount made available. In such cases, it is necessary to provide supplemental iron.

Some obstetricians believe it is advantageous to provide the mother with iron therapy as a prophylaxis against iron deficiency anemia, especially those with a history of anemia or frequent pregnancies. Others maintain that an adequate diet for pregnancy is sufficient. Ferrous sulfate preparations are the most effective but other forms of medical iron are less irritating for the patient.

The significance of low serum folate levels in the mother for the health of the fetus is not clear. Normal hemoglobin levels have been reported in newborns whose mothers had severe folate deficiency-induced megaloblastic anemia.[30] Placental transfer of folate is an active process, so that fetal folate supply is maintained even though the mother is severely depleted. Fetal storage of folate seems to be enhanced by administration of folate supplements to the mother, but this may be advantageous only to the low birth weight or premature infant. Such an infant does not have as much intrauterine time or nutrition as the term infant to build up his body stores to the normal level and would benefit from a high maternal level.[36]

CARDIAC DISEASE

Cardiac diseases during pregnancy are treated in much the same fashion as in the non-pregnant state. Dietary regulation in pregnant cardiac patients is concerned mainly with obesity and vascular congestion as contributory causes of failure (Chapter 28). Overweight must be avoided to minimize the work of the heart, and adequate rest is essential.

Sodium and Fluids. The relation of vascular congestion to fluid balance is discussed in Chapter 28, Nutritional Care for Patients with Cardiovascular Diseases. Since sodium and fluids are frequently restricted in certain cardiac diseases, the diet of the pregnant woman requires careful, supervised planning. It must also be kept in mind that sodium retention and intravascular volume expansion are normal in the pregnant woman.

Because milk is high in sodium chloride content, the daily three-fourths to one quart of milk necessary for calcium requirements may have to be restricted. If it is necessary to reduce the amount of milk to less than three-fourths of a quart a day, it may be advisable to use a low sodium milk or to supply part of the needed calcium by medication.

Iodine. The iodine content of the diet needs special evaluation when iodized salt cannot be used because of sodium restriction. Iodine may have to be prescribed if the iodine content of the diet and of the local drinking water is in-

adequate, as it is in areas of the world termed the "goiter belt."

Cholesterol. With the current emphasis on the influence of cholesterol as a cause of vascular sclerosis, it seems appropriate to mention that serum cholesterol values may rise to as high as 350 to 400 mg. per 100 ml. serum during the last trimester of *normal* pregnancy. (The normal serum cholesterol range is approximately 150 to 250 mg. per 100 ml. serum, with an average of 180 mg. per 100 ml. serum in the nonpregnant state.)

DIABETES

The diet of the pregnant diabetic woman must be adequate to meet maternal and fetal nutritional needs. Statistics reveal that pregnancy may aggravate uncontrolled cases or may initiate imbalance in controlled ones. Diabetes may exist only during the stress of pregnancy and resolve itself after delivery, a condition called "gestational diabetes." The etiology of "gestational diabetes" is not understood, but it usually can be controlled by diet alone. In the diabetic who is pregnant the instance of toxemia is high, and fetal morbidity and mortality are significantly greater than in normal pregnancy. It has been found, for instance, that respiratory distress symptoms are five to six times more likely to develop in infants of diabetic mothers than in infants of non-diabetic mothers, and that maternal diabetes mellitus predisposes the infant to newborn respiratory distress syndrome.[32] Successful pregnancy depends upon adequate dietary and insulin management to meet the growth needs of the fetus and to prevent depletion of the mother's nutritional stores. Needs for increased intake go hand in hand with needs for increased insulin. The demands of pregnancy may impose a need for insulin in a diabetic gravid woman whose condition was adequately controlled by diet alone in the non-pregnant state.

There is no fixed rule to determine the amount of insulin administered during pregnancy. Insulin requirements usually increase, but only temporarily. The increase occurs rather abruptly during the fifth month and may last through the ninth month. Frequent changes in the diet and the insulin dosage may be necessary.

In women who have been diabetic for several years, pregnancy frequently affects the eyes by aggravating existing retinopathy. Occasionally, abortion is necessary to prevent blindness.[9]

Infants born to diabetics are, as a rule, larger than those of non-diabetics. At least 25 per cent of these infants weigh more than 10 pounds at birth. The reason for this is most likely the exposure of the infant in utero to supernormal levels of its own insulin, which in fact is a growth hormone.[2] High insulin levels are caused by the hyperglycemia of the mother, which crosses the placenta. Infants of diabetic mothers also tend to become hypoglycemic shortly after birth. The probability of the infant becoming hypoglycemic is directly related to the maternal glucose intolerance.

The hazards of labor are increased and in many cases cesarean section is advised. It must be emphasized that unfavorable effects are in proportion to the care the mother receives; when the diabetes is under control, complications are rare. Early prenatal care is an important factor.

TOXEMIA

For many years nutrition has been related to the occurrence of toxemias of pregnancy. Because no toxins have been found to cause this disorder, as was first thought, the term "toxemia" is actually a misnomer. Prevention and treatment have been largely empirical. The Committee on Maternal Nutrition, Food and Nutrition Board, National Research Council in a report of their review of the literature considered toxemia under two classifications: preeclampsia and eclampsia. *Pre-eclampsia* is defined as acute hypertension with proteinuria or edema or both appearing after the twentieth week of pregnancy. *Eclampsia* is defined as the occurrence of one or more convulsions with the criteria for the diagnosis of pre-eclampsia.

A dramatic decline in maternal mortality from toxemias has occurred in the United States during the past 25 years. The mortality rates by state have varied widely. The most striking association of the differences is related to per capita income. In those states with low per capita income the incidence of maternal mortality from toxemia is higher than in those states with higher per capita income. Since severe toxemia of pregnancy occurs most frequently among women in the lower socioeconomic strata, whose diets are often substandard, the hypothesis has been generally advanced that malnutrition may be a causative factor.

Pre-eclampsia tends to be more severe when it develops in markedly underweight women at conception and when they fail to gain weight

normally during the prenatal period. Pre-eclampsia is more common among the very young primigravidas and those over age 30, diabetics, those with multiple pregnancies and those with a hypertensive disorder. The Committee reported that little scientific evidence was found to indicate calorie restriction and the restriction of accumulation of fat as means for preventing toxemia. Since the work of Strauss, protein deficiency resulting in hypoproteinemia and water retention is considered by many to be a primary factor in the cause of toxemia.[19, 35] In the United States the decreased incidence of toxemia may be attributed to improvement in diet, especially in the protein intake. Although the proportion of calories from protein has remained at 11 to 13 per cent over the past half century, two thirds of the protein now comes from animal sources compared with one half in the 1904 to 1913 period. In order to avoid protein depletion, appropriate dietary regulation is required. It may be necessary to increase the protein to as much as 120 gm. or more. However, when nitrogen retention is present, as in certain renal diseases, the protein intake must be individualized and this may even necessitate less than the normal requirement.

The edema of pre-eclampsia is largely extracellular sodium retention. Even before the edema develops there is an increased response of the vascular system to angiotensin, which develops into hypertension and edema. However, the intravascular volume is less than that of normal gravid women, which leads to a compromise of the placental and fetal circulation. It is still unclear whether the treatment of this condition should be sodium restriction.[28] The Committee on Maternal Nutrition believes that the matter of routine salt restriction in pregnancy as a means of preventing pre-eclampsia requires further research and assessment. Others report equal or better results in treating toxemia when the salt intake was high. Gray et al.[15] studied 28 normal pregnant women in an attempt to define the role of dietary sodium in salt and water retention during normal pregnancy. They report that the amount of sodium retained could not be influenced by differences in the average quantity of sodium ingested during this time.

In the studies of Klieger and associates, placentas from patients with toxemia contained one third the normal content of B_6 and decreased pyridoxal kinase activity. This would result in insufficient enzymes available to convert pyridoxal to the active enzyme pyridoxal phosphate. The relationship between insufficient B_6 metabolism and toxemia needs further study.[20]

EDEMA

The pregnant woman has a different sodium balance that results in a tremendous reabsorption of sodium. This is probably necessary to maintain the expanded blood volume needed to perfuse the placenta and fetus. There is a physiological edema of pregnancy that does not seem to develop into pre-eclampsia and should not be treated with sodium restriction or diuretics.

NAUSEA AND VOMITING IN PREGNANCY

Morning sickness or nausea is common during the early months of pregnancy, and the condition usually disappears just as spontaneously as it appears. However, when early pregnancy is characterized by excessive vomiting, an acute protein and calorie deficit and the loss of minerals, vitamins and electrolytes may result.

In cases of *pernicious vomiting*, fats are a fairly common offender. Many obstetricians achieve benefits for women by advising the withholding of fluids from one to two hours before and following meals, in addition to the prescription of a dry diet. If the fat in whole milk is not well tolerated, skim milk may be used.

Frequent small meals consisting of such foods as thickly cooked cereal, Melba toast with jelly, saltines and baked potato, served at two-hour intervals, usually are well tolerated initially. If the food is retained, fluids may be tried one hour before and after the serving of food. A dry, soft diet may be given as soon as all fluids and foods are retained. Fats and fluids, as tolerated, are gradually added to the meals.

Dry Diet
FOODS ALLOWED
Meats: Lean meat, fish, chicken and crisp bacon (prepared by broiling or roasting methods).
Eggs: Hard cooked.
Cheese: American, Cheddar and Swiss cheese.
Breads: Toasted enriched white bread and saltines.
Cereals: Thick cooked cereals and the dry ready-to-eat variety.

Potatoes: Baked, boiled or mashed.

Fats: Butter or fortified margarine and peanut butter in limited amounts.

Desserts: Arrowroot cookies, sponge cake, pound cake, angel food cake, baked custard, vanilla ice cream (if tolerated).

Sugar: Sugar, jelly, jam and honey.

Liquids: At the beginning of the diet regimen, all liquids are served between meals; later on, if tolerated, liquids may be allowed with the meals.

MEAL PLAN

8:00 A.M.	Cereal with sugar, fortified margarine or butter.
	Toasted enriched white bread with jelly
	Crisp bacon or hard cooked egg
10:00 A.M.	Orange juice
11:00 A.M.	Milk
12:00 NOON	Lean meat, small serving
	Baked potato
	Toasted enriched white bread, lightly buttered
	Jelly
	Dessert
2:00 P.M.	Milk
4:00 P.M.	Fruit juice
6:00 P.M.	Meat or cheese, small serving
	Potato or dessert
	Crackers or toast
	Jelly, jam or peanut butter
8:00 P.M.	Milk

In summary, the pregnant woman should be told of the importance of eating during this period and be encouraged to eat as much as possible when she is not nauseated. She can be told about ways to include concentrated sources of calories in her diet. See Chapter 27 on Underweight.

CONSTIPATION AND HEARTBURN

As pregnancy progresses, constipation can become a problem because of decreased gastrointestinal motility, pressure of the enlarged uterus on the gastrointestinal tract, decreased exercise and iron supplementation. Suggestions to increase the intake of fibrous foods, fluids and prunes or prune juice should help. Increased exercise, such as additional walking, may also help. See Table 23–1.

Heartburn can also result from the pressure of the uterus on the stomach. An antacid may be necessary, and suggestions to omit alcohol, coffee, tea and other caffeine-containing drinks that increase gastric acid secretion and to eat frequent small amounts should relieve the problem.

PICA

Cravings for unusual foods and the eating of non-food substances (pica) are relatively common occurrences of pregnancy. These practices are deleterious only when they interfere with the intake or absorption of other foods and nutrients. Some clay eating *(geophagia)*, frequently seen among black women, may reduce the absorption of iron.[25] However another commonly eaten substance, cornstarch, has no effect on iron absorption. It can be detrimental because it is a non-nutritious pure carbohydrate that provides calories, satiates appetite and interferes with the intake of more nutritious foods.

Pica, particularly *pagophagia* (excessive ice eating), seems to be correlated with and may be indicative of iron deficiency. It seems to resolve itself after repletion of iron nutrition.[31] When dietary histories are taken, the nurse or dietitian should ask about the eating of such substances as clay, dirt, cornstarch, laundry starch, plaster, cigarette ashes, flour and ice. These forms of pica are important to an understanding of the dietary habits and nutritional status of the patient and may indicate potential nutritional deficiencies.

LEG CRAMPS

Pregnant women frequently complain of leg cramps (cramping of the gastrocnemius muscle), usually at night. This is thought to be due to a neuromuscular irritability caused by low serum calcium and high serum phosphate. Although the relationship of calcium and phosphorus to leg cramps is not completely understood, recommendations proposed in the 1950's are still effective and valid today: (1) reduction of milk intake (milk contains large amounts of phosphorus), (2) supplementation with calcium salts such as calcium lactate or carbonate and (3) regular ingestion of aluminum hydroxide to prevent phosphate absorption.[27] These suggestions usually work and may need to be followed only temporarily until the cramping is gone.

FOOD INTAKE DURING LABOR

Patients who are in early labor frequently make the mistake of eating a hearty meal before

entering the hospital. They believe erroneously that large amounts of food are required to give strength for parturition.

It has been demonstrated that during labor the stomach does not readily empty itself. It is not uncommon for patients at delivery to vomit food which was ingested 24 to 48 hours previously.

The pregnant patient should be warned against ingestion of solid foods or liquids once labor has commenced. Food particles may remain in the stomach and later on be vomited and aspirated if the woman is anesthetized, thereby causing serious obstructive reactions of the respiratory tract. Suffocation and massive atelectasis may result.

The work of Mendelson,[16, 24] which showed the possibility of aspiration of liquid stomach contents during anesthesia, has resulted in the hospital practice of omitting all oral feedings during the first stages of labor. If the patient has ingested solid or liquid food recently, he suggests the alkalinization and emptying of the stomach contents prior to the administration of general anesthesia, if the woman has elected to have it during delivery. Should fluid and calorie balance be disturbed in the event of prolonged labor, parenteral feedings may be given.

DIET DURING LACTATION

The preparation for assuring an adequate supply of good quality breast milk must begin with the onset of pregnancy. Most of the dietary essentials are increased, over and above the requirements during pregnancy, to meet the demands of milk production for an infant who doubles its birth weight in five months. These increased requirements are expressed by the allowances recommended by the Food and Nutrition Board of the National Research Council in Table 13–1.

Calories

The actual mechanism involved in the production of milk by the maternal organism demands a daily energy *expenditure* of an extra 600 to 800 kcalories above the normal intake. The additional *food* necessary for the maternal organism to produce and secrete milk is about 500 extra kcalories when an adequate diet and an 11 to 12.5 kg. weight gain has been achieved during pregnancy. Because about 4 kg. (9 lb.) of fat has been stored in the mother's body in preparation for lactation and for use in milk production, the RDA for additional calories for

lactation is 500 kcalories per day for the first three months, with the other 100 to 300 kcalories coming from fat stores. Daily energy requirements have to be greater for mothers nursing longer than three months, especially if their weight falls below what is normal for their height or if they are suckling more than one infant. Extra calories also may be needed for the additional activity necessitated by caring for the infant.

The number of extra calories required for lactation depends on the amount of milk produced. Food requirements are not uniform during the entire period of lactation but depend on the demands of the infant. See Table 13–5.

Protein

An adequate intake of protein of high biological value during pregnancy is essential in the preparation for lactation. Lactation makes large demands on human nitrogen stores. The food intake of a nursing mother must contain sufficient protein to supply both the maternal needs and the essential amino acids to be transferred through her breast milk to the baby. Human milk contains 12 mg. of protein per ml. The amount of protein in 850 ml. is 10 gm. If the protein in the mother's diet is inadequate both to meet her body maintenance needs and to provide the protein for the milk secreted, a loss of maternal body tissue will result. The protein content of the milk will not be reduced. An increase of 20 gm. of protein daily in addition to the usual 0.8 gm. per kg. body weight require-

Table 13–5   ENERGY COST OF PRODUCING BREAST MILK*

AGE OF BABY (*Months*)	VOLUME OF MILK TAKEN (*ml./day*)	ENERGY VALUE OF MILK (*Kcal.*)	TOTAL ENERGY COST† (*Kcal./day*)
0–1	600	402	446
1–2	840	563	626
2–3	930	623	692
3–4	960	643	714
4–5	1010	677	752
5–6	1100	737	819

*From: Winick, M.: Nutritional disorders of American women. Nutrition Today, *10*:26, 1975.
†Assuming 90% efficiency.

ment of the nonlactating woman is the amount recommended by the Food and Nutrition Board of the National Research Council (Table 13–1). The diet properly provides this only if it is otherwise well balanced in mineral and vitamin content and adequate in calories.

Fat

The kind of fat in the breast milk reflects the composition of fat in the maternal diet. Polyunsaturated fatty acids predominate in human milk. The polyunsaturated fatty acids in the mother's diet contribute about 6 to 9 per cent of the calories in human milk as linoleic acid.

Calcium and Vitamin D

In order to prevent depletion of calcium, the mother needs approximately 400 mg. above the normal amount of 800 mg. during lactation. (A total of approximately 4 cups of milk.) The intake of 400 I.U. of vitamin D for the utilization of calcium and phosphorus in bone formation is recommended and this can also be obtained from 4 cups of vitamin D-fortified milk.

Iron

Some lactating women tend to become anemic unless the iron allowance in their diet is maintained at the same level as during pregnancy. During lactation there is loss of iron which, if considered on an annual basis, is probably similar in quantity to that lost in the menstrual flow.

Vitamins

There is an increased demand for vitamin A, vitamin E, riboflavin, thiamin, niacin, vitamin B_6, folic acid, vitamin B_{12} and ascorbic acid during lactation. (See Table 13–1.) Breast milk reflects the mother's intake of water-soluble vitamins. For example, infants nursed by mothers who have beriberi develop infantile beriberi. Breast milk does not reflect the intake of fat-soluble vitamins. See Chapter 14, Nutrition in Infancy, for further discussion of human milk.

FOOD ALLOWANCES FOR THE NORMAL LACTATING WOMAN

The increased nutritional requirements during lactation can be supplied by adding another cup of whole milk and another serving from the bread and cereal group to the foods necessary for pregnancy. (Table 13–3.) Five or six small meals daily are recommended. See the pattern suggested in Table 13–4. The volume of milk produced is reduced when the maternal diet is inadequate. However, the milk remains balanced because the underfed mother draws on her own tissues. Smoking and oral contraceptives may reduce the volume of milk. Oral contraceptives should not be started earlier than six weeks postpartum. It is still not clear how the different oral contraceptives affect lactation or which, if any, are preferred for lactating mothers. Nicotine, a highly toxic drug, is fat-soluble and is transmitted through milk to the infant.

Breast milk reflects the environment of the mother. The kinds and amounts of drugs, pesticides and toxicants a baby can be exposed to and their effect on the composition of maternal milk and on infant health are not well known. Pesticide residues have been found in breast milk at many times the WHO-recommended maximum level for cow's milk.[3, 21, 37] Just because a drug the mother is taking is found in her milk does not mean it will have a harmful effect on the infant (Table 13–6.)

Fluids. The total daily intake of fluids should be at least two quarts, because fluids tend to increase the volume of milk.

NUTRITIONAL IMPLICATIONS OF ORAL CONTRACEPTIVES

Millions of women take oral conceptives as a convenient way to extend the interconceptional period, prevent unwanted pregnancies or delay the starting of a family. Oral contraceptives appear to increase the requirement for several nutrients, in particular folic acid and vitamin B_6, and to a lesser extent riboflavin, thiamin and ascorbic acid. Clinical evidence of deficiency is rare, although vitamin B_6-responsive depression and folate-responsive megaloblastic anemia have been reported. Subclinical deficiency, identified as lowered serum levels of these nutrients, is more common. See Table 13–7.

On the other hand, plasma levels of some nutrients such as vitamin A, iron and copper increase. The implications for nutritional requirements in women taking oral contraceptives are unclear. Serum iron may increase because of decreased iron loss that accompanies reduced menstrual flow, commonly associated with oral contraceptive use. See Chapter 21, Interactions Between Drugs, Nutrients and

Table 13–6   DRUGS EXCRETED IN HUMAN MILK*

DRUG	IMPLICATION FOR MOTHER	IMPLICATION FOR NURSING INFANT
Antibiotics (broad- and medium-spectrum)	Mother should not take certain ones	Sensitization of baby may occur, especially with penicillin Anemia, shock, death Hepatotoxic
Anticoagulants	Mother should not take	Infant can develop serious hemorrhage
Anticonvulsants	No problem except with primidone (Mysoline)	Drowsiness in infant
Antimigraine agents, e.g. ergotamine (Cafergot)	Mother should not take	May cause vomiting, diarrhea, shock and hypertension
Antitumor drugs	Mother should not take	May harm infant's developing cells
Antispasmodics and anti- cholinergics, e.g. tri- hexyphenidyl (artane) and nylidrin (Arlidin)	Mother should not take	Diminish lactation and may cause heart irregularities in baby
Aspirin, phenacetin and combinations	Mother should not take	May cause bleeding in infant May cause a macular rash
Hypotensives in combina- tion with diuretics	Mother should not take; may cause galactor- rhea	Hazardous to infant because may cause increased respiratory tract secre- tions, cyanosis, and anorexia
Isoniazid	Mother should not take	Causes mental retardation in infant
Laxatives	Present in milk	Can cause diarrhea in baby
Propanol	Mother should not take	May cause bronchospasm, brady- cardia, hypotension, congestive heart failure and hypoglycemia in baby
Psychotropic drugs	Mother should not take	Drowsiness, other unknown effects in infant
Radioactive iodine	Mother should not be given	Suppresses infant's thyroid
Steroids	Mother should not take; decrease lactation	Decrease lactation and thus infant growth Cause gynecomastia in baby
Thiazide diuretics	Present in milk	May cause dehydration in infant
Urinary anti-infectives	Present in milk; mother should not take sul- fonamides	May be noxious to infant if taken by mother continuously Sulfonamides noxious to infants less than 2 months old.
Vaginal medications (Flagyl vaginal inserts, AVC cream, other sul- fonamides)	Mother should not use	Cause jaundice of newborn

*Adapted from: Rothermel, P. C., and Faber, M. M.: Drugs in breastmilk—A consumer's guide. Birth Fam. J., 2:76, 1975.

Table 13–7 NUTRITIONAL ABERRATIONS ATTRIBUTED TO CONTRACEPTIVE STEROIDS

NUTRIENT	CLINICAL EFFECTS
Folacin	Serum level ↓ Erythrocyte level ↓ Megaloblastic anemia (rare)
Vitamin B$_{12}$	Serum level ↓
Riboflavin	Erythrocyte level ↓ Glossitis (rare)
Vitamin B$_6$	Disturbed tryptophan metabolism Plasma PLP ↓ Depression
Ascorbic acid	Leukocyte content ↓ Platelet level ↓
Vitamin A	Plasma level ↑
Iron	Serum level ↑ TIBC ↑
Copper	Plasma copper ↑ Ceruloplasmin ↑
Zinc	Plasma zinc ↓

Nutritional Status, for additional discussion of the processes involved in the effects of these drugs on nutritional status.

The interconception period should be a time of good nutrition not only to offset the effects of oral contraceptives, but also to maintain lactation with no nutritional cost to the mother and to replace any calcium, iron, protein or vitamin stores that may have been reduced during pregnancy. An equally important reason is to provide good nutrition for the entire family and to initiate good eating habits in the new family member.

PROBLEMS AND SUGGESTED TOPICS FOR DISCUSSION

1. What are the special nutritional needs during pregnancy? What kinds and amounts of food supply these needs?
2. Why are diet and good nutrition important during the prenatal period? During lactation?
3. Visit a patient in the prenatal clinic and obtain an average dietary intake for a day. Check diet for nutritional adequacy. How does it need to be nutritionally improved?
4. Visit a patient in the postnatal clinic and obtain an average dietary intake for a day. Check diet for nutritional adequacy. Is her weight normal? Help her with the necessary corrections.
5. Visit a patient in your hospital who has toxemia compli-

cations in her pregnancy. Obtain a typical dietary intake. Calculate it to determine adequacy of proteins. Plan a correct diet with mild sodium restriction for this patient that is adequate in all nutrients. Follow the progress of the patient.
6. Survey the complications of pregnancy in your hospital. What part does diet play in each?
7. How does the diet during lactation differ from that of a non-lactating woman? Take a diet history of a lactating woman and assist her with the changes she needs to make in her dietary pattern.

CITED REFERENCES

1. Baird, D.: Variations in fertility associated with changes in health status. J. Chronic Dis., *18*:1109, 1965.
2. Baird, J. D., and Farquhar, J. W.: Insulin-secreting capacity in newborn infants of normal and diabetic women. Lancet, *1*:71, 1962.
3. Bakken, A. F., and Seip, M.: Insecticides in human breast milk. Acta Paediatr. Scand., *65*:535, 1976.
4. Blackburn, M. W., and Calloway, D. H.: Energy expenditure and consumption of mature, pregnant and lactating women. J. Am. Diet. Assoc., *69*:29, 1976.
5. Burke, B. S.: Nutrition during pregnancy: A review. J. Am. Diet. Assoc., *20*:735, 1944.
6. Burke, B. S., et al.: Nutrition studies during pregnancy. Am. J. Obstet. Gynecol. *46*:38, 1943.
7. Burke, B. S., Harding, V. V., and Stuart, H. C.: Nutrition studies during pregnancy. Relation of protein content of mother's diet during pregnancy to birth length, birth weight and condition of infant at birth. J. Pediatr., *23*:506, 1943.
8. Burke, B. S., et al.: Nutrition studies during pregnancy. Relation of maternal nutrition to condition of infant at birth: Study of siblings. J. Nutr., *38*:453, 1949.
9. Cahill, G.: Microvascular lesions. *In* Wolf, S., and Berle, B. B. (eds.), Advances in Experimental Medicine and Biology, Vol. 65: Dilemmas in Diabetes. New York, Plenum Press, 1975.
10. Dieckmann, W. J., et al.: Observations on protein intake and the health of the mother and baby. Clinical and laboratory findings. J. Am. Diet. Assoc., *27*:1046, 1951.
11. Eaves, L. C., et al.: Developmental and psychological test scores in children of low birth weight. Pediatrics, *45*:9, 1970.
12. Ebbs, J. H., Tisdall, F. F., and Scott, W. J.: The influence of prenatal diet on the mother and child. J. Nutr., *22*:515, 1941.
13. Felig, P.: Maternal and fetal fuel homeostasis in human pregnancy. Am. J. Clin. Nutr., *26*:998, 1973.
14. Fitzhardinge, P. M., and Stevens, E. M.: The small-for-date infant. II. Neurological and intellectual sequelae. Pediatrics, *50*:50, 1972.
15. Gray, M. J., et al.: Regulation of sodium and total body water metabolism in pregnancy. Am. J. Obstet. Gynecol., *89*:761, 1964.
16. Haussman, W., and Lunt, R. L.: The problems of the treatment of peptic aspiration pneumonia following obstetric anesthesia. "Mendelson's syndrome." J. Obstet. Gynaecol. Brit. Emp., *62*:509, 1955.
17. Hogan, A. G.: Nutrition: Maternal nutrition and congenital malformations. Annu. Rev. Biochem., *22*:299, 1953.
18. Jacobson, H. N. (ed.), Report of a Workshop on Nutritional Supplementation and the Outcome of Preg-

nancy. Washington, D.C., National Research Council, National Academy of Sciences, 1974.

19. Kaminetsky, H. A., et al.: The effect of nutrition in teen-age gravidas on pregnancy and the status of the neonate. Am. J. Obstet. Gynecol., *115*:639, 1973.

20. Klieger, J. A., et al.: Abnormal pyridoxine metabolism in toxemia of pregnancy. Am. J. Obstet. Gynecol., *94*:316, 1966.

21. Kroger, M.: Insecticide residues in human milk. J. Pediatr., *80*:401, 1972.

22. Lechtig, A., et al.: Effect of food supplementation during pregnancy on birthweight. Pediatrics, *56*:508, 1975.

23. McCance, R. A., Widdowson, E. M., and Lehman, H.: The effect of protein intake on the absorption of calcium and magnesium. Biochem. J., *36*:686, 1942.

24. Mendelson, C. L.: The aspiration of stomach contents into the lung during obstetric anesthesia. Am. J. Obstet. Gynecol., *52*:191, 1946.

25. Minnich, V., et al.: Pica in Turkey. II. Effect of clay upon iron absorption. Am. J. Clin. Nutr., *21*:78, 1968.

26. Ounsted, M., and Ounsted, C.: Maternal regulation of intrauterine growth. Nature, *212*:995, 1966.

27. Page, E. W., and Page, E. P.: Leg cramps in pregnancy: Etiology and treatment. Obstet. Gynecol., *1*:94, 1953.

28. Pike, R. L., and Smiciklas, H. A.: A reappraisal of sodium restriction during pregnancy. Int. J. Gynaecol. Obstet., *10*:1, 1972.

29. Primrose, T., and Higgins, A.: A study of human antepartum nutrition. J. Reprod. Med., *7*:257, 1972.

30. Pritchard, J. A., Whalley, P. J., and Scott, D. E.: The influence of maternal folate and iron deficiencies on intrauterine life. Am. J. Obstet. Gynecol., *104*:368, 1969.

31. Reynolds, R. D., et al.: Pagophagia and iron deficiency anemia. Ann. Intern. Med., *69*:435, 1968.

32. Robert, M. F., et al.: Maternal diabetes and the respiratory distress syndrome. N. Engl. J. Med., *294*:357, 1976.

33. Semmens, J. P.: Implications of teen-age pregnancy. Obstet. Gynecol., *26*:77, 1965.

34. Smith, C. A.: The effect of wartime starvation in Holland upon pregnancy and its product. Am. J. Obstet. Gynecol., *53*:599, 1947.

35. Strauss, M. B.: Observations on the etiology of the toxemias of pregnancy. The relationship of nutritional deficiency, hypoproteinemia and elevated venous pressure to water retention in pregnancy. Am. J. Med. Sci., *190*:811, 1935.

36. Strelling, K. M.: Transfer of folate to the fetus. Dev. Med. Child Neurol., *18*:533, 1976.

37. Wilson, D. J., et al.: DDT concentrations in human milk. Am. J. Dis. Child., *125*:814, 1973.

38. Woodhill, J. M., et al.: Nutrition studies of pregnant Australian women. Am. J. Obstet. Gynecol., *70*:987, 1955.

39. Zamenhoff, S., Marthens, E. van, and Grauel, L.: DNA (cell number) in neonatal brain: Second generation (F_2) alteration by maternal (F_0) dietary protein restriction. Science, *172*:850, 1971.

ADDITIONAL REFERENCES

Anemia during pregnancy. Lancet, *2*:1429, 1974.

Arena, J. M.: Contamination of the ideal food. Nutrition Today, *5*:2, 1970.

Barness, L. A., and Pitkin, R. M. (eds.): Nutrition. Clin. Perinatol., *2*(2), 1975.

Burke, B. S.: Diet and nutrition during pregnancy. Am. J. Nurs., *52*:1378, 1952.

Canosa, C. A. (ed.): Modern Problems in Pediatrics, vol. 14: Nutrition, growth, and development. Basel, S. Karger, 1975.

Cheek, D. B. (ed.): Fetal and Postnatal Cellular Growth: Hormones and Nutrition. New York, John Wiley and Sons, 1975.

Committee on Maternal Nutrition: Maternal Nutrition and the Course of Pregnancy. Washington, D.C., Food and Nutrition Board, National Academy of Sciences, 1970.

Committee on Nutrition: Nutrition in Maternal Health Care. American College of Obstetricians and Gynecologists, Suite 2700, One East Wacker Drive, Chicago, Illinois, 60601, 1974.

Corruccini, C. G., and Cruskie, P. E.: Nutrition during pregnancy and lactation. Maternal and Child Health Unit, California Department of Health, 714 P Street, Sacramento, California, 95814, 1975.

David, M. L., and Doyle. E. W.: First trimester pregnancy. Am. J. Nurs., *76*:1945, 1976.

Davies, A. M., et al.: Toxemia of pregnancy in Jerusalem. II. The role of diet. Isr. J. Med. Sci., *12*:508, 1976.

Fetal malnutrition. Nutr. Rev., *31*:179, 1973.

Food and Nutrition Board, NRC/NAS: The relationship of nutrition to brain development and behavior. National Academy of Sciences, 2101 Constitution Avenue, N.W., Washington, D.C., 20418, 1973.

Gal, I., and Parkinson, C. E.: Effects of nutrition and other factors on pregnant women's serum vitamin A levels. Am. J. Clin. Nutr., *27*:688, 1974.

Gold, E. M.: Interconceptional nutrition. J. Am. Diet. Assoc., *55*:27, 1969.

Gordon, J. E.: Nutritional individuality. Am. J. Dis. Child., *129*:422, 1975.

Growth of the human brain: Some further insights. Nutr. Rev., *33*:6, 1975.

Haworth, J. C., and Dilling, L. A.: Relationships between maternal glucose intolerance and neonatal blood glucose. J. Pediatr., *89*:810, 1976.

Hytten, F. E.: Is breast feeding best? Am. J. Clin. Nutr., *7*:259, 1959.

Jacobson, H. N., et al.: Effect of weight reduction in obese pregnant women on pregnancy, labor, and delivery, and on the condition of the infant at birth. Am. J. Obstet. Gynecol., *83*:1609, 1962.

Jacobson, H. N.: Weight and weight gain in pregnancy. Clin. Perinatol., *2*:233, 1975.

Jacobson, H. N., and Mills, S. H.: Pregnant and lactating women. *In* Mayer, J. (ed.), U.S. Nutrition Policies in the 70's, San Francisco, W. H. Freeman and Co., 1973.

Jones, C. J. P., and Fox, H.: Placental changes in gestational diabetes. Obstet. Gynecol., *48*:274, 1976.

King, J. C., Calloway, D. H., and Margen, S.: Nitrogen retention, total body K^{40} and weight gain in teenage pregnant girls. J. Nutr., *103*:772, 1973.

King, J. C., et al.: Assessment of nutritional status of teenage pregnant girls. I. Nutrient intake and pregnancy. Am. J. Clin. Nutr., *25*:916, 1972.

Lactation and composition of milk in undernourished women. Nutr. Rev., *33*:42, 1976.

Larson, R. H.: Effect of prenatal nutrition on oral structures. J. Am. Diet. Assoc., *44*:368, 1964.

Lasky, R. E., et al.: Birthweight and psychomotor performance in rural Guatemala. Am. J. Dis. Child., *129*:566, 1975.

Layrisse, M., Roche, M., and Baker, S. J.: Nutritional anemia. *In* Beaton, G. H., and Bengoa, J. M. (eds.),

Nutrition in Preventive Medicine, WHO Monograph Series No. 62. Geneva, WHO, 1976.

Lechtig, A., et al.: Influence of maternal nutrition on birth weight. Am. J. Clin. Nutr., *28*:1223, 1975.

Lind, T., and Harris, V. G.: Changes in the oral glucose tolerance test during the puerperium. Br. J. Obstet. Gynaecol., *83*:460, 1976.

Lindheimer, M. D., and Katz, A. I.: Sodium and diuretics in pregnancy. N. Engl. J. Med., *288*:891, 1973.

Lumeng, L., et al.: Adequacy of vitamin B supplementation during pregnancy: A prospective study. Am. J. Clin. Nutr., *29*:1376, 1976.

Macy, I. G., et al.: The Composition of Milks. Washington, D. C., National Research Council, Publ. No. 254, 1953.

Maternal nutrition and fetal growth. Nutr. Rev., *32*:241, 1974.

McGanity, W. J., et al.: The Vanderbilt cooperative study of maternal and infant nutrition. VIII. Some nutritional implications. J. Am. Diet. Assoc., *31*:582, 1955.

McGanity, W. J., et al.: The Vanderbilt cooperative study of maternal and infant nutrition. XII. Effect of reproductive cycle on nutritional status and requirements. JAMA, *168*:2138, 1958.

Metabolic adaptation to pregnancy. Nutr. Rev., *32*:270, 1974.

Metcoff, J.: Maternal nutrition and fetal growth. *In* McLaren, D. S., and Burman, D. (eds.), Textbook of Pediatric Nutrition. Edinburgh, Churchill Livingstone, 1976.

Mullick, S., et al.: Serum lipid studies in pregnancy. Am. J. Obstet. Gynecol., *89*:766, 1964.

Munro, H. M.: Report of a conference on protein and amino acid needs for growth and development. Am. J. Clin. Nutr., *27*:55, 1974.

Naeye, R. L., et al.: Relation of poverty and race to birth weight and organ and cell structure in the newborn. Pediatr. Res., *5*:17, 1971.

Naeye, R. L.: Malnutrition, a probable cause of fetal growth retardation. Arch. Pathol., *79*:284, 1964.

Niswander, K. R., and Gordon, M.: The Women and Their Pregnancies: The Collaborative Perinatal Study of the National Institute of Neurological Diseases and Strokes. Philadelphia, W. B. Saunders Co., 1972.

Nutritional needs during pregnancy. Dairy Council Digest, *45*:19, 1974.

Oakes, G. K., Chex, R. A., and Morelli, I. C.: Diet in pregnancy: Meddling with the normal or preventing toxemia? Am. J. Nurs., *75*:1134, 1975.

Pike, R. L.: Sodium intake during pregnancy. J. Am. Diet. Assoc., *144*:176, 1964.

Pike, R. L., and Gursky, D. S.: Further evidence of deleterious effects produced by sodium restriction during pregnancy. Am. J. Clin. Nutr., *23*:883, 1970.

Pitkin, R. M.: Calcium metabolism in pregnancy: A review. Am. J. Obstet. Gynecol., *121*:724, 1975.

Pregnancy and Nutrition (bibliography). Nutrition Education Resources Series No. 2, National Nutrition Education Clearing House, Society for Nutrition Education, 2140 Shattuck Avenue, Suite 1110, Berkeley, California, 94704.

Rush, D., et al.: Dietary services during pregnancy and birthweight: A retrospective matched pair analysis. Pediatr. Res., *10*:349, 1976.

Scott, K. E., and Usher, R.: Fetal malnutrition: Its incidence, causes and effects. Am. J. Obstet. Gynecol., *94*:951, 1966.

Requirement of vitamin B_6 during pregnancy. Nutr. Rev., *34*:15, 1976.

Shank, R. E.: A chink in our armor. Nutrition Today, *5*:2, 1970.

Thomson, A. M., et al.: The energy cost of human lactation. Br. J. Nutr., *24*:565, 1970.

Usher, R. H.: Clinical and therapeutic aspects of fetal malnutrition. Pediatr. Clin. North Am., *17*:169, 1970.

Warkany, J.: Production of congenital malformations by dietary measures (Experiments in mammals). JAMA, *168*:2020, 1958.

Weigley, E. S.: The pregnant adolescent. J. Am. Diet. Assoc., *66*:588, 1975.

White, H. S.: Iron deficiency in young women. Am. J. Public Health, *60*:659, 1970.

Winick, M. (ed.): Nutrition and Fetal Development. New York, John Wiley and Sons, 1974.

Chapter 14

NUTRITION IN INFANCY

Nutritionally, the first year or two of life mark in major degree a continuum of fetal conditions, a transitional stage to be sure, but with maintained dependence on a largely maternal environment for food and protection, and a social adaptation in food habits and otherwise that permits successful coexistence with fellow humans.

John E. Gordon*

The infant continues to grow and develop rapidly after birth. Postnatal life is a continuum in human development. Normal growth and development depend largely upon the nutritional status of the infant. Nutritional status is related directly to the nutrition of the mother, to inherited characteristics and to a dietary intake of the essential nutrients. The infant born with a poor nutritional rating is handicapped from the beginning of life. Stunted growth and depressed brain and neurological development may result from dietary inadequacies or restrictions at the early stage of physical development. In many underdeveloped countries where infant mortality is high, nutritional status is poor largely because of an inadequate intake of dietary essentials at the appropriate stage of development. Infant mortality in the United States has declined but ranks thirteenth among the nations of the world.

NUTRITIONAL ALLOWANCES FOR THE INFANT

During the first few days of life, the infant usually loses a few ounces, which is of no serious consequence. A daily intake of the dietary essentials, without feeding problems, will result in a gain in weight within a week or 10 days.

Calories

During infancy the body grows faster than at any other time of life, and the caloric require-

ments per unit of body weight are high. While the calorie allowance *per kg.* decreases progressively from birth, the total caloric needs of the infant increase from month to month. About one quarter of the calories taken in the first three months of life are used for growth, while at 9 to 12 months of age only 6 per cent of the calories are used for growth.[16]

At birth a baby requires about 350 to 500 kcalories, and at one year from 800 to 1200 kcalories. Milk provides all the calories at birth. At six months, it supplies 50 to 70 per cent of the calories. Cereal, vegetables, fruit, meat and egg, when introduced, provide the remaining energy needs. The Food and Nutrition Board of the National Academy of Sciences—National Research Council recommends that during the first year of life calorie allowances be reduced in suitable steps from a level of 117 kcalories per kg. of body weight at birth and for the first six months to 108 kcalories per kg. by the end of one year. (See Table 14–1.) There are wide individual variations in physical activity and individual adjustments must be made.

Weight Gain as an Indicator of Dietary Adequacy

The infant requires approximately 2½ to 3 ounces of breast milk or formula per day per pound of body weight. However, this is a *general rule,* and it is better to allow the infant to regulate his own intake. Ounsted and her colleagues found that infants do this very well, and that those born small-for-date (small for gestational age) will have a larger intake on a per kg. basis than those born large-for-date, who will

---

*Am. J. Dis. Child., *129*:422, 1976.

Table 14–1   DAILY DIETARY ALLOWANCES FOR INFANTS AND NUTRIENT CONTENT OF HUMAN MILK, COW'S MILK AND INFANT FORMULA*

| NUTRIENT | DAILY ALLOWANCES | | HUMAN MILK | COW'S MILK | TYPICAL FORMULA |
	0–6 mo.	6–12 mo.	(per liter)		
Kilocalories	117/kg.	108/kg.	750	670	680
Protein (gm.)	2.2/kg.	2.0/kg.	11	36	16
Casein (gm.)	—	—	4.4	29.5	13.1
Lactalbumin (gm.)	—	—	6.7	6.5	2.9
Lactose (gm.)	—	—	68	49	72
Fat (gm.)	—	—	45	36	36
Polyunsaturated (gm.)	—	—	7	1.4	8
Monounsaturated (gm.)	—	—	21	11	5
Saturated (gm.)	—	—	17	21	21
Cholesterol (mg.)	—	—	200	113	160
Vitamin A (I.U.)	1400	2000	1898	1447	2500
Vitamin D (I.U.)	400	400	22[a]	400	400
Vitamin E (I.U.)	4	5	2.7	1.5	15
Vitamin C (mg.)	35	35	43	10	55
Folacin (μg.)	50	50	52	55	50
Niacin (mg. equiv.)	5	8	1.5	9.5	7.0
Riboflavin (mg.)	0.4	0.6	0.36	1.8	1.0
Thiamin (mg.)	0.3	0.5	0.16	0.3	0.6
Vitamin B_6 (mg.)	0.3	0.4	0.1	0.5	0.4
Vitamin B_{12} (μg.)	0.3	0.3	0.3	5.3	1.5
Vitamin K (μg.)	15[b]	15[b]	15	60	65
Calcium (mg.)	360	540	340	1220	510
Phosphorus (mg.)	240	400	140	960	390
Iodine (μg.)	35	45	30	47	68
Iron (mg.)	10	15	0.2[c]	0.5	1.5[d]
Magnesium (mg.)	60	70	40	120	41
Zinc (mg.)	3	5	1.6[c]	4	5
Copper (μg.)	60/kg.[e]	60/kg.[e]	240[c]	300	400
Sodium (mEq.)[g]	8[f]	6[f]	7	22	10
Potassium (mEq.)	7[f]	6[f]	13	38	18
Chloride (mEq.)	7[f]	6[f]	11	28	15
Renal solute load (mOsm/l)[h]			79	232	105

[a] May be higher if vitamin D sulfate is included (360 I.U.). Lakdawala and Widdowson, Lancet, *1*:167, 1977. Not known if vitamin D sulfate form is biologically active in the neonate.
[b] Advisable intake.
[c] Picciano and Guthrie, Am. J. Clin. Nutr., *29*:242, 1976.
[d] Also available with 12.6 mg. per liter.
[e] Estimated requirement.
[f] Advisable intakes.
[g] Milliequivalents.
[h] Milliosmoles per liter.
*Sources: Fomon, S. J.: Infant Nutrition. Philadelphia, W. B. Saunders Co., 1974, pp. 362–63, 222, 326–29. Composition literature of infant formulas from Ross Laboratories, Columbus, Ohio. Macy, I. G., and Kelly, H. J.: Human milk and cow's milk in infant nutrition. In Kon, S. K., and Cowie, A. T. (eds.): Milk: The Mammary Gland and Its Secretion, vol. II. New York, Academic Press, 1961, p. 268. National Dairy Council: Newer Knowledge of Milk, 3rd ed. Chicago, 1972.

have a smaller intake per kg. of body weight. It seems that the small-for-date infant (that is, an infant weighing less than the tenth percentile of the standard weight for his gestational age) has a built-in feedback system that promotes greater caloric intake to allow for "catch-up" growth, and the large-for-date infant has the opposite tendency.[21] For babies born the appropriate size (between the tenth and ninetieth percentiles),

the caloric intake on a per kg. basis is directly related to the size of the baby. The heavier the baby, the greater the caloric intake per kg. of body weight. (See Chapter 37 for full discussion of nutritional care for the low birth weight infant.)

To determine whether the infant is getting an adequate amount of milk, it is possible to weigh the baby before and after each feeding during a

24-hour period about once a week. The differences in weight at each feeding are totaled, which gives an accurate, quantitative figure for the amount of breast milk consumed within the 24-hour period. Insufficient intake is also indicated by the infant's reactions after completion of the feeding. If he is restless, cries and fails to fall asleep after nursing, the feeding may be inadequate and the infant may require supplementary bottle feedings or food. Between the fourth and fifth month the weight of the baby should double, and at the end of the year the birth weight of the baby has usually tripled. See Appendixes 24 to 27.

Overweight. An excessive weight gain is undesirable, and a large, overweight baby is not considered to be in the best state of health. In 1969 at the White House Conference on Nutrition it was stated that obesity in infants is one of the most common problems of infant feeding in this country. A baby who is overweight during the first year of life is more likely to grow up to be an obese adolescent or adult than is one weighing within the normal range.

Early feeding of solids is a common and easy way to overfeed an infant. The infant has not developed sufficiently to be able to adjust to the intake of food and liquid of a different caloric density than breast milk, which is frequently the case with infant foods, table foods and improperly mixed infant formulas. Solids frequently supplement milk intake rather than substitute for it, and an excess of calories is consumed.

It is also easy to overfeed the bottle-fed infant even when only formula is given. The mother may feel it is important for the infant to take the last ounce in the bottle even though the infant doesn't really want it. The infant does not have complete control over his intake as he does when he feeds at the breast.

Hirsch and Knittle in their work with rats and young children have found that overfeeding in early life produces excess and large fat cells that are needed for the storage of fat. These cells are permanent. The regulation of

weight is made more difficult because these cells remain filled with fat.[14] There appear to be two periods during growth when the child is most susceptible to the hypercellularity of adipose tissue—during the first few years of life and during the period between 9 and 13 years of age.[26]

Protein

Protein requirements during infancy, when there is rapid growth, are higher on a per kilogram basis than those of the adult or older child; nitrogen must be provided for the formation of new tissue, the maturation of tissue and the maintenance of tissues. In early infancy, some form of milk constitutes the only protein food. Since the protein of milk contains all the amino acids essential for growth, the protein needs of the infant are believed to be met automatically through human milk or formulas designed to simulate human milk.

The utilization efficiency of the protein of mother's milk by the infant is assumed to be 100 per cent. Based on the composition of human milk (see Table 14–1), the requirements for protein are 1.6 gm. per 100 kcal. from birth to age four months, 1.4 gm. per 100 kcal. from 4 to 12 months of age and 1.2 gm. per kg. per day from 12 to 36 months of age.[4] The RDA on the basis of body weight (kg.) for the first six months is 2.2 gm. and from six months to one year 2.0 gm. Histidine, an essential amino acid for the infant, is needed in addition to the eight required by the adult. The minimum requirement is 34 mg. per kg. per day[15] and is amply supplied by human and cow's milk as well as by the standard formulas. Tyrosine and cystine may also be essential for the premature infant.[5] To allow for proteins of lower biological value than those of human milk, the advisable intakes of protein are higher: 1.9 gm. per 100 kcal., 1.7 gm. per 100 kcal. and 1.4 gm. per kg. per day for the age categories referred to previously.[5] See Table 14–2.

If the dietary protein is more than 8 per cent

Table 14–2 ESTIMATED REQUIREMENTS AND ADVISABLE INTAKES FOR PROTEIN FOR NORMAL FULL-SIZE INFANTS AND CHILDREN*

AGE	REQUIREMENT	ADVISABLE INTAKE
Birth to 4 months (gm/100 kcal)	1.6	1.9
4 to 12 months (gm/100 kcal)	1.4	1.7
12 to 36 months (gm/kg/day)	1.2	1.4

*From: Fomon, S.J.: Infant Nutrition, 2nd ed. Philadelphia, W. B. Saunders Co., 1974, p. 141.

of calories as provided by human milk, the protein requirement is usually met. Below 8 per cent it is impossible to feed the infant enough food to meet his protein requirements. Higher than 10 per cent of the calories from protein of high biological value makes no difference in nitrogen retention, but increases the *renal solute load*. Any protein not needed for growth and maintenance undergoes deamination in the liver, and the non-nitrogenous residue can be oxidized to provide energy or converted to fat and stored as energy reserve. The nitrogenous end products must be excreted. This requires a sufficient quantity of water in the diet.

Fat

A small amount of an essential fatty acid, *linoleic acid,* has been found to be necessary for growth and dermal integrity in human infants. Both human milk and cow's milk contain it, but human milk normally contains about three times as much linoleate as cow's milk. Human milk contains 6 to 9 per cent of calories as linoleate, and linoleic acid in the range of 3 per cent of total calories is reported to meet the infant requirement. The linoleic acid content of breast milk reflects the linoleic acid intake of the mother. Infants and children probably have a greater need for fats than do adults. During the first three months of life, infants store large amounts in the skin and internal organs. Tests show that fat is added until the age of one, when the situation changes; during the next four years there is a steady loss of this tissue. From the fifth to the eighth year there is neither loss nor gain. Thereafter, fat is added gradually until adult life. The only exception is the year or two before the adolescent growth spurt.

Young infants lacking fat in their diet have been reported to develop certain types of eczema (see Fig. 14–1). Hansen[13] reported thickening and dryness of the skin, oozing in the body folds and eruption in the diaper region (Fig. 14–1) in infants on low fat intake and has established the abnormalities as a manifestation of linoleic acid or essential fatty acid deficiency, not of the total fat content. The principal sources of fat in human milk and in standard formulas are shown in Table 14–1.

Fat is less well absorbed by the newborn than by the older infant, and the low birth weight infant has even less efficient fat absorption. However, human milk fat is better absorbed and more easily tolerated by all infants than cow's milk fat because human milk fat contains fatty acids of shorter chain length,

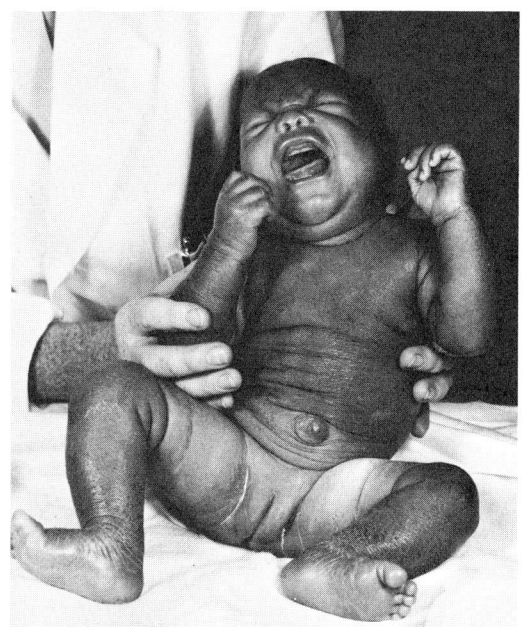

Figure 14–1 Thickening and dryness of the skin, oozing in the body folds and eruption in the diaper region caused by linoleic acid deficiency in infant having a low fat intake. (Photo courtesy of Dr. A. E. Hansen and The National Live Stock and Meat Board Food and Nutrition News, *29,* No. 5, 1958.)

which are also less saturated. Proprietary formulas, on the other hand, do not contain butterfat but mixtures of corn and coconut oils, which provide a fat almost as well absorbed as human milk fat.

The infant should receive about 35 to 55 per cent of his or her calories from fat. If the fat intake is significantly less than this, as in the case of skim milk feedings, the infant may have a deficient intake of calories. He or she may try to make up the caloric deficit by increasing the volume of milk taken, but usually cannot make up the entire amount. Even if the infant can take the increased volume needed to make up the calories, he or she will probably become dehydrated because of the high renal solute load resulting from excessive protein, calcium and phosphorus intake. A high fat intake (40 per cent or more of the calories), particularly from poorly absorbed butterfat, will also result in an inadequate caloric intake. The infant loses the calories from the unabsorbed fat and becomes hungry and cranky, with fatty, foul-smelling stools. This typically happens in the infant who, at an early age (less than six months), is fed only homogenized milk or evaporated milk without carbohydrate. Corn syrup is added to evaporated milk when making formula to bring the percentage of calories from

fat down to about 40 per cent. If homogenized milk is to be used, it should not be started until the infant also begins taking additional carbohydrate in the form of at least two jars of commercially prepared baby food or its equivalent in table foods.[6]

Atherosclerosis Prevention. Because of the early appearance of "fatty streaks" in the arteries of U.S. school children, the kinds of fat and cholesterol in the diet of infants have received attention as a possible factor in the later development of atherosclerosis. These "fatty streaks" presumably arise from blood lipids and progress toward atherosclerosis. However, there is no evidence to recommend changing the diet of infants during the first year or two of life from the model of the breast-fed infant.

The cholesterol content of breast milk is one-third higher than that of cow's milk and six to seven times higher than that of commercial formula. It has been suggested that the high cholesterol content of breast milk is necessary for proper development and that the absence of cholesterol in infancy may limit the infant's ability to synthesize steroid hormones and bile acids; and that cholesterol is necessary to develop enzyme systems for feedback control of cholesterol synthesis and catabolism later in life. However, this has been substantiated only in rats and pigs and not in humans. Studies comparing the cholesterol content of early infant feedings with later serum cholesterol levels have been made in children throughout childhood and adolescence, and no significant differences have been shown between those who were breast-fed and those who were formula-fed.[10, 11] However, it may be that (1) the period of breast feeding was not continued long enough, (2) the protective effect of early high cholesterol feeding is not seen until even later in life, or (3) the fatty acid content of each mother's breast milk was different; this was not controlled. The fatty acid composition of the fat in breast milk does affect the serum cholesterol level of the infant, and the mother's breast milk reflects to some extent her dietary fat intake.[23]

Carbohydrate

As a rule, approximately half of an infant's calorie allowance is supplied as carbohydrate. The disaccharide lactose, which is found only in milk, appears to be the carbohydrate of choice in infant feeding. Dextrose, maltose, dextrins, sucrose and lactose are used in for-

mulas and are digested and absorbed to a lesser extent than lactose alone but are better utilized than starch. Starch is not well digested or absorbed by the very young infant because of the low activity of pancreatic amylase, which is needed for its digestion. This is another reason to postpone the introduction of infant cereals and other starch-containing infant foods until the child is at least three months old. Table 14–3 shows the carbohydrate composition of commonly used infant formulas.

Minerals

Calcium and Phosphorus. An infant fed with standard formula receives about 170 mg. of calcium per kg. but retains only 35 to 50 per cent of it. Although the calcium available to the breast-fed infant is less, it is assumed that his calcium needs are met fully. The calcium in breast milk is better absorbed. The high recommended daily allowance of 360 to 450 mg. of calcium during the first year of life applies only to the bottle-fed infant.

A ratio of approximately 1.2:1.0 calcium to phosphorus occurs in cow's milk and formulas compared with the ratio of 2:1 in human milk. It is recommended that the calcium to phosphorus ratio in an infant's diet be maintained at a 1.5:1.0 ratio. Later the amount of phosphorus can be raised to a ratio similar to that of cow's milk.

Iron. If the mother's diet is adequate during pregnancy, the baby has adequate stores of iron at birth to permit maintenance of a normal hemoglobin level for about six months. The RDA for infants zero to six months old is set at 10 mg. per day or 1 mg. per kg. per day. At four to six months, when iron reserves are depleted, approximately 15 mg. of iron per day is recommended, until the age of three years. Enriched cereals, iron-fortified formula, meat and egg yolk provide the iron needed. The low birth weight infant (under 2500 gm.) and the infant of a multiple birth with significant reduction in total hemoglobin levels require 2 mg. per kg. per day beginning about two months after birth. This will necessitate the use of an iron supplement in addition to breast milk or the use of an iron-fortified formula. This group of infants is especially prone to iron deficiency anemia.

Iron deficiency anemia commonly appears in children 9 to 24 months old and is most prevalent in children from lower socioeconomic populations.

Fresh cow's milk has been shown to be associated with a small but chronic gastrointesti-

nal blood loss. Therefore, it should not be used before six months of age and preferably not until after the first year of life. Intake should not exceed 3 cups when the child is six months to one year old.

Fluoride. Fluoride is considered to be an essential nutrient in the structure of teeth and is necessary for resistance to tooth decay. It has a protective role during the period of calcification of dental tissues. A lactating mother drinking fluoridated water or the use of formulas made with fluoridated water will protect the infant. See Table 14–1 for recommended allowances.

Zinc. Although there are not sufficient data to determine the zinc requirement for the human infant, the RDA has been set at 3 mg. for the first six months of life and 5 mg. for the second six months. For the second year, the RDA is increased to 10 mg. and remains at this level throughout childhood. The RDA for infancy has been based on the zinc concentration of human milk, which is 1.4 to 3.95 mg. per liter.[22] Breast milk is assumed to be the model food during infancy and the one that best meets the infant's requirements. Therefore, the amount of zinc supplied by breast milk can be used to establish the RDA and the standards for feedings using other than human milk. (See Table 14–1.)

Water

Special attention must be given to the water needs of bottle-fed infants. The recommendation for infants is 1.5 ml. per kcal. The infant's surface area per unit of body weight and basal metabolic rate are each twice that of an adult. Therefore there are greater heat and water losses and more metabolic wastes with the infant than the adult. A high protein formula, excess sodium and potassium intake and high environmental temperature or fever require more water to eliminate body metabolic wastes and replace water loss.

Vitamins

If the diet of a nursing mother is nutritionally adequate, the vitamins necessary for the infant will be contained in her milk, with the possible exception of vitamin D and ascorbic acid. The ascorbic acid content of her milk reflects her vitamin C intake and may have to be supplemented. A vitamin D supplement may be needed if the infant is not exposed to sunlight. However, it is now known that human milk contains much more vitamin D than was thought previously, and most of it is present in water-soluble form.[17] It is not known whether this water-soluble form has the same biological activity as the lipid-soluble form, but if it does breast-fed infants would not need vitamin D supplements. This could explain why breast-fed infants, even those in northern climates with little sun exposure, do not seem to get rickets.

Cow's milk contains considerably less vitamin D in the water-soluble form and cannot meet the needs of the human infant unless it is fortified. Ascorbic acid in cow's milk is also inadequate. The infant being fed with evaporated milk formula should have a vitamin C supplement but vitamin D supplementation will not be necessary, since evaporated milk is fortified with vitamin D. All proprietary formulas contain the necessary amounts of vitamins C and D, and no supplementation is necessary.

Vitamin A. The vitamin A requirement of human infants has not been determined. The amount stored in the infant's liver at birth depends largely on the vitamin A intake of the mother. The infant consuming 850 ml. of human milk receives about 1500 I.U. of vitamin A per day. The recommended daily allowance for the first year of life has been set at 1400 to 2000 I.U. (about 300 to 400 R.E.).

Vitamin D. The recommended allowances (RDA) for vitamin D in infancy are well established. An intake of 100 I.U. per day will prevent rickets and 300 I.U. per day will cure rickets. With a sufficient calcium intake, the recommended ingestion of 400 I.U. per day promotes calcium absorption and metabolism, provides for skeletal growth and prevents rickets in normal full-term and premature infants. Excessive intake of vitamin D (1000 to 3000 I.U. per kg. per day) may be toxic and may lead to hypercalcemia.

Vitamin E. Very little placental transfer of vitamin E occurs and infants have low tissue concentration of that vitamin. Low birth weight infants have an even greater tendency to low plasma vitamin E levels and may develop hemolytic anemia. A vitamin E supplement (alpha-tocopherol) of 0.5 mg. per kg. per day is recommended for them.[7] The content in human milk ranges from 2 to 5 I.U. per liter. This amount meets the RDA of 4 to 5 I.U. Cow's milk contains about one tenth to one half the amount in human milk. A supplement to cow's milk formula of 5 I.U. is needed during the first year of life. Proprietary formulas, which con-

Table 14–3 COMPOSITION OF INFANT FORMULAS PER LITER

MILK OR FORMULA	KCAL.	PRO-TEIN (gm.)	FAT (gm.)	CHO (gm.)	ASH (gm.)	CAL-CIUM (mg.)	PHOS-PHORUS (mg.)	SODIUM (mg.)	SODIUM (mEq.)
Human milk	750	11	45	68	2.0	340	140	161	7
Proprietary formulas									
Similac	680	15.5	36	72	3.7	510	390	220	10
Enfamil	670	15	37	69	3.4	550	460	280	12
SMA	670	15	36	72	2.5	440	330	150	6
Advance	540	28	20	62	5.0	800	600	450	20
Cow's Milk									
Evaporated milk formula[b]	660	28	32	69	7.0	1027	827	498	22
Skim	360	36	1	51	7.0	1210	950	520	23
2%	590	42	20	60	8.0	1430	1120	610	27
Whole	670	36	36	49	7.0	1220	960	498	22
Special formulas									
ProSobee	680	25	34	68	5.0	790	530	420	18
Neo-Mull-Soy	680	18.6	36	66	5.0	850	630	360	16
Isomil	680	20	36	68	3.8	700	500	300	13
Meat base formula	650	28	33	62	4.0	980	650	180	8
Nutramigen	670	22	26	88	5.6	630	470	315	14
Cho-Free	670	19	36	—	5.0	892	682	367	16
Pregestimil	670	22	28	88	6.0	630	470	315	14
Portagen	670	24	32	78	7.0	630	470	315	14
Lofenalac	670	22	27	87	6.0	470	470	483	21
Lonalac	670	34	35	48	6.0	560	570	25	1.1
Similac PM 60/40	670	15	35	75	2.0	200	120	161	7
Enfamil Premature	810	18	45	83	4.5	660	560	340	15

[a] Available with iron supplement (12–13 mg./liter).
[b] Formula: 10 oz. evaporated milk
       1 oz. corn syrup
      14 oz. water

      25 oz. formula
[c] Medium-chain triglyceride.

Table 14–3 COMPOSITION OF INFANT FORMULAS PER LITER *(Continued)*

POTASSIUM (mg.)	(mEq.)	IRON (mg.)	PROTEIN SOURCE	FAT SOURCE	CHO SOURCE	COMMENT
507	13	0.2	lactalbumin, casein	human	lactose	Protein readily digested. Adequate in all vitamins and minerals except possibly vitamins C and D, and fluoride.
700	18	tr.[a]	casein	soy, coconut and corn oils	lactose	Vitamins and minerals added.
700	18	1.4[a]	casein	soy and coconut oils	lactose	Vitamins and minerals added.
560	14	13	casein, de-mineral-ized whey	oleo, soybean, safflower and coconut oils	lactose	"Humanized" formula—close to human milk. Vitamins and minerals added.
1100	28	18	casein, soy protein	soy and corn oils	lactose, corn syrup solids	Formula for infants 9–12 months old.
1212	31	2	casein	butterfat	lactose, sucrose	Inadequate in iron, vitamin C and possibly fluoride.
1450	37	tr.	casein	none	lactose	Inappropriate for infants.
1750	45	1	casein	butterfat	lactose	Inappropriate for infants.
1440	37	tr.	casein	butterfat	lactose	Inappropriate for infants less than 6 months of age.
740	19	12.6	soy protein	soy oil	sucrose, corn syrup solids	Vitamins and minerals added. For infants allergic to cow's milk.
900	23	10.4	soy protein	soy oil	sucrose	Vitamins and minerals added. For infants allergic to cow's milk.
710	18	12	soy protein	coconut and soy oils	sucrose, corn syrup solids	Vitamins and minerals added. For infants allergic to cow's milk.
380	10	13.7	beef hearts	sesame oil	modified tapi-oca, cane sugar, sucrose	Vitamins and minerals added. For infants allergic to soy protein.
680	17	12.6	casein hy-drolysate	corn oil	modified tapi-oca, sucrose	Protein more easily digested. Non-allergenic. Lactose-free.
892	23	8.4	soy protein	soy oil	none	For infants with a carbohydrate intolerance. Iron needed.
680	17	12.6	casein hy-drolysate	MCT[c] oil, corn oil	dextrose, modified tapioca	Protein and fat easily digested. Non-allergenic protein. Used in mal-absorption.
840	22	12.6	sodium caseinate	MCT oil, corn oil	sucrose, corn syrup solids	Lactose-free. Used in malabsorp-tion. Vitamins added.
1053	27	12.7	amino acids		lactose, tapi-oca starch	Low in phenylalanine. Used in PKU. Vitamins added.
1053	27	1			lactose	Low in sodium. Vitamins added.
585	15	12	casein, de-mineral-ized whey	coconut and corn oils	lactose	"Humanized" formula—close to human milk. Vitamins and minerals added.
830	21	15	casein	soy and coconut oils	lactose, sucrose	Higher caloric and protein con-centration. Vitamins and minerals added.

tain higher amounts of polyunsaturated fat, are adequately fortified with vitamin E.

Vitamin K. The vitamin K nutriture of the newborn requires special attention. A deficiency may develop and result in bleeding or "hemorrhagic disease of the newborn." This is more common in breast-fed infants because breast milk contains only 15 μg. of vitamin K per liter, while cow's milk and cow's milk formulas contain approximately four times that amount. Breast-fed infants consume less milk during the first few days of life than do formula-fed infants, which also accounts for their low vitamin K intake. It is recommended that every newborn infant receive a vitamin K supplement soon after birth in the form of 3-phytylmenaquinone (vitamin K_1).

Ascorbic Acid. The recommended allowance (RDA) of 35 mg. of ascorbic acid is supplied daily in 850 ml. of human milk. Infants fed formulas will have their requirements met by the vitamin C in the formula. Infants fed cow's milk need a daily dietary supplement.

Thiamin. Thiamin content of human milk is usually adequate if the dietary intake is adequate. Human milk contains an average of 0.01 mg. of thiamin per 100 ml. as compared with 0.03 mg. per 100 ml. in cow's milk. The minimum thiamin requirement for the human infant based on intake from mother's milk or formula and urinary excretion studies seems to be approximately 0.27 mg. per 1000 kcal., and the recommended daily allowance (RDA) is 0.5 mg. per 1000 kcal. Enriched cereals are good sources of thiamin in the infant's diet. Proprietary formula or evaporated milk formula will meet the infant's thiamin requirements.

Riboflavin. The riboflavin RDA for infants to six months of age is 0.4 mg. and for those aged 6 to 12 months, 0.6 mg. Human milk and proprietary formulas contain 0.04 mg. per 100 ml. and cow's milk 0.17 mg. per 100 ml.

Niacin. The niacin allowance recommended for infants up to six months old is 8 mg. per 1000 kcal., about two thirds of which will come from tryptophan. The older infant requires 6.6 mg. per 1000 kcal. but not less than 8 mg. of niacin equivalents daily. An average of 0.17 mg. of niacin and 22 mg. of tryptophan, or a niacin equivalent of 0.50 per 100 ml., is contained in human milk and formula. One hundred ml. of cow's milk contains 0.92 niacin equivalents.

Pyridoxine. The infant's storage of pyridoxine (B_6) at birth protects him against a diet containing very little of the vitamin. The RDA is 0.3 mg. to six months of age and 0.4 mg. from six months to one year. The amount of B_6 in human milk gradually increases from 0.01 to 0.02 mg. per liter during the first month of lactation to 0.10 mg. per liter from then on. If the mother is undernourished and the B_6 content of her milk falls below 0.06 to 0.08 mg. per liter, chemical and biochemical abnormalities may occur in the infant. The extreme manifestation of B_6 deficiency in the infant is convulsions. Cow's milk contains 0.35 to 0.60 mg. of vitamin B_6 per liter. The higher content of vitamin B_6 correlates with the higher protein found in cow's milk as compared to human milk. Formulas contain more than adequate amounts of pyridoxine in relation to the protein provided by them. Meats in general are a good source of B_6, fish is a fair to good source and dairy products are a poor to good source.

Folacin. The RDA for folacin is 50 μg. for the infant to the age of 12 months. This need is adequately supplied by breast milk or formulas, except those made from goat's milk. If the infant's formula is goat's milk a daily folic acid supplement (50 μg.) is necessary.

Vitamin B_{12}. The infant serum levels of cobalamin (vitamin B_{12}) are approximately twice that of the mother. The RDA for infants during the first year of life is 0.3 μg. (See Table 14–1.)

The Committee on Nutrition of the American Academy of Pediatrics, concerned about the composition of proprietary infant formulas, made a policy statement on standards for these products.[3] These standards are based on the composition of milk from a healthy mother. The minimum amount for each nutrient is close to that in human milk and thus is the preferable quantity. The maximum amount is given for formulas intended for low birth weight or sick infants, who take less formula and therefore need the higher nutrient content.

BREAST FEEDING VERSUS FORMULA FEEDING

Although advancement in the planned formula nutrition of newborn infants has been made, breast milk is still considered the optimal food for the human infant.[3] Moreover, as the world supply of animal protein (milk protein in this case) becomes more precious, it is ecologically wise to breast feed an infant if at all possible. Holt and Snyderman[28] report the results of ideal artificial feeding as being comparable to breast feeding, but there are additional advantages to breast feeding that we are either dis-

covering or cannot measure. The healthy woman with firm, healthy nipples who prefers to nurse her baby should be encouraged to do so. The mother with small, delicate or inverted nipples should be taught during her pregnancy how to prepare them for breast feeding. However, she may still elect to bottle feed her baby. Regardless of the mother's physical condition, a woman who has an aversion to nursing or who must return to work should not be threatened about the future welfare of her baby if she does not breast feed. A mother and her baby are a nursing couple, and the method of feeding must meet the needs of both.

POSSIBLE CONTRAINDICATIONS FOR BREAST FEEDING

If the mother has a chronic illness, it may not be wise for her to breast feed her baby. All drugs ingested by the lactating mother are found in breast milk to some degree. Little is known about the kind and amount of drugs and toxicants an infant can safely tolerate. Estrogen-containing contraceptives may reduce the quantity of milk, so progestogen-containing contraceptives are preferred.[25] Heavy cigarette smoking may reduce the volume of milk excreted. Nicotine is highly toxic, is fat-soluble and is transmitted through breast milk to the infant. (See Table 13–8.) In other cases, nursing may interfere with the mother's well-being, especially if labor has been complicated by severe hemorrhage or sepsis.

Breast feeding may have to be discontinued temporarily if hyperbilirubinemia develops in the infant. After 24 to 48 hours, the infant's blood bilirubin level drops and breast feeding can be resumed. Another situation requiring temporary discontinuation of breast feeding is acute illness in the mother. The breast should be pumped during this period to maintain milk supply until the mother is ready to resume nursing.

ADVANTAGES OF BREAST FEEDING

The advantages of breast feeding are many. It is free from bacterial contamination, is economical and requires no elaborate preparation, may improve the parent–child relationship and is less likely to be associated with infant allergic manifestations. Breast feeding also has the advantage of immunizing the baby against certain infectious diseases through the action of the antibodies (particularly immunoglobulin A), antimicrobial enzymes, T cell lymphocytes, macrophages, complement and lactoferrin received in the mother's milk and colostrum. It is not known to what extent these immunological factors are absorbed but they certainly have a protective effect against gastrointestinal infection. In addition, human milk contains a "bifidus factor," a group of nitrogen-containing polysaccharides, which promotes the growth of bifidobacterial flora in the gut. This, combined with the low pH of breast milk, creates an environment that is not conducive to the growth of E. coli, Shigella and other potentially harmful bacteria. There is evidence that breast milk may also protect against necrotizing enterocolitis.[27] (See Chapter 37.)

Human milk protein, being largely in the form of lactalbumin rather than the casein of cow's milk and cow's milk-based formula, is easier to digest and is better tolerated and absorbed. Because the protein is better utilized, and because the human infant does not grow as rapidly as the calf, the protein content is less than that of cow's milk. For this reason, and because the mineral content is also lower, breast milk results in a lower renal solute load for the infant.

There is evidence that the iron in breast milk is better and more fully absorbed by the infant than the iron in cow's milk, and that the infant solely breast fed even until the age of 18 months can maintain a sufficient iron balance.[20] However, since the exclusively breast-fed infant of that age is a rarity, it is recommended that breast-fed infants be given some form of iron supplement after six months of age. It has long been the impression of pediatricians that exclusively breast-fed infants have higher hemoglobin concentrations than do bottle-fed infants. Some theories to explain this increased iron absorption are that (1) human milk contains more lactose, which is known to enhance iron absorption, (2) human milk contains more ascorbic acid, which also enhances iron absorption, and (3) phosphorus is present in higher quantities in cow's milk and is known to decrease iron absorption.[20]

It is less likely that a mother will overfeed her infant when she is nursing because the infant controls his or her own intake. This may vary from feeding to feeding and from day to day. In addition, the composition of human milk, unlike that of a formula, changes from being thin and watery to a more concentrated form as the feeding progresses. Thus, an infant who

finishes at one breast with milk rich in fat and protein will begin at the second breast with a thin, watery milk that can satisfy thirst as well as hunger. Hall postulates that such changes in milk concentration are associated with the development of an appetite control mechanism in breast-fed babies.[12]

TECHNIQUES OF BREAST FEEDING AND BOTTLE FEEDING

Details on the techniques of breast and bottle feeding will be acquired in the pediatric lectures and by experience and therefore will not be duplicated in this text. See Applebaum references at the end of this chapter for good discussions of the techniques of breast feeding. La Leche League, a group that promotes breast feeding, also has many materials to help with understanding breast feeding and aiding the new mother. Babies instinctively know how to suck but may need some help in getting started. The infant is laid close to the mother with his cheek against her breast. The mother can help by holding the breast so that the baby can easily get the nipple into his mouth. (See Figure 14–2.) The bottle-fed baby should be held as though he is being breast fed in order to establish security and companionship.

Complemental Feeding. When the mother's milk supply is inadequate to meet the entire nutritional needs of the infant, the baby is given one or more supplementary bottle feedings. This is known as complemental or mixed feeding.

INFANT FORMULAS

Cow's Milk Formulas

Usually either whole cow's milk, canned evaporated milk or dried milk is used as the basis for feeding the infant who is not breast-fed. The infant may tolerate evaporated milk or dried milk more easily than whole cow's milk because the curd formed in digestion is very fine. Fresh cow's milk is not recommended as an infant feeding for many reasons, already discussed. Advantages of canned evaporated milk and dried milk are economy, consistency of the product, convenience and availability. Canned evaporated milk, which has no additional sugar, should not be confused with sweetened condensed milk!

Commercial Formulas

The common formulas today are available in powdered, concentrated or ready-to-feed form. These prepared formulas have vegetable oils as their fat, contain lactose and added sucrose, and use non-fat dry milk as their protein source, largely in the form of casein. They are fortified to meet all the vitamin and mineral requirements of the infant. For those infants requiring iron supplements, formulas containing 12 to 13 mg. of iron per 100 ml. are also available. When breast feeding is not possible, prepared commercial formulas are the most similar to human milk and are the next best choice. (See Table 14–3.)

Soybean-based Formulas

Soybean protein is unique among vegetable proteins by virtue of its high biological value. While soy protein is biologically inferior to milk protein, growth rates and general development of infants on this formula are normal. The protein content must be higher to make up for the lower PER (protein efficiency ratio) of soy protein. See Chapter 5 for definition of PER.

At a time when animal sources of protein are becoming less plentiful, infant formula manufacturers are beginning to develop formulas based on vegetable protein to be used in the feeding of all healthy infants who are not breast-fed. Usually, this type of formula is used

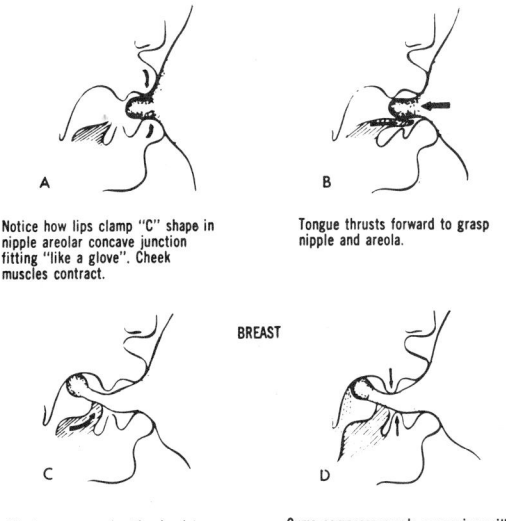

A
Notice how lips clamp "C" shape in nipple areolar concave junction fitting "like a glove". Cheek muscles contract.

B
Tongue thrusts forward to grasp nipple and areola.

BREAST

C
Nipple moves against hard palate as tongue whips backward bringing areola into mouth. NEGATIVE pressure is created by tongue and cheeks against nipple. Suction effect is created.

D
Gums compress areola squeezing milk into back of throat where suction occurs against nipple. Milk flows against hard palate from high pressure system to negative pressure at back of throat.

Figure 14–2   How the infant breast feeds.

for infants with an allergy to cow's milk protein.

Special Infant Formulas

In cases of digestive disturbances, diarrhea or allergy, special milk preparations are available. (See Table 14–3.) Since babies with diarrhea experience more difficulty digesting fats than proteins, boiled skim milk is often used in the basic formula. Or the formula may contain MCT (medium chain triglyceride) oil, which is a better-absorbed source of fat. Acid milk is sometimes used in cases of digestive disturbances, because it produces a very fine curd that is readily digested in the stomach.

PREPARATION OF INFANT FORMULAS

Milk and Fluid Allowance. The amount of milk should be sufficient to meet the infant's individual needs and satisfy his hunger. During a 24-hour period an infant will take 2 to 3 ounces per pound of body weight (120 to 210 ml. per kg.) of a 20 kcal. per oz. formula. This supplies an intake of 40 to 60 kcal. per pound or 90 to 130 kcal. per kg. The baby is his own best regulator of his intake. He can judge it fairly well as long as the formula is of the proper strength—20 kcal. per oz. (67 kcal. per 100 ml.), or the same as that of breast milk. In the first few weeks of life he or she will take 2 to 3 ounces at a feeding, by two months of age will take 4 to 5 ounces and by six months will take 7 to 8 ounces at a feeding.

The fluid requirement is approximately 150 ml. (5 ounces) per kg. of body weight per 24-hour period, or 1.5 ml. per kcal. This amount of fluid is provided by the usual 67 kcal. per 100 ml. formula. However, an infant should be offered additional water in hot weather. See Table 14–4 for fluid requirements of infants.

Sugar Added to Formula. The carbohydrate content of cow's milk is increased to meet the energy requirements and reduce the renal solute load of whole cow's milk. Five to 6 per cent of the total formula volume is the quantity of sugar added. The forms of sugar used are white corn syrup, milk sugar, malt sugar (Dextri-Maltose), lactose, granulated sugar, brown sugar and thick cereal preparations. A typical formula is:

Evaporated milk   1 oz. per lb. body
                  weight of infant.
                  (66 ml. per kg.)

Table 14–4   FLUID REQUIREMENTS OF INFANTS AND CHILDREN*

| AGE | AMOUNT OF WATER |
	(ml./kg./day)
1 week	80–100
2 weeks	125–150
3 months	140–160
6 months	130–155
9 months	125–145
1 year	120–135
2 years	115–125

*Adapted from: Vaughan, V. C., and McKay, R. J. (eds.): Nelson Textbook of Pediatrics, 10th ed. Philadelphia, W. B. Saunders Co., 1975.

Cane sugar or corn syrup	0.5 oz. or 1 tablespoon (15 ml.) for every 5 oz. (150 ml) of evaporated milk used.
Water	Added to make 2½ oz. (75 ml.) of total formula per pound of body weight of the infant. (165 ml. per kg.)

Example: For a 10 pound baby this would mean mixing 10 ounces of evaporated milk with 2 tablespoons of corn syrup and 14 ounces of water to make a total of 25 ounces of formula. See Table 14–3 for an analysis of this formula.

Economy in infant feeding is especially important to families on limited incomes. In low income groups, the lowest cost combination of foods and supplements consistent with safety and availability of facilities for home preparation is desirable, especially if other members in the family are deprived of adequate food. See Table 14–5 for comparative costs of the various methods of infant feeding. Evaporated milk formula is the least expensive acceptable method, followed by breast feeding and the powdered forms of formulas.

TECHNIQUE OF FORMULA PREPARATION

The amount of formula needed for a 24-hour period or longer can be prepared at one time and divided into the number of bottles that will be used for feedings. The bottles are stoppered and kept in the refrigerator until feeding time. When needed, a bottle of formula is placed in warm water until body temperature is reached.

Table 14–5 COSTS OF SEVERAL COMMONLY USED MILK-BASED INFANT FEEDINGS*

FEEDING	FOOD COST PER OUNCE FED	PRICE RANGE BY SOURCE OF SUPPLY[1]	ESTIMATED FOOD COST FOR FIRST YEAR OF LIFE[2]
Whole milk	$.0123	$.0117–.0131	$116
Evaporated milk–corn syrup (Karo) formula[3]	.0142	.01389–.0142	133
Lactation on moderate cost foods[4]	.0180	—	167
Commercial formula			
Concentrated form[5]			
Enfamil	.0242	.0242	227
Similac	.0235	.0227–.0242	221
Advance (formula for older infants)	.0234	—	220
Powdered form[5]			
Enfamil	.0263	—	247
Similac	.0252	—	237
Ready-to-serve form			
Enfamil	.0294	.0291–.0297	276
Similac	.0288	.0278–.0297	271
Advance (formula for older infants)	.0278	—	261

[1] Stores inventoried included three to four supermarkets, drugstores, etc. in Boston, June 1976.

[2] Assumes that this was the only milk-based feed that was fed. The estimates for amounts of formula or milk fed are taken from standard hospital instructions for ounces of formula to be fed per day: up to one month, 18 oz.; one to two months, 21 oz.; two to three months, 24 oz.; three to six months, 30 oz.; six to seven months, 28 oz. (Beikost increasing sharply); seven to nine months, 28 oz.; nine to twelve months, 24 oz.; or a grand total of 9394 oz. for one year.

[3] A 13 oz. can of evaporated milk varied in price from 33 to 34 cents; corn syrup was 59 cents per 16 oz., and the evaporated milk was diluted 1 to 1 with water; so 28 oz. formula cost $.3989 or $.0142 per ounce at 34 cents per can; or $.01389 if can was 33 cents.

[4] Assumes 800 ml. or 26.7 oz. of milk produced per day.

[5] Concentrate and ready-to-serve formulas are readily available in many retail outlets, including pharmacies and supermarkets in the Boston area. However, powder is difficult to obtain except at pharmacies and drugstores, which generally sell all products at a higher price. Thus it is not as inexpensive as might be expected.

*From: Lamm, E., Delaney, J. and Dwyer, J.T.: Economy in the feeding of infants. Pediatr. Clin. North Am., *24*:71, 1977.

The formula and bottles are sterilized, either during preparation of the formula or at some other time before the infant is fed.

Formula Making Equipment[29]

The nurse is frequently responsible for teaching a new mother how to make her baby's formula. There are several good teaching publications on this subject available from local health departments or the Office of Child Development of the U.S. Department of Health, Education and Welfare. Keeping a set of equipment to use only for preparing the formula will make the sterilizing and formula preparation easier.

Kettle for sterilizing. Such a kettle has a tight-fitting cover and a rack inside to hold the bottles.

A wire rack or a pie tin punched with holes (upside down) that fits the bottom of the kettle for holding the bottles.

A bottle brush with a long handle and with stout bristles to scrub the inside of the bottles. It should be one that is bent at the tip, so that the bristles clean the bottom of the bottle and not just the sides.

A measuring tablespoon.

A measuring cup, marked in ounces, with a pouring lip.

A 2 quart saucepan or jar with a pouring lip in which to mix the formula.

A small saucepan with a lid, in which to boil and keep the nipples (if you use the aseptic technique, p. 309).

A funnel makes it easier to pour the formula into the bottles. If you get a plastic funnel, make sure it is the kind that can be boiled.

A long-handled spoon.

A can opener that punches holes (if you use canned milk).

A small wide-mouthed jar with a cover, for used nipples.

Bottles to hold a 24-hour supply of formula.

Nipples and nipple caps.

A pair of tongs is convenient to handle hot bottles and other sterile equipment.

Nursing bottles. The standard-sized nursing bottle holds 8 oz. Ounces are marked, so there need be no guesswork when you pour the formula. Wide-mouth bottles are easiest to clean.

Bottles of heat-resistant glass or of boilable plastic cost more but will probably be cheaper in the long run.

Have as many bottles as are needed in a 24-hour period, plus extras to allow for possible breakage. Two to three extra 4-oz. bottles will be needed for water and orange juice.

Bottles are easier to clean if rinsed after each feeding and filled with cold water.

Nipples. Have one nipple for each feeding, and one for each drink of water or orange juice.

The holes in the nipples may have to be made larger. Try out the nipple by putting it on a bottle with water in it, and turning it upside down. Watch to see if there is a steady drip. Remember that water will come through faster than milk because it is thinner. If the holes seem too small, heat the point of a fine needle in the flame of a match. While the point is red hot, poke it through one or more holes in the nipple.

After each feeding, wash the nipple and squeeze water through the holes. Dry it, and keep it in a covered jar until ready to sterilize the day's supply.

Nipple covers. Nipple caps or covers are made of glass, plastic, aluminum or paper. Paper caps are inexpensive but can be used only once.

Methods of Formula Sterilization

In a country such as the United States, where the water is not contaminated and the environment is relatively free from carriers of enteric pathogens, it is probably not necessary to sterilize an infant's formula. In fact, many mothers do not sterilize formula, seemingly with no adverse effects to their infants. In most situations, thorough cleaning with soap and hot water followed by rinsing and drying of bottles and nipples is probably adequate to prevent formula contamination.[9]

In general there are two methods of preparing sterile formula, namely, terminal heating and aseptic technique. The first method is to mix the formula, pour it unboiled into bottles that have been washed but not sterilized, put on the nipple and last, sterilize the filled bottles. This method eliminates the possibility of contamination and is simple to carry out. It allows less chance for contamination and is the method of choice for formulas that must be prepared or diluted. It is suitable for all types of formulas.

The second or aseptic method is to sterilize the equipment, bottles, nipple collars, nipple covers or disc seals and measuring equipment and then pour the boiled or sterile formula into the sterilized bottles. Any water added must first be boiled. This method is suitable for all types of formulas.

Following is a detailed description of the technique of each method.

Terminal Heating Method. (See Fig. 14–3.)

1. Wash thoroughly with hot water and detergent all the articles to be used. Scrub the insides of the bottles and nipple covers and the insides and outsides of the nipples with the bottle brush.

2. Rinse all articles well. Drain. Squeeze clean water through nipple holes.

3. Measure the milk, water and sugar (or syrup) into the large saucepan. If granulated sugar is used, level off the measuring spoon with the back of a table knife. If syrup is used, pour from the bottle into the measuring spoon. If the milk used is not homogenized, shake the bottle well to mix the cream before measuring. If evaporated milk is used, wash the top of the can with soap and water and rinse it off well before opening. If dried milk is used, mix powder with water according to the amounts prescribed and beat with an egg beater to blend.

4. Divide the milk mixture among the number of bottles needed in 24 hours.

5. Put nipples and nipple covers on the bottles. Do not push or screw nipple covers down tight, because during sterilization the hot air may blow the caps off.

6. Put the bottles of formula on the rack in the kettle. Put one or two bottles of drinking water, covered with nipple and cap, in at the same time. Pour water into the kettle until it comes about half way up on the bottles. Cover the kettle.

7. Bring the water in the kettle to a boil. *Boil actively for 25 minutes.* As soon as the bottles are cool enough to handle, take them out of the kettle. Tighten nipple caps.

8. After the bottles cool, put them in the refrigerator at once. A rack to hold the bottles upright is very convenient.

Aseptic Technique

1. Wash the bottles, nipple covers, funnel and nipples thoroughly in hot water with a detergent. With the bottle brush, scrub the insides of the nursing bottles and nipple covers, disc seals and collars and the insides and outsides of the nipples.

2. Rinse all these articles well. Squeeze clean water through the nipple holes.

3. If the sterilizing kettle has a rack to hold the bottles, set each bottle in it, upside down. Fit nipple covers, funnel, tongs, can opener, measuring

a good way to make the baby's formula is

HEATING AFTER BOTTLING

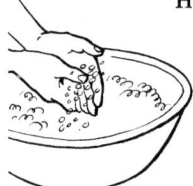

① Wash your hands with soap and water.

② Wash a 1½ to 2-quart jar, jar top, baby bottles, bottle caps or nipple covers, tablespoons, nipples and can opener with soap and hot water.

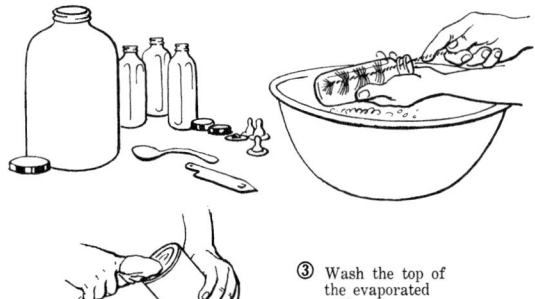

③ Wash the top of the evaporated milk can.

④ Rinse all with clean water.

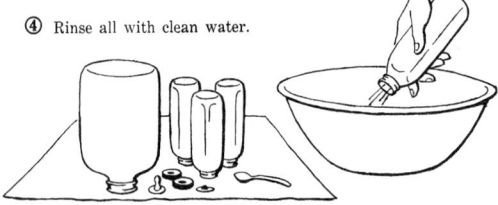

⑤ Put the needed amount of water, evaporated milk, syrup or sugar into the jar.

⑥ Stir with the clean spoon.

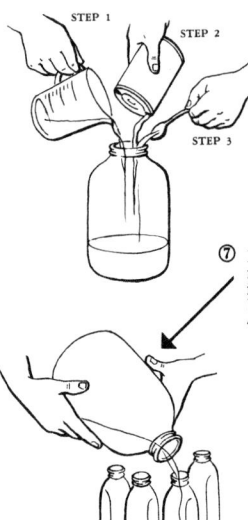

STEP 1

STEP 2

STEP 3

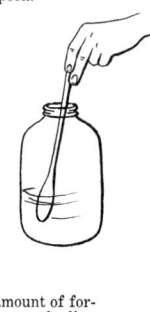

⑦ Pour the amount of formula for one feeding into each of the clean bottles. Usually this is 4, 6, or 8 ounces.

⑧ Put the nipples and bottle caps or nipple covers on the bottles.

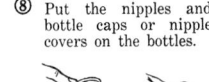

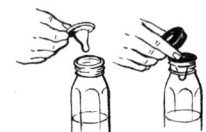

⑨ Put a wire rack, or a clean cloth in the bottom of a large pot and add about 3 or 4 inches of water.

⑩ Put bottles filled with the formula into the pot. Be sure the bottle caps are loose.

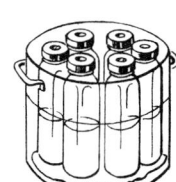

⑪ Cover the pot. After the water starts to boil, boil for 25 minutes.

⑫ Remove the pot from the fire. Leave cover on. Let cool slowly so that milk won't clog the nipples. When you can hold your hands against the sides of the pot remove the bottles. Tighten the caps and place the bottles in the refrigerator or icebox.

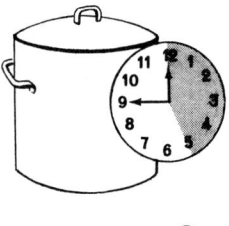

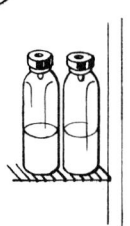

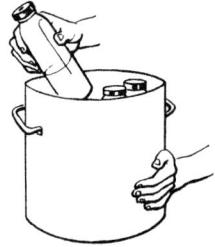

Figure 14–3 Basic steps in the terminal heating method of making a baby's formula. (Courtesy of the Office of Child Development, U.S. Department of Health, Education and Welfare.)

cup and spoons between the bottles. If the kettle has no rack, lay the bottles on their sides in the kettle with the other equipment on top.

4. If the kettle has a rack and a tight-fitting cover, pour in about 5 inches of water and put on the cover. When the water boils actively, steam will form and will sterilize the equipment. Keep the water boiling for at least *five minutes*. If the kettle does not have a tight-fitting lid, put in enough water to completely cover the bottles and all the other things to be sterilized. Boil for at least five minutes after the water has come to a boil.

5. Drain off some of the water. Leave the things in the covered kettle until ready to use them or remove with tongs and place bottles on clean towel or rack.

6. Drop the nipples into boiling water in a small pan, cover and let boil for five minutes. Then pour the water off, let the steam escape and leave the nipples in the covered pan until needed. Boiling nipples too long or letting them stand in water wears them out.

7. Boil water for formula (and drinking water) for five minutes and measure required amount.

8. Add evaporated milk* and carbohydrate or a commercially processed formula to the boiled water. Wash top of container with soap and water and rinse.

9. Pour into bottle. If funnel is used, remove it from the sterilizer without touching its rim or stem and set it in one of the bottles. Attach nipples and cover. For disc seals invert nipples in bottle, apply disc and screw collar down tight. Do not touch any part of the nipple that goes into baby's mouth. Use tongs. (Follow the directions that come with the kind of nipple and bottle used.)

10. Store in refrigerator.

Previously sterilized bottles, nipples and nipple covers are required for use with the commercial ready-to-use formulas, which are sterile in the cans and bottles. For the concentrated liquid and powdered forms, which require mixing, sterilized water is also required. Tops should be washed and rinsed before opening the can. When opened, canned or bottled formulas should be refrigerated and used within 48 hours. Follow instructions given on the bottle or can for best procedure.

Warming the Prepared Feeding

Formulas are generally warmed before each feeding, but several investigators believe that this practice may be unnecessary. Ice-cold formulas apparently are well tolerated by 50 per cent of very young infants and 75 per cent of older infants. However, studies indicate that feedings given directly from the refrigerator tend to lower gastric temperature, decrease

proteolytic enzyme activity and delay digestion. For heating the bottle before feeding, the following directions should be followed: Remove the formula-filled nursing bottle from the refrigerator and set it upright in a small deep saucepan with 3 to 4 inches of warm water. Place the pan over high heat and leave until the water is ready to boil. Shake the bottle several times so that milk is warmed through.

Remove nipple cover, being careful not to contaminate the nipple.

Test the temperature of the milk by letting a few drops trickle onto the inner side of the wrist. It should feel warm but not hot.

FEEDING SCHEDULE

The following feeding schedules for infants are typical and are dependent upon the number of required daily feedings.

Five feedings per day:
6 and 10 A.M.; 2, 6 and 10 P.M.
Six feedings per day:
2, 6 and 10 A.M.; 2, 6 and 10 P.M.
Seven feedings per day:
6, 9 and 12 A.M.; 3, 6, 9 and 12 P.M.
Eight feedings per day:
3, 6, 9 and 12 A.M.; 3, 6, 9 and 12 P.M.

Babies thrive better when fed regularly. However, this does not mean rigidly set intervals of three to four hours, regardless of how much sooner or later they get hungry. The baby should be allowed to develop a feeding schedule of his own, known as "self-regulation," or "self-demand feeding." A baby's hunger is considered the best clock to go by. It is best for a mother and her baby to develop their own nursing "schedule." During the first few weeks, a baby may wake up and appear to need food a dozen times in 24 hours. By the end of the first month, there may be three hours between feedings. By the time the baby is two months old, he frequently sleeps through the night after a late evening feeding. When they are between two and three months old, the majority of babies are on a four-hour feeding schedule.

SUPPLEMENTARY FOODS

Infants have supplementary foods added to the formula or breast feeding during the first year of life to provide the essentials that milk does not supply in adequate amounts, especially iron and vitamin C. These supplements are added gradually, guided by the age, developmental growth and condition of the in-

---

*Whole milk or other unsterilized milk is boiled with the water. Stir constantly while it is boiling.

fant. The age at which solid foods are given varies widely, reflecting divergent opinions on the ability of the infant's gastrointestinal tract to process the food properly. It also depends upon the culture and the social pressures that the mother feels to start feeding solid foods.

The Academy of Pediatrics Committee on Nutrition states that a normal full-term infant can thrive on human milk or formula for the first four to six months of life when diet is appropriately supplemented with vitamins (ascorbic acid and vitamin D). Occasionally, milk is the only food the infant or child receives, and in such excessive amounts that other essential foods, notably foods containing iron, may be excluded, causing one or more deficiencies. Although milk is an excellent food for all ages, especially infants and children, it should not be given to the exclusion of other equally necessary foods.

The proper time to introduce solid foods is determined by changes in the behavior of the oral musculature and by gastrointestinal development, although many babies are fed semisolid food before one month of age. At about four to six months of age when the spoon is inserted between the lips, the lips part, the tongue depresses and food placed at the tip forms into a ball. It is then thrown to the back of the pharynx and swallowed. Earlier, when the spoon is placed between the lips, the baby purses his lips, raises his tongue and pushes against the spoon. Few infants are ready for anything but liquid food until about 16 weeks of age. Salivary enzymes necessary for the digestion of complex starches, such as salivary amylase, are not present until two to three months of age. Lactose and sucrose (added to formulas but not present in breast milk) do not require the salivary enzymes. Forcing solid foods before he is ready for them may be frustrating to the infant as well as to the mother, may result in an unpleasant experience and may possibly be the beginning of food problems.

One indication that the infant may be ready for solid food is when he still seems hungry after nursing or after taking 26 to 30 ounces of formula in 24 hours. It appears that the best time to begin feeding solid food is between four and six months of age. When chewing movements begin (about seven to nine months) table foods requiring chewing should be introduced.

The sequence given here is the usual order in which the formula supplements are added. There may be considerable variation, depending upon the physical and physiological development of the infant and the attitude and needs of the mother. No set guideline is feasible. The eating process is a learning experience and each child develops at his particular rate. If the child were known to have an allergic background, such foods as orange juice and eggs and foods containing cow's milk could be introduced in small quantities and increased gradually as tolerated.

FOOD	AVERAGE AGE WHEN ADDED
Orange juice if infant is on evaporated milk formula	2 weeks
Cereal (whole grain or enriched)	3 to 4 months
Vegetable purée, meat purée	4 to 5 months
Fruit purée	5 to 6 months
Potatoes, boiled or baked, may sometimes be used in place of cereal	6 months
Zwieback or dried bread	8 months
Egg yolk	7 to 8 months (or 2 to 4 months)
Meat	6 to 10 months

Some infants may also need iron supplements from this early point in life. Formulas with added iron are available. One fourth to one third of a cup of orange juice supplies approximately 35 mg. of ascorbic acid. If either orange or tomato juice is not tolerated, a supplement containing 35 mg. ascorbic acid should be given daily. Because tomato juice is only half as rich in ascorbic acid as orange juice, it is necessary to give twice as much tomato juice to meet the daily requirement. If a prepared formula is being used, vitamin C does not need to be given, since it has been added to the formula in the recommended amounts. Milk fortified with vitamin D is a good source of that vitamin if the intake of milk provides 400 units daily of vitamin D. Infants regularly exposed to sunlight will receive enough vitamin D. Commercial formulas are fortified with vitamin D.

Cereals

Cooked cereal is the customary first supplementary food added to the infant's diet. Because the infant's storage of iron is depleted after the first three or four months of life, one of

the reasons for introducing solid foods is to replenish iron. It is best to begin with infant cereals because of their high iron content, about 4 mg. per 100 gm. (See Table 38–4.) Toward the end of the first year, regular iron-fortified cereals can be used. The ready-prepared baby cereals need only to be mixed with a little warm formula, warm boiled milk or warm boiled water. Anderson and Fomon[1] found that mothers generally fed infants less than one third of an ounce of dry cereal to approximately two ounces of cereal–milk or cereal–formula mixture (one part dry cereal, six parts milk). The dry infant cereals are more economical than the "wet pack" type.

Regardless of the grain used, the cost of the cereals is approximately the same. In situations in which cost per unit of protein is important, one would choose the high protein cereals. The labels on many baby foods give the nutritional content of the jar, expressed as a percentage of the U.S. RDA for that nutrient. See Chapter 10 for an explanation of the U.S. RDA, particularly Table 10–9.

Eggs

Only the egg yolk in very small amounts of one-fourth teaspoon is offered to the young baby. Because some infants are sensitive to the protein of egg yolk, it is advisable to increase gradually the amount of whole yolk served daily. The raw yolk may be given alone, or may be added to the milk, cooked with milk into a custard, added to vegetables or cereals; or the yolk may be coddled, poached or cooked. Egg yolk simmered for about 10 minutes and put through a sieve is an easy method of preparation. The sieved yolk can be mixed with a small amount of milk or added to the cereal. Allergy to egg white seems to be more prevalent than to the egg yolk. Until about the end of the first year, care should be exercised in separating the egg yolk from the egg white.

Vegetables and Fruits

Opinions differ as to which should be introduced first—fruits or vegetables. Some believe that if fruit (especially sweetened) is introduced first, vegetables will be poorly accepted. The fruits and vegetables served to the baby may be either canned or freshly cooked and strained. Use green or deep yellow vegetables such as carrots, squash, spinach, green beans or turnip greens. Mashed raw banana is acceptable. In the beginning only a teaspoonful is given; the amount is increased gradually until the year old baby receives 3 to 4 tablespoons of fruits and vegetables. To familiarize the child with different flavors, a variety of fruits (such as applesauce, peaches, apricots, pears and cooked prunes) and vegetables should be offered. By six months, boiled or baked potatoes may sometimes take the place of cereal. Before the end of the first year, more coarsely mashed or chopped vegetables should be substituted for the strained varieties. Near the end of the year, butter or fortified margarine can be added to vegetables for flavor.

Meat and Fish

Scraped lean meat or liver cooked in little or no fat can be added before the baby has teeth. Leverton and associates[18] conducted a study in which they included strained meat in the diet as early as six weeks with favorable results. They report that the infants who received a dietary supplement of strained meat showed higher hemoglobin values as a result. However, meat is usually added to the diet between the fourth and sixth month. When the secretion of the proteolytic enzymes in the intestinal juice increases, the infant is able to digest most proteins. Canned puréed and chopped varieties, as well as meat soups, prepared for babies and ready to use, save time and effort.

Toward the end of the first year, white-fleshed fish such as cod or haddock (baked, steamed or broiled) can be served in place of meat once or twice a week. Canned salmon or tuna with fat removed can also be used. Start with a teaspoon and gradually increase. When teeth and chewing movements appear, the baby may have thinly sliced liver, chicken or other fowl, beef, veal or well-cooked lean pork.

Bread

Bread dried in the oven or zwieback can be added when the baby's first teeth have come in. He can have it after meals or for midmorning or midafternoon snacks. The main purpose of the dried bread is to exercise his jaws.

Other Factors

The renal solutes (nitrogenous substances and electrolytes) must be excreted from the kidney. Infants fed strained meats, egg yolk and high meat dinners have comparatively high renal solute excretion (loads). Those infants fed fruit juices, fruit puddings and desserts

have low renal solute loads and the other infant foods cause intermediate renal solute loads. The choice of infant foods is important at various times when the volume of food is low, when extrarenal losses of fluid are abnormal and when renal concentrating ability is low. Kidney function generally becomes efficient by six to eight weeks, after which protein foods, in addition to formula or breast milk, can be handled.[1]

Sodium and monosodium glutamate have been used in commercially strained and junior foods. Salt is still added to some but the amount is limited. These seasonings were probably added to the foods primarily to satisfy the tastes of mothers. A study was conducted by Fomon and co-workers[8] to compare the consumption of salted and unsalted strained foods by four month old and seven month old infants. On the basis of an average daily food intake, infants appeared to accept the unsalted foods as well as the salted ones. The unsalted foods usually fed to infants contain sufficient sodium to meet the infant's need. From a nutritional point of view there is no justification for adding salt to strained foods for infants. Animal studies have suggested that large amounts of sodium in infant foods may predispose susceptible infants to development of hypertension later in life. (See Chapter 28.) Studies on the salt intake of infants in the first year of life varied widely but results were rather high. About 60 per cent of the total sodium in the diet of the infant is contributed by processed vegetables, meats and eggs. An infant eating foods to which salt has been added commercially or by the mother at four months of age may be receiving three times the amount of sodium recommended. The issue of the safety of added sodium chloride and monosodium glutamate in infant food is not resolved. In 1970 the National

Table 14–6 AVERAGE CALORIC DISTRIBUTION OF FOODS FED TO INFANTS*

| FOOD | TOTAL SOLIDS (%) | KCAL PER 100 GM. | PER CENT OF CALORIES FROM | | |
			Protein	Fat	Carbohydrate
Human milk	13	75	6	56	38
Prepared infant formulas					
[1]Milk-based	13	67	9	48	43
[2]Soy-based	13	67	13	47	40
Cow's milk					
Whole	13	65	22	48	30
2 per cent	13	59	28	31	41
Skim	10	36	40	3	57
[3]Strained foods					
Egg yolks	29	192 (184–199)	21 (20–23)	76 (69–80)	3 (0–8)
Meats	21	106 (86–194)	53 (20–72)	46 (28–80)	1 (0–8)
Desserts and puddings	23	96 (71–136)	4 (0–18)	7 (0–31)	89 (51–99)
Fruits	22	85 (79–125)	2 (0–10)	2 (1–7)	96 (87–99)
High-meat dinners	17	84 (63–106)	29 (20–42)	47 (20–57)	24 (19–40)
Fruit juices	16	65 (45–98)	2 (0–5)	2 (0–7)	96 (89–100)
Creamed vegetables	16	63 (42–94)	13 (5–26)	13 (3–25)	74 (57–90)
Soups and dinners	13	58 (39–94)	16 (7–33)	28 (2–54)	56 (34–86)
Plain vegetables	12	45 (27–78)	14 (5–32)	6 (1–19)	80 (62–92)
[4]"Typical" baby food	20	75	8	12	80
Average U.S. diet	—	—	12	42	46

[1]Average of Similac, Enfamil and SMA.
[2]Average of Isomil, ProSobee, Neo-Mull-Soy, i-Soyalac and Nursoy.
[3]Range is in parentheses.
[4]Average composition weighted by sales by product category.
*From Anderson, T.A.: Commercial infant foods: Content and composition. Pediatr. Clin. North Am., 24: 1, 1977.

Academy of Sciences recommended to the Food and Drug Administration that the level of salt added to strained and junior foods not exceed 0.25 per cent, and all baby food manufacturers comply with this recommendation. See Table 14–6 for a summary of the caloric distribution of various baby foods. Baby foods that are made at home are economical but should be prepared carefully. (See Table 14–7.)

MEAL PLAN

At the age of 12 months, the infant should be consuming a varied diet and eating from the family table. The transition from strained to coarser textured foods begins around six months of age. The following list shows the foods infants who are nine to 12 months old usually eat. The amount and type of foods served are adjusted to the child's age.

Foods

Milk: Homogenized.

Eggs: Poached, scrambled or soft cooked.

Meats, fish or poultry: Beef juice; ground beef, lamb, veal, liver, well-cooked lean pork or chicken; chopped bacon, flaked fish.

Cheese: Cottage cheese.

Breads: Fine whole grain or enriched white bread; toast; crackers; zwieback.

Cereals: Fine-grained cooked cereal, or fortified ready-to-eat (without sugar).

Cereal products: Plain cooked spaghetti, macaroni, noodles, rice or grits (enriched).

Fats: Butter and fortified margarine.

Vegetables: Mashed vegetables, vegetable purée or cooked vegetables of low fiber.

Fruits: Cooked fruit purée; cooked fruit without skins or seeds; mashed ripe banana; fruit juices.

Soups: Vegetable and cream soups.

Desserts: Custard, rennet pudding, gelatin, bread, cream, rice and tapioca puddings; plain ice cream.

The meal plan may look something like this:

Breakfast: Cereal, egg, milk (orange juice).

Midmorning: Orange juice if not given at breakfast or crusty bread or both.

Noon meal: Vegetables, meat, milk.

Midafternoon: Milk, crusty bread or crackers.

Evening meal: Vegetables, meat, potato, milk.

WEANING

In a 1971 milk consumption survey of over 2000 infants from New York City and San

Table 14–7 DIRECTIONS FOR HOME PREPARATION OF BABY FOOD

1. Start with only single-ingredient foods, introduced one at a time.
2. Choose different foods from the four basic food groups so that their nutritional contributions will be complementary.
3. Select fresh fruits and vegetables from reliable sources that are not damaged or spoiled.
4. Thoroughly clean, wash and trim all foods.
5. Properly cook foods to provide tenderness, inactivate undesirable enzymes, improve digestibility and destroy undesirable or dangerous bacteria.
6. Use as little cooking water as possible to avoid discarding water-soluble nutrients.
7. Cook foods no longer than necessary to avoid destroying heat-sensitive nutrients.
8. Leftovers should be used very carefully since they may be contaminated with bacteria. They may also lose some of their nutrient value when reheated.
9. To avoid salt and curing agents, do not use ham, bacon, cold cuts or similar meats.
10. Do not add salt to the food until the baby's portion has been removed.
11. Sugar or honey may be added, but use only enough to take away the tartness of some fruits.
12. Add enough liquid to achieve a consistency that the baby can swallow easily.
13. A blender or food mill is good for preparation but must be thoroughly cleaned after each use, because it can be a source of bacteria.
14. Carefully clean utensils, pans and storage containers for the baby foods before preparing them.
15. Prepare baby foods in amounts that can be fed at one meal. If prepared in large amounts, freeze food in containers the size of one portion, such as an ice cube tray.
16. Food should be stored in single portion containers to avoid thawing and refreezing, which can lead to bacterial contamination and poor texture.
17. Food not eaten by the baby at a feeding should be refrigerated immediately.
18. Food poisoning in an infant can be more serious than in an adult, so extra caution is necessary when preparing baby foods.

Francisco, Riveria[24] reported that canned formulas were the most common sources of milk used during the first three months of life. Among middle income families, about 25 per cent were breast-fed during the first month. Among low income families, less than 5 per cent of mothers breast fed their infants. After six months the majority of the infants drank fresh cow's milk. Infants under six months of age from lower income families used evaporated milk more often than did infants from higher income families.

The breast-fed baby is usually weaned by the sixth month. Many mothers wean their babies earlier and many extend the nursing period. It is an individual choice made by the mother and her baby. Preparation for weaning begins when

supplementary foods are served to the baby. The addition of semi-solid foods to the diet teaches the baby to rely less on the breast as a food source. Cow's milk from a bottle or cup eventually replaces all the breast feedings. The mother's mammary glands respond to the decreased demand and secrete smaller amounts until the flow finally stops. Through gradual weaning, the mother's discomfort is minimized and the infant rarely experiences any indigestion.

The bottle-fed baby is weaned to milk in a cup when he is ready, usually before the end of the first year. It is wiser to diminish gradually the number of bottle feedings, although the morning and bedtime feedings may be continued for some time. The addition of solid foods to the baby's diet decreases the need for bottle feedings, and ultimately the bottle feedings are abandoned for whole milk and solid foods.

Nursing Bottle Syndrome

One danger in providing older infants with a bottle "to go to sleep with" is the development of dental caries. The child often will fall asleep with milk in his mouth. Oral bacteria will grow in this nice medium of milk sugar and will produce acid, which acts on the infant's teeth to produce caries. It would be better to put the child to bed with a bottle of water instead of milk. (See Chapter 33.)

FEEDING OF THE LOW BIRTH WEIGHT OR HIGH RISK INFANT

The feeding of these infants is thoroughly discussed in Chapter 37, Nutritional Care for the Low Birth Weight and High Risk Infant.

EATING HABITS AND THE PSYCHOLOGY OF INFANT AND CHILD FEEDING

Eating patterns begin with the first introduction to food and they follow development emotionally, physically and socially.

Anorexia is one of the most common complaints about child feeding. Frequently, the origin of the indifferent appetite displayed by a child can be traced to the food habits started in infancy. The feeding formula prescribed by the physician may be the initial cause. The conscientious parent may overlook the variation in appetite, being too zealous in fulfilling the prescribed time schedule and amount of feedings. Rebellion against food can begin because of a rigid instead of a flexible feeding schedule.

Feeding problems often are not recognized until age two when a child's growth rate slows, his appetite lessens and his burgeoning sense of independence leads him to balk at many requests and expectations for the sheer assertive joy of refusal to secure attention. Because appetite can be strongly influenced by emotions and attitudes, as well as by physical hunger, the first aim is to keep eating enjoyable. The feeling of being loved and the feeding process are closely intertwined. One does not give the child food alone; attitudes are also being fed. An unloved child may lose his appetite, and nutritional deficiency may cause retarded growth. Too much excitement or distraction at mealtime, particularly in the early stages of learning, may cause a child to neglect eating. The nurse's approach is important in the formation of good eating habits. She, as well as the child's parents, needs to understand the child and his feelings about food. It is important to see food as a child sees it and to maintain respect for the child. Focus attention on the learner as well as on what is to be learned.

LEARNING TO EAT

In the weaning stage an infant has to learn many things: not to suck food, to want solid food, not to be held during eating and how to eat—new manipulative skills that include chewing and swallowing solid food. Introducing solid food before three to four months of age is not necessary for nutrition and may present difficulties because the food-swallowing reflex is not developed. First experiences at eating usually result in the baby pushing the food out into his cheeks or out of his mouth with his tongue. He does this because he is learning to master pushing food to the back of his mouth with his tongue in preparation for swallowing. Also, pushing the food into his cheeks allows him to taste it better, since an infant's tastebuds are on the inside of the cheeks as well as on the tongue.

Babies are individuals! Baby John's gluttonous appetite is no criterion for judging baby Mary's diminutive one. Some babies will gulp down a large feeding to satiate their appetites, while other babies enjoy frequent small feedings.

Pushing a fist full of food into his mouth is the cue a baby usually gives when he wants to feed himself. If the doting parent misses the cue, a

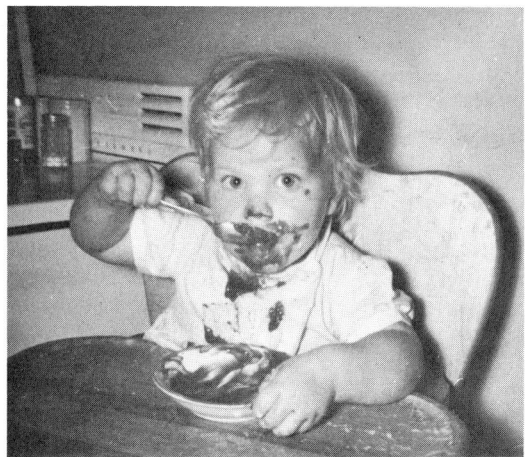

Figure 14–4 Very young children should be encouraged to feed themselves. They will spill and scatter the food at first but should be encouraged to keep on trying. This youngster is learning to eat with a spoon. She is making a mess but will gradually make a go of it.

feeding problem can easily develop. Very young children should be encouraged to feed themselves. They will spill and scatter the food at first but should be encouraged to keep on trying (see Fig. 14–4). Too much help and attention from the mother or nurse will slow down the child's efforts because he dislikes being interfered with and will build up his resistance to eating. Eating will cease to be fun.

At the beginning of a meal the child is hungry and should be allowed to feed himself; when he becomes tired, he can quietly be helped. Emphasis on table manners and the fine points of eating should be left until later when he has matured and developed enough to be ready for it. If he wants to eat with his fingers instead of the spoon—let him! But if he plays with the food, just squeezing it or daubing it on himself and the furniture, it should be put out of reach. He has probably had enough.

The food should be in a form that is easy to handle and eat. Meat should be cut into bite-sized pieces, potatoes and vegetables mashed so that a spoon can be used easily. Raw fruits and vegetables should be in sizes that can be picked up in the hands. In addition, the dishes and silver should be small and easy to handle. The cup should be easy to hold and other dishes so designed that they do not tip over easily. (See Fig. 14–5.) Child psychologists agree that the food habit pattern is established, for better or worse, when the first bottle is fed to the newborn infant. It is important to establish good food habits during infancy because they

form the basis of the individual's food habits carried throughout life.

Size of Servings

The size of servings offered a child is very important. A baby's stomach at birth holds about two tablespoons of food, and at one year the stomach holds about a cupful of food. The stomach enlarges gradually until in adult life it holds approximately two quarts. A child cannot be expected to eat as much as an adult. A large serving of food will often discourage the dainty, fastidious eater. At one year, the baby will eat one third to one half, at three years, one half or a little more, and at six years he will eat about two thirds of the amount an adult consumes. A little child should not be served a large plate full of food; the size of the plate and amount should be kept in proportion to his age. A tablespoon (not heaping!) of each food offered for each year of age is a good guide to follow. Serving him less than you think or hope he will eat helps a child to eat successfully and happily. He will ask for more food if his appetite is not satisfied.

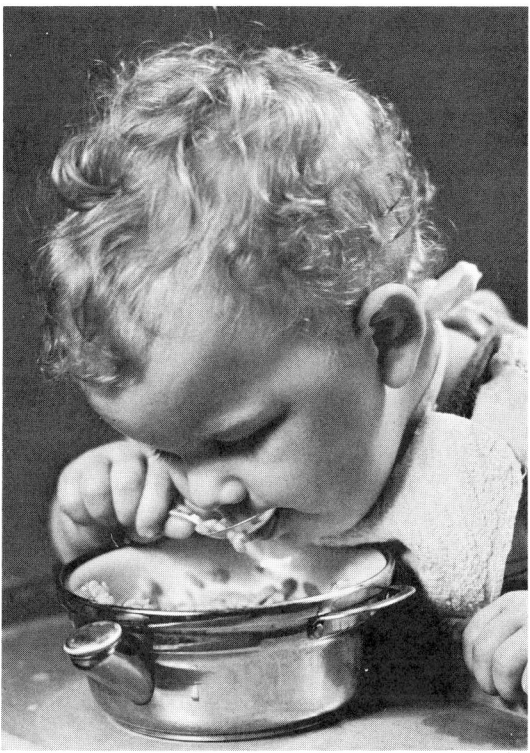

Figure 14–5 The child's spoon is easy to handle and the dish will not easily tip over. (Harold M. Lambert Studios.)

Type of Food

Because the baby's stomach is so small, there is no room there for foods that do not serve a purpose. Pastry, candy, sweet drinks and highly sweetened foods take the place of nourishing ones. Instead, strained fruits and vegetables, chopped meats, eggs and milk should be served. At the age of six months the baby may be fed chopped or mashed vegetables so that he will become accustomed to the coarser foods early in life and will start the mechanism of chewing along with swallowing. Children in general prefer simple, uncomplicated foods. Lowenberg[19] found that a stew in which vegetables and meat were ground and cooked together was considerably more popular with young children than one with separate pieces of vegetables and meat. It was found that children of ages two to six years often prefer raw to cooked vegetables and fruits. Food from the meal planned for adult members of the family may be adapted for the child and served in child-size portions. Highly seasoned sauces should be omitted from the child's plate, and the filling of pies can be served as pudding. Children under six usually prefer very mild-flavored foods, even those which an adult would consider too bland. Because the child's stomach is small, he may require a supplement between meals of milk, fruit, milk and crackers or a sandwich.

Variety of Foods

It is especially desirable that the baby receive foods varied both in texture and flavor. The infant who is accustomed to many kinds of foods is less likely to grow up with definite food dislikes. To add variety to the infant's diet, one of the two cereal feedings during the day may be supplemented with different sieved vegetables and fruits.

Food attitudes do not change markedly during childhood. Many factors influence preferences. It is important to offer a variety of dishes and not allow the youngster to continue on a diet consisting of one or two favorite foods.

New Foods

Introduction of new foods may be a problem with some children. The old advice was to encourage the child to "try just a taste." At Merrill-Palmer Institute, Detroit, the researchers found that children did exactly that—nibbled one leaf of a Brussels sprout or took a "lick" of a beet and no more. More successful is an approach that intrigues a child's curiosity about a new food—the look, smell and feel of it—even before it is cooked, perhaps at the marketing stage. Give only a small portion of an unfamiliar food the first time. If rejected, do not force, but wait a few days and give it another trial. If he himself asks for a bite of it when it is served the next time he is closer to learning to like it, according to Lowenberg, than if he is forced to eat even a bite of it. The less said the better. A child will find it much easier to learn to like beets, for example, if he does not have to live up to the reputation of being a beet hater. Any new food should be given along with a familiar food the infant likes, at a time when he is hungry, happy and not tired.

Many studies on food attitudes have been made. Breckenridge[2] made a survey of the preferences of 51 grammar school pupils. They were questioned first about 25 specific food items. Fatty meat was the one food disliked by more than half the children. All but one liked meat when prepared alone (not in a stew) and ice cream. Fish was the second least popular; cheese and meat mixtures were not far behind. Potatoes, bread, crackers, milk, raw fruits and cereal were high on the list of favorites. Candy and sweets were liked by 86 per cent of the children. Raw vegetables were more popular than cooked, and raw fruits and juices were preferred to the canned or cooked products.

The largest number of specific dislikes was among the cooked vegetables, with carrots and cabbage heading the list. This may be reduced by cooking vegetables for longer periods of time, which reduces the flavors children find disagreeable but also removes nutrients. This might be worthwhile when first introducing a vegetable.

Eggs were next on the list of disliked foods, especially soft-cooked. Grapefruit juice was not too popular. Antipathies to fish were common, but some admitted that what they objected to was "fish with bones."

Forced Feeding

A child should not be forced to eat; instead, the cause for the unwillingness to eat should be determined. He may have a very good reason. A normal, healthy child will eat without coaxing. Sometimes refusal of food is due to a child's being too inactive to make him hungry or too active and overtired (Fig. 14–6). Over-fatigue can be avoided by planning a short rest

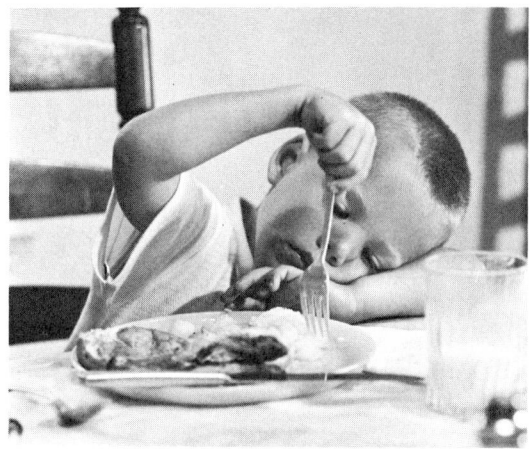

Figure 14–6   "Really tired or just dawdling?" (From: Good Housekeeping magazine, Feb., 1960. Courtesy of Suzanne Szasz.)

before meals or quiet enjoyment of a picture book (Fig. 14–7). An over-anxious parent can affect the appetite of the infant or child. Emotions can retard the flow of gastric juice and inhibit digestion.

If the child refuses to eat, the reason may be too much attention. Children enjoy the attention of their parents and soon learn that refusal to eat is one way to obtain it. Seeking of attention is necessary to satisfy the need for affection, a feeling of belonging. Food and eating contribute to cultural and emotional life as well as to physiological needs. Through food, the infant and child form a basic concept of the world in which they live, the people in it and their relationship to them.

If a child refuses to eat, the meal should be completed without comment and the child's plate removed. At the next mealtime he will be hungry enough to enjoy meat, vegetables and milk. Such denial and discipline is usually harder on the parent than on the child. However, the parent can display affection toward the child to prevent a feeling of not belonging.

Where the Child Should Eat

The child should eat his meals at the family table. Child psychologists contend that it seems unfair to set the child apart from the family group. The child has an opportunity to learn table manners while enjoying meals with a happy, well-established family group. Sharing the family fare strengthens ties and makes mealtime a pleasure period. However, if the adult meal is delayed or there are adult guests, the child should receive his meal at the usual

time. If the child has young visitors, he may wish to entertain them at his own little table at the usual meal hour.

As the child eats with the family, everyone must be careful not to make unfavorable comments about any food. Children are great imitators of someone they admire, so if father turns up his nose at squash, for example, they are likely to do the same. Parents sometimes have to learn to eat what they want their infant to like.

So much has been written about feeding both the problem child and the well child that nursery school bulletins and government-sponsored pamphlets should be consulted.

Family Focus in Feeding

From the nutritional standpoint the infant or child is not an isolated member of the family. While guiding parents in feeding the young, the nurse indirectly improves the entire family's diet for the present and the future. By choosing and adapting suitable family foods for the baby and growing children, the whole family benefits by being well fed. Simple, wholesome foods, so good for the young members, can prove economical and adaptable when part of an overall food plan, especially when the budget is restricted. Most normal, healthy children do best when their feeding is integrated with the total family food plan. This is sound child care as

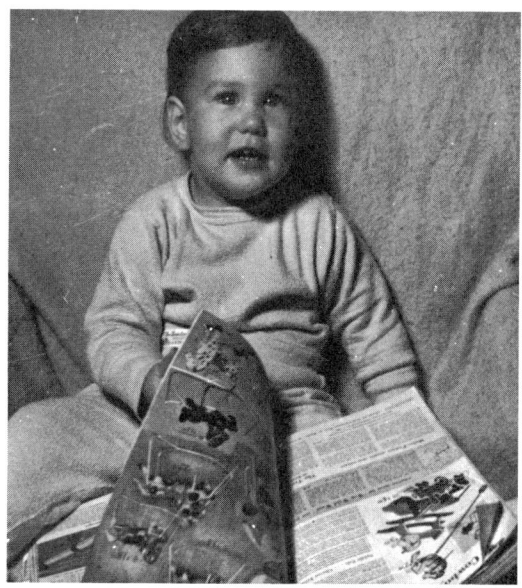

Figure 14–7   Overfatigue at mealtime can be avoided by planning a short rest or quiet enjoyment of a picture book before meals.

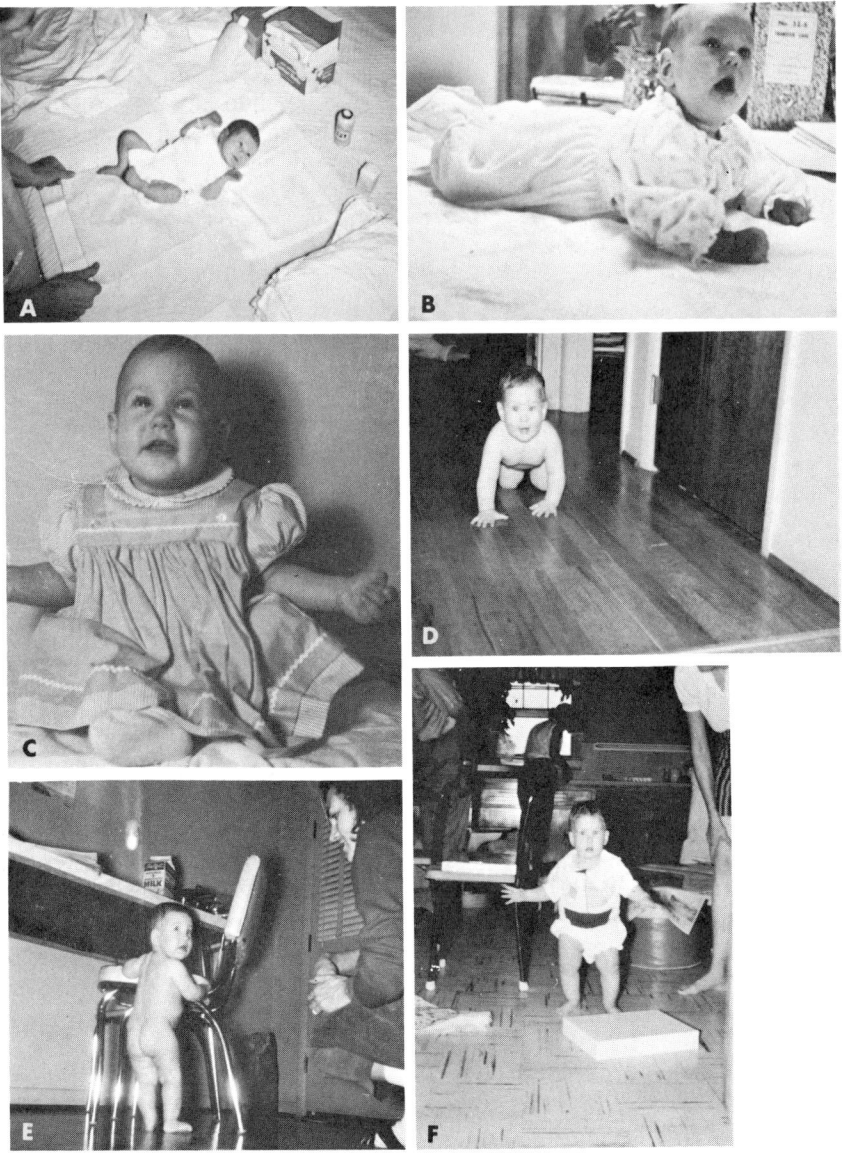

Figure 14–8 Stages in developmental growth of an infant during the first year. *A,* A newborn infant stays in the position in which he is placed. *B,* Lifting his chin and finally his head when lying on his stomach, a baby shows early signs of beginning muscle control, usually around three to five months. *C,* Sitting up unaided is the next big achievement, commonly made between six and eight months. *D,* Crawling starts between seven and nine months. *E,* The baby pulls himself up to a standing position at about nine to 10 months. *F,* Standing alone and then walking alone may begin anywhere from nine to 15 months.

well as sound family economics. Each age and stage in life has its special nutritional requirements, and a family well-fed has all its members on the road to good health. Infant feeding should be aimed toward life-long healthful living. In choosing the baby's diet, selection should be based on the whole family's foods.

DEVELOPMENTAL GROWTH

As the infant grows in size, height and weight, he is also making progress in what he does with his body and mind. He gains in understanding and body coordination. This is developmental growth. No two babies develop at the same rate; each sets his own pace. Each is influenced by his environment, to which he reacts according to his own capacities. However, all babies follow the same general pattern. Figure 14–8 illustrates the usual order of a few of the significant physical achievements of a healthy, well-nourished infant during the first year. All stages are influenced by the diet and

are subject to setbacks and deformities, both physical and mental, if the child is not properly nourished. (See Chapter 12, Nutritional Deficiency Diseases, and Chapter 38, Nutritional Care in Diseases of Infancy and Childhood.)

Infants should be encouraged to develop their natural desire to explore by being given surroundings and care that allow freedom for using their abilities. Let a baby finger and explore the food as much as he wishes. It is part of his development to find out the feel of scrambled eggs and oatmeal as well as their taste and smell. Food texture is important in forming likes and dislikes. The crispness of lettuce and carrots makes chewing fun; it is possible that infants consider whether this or that food is worth chewing by feel and appearance, in much the same way as we look upon taste as a criterion in judging a meal.

PROBLEMS AND SUGGESTED TOPICS FOR DISCUSSION

1. Make a survey of the feeding formulas ordered for babies in your hospital. List the contents of the various formulas. What type of milk is used most frequently as the basis of the formula?
2. Observe for one week the feeding habits of a newborn baby who is bottle-fed. How often is the infant fed and how much food is taken at each feeding? Observe and record the feeding habits of a breast-fed baby. Compare.
3. List the benefits of breast feeding over bottle feeding. Explain. When should formula feeding take precedence over breast feeding?
4. Make a study of the following proprietary foods: dried milk, vegetable-protein formulas, liquid whole milk and meat base formula. Compare cost and food values. What are the major factors that determine the feeding used?
5. What procedure is used in your hospital for calculating infant formulas for the well baby? Calculate a feeding formula for a newborn baby in your hospital, using whole cow's milk as the basis for the formula.
6. When are supplementary foods usually added to the infant's diet? List the order in which the various foods may be introduced and the reason for giving each.
7. How much food is a one year old infant in your hospital eating? Check the diet for nutritional adequacy.
8. How can you help the children in your family or a friend's family form good food habits?
9. What special techniques and precautions need to be observed in the preparation of infant formulas? What method of formula preparation and sterilization is used in your hospital? Why? What is used in the outpatient well baby clinic?
10. At what age are feeding problems likely to occur? What effect do emotions and attitudes have on an infant's eating habits?
11. What is meant by developmental growth? Do all infants develop at the same rate? Explain.

CITED REFERENCES

1. Anderson, T. A., and Fomon, S. J.: Commercially prepared infant cereals. J. Pediatr., 78:789, 1971.
2. Breckenridge, M. E.: Food attitudes of five to twelve year old children. J. Am. Diet. Assoc., 35:704, 1959.
3. Committee on Nutrition, American Academy of Pediatrics: Commentary on breast-feeding and infant formulas, including proposed standards for formulas. Pediatrics, 57:278, 1976.
4. Fomon, S. J.: Infant Nutrition, 2nd ed. Philadelphia, W. B. Saunders Co., 1974, pp. 140–141.
5. Fomon, S. J., Infant Nutrition, p. 121.
6. Fomon, S. J., Infant Nutrition, p. 166.
7. Fomon, S. J., Infant Nutrition, p. 221.
8. Fomon, S. J., Thomas, L. N., and Filer, L. J.: Acceptance of unsalted strained foods by normal infants. J. Pediatr., 76:242, 1970.
9. Fomon, S. J., Ziegler, E. E., and O'Donnell, A. M.: Infant feeding in health and disease. In Fomon, S. J.: Infant Nutrition, 2nd ed. Philadelphia, W. B. Saunders Co., 1974, p. 478.
10. Friedman, G., and Goldberg, S. J.: Concurrent and subsequent serum cholesterols of breast- and formula-fed infants. Am. J. Clin. Nutr., 28:42, 1975.
11. Glueck, C. J., et al.: Plasma and dietary cholesterol in infancy: Effects of early low or moderate dietary cholesterol intake on subsequent response to increased dietary cholesterol. Metabolism, 21:1181, 1972.
12. Hall, B.: Changing composition of human milk and early development of an appetite control. Lancet, 1:779, 1975.
13. Hansen, A. E., et al.: Role of linoleic acid in infant nutrition. Pediatrics, 31:171, 1963.
14. Hirsch, J., and Knittle, J. L.: The cellularity of obese and non-obese human adipose tissue. Fed. Proc., 29:1516, 1970.
15. Holt, L. E., and Snyderman, S. E.: Report to the council: The amino acid requirements of infants. JAMA, 175:100, 1961.
16. Joint FAO/WHO Ad Hoc Expert Committee: Energy and Protein Requirements. WHO Technical Report No. 522, Geneva, WHO, 1973, p. 33.
17. Lakdawala, D. R., and Widdowson, E. M.: Vitamin D in human milk. Lancet, 1:167, 1977.
18. Leverton, R. M., et al.: Further studies of the use of meat in the diet of infants and young children. J. Pediatr., 40:761, 1952.
19. Lowenberg, M. E. F.: For the young child—Success in eating. Food and Nutrition News, 40(6), 1969.
20. McMillan, J. A., Landaw, S. A., and Oski, F. A.: Iron sufficiency in breast-fed infants and the availability of iron from human milk. Pediatrics, 58:686, 1976.
21. Ounsted, M., and Sleigh, G.: The infant's self-regulation of food intake and weight gain. Lancet, 1:1393, 1975.
22. Picciano, M. F., and Guthrie, H. A.: Copper, iron and zinc contents of mature human milk. Am. J. Clin. Nutr., 29:242, 1976.
23. Potter, J. M., and Nestel, P. J.: The effects of dietary fatty acids and cholesterol on the milk lipids of lactating women and the plasma cholesterol of breast-fed infants. Am. J. Clin. Nutr., 29:54, 1976.
24. Riveria, J.: The frequency of use of various kinds of milk during infancy in middle and lower income families. Am. J. Public Health, 61:277, 1971.
25. Rosa, F. W.: Resolving the "public health dilemma" of steroid contraception and its effect on lactation. Am. J. Public Health, 66:791, 1976.

26. Salans, L. B., Cushman, S. W., and Weismann, R. E.: Studies of human adipose tissue: Adipose cell size and number in non-obese and obese patients. J. Clin. Invest., 52:929, 1973.
27. Santulli, T. V., et al.: Acute necrotizing enterocolitis in infancy: A review of 64 cases. Pediatrics, 55:376, 1975.
28. Snyderman, S. E., and Holt, L. E., Jr.: Nutrition in infancy and adolescence. In Goodhart, R. S., and Shils, M. E.(eds.), Modern Nutrition in Health and Disease. Philadelphia, Lea & Febiger, 1973.
29. U. S. Department of Health, Education and Welfare, Children's Bureau: Infant Care. Publication No. 8, 1963.

ADDITIONAL REFERENCES

Applebaum, R. M.: Techniques of breastfeeding. J. Trop. Pediatr., 21:273, 1975.
Applebaum, R. M.: Modern management of successful breast feeding. Pediatric Clin. North Am., 17:203, 1970.
Anderson, T. A., and Fomon, S. J.: Commercially prepared strained and junior foods for infants: Nutritional consideration. J. Am. Diet. Assoc., 58:520, 1971.
Arena, J. M.: Contamination of the ideal food. Nutrition Today, 5:2, 1970.
Beal, V. A.: An acceptance of solid foods and other food patterns of infants and children. Pediatrics, 20:448, 1957.
Beal, V. A.: Breast and formula feeding of infants. J. Am. Diet. Assoc., 55:31, 1969.
Citizen's Committee on Infant Nutrition: White Paper on Infant Feeding Practices. Washington, D. C., Center for Science in the Public Interest, 1974.
Committee on Nutrition, American Academy of Pediatrics: Iron supplementation for infants. Pediatrics, 58:765, 1976.
Ferguson, B. B., Wilson, D. J., and Schaffner, W.: Determination of nicotinic concentrations in human milk. Am. J. Dis. Child., 130:837, 1976.
Fomon, S. J.: Infant Nutrition, 2nd ed. Philadelphia, W. B. Saunders Company, 1974.
Fomon, S. J., and Anderson, T. A. (eds.): Practices of Low-Income Families in Feeding Infants and Small Children. Rockville, Maryland, U. S. Dept. of HEW, Public Health Service, Maternal and Child Health Service, 1972.
Fomon, S. J., et al.: Skim milk in infant feeding. Acta Paediatr. Scand., 66:17, 1977.
Fresh cow's milk and iron deficiency in infants. Nutr. Rev., 31:318, 1973.
Fries, J. H.: Milk allergy—Diagnostic aspects and the role of milk substitutes. J.A.M.A., 165:1542, 1957.
Guthrie, H. A.: Infant feeding practices—a predisposing factor in hypertension? Am. J. Clin. Nutr., 21:863, 1968.
Guthrie, H. A.: Nutritional intake of infants. J. Am. Diet. Assoc., 43:120, 1963.
Heinstein, M. I.: Influence of breast feeding on children's behavior. Children, 10:93, 1963.
Holt, L. E., Jr., et al.: A study of premature infants fed a cold formula. J. Pediatr., 61:556, 1962.
Holt, L. E., and Snyderman, S. E.: The effect of high caloric feeding on premature infants. J. Pediatr., 58:237, 1961.
Holt, L. E., and Snyderman, S. E.: Protein and amino acid requirements of infants and children. Nutr. Abstr. Rev., 35:1, 1965.
Jelliffe, D. B., and Jelliffe, E. F. P.: Nutrition and human milk. Postgrad. Med., 60:153, 1976.
Lamm, E., Delaney, J., and Dwyer, J. T.: Economy in the feeding of infants. Pediatr. Clin. North Am., 24:71, 1977.
Lowenberg, M. E.: Philosophy of nutrition and application in maternal health services. Am. J. Clin. Nutr., 16:370, 1965.
Matoth, Y., et al.: Studies on folic acid in infancy. III. Folates in breast fed infants and their mothers. Am. J. Clin. Nutr., 16:356, 1965.
Meyer, H. F.: Breast feeding in the United States. Clin. Pediatr., 7:708, 1968.
Muto, S., et al.: Soybean products as protein sources for weaning infants. J. Am. Diet. Assoc., 43:451, 1963.
Ounsted, M.: Infant feeding. Nurs. Times, 72:700, 1976.
Overfeeding in the first year of life. Nutr. Rev., 31:116, 1973.
Owen, G. M.: Modification of cow's milk for infant formulas. Current practices. Am. J. Clin. Nutr., 22:1150, 1969.
Pipes, P.: When should semisolid foods be fed to infants? J. Nutr. Educ., 9:57, 1977.
Polansky, M. M., and Toepfer, E. W.: Vitamin B_6 components in some meats, fish, dairy products and commercial infant formulas. Agricultural and Food Chemistry, 17:1394, 1969.
Pratt, E. L.: Dietary prescription of water, sodium, potassium, calcium and phosphorus for infants and children. Am. J. Clin. Nutr., 5:555, 1957.
Review. Cow's milk versus human milk protein in infant feeding. Nutr. Rev., 20:67, 1962.
Review. Growth failure associated with maternal deprivation. Rev., 21:229, 1963.
Review. Histidine requirement in infancy. Nutr. Rev., 22:114, 1964.
Review. Linoleic acid in infant nutrition. Nutr. Rev., 22:45, 1964.
Schulman, I.: Iron requirements in infancy. J.A.M.A., 175:118, 1961.
Siegenthaler, E. J., Byrne, A. M., and Ekpenyong, I.: An evaluation of the effectiveness of sterilization of infant formulas by thermal heating and an aseptic method. Ecology of Food and Nutrition, 4:215, 1976.
Stitt, P. G., and Heseltine, M. M.: Some practical consideration of economy and efficiency in infant feeding. Am. J. Public Health, 52:125, 1962.
Vaughan, V. C., III, et al.: A study of techniques of preparation of formulas for infant feeding. J. Pediatr., 61:547, 1962.
Witten, C. F.: T.L.C. and the hungry child. Nutrition Today, 7:10, 1972.
Wood, A. L.: The history of artificial feeding of infants. J. Am. Diet. Assoc., 31:474, 1955.
Woodruff, C. W., and Clark, J. L.: The role of fresh cow's milk in iron deficiency. I. Albumin turnover in infants with iron deficiency anemia. Am. J. Dis. Child., 124:18, 1972.
Woodruff, C. W., Wright, S., and Wright, R. P.: The role of fresh cow's milk in iron deficiency. II. Comparison of cow's milk with a prepared formula. Am. J. Dis. Child., 124:26, 1972.

Chapter 15

NUTRITION IN CHILDHOOD AND ADOLESCENCE

HEALTHY GROWTH AND DEVELOPMENT

Heredity and environment determine the way children grow and the size and shape that they become. Their genetic inheritance specifies how much their bones will grow and what kind of physique they will have, but their environment during the period of growth when cells multiply and increase in size may encourage or inhibit genetic possibilities. Growth of the young reflects individual health. Adequate nutrition and freedom from disease play important roles in determining whether an individual attains his or her potential. Harmful environmental factors such as malnutrition and disease disrupt normal growth patterns. Development, that is, the changes in growth of an individual, is a continuous, orderly process that leads eventually to maturity. The rate (or age) at which growth and development take place varies with each individual. The danger of accepting any "standard measurement" of growth and development is the tendency to hold too rigidly to exact figures. An individual must be assessed according to many factors attributing to his growth and development. The nutritional requirements of the child vary with chronological age, growth rate, maturational stage, physical activity, and the efficiency of absorption and utilization of the nutrients.

Healthy growth and development depend more upon good nutrition than upon any other factor. "From the beginnings of growth in the prenatal period to the time when the child attains his full size as an adult, the food that he eats and his ability to convert that food into energy and new body tissues will influence the state of his health not only as a child but throughout life."[6]

For convenience in classification, the following age grouping is used in this text to designate the various *stages of growth and development* of the child:

Infant—Birth to one year.
Preschool child—one year to five years.
School child—six years to 12 years.
Adolescent—13 years to 19 years.
Adult—20 years and older.

Rates of Growth

There are four phases of growth in height and weight: a period of very rapid growth during infancy; a period of slower but fairly uniform gain throughout early and middle childhood; a period of marked acceleration during adolescence; and a period of gradual decline of growth until its cessation.

Throughout infancy and early middle childhood, boys are usually taller and heavier than girls, but during early or pre-adolescence the reverse is true. When girls are 9 to 13 years old they grow very rapidly and, during this period, are actually larger than boys of the same age. However, during their growth period their growth velocity is never as fast as that of boys, and their nutritional needs are not quite as great. Their growth impulse reaches its maximum at approximately 13 years of age and starts to slacken at about the time boys start their accelerated growth. Boys grow rapidly when they are about 15 years old and soon regain their advantage in size. Median age for termination of stature growth is about 17 years in girls and 21 years in boys. Weight gain may continue for another year or so after that. Some of the girls' weight gain during adolescence is from fat, which they retain. Boys gain fat also but tend to lose it later. A much greater proportion of their weight gain is in the form of lean body mass, and by the end of adolescence they have one third more muscle cells than females. The fact that their growth patterns are different

323

should have implications for the nutritional requirements of boys and girls, but this is not completely understood.

All the body organs do not develop at the same rate of speed. After infancy, height assumes greater importance than weight. Although heredity determines stature, diet and disease exert a marked influence. The progressive increase in height of children over the years is believed to be owing, in part, to improved economic conditions, better diets and advances in medical care and health services.

NUTRITIONAL ALLOWANCES

It is very important that the diet be nutritionally adequate throughout childhood. (See Table 10–1, Chapter 10.) The recommended dietary allowances (RDA) established by the Food and Nutrition Board of the National Research Council–National Academy of Sciences represent the level of intake of the nutrients that children in each age group require for optimal health. They are designed to provide a margin above the physiological requirements of individuals in the general population, and therefore the recommendations applied to an individual child may be misleading. One cannot assume that a child is inadequately nourished if his intake falls below the recommended allowances. Another child's intake of the nutrients may come close to the recommended allowances and yet the child may be overweight.

The requirements of children vary widely even within the same age group—the short versus the tall, the small frame versus the large frame, the boy versus the girl. For instance, Hepner has shown that the dietary allowance for iron in a male 10 to 16 years of age in the third percentile is 6.6 mg. but is 12.9 mg. for the male in the ninety-seventh percentile.[5]

There are three functions of the diet for the child: The food must (1) provide fuel for muscular activity, (2) supply the necessary chemical elements and compounds the child's body requires for building new tissues (growth) and the repair of worn-out tissues and (3) give pleasure and satisfaction to the child.

Because growing children are building bones, teeth, muscles and blood, they need more nutritious food in proportion to their weight than adults. For instance, during the period of adolescence the nutritional requirements are increased to such an extent that it is sometimes difficult to meet them. To provide

for this accelerated growth, the diet must include foods that are concentrated sources of vitamins and minerals. If children are to grow strong and be normal and healthy, they must eat, digest and absorb enough proteins, fats, carbohydrates, minerals and vitamins to meet their body needs.

Calories

The energy or calorie requirements of the child are determined by his basal metabolism, age and activity. To simplify the process of calculation, consult Table 10–1, which gives the recommended calorie allowances for all age groups. Of the total calorie intake, a suggested proportion is 50 to 60 per cent in carbohydrates, 25 to 35 per cent in fats and the remaining amount (10 to 15 per cent) in protein.

The Recommended Daily Allowances for children of different ages serve as a guide to the calorie needs of children for the heights and weights given in the table. However, variations for children of different heights and weights than those in the RDA table must be considered. The RDA on a per kg. basis for protein and kcalories is given in Table 15–1. The calorie allowance gradually decreases from 100 kcal. per kg. (46 kcalories per lb.) of body weight at ages one to three years to 36 kcal. per kg. and 45 kcal. per kg. for women and men, respectively, at ages 19 to 22 years.

Because of the wide individual variation in physical activity in children, it is difficult to determine a standardized amount of food for them. However, checking on the child's weight, growth and general state of well being will help to serve as a guide.

Fluids

The total daily fluid requirement for a normal healthy child is four to six glasses, 1 to 1½ quarts or 1000 to 1500 ml.

Protein

The child's protein requirements are higher on a per kg. basis than those of an adult. (See Table 15–1.) The recommended daily allowances indicate that the protein need per kg. of body weight decreases from approximately 1.8 gm. in early childhood to 1.2 gm. in late childhood to 0.9 gm. in late adolescence. The protein recommendation is higher in early life because of the large amount required for tissue growth.

Table 15–1 RECOMMENDED DIETARY ALLOWANCES OF CALORIES AND PROTEIN FOR CHILDREN AND ADOLESCENTS*

AGE AND SEX	KCALORIES		GM. OF PROTEIN		CALORIE: PROTEIN RATIO
	Per kg.	*Per lb.*	*Per kg.*	*Per lb.*	
1–3 yr.	100	46	1.8	0.9	55:1
4–6 yr.	90	41	1.5	0.7	60:1
7–10 yr.	80	36	1.2	0.5	67:1
11–14 yr.					
girls	55	25	1.0	0.5	55:1
boys	64	29	1.0	0.5	64:1
15–18 yr.					
girls	39	18	0.9	0.4	43:1
boys	50	22	0.9	0.4	56:1
19–22 yr.					
women	36	16	0.8	0.37	45:1
men	45	20	0.8	0.37	56:1

*From: Food and Nutrition Board: Recommended Dietary Allowances, 8th ed. Washington, D.C., National Academy of Sciences, 1974.

There is considerable variation in the occurrence of growth phases among individuals, but all phases follow the same general pattern. An adequate protein intake for the child is one that contains sufficient amounts of all the known essential amino acids in palatable and digestible form to cover maintenance needs, besides providing an extra amount for protein deposition compatible with normal growth. Therefore, the protein should be of high biological value.

Unfortunately, we do not have sufficient knowledge about the amino acid requirements of children after infancy, which makes the establishment of an RDA for protein precarious. We do not know how efficiently growing children utilize protein nor exactly what percentage of the protein should be in the form of essential amino acids. This lack of knowledge makes the use of complete proteins and complete mixtures of protein extremely important in the child's diet. When any of the essential amino acids is not present or not present in the right amount, normal growth is affected.

The Food and Nutrition Board protein allowances recommended for children after infancy provide approximately 10 to 15 per cent of the child's total calorie intake as protein, one half to two thirds of which is derived from animal or other high quality sources. These allowances are estimated to provide approximately twice the minimal need for the average child and to allow a reasonable margin for the rapidly growing child.

Milk is one of the important foods needed to meet the protein requirements. Children under nine years should have two to three cups daily, and those from nine to 12 years of age, three or more cups; teenagers need one quart or more. The child two, three or even four years old prefers his milk lukewarm and not icy cold. It has been observed that the amount of food a child takes is related to its temperature. Meats and eggs are equally important foods that provide protein in the diet. The remainder of the protein requirements can be met by including breads, cereals, potatoes, fruits, vegetables and desserts.

Minerals and Vitamins

Minerals and vitamins are necessary for normal growth and development. Insufficient vitamin and mineral intake can cause a variety of deficiency diseases, which are described in Chapter 12, Nutritional Deficiency Diseases, and Chapter 38, Nutritional Care in Diseases of Infancy and Childhood. Adequate milk intake will cover many of the mineral and vitamin requirements. Three cups of milk contain approximately 0.8 gm. of calcium and enough phosphorus to ensure proper bone and tooth formation. This amount also adds a rich supply of vitamin A, riboflavin, vitamin D, vitamin B_{12} and some thiamin and niacin.

The iron requirement will be met by an adequate intake of protective foods, but this calls for careful attention to the selection of foods that are good sources of iron and foods that are fortified with iron. Children of ages one to three years should have 15 mg. of iron daily, while children four to 10 years old should have 10 mg. daily. Adolescents 11 to 18 years old should have 18 mg. daily. After 18 years of age, 10 mg. is believed to be sufficient for males. The allowance remains at 18 mg. for females to

provide adequate storage of iron against the drain on iron reserves during the menses or during pregnancy and lactation. The need for iodine is increased during puberty and should be given consideration also.

Some source of vitamin D (400 I.U. daily) is needed throughout the growth period, and continued use of fortified milk is recommended through the school years and adolescence. The Recommended Dietary Allowances for different age groups, set up by the Food and Nutrition Board, National Academy of Sciences—National Research Council, list the various mineral and vitamin requirements. (See Table 10–1.)

Possible Nutritional Deficiencies

In a study[4] concerning the nutritive value of food fed to 40 infants ranging in age from nine months to two years, ascorbic acid, thiamin and iron were the nutrients most frequently found to be below the recommended allowances. In young children calcium, iron, ascorbic acid and vitamin A are the most common deficiencies. This was also shown in the Ten-State Nutrition Survey.[2] These deficiencies are found in older children as well.

THE ADEQUATE DIET

The nucleus of an adequate diet for the child is presented here. Such a pattern is the basis for all normal and therapeutic diets for children. If these foods are included in the daily diet, the child's protein, mineral and vitamin requirements will be met. Additional foods are added to this nucleus to meet individual energy requirements.

THE NUCLEUS OF AN ADEQUATE DIET PATTERN FOR A CHILD

FOOD	AMOUNT
Milk, vitamin D fortified	Children: 1 pt. to 1 qt. daily depending on age Adolescents: 1 qt. or more per day
Butter or fortified margarine and vegetable oil	At least 4 teaspoons daily
Eggs	3 per week
Meat, fish, poultry or equivalent	1 or 2 servings per day
Whole grain or enriched cereals and breads	4 or more servings per day
Vegetables	2 servings daily besides potatoes, 1 dark green, leafy or deep yellow
Fruits	2 servings, 1 of them a citrus fruit, per day

THE PRESCHOOL CHILD (AGE ONE TO FIVE YEARS)

By the time the baby is one year old, good feeding habits should be established. The baby's meals have been increased to include milk, cereals, eggs, breadstuffs, butter or fortified margarine, meats, soups, vegetables, fruits and puddings. (See Chapter 14, Nutrition in Infancy.) Because the baby's teeth have developed, the selection of food should include those that will encourage chewing. Although the baby's size and individual requirements govern the amount given, the food for daily meals should be selected from whole grain or enriched breads and cereals, milk, egg, meat, fish or poultry, butter or fortified margarine, vegetables, fruits, fruit juices, cheese and ice cream or milk puddings. If good eating habits are established early in the child's life, many bothersome complaints can be avoided. Protein foods containing iron (meat, eggs) should be fed along with milk. Unlimited milk consumption that leads to neglect of other necessary foods should be discouraged. A wide variety of foods is the best plan to assure an adequate diet at all ages. (See Table 15–2.)

As the child passes from the fast-growing period of infancy into the one to three year age, he becomes more selective and more independent about food. This period is sometimes difficult for parents because the appetite wanes, the rate of growth is slow and irregular, weight often drops, and the child begins to find wider horizons of activity offering greater interests. Desire for food becomes erratic, and there is a noticeable drop in consumption of food between the second and third years. The child may go for weeks or even months without gaining an ounce. The "won't eat" era is a normal phase of development and is much harder on the parents than the child. Many problems can be avoided if parents are told that this decline in eating is to be expected. It is during this period that the nurse and parents must be careful not to foster poor eating habits by over-anxious urging or by bribing the child to eat. It is also during this period that the nurse, nutritionist or physician is often asked, "Shouldn't we be giving our child a vitamin pill?" The decrease in appetite usually is brief and the child's health is not in jeopardy. However, it is still a good idea to assess his nutritional intake before answering the parents' question. If the child's diet is extremely inadequate, the use of a multivitamin and mineral supplement that meets the RDA is justified temporarily. It can be emphasized to parents

Table 15–2 FOODS INCLUDED IN A GOOD DAILY DIET (AVERAGE AMOUNTS FOR EACH AGE)*

FOOD	PRESCHOOL 3–5 Years Old	EARLY ELEMENTARY 6–9 Years Old	LATER ELEMENTARY 10–12 Years Old	EARLY ADOLESCENCE 13–15 Years Old
Milk	2 cups	2–3 cups	3 cups or more	3–4 cups or more
Eggs	1 whole egg	1 whole egg	1 whole egg	1 or more whole eggs
Meat, poultry, fish	2 ounces (¼ cup) (1 small serving)	2–3 ounces (1 small serving)	3–4 ounces (1 serving)	4 ounces or more (1 serving)
Dried beans, peas (Also an occasional replacement for meat, poultry or fish)	3–4 tablespoons	4–5 tablespoons	5–6 tablespoons	½ cup or more
Potatoes (May occasionally be replaced by equal amount enriched macaroni, spaghetti or rice)	3–4 tablespoons	4–5 tablespoons	½ cup or more	¾ cup or more
Other cooked vegetables (Often a green leafy or deep yellow vegetable)	3–4 tablespoons at one or more meals	4–5 tablespoons at one or more meals	⅓ cup or more at one or more meals	½ cup or more at one or more meals
Raw vegetables (Lettuce, carrots, celery, etc.)	2 or more small pieces	¼ cup	⅓ cup	½ cup or more
Vitamin C source (Citrus fruits, tomatoes, etc.)	1 medium-sized orange or equivalent	1 medium-sized orange or equivalent	1 medium-sized orange or equivalent	1 large orange or equivalent
Other fruits	⅓ cup at one or more meals	½ cup or more at one or more meals	½ cup or more at one or more meals	2 servings
Cereal, whole grain restored or enriched	½ cup or more	¾ cup or more	1 cup or more	1 cup or more
Bread, whole grain or enriched	2 or more slices	2 or more slices	2 or more slices	2 or more slices
Butter or fortified margarine	1 tablespoon	1 tablespoon	1 tablespoon or more	1 tablespoon or more
Sweets	⅓ cup simple dessert at 1 or 2 meals	½ cup simple dessert at 1 or 2 meals	½ cup or more simple dessert at 1 or 2 meals	½ cup or more at 1 or 2 meals
Vitamin D source	Enough to provide 400 I.U. of vitamin D daily			

*From: Foods for Growing Boys and Girls. Battle Creek, Mich., The Kellogg Company, Department of Home Economics Services, 1964.

that what the child does eat should be as nutritious as possible. Appetite usually tends to improve as the child approaches school age, and an increase in growth and weight is bound to follow.

Protein–calorie malnutrition—as pointed out in Chapter 12—is prevalent in preschool children around the world. The preschool child belongs to the most vulnerable age group with respect to certain physical and social needs. Unfortunately, this is the age group being reached least effectively. Younger children in the home place priority demands on the mother and are the most difficult to reach with services from outside the home. The World Food Program (WFP), UNICEF, FAO, WHO and government projects have organized a program[8] to establish permanent distribution channels (mainly commercial) that provide special food mixtures for preschool children. (See Fig. 15–1.) These mixtures are cereal-based, precooked foods designed for children and are similar to those available in supermarkets of developed countries. The projects are

planned to provide a vehicle for the use of new protein-rich foods.

Two, three and four year olds want to identify food. They seem to prefer simple foods that they can handle ("finger foods") rather than mixed dishes. Gravies and cream sauces are not popular. Exclusive eating of a few favorite foods is common with the four and five year old. The five and six year old youngsters are imitators. Children can perceive food as conflict, praise or scold food according to the authority in the home. Food aversions develop for many reasons. Emotional experiences at the table, unpleasant associations aroused by food and fear of new and strange foods are some of the attitudes toward food that are learned in childhood. They need to be recognized and either understood or prevented early in life.

Colorful, attractive foods that are easy to handle and eat are appealing to children. An environment and utensils that are conducive to enjoyment and ease in handling food encourage curiosity and successful eating patterns.

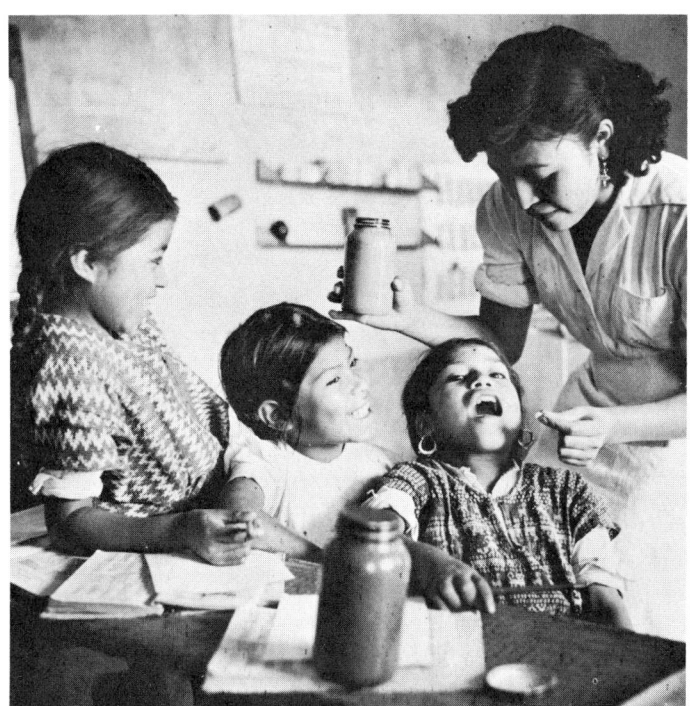

Figure 15–1 Babies, young children, expectant and nursing mothers are the first victims of the shortage of certain key foods. Under the direction of INCAP, field workers carry out surveys and initiate measures to combat deficiency diseases. In an Indian village, a nurse gives prophylactic vitamin B_{12} tablets to the schoolchildren. (Courtesy of Pan-American Sanitary Bureau, Regional WHO Office.)

An adequate meal contains sufficient calories for energy needs and a complete protein (one protein food or a combination of foods that supply all essential amino acids). A good meal may be obtained from a wide selection of foods to provide the necessary nutrients.

The following is a suggested meal plan for a preschool child that would require very little, if any, adjustment in the pattern to use for the whole family.

BREAKFAST

Fruit or juice
Cereal with milk
Toast or roll
Butter or margarine
Milk

Table 15–3 MOTHERS' CONCERNS ABOUT EATING BEHAVIOR OF PRESCHOOL CHILDREN*

CONCERNS	0 TO 3 MO. (%)	3 TO 6 MO. (%)	6 TO 9 MO. (%)	9 MO. TO 1 YR. (%)	1 TO 1½ YR. (%)	1½ TO 2 YR. (%)	2 TO 3 YR. (%)	3 TO 4YR. (%)	4 TO 5 YR. (%)	5 TO 6 YR. (%)	TOTAL (%)
Chooses limited variety	2.6	8.7	12.0	24.6	34.1	37.6	40.3	41.2	44.8	34.2	35.8
Dawdles with food	10.3	3.1	15.5	14.6	34.1	25.7	36.8	43.8	39.7	33.3	33.5
Eats too little fruits and vegetables	0.0	2.4	12.9	14.5	15.8	29.4	27.2	27.5	27.9	27.1	23.9
Eats too many sweets	0.0	0.0	0.0	1.4	4.7	7.8	26.3	28.9	27.9	26.4	20.7
Eats too little meat	0.9	4.7	7.2	22.5	22.6	30.3	22.3	21.6	24.0	17.7	20.5
Eats too little food	8.5	2.4	8.2	10.1	14.7	13.8	21.6	28.3	21.1	22.8	19.9
Drinks too little milk	0.0	3.9	4.8	10.9	10.8	16.5	20.1	18.6	18.7	18.5	16.3
Drinks too much milk	9.4	7.9	7.1	5.1	10.0	13.8	10.0	7.1	7.1	5.9	8.0
Eats too much food	7.7	4.7	8.2	8.7	5.1	3.7	2.7	3.1	5.4	6.4	4.9
Eats too much meat	0.0	0.0	0.0	0.0	1.4	5.0	3.5	4.4	4.3	5.9	3.7
Number of children	117	127	84	138	279	218	551	610	691	628	3444

*From Eppright, E. S., et al.: Eating behavior of preschool children. J. Nutr. Ed., *1*:16, 1969. (This paper is published as Journal Paper No. J-5983 of the Iowa Agriculture and Home Economics Experiment Station, Ames, Iowa. Project No. 1532 contributing to North Central Regional Project No. 75.)

LUNCH OR SUPPER

Main dish—chiefly meat, eggs, fish, poultry,
  dried beans or peas, cheese, peanut butter
Vegetable or salad
Bread
Butter or margarine
Dessert or fruit
Milk

DINNER

Meat, poultry or fish
Cooked vegetable
Potato or substitute
Raw vegetable
Bread
Butter or margarine
Fruit or pudding
Milk

Midmorning and midafternoon snacks usually continue for this age group unless they interfere with the appetite at mealtime. Good snacks, which are part of the whole day's meal plan and will make a real contribution to nourishment, might include the following:

Dry cereal, with milk or out of the box
Simple cookie or Graham cracker
Raw vegetables
Canned, fresh or dried fruit
Toast, plain or cinnamon
Cheese wedge
Fruit sherbet or ice cream
Fruit juice
Milk
Fruit drinks made with milk and juice

A survey[3] of the eating behavior of over 3000 preschool children ranging in age from birth to six years, representing 2000 households of moderate to marginal income living in the North Central region of the United States, revealed that mothers have many concerns about the eating habits of their preschool children. The major concern about the greatest percentage of the children was their choice of a limited variety of foods (Table 15–3). The concern about dawdling, playing with food and eating too little food reached the highest peak in the three to four year olds. An appreciable concern for eating too many sweets appeared in mothers of children two years of age and remained through the sixth year in over 25 per cent of the group surveyed. Consumption of milk for children less than one year of age averaged 3 or more cups daily. From one year of age on, the mean daily milk intakes approximated 2½ cups. The peak of the consumption of milk reported in this survey and others[1] appeared around six months of age and decreased toward the end of the first year or early in the second year. Boys averaged greater intake of milk than did girls. The vegetables most frequently disliked were spinach, carrots, green beans and peas (in the order listed). Dislikes of vegetables were closely associated with those of older siblings. Children's food dislikes were associated more with the dislikes of their fathers and older brothers than with those of mothers and older sisters. Preschool children, beginning in the two to three year old group, in this survey made food selection decisions more often at breakfast and snack periods than at other times. However, this study indicated that almost half the children enter school with little experience in making decisions about food selection.

Beal observed that a smooth curve representing nutrient requirements by age tends to correspond to weight and height curves. Early in infancy the curve rises rapidly but with decreasing acceleration. Appetite, food intake and weight gain are usually erratic in the preschool years. These have been associated with changes in growth rate. Much more investigation of the eating behavior of children is needed. A lack of understanding of the physiological and psychological changes taking place in children as they pass through the toddler phase into the early preschool years may cause problems. The resolution of the problems and concerns of mothers has implications for nutrition education.

THE SCHOOL CHILD (AGE SIX TO 12 YEARS)

During the early school years growth in height and weight is slow but steady. A child may add 10 or 12 inches to his height and 30 to 35 pounds to his weight. There is a relatively constant increase in food intake.

Going to school brings new problems. The meal schedule must be spaced in relation to the school routine rather than to the child's needs or desires. He has to decide whether he wants to eat lunch in the school cafeteria or carry it from home. The decision often rests on the practices of his peers. However, the excitement of school, new contacts and routine, when approached as a new challenge, helps to continue or promote good eating habits and regular meals. There should be sufficient time for eating all meals, including an adequate breakfast. Calm, unhurried meals contribute to good digestion and appetite.

The school child, six to 12 years of age, re-

quires the same basic foods as when he was younger, but the quantities are increased to take care of his greater needs. His energy needs gradually increase and approach those of adults during this period. His eating habits and attitudes toward food vacillate. Teachers and other leaders as well as peers influence the selection of food positively and negatively. The child seems to prefer meat, potatoes, bread, crackers, milk, ice cream, cereals and raw fruit and to dislike fat meat, fish, cooked vegetables, cheese, and mixed meat and egg dishes. His intake of protein, calcium, vitamin A and ascorbic acid is apt to be low. The eating of highly seasoned or poorly fried foods, pastries, tea, coffee, chocolate and sweets should be discouraged. They provide empty calories and usually take away appetite for nutritious foods.

At school the child should have a hot meal from the school lunch program or a lunch brought from home, rather than candies, cookies and sweetened bottled beverages from a snack bar. (See section on School Lunch Programs in Chapter 19.) Instruction in how to select a good lunch—the kinds and amounts of foods needed daily to develop a healthy body—should be started early in the home and continued at school. One way to help a child want to eat wisely is to convince him that what he eats really does make a difference in the way he grows. Children at this age desire to grow normally and to be like their peers. They are ready to learn about the relationship of food to a healthy body.

THE ADOLESCENT OR TEENAGER (AGE 12 TO 18 YEARS)

As previously stated, the adolescent years are the second period of rapid growth, but this varies greatly even for individuals of the same chronological age. Because the growth spurt varies with the individual, so should the quantity of the nutritional intake. Just such a relationship has been shown—the calorie and nutrient intake are highest when the velocity of growth is most rapid, and this is dependent on *physiological,* not chronological, age.

These years are also the most active period of life. Because of the double demands of activity and growth, food needs are high and extremely important. (See Table 15–4 for daily dietary requirements for ages 11 to 18 years.)

During his growth spurt, the adolescent boy usually has a tremendous appetite and, if provided with adequate amounts of protective foods, will have no trouble meeting his dietary needs. Adolescent girls sometimes are watching their weight and restricting calories, so nutritional counseling is advisable to help them improve their dietary intake. Both sexes tend to assert their independence as "almost adults," and as a demonstration of their rejection of parental restriction may ignore the basic

Table 15–4 RECOMMENDED DAILY ALLOWANCES FOR ADOLESCENTS*

NUTRIENT		BOYS		GIRLS	
		Age 11–14	*Age 15–18*	*Age 11–14*	*Age 15–18*
Calories	(kcal.)	2800	3000	2400	2100
Protein	(gm.)	44	54	44	48
Vitamin A	(I.U.)	5000	5000	4000	4000
Vitamin D	(I.U.)	400	400	400	400
Vitamin E	(I.U.)	12	15	12	12
Ascorbic acid	(mg.)	45	45	45	45
Folacin	(mg.)	0.4	0.4	0.4	0.4
Vitamin B$_{12}$	(μg.)	3	3	3	3
Niacin	(mg.)	18	20	16	14
Riboflavin	(mg.)	1.5	1.8	1.3	1.4
Thiamin	(mg.)	1.4	1.5	1.2	1.1
Vitamin B$_6$	(mg.)	1.6	2.0	1.6	2.0
Calcium	(gm.)	1.2	1.2	1.2	1.2
Phosphorus	(gm.)	1.2	1.2	1.2	1.2
Iodine	(μg.)	130	150	115	115
Iron	(mg.)	18	18	18	18
Magnesium	(mg.)	350	400	300	300
Zinc	(mg.)	15	15	15	15

*From: Food and Nutrition Board, National Research Council: Recommended Dietary Allowances, 8th ed. Washington, D.C., National Academy of Sciences, 1974.

foods in favor of sweets, soft drinks and "snack" foods with empty calories. Of particular concern are those teenagers who decrease their food intake when their need for nutrients is greatest. Girls, more often than boys, are likely to omit or restrict essential foods, particularly milk, bread and potatoes, in an effort to reduce or to stay thin for the sake of appearance. Skipping breakfast and other meals often results from the teenager's time schedule not coinciding with the family meal schedule. For example, meeting friends or being on time for a date are more important to them than meals. Teenagers want to be popular with their peers.

Findings from the Ten-State Nutrition Survey and the Texas Nutrition Survey showed that adolescents had the highest prevalence of unsatisfactory nutritional status among the various age groups. Both of these studies were made of low income populations, so the poor nutritional status may be a result of many factors, including infection, lack of health care, and psychological stress as well as reduced nutrient intake. Poor nutritional status is even more prevalent in black and Spanish-American groups.

Nutritional counseling of teenagers requires a careful approach in order to arouse their interest and motivate them to do something about their nutritional status. They welcome challenging problem-solving situations. Efforts to involve them in the problems of obtaining and maintaining good nutritional status are rewarding and usually have a lasting effect. Teenagers respond to your acceptance of what they eat, emphasis on what is good about their diet and eating habits and involvement in the solution of their own problems. When given the information needed to improve their own diet, teenagers are apt to convince themselves of the relationships between good nutrition and appearance, energy, growth and development. Appearance is important to adolescents. Girls are interested in their size, skin, hair and eyes; boys are interested in their skin, muscle development and stamina. With an understanding of the relationship of nutrition to appearance and physical prowess, these motivating forces play an important role in improving nutritional status. Teenage leaders who exemplify good nutritional appearance are more effective counselors with their peers than are adults. Cooperative efforts on the part of parents, teachers, community leaders, school lunch supervisors, nurses, doctors, nutritionists, extension agents and others are essential for meaningful nutrition education that will bring about effective changes in the behavior of teenagers.

Underweight and Overweight. Weight problems are of considerable concern to the adolescent. A significant number of them are underweight or overweight with more girls than boys having such problems. Undernutrition implies that the individual has not had a sufficient supply of calories and one or more of the essential nutrients over a long period of time. His nutritional status is poor as the result of several factors. When an individual is 10 per cent or more below the standard appropriate for his height and body frame, he is considered to be underweight.

About one third of adolescents studied are overweight. Overnutrition implies that the individual's caloric intake has been in excess of energy needs over a period of time. It can be a result of too large an intake or too little physical activity. The problem of teenage obesity is a very real one in the United States and is a subject for considerable physiological and psychological study, especially since the period between ages 10 and 14 is a time of adipose tissue cellular development in both obese and non-obese individuals. Adipose cell number increases permanently during this period.

On the other hand, some teenagers are "dieting" whether they need to or not. Many who are not overweight as well as those who are put themselves on diets and are easy marks for current reducing fads. The resulting erratic eating habits lead to a poor nutritional status. The fluctuation in weight experienced by many overweight teenagers when dieting is physiologically unsound and psychologically frustrating. Inadequate levels of nutrients are unavailable to the body at times when many of them are needed for growth, and the inability to maintain weight loss is discouraging. When calories and activity balance, weight is maintained. The inactivity of the overweight teenager plays a role in the weight control problem. Because of embarrassment about their size, overweight teenagers usually do not participate in active sports or exercise, which further reduces their caloric expenditure and completes the vicious cycle of inactivity–overweight–embarrassment–inactivity. (See Fig. 27–4.) Consideration of both calorie restriction, including all essential nutrients, and suitable activity for the overweight individual is important in any weight reduction program. (See Chapter 27, Nutritional Care in Conditions of Overweight and Underweight.)

Food Habits. The nutritional problems of teenagers appear to be correlated or related to eating habits. Their dietary intake is cause for much concern for several reasons. During this period of accelerated physical and emotional growth the adolescent is very often under considerable stress and anxiety, which are reflected in physiological, psychological and social behavior. These interrelated behaviors can be manifested in poor eating habits, poor selection of foods, irregular hours of eating and omission of meals. Between-meal snacking does not in itself seem to be a cause of poor nutritional intake. Teenagers eat about one third to one quarter of their total calories as snacks, which contribute significantly to their nutrient intake. With a little guidance in selecting foods that contain more vitamin A, iron and calcium, the teenager's diet could easily be improved within the snacking pattern.[9]

Pregnancy. The adolescent who becomes pregnant during this period of growth and development faces many more physiological and psychological stresses than do older females. Most of these are a result of the fact that her own body growth and development between the ages of 12 and 17 is not completed. (After 17 years of age, growth in the majority of girls has generally stopped.) When the younger teenager becomes pregnant she has difficulty providing for her own physical (and psychological) needs as well as the demands of the growing fetus, especially if her nutritive intake has been inadequate. Pregnancy at this time presents many risks that are related to nutrition. (See Chapter 13.)

Nutrition in Athletics. Athletes eagerly rely on food to provide the physical stamina they need to participate in school sports. Belief that certain foods will enable the athlete to do more and better work, win more medals or gain a greater number of victories has existed for some time. Coaches have been known to promote special regimens. Some of these pertaining to glycogen stores are valid. Theories have been advanced that certain diets, such as a high protein diet or diets including no milk or a considerable amount of milk, will promote better performance. These have no validity. The athlete's only increased needs are for water, calories and electrolytes. A well-balanced diet of normal foods provides all the protein an athlete requires for maximum performance. He or she may need 3000 to 4000 or more kcalories daily to meet energy needs, and the foods used to supply energy will probably increase the protein intake. Exercise does not lead to a sig-

nificant increase in the amount of protein metabolized, even after glycogen stores have been used. The protein requirement for increasing muscle mass will be met by the increased intake of calories. An excessive protein intake will increase the water requirement, because additional fluid is required to eliminate the nitrogen by-products of protein digestion as urine.

During short periods of exercise, ATP (adenosine triphosphate) and phosphocreatine provide energy supplies for the body. These first sources are exhausted in a matter of minutes, and then glycogen in the liver and muscle is used for energy. Through a well-designed nutrition program these glycogen stores can be increased. This may be valuable for an athlete competing in events lasting more than several minutes. The last sources of energy used are the fat and glucose in the body, which unlike the first two require oxygen for their metabolism. They are needed for prolonged, heavy exercise. Rapid metabolism of body fat is dependent upon the conditioning and training of the athlete. The intensively trained athlete can utilize fat for energy more efficiently.

Eating a high carbohydrate diet for a week will increase the glycogen stores. They can be increased even further if, during the week before the event, the athlete takes a very low carbohydrate diet (100 gm. carbohydrate) and exercises vigorously for two days, then takes a very high carbohydrate diet for three to four days. In this way, the glycogen stores are first depleted and then restored to an even higher level.[7] These diets should always be adequate in protein, energy and other nutrients for the teenager and should be used only with the advice of a physician.

Weight reduction in the adolescent athlete should not be achieved through severe calorie restriction but by moderate calorie restriction and increased exercise. Calories should not be limited to less than 2000 kcal per day. During training, the initial weight loss is the result of loss of fat and tissue fluids, since fat tissue contains water. However, as training progresses and the body develops protein tissue and muscle mass, there may be no further weight loss but possibly a weight gain. At this point, continued weight loss would involve body protein and not body fat and would be detrimental. A lower than normal body weight maintained for three to four years of high school athletics could prevent maximal growth and performance.

Water and salt intake are important during

strenuous exercise, and it is wrong and dangerous to restrict or avoid water intake at that time. Even the loss of as little as 3 per cent of total body water results in dehydration exhaustion syndrome or decreased work or exercise performance. Lost water must be replaced periodically throughout the exercise period. Restricting water intake to induce weight loss, as wrestlers frequently do, is just as detrimental and dangerous.

Breakfast

An important meal of the day most often skipped or hurried is breakfast. Studies conducted at the University of Iowa show that it is difficult to supply the recommended nutrients for the day without a morning meal. Foods usually eaten for breakfast provide nutrients such as calcium, riboflavin and ascorbic acid that may not be obtained at any other time of the day either in meals or as snack foods. Children who did not eat breakfast or had inadequate breakfasts were more fatigued, less attentive and unable to achieve as much as those who had better breakfasts. Those who ate breakfast worked, played and thought better during the late morning hours. Breakfasts of equal calorie value but low in protein and high in fat or carbohydrate do not have this effect. Breakfasts with adequate protein elevate the blood glucose level above fasting level for approximately four hours after the meal, while meals with less than adequate protein but high in fat and carbohydrate elevate the glucose level for about two and three hours, respectively. Within approximately one hour after a carbohydrate breakfast of the same isocaloric value the blood glucose rises to a peak, and by the end of the second hour it falls to the fasting level. One fourth to one third of the day's food allowance is recommended at breakfast. A variety of foods other than the traditional breakfast foods could meet the criteria of an adequate breakfast. Many rationalizations are given for not eating breakfast—lack of time, lack of appetite in the morning, preference for sleeping longer, no one to prepare food.

Snacks

Snack time is an important social occasion, especially to teenagers, and seems to be here to stay. The choice of foods eaten at snack time is influenced by members of the group. They often may not improve a diet that needs improvement. Choice of food for snacks can be those that supply essential nutrients and need not spoil the appetite for meals. Sandwiches, fruits and milk products are appropriate snack foods. Foods such as candy, carbonated beverages and concentrated sweets supply empty calories and usually take away appetite for other foods. Snacks should be considered as a part of the day's food and should contribute to the total nutrient supply.

Dietary Allowances

Determining the nutritional allowances for adolescents is difficult because it is an age when the rate of growth varies widely. During the five to seven year period of rapid growth, there are 18 to 24 months when the rate of growth is at its peak and may approach the growth rate of infancy. During this time girls and boys have nutritional needs twice the average for the entire adolescent period. Usually the increased caloric intake during the months of most rapid growth will also result in an adequate intake of nutrients.

Up to 10 years of age the calorie allowance for children of both sexes is 80 to 90 kcalories per kg. of body weight. After 10 years of age the kcalorie values gradually decline to 50 for adolescent males and 39 for adolescent females (RDA). (See Table 15–1.) After nine years of age, there are major differences in growth rates between the sexes, and therefore separate recommended allowances are given for boys and girls.

Interpretation of these values requires caution. Physical activity of individuals varies considerably. Inactive children may become obese even when their calorie intake is below the recommended allowances, and extremely active children need larger allowances.

Approximately 15 per cent of the total calories should be derived from protein in order to maintain a positive nitrogen balance. Approximately one half to two thirds of the protein should be supplied from complete protein foods—milk, eggs, meat, cheese or complete protein mixtures—in order to supply all of the essential amino acids.

Retention of 400 mg. per day of calcium may be needed for adequate mineralization of the rapidly growing skeleton during prepubertal and pubertal growth. Diets supplying the recommended 1200 mg. of calcium permit adequate retention. A quart of milk supplies this amount of calcium. Milk also contains vitamin D (400 I.U. per quart), which is necessary for the absorption of calcium.

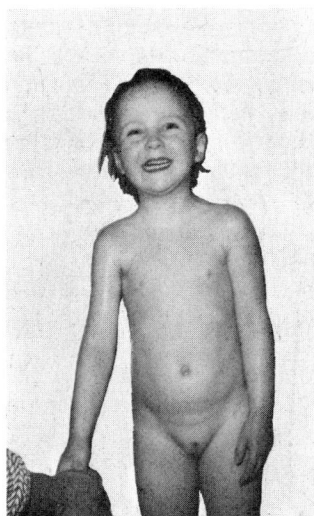

Figure 15–2 Growth, muscular development and general appearance reflect good nutrition in a five year old.

The amount of iron recommended (18 mg.) probably cannot be supplied in the food usually ingested. This requires education about choosing foods that are fortified with iron, such as breakfast cereals and bread, and possibly the recommendation of an iron supplement. Anemia develops during periods when the growth rate is very high if the intake cannot provide for the iron needs. See Chapter 29. (Appendix Table 8 lists foods high in iron.)

Dietary surveys indicate that many adolescents obtain less than two thirds of the Recommended Dietary Allowances (RDA) for ascorbic acid, vitamin A, calcium and iron.

NUTRITION AND THE YOUNG ADULT

With the end of adolescence physical growth is usually complete, although sometimes, particularly in males, it may continue into the early twenties, thus requiring continued high nutrient intake.

Emotional, social and psychological growth are never complete, and young men and women are still concerned with establishing their own sense of identity and developing a sense of responsibility. They are eager to try new experiences, and frequently this means experimenting with unfamiliar foods, different patterns of eating and new diets as part of new and different lifestyles. In addition, without parents or others monitoring their intake,

young adults can develop erratic or religiously fanatical eating habits. This is a period of flexibility in eating patterns, making it an excellent time for nutrition education and the establishment of healthful eating and exercise patterns for the rest of adult life.

Good eating habits and optimal nutritional status should be encouraged in young women in preparation for pregnancy, should they decide to have children. Equally important is attention to the nutritional requirements of women who take oral contraceptives. The metabolism of vitamin B_6, folic acid, glucose and triglycerides can be modified by the use of these drugs, which might change nutritional requirements. (See Chapter 21.) Good eating habits for young men and women are needed to maintain energy, stamina and alertness at this very active, competitive time of life. Finally, if they decide to have children their own good eating habits will be a natural influence on the development of good eating habits in their children.

INDICATIONS OF GOOD OR POOR NUTRITION

Growth, muscular development and appearance are the hallmarks of good or poor nutrition (Fig. 15–2). Careful observation of the child will reveal many facts about his state of nutrition.

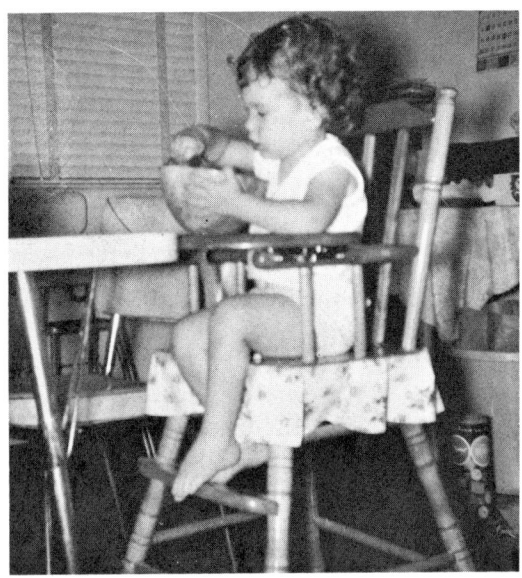

Figure 15–3 This child exhibits good posture while eating.

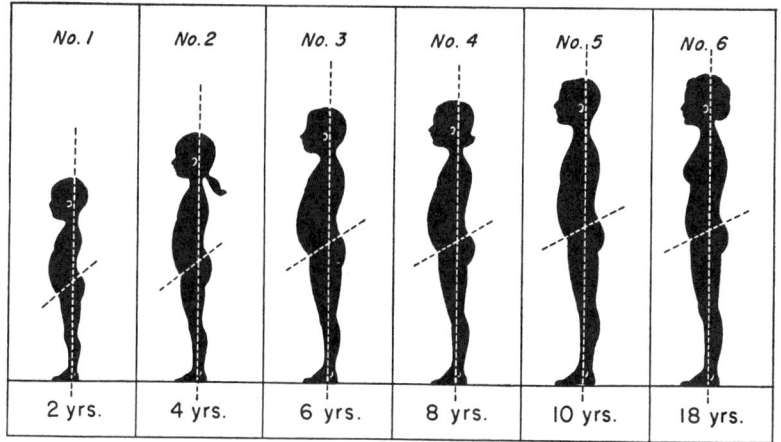

Figure 15–4 Silhouette copies of photographs of children of various ages who were considered to have acceptable posture. These illustrations are not drawn to scale. The apparent kyphosis at ages six and eight is caused by scapular winging, which is commonly seen at these ages. The relative tilt is illustrated. (McMorris, R. O.: Faulty posture. Pediatr. Clin. North Am., *8*(1), 1961.)

Height and Weight

There are many height-weight-age tables available to consult and note whether the child is within normal limits. (See Appendix Tables 16, 17 and 24 through 27.) Obviously not all children have the same body build. Some are large-boned and anatomically robust, while other children are small-boned and appear more delicate and dainty. This differentiation is important to consider when checking the child's weight and height. A deviation from the average weight for height and age may be perfectly normal for a particular child. All healthy children grow but each child has his own pathway of development. Thus, height and weight are best evaluated in terms of the child's previously periodic records. Growth is subject to many different influences; disease, sex, heredity, hormonal activity, physical condition, seasonal fluctuations and nutrition (food) are some of the factors.

Appearance

Does the child look healthy? The color and turgor of skin and the condition of the musculature are revealing factors. The skin should look firm, healthy, smooth and elastic and not appear flabby nor fat. A fat child is not a healthy child! He may be in a poor state of nutrition. A child or adult can be overweight from a diet composed of fats and carbohydrates that lacks minerals, vitamins and proteins.

A child in a good state of nutrition whose emotional needs are satisfied tends to be happy, active, alert and playful, while a child in a poor state of nutrition will be listless and apathetic or unhappy and whiney.

Posture

The healthy child experiences little difficulty in exhibiting good posture traits (Fig. 15–3); head and chest held high, abdomen in, weight distributed evenly on the balls of the feet, knees flexed, no curvature of the back and all parts of the skeleton in good alignment (Fig. 15–4). The

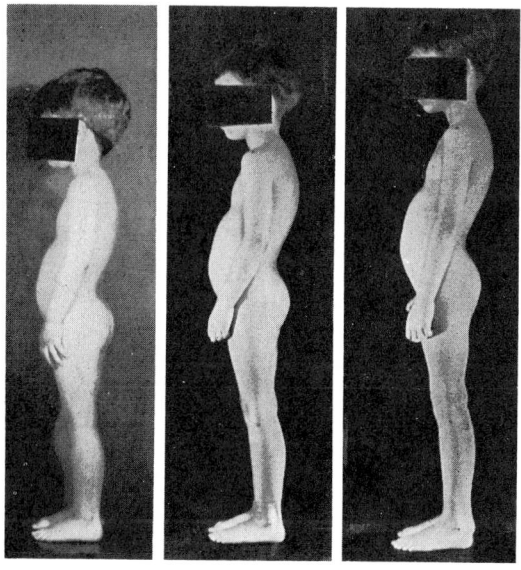

Figure 15–5 Poor postural pattern of a child persisting at different age levels. Note sharp angle of pelvic tilt, prominent abdomen, lordosis, round back, flat chest, forward shoulders and forward head.

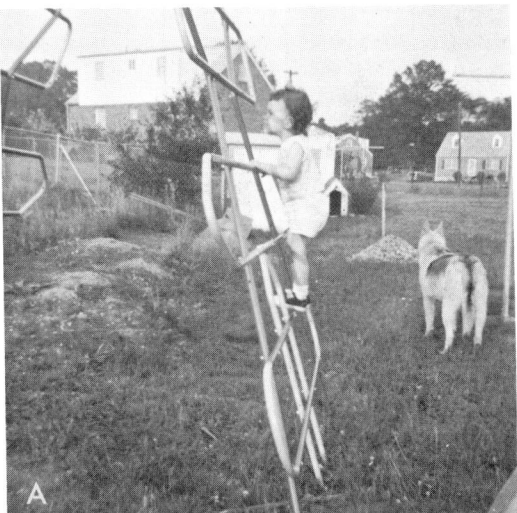

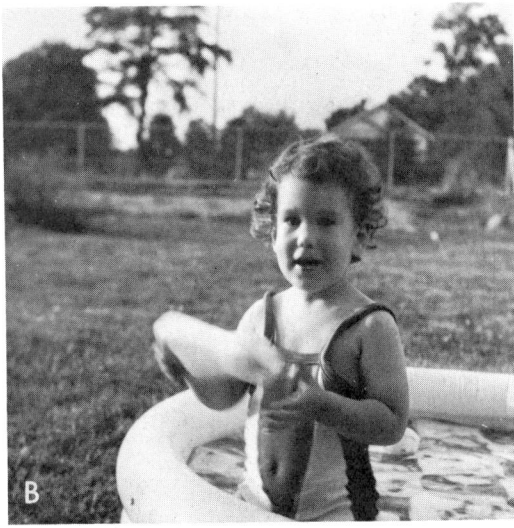

Figure 15–6 Along with a well-balanced, nutritious diet, this 23 month old child enjoys ample outdoor play. Sun, air, water and fun all contribute toward a healthy body and a good appetite.

child in a poor state of nutrition has a difficult task to show good posture. He is listless, pale, weak, chronically tired and slouches (Fig. 15–5). A continuous infection of tonsils and adenoids may add to the poor state of health. Along with the well balanced, nutritious diet, the child should receive ample rest and sleep, fresh air, sunshine and exercise to stimulate the appetite. (See Fig. 15–6).

Muscle Control

Children should have good control of their muscles either at play (Fig. 15–7) or at the table

(Fig. 15–8). There will be noticeable posture changes as the baby grows into childhood. The infant of a few months will squirm, kick and wave his arms for exercise. At the age of six months, the average baby will roll about and attempt to sit up. This is followed by crawling, creeping and attempts to stand (Fig. 14–8). After the first wobbly steps are taken, practice is needed before the muscles are strong enough to permit running and jumping. Children should stand and walk erect. The legs should not be bowed and the head should be of normal shape and size. Children who suffer from avitaminosis D, the condition described in Chapter 12, Nutritional Deficiency Diseases, have bowed legs and abnormal head and chest development, and in extreme cases the result is rickets. (See Figs. 12–16 to 12–19.)

Also make these observations.

Does the child sleep well?

Does the child eat well?

Does the child have good daily elimination?

Does the child's hair look glossy and healthy instead of stringy and lifeless?

Are the eyes clear and bright?

Does the child have an alert and happy expression?

The child's teeth and gums are also a good indication of either desirable or poor nutrition. The gums should be firm, hugging the teeth, and light pink in color, with no bleeding tendencies. The approximate number of teeth expected for his age are listed:

6 teeth at one year of age

12 teeth at one and one half years of age

16 teeth at two years of age

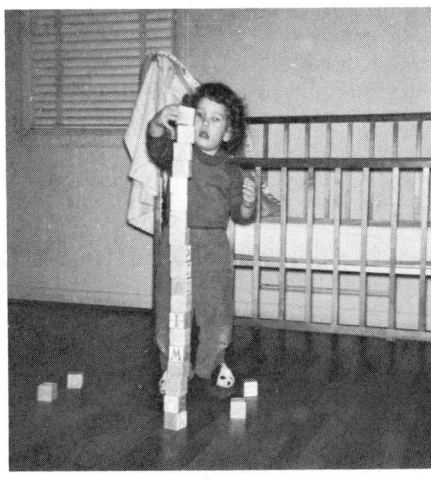

Figure 15–7 Good muscle control and coordination reflect a well-nourished, well-adjusted child. This child is two and one half years old.

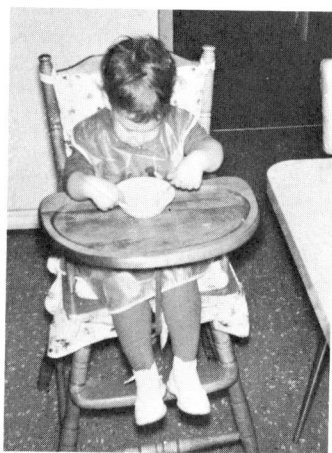

Figure 15–8 This 19 month old child shows good muscle control in feeding herself. She can use either hand and do a good job!

20 teeth at two and one half years of age

24 teeth at six years, 4 of which are permanent molars

For further discussion of the evaluation of growth and nutritional status of a child see Chapter 11, Assessment of Nutritional Status.

PROBLEMS AND SUGGESTED TOPICS FOR DISCUSSION

1. Check the children in your pediatric unit against the height-weight-age tables. Explain any variations.
2. What and how much are a one year old, a two year old, a six year old, and a 14 year old eating? Check the food record for nutritional adequacy.
3. Obtain a list of an average day's intake of food from a boy in the clinic who is 15 years old. How does he rate his diet? How may it be improved?
4. Follow the same procedure suggested in problem 3 for a child who is 10 years old.
5. Follow the same procedure suggested in problem 3 for an adolescent girl who is 14 years old.
6. How does nutrition affect healthy growth and development? What are the visible signs of poor nutrition? How does a girl's growth and development differ from that of a boy? Give the general growth and development pattern of a child from ages one to 18.
7. What changes in eating habits take place from ages one to 18? Account for the changes.
8. Milk is an excellent food for children, but under what circumstances may it need to be limited?
9. Why is malnutrition prevalent in preschool children? What is being done about it?
10. What are the food needs of teenagers? What nutrients have been found to be inadequate or low in the diets of adolescent girls? Adolescent boys? Give reasons for the poor diets of teenagers.
11. How can you help a teenage girl to improve her nutrition and health habits?
12. Why are adequate breakfasts and lunches of importance to the school child? What is a good breakfast? What is a good lunch?
13. What would you teach mothers concerned about the eating behavior of their preschool children?

CITED REFERENCES

1. Beal, V.: Dietary intake of individuals followed through infancy and childhood. Am. J. Public Health, *51*:1107, 1961.
2. Center for Disease Control: Ten-State Nutrition Survey, 1968–70. Washington, D.C., U.S. Department of Health, Education and Welfare, Health Services and Mental Health Administration, 1972, DHEW Publication No. (HSM) 72–8130–34.
3. Eppright, E. S., et al.: Eating behavior of preschool children. J. Nutr. Educ., *1*:16, 1969.
4. Guthrie, H.A.: Nutritional intake of infants. J. Am. Diet. Assoc., *43*:120, 1963.
5. Hepner, R.: Discussion. In McKigney, J. I., and Munro, H. N., Nutrient Requirements in Adolescence. Bethesda, Maryland, National Institutes of Health, NICHD Office of Research Reporting, 1976, DHEW Publication No. (NIH) 76–771.
6. Oettinger, K. B.: Nutrition and Healthy Growth. Washington, D.C., U.S. Department of Health, Education and Welfare, Children's Bureau Publication No. 352, 1955, p. ii.
7. Smith, N. J.: Food for Sport. Palo Alto, California, Bull Publishing Co., 1976, pp. 74–88.
8. Teply, L. J.: Nutritional needs of the pre-school child. Nutr. Rev., *22*:65, 1964.
9. Thomas, J. A., and Call, D. L.: Eating between meals—A nutrition problem among teenagers?. Nutr. Rev., *31*:137, 1973.

ADDITIONAL REFERENCES

Astrand, P.: Something old and something new (glycogen loading). Nutrition Today, *3*:9, 1968.

Breckenridge, M. E.: Food attitudes of five-to-twelve-year-old children. J. Am. Diet. Assoc., *35*:704, 1959.

Bryan, M. S., and Lowenberg, M. E.: The father's influence on young children's food preferences. J. Am. Diet. Assoc., *34*:30, 1958.

Burke, B. S., et al.: A longitudinal study of animal protein intake of children from one to eighteen years of age. Am. J. Clin. Nutr., *9*:616, 1961.

Burke, B. S., et al.: A longitudinal study of the calcium intake of children from one to eighteen years of age. Am. J. Clin. Nutr., *10*:79, 1962.

Burke, B. S., et al.: Relationship between animal protein, total protein, and total caloric intakes in the diets of children one to eighteen years of age. Am. J. Clin. Nutr., *9*:136, 1961.

Caghan, S. B.: The adolescent process and the problem of nutrition. Am. J. Nurs., *75*:1728, 1975.

Committee on Nutrition, American Academy of Pediatrics: Factors affecting food intake. Pediatrics, *33*:135, 1964.

Committee on Nutritional Misinformation: Water Deprivation and Performance of Athletes. Washington, D.C., Food and Nutrition Board, National Academy of Sciences, 1974.

Daniel, W. J.: Nutrition and adolescence. Dietetic Currents, *3*(4), 1976. (Published by Ross Laboratories, Columbus, Ohio.)

Eppright, E. S., and Swanson, P. P.: Distribution of calories in diets of Iowa school children. J. Am. Diet.,

31:144, 1955; II. Distribution of nutrients among meals and snacks of Iowa school children. *31*:256, 1955.

Everson, G. J.: Bases for concern about teenagers' diets. J. Am. Diet. Assoc., *36*:17, 1960.

Gross, I., Wheeler, M., and Hess, K.: The treatment of obesity in adolescents using behavioral self control. Clin. Pediatr., *15*:920, 1976.

Gyorgy, P.: Conference notes (preschool child). Am. J. Clin. Nutr., *14*:65, 1964.

Hathaway, M. L.: Heights and Weights of Children and Youth in the United States. Washington, D.C., U.S. Department of Agriculture, Home Economics Research Report No. 2, October, 1957.

Hinton, M. A., et al.: Eating behavior and dietary intake of girls 12 to 14 years old. J. Am. Diet. Assoc., *43*:223, 1963.

Kerry, E., et al.: Nutritional status of preschool children. Dietary and biochemical findings. Am. J. Clin. Nutr., *21*:1274, 1968.

Leverton, R. M.: The paradox of teenage nutrition. J. Am. Diet., *53*:13, 1968.

Lowenberg, M. E.: Food preferences of young children. J. Am. Diet. Assoc., *24*:430, 1964.

Mitchell, H. S.: Nutrition in relation to stature. J. Am. Diet. Assoc., *40*:521, 1962.

Nutrition and athletic performance. Dairy Council Digest, *46*(2), 1975. (Published by National Dairy Council, Chicago, Illinois.)

Ohlson, M. A., and Hart, B. P.: Influence of breakfast on total day's food intake. J. Am. Diet. Assoc., *47*:282, 1965.

Owen, G. M., et al.: A study of nutritional status of pre-school children in the United States, 1968–70. Pediatrics, *53* (Suppl.):597, 1974.

Pate, M.: The preschool child protection program (P.P.P.). Am. J. Clin. Nutr., *14*:63, 1964.

Peckos, P. S., and Heald, F. P.: Nutrition of adolescents. Children, *11*:27, 1964.

Review. Growth standards for infants and children. Nutr. Rev., *21*:141, 1963.

Review. The effects of a balanced lunch program on the growth and nutritional status of school children. Nutr. Rev., *23*:35, 1965.

Roche, A. F.: Some aspects of adolescent growth and maturation. In McKigney, J. I., and Munro, H. N. (eds.), Nutrient Requirements in Adolescence. Cambridge, Mass., MIT Press, 1976.

Roth, A.: The teen-age clinic. J. Am. Diet. Assoc., *36*:27, 1960.

Smith, C. A.: Overuse of milk in the diets of infants and children. JAMA., *172*:567, 1960.

Smith, N. J.: Gaining and losing weight in athletics. JAMA, *236*:149, 1976.

Spindler, E. B., and Acker, G.: Teen-agers tell us about their nutrition. J. Am. Diet. Assoc., *43*:228, 1963.

U.S. Department of Agriculture: Food, the Yearbook of Agriculture, 1959. Lowenberg, M. E.: Between infancy and adolescence, pp. 296–302; Storvick, C. A., and Fincke, M. L.: Adolescents and young adults, pp. 303–310.

Zambrawski, E. J., et al.: Iowa wrestling study: Weight loss and urinary profiles of collegiate wrestlers. Med. Sci. Sports, *8*:105, 1976.

Chapter 16

NUTRITION IN ADULTHOOD AND LATER YEARS

THE PROCESS OF AGING

Aging is a normal process. It begins with conception and ends only with death, but may progress at varying rates, depending upon several factors—among them nutrition. The best preparation for healthy later years begins in early childhood and possibly *in utero*.

From conception and during the period of growth, anabolic processes exceed catabolic or degenerative changes. When the body has reached physiological maturity, the rate of degenerative change becomes greater than the growth process. These changes impair the function of any organ to some degree. The decreased efficiency is caused by a loss of cells, leaving the functioning capacity of the organ to the remaining cells.

Studies of cultures of human cells *in vitro* have shown that there is a limit to their proliferative capacities. The cells divide and produce new cells a specific number of times and then slow down or stop dividing. How this process is controlled *in vivo* is not understood.[3]

Table 16–1 PERCENTAGE OF FUNCTIONS OF TISSUES REMAINING IN A 75 YEAR OLD MALE*

TISSUE	PER CENT REMAINING IN 75 YEAR OLD MALE
Body water content	82
Number of glomeruli in kidney	56
Number of nerve trunk fibers	63
Brain weight	56
Number of taste buds	36

*From: Shock, N. W.: The physiology of aging. Scientific American, *206*:100, 1962. Copyright © 1962 by Scientific American, Inc. All rights reserved.

One theory of aging states that the cells form defective RNA from the DNA. The defective RNA then designates the synthesis of defective proteins and defective enzymes. Cells are unable to function, so they die and are permanently lost. Tissues vary in their loss of functions. The percentages of remaining cells of some tissues are shown in Table 16–1.

A decrease in the number of mitochondria with age has been reported. This results in diminished function of a cell to release energy. Structural changes associated with collagen occur. Collagen becomes less elastic and stiffer as the cell ages. It is likely that changes in collagen structure are involved in many of the diseases and disabilities associated with aging. The aging appearance of the skin may be due to the accumulation of collagen.

A deterioration of the body's immune system may cause the changes of aging. Antibody synthesis may become defective, so that antibodies against the body's own tissues are produced with damaging results.

The aging process, according to another theory,[12] depends upon the way vitamin E and ascorbic acid are used by the body. Aging seems to be influenced by an intracellular struggle between two factors acting on the third: the duration and intensity of radiation, which can penetrate every cell and produce *free radicals* (intermediates with at least one unpaired electron), the polyunsaturated lipids upon which they act and the available *vitamin E* present to protect the lipids from excessive oxidation. Vitamin E is a potent antioxidant.

When a free radical strikes a polyunsaturated lipid, it will have little effect if enough vitamin E is present. If there is an intracellular deficiency of vitamin E, the free radical will strike a lipid molecule, release a hydrogen atom and initiate peroxidation of polyunsaturated lipid, which produces nonfunctional peroxide molecules. These peroxide molecules can cause considerable cell damage. The mitochondria and endoplasmic reticulum are vulnerable to peroxidation. The energy-generating processes of electron transport and phosphorylation cease. The cell dies and only a "clinker" remains. Cell age of a tissue is determined by the ash or "clinker" that remains when the cell has been burned out by peroxidation.

Ascorbic acid plays a role in the enzyme functions relating to the hydroxylation of proline in collagen biosynthesis. It reacts with glutathione and through antioxidant synergism ascorbic acid increases its protective role. It has the ability to act as a synergist with vitamin E. Both vitamin E and ascorbic acid appear to be important in retarding the process of cellular aging.

Selenium, present in trace amounts in a wide variety of foods, seems to have an important antioxidant role, although it is not defined in humans. *Glutathione peroxidase,* an enzyme that detoxifies harmful oxidation products, contains selenium. Further research is in progress. Although the causes of aging are not fully understood, it is agreed that the changes that occur are irreversible.

LONGEVITY AND NUTRITION

Since 1950 there has been no increase in the life expectancy of a person 20 years old, even though Americans spend several times more money on health care now than they did in 1950. Our progress in medical care has resulted in a reduction of the death rate from bacterial disease, and this is reflected in our lower rates of infant and child mortality. However, as mortality from these diseases has declined, mortality from degenerative diseases such as atherosclerosis and diabetes mellitus has increased. We know that the diseases of old age can be delayed somewhat by dietary changes, but is it possible that diet can affect the aging process itself?

Calories

The hope of prolonging the period during which the characteristics of youth can be maintained is the impetus for a great deal of nutrition research. McCay and co-workers[5] contributed a series of studies on longevity, in which it was shown that restriction of calories, if started

early in life, is the single most important factor for extending the life span. Ross, in experiments with rats, extended some life spans to 1800 days (normal lifespan is 700 to 1000 days) through severe underfeeding. This extended age corresponds to 180 years in human beings.[8] There is general agreement that lean rats live longest, and statistics for humans indicate that overweight in adults is associated with shortened life span. However, early caloric restriction cannot be applied to humans at this point because the division between beneficial and detrimental caloric deprivation is not yet clear.

Fat

The amount of fat in the diet seems to be related to longevity. Results from a long-term study of women indicate that the greater the amount of fat in the diet at middle age, the shorter the life span, even when fat intake was not related to obesity.[9] This same finding has been reported in rats fed high-fat diets early in life. We do not know how dietary intake affects growth and the life span, but the mechanism appears to be centered in the neuroendocrine and immunological systems of the body.

NUTRITIONAL NEEDS IN THE MIDDLE YEARS

Middle age is defined for the purposes of this text as the years from the late twenties to the early sixties—the largest portion of a person's lifespan. During this period human beings are usually most productive. It is a time of job achievement and recognition, child rearing and the establishment of lifestyle, values and attitudes that will be transmitted to one's children. Most people are in relatively good health at this age, but bad habits can lead to poor health later. Cigarette smoking, stressful employment, little exercise, excessive alcohol intake and a diet high in saturated fat, cholesterol, sodium and sugar and low in fiber can be factors in the development of hypertension, overweight, atherosclerosis, diabetes mellitus and gastrointestinal problems. The middle years are an important time for education and medical care to preserve health and prevent or delay the onset of chronic disease. During these years, individuals are most able to afford the proper food and medical care necessary to maintain their health, but they are also more likely to say, "I don't have time to see a doc-

tor" or "I don't have time to think about my eating habits."

The preventive nutritional care most likely to be required by this group is that for hypertension, overweight, atherosclerosis, diabetes mellitus, gastrointestinal problems and periodontal disease, all of which are discussed in other chapters. It is important when caring for individuals in this age group to remind them that neglect of their health now is detrimental. Attention to the improvement of exercise and eating habits can make a difference and make them feel their best now as well as later. The recommended dietary allowances for the majority of this group are defined as allowances for persons aged 23 to 50. (See Table 10–1.)

NUTRITIONAL NEEDS IN THE LATER YEARS

The physical, physiological and psychosocial factors of aging become more prominent and debilitating as the person gets older. For this reason the elderly person has particular nutrient needs related to his or her process of aging in a specific situation, just as the child has particular needs related to the individual process of growth. These needs are attracting more attention and research as the number of aged in our population increases. At present, people aged 65 and over constitute about 10 per cent of the U.S. population, but if the U.S. birth rate continues to decline, the elderly are expected to constitute about 15 per cent of the population in the year 2000.

The elderly population is *not a homogeneous group,* and no general statements can be made about them. Each elderly person is an individual, and the health professional must be very conscientious to avoid the pitfall of stereotyping older people. The information presented in this chapter should function only as a flexible guideline for providing nutritional care for an elderly person.

THE EFFECT OF AGING ON NUTRITIONAL STATUS

Physiological Factors

Sensory. As a person ages, the senses of taste, smell, sight, hearing and touch diminish at individual and different rates. For example, the number of taste buds per papilla drops from 245 in children and young adults to 88 in people 74 to 85 years old.[1] The decreased sense of

taste in particular can greatly affect food intake. Decreased eyesight makes the buying of food and the reading of food labels difficult, and the preparation of food can be hazardous. As the sense of smell decreases, much of the sensual pleasure from food is gone, and the detection of spoiled food is not as easy. The result of sensory decline can be a tendency to neglect food and eating, and frequently there is also a loss of appetite.

Gastrointestinal. The following changes take place in the gastrointestinal system with age:

1. Decreased salivary secretion makes mastication and the swallowing of food more difficult. This can be worsened by breathing through the mouth and by certain medications. The severe saliva depletion of individuals in their late seventies and older can also result in rampant dental caries, because the teeth-cleansing effect of saliva is reduced.

2. About 50 per cent of persons over 65 years of age have lost all their teeth, and only 75 per cent of this group have satisfactory dentures. Those over 65 years of age who still have their teeth may be plagued by periodontal diseases and by dental caries resulting from years of dental neglect. Chewing and eating can become painful and embarrassing. There is a tendency to eat softer, blander foods, which often have more calories in relation to their nutritive value than do the fruits and vegetables that they tend to replace. These softer foods usually have less vitamin A, vitamin C, folic acid and fiber, and the change in eating pattern can lead to a deficient nutrient intake and to constipation.

3. Decreased gastric secretion of hydrochloric acid, pepsin and intrinsic factor results in impaired protein digestion, less efficient absorption of vitamin B$_{12}$ and a greater possibility of bacterial contamination of gastric juice.

4. Decreased secretion of most digestive enzymes and bile makes digestion and absorption of food slower and less efficient. Absorption of fat, fat-soluble vitamins and calcium is reduced.

5. The increased amount of residue that results from poor digestion and absorption can cause increased flatulence.

6. Decreased gastrointestinal movement makes constipation a frequent problem in the elderly. It should always be evaluated and treated if it is a real problem.

Metabolic. With age, *glucose tolerance* appears to decrease. This can be a result of two factors: (1) a diminished insulin secretion in response to a glucose challenge or (2) a decreased tissue response to the action of insulin. The latter may be owing to an increased proportion of fat tissue in the elderly person regardless of whether he or she is overweight. Adipose tissue has a certain "insulin resistance." Whether diminished glucose tolerance is a natural process of aging or whether the person is truly a diabetic is difficult to determine. Authorities question the use of glucose tolerance curves developed for younger adults to diagnose diabetes in an elderly person. Treating glucose-intolerant persons as diabetics, with the attendant lifestyle changes that include insulin injection, change of diet and social or economic stigma, may be unjustified.

Basal metabolic rate decreases by 10 to 15 per cent or more after the age of 50, largely because of the decrease in lean body mass, since adiposity increases even in the presence of stable body weight.

The presence of *chronic disease* can affect nutritional requirements by altering metabolic processes and by affecting digestion and the absorption, utilization and excretion of nutrients.

Cardiovascular and Renal. The capacity of the lungs and the amount of blood the heart can pump diminish as total peripheral resistance increases with age. The rate of blood flowing through the kidneys decreases and the number of nephrons diminishes. The composition of the blood may be modified, depending upon the functioning of the cells. The handling of excessive amounts of protein waste products or electrolytes becomes more difficult, and ample fluid intake is very important. The elderly individual. is not able to respond as quickly to metabolic challenges to the acid–base balance.

Psychosocial Factors

As a rule, the aged individual is set in his ways. Radical changes in eating habits, as well as changes in foods, are not always welcome. Food habits are firmly established by this age and, if faulty, are difficult to replace with better ones. Superstitions and fallacies about food are relinquished reluctantly. The familiar is comfortable. Many of the elderly do not know how to prepare foods and claim that new foods do not taste good.

Special problems arise when the aged lack variety in their diet or become uninterested in food. The primary causes for the failure to obtain an adequate diet are social isolation (sep-

aration) and retirement (reduced income). Because of his greater amount of leisure time, the person has time to think about his next meal and either may relish the idea of eating or may become critically despondent over its monotony. This is most likely to happen with persons who live alone or who have to do their own cooking. They find it easier to eat the same thing day after day and, unless watched carefully, may suffer from malnutrition even though overweight. In general, a more varied diet provides more nutrition. (See Fig. 16–1.)

Depression. The person who refuses to eat may be anxious or depressed and thus have a poor appetite and an inadequate intake. Depression is usually from a sense of loss—loss of loved ones, productivity, a sense of worth, mobility, income and finally, body image. He or she may avoid food to obtain attention that will overcome the sense of loss or may become a compulsive nibbler and overeat to compensate. Eating patterns are very erratic in some older persons. They may overeat one day and

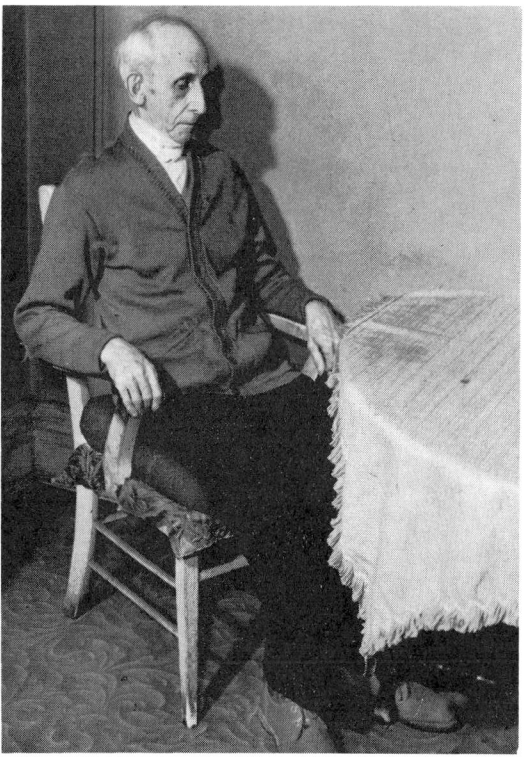

Figure 16–1 The chronically ill, elderly person who fails to eat becomes listless and apathetic and may spend his days vegetating. Remarkable changes can be effected by an abundant diet. (From Halpern, S. L.: Nutrition and chronic disease. Reprinted from Health News, monthly publication of the New York State Department of Health, September, 1955.)

nibble on foods the next. Swanson found one case in which a woman's daily intake varied from 800 to 3700 kcalories.

Reduced Income. Most people retire at age 60 to 65 and usually have several more years of life, during which they may be supported only by Social Security payments or by an employee pension plan. Frequently this income is inadequate and the elderly individual becomes poor. Unfortunately, food intake suffers. Although most poor elderly people are eligible for food stamp programs, they frequently do not use them. A survey of an urban population composed of low to moderate income elderly persons found that, while two thirds of the respondents were aware of the food stamp program, only 10 per cent said they used it, even though most of them would have been eligible.[10] Some reasons why an elderly person may not use food stamps are:

1. A feeling that food stamps are a form of charity.

2. The monthly trip to the food stamp office is inconvenient, dangerous or impossible.

3. The purchase of food stamps requires a large expenditure of money, leaving little for other necessities or emergencies.

4. The use of food stamps may stigmatize the person in the grocery store as poor and a recipient of charity.

Physical Factors

When plagued by decreased sight and physical handicaps the elderly are trapped by immobility. Food shopping is difficult. Some are confused by the variety of items in the stores. The distance from the stores and the inability to carry groceries are handicaps. Transportation to and from the market or the food stamp centers may be a problem. The trend for small neighborhood grocery stores to close and be replaced by large supermarkets in shopping centers presents a great inconvenience to the urban dweller without a car. Walking long distances, having to cross busy highways and carting or carrying groceries can make the trip forbidding and hazardous. (See Fig. 16–2.) Using buses can be difficult when carrying groceries, assuming a bus system exists.

Because of reduced income the elderly person may be forced to live in poor, crime-ridden areas. This adds to the problem of isolation, making him or her fearful of leaving the home or apartment. A stroke, fracture or heart condition may decrease mobility even more. Moving to a smaller house, a first floor apartment or a

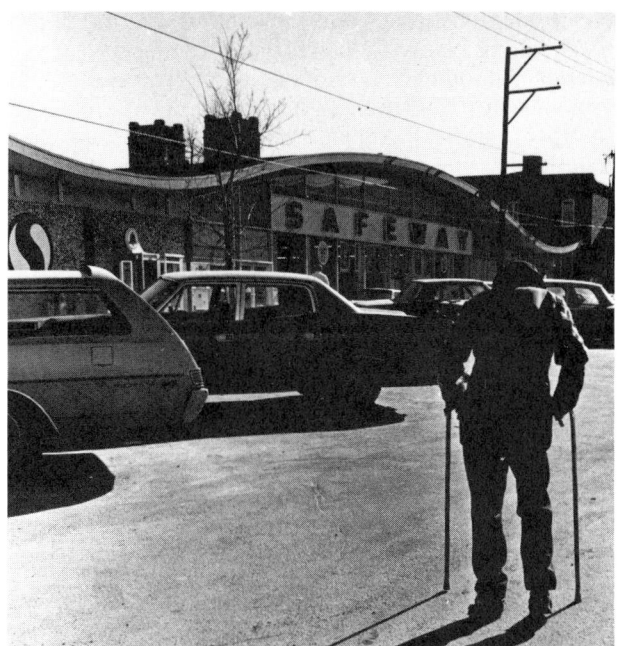

Figure 16–2 How will he carry groceries home? (From Sherman, E. M., and Brittan, M. R.: Contemporary food gatherers.Gerontologist, *13*:358, 1973. Photo courtesy of Barbara Caley, ACSW, St. Luke's Geriatric Clinic, Denver, Colorado.)

house without stairs could help, but the poor elderly person is trapped financially; he or she cannot afford to pay for a move or to leave a house which is already paid for. See Table 16–2 for a summary of the factors that may cause undernutrition in the elderly.

NUTRITIONAL REQUIREMENTS OF THE ELDERLY

Calories

There is a decrease in caloric requirements with age. In addition to a normal decline in metabolism of some 10 to 15 per cent (or more) after the age of 50, there is almost always a slackening of physical activity, which lowers the need for calories still further. It is difficult,

Table 16–2 POSSIBLE CAUSES OF UNDERNUTRITION IN THE ELDERLY

Loss of income—poverty
Social isolation
Diseases that reduce appetite, decrease absorption or utilization of nutrients or increase requirements for nutrients
Drugs that affect food intake, or the absorption, utilization or excretion of nutrients
Ignorance about good nutrition or food preparation
Dental problems
Depression or mental problems
Decreased physical ability to buy food or prepare a meal
Alcoholism

however, to estimate the degree of reduction in physical activity of individuals in the later years of life. Both the reduction of physical activity and the decline in basal metabolic needs vary with individuals. The Food and Nutrition Board (FNB), in the 1974 RDA, proposed that calorie allowances be reduced at age 50 to 90 per cent of the amount required as a mature adult of age 23 or so. If the person remains physically active after age 50, however, this reduction may not need to be as great.

The reference man and woman at age 23 need approximately 2700 and 2000 kcal., respectively. Assuming that they maintain good health, normal activity and approximately the same weight, at age 65 they need approximately 2400 and 1800 kcal. per day, respectively. If their weight is greater at age 65 than it was at age 23, there has probably been addition of fat tissue.

It seems advisable that most of the reduction in calories should come from a reduction in the carbohydrate and fat in the diet. Since aged persons require fewer calories but not less protein, vitamins or minerals, the foods eaten should obviously be good sources of these nutrients. Calories should not be wasted on low-nutrient foods such as candy, cola drinks, rich pastries and desserts. When calories are limited to less than 1800, careful planning is required to provide an adequate diet, as was

clearly demonstrated by Swanson.[11] Food intakes falling below 1800 calories provided inadequate amounts of protein, calcium, iron and vitamins for nutritional safety. Too often "empty calories" replace nutritious foods, e.g., tea with cream and sugar instead of a nutrient-rich food such as milk, or cake instead of a fresh or cooked fruit for dessert.

Protein

Body protein mass decreases with age. This is probably due in large part to a decrease in skeletal muscle mass. Visceral protein metabolism (for the internal organs) becomes more important. Total body protein increases from birth and reaches a maximum in the twenties, then slowly decreases throughout the middle and later years. The decrease seems to occur more rapidly in men than in women. Total body protein breakdown and synthesis also decreases with age, so that in healthy elderly people body protein is 60 to 70 per cent of that of young adults. Although it seems that the protein needs of the old person would be less than those of a young adult, there is not enough information on the amino acid and protein needs of the elderly to make this statement. The requirements for certain amino acids (threonine, tryptophan and methionine) may be different than for young adults, and the optimal pattern of essential amino acids may change with age.[15] In 1974 the FNB concluded that the protein RDA of 0.8 gm. per kg. per day for younger adults is appropriate for the healthy elderly person.

Stressful physical and psychological stimuli can induce a negative nitrogen balance. Infection, altered gastrointestinal function and metabolic changes caused by chronic disease can reduce the efficiency of dietary nitrogen utilization. Even without disease the aging gastrointestinal tract has reduced protein digestion and absorption. The elderly person should be assessed for these problems to determine the appropriate protein intake. Young and Scrimshaw recommend a protein intake of 1 gm. per kg. per day.[16]

Dietary studies of older people frequently show low intakes of the foods that are good sources of protein. A low protein intake usually occurs with a low caloric intake. Meat consumption decreases because of financial restraints, lack of cooking facilities, poor advice, lack of teeth and a number of other reasons. Negative nitrogen balances are often found when balance studies are made, and clinical

protein deficiencies are also frequently observed. Such deficiencies contribute to edema, itching of the skin, chronic eczema, fatigue, muscle weakness and tissue wastage. Wounds heal slowly and body resistance is lowered. However, the question arises as to whether the protein deficiencies seen are caused solely by low intake or by a combination of low intake, incomplete digestion and assimilation and insufficient calories. A low intake of protein usually means a low vitamin and mineral intake, and vitamin deficiency could be present with protein deficiency.

Carbohydrate

As mentioned, elderly people have a reduced glucose tolerance and therefore are more subject to temporary hypo- or hyperglycemia than a younger person is. When the blood sugar levels are increased by a large load of sugar, the rate of return to lower values is significantly slower in an older person. The use of sugar and sweets may well be restricted to prevent an undue load on the sugar-regulating mechanism of the body. Starchy foods should be included because they are mobilized and burned more slowly than sugar, and in many instances the starchy foods, such as whole grains or enriched cereals, potatoes and dried beans, carry B vitamins, iron, fiber and other essential food elements.

Fat

Because of current research concerning a possible relationship between serum cholesterol, saturated fatty acids and atherosclerosis (see Chapter 28), and because of the possible correlation between dietary fat and the level of serum cholesterol, it may prove advisable to decrease the proportion of fat in the diet. From epidemiological evidence, serum cholesterol levels seem to peak in men between 50 and 59 years of age and in women between 60 and 69 years of age, and then to fall in the later years. Serum triglycerides rise with continuing age and probably reflect the decreased capacity of elderly persons to remove dietary fat from the blood. Restricting dietary fat, particularly saturated fat, may be helpful but fat intake should still be about 30 per cent of total calories.

Food sources of cholesterol include many protective foods (egg yolk, whole milk, liver and beef), and rigid restriction of these might lead to deficiencies of other nutrients. It would

not seem advisable to restrict these foods rigidly in the daily diet of the person over 75 years of age, since the atherosclerosis prevention aspect for them would seem to be slight.

Fats are often a cause of indigestion, which may be due to the reduction of gastric, liver and pancreatic activity. The fats that are used in the diet for flavor and satiety value should be largely those that are low in saturated fatty acids and those that carry vitamins A and D. Distributing the fat intake among all the meals also helps in its digestion and absorption. The recommended daily intake of the essential fatty acids is 2 per cent of the calorie intake. This is supplied by polyunsaturated fats (also a good source of vitamin E). An excessive or severely restricted intake of fat interferes with the already decreased absorption of calcium.

Minerals

Of the minerals, *calcium* and *iron* are probably of greatest importance in the nutrition of the aged. Fragility of bones and capillaries may be attributed to a low intake of calcium-rich foods such as milk. The 1965 U.S.D.A. Nationwide Food Consumption Survey showed that diets of people aged 65 and over averaged more than 30 per cent (women) and 24 per cent (men) below the RDA for calcium. The women studied in the survey used the equivalent of less than 1 cup of milk daily. The men used slightly more. Women showed below-average amounts for iron.

Many of the symptoms attributed to senile weakness may be due to dietary deficiencies over a period of years. In many older persons, nutritional deficiency may even be found in the presence of an adequate diet if there is impaired digestion and absorption, impaired circulation, nutritive loss, endocrine imbalance, chronic infection or psychological stress, thus increasing the nutritional needs.

Osteoporosis. This is a condition of *reduced bone mass* that develops when more calcium is lost from bones than is taken in. It is more common in the later years of life. Although other factors are present in osteoporosis, one factor may be inadequate calcium intake over a period of years. A gradual decrease in bone mass takes place until finally there is pain and possibly fracture after a fall. The best protection against osteoporosis in old age is to include an adequate amount of calcium and vitamin D in the daily diet during adulthood. Osteoporosis is discussed more fully in Chapter 12, Nutritional Deficiency Diseases.

Osteomalacia. This condition of *decreased bone mineralization,* commonly referred to as adult rickets, is caused by poor utilization of calcium induced by a severe lack of vitamin D. Elderly individuals who do not drink milk or who have had a gastrectomy, who suffer from malabsorption, liver disease or kidney disease, who are taking anticonvulsant drugs or who do not get adequate exposure to sunlight can develop vitamin D deficiency and osteomalacia. Not enough calcium and vitamin D are available for normal bone upkeep, so the bones gradually weaken and fractures frequently result. Osteomalacia is further discussed in Chapter 12.

Nutritional Anemia. This is frequently found in older persons and may be caused by deficiencies of iron, protein, vitamin B_{12}, folacin, ascorbic acid or, more likely, by a combination of factors including reduced gastric acidity. The Ten-State Nutrition Survey revealed that iron deficiency anemia is more prevalent in adults over 60 years of age than in younger people, regardless of income or race. Folic acid deficiency, which can result in a hyperchromic megaloblastic anemia, is frequently seen in an elderly population. This vitamin is not widely present in food, is easily destroyed during cooking, and may not be absorbed from the gastrointestinal tract, which may be the problem for many elderly persons. (See Nutritional Anemias in Chapter 29.)

Periodontal Disease. Periodontal disease is characterized by demineralization of the alveolar bore of the mandible, which leads to loosening of the teeth, traumatization of the gingivae, hemorrhage and infection of the gums. It is thought that periodontal disease may be an early form of osteoporosis, in which case adequate calcium intake and the ratio of dietary phosphorus to calcium during the lifetime may be important. Periodontal disease is the most common cause of loss of teeth in Americans over the age of 35. (See Chapter 33.)

Vitamins

A number of studies have shown that increases in the vitamin intake of the aged give general health improvement. This could mean that the present allowances, which are the same as the allowances for younger adults, are not adequate for elderly people. More likely it reflects the fact that the elderly tend to have low intakes of vitamins. The Health and Nutrition Examination Survey, 1971–72 (HANES) showed that 61 to 62 per cent of poor black and

Table 16–3   CALCIUM, IRON, VITAMIN A AND VITAMIN C INTAKE OF PEOPLE 60 YEARS AND OLDER*

| | HANES STANDARD (Per Day) | PER CENT OF PEOPLE HAVING NUTRIENT LEVELS LESS THAN STANDARD | | | |
| | | Income Below Poverty | | Income Above Poverty | |
NUTRIENT		White	Black	White	Black
Calcium	[a](F) 600 mg. (M) 400 mg.	40	45	34	48
Iron	10 mg.	63	67	47	65
Vitamin A	3500 I.U.	61	62	56	52
Vitamin C	(F) 55 mg. (M) 60 mg.	59	54	39	44

*Adapted from: Preliminary Findings of the First Health and Nutrition Examination Survey (HANES), United States, 1971–72. Rockville, Maryland, U.S. Department of Health, Education and Welfare, National Center for Health Statistics, 1974. DHEW Publication No. (HRA) 74–1219–1.

[a]F = females, M = males.

white people 60 years of age or older who were examined had vitamin A intakes below 3500 I.U. per day. (RDA is 5000 I.U. for males and 4000 I.U. for females.) Vitamin C intakes were also low. (See Table 16–3.)

Some workers have shown that health is improved by giving B vitamins and vitamin C, while others have found that it takes large doses of the water-soluble vitamins to correct deficiencies of long standing in older people. Many of the so-called "normal" or "typical" characteristics of aging, such as slow adaption of the eyes to darkness, follicular hyperkeratosis and certain conjunctival lesions, have been improved by prolonged and increased administration of vitamin A.

Mental faculties can be deranged by vitamin B deficiencies. Deficiency of B_{12} may be the cause of disorientation, confusion and fatigue in elderly persons. Frequently these symptoms are thought to be natural characteristics of aging, or some organic brain lesion is suspected. Low serum B_{12} levels, which occur before megaloblastic anemia or neurological changes, can result from a poor dietary intake of vitamin B_{12} (as may happen with a person following a strict vegetarian diet), may be secondary to folic acid deficiency or may result from undiagnosed pernicious anemia. Low serum vitamin B_{12} levels seem to be fairly common in a geriatric population, and the elderly person should be assessed for the adequacy of vitamin B_{12} and folic acid nutrition and treated accordingly.[2]

Some individuals may need to supplement their diet with vitamin concentrates. However, with the accessibility and widespread use of vitamins, studies have shown that many people take vitamins that are already in their diet in sufficient amounts and do not take those that

they need. It is necessary to look at the diet before recommending a vitamin or mineral supplement. Guidance in selecting the right supplementary vitamins is needed. In many cases, a maintenance level multivitamin and mineral supplement may be well worth the expenditure and may cure latent nutritional deficiency states, the basis for many chronic complaints. It is important to remember that foods containing vitamins provide calories, protein and minerals. Vitamin supplements do not. (See Chapter 8, Vitamins.)

Elderly people are often swayed by the claims made for health food and can waste money on organic vitamins, mineral supplements and special foods that are supposed to make them feel better. They may feel better, in fact, because of the improved nutrient intake. However, it would be better for them to spend their money on a general vitamin and mineral supplement than on health foods. The supplement would give the same results at a fraction of the cost.

Water

The importance of water in the diet increases with age. With diminished kidney function, water becomes increasingly important as a carrier and is reported to ease rather than burden the kidney. Drinking adequate amounts of fluids (five to eight glasses daily) also aids digestion and helps in the control of constipation, which so frequently plagues older people.

REQUIREMENTS DURING CRITICAL ILLNESS

During the aging process, the cytoplasm of cells undergoes regressive and degenerative

changes that lead to a depression of basic cellular mechanisms. The result is that the energy pathways that are so crucial in times of stress do not function efficiently in old cells. Second, the cellular potassium-sodium pump is not as efficient, which means that the aging body is less able to correct fluid and electrolyte imbalances quickly. Third, the aging cell does not have metabolic enzyme reserves that allow it to switch on new metabolic pathways and respond to challenges to homeostasis. Therefore, nutritional support for critically ill aged patients should include early and aggressive infusion of glucose, amino acids, electrolytes, vitamins and insulin.

NUTRIENT INTAKE AND NUTRITIONAL STATUS OF THE ELDERLY

The results of the Ten-State Nutrition Survey of low income people revealed that some of the elderly show evidence of general undernutrition. Some of the findings were:

1. Obesity was prevalent, especially among women.

2. Low serum vitamin C levels were more prevalent in women than in men and gradually decreased with age.

3. Iron deficiency anemia was present in a large number of the elderly, regardless of ethnic background.

Surveys of the nutrient intake of the elderly, although incomplete, have given us some information on their eating habits. Some studies show that the consumption of green leafy and yellow vegetables, rich in vitamin A, is low, along with consumption of foods rich in vitamin C. Other studies have shown that elderly people reduce their caloric intake with age, especially after age 75.

However, it is a mistake to assume that the eating habits of all elderly are poor ones or that they all have poor nutritional status. In a 1973 study of 529 non-institutionalized elderly persons of all economic backgrounds aged 60 to 102 years, Todhunter found that although over 50 per cent lived alone, their dietary adequacy when compared to that of those living with others did not differ significantly.[13]

Although the Ten-State Nutrition Survey revealed biochemical and clinical signs of nutritional deficiency, it was found that the nutrient quality of the diet of the elderly per 1000 kcal. was higher than that for adolescents. The quality of the diet does not seem to be the problem, but rather the *amount* of the intake. This was also noticed in the Todhunter study; the size of servings rather than the choice of foods was a major factor influencing nutrient intake.[13]

From her study of elderly people, Todhunter concludes: "Their food habits and beliefs were free from faddism, they were willing to try new foods and to change at least some of their food habits, and they had a good appetite."[14]

FOOD FOR THE ELDERLY

Assisting older persons to provide an adequate diet for themselves often presents many problems. Chronic disease, combined with economic and psychological factors, operates to develop an oversimplified dietary program—one that is too frequently inadequate in protective foods. Education about a modified diet, usually as a valid part of medical care, frequently worsens the situation by further limiting the elderly person's food choices.

The nurse should consider all problems before attempting to help an aged person with his diet. The nurse works *with* the food pattern of the person. Together *with* the individual she helps plan a pattern, that he can live with. Helpful pamphlets, charts and booklets giving hints and simple information about food for the aged are available from state health departments, offices of aging and Title VII nutrition programs for the elderly.

Older people, just like people in other age groups, need a well-balanced diet that includes the protective foods. (See Chapter 10.)

The protective protein from meat, fowl, fish, eggs, milk and products made from milk is essential, along with the provision of vitamins and minerals. Fruits and vegetables are other important protective foods. Dentures may limit consistency of food to the softened varieties such as mashed, chopped or strained. Whole-grain bread and cereals are encouraged because they aid in maintaining normal bowel functions, as well as adding valuable food nutrients. In the aged it is quite likely that, under conditions of restricted activity and the associated diminished food intake, the resultant intestinal residue will not stimulate normal bowel movement. Thus, the older adult should be protected from the alluring claims of the food faddist and be reassured that the natural roughage in the fruits, leafy vegetables and whole-grain cereals of a good diet will promote satisfactory intestinal evacuation.

Milk is an important food in the diet of the

aged. Yet too frequently it is omitted or replaced by tea or coffee. Some older people even resent being encouraged to drink milk, while others dislike it. It is frequently thought to cause gas, which may be true if lactase, the enzyme needed to digest milk, is absent. See section on lactase deficiency, Chapter 23. As has been pointed out, milk is the chief source of calcium, is a good source of protein, a rich source of riboflavin and, when fortified, an excellent source of vitamin D. The consensus seems to favor the use of at least two glasses (16 oz.) or more daily, which can be served as a beverage as well as being used in cream soups and milk desserts. If this is not possible, the nurse or nutritionist should look for other sources of vitamin D, calcium and riboflavin in the diet. If the diet still appears low in these nutrients, and ingestion of milk or milk products seems impossible, then dietary supplementation is recommended.

Foods that furnish few or no essential nutrients but many calories, such as rich sauces, gravies, pies, frosted cakes, sugar, preserves, candies, oils, fried and fatty foods, are all on the list of products that are better decreased if not actually eliminated. These provide empty calories that the elderly person cannot usually afford either economically or physiologically. However, such foods frequently offer a tremendous psychological boost and may be included for this reason.

For those with sensitive digestive systems the suggestions are to eat something hot at each meal, four or five light meals rather than three substantial ones and the larger dinner meal at noon rather than at night. Concentrated foods in liquid mixtures may be necessary as supplements between meals.

The general principles governing the planning of a diet for the aged are not fundamentally different from those for the mature younger adult. However, modifications may be necessary because of certain characteristics inherent in the process of aging and peculiar to the elderly, such as poor dentures, lack of appetite, diminished sense of taste and smell, physical inability to get around with ease to obtain proper food, difficulties in manipulating eating utensils or in swallowing or inadequate cooking and refrigeration facilities. False notions about economy frequently misguide the aging person into a deficient, monotonous diet of tea and toast or their equivalents. Some aged persons do not know how to choose a good diet. Many eat snacks instead of regular meals and include only a small variety of food in the daily diet.

FOOD PLANS FOR THE AGED

With many elderly persons, income is a major factor in determining the adequacy of their diets. In many cases, Social Security is the major source of income.

The lowest estimated cost of food (October, 1976) at home for the thrifty food plan calls for $20 per week or $86.50 per month to provide an adequate diet for a couple 55 years of age or older. Table 16–4 gives the costs of three other food plans for a couple 55 years of age or older. All four food plans were designed by the U.S. Department of Agriculture. This represents 50

Table 16–4   COST OF FOOD AT HOME ESTIMATED FOR FOOD PLANS FOR THE ELDERLY 55 YEARS OR OLDER (OCTOBER, 1976)[*a]

	THRIFTY PLAN[b]	LOW COST PLAN	MODERATE COST PLAN	LIBERAL PLAN
Elderly couple, living together[c]				
Cost for 1 week	$20.00	$26.00	$32.30	$38.70
Cost for 1 month	86.50	112.80	139.70	167.40
Elderly male, living alone[d]				
Cost for 1 week	11.88	15.48	19.32	23.28
Cost for 1 month	51.36	67.20	83.52	100.68
Elderly female, living alone[d]				
Cost for 1 week	9.96	12.84	15.96	18.96
Cost for 1 month	42.96	55.80	68.88	81.96

[*]From: U.S. Department of Agriculture, Agricultural Research Service, Consumer and Food Economics Institute, Hyattsville, Maryland, 20782.

[a]Assumes that food for all meals and snacks is purchased at the store and prepared at home.

[b]See footnote *a* of Table 16–5 for the amounts of *edible* food waste allowed with each plan.

[c]Adjustment for two-person family included.

[d]If elderly person is living as part of a two-person family subtract 10 per cent, if part of a three-person family subtract 15 per cent, if part of a four-person family subtract 20 per cent.

Table 16–5 FOUR FOOD PLANS—QUANTITIES FOR AN ELDERLY PERSON FOR ONE WEEK, 1974–75*[a]

KIND OF FOOD	THRIFTY PLAN		LOW COST PLAN		MODERATE COST PLAN		LIBERAL PLAN	
	Man	*Woman*	*Man*	*Woman*	*Man*	*Woman*	*Man*	*Woman*
Milk, cheese, ice cream (qt.)[b]	2.37	2.85	2.61	3.01	2.97	3.35	3.24	3.65
Meat, poultry, fish (lb.)[c]	2.45	1.84	3.63	2.45	4.64	3.21	5.54	3.79
Eggs	4	4	4	4	4	4	4	4
Dry beans and peas, nuts (lb.)[d]	0.25	0.19	0.21	0.15	0.19	0.14	0.19	0.15
Dark green, deep yellow vegetables (lb.)	0.51	0.60	0.61	0.62	0.70	0.72	0.76	0.76
Citrus fruit, tomatoes (lb.)	1.85	2.02	2.38	2.54	2.91	3.09	3.52	3.71
Potatoes (lb.)	1.75	1.26	1.72	1.22	1.69	1.17	1.68	1.14
Other vegetables, fruit (lb.)	3.77	3.73	4.92	4.57	5.88	5.50	6.97	6.42
Cereal (lb.)	1.09	1.12	1.02	0.97	0.89	0.81	0.89	0.74
Flour (lb.)	0.80	0.68	0.62	0.58	0.53	0.52	0.54	0.54
Bread (lb.)	1.90	1.30	1.73	1.24	1.58	1.20	1.49	1.17
Other bakery products (lb.)	1.12	0.58	1.23	0.86	1.45	0.98	1.57	1.12
Fats, oils (lb.)	0.79	0.37	0.77	0.38	0.87	0.45	0.94	0.48
Sugar, sweets (lb.)	0.94	0.45	0.90	0.64	1.05	0.73	1.09	0.77
Accessories[e] (lb.)	0.73	0.66	1.16	1.11	1.50	1.39	1.82	1.66

*From: Consumer and Food Economics Institute, Agricultural Research Service, U.S. Department of Agriculture, Hyattsville, Maryland, 20782.

[a] Amounts are for food as purchased or brought into the kitchen from garden or farm. Amounts allow for a plate waste, spoilage or discard of one-fourth of *edible* food with the liberal plan, one-sixth of *edible* food with the moderate cost plan, one-tenth of *edible* food with the low cost plan and one-twentieth of *edible* food with the thrifty plan.

[b] Fluid milk and beverage made from dry or evaporated milk. Cheese and ice cream may replace some milk. Count as equivalent to a quart of milk: natural or processed Cheddar-type cheese, 6 oz.; cottage cheese, 2½ lb.; ice cream, 1½ qt.

[c] Bacon and salt pork should not exceed ⅓ lb. for each 5 pounds of this group.

[d] Weight in terms of dry beans and peas, shelled nuts and peanut butter. Count 1 lb. of canned dry beans — pork and beans, kidney beans, etc. — as 0.33 lb.

[e] Includes coffee, tea, cocoa, punches, ades, soft drinks, leavenings and seasonings. The use of iodized salt is recommended.

per cent of the total income for some older persons who are unable to buy the food they need. Food stamps, available to supplement incomes, assist in obtaining food to be prepared at home.

For individuals who prepare food at home, the four food plans in Table 16–5 are guides for weekly shopping and meal planning. The amounts listed are for foods as purchased. They allow for discarding inedible parts such as rinds, but not for careless waste. The amounts in each food group, namely, Thrifty Plan, Low Cost Plan, Moderate Cost Plan and Liberal Plan, are for a healthy man and woman at least 55 years of age who, it is assumed, are somewhat less active than in younger years. The amounts can be adjusted for more or less activity.

Each plan will provide for nutritional requirements. The main difference is that meals will be less varied on the Thrifty and Low Cost Plans. The Moderate Cost and Liberal Plans provide for larger amounts of meat, eggs, fruit and vegetables. In addition, more expensive items within the groups, such as foods out of season and more highly processed foods, can be included.

An adequate meal contains foods supplying sufficient calories and a complete protein or a combination of foods to provide all the essential amino acids. Wise selection of foods for the day provides the necessary minerals and vitamins. A suggested meal pattern for senior citizens is shown in Figure 16–3.

Feeding Programs

In Title VII of the 1973 Older Americans Act, the National Nutritional Program for the Elderly authorized funds for group feeding programs for the aged. These local programs are administered by health centers, church groups and senior citizen groups, and frequently are run by the elderly participants themselves. The daily meal provided is meant to be a pleasant social experience in addition to

BREAKFAST

Citrus fruit or juice
Cereal or egg
Toast and spread*
Tea, coffee or cocoa (made
with skim milk)

LUNCH

Soup or juice
Sandwiches (meat, fish, cheese, egg
or peanut butter)
Raw salad or cooked vegetable
Simple dessert**
Skim milk

DINNER

Fish, meat, poultry, cheese or egg
Potato
Green or yellow vegetable
Bread or roll and spread*
Simple dessert**
Tea or coffee

IN-BETWEEN SNACKS

Skim milk
Fruit or juice

* Spread: Margarine containing a significant amount of *liquid vegetable oil*, mayonnaise, cottage cheese, or a little jam or jelly, if desired.

** Simple dessert: Fruit, plain cake, or pudding (made with skim milk)

Figure 16–3   This is a suggested meal pattern for senior citizens, based on a guide to good meal planning. (Courtesy of Bureau of Nutrition, Department of Health, City of New York.)

being nutritious. (It should provide one third of the RDA.) Outreach, transportation, nutrition education and social counseling are part of the program, in addition to the recreation and socialization surrounding the meal.

Participants who were interviewed gave equal importance to the food and the social aspects of the program. The group meals act as a catalyst for involving the elderly in social activities and in community responsibilities. It becomes very important to reach out *actively* to the elderly to participate, as is illustrated by this excerpt:

The older American presents difficulties in outreach simply not found in other populations. He ordinarily pays his bills, lives within his means, obeys the laws, and is seldom found in the courts. He does not ordinarily march in the streets protesting his low pension, inadequate housing, or poor transportation. He gradually drops away from his social clubs and churches and stays within his own small circle of acquaintances and activities, calling no particular attention to his needs until he becomes ill enough to be hospitalized. In short, he is almost deliberately inconspicuous.[7]

Nutrition education in these settings is more effective if presented by an informal group discussion approach than by the lecture approach. Nutrition education is also effective if utilized in the designing of program menus by a group of participants.[4]

Food Stamp Program

The present food stamp program has been modified so that it is useful to the elderly person who cannot get to the food stamp office. A proxy can be sent to enroll in the program and pick up the stamps. In some states food stamps can be purchased by mail and can be used to pay for "Meals on Wheels" delivered to the elderly person's home. See Chapter 18, Food and Nutrition in the Community, for more discussion of food programs.

NUTRITION EDUCATION

For the elderly person to be motivated to change lifetime eating habits, the reason must be a good one and the approach humane. The traditional methods of presenting nutrition information in lecture or pamphlet form, with admonitions about illness or earlier mortality or promises of improved appearance and vigor, are not likely to be effective with this population. More appropriate are group discussions among elderly people who initiate questions or topics that they would like discussed.

During individual counseling, try to understand *why* an elderly patient is or is not eating correctly or is not responsive to your nutrition counseling. There may be a reason unrelated to food, cooking facilities, income or the ability to make a meal. It may not be a rational one. The environment of an aged person is complex and changing as he or she accepts a new role in society. The ways in which each individual elderly person reacts to this change of life must be thoroughly understood before nutrition counseling or education can be meaningful and accepted.

Nutritional studies indicate that the elderly are relatively uninformed about nutrition compared with other age groups. When most of today's elderly people were in school, they received very little information about nutrition. While younger adults are receptive to changes in their eating habits, older adults do not think this information applies to them. They may delude themselves into believing that nutrition does not matter for them. However, one important concern of elderly persons is their health. Once they accept the fact that proper nutrition is essential to good health, they are eager to learn how it can keep them healthy and living independently.[6]

NUTRITIONAL CARE IN NURSING HOMES

The nutritional care of the elderly in nursing homes must be directed toward meeting their physiological and psychological needs over a long period of time. These needs change depending upon the aging process, degenerative disease process and the emotional and mental status of the patient. It becomes very important to reassess the nutritional status and needs of the patient periodically to avoid continuing an unnecessary diet modification or missing an important but unmet nutritional need.

Weight history is an important record of nutritional status, and each patient should be weighed weekly and his or her weight recorded. Other clinical signs of malnutrition should be noted. This is especially important for the bedridden patient, who may be difficult to weigh. For example, a bedridden person's legs should be examined periodically. They can exhibit signs of thiamin deficiency (Fig. 16–4) or vitamin C deficiency (Fig. 16–5).

The most important nutritional care activity

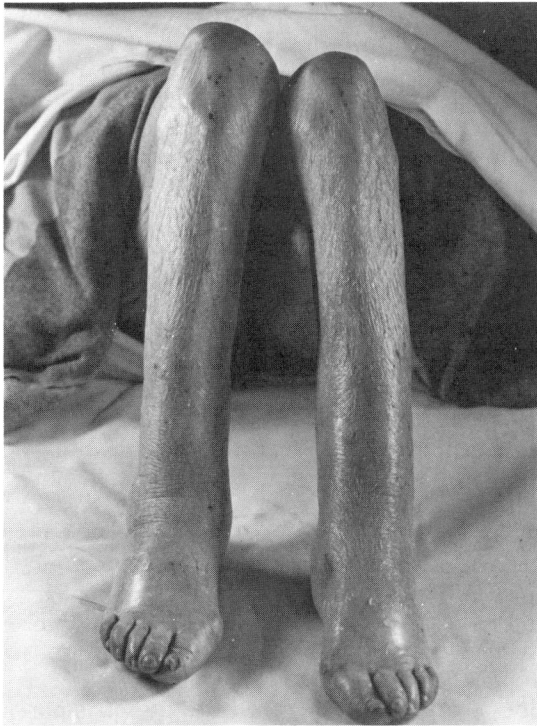

Figure 16–4 Thiamin deficiency edema. (From: Dreizen, S.: Clinical manifestations of malnutrition. Geriatrics, 29:97, 1974. Reprinted from Geriatrics © 1974 by Harcourt Brace Jovanovich, Inc.)

may be the same, but the older person has less efficient mechanisms for coping with stress. The provision of good food for the elderly patient in a pleasant sociable setting can do a great deal to boost morale. Whom he eats with is as important to the elderly person as what he eats.

Mental status is affected by nutritional intake and unfortunately, the possibility of malnutrition as a factor in mental health is frequently overlooked. Clinical vitamin deficiency states, particularly of the B vitamins, can result in behavior changes such as depression, anorexia, irritability, forgetfulness, insomnia, delirium and hallucinations (the dementia of niacin deficiency). To what extent latent or subclinical deficiencies of thiamin, niacin, folic acid or vitamin B_{12} affect behavior is still very unclear. Mental illness is the result of the interaction of many factors, and a vitamin deficiency state is just one of these variables that may predispose a person to mental illness in the presence of enough other adverse stimuli. It is difficult to separate the effects of vitamin deficiency from organic changes due to aging or from the influences of the social environment surrounding an elderly person. It is usually only in states of severe vitamin depletion that mental changes are seen. Drugs can also affect the mental functions of an elderly person more than those of a younger person.

Some inappropriate mental behavior may result from the fact that the elderly individual cannot properly perceive his environment because of decreased sight, hearing and touch. Signs of senility are seen in lagging memory and chronic degenerative diseases.

Low blood pressure or an infection may make a person acutely confused. Mild strokes or atherosclerosis impairing the blood supply to the brain can result in chronic dementia. We

performed by a nurse in a nursing home is noticing and recording the quantity and quality of fluid and food intake by the elderly patient. Old people in a nursing home may not eat for various reasons, including the strangeness or unpalatability of the food. Improving the eating behavior of the elderly patient requires a special effort by the dietitian to make the foods he likes available in an attractive and palatable way, and an effort by the nurse to create a pleasant atmosphere, encourage independence in eating or, if necessary, help him eat. The attitudes of the nurse and the dietitian can be supportive or destructive and are reflected in the nutritional health of the elderly in the institution.

EMOTIONAL AND MENTAL HEALTH OF THE ELDERLY

Depression in an elderly person is frequently overlooked and is regarded as a common occurrence with senescence. However, depressive illness in the aged is similar to that in younger persons, and can be treated with a favorable outcome. The causes of depression

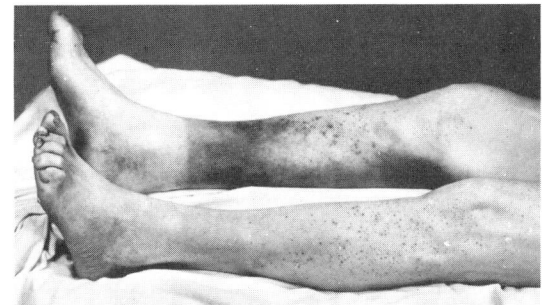

Figure 16–5 Ecchymosis and petechiae resulting from vitamin C deficiency. (From: Dreizen, S.: Clinical manifestations of malnutrition. Geriatrics, 29:97, 1974. Reprinted from Geriatrics © 1974 by Harcourt Brace Jovanovich, Inc.)

still do not know how much of intellectual loss is due to mental disease and how much to the process of aging.

The aged must help to minimize the incidence of disease by following the same rules of hygiene that are recommended for younger people. This includes weight control, more sleep and moderation in exercise and other endeavors. To be well adjusted, the aged person needs some interests and activity—both mental and physical—plus a feeling of usefulness and of being wanted.

PROBLEMS AND SUGGESTED TOPICS FOR DISCUSSION

1. List the ways in which the nutritional needs and food intake of a senior citizen may differ from those of a normal younger mature adult.
2. What are the main food habits and problems of the aged?
3. Interview an aged man living alone. Identify the problems that he encounters in providing meals. Help him to plan an adequate diet.
4. Take a diet history from an elderly woman in the hospital or clinic. Assist her with improvements in her dietary program, taking into consideration any problems she may have connected with her diet. Check for adequacy.

CITED REFERENCES

1. Arey, L. B., Tremaine, M. J., and Monzingo, F. L.: The numerical and topographical relations of taste buds to human circumvallate papillae throughout the life span. Anat. Rec., 64:9, 1935.
2. Elsborg, L., Lund, V., and Bastrup-Madsen, P.: Serum vitamin B_{12} levels in the aged. Acta Med. Scand., 200:309, 1976.
3. Hayflick, L.: The cell biology of human aging. N. Engl. J. Med., 295:1302, 1976.
4. Holmes, D.: Nutrition and health screening services for the elderly. J. Am. Diet. Assoc., 60:301, 1972.
5. McCay, C. M., et al.: Nutrition requirements during the latter half of life. J. Nutr., 21:45, 1941.
6. Pelcovits, J.: Nutrition education in group meals programs for the aged. J. Nutr. Educ., 5:118, 1973.
7. Pelcovits, J.: Nutrition to meet the human needs of older Americans. J. Am. Diet. Assoc., 60:297, 1972.
8. Ross, M. H.: Nutrition and longevity in experimental animals. In Winick, M. (ed.), Nutrition and Aging. New York, John Wiley and Sons, 1976, pp. 43–57.
9. Schlenker, E. D., et al.: Nutrition and health of older people. Am. J. Clin. Nutr., 26:1111, 1973.
10. Sherman, E. M., and Brittan, M. R.: Contemporary food gatherers. A study of food shopping habits of an elderly urban population. Gerontologist, 13:358, 1973.
11. Swanson, P.: Adequacy in old age. I. Role of nutrition. J. Home Econ., 56:651, 1964.
12. Tappel, A. L.: Where old age begins. Nutrition Today, 2:2, 1967.
13. Todhunter, E. N.: Life style and nutrient intake in the elderly. In Winick, M. (ed.), Nutrition and Aging. New York, John Wiley and Sons, 1976.
14. Todhunter, E. N.: Life style and nutrient intake in the elderly. In Winick, M. (ed.), Nutrition and Aging. New York, John Wiley and Sons, 1976, p. 127.
15. Young, V. R., et al.: Protein and amino acid requirements of the elderly. In Winick, M. (ed.), Nutrition and Aging. New York, John Wiley and Sons, 1976.
16. Young, V. R., and Scrimshaw, N. S.: Protein needs of the elderly. Nutrition Notes, Dec., 1975, p. 6. (Published by the American Institute of Nutrition, Rockville, Maryland.)

ADDITIONAL REFERENCES

Albanese, A. A.: Nutrition and health of the elderly. Nutrition News, 39(2), 1976. (Published by the National Dairy Council, Chicago, Illinois).
Beeuwkes, A. M.: Studying the food habits of the elderly. J. Am. Diet. Assoc., 37:215, 1960.
Bozian, M. W.: Nutrition for the aged or aged nutrition. Nurs. Clin. North Am., 11:169, 1976.
Bymers, G. J., and Murray, J.: Food marketing practices of older households. J. Home Econ., 52:172, 1960.
Campbell, V. A., and Dodds, M. L.: Collecting dietary information from groups of older people. J. Am. Diet. Assoc., 51:29, 1967.
Carlson, L. A. (ed.): Nutrition in Old Age. Symposium X of the Swedish Nutrition Foundation. Uppsala, Sweden, Almqvist and Wiksell, 1972.
Consumer and Food Economics Research Division, Agricultural Research Service: Food Guide for Older Folks. Home and Garden Bulletin 17. Washington, D.C., U.S. Department of Agriculture, Revised 1963.
Davidson, C. S., et al.: The nutrition of a group of apparently healthy aging persons. Am. J. Clin. Nutr., 10:181, 1962.
Davies, L.: Nutrition education for the elderly. Proc. Nutr. Soc., 35:125, 1976.
Dreizen, S. (ed.): Symposium on nutrition. Geriatrics, 29:55, 1974.
Elwood, T. W.: Nutritional concerns of the elderly. J. Nutr. Educ., 7:50, 1975.
Epstein, L. J.: Depression in the elderly. Symposium on age differentiation in depressive illness. J. Gerontol., 31:278, 1976.
Exton-Smith, A. N.: Physiological aspects of aging: Relationship to nutrition. Am. J. Clin. Nutr., 25:853, 1972.
Goodman, J. I.: The problem of malnutrition in the elderly. J. Am. Geriatr. Soc., 5:504, 1957.
Goodman, J. I.: Nutrition, life tenure, and the degenerative diseases. Geriatrics, 13:359, 1958.
Gregor, J. L., and Sciscoe, B. S.: Zinc nutriture of elderly participants in an urban feeding program. J. Am. Diet. Assoc., 70:37, 1977.
Howell, S. C., and Loeb, M. B.: Nutrition and Aging: A Monograph for Practitioners. St. Louis, Mo., St. Louis Gerontological Society, 660 South Euclid St., 1969. Also in Gerontologist, 9:1, 1969.
Jukes, T. H., and Borsook, H.: Nutritional management of the anemic geriatric patient. Geriatrics, 29:147, May, 1974.
Justice, C. L., Howe, J. M., and Clark, H. E.: Dietary intakes and nutritional status of elderly patients. J. Am. Diet. Assoc., 65:639, 1974.
Kent, S.: Is diabetes a form of accelerated aging? Geriatrics, 31:140, November, 1976.
Kent, S.: What nutritional deprivation experiments reveal about aging. Geriatrics, 31:141, October, 1976.
Lipolysis, aging and hormones. Nutr. Rev., 32:312, 1974.
Lutwak, L.: Periodontal disease. In Winick, M. (ed.), Nutrition and Aging, New York, John Wiley and Sons, 1976.
Mitchell, D. L., and Goldfarb, A. I.: Psychological needs

of aged patients at home. Am. J. Public Health, 56:1716, 1966.

Nutrition and Human Needs. Part 14: Nutrition and the aged. Hearings before the Select Committee on Nutrition and Human Needs of the United States Senate, Ninetieth Congress (Second Session) and Ninety-first Congress (First Session), Washington, D.C., Sept. 9–11, 1969.

Pelcovits, J.: Nutrition in older Americans. J. Am. Diet. Assoc., 58:17, 1971.

Piven, F. F., and Coward, R. A.: Regulating the Poor. New York, Vintage Books, 1971.

Ravetz, E.: The effect of a protein supplement in the nutrition of the aged. Geriatrics, 14:567, 1959.

Ross, M. H., Lustbader, E., and Bras, G.: Dietary practices and growth responses as predictors of longevity. Nature, 262:548, 1976.

Schumer, W.: The effect of aging on cellular and respiratory mechanisms—Metabolic mechanisms of aging cells. In Siegel, J. H., and Chodoff, P. (eds.), The Aged and High Risk Surgical Patient: Medical, Surgical, and Anesthetic Management. New York, Grune & Stratton, 1976, pp. 149–152.

Shagan, B. P.: Diabetes in the elderly patient. Med. Clin. North Am., 60:1191, 1976.

Shock, N. W.: Physiologic aspects of aging. J. Am. Diet. Assoc., 56:491, 1970.

Steinkamp, R. C., Cohen, N. L., and Walsh, H.: Resurvey of an aging population—fourteen year follow-up. J. Am. Diet. Assoc., 46:103, 1965.

Tappel, A. L.: Will antioxidant nutrients slow aging processes? Geriatrics, 23:97, October, 1968.

Wallace, D. J.: The biology of aging: 1976, an overview. J. Am. Geriatr. Soc., 25:104, 1977.

Wallace, P. W., and Westmoreland, B. F.: The electroencephalogram in pernicious anemia. Mayo Clin. Proc., 34:281, 1976.

Watkin, D. M., and Mann, G. V. (eds.): Nutrition and aging symposium. Am. J. Clin. Nutr., 26:1095, 1973.

Watkin, D. M.: The aged. In Mayer, J. (ed.), U.S. Nutrition Policies in the Seventies. San Francisco, W. H. Freeman and Co., 1973.

UNIT FOUR

NUTRITION, PEOPLE AND THE COMMUNITY

Chapter 17

GEOGRAPHIC AND CULTURAL DIETARY VARIATIONS

FOOD PATTERNS

Food patterns of a country are molded by its agricultural resources, technical progress, buying power and cultural patterns. Some factors influencing the food habits of individuals are race, religion and regional locality. When people come to the United States to make their homes, they bring along the food tastes of their native lands. An example is in the many varieties of breads in this country, which vary with national heritage. The firmly rooted habits of social groups are not readily relinquished, nor should they be. The regional availability of food is another strong influence on food selection. Sometimes the familiar foods are not available and the adjustment to different tastes is not made willingly. Many food customs of the foreign-born are excellent both nutritionally and economically and contribute to our pattern of living in the United States. Familiarity with the food patterns of the various nationality groups may help us to better understand and appreciate those from that culture who live in the United States.

Since World War II, many people from European and Asiatic countries have migrated to Canada. Most large Canadian cities contain a variety of ethnic groups. The Toronto Nutrition Committee compiled a food customs guide to assist nutrition workers in Canada in evaluating traditional eating habits in terms of Canada's Food Rules and in establishing good eating habits among the new Canadians.[5]

Social and cultural influences on food patterns are not well understood but the habit of eating is culturally based. Some cultures, such as the middle class urban American, generally have the largest meal of the day in the early evening and consider it a social occasion. It is served on a table on plates with utensils and napkins and with a minimum amount of eating sounds. In some cultures, people eat on the floor, use their fingers and smack their lips to show appreciation of what they are eating. Food patterns are interwoven with the culture of a people, and these must be recognized and considered by anyone in charge of feeding people or involved in diet modification, nutrition counseling or education. Whenever changes are desired in nutritional behavior they must be accomplished with a minimum of disruption in the lifestyles of individuals and their families.

Food patterns are based on the type of food production and service in a culture. Distinct differences are apparent when the diets of areas where almost all food (plant and animal) is self-produced or gathered are compared with diets in those areas where the food is supplied from large-scale commercial agriculture (domestic and foreign). One of the differences is the ability of a people to *preserve* food, and this is reflected in the food pattern. Some cul-

tures preserve food for future needs or for periods of scarcity. Other cultures do not preserve food and thereby experience a "feast or famine" way of life. The *distribution* of food (transportation, storage and marketing facilities) affects the food pattern. In some countries, the foods available in the cities are different from those available in the rural areas. Different methods of *food preparation* influence food patterns as well as the nutritive value of foods. (See Fig. 17–1.) One-pot dishes are used by some cultures, while in other cultures baking and roasting in an oven are the familiar ways of preparing food. Scarcity of fuel also affects the method of cooking.

Food patterns are based on *edible* materials one's culture considers to be food. For instance, while most Americans shy away from eating insects, fat crickets are sold at the market in Bangkok and sun-dried termites are a delicacy in Rhodesia.[7] Many foods may not be considered food by some cultures, but others eat them. In almost every culture, the people eat only a portion of the food supply available to them.

FOOD AND BEHAVIOR

Investigators realize the close relationships between food habits and social and religious beliefs. They define the study of food habits as "the study of the way in which individuals or groups of individuals, in response to social and cultural pressures, select, consume and utilize portions of the available food supply." One school of thought may condemn a practice that another praises. People like what they eat, and to understand the behavior of individuals within social groupings, their reactions to environment and their survival at different levels of efficiency and reproduction requires the integration of various sciences: anthropology, psychology, biochemistry, agriculture, economics, genetics, physiology and sociology.

Food has varying values to the members of different social groupings. To some, food is a means of disciplining children or exhibiting maternal affection, while adolescents may use food to show independence. In other families, the daily meals are important as a get-together, and lavish expenditures may be made on food to compensate for deprivations in other areas. Individuals may eat food for pleasure, from a sense of duty or for the nourishment derived. The amount of food consumed, the number of meals per day and the distribution of meals through the day often are based on traditions of the culture. The afternoon tea of the English and the early and late breakfasts of other nationalities influence the quantity of food consumed. See Food Habits, Chapter 19.

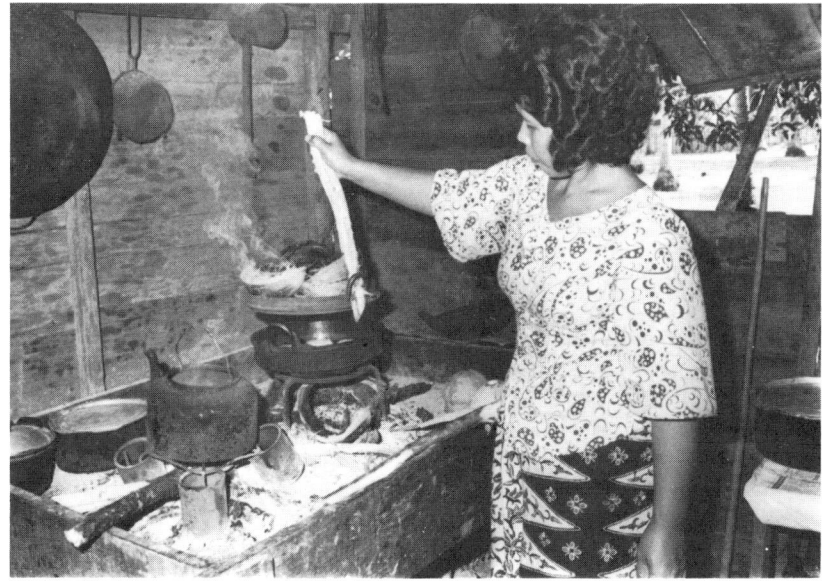

Figure 17–1   Food preparation in Malay kitchen. (From: Wilson, C. S.: J. Nutr. Educ., Winter 1971, p. 97.)

REGIONAL DIETARY VARIATIONS IN THE UNITED STATES

The South

Traditionally, hot breads have been one of the characteristic features of the Southern diet. Vegetable greens of all kinds are used. Vegetables are usually cooked a long time and often with fat pork. Much of the vitamin content is destroyed in this long cooking; however, a saving factor is the general use of the pot liquor. Sweet potatoes seem to be preferred to white potatoes. Southern fried chicken is a favorite, as are hominy grits and corn pone. Fish is used abundantly along the coast, fried shrimp and raw oysters being especially popular. Nuts are abundant. Buttermilk, canned evaporated milk and dried milk are used.

The elegance of entertaining still prevails in Southern homes. In New Orleans and the neighboring area the early influence of French cookery is still prevalent. New Orleans is considered one of the cities in the nation where gourmets may relish French cuisine.

Blacks in the South are apt to use cornmeal, hominy, hominy grits, rice, cornbread, hoecakes and hot biscuits extensively. Mustard, collard and turnip greens are favorites.

Salt pork, fatback, ham hocks or bacon ends are cooked with the greens and other vegetables such as kale and cabbage. This gives them additional flavor. Black-eyed peas and kidney beans are also popular. All fresh fruits are favored. Pork in all forms, chicken, fish and, when available, rabbit, squirrel and raccoon are used.

A typical main meal is a boiled dinner: fresh or smoked pork, fish or chicken, greens, sweet potatoes and cornbread. Butter, margarine and drippings from pork are used. Sorghum or molasses is used frequently on the hot bread. Blacks usually take these food habits with them if they move to the North.

With the new emphasis on black people's contribution to the American culture, "soul food" has gained prominence. Food discarded or disfavored by the owners of slaves during pre-Civil War years was prepared in slave kitchens. Such foods included pork snout and tail, bacon ends, ribs, chitlins and chicken wings. Animals from the field, such as opossum, squirrel and rabbit, and fish and turtles from the waters were used, along with local vegetables. Much originality and feeling or "soul" went into the preparation of these foods. Currently they are served on special occasions. (See Fig. 17–2.)

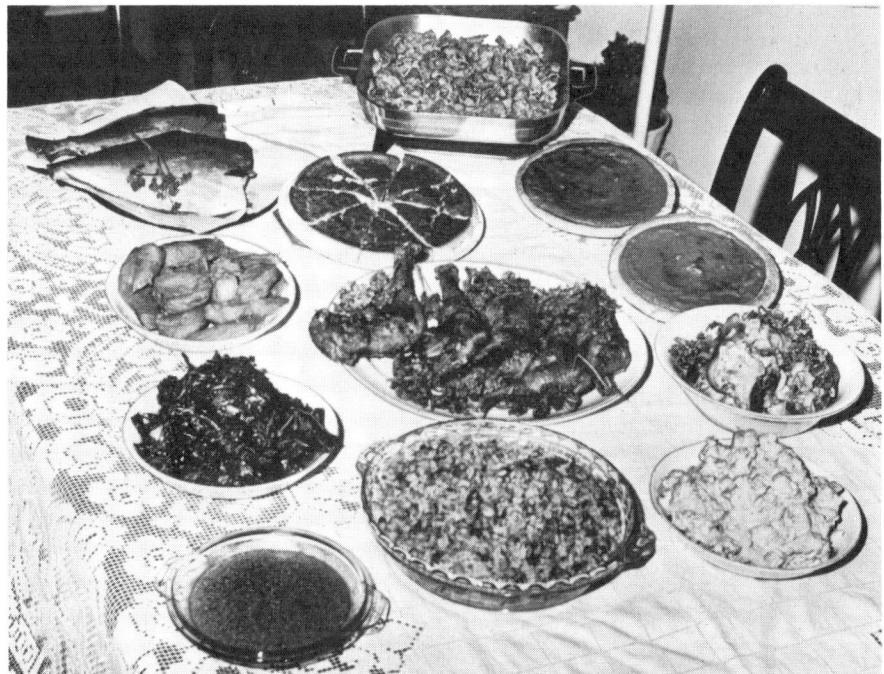

Figure 17–2 These dishes are considered to be the *pièce de résistance* of soul food cookery. From top, clockwise: chitlins or wrinkled steak, sweet potato pies, pigs' feet, potato salad, hopping John, pot liquor, collard greens, candied yams, porgies and (center) cornbread and fried chicken. (Courtesy of the Evening and Sunday Bulletin, Philadephia.)

The Southwest

In the Southwestern states and along the Pacific coast the influences of several cultures are noticeable, namely the early nomadic tribes of Indians, the Spanish and Mexicans from Central and South America and the Chinese, Japanese, Filipinos and Hawaiians from across the Pacific Ocean. The vegetarian habits of the Chinese, Japanese, Filipinos and Hawaiians have been brought along and are reflected in their garden produce.

Foods that have been used for generations and are therefore considered typical of the region are tortillas, tamales, pinto beans, chili and certain forms of corn. Spanish and Mexican influences are strong in Texas, Arizona, New Mexico and Southern California. More recently, Oriental and Hawaiian dishes have become popular in California. Recipes for saffron buns and Cornish pasties were brought to Nevada from England by Cornishmen who came to work in the mines. Cookouts, with the menu ranging anywhere from poultry, such as turkey, to a whole steer barbecued over an open fire, date back to the early days of ranching and cattle raising. Along the varied coastline and terrain can be found native products such as sand dabs, Gulf shrimp, Dungeness crab, avocados, almonds and ripe olives, which are used in ingenious ways and distinctive dishes. The custom of serving the salad as a first course originated in California, which is especially famous for Caesar salad.

The hot spiced foods from Mexico are reflected in the seasoning of foods.

The Middle West

Into the fertile, widespreading valley of the Mississippi and its tributaries and along the shores of the Great Lakes, the Scandinavians, Swiss, Germans, English and other nationalities have migrated. First generation families maintain many of their native eating habits, while second and third generation offspring, born in this country, adjust to the social grouping, and their diet becomes a blend of American and traditional native food. The third generation homemakers prepare some of the characteristic native dishes, and on festival days the menus often are replicas of former eating customs. Taking advantage of available ingredients and using some ingenuity, the people created a number of distinctive regional dishes. Fish from the Great Lakes and the rivers is a favorite food, as is the game hunted in marshes, plains and forests. Wisconsin has become famous as a dairy state and ranks with California, New York and Texas as a big vegetable producer. Iowa agriculture is the epitome of high-protein production. This is the heart of the great American corn belt, and here, more than in any other area in the world, food producers concentrate on the conversion of feed grains and forage crops into meat, milk and eggs. The homemakers of the Middle Western states take pride in their cookery skills, and their hospitality is reflected by a bountiful table.

The Middle Western states are now regarded as industrial states, and agriculture is no longer the chief occupation.

The Eastern Seaboard

Historical events are reflected in the food characteristics of the people who reside in New England and other states along the Eastern seaboard. Every schoolchild knows the story of the Pilgrims and the education they received from the Indians in the use of available fowl, fish, corn and other products. Baked beans, fish or clam chowder, fish cakes, lobster and turkey for holidays or special occasions are some of the old New England customs. The molasses and spices shipped from the West Indies, the retention of some of the food habits from the countries of Europe plus the acquisition of new food tastes characterize the meals of easterners, with the exception of the metropolitan areas, New York, Philadelphia and Washington. Philadelphia is known for "sticky buns" and scrapple.

In the large seaboard cities, immigrants arrive and stay with relatives until they are familiar with the ways of their new home. Gradually an adjustment is made to dress and living conditions, while eating habits become a blend of the traditional and the current trends. For example, New York has areas that have food shops and restaurants catering to the food tastes of Jews, Italians, Spanish, Puerto Ricans, French, Germans, Irish, Armenians and many others.

DIETARY PATTERNS OF NATIONALITY GROUPS

National Recipes

There are a number of regional and national recipe books available for those who wish to prepare and eat dishes of other cultures.

Food Plans

Following are the dietary patterns of a number of countries to help the student obtain a better understanding of various foreign-born individuals and families who may need aid in meal planning, food budgeting and dietary instruction. It is a very large undertaking to provide food and dietary information for persons who immigrate to the United States under conditions of stress. The rapid influx of Cubans to Florida and Vietnamese to California, for example, led to crowded conditions, linguistic problems and unfamiliar foods for the newcomers.

Rapid change is taking place in all countries, and it should be kept in mind that, while the dietary patterns listed here consist of typical native foods and customs, all nations are recipients of the United Nations educational programs on food and agricultural practices. Thus, what is typical today may not be in a few years. Also remember that when people immigrate to another country, for example the United States, they pick up American eating habits just as Americans pick up the eating habits of other countries. The best way to learn the eating patterns of a people is to talk with them, eat with them and ask about their foods.

DIETARY RESTRICTIONS AND PATTERNS OF RACIAL AND RELIGIOUS GROUPS

JEWISH FOOD CUSTOMS AND DIETARY LAWS[6]

The Jewish dietary laws are biblical ordinances codified and interpreted into rules regarding food. The rules pertain chiefly to the selection, slaughter and preparation of meat. Animals allowed to be eaten for food are the quadrupeds having a cloven hoof that chew a cud, specifically cattle, sheep, goats and deer; they are considered "clean." Permissible fowl are chicken, turkey, goose, pheasant and duck. All animals and fowl must be inspected for disease and killed by a ritual slaughterer according to specific rules. Only the forequarter of the quadruped may be used. If the hip sinew of the thigh vein can be removed, the hindquarter is also allowed.

Blood is forbidden as food, since blood is synonymous with life. Thus, the traditional process of "koshering" the meat and poultry removes all blood before cooking. Koshering involves soaking the meat in water, salting it thoroughly, allowing it to drain and then washing it three times to remove the salt.

Meat and milk cannot be combined in the same meal. Milk or milk foods may be eaten immediately before the meal, but not with it. After meat has been eaten, six hours must elapse before milk products may be used. Because of this rule, traditional orthodox Jewish homes must keep two completely separate sets of dishes, silver and cooking equipment, one for meat meals and one for dairy meals.

Fish allowed are only those having fins and scales. This bars all shellfish and eels. Fish may be eaten with either dairy or meat meals.

Eggs, too, may be used with either meat or milk. However, any egg yolk containing a drop of blood may not be used, since the blood is considered to be chick embryo or a sign of a new life.

Fruits, vegetables, cereal products and all of the other foods that make up a normal adequate diet may be used without restriction.

Bakery products and prepared food mixtures must be produced under acceptable kosher standards to satisfy the orthodox Jew.

Holiday Observance. The most important of the holy days is the Sabbath, or day of rest, observed on Saturday. The meal on Friday night is the choicest of the week and usually includes both fish and chicken. No food is allowed to be cooked or heated on Saturday, so all food eaten on the Sabbath is cooked the previous day and either kept warm in the oven or eaten cold.

The festival holidays are Rosh Hashanah, the New Year, in September; Succoth, the fall harvest holiday; Chanukah, the feast of lights, in midwinter; and Purim, a gay holiday in spring. Each holiday has delicacies associated with it.

Yom Kippur, or the Day of Atonement, occurs 10 days after Rosh Hashanah and is a day of fasting, with abstinence from all food and drink, including water, from sundown on the eve of the holiday to sundown on the holiday. Pregnant women and those who are ill are urged to refrain from fasting.

Passover, a spring commemorative festival lasting eight days, requires special dietary consideration. During this period, leavened bread or cake is prohibited. Matzoth, an unleavened bread, is eaten and all cake and baked products are made from flour of ground-up matzoth or

THE CHINESE FOOD PLAN

FOODS	PREPARATION
Meats: Pork (favorite), lamb, goat and poultry. Entire animal is eaten, including organs, brain, spinal cord, skin and coagulated blood.	Quantity is small and usually cut into small thin slices about 2 inches long and cooked in sesame or peanut oil with soy sauce, spices and a little water and served mixed with vegetables. Many methods for preserving and drying. Sweet and pungent pork or duck is a favorite (meat cubes rolled in batter and fried in oil, then simmered in sauce made of pineapple, green peppers, molasses, brown sugar, vinegar and seasonings.)
Fish: Fish and shellfish liked.	Fish is frequently baked with native spices or prepared in sweet-and-sour dishes. Many dried.
Other proteins: Hen, duck and pigeon eggs in abundance when afforded; soybean products; legumes.	Eggs are preserved and dried; also combined with chicken, mushrooms and bean sprouts and served with soy sauce (looks like vegetable omelet), termed *egg foo yong.* Egg roll served at beginning of meal is made of shrimp or meat and chopped vegetables rolled in thin dough and fried in deep fat. Soybeans used as sauce, as milk for infants in China and in many products. Legumes as substitute for meat.
Vegetables: Many plants such as carrots, onions, leeks, peas, cabbage, white turnips, corn, cucumbers, green and yellow beans, squash, shepherd's purse, radish leaves, sprouts (bean, bamboo, etc.), some white but more sweet potatoes.	Cut into uniform pieces and simmered or steamed with eggs or meat or added to meat and widely used in soups.
Fruits: Kumquat is favorite.	Preserved dessert.
Cereals and breads: Rice used freely. Some wheat, barley, corn and millet seed. Noodles are popular. Rice is main dish; others are side dishes.	Rice is used as main dish, plain or fried. Millet seed is made into cakes or used in a gruel. Noodles are small and fried. Steamed bread is eaten at breakfast.
Milk: Very little and generally not used. Given to children and invalids.	
Cheese: Little used.	
Fats: Chief oil is peanut oil. Some soy oil, rice oil, sesame oil or lard. Practically no butter or cream used.	Used in cooking.
Seasonings: Sesame seed, salt, ginger, garlic, fresh herbs, red pepper.	
Beverage: Tea is the national beverage.	Beverage at all meals, when afforded.

THE CUBAN FOOD PLAN
(PRE-CASTRO REGIME)

FOODS	PREPARATION
Meats: Beef, pork, lamb, veal, poultry, sausages.	Pork is either roasted or fried. Beef and chicken are used in soups, stewed, roasted, broiled or barbecued. The sausages are used with beans.
Fish: All varieties of fish (fresh, salted, smoked and canned).	Fried, boiled, marinated, roasted or grilled.
Other proteins: Beans (black, red, kidney, navy, yellow, lima, green); split peas; eggs.	Black beans with rice and roast pork is a favorite dish and is eaten on Christmas day. Eggs are eaten daily: fried, scrambled or in dessert.
Vegetables: Native tubers such as *yuca, ñame, malanga* (white and yellow), *boniato* (white yams), *chayote, berenjena,* plantain, potatoes, lettuce, tomatoes, carrots.	The tubers are boiled and served with *mojo* (made with sour orange, crushed garlic, sliced onions and hot oil), or mashed with butter and milk. Fried ripe or green plantains are a favorite side dish.
Fruits: Anona, *mamey, guanábana, chirimoya,* papaya, banana, *zapote, marañón,* mangoes, grapefruit, oranges (sweet and sour), coconuts, *caimito.*	Eaten fresh, in juice, or in desserts such as pastes, jellies, puddings.
Cereals: Rice, cornmeal, cornstarch, imported breakfast cereals such as oatmeal, corn flakes.	The favorite is white (long grain) steamed rice; sometimes *bijol* is added to make it yellow as in *arroz con pollo* (yellow rice with chicken). White rice is eaten daily for dinner and supper.
Milk: Fresh cow's milk (whole, skimmed), condensed, evaporated, dry; sour cream; goat's milk for the sick, usually.	Adults use it in coffee; children use as beverage. Also used in cream sauces, gravies, desserts, etc.
Cheese: Gouda, cream, *queso de mano.*	The native cheese is *queso de mano* (hard cheese) made from milk, lactate of calcium and salt, which looks like compressed cottage cheese; usually eaten with guava paste.
Fats: Pork lard, olive oil, peanut oil, soy oil, butter, margarine and shortening.	Pork lard is most popular. Oil is used in salads and beans.
Desserts: Fruits, ice cream, cakes, pies, custards, puddings; guava, prune and mango pastes; *morón* cookies, *terrejas, boniatillo, buñuelos, cafiroleta.*	Eaten after each meal and also as snacks. *Raspadura* is very sweet and the most typical native dessert.
Seasonings: Oil, vinegar, cumin, oregano, *bijol,* salt, pepper, garlic, onion, green peppers.	
Beverages: Coffee, beer, wines, tea, carbonated beverages.	Dark strong coffee served demitasse, with or without sugar.

THE GREEK FOOD PLAN

FOODS	PREPARATION
Meats: Lamb is main meat. Some beef, goat, mutton, pork products; poultry is popular.	Meat is either cut into small pieces or ground. Poultry is cooked into broth. Lamb is cooked on skewers or cut up and browned in oil or fat with rice or flour and vegetables.
Fish: Salt-water fish (fresh, smoked or salted), shellfish, smoked roe, squid and octopus.	Fish is fried or steamed with vegetables. Used frequently.
Other proteins: Eggs, white beans and legumes.	Legumes are boiled, mashed or stewed and eaten either hot or cold. Soup made of dried beans, onions, celery and carrots is a national dish. Eggs are popular.
Vegetables: Cabbage, cauliflower, cucumbers, eggplant, greens, okra, onions, peppers, some potatoes, vine leaves, zucchini, tomatoes, salad greens, oranges and lemons.	Vegetables are boiled or fried in a small amount of olive oil and served hot or cold. Many vegetables are stuffed. Potatoes or vegetables are cooked with meat or fish. Lemon juice is used to dress salads and cold foods.
Fruits: Apricots, cherries, dates, figs, grapes, melons, nuts, plums, peaches, pears, quinces and raisins.	Fruits in season are eaten raw, grapes are pressed into wine or dried as raisins. Fruit for dessert.
Cereals and breads: Maize, rice and wheat.	Maize is used in polenta; rice is an ingredient for *pilawi* and stuffing for vegetables; wheat is made into bread. Bread used abundantly and white is preferred.
Milk: Cow's, goat's and sheep's milk.	Milk is boiled for children. Fermented milk or *yaourti* is eaten as dessert or with pastry.
Cheese: Soft and mild, hard and dry cheeses.	Cheese is popular.
Fats: Olive oil, seed oils, salted black olives and little butter.	Olive oil is used to dress salads and hot or cold vegetables and in cooking.
Seasonings: Caraway and pumpkin seeds, herbs, honey, nuts (hazel, pignolia and pistachio) and sesame.	Seeds are eaten between meals, and nuts are served as dessert.
Beverages: Coffee and wine.	Coffee (American) is the beverage served in the mornings. At other meals it is made and served Turkish style. Wine is served at meals.

THE JAPANESE FOOD PLAN

FOODS	PREPARATION
Meats: The Buddhist tradition of not eating meat conforms with the physical necessities of agriculture. The Japanese consume very little meat, except beef. Since World War II, however, protein intake has increased; from 1950 to 1960 it increased 10 per cent and animal protein almost doubled.	Quantity is small. Usually cut into small pieces and served mixed with vegetables and cereal products. (See Fig. 17–3.)
Fish: Liked and one of the staple foods.	Prefer fish, shellfish and other marine life to meats of all types. Certain kinds of raw fish are considered great delicacies. Others cooked or dried.
Other proteins: Soybean preparations used freely. Eggs used when available.	Variety of soybean preparations.
Vegetables: Prefer plants such as seaweed, bamboo shoots, onions, large radishes, dried mushrooms *(shiitake)* and beans. Potatoes and others when available.	Pickled is the favorite form. Others cooked with meat or fish.
Fruits: Principal fruit is *nasi* (tastes somewhat like pear, shaped like an apple; yellow, rough skin). Some persimmons and mulberries. Tangerines in mountain regions. Postwar increase in variety.	Dessert.
Cereals and breads: Rice is main food. Some barley, oats and rye.	Rice is mixed with barley by farmers and the poorer classes. Wheat bread, especially in urban communities.
Milk: Enjoy when available; mainly import evaporated or dry milk powder.	Mostly for children.
Cheese: Very little.	
Fats: Soy oil. Rice oil. Suet when available. Practically no butter and cream.	Used in cooking.
Seasonings: Salt, *sake* (liquor distilled from rice).	
Beverages: Tea, *sake.*	Tea freely used when afforded.

Figure 17–3 A Japanese meal. Sukiyaki, made with beef and vegetables, may be served with tea, rice and a small marinated salad.

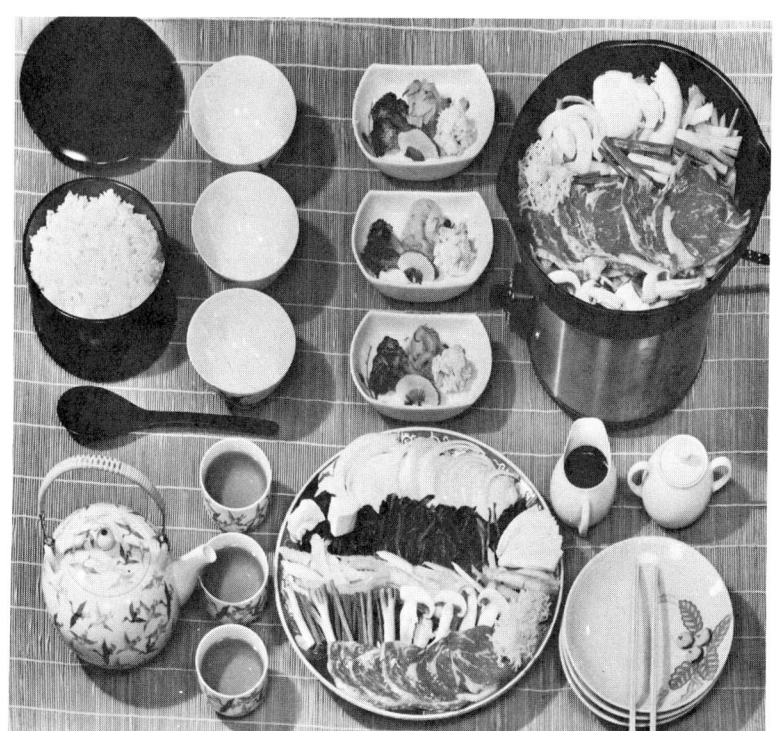

This is an example of a meal that is Japanese in inspiration, American by adaptation. The ingredients of sukiyaki are beef suet, paper-thin sliced tender beef, sliced onions, sliced celery, steamed spinach, scallions, sliced mushrooms, sliced bamboo shoots, cubes of soybean curd, vermicelli, sugar, soy sauce and *sake*. A very hot skillet is rubbed with the suet, and meat is seared on both sides. The heat is turned low, and the remainder of ingredients are added. The entire contents of the skillet are then simmered five to seven minutes longer. Vegetables should be crisp when eaten. In preparing sukiyaki, Japanese often use dried mushrooms (*shiitake*) of very intense flavor and fragrance. These are soaked several hours before they are added to the dish. They are available in Japanese groceries.

"Suki" means plow and "yaki" means roasted. According to a story, probably apocryphal, this dish originated in Japan a century or more ago at a time when Buddhism forbade the eating of beef. A farmer slaughtered a steer in secret on a lonely mountain and then cooked it, using part of his plow as a grill over the fire. Hence the term "plow-roasted"—sukiyaki. (From: New York Times Magazine, April 24, 1955.)

THE FOOD PLAN OF SOUTHEAST ASIA AND SOUTH VIETNAM

FOODS	PREPARATION
Meats: Poultry, pork back, very little beef.	Poultry and pork back served two or three times a week. Beef is very expensive and seldom served.
Fish: Many kinds of fish used regularly.	*Nuoc mam*, a fish sauce made by a salt pickling process, is served with most foods.
Other proteins: Soybeans, peanuts.	
Vegetables: Cabbage, *manioc*, maize, sweet potatoes, spinach, squash, watercress.	
Fruits: Coconuts, sugar cane.	Juice of sugar cane used to sweeten foods; cane is eaten raw.
Cereals and breads: Rice	Rice is the principal food, eaten at least once a day.
Milk: Little fresh milk is used.	
Beverage: Tea	Served at all meals. Chinese influence on choice and preparation of foods prevails; some French influence.

THE SPANISH-AMERICAN–MEXICAN FOOD PLAN[2]

FOODS	PREPARATION
Meats: Chicken, pork chops, weiners, cold cuts and hamburger.	Used only once or twice a week.
Other proteins: Eggs, beans.	Eggs used frequently and usually fried. In rural areas, chickens are kept for their eggs. Beans usually eaten mashed and refried with lard.
Vegetables: Potatoes, red and green chilies, fresh and canned tomatoes, pumpkin, corn, field greens, onions, carrots.	Potatoes are basic item, usually fried; may be used three times a day. Chilies are popular at each meal and are good source of vitamin A even when dried. Fresh tomatoes are very popular. Other vegetables used frequently.
Fruits: Bananas, melons, peaches, canned fruit cocktail, oranges, apples.	Oranges, apples used occasionally as snacks. Others are the more popular fruits.
Cereals and breads: Oatmeal, enriched white flour, packaged breakfast cereals, macaroni, white bread, tortillas, sweet rolls.	Sugar-coated packaged cereals are popular; oatmeal used occasionally. Macaroni is fried and served with beans and potatoes. Tortillas are homemade daily. Both purchased and homemade breads are used frequently. Purchased sandwich bread is a status symbol.
Milk: Limited availability, expensive. *Cheese:* Limited amounts used. *Fats:* Lard, salt pork, bacon fat. *Beverages:* Soft drinks; other sweets very popular.	Used liberally. Most foods are fried.

potato starch, leavened only with beaten egg whites. No salt is allowed in traditional Passover matzoth. Variations of fried matzoth or matzoth meal pancakes are prepared with generous amounts of fat.

MUSLIM RELIGIOUS DIETARY CODE

The following dietary restrictions are followed by the Muslim:
1. Pork and pork products such as gelatin are prohibited.
2. Alcoholic beverages and alcohol products (such as vanilla extract) are prohibited.
3. All meat used for food must be slaughtered according to ritual letting of blood and while speaking the name of God. This may be done by anyone since there is no special person designated for this function. Muslims use Kosher meat products because they know they have been slaughtered in the proper manner.
4. Although all foods not specifically prohibited are allowed, certain foods are recommended: milk, dates, meat, seafood, sweets, honey and vegetable oil, especially olive oil.
5. Fasting is practiced for one month of every year, which varies with the Islamic lunar calendar. Muslims will fast completely from dawn to sunset and will only eat twice a day—before dawn and after sunset. They are also encouraged to fast three days of every month. Menstruating, pregnant or lactating women are not required to fast, but must make up the fasting days at some other time.
6. Muslims are advised not to eat to capacity and always to share food.

ROMAN CATHOLIC DIETARY LAWS*

On Abstinence
1. Everyone, after the 7th birthday, is bound to observe the law of abstinence.
2. On days of complete abstinence, meat and soup or gravy made from meat may not be used at all. At the present time, these days are Ash Wednesday and the Fridays during Lent.

On Fast
1. Everyone, from the 21st birthday to the 59th birthday inclusive, is also bound to observe the law of fast except pregnant women and nursing mothers.
2. The days of fast vary because church laws have been changed in recent years.

---

*The dietary restrictions governing abstinence and fast have been liberalized. Customs vary in different localities and with individuals.

3. On days of fast, only one full meal is allowed. Two other *light meatless* meals, sufficient to maintain strength, may be taken according to each one's needs. Meat may be taken at the principal meal on a day of fast, except on Ash Wednesday.
4. When health or ability to work would be seriously affected, the law does not apply.

VEGETARIANS

The cultural philosophies of so-called pure vegetarians are based mainly on Eastern religions and have many similarities, yet they are distinctly different.[3] Some regimens are nutritionally adequate and others are not.

Lacto-ovo-vegetarian dietary consists of vegetables supplemented with milk, cheese and eggs. Many legumes and nuts are included and used in a variety of ways. Meat of all kinds, fish and poultry are prohibited. The Seventh Day Adventists follow this program. Lactovegetarians eat all vegetables supplemented with milk and cheese only. No other animal protein is permitted. Pure vegetarians ingest vegetables only and prohibit the use of animal foods, dairy products and eggs. The fruitarian diet consists of raw or dried fruits, nuts, honey and olive oil.

Pure vegetable and fruit diets without legumes, nuts and grains are nutritionally inadequate in protein, iron, calcium, riboflavin, vitamin B_{12} and possibly vitamin D. Mutual protein supplementation using mixtures of vegetables, beans, grains and nuts can, if properly planned, supply a good balance of essential amino acids and adequate amounts of calcium, riboflavin, iron, vitamin A and vitamin D. Vitamin B_{12} would have to be given in supplement or obtained from a B_{12}-fortified soy milk. See Table 10–5 and Chapter 5, Proteins.

The Zen Buddhist believes that one's health and happiness depend on a proper balance between the "yin and yang" foods. This way of eating is known by some American groups as the Zen Macrobiotic diet. The dietary pattern progresses through ten steps ranging from the lowest level diet, which includes 30 per cent vegetables, 30 per cent animal products, 15 per cent salad and fruits, 10 per cent soups, 10 per cent cereals and 5 per cent desserts, to the highest level, which contains 100 per cent cereals.[1] Erhard[4] explains how the philosophy of eating can be used in a nutrition program to improve the dietary pattern.

SOUL FOODS

Soul foods in present-day meals do not refer to any particular food or group of foods. They can include chicken wings, plantain, apple pie, a famous jelly layer cake, jams, shrimp or any food into which the person who cooks the food puts a great deal of feeling and pride during its preparation and serving. It is a "natural" feeling and if one's attitude is natural, imaginative and creative, soul food will be served at the table, regardless of nationality, race or creed.

PROBLEMS AND SUGGESTED TOPICS FOR DISCUSSION

1. What changes in food patterns have taken place in the United States? What caused these changes?
2. Interview someone with a different ethnic origin from your own and find out about his or her native food habits and social customs.
3. Evaluate one of the dietary patterns given previously to make sure it contains the basic foods.
4. Plan field trips to restaurants and food shops offering foods of various nationalities.
5. From the suggested reading list, select references and report on topics pertaining to the regional food habits in the United States.
6. Select a family representing the most prevalent nationality in your neighborhood. Interview the home-maker of this family to determine the quality of the menus served for one week. How do they rate? What improvements in them are needed? How does the homemaker perceive the changes?
7. Design a menu for two days for an adequate vegetarian diet.

CITED REFERENCES

1. Council of Foods and Nutrition: Zen macrobiotic diets. JAMA, *218*:397, 1971.
2. Cultural Food Patterns in the U.S.A. Chicago, American Dietetic Association, 1976.
3. Erhard, D.: The new vegetarians, pt. 1 and 2. Nutrition Today, *8*:4, 1973 and *9*:20, 1974.
4. Erhard, D.: Nutrition education for the "now" generation. J. Nutr. Educ., *2*:135, 1971.
5. Food Customs of New Canadians. Toronto, Toronto Nutrition Committee, Box 744, Terminal A, 1967.
6. Kaufman, M.: Adapting therapeutic diets to Jewish food customs. Am. J. Clin. Nutr., *5*:676, 1957.
7. Trager, J.: The Foodbook. New York, Grossman Publishers, 1970.

ADDITIONAL REFERENCES

Adolph, W. H.: Nutrition in the Near East. J. Am. Diet. Assoc. *30*:753, 1101, 1954.
Cantoni, M.: Adapting therapeutic diets to the eating patterns of Italian-Americans. Am. J. Clin. Nutr., *6*:548, 1958.
Cassel, J.: Social and cultural implications of food and food habits. Am. J. Public Health, *47*:732, 1957.
Chang, B.: Some dietary beliefs in Chinese folk culture. J. Am. Diet. Assoc., *65*:436, 1974.

Committee on Nutrition, American Academy of Pediatrics: Nutritional aspects of vegetarianism, health foods and fad diets. Pediatrics, 59:460, 1977.

Community Nutrition Section, American Dietetic Association: Selected List of References of National Food Patterns and Recipes, 1954.

Cornely, P. B., et al.: Nutritional beliefs among a low-income urban population. J. Am. Diet. Assoc., 42:131, 1963.

Drummond, J. C.: The Englishman's Food: A History of Five Centuries of English Diet. London, J. Cape, 1939.

Ellis, F. R., and Montegriffo, V. M. E.: Veganism, clinical findings and investigations. Am. J. Clin. Nutr., 23:249, 1970.

Gifft, H. H., Washbon, M. B., and Harrison, G. G.: Nutrition, Behavior and Change. Englewood Cliffs, New Jersey, Prentice-Hall, Inc., 1972.

Hacker, D. B., and Miller, E. D.: Food patterns of the Southwest. Am. J. Clin. Nutr., 7:224, 1959.

Hardinge, M. G., et al.: Nutritional studies of vegetarians. J. Am. Diet. Assoc., 43:550, 1963, and 48:25, 1966.

Harris, R. S. et al.: The composition of Chinese foods. J. Am. Diet. Assoc., 25:28, 1949.

Hegsted, D. M.: World wide opportunities. J. Am. Diet. Assoc., 31:236, 1955.

Jerome, N. W.: Northern urbanization and food consumption patterns of southern-born Negroes. Am. J. Clin. Nutr., 22:1667, 1969.

Joseph, S., et al.: Composition of Israeli mixed dishes. J. Am. Diet. Assoc., 40:125, 1962.

Judd, J. E.: Century-old dietary taboos in 20th century Japan. J. Am. Diet. Assoc., 33:489, 1957.

Koroff, S. I.: The Jewish dietary code. Food Technology, 20:76, 1966.

Lee, D.: Cultural factors in dietary choice. Am. J. Clin. Nutr., 5:166, 1957.

Lowenberg, M. E. et al.: Food and Man, 2nd ed. New York, John Wiley & Sons, Inc., 1974.

Marsh, A. G., et al.: Metabolic response of adolescent girls to lacto-ovo-vegetarian diet. J. Am. Diet. Assoc., 51:441, 1968.

Mead, M.: Food habits research: Problems of the 1960's. National Academy of Sciences, National Research Council, Pub. No. 1225, 1964.

Mitchell, H. S., and Joffe, N. F.: Food patterns of some European countries: Background for study programs and guidance of relief workers. J. Am. Diet. Assoc., 20:676, 1944.

Molony, C. H.: Systematic valence coding of Mexican "hot"–"cold" food. Ecol. Food Nutr., 4:67, 1975.

Natow, A. B., Heslin, J., and Raven, B. C.: Integrating the Jewish dietary laws into a dietetics program. J. Am. Diet. Assoc., 67:13, 1975.

New, P. K-M., and Priest, R. P.: Food and thought: A sociologic study of the food cultist. J. Am. Diet. Assoc., 51:13, 1967.

Pongborn, R. M., and Bruhn, C. M.: Concepts of food habits of other ethnic groups. J. Nutr. Educ., 2:106, 1971.

Queen, G. S.: Culture, economics, and food habits. J. Am. Diet. Assoc., 33:1044, 1957.

Report of the Committee on Food Habits. Manual for the Study of Food Habits. National Academy of Sciences, National Research Council, Bull. No. 111, 1943. Reprinted 1964.

Roberts, L. J.: Basic food pattern for Puerto Rico. J. Am. Diet. Assoc., 30:1097, 1954.

Sakr, A. H.: Dietary regulations and food habits of Muslims. J. Am. Diet. Assoc., 58:123, 1971.

Sakr, A. H.: Fasting in Islam. J. Am. Diet. Assoc., 67:17, 1975.

Stitt, K. R.: Nutritive value of diets today and fifty years ago. Nutr. Rev., 21:257, 1963.

Torres, R. M.: Dietary patterns of the Puerto Rican people. Am. J. Clin. Nutr., 7:349, 1959.

Valassi, K. V.: Food habits of Greek-Americans. Am. J. Clin. Nutr., 11:240, 1967.

White, H. S., et al.: Dietary surveys in Peru. J. Am. Diet. Assoc., 30:856, 1954.

Chapter 18

FOOD AND NUTRITION IN THE COMMUNITY

FOOD SURVEYS

Food Supply Data

A summary of food consumption surveys made by the United States Department of Agriculture[11] covering a period of 47 years, is shown in Table 18–1, which lists the nutritive value of diets per person in the United States from 1910 to 1976. The figures are based upon total available food and not on actual consumption and thus are difficult to interpret accurately, particularly because waste is not considered. However, they do give some insight

Table 18–1 NUTRITIVE VALUE OF DIETS PER PERSON IN THE UNITED STATES*

YEAR	KCALORIES	PROTEIN (gm.)	FAT (gm.)	CARBO-HYDRATE (gm.)	CALCIUM (gm.)	IRON (mg.)	VIT. A (I.U.)	THIAMIN (mg.)	RIBO-FLAVIN (mg.)	NIACIN (mg.)	ASCORBIC ACID (mg.)
1910	3500	101	123	498	0.84	15.3	7000	1.63	1.86	17.8	107
1920	3280	93	122	460	0.88	14.9	7400	1.53	1.86	16.2	107
1930	3450	92	134	477	0.90	14.3	7800	1.55	1.89	15.9	108
1940	3340	92	142	432	0.96	14.8	8200	1.55	1.95	16.5	122
1950	3250	95	144	401	1.03	17.1	8200	1.90	2.31	19.4	112
1955	3220	96	148	386	1.04	16.4	7400	1.85	2.34	19.7	108
1957–59[a]	3130	95	143	374	0.98	16.3	8100	1.85	2.31	21.1	105
1967	3210	99	150	373	0.95	17.4	7900	1.92	2.36	23.0	108
1974	3280	100	156	376	0.92	18.3	8200	1.99	2.37	23.9	117
1976[b]	3290	102	157	376	0.93	18.6	8100	2.06	2.47	25.3	123

[a] Average
[b] Preliminary

*Sources: Trulson, M. F.: The American diet—Past and present. Am. J. Clin. Nutr., 7:93, 1959. Compiled from: Supplement for 1956, Consumption of Food in the United States, 1904–1952. Washington, D.C., U.S. Department of Agriculture, Agriculture Handbook No. 62, 1956.
"Dietary Levels of Households in the United States". Washington, D.C., U.S. Department of Agriculture, Agriculture Marketing Service and Agricultural Research Service Report No. 6.
Marston, R., and Friend, B.: Nutritional Review. National Food Situation, 158:25, November, 1976.

into trends. A marked decrease in carbohydrate intake, particularly from grain products and potatoes, occurred during this period. Sugar and syrup consumption increased sharply until 1930, fell during World War II when it was rationed and remained fairly stable during the rest of this period. Fat consumption increased in spite of the decrease in total calories, with a concurrent increase in the use of hydrogenated fats. Increased consumption of meat, poultry, fish and dairy products resulted in more animal protein in the diet to compensate for the vegetable protein lost with decreased grain consumption. The drop in calories was reflected in the sharp curtailment in consumption of cereals, breads and potatoes. A noticeable change in the selection of a greater variety of foods was noted. Enrichment and fortification of staple products resulted in a marked rise in essential nutrients—thiamin, riboflavin, niacin and iron—in the early 1950's.

Food Consumption Survey 1965[13]

In the spring of 1965, over a period of 13 weeks, a survey of the food intake and of the nutritive value of diets of men, women and children in the United States was made. Information was obtained on the food intake for one day of individual members of the households interviewed. This represents the first time an estimate of the food eaten by individuals has been obtained on a nationwide basis. Approximately 15,000 reports on food eaten at home and away from home by men, women and children living in households were collected.

The 1965 survey showed that men and boys eat larger quantities of most types of foods than women of the same age. This is especially true for cereals, bread and other baked goods, meat, fish and poultry, fats and oils, and sweets and sugars. For vegetables and fruits, namely, tomatoes and citrus fruit, dark green and deep yellow vegetables and fruit, the average quantities eaten by women and girls equaled or exceeded the quantities eaten by men and boys at the same ages. Average amounts of all foods eaten by men and women 20 to 34 years of age are shown in Table 18–2.

The highest level of consumption of milk and milk products (butter not included) was by children under one year old, and the next highest was by boys aged nine through 19. Boys and men used more milk products than girls and women at all ages past nine years. As noted in Figure 18–1, the milk consumption of females decreased from age 12 and was lowest in the 35

Table 18–2 AVERAGE AMOUNTS OF FOOD EATEN IN ONE DAY*

FOOD (AS SERVED)	MEN	WOMEN
Milk and milk products		
Milk, milk drinks (cups)	1¼	¾
Cream, ice cream (cups)	¼	¼
Cheese (oz.)	⅓	⅓
Eggs (each)	1	½
Meat, poultry, fish (oz.)		
Beef	4	2¼
Pork	3½	2
Other meat	¼	¼
Poultry	1¼	¾
Fish, shellfish	½	¼
Mixtures	2¾	1¾
Legumes, nuts (tbsp.)		
Legumes, mixtures	2	1¼
Nuts, nut butter	½	¼
Grain products		
Bread, rolls, biscuits (slices)	5¼	3
Other baked goods (oz.)	2¾	1¾
Cereals, pastas (oz.)	1½	1¼
Mixtures (oz.)	1½	1½
Tomatoes, citrus fruit (cups)		
Tomatoes	¼	¼
Citrus fruit	¼	¼
Dark green and deep yellow vegetables (tbsp.)	1¼	1¼
Potatoes (cups)	½	¼
Other vegetables and fruit (cups)		
Other vegetables	½	½
Other fruit	½	¼
Sugars, sweets		
Sugar (tsp.)	4¼	3¼
Syrup, honey, molasses (tsp.)	1	½
Jelly, jam, gelatin desserts (tsp.)	2¾	2¼
Candy (oz.)	¼	¼
Fats, oils (tbsp.)		
Table fats	1¼	¾
Other fats, oils	1¾	¾
Beverages other than milk, juices and alcoholic drinks		
Tea (6-oz. cups)	¾	¾
Coffee (6-oz. cups)	2¼	2¼
Soft drinks (12-oz. bottles)	½	½

*Average amounts of food eaten in one day (Spring 1965) by men and women 20 to 34 years of age. (From: Food for Us All, 1969 Yearbook of Agriculture. Washington, D.C., U.S. Department of Agriculture, 1969, p. 272.)

to 54 age group, when the average milk or the calcium equivalent of milk products used was less than one cup per day. Males showed a sharp decrease in consumption of milk and milk products to about one cup between the ages of 20 to 34 and 35 to 54.

There was a steady increase in the consumption of meat, poultry and fish until the 20 to 34 age group and thereafter the consumption declined. The amounts of meat, poultry and fish

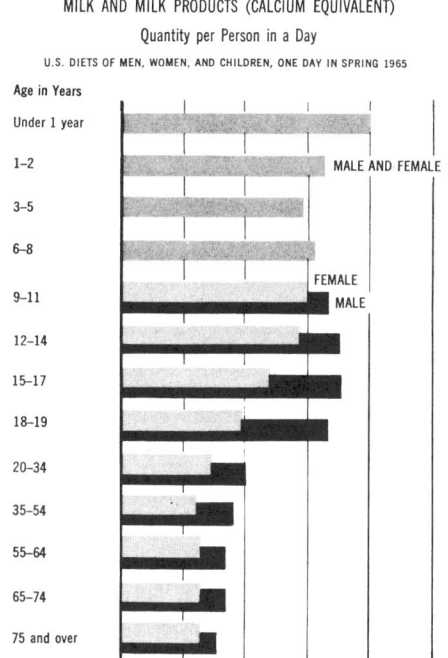

MILK AND MILK PRODUCTS (CALCIUM EQUIVALENT)

Quantity per Person in a Day

U.S. DIETS OF MEN, WOMEN, AND CHILDREN, ONE DAY IN SPRING 1965

Figure 18–1 U.S. diets of men, women and children one day in spring, 1965. (From: Food For Us All, 1969 Yearbook of Agriculture, Washington, D.C., U.S. Department of Agriculture, 1969, p. 269.)

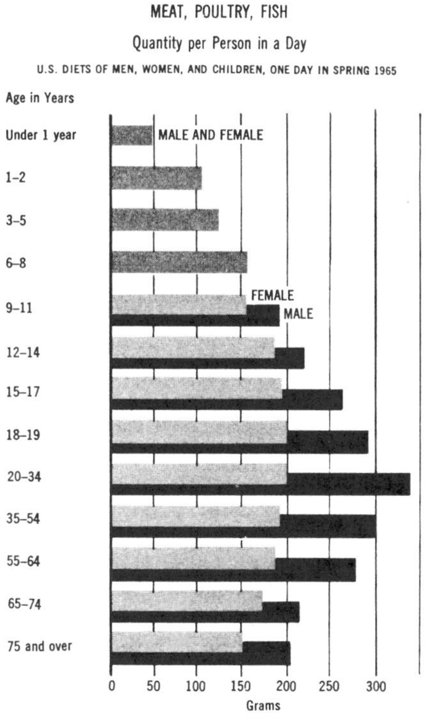

MEAT, POULTRY, FISH

Quantity per Person in a Day

U.S. DIETS OF MEN, WOMEN, AND CHILDREN, ONE DAY IN SPRING 1965

Figure 18–2 U.S. diets of men, women and children one day in spring, 1965. (From: Food For Us All, 1969 Yearbook of Agriculture. Washington, D.C., U.S. Department of Agriculture, 1969, p. 268.)

eaten by males were considerably higher than those eaten by females. (See Fig. 18–2.) On the day of the survey, over 85 per cent reporting (except the very youngest children) used one or more of these foods.

The peak years for consumption of grain products by boys were ages 15 through 19. Their average consumption of grain products was the equivalent of six slices of bread per day plus 7 ounces of other grain cereals. Bread products (including rolls and biscuits) were preferred by more persons and in larger quantities than other items in this group of foods. Larger quantities of grain products were used by boys and men than by girls and women in all age groups above nine years. (Fig. 18–3.)

Use of dark green and deep yellow vegetables was low. Only 10 to 20 per cent of all persons in the various age groups ate any of these vegetables on the day of the survey. On that day more than 75 per cent of most groups used one or more foods from other vegetable and fruit groups. The total quantity of vegetables and fruits used on this day is shown in Figure 18–4.

Beverages other than milk and fruit juices included coffee, tea, soft drinks and alcoholic beverages. Almost one third of the children and one half of the adolescents reported having soft

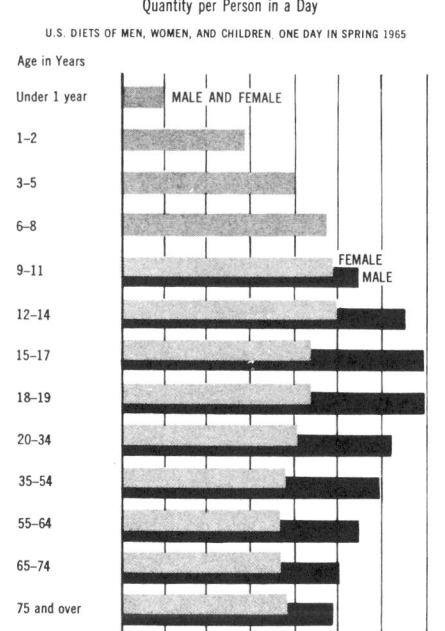

GRAIN PRODUCTS (FLOUR EQUIVALENT)

Quantity per Person in a Day

U.S. DIETS OF MEN, WOMEN, AND CHILDREN, ONE DAY IN SPRING 1965

Figure 18–3 U.S. diets of men, women and children one day in spring, 1965. (From: Food For Us All, 1969 Yearbook of Agriculture. Washington, D.C., U.S. Department of Agriculture, 1969, p. 268.)

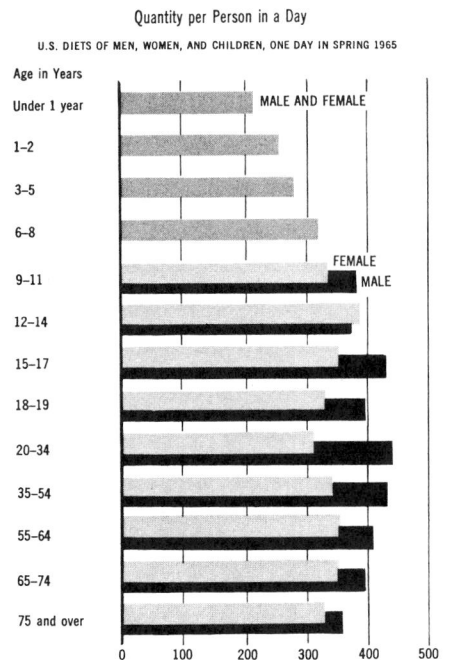

VEGETABLES AND FRUITS
Quantity per Person in a Day
U.S. DIETS OF MEN, WOMEN, AND CHILDREN, ONE DAY IN SPRING 1965

Figure 18–4 U.S. diets of men, women and children one day in spring, 1965. (From: Food For Us All, 1969 Yearbook of Agriculture. Washington, D.C., U.S. Department of Agriculture, 1969, p. 269.)

drinks on the day of the survey. The average quantities of milk and milk products generally ingested by persons in different age groups varied inversely with the average quantities of other beverages used.

The average nutritive content of the food and beverages consumed by the different sex and age groups in the 1965 survey was compared with the 1968 Recommended Dietary Allowances. Average diets approached (90 to 100 per cent) or were above the recommended allowances for calories and five of the seven nutrients studied: protein, vitamin A, thiamin, riboflavin and ascorbic acid. Calcium and iron were the nutrients that fell below the recommended allowances. (See Fig. 18–5.)

Calcium and iron (Figs. 18–6 and 18–7) in the day's food were more than 30 per cent below the Recommended Dietary Allowances for girls and women especially. The average diets of girls (15 to 17 years) and of women (from 35 years on) were about 35 per cent below Recommended Dietary Allowances for calcium. Diets of girls and women nine through 54 years were, on the average, approximately 40 per cent below the amounts suggested for iron. The iron in diets of children under three years was about 50 per cent below recommended

NUTRIENT INTAKE BELOW RECOMMENDED ALLOWANCE
Average Intake of Group Below Recommended Dietary Allowance, NAS–NCR, 1968
U.S. DIETS OF MEN, WOMEN, AND CHILDREN, ONE DAY IN SPRING 1965

Sex-Age Group	Protein	Calcium	Iron	Vitamin A value	Thiamin	Riboflavin	Ascorbic acid
MALE AND FEMALE:							
Under 1 year			• • • •				
1– 2 years			• • • •				
3– 5 years			• •				
6– 8 years							
MALE:							
9–11 years		•					
12–14 years		• •	• • •		•		
15–17 years		•	•				
18–19 years							
20–34 years							
35–54 years		•					
55–64 years		• •					
65–74 years		• •					
75 years and over	• • •		•		• •	•	
FEMALE:							
9–11 years		• • •	• • • •		•		
12–14 years		• • •	• • • •	•	•		
15–17 years		• • • •	• • • •		• •		
18–19 years		• • •	• • • •	•	•		
20–34 years		• • •	• • • •		•	•	
35–54 years		• • • •	• • • •		•	• •	
55–64 years		• • • •			•	•	
65–74 years		• • • •	•	•	• •	• •	
75 years and over		• • • •	•	• •	• •	• • •	

BELOW BY:
1–10%   •
11–20%   • •
21–29%   • • •
30% OR MORE • • • •

Figure 18–5 Average intake of nutrients below Recommended Dietary Allowance. U.S. diets of men, women and children one day in spring, 1965. (From: Food For Us All, 1969 Yearbook of Agriculture. Washington, D.C., U.S. Department of Agriculture, 1969, p. 270.)

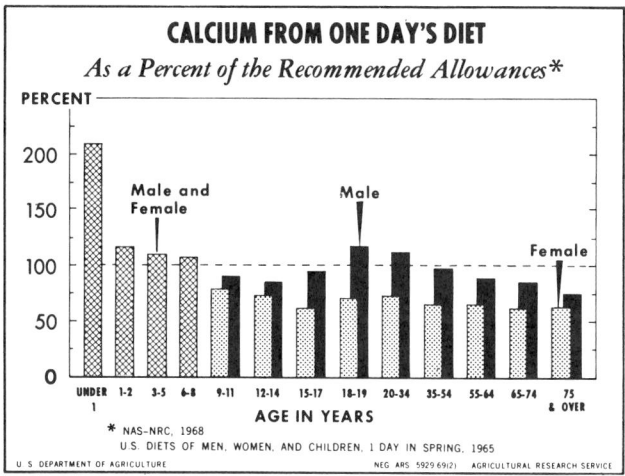

Figure 18–6   Calcium from one day's diet. (From: Nutrition Program News, Washington, D.C., U.S. Department of Agriculture, September–October, 1969.)

amounts, but the average amounts of calcium for this age group were above recommendations. The Food and Nutrition Board indicates that the recommended allowances for iron cannot be met with ordinary food products by all sex and age groups.[14] Ordinary diets provide about 6 mg. of iron per 1000 calories of food. That level was not reached in the diets of children under six years of age, boys 12 to 14 years or females under 55 years.

Males consumed approximately the same number of calories as recommended by the Food and Nutrition Board and females about 10 per cent below the recommendations.

The fat in the diets ranged from an average of 39 per cent for infants to 45 per cent of the calories for men 20 to 64 years of age.

The average intake of protein for all age groups in the study was over 100 per cent of the recommended amounts. The average intakes of vitamin A, thiamin and riboflavin in the diets of several groups of females were 5 to 15 per cent below the recommended allowances. The amounts of these vitamins in the diets of men were well above the recommended amounts. Men 75 years and over had an intake below the recommended allowance for ascorbic acid.

Nutritive content of vitamin supplements was not recorded and was not taken into account in the calculation of the nutritive value of the diets. Approximately 55 per cent of the infants under one year of age and 43 per cent of children one through two years received vitamin or mineral supplements. The elderly also tended to have a high intake of vitamin supplements.

Figure 18–7   Iron from one day's diet. (From: Nutrition Program News, Washington, D.C., U.S. Department of Agriculture, September–October, 1969.)

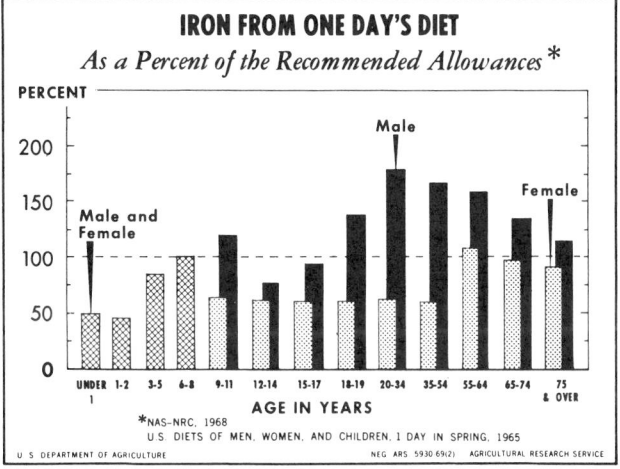

On the basis of this survey one can summarize the nutrient intake of several groups:

1. Infants and children under three years of age had an average iron intake 50 per cent below the RDA, and some nutrients, including calories, were found to be in excess of recommended amounts.
2. Adolescent girls and women aged nine through 64, with the exception of women aged 55 to 64, had average calcium intakes 20 per cent below the RDA and average iron intakes 30 per cent below the RDA.
3. Women aged 65 years and older had intakes of thiamin, riboflavin, vitamin A and iron below the RDA.
4. The diets of men 75 years and older were below the RDA for calcium, vitamin A, riboflavin and ascorbic acid.

The quality of the diet and income are closely related[7] (See Fig. 18–8.) In the 1965 household survey about one third of the families with incomes under $3000 had poor diets. However, education and knowledge of nutrition is also a factor, since about one tenth of the families with incomes over $10,000 had poor diets. Ignorance of or indifference to the selection of good diet was observed at almost all income levels.

The findings of the 1965 survey demonstrate the need to develop and intensify nutrition education programs. The survey indicates that there are individuals in many families at all income levels who need guidance in meeting their nutritional needs. The age groups that need special emphasis are teenage girls, women and older men. They need assistance in selecting foods that will provide increased amounts of calcium, iron, thiamin, riboflavin and vitamin A. Some low-income families need guidance in extending their purchasing power through food assistance and education programs that help make better use of their money spent for food. Nutrition education programs need to be adapted to (1) different age groups, (2) different income groups, (3) the food habits and lifestyles of individuals and groups of people and (4) mass media and other communication systems. Emphasis must be placed on (1) nutrients most often found to be below the daily recommended allowance in the age group, (2) extension of purchasing power through food assistance programs, (3) energy-saving methods of preparing and serving foods and of obtaining nutrients, (4) foods of high nutrient density to meet the recommended dietary allowances within calorie restrictions in a society with a large number of overweight persons and (5) eating habits and lifestyles that will prevent chronic degenerative diseases such as obesity, atherosclerosis, diabetes mellitus and dental caries.

Food Consumption Survey 1977–78

In 1977, the U.S.D.A. began its sixth food consumption survey of 15,000 households. Two studies in addition to the usual one will include consumption information from Alaska, Hawaii and Puerto Rico and information on 5000 households of elderly persons.

National Nutrition Survey 1968–70

The National Nutrition Survey or Ten-State Nutrition Survey conducted by the U.S. Department of Health, Education and Welfare was designed to evaluate not only the dietary intake but also the nutritional status of the people. In addition to dietary intake information, data included socioeconomic information, anthropometric measurements, clinical findings and biochemical data. According to its reports, the findings of surveys conducted in 10 states indicate that many people in low-income areas are seriously malnourished. The trends in this survey suggest that economic status may be an important underlying factor in the families' nutritional patterns, along with lack of con-

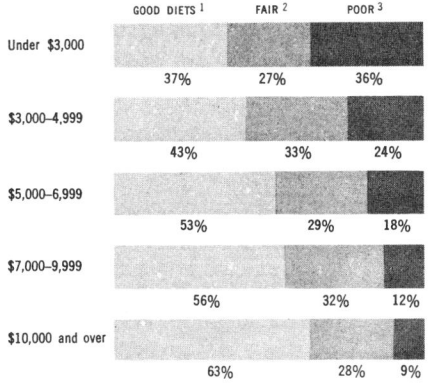

DIETS AT 3 LEVELS OF QUALITY, BY INCOME, 1965

U.S. households, one week in Spring

	GOOD DIETS [1]	FAIR [2]	POOR [3]
Under $3,000	37%	27%	36%
$3,000–4,999	43%	33%	24%
$5,000–6,999	53%	29%	18%
$7,000–9,999	56%	32%	12%
$10,000 and over	63%	28%	9%

[1] Met recommended dietary allowances (1963) for 7 nutrients.
[2] Met at least ⅔ RDA for 7 nutrients but less than RDA for 1 to 7.
[3] Met less than ⅔ RDA for 1 to 7 nutrients; is not synonymous with serious hunger and malnutrition.

Figure 18–8 Diets in U.S. households for one week in spring, 1965, showing three levels of quality by income. (From: Food For Us All, 1969 Yearbook of Agriculture. Washington, D.C., U.S. Department of Agriculture, 1969, p. 271.)

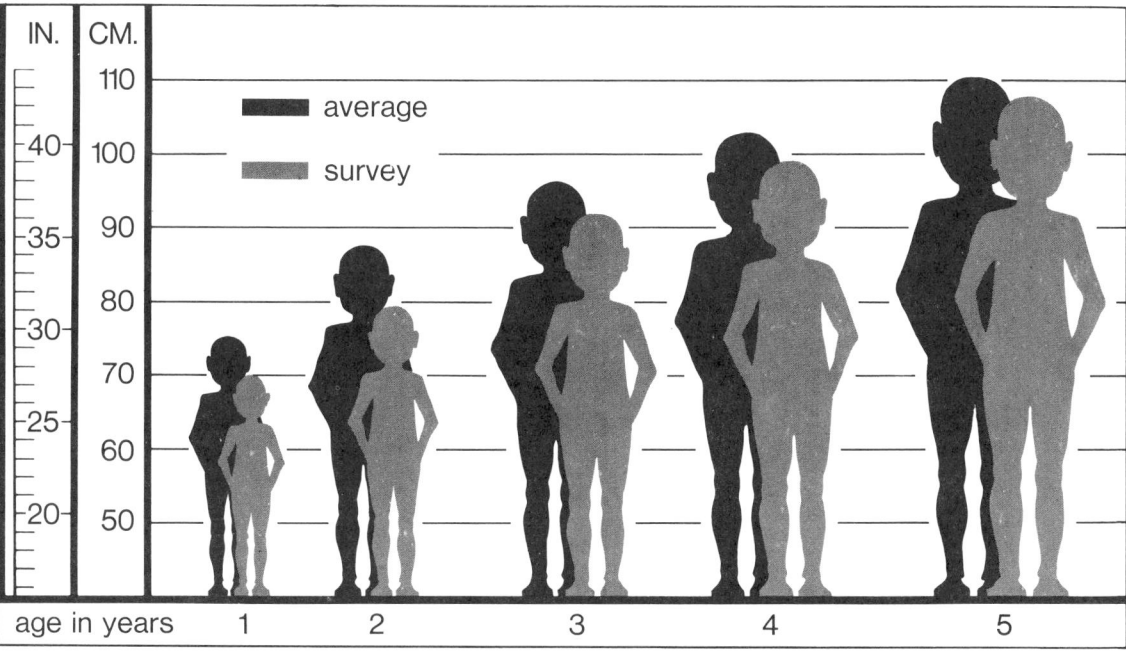

Figure 18–9 Height and age relationship for boys five years of age and under, from the National Nutrition Survey, 1968, of low income groups. (From: Nutrition Today, 4:No. 1, 1969, p. 10.)

cern, lack of knowledge of the right foods to eat or buy and ignorance of health care. The clinical findings of the prevalence of anemia and reduced levels of serum albumin, vitamin A, ascorbic acid and urinary thiamin and riboflavin clearly indicate the seriousness and magnitude of the problem. In general, adolescents had the greatest prevalence of unsatisfactory nutritional status. Obesity was a major problem, particularly among black women.[5] Children from poor families were smaller than children from families with higher economic status. (See Fig. 18–9).

Preschool Nutrition Survey 1968–70

In this survey, 3400 children between one and six years of age from 36 states and the District of Columbia, representing whites, blacks, Spanish-Americans and American Indians, were evaluated for nutritional status. Family incomes were at three levels, and one third of the families had incomes more than three times the poverty level. Some of the findings from this survey were:[26]

1. Low socioeconomic status was systematically associated with smaller size in white children.
2. Blacks tended to be smaller at birth than whites and remained smaller for the first two to three years of life. Thereafter, blacks tended to grow more rapidly.
3. As the socioeconomic status of the family increased, the nutrient intakes of the children improved. This was most evident for vitamin C.
4. Protein intakes of the subgroups averaged 1.5 to two times the RDA. All children seemed to have adequate protein intakes, as evidenced by adequate serum albumin levels.
5. Ten to 15 per cent of the children had borderline low intakes of ascorbic acid.
6. Twelve per cent of black preschool children, 10 per cent of Spanish-American and 7 per cent of white preschool children were classified as being anemic.

Most of these findings tended to confirm those related to children in the Ten-State Nutrition Survey.

Health and Nutrition Examination Survey (HANES) 1971–74

This survey of over 20,000 persons, representing the first health survey of the U.S. population with a nutrition component, was meant to assess and monitor the nutritional status of the American people over a period of time. Population subgroups were defined according to two levels of poverty, sex, age and race.

Preliminary clinical data suggest that signs of clinical deficiency such as tongue changes, bowed legs and knock knees, bleeding or swollen gums, goiter and low urinary excretion of thiamin and riboflavin are more common in blacks than in whites. In terms of a high risk of suffering and dying from certain diseases, e.g., hypertension, heart disease and diabetes, obese black women are in the highest risk group, and thus probably deserve special attention in both control and preventive programs.[24]

Dietary intake data obtained by the 24-hour recall method show:

1. Some population groups had mean intakes of protein, calcium, vitamin A and ascorbic acid that were lower than the RDA.
2. For the nutrients thiamin and riboflavin, adequate or more than adequate mean intakes were reported for all population groups.
3. For most population subgroups, the mean intakes for iron and calories were below the RDA.

However, without further biochemical and clinical evidence, it is impossible to say to what extent malnutrition exists in these populations.[19]

Copies of hearings on U.S. malnutrition before the Select Committee on Nutrition and Human Needs of the United States Senate; Reports on the White House Conferences on Food, Nutrition and Health; and the White House Conferences on Children and Youth and Aging are available from the U.S. Government Printing Office, Washington, D.C. These reports indicate a need for more effective nutrition education in community health programs and more extensive food assistance programs.

FOOD ECONOMICS

Economics may be defined as the science dealing with the production, distribution, exchange and consumption of wealth. This section will deal with economics as it relates to food, with special emphasis on food economy. During the past half century the science of food economics has made tremendous progress. The growing, processing and packaging of food so that it can be transported for thousands of miles and remain in good condition for months or even years is one of the wonders of modern living.

However, in 1973 Americans were faced for the first time with soaring food costs and food production shortages instead of surpluses. In that year alone, food prices increased 22 per cent over those of the previous year, while wages increased only half that amount. The trend of rapidly increasing food prices will probably continue as the United States feels the effect of the dry years of 1975 through 1977 and the effect of the increasing price of oil and petroleum products, which are necessary in food production. A greater percentage of the family budget will be spent on food, and knowledge regarding ways to eat well for less money will become more necessary for the health professional who is helping families improve their diets. In general, during periods of rapidly increasing food costs, American consumers tend to eat less; to eat meat less frequently, in smaller portions, and as cheaper cuts; and to eat fewer prepared or convenience items.

The food plans, menu planning suggestions and examples, market order and economy hints for planning, marketing and cooking to be discussed here are basic guidelines primarily. They provide the information and tools helpful to those who counsel individuals and families. The counselor, using the principles of teaching and learning, assists people in improving their dietary patterns, in changing improper habits and in providing adequate nutrition. The problem-solving begins with the amount of money the individual has to spend for food and the kind of food purchased. From this data, the counselor and the person together plan the appropriate steps toward the goals desired.

THE COST OF AN ADEQUATE DIET

Budget Allowance for Food

Food takes the greatest share of the family budget at a low or moderate income level. This is particularly true of the large family, which may allot as much as half or even more of income to food. In 1976, according to the Bureau of Labor Statistics, the urban working poor family spent almost 40 per cent of its disposable income on food.[8] It costs more to feed a large family, but the average cost per person is less, because the small family generally cannot buy and prepare the meals as economically as the large one.

In the United States almost 200 billion dollars a year is spent for food. This represents about 17 per cent, on the average, of take-home pay (about 5 per cent less than that spent for food in 1950). A larger share of food prepara-

tion is done outside the home than it was two decades ago. The highest income group used approximately one third of the money spent for food on meals and snacks eaten away from home.[17]

Food prices tend to follow the general economic trend in the nation. They represent costs and profits earned by farmers, processors and retail operators. One way in which the U.S. Department of Agriculture measures trends in food prices in the United States is by recording changes in the cost of a "market basket." The quantities and qualities of foods in this market basket are kept constant. The market basket is based upon the average quantities of food purchased per year by the families of the urban wage earner and clerical worker and by single workers living alone. The cost is estimated using retail prices that are published by the Bureau of Labor Statistics. The retail cost of the market basket has increased steadily. Rising marketing costs have been the main cause for higher prices. Currently the populace tends to purchase more expensive and higher quality foods than it did a decade ago.

The average family will spend approximately one half its budget for milk, meat and eggs and about one fifth for vegetables and fruits. The rest is almost equally divided among grain products, oils, sugars and miscellaneous. Nearly one fifth of the money spent in supermarkets is not for food, but for something to wear, read, clean with, listen to or smoke, or for alcoholic beverages and drugs.

The Food Plan

To assure adequate nutrition for each member of the family, it is wise to use a plan. The Recommended Daily Dietary Allowances of the Food and Nutrition Board are used as the yardstick for planning the adequate diet as described in Chapter 10, and can also serve as the basis for determining the cost of an adequate diet as shown in Tables 18–3 to 18–6. These four food plans—a thrifty, a low cost, a moderate cost and a liberal plan, based on the latest information on food consumption and nutritional recommendations—were worked out and published in booklet form by the Consumer and Food Economics Research Division, Agricultural Research Service, U.S.D.A. Each plan can be used as a guide for weekly budgeting, marketing and individual or family food planning, as it shows the approximate amount of food needed by each member of a family. Table 18–7 shows the estimated cost of each of

the four food plans for one week's and one month's food supplies for four family groups, as well as for sex and age groups and pregnant and lactating women, estimated on the basis that all meals are served at home or from the home food supply. Meals away from home cost about twice as much as those prepared in the home. Table 18–8 recommends the applicable budget level according to family size and income. These food plans are only a few of the many possible ones that could be developed for various cost levels. Other plans at the same cost and of similar nutritional adequacy could be designed to fit the food consumption patterns of an individual household more closely.

Characteristics of Diets at Different Cost Levels

The *thrifty* plan (the least costly) is used as the basis for coupon allotment by the Food Stamp Program. It includes an assortment of foods that conforms to the average food consumption of families with small food expenditures and yet it provides nutrition and controls cost. The low cost and especially the thrifty plans require skill in buying, storing and preserving food to ensure that the family is well fed nutritionally. The *moderate cost* plan is suitable for the average American family. It includes larger quantities of milk, eggs, meats, fruits and vegetables than the low cost plans. It also has more variety and less home preparation. The *liberal* plan allows for more variety, more animal products and more fruits and vegetables.

In general, the quantity of milk and milk products, leafy green and yellow vegetables, tomatoes and citrus fruits should not be changed very much, regardless of the amount to be spent for food. The greatest reduction in the cost of food can be made by reducing somewhat the quantities of meat, fish, poultry and the group described as "other vegetables and fruits" and by increasing the intake of potatoes, cereals, dry beans and peas. Within any food group there are both expensive and less expensive sources of the essential nutrients. For example, evaporated or powdered milk can be used in place of fresh fluid milk; cereals cooked or made at home cost less than the ready-to-eat varieties; lower grades and cheaper cuts of meat can be used and fruits and vegetables can be grown at home, purchased in season or purchased in bulk from a food co-op. Additional adjustments are listed in this chapter under "Economy Hints." Knowing how to

Text continued on page 381.

Table 18-3   THRIFTY FOOD PLAN*

Amounts of Food for a Week[a]

FAMILY MEMBER	MILK, CHEESE, ICE CREAM[b] (Qt.)	MEAT, POULTRY, FISH[c] (Lb.)	EGGS (No.)	DRY BEANS AND PEAS, NUTS[d] (Lb.)	DARK GREEN, DEEP YELLOW VEGETABLES (Lb.)	CITRUS FRUIT, TOMATOES (Lb.)	POTATOES (Lb.)	OTHER VEGETABLES, FRUIT (Lb.)	CEREAL (Lb.)	FLOUR (Lb.)	BREAD (Lb.)	OTHER BAKERY PRODUCTS (Lb.)	FATS, OILS (Lb.)	SUGAR, SWEETS (Lb.)	ACCESSORIES[e] (Lb.)
Child															
7 mo.–1 yr.	4.95	0.39	1.2	0.15	0.41	0.55	0.09	2.49	1.02[f]	0.02	0.08	0.04	0.04	0.19	0.05
1–2 yr.	3.30	0.83	3.3	0.17	0.22	0.89	0.65	2.26	1.02[f]	0.31	0.78	0.24	0.11	0.30	0.37
3–5 yr.	3.54	0.95	2.5	0.28	0.20	0.92	0.88	2.28	1.03	0.37	0.94	0.53	0.38	0.74	0.59
6–8 yr.	4.22	1.27	2.4	0.49	0.22	1.10	1.23	2.50	1.12	0.62	1.42	0.79	0.51	0.94	0.84
9–11 yr.	4.92	1.61	3.4	0.53	0.28	1.52	1.48	3.38	1.34	0.81	1.82	1.10	0.60	1.20	1.10
Male															
12–14 yr.	5.18	1.79	3.6	0.67	0.33	1.45	1.59	3.30	1.22	0.81	2.07	1.13	0.77	1.21	1.45
15–19 yr.	5.08	2.35	4.0	0.43	0.32	1.70	2.10	3.43	0.98	0.99	2.36	1.46	1.00	1.05	1.73
20–54 yr.	2.57	3.03	4.0	0.44	0.39	1.80	2.02	3.69	0.89	0.92	2.29	1.33	0.95	0.86	1.24
55 yr. and over	2.37	2.45	4.0	0.25	0.51	1.85	1.75	3.77	1.09	0.80	1.90	1.12	0.79	0.94	0.73
Female															
12–19 yr.	5.35	1.80	3.8	0.28	0.42	1.74	1.22	3.61	0.72	0.76	1.49	0.84	0.51	0.74	1.36
20–54 yr.	2.81	2.41	4.0	0.27	0.52	1.86	1.51	3.39	0.90	0.67	1.41	0.67	0.57	0.57	1.18
55 yr. and over	2.85	1.84	4.0	0.19	0.60	2.02	1.26	3.73	1.12	0.68	1.30	0.58	0.37	0.45	0.66
Pregnant	5.25[g]	2.69	4.0	0.42	0.56	2.17	1.89	4.03	1.13	0.58	1.41	0.66	0.59	0.58	1.48
Nursing	5.25[g]	3.00	4.0	0.38	0.57	2.36	1.92	4.27	0.98	0.63	1.56	0.82	0.80	0.75	1.54

[a] Amounts are for food as purchased or brought into the kitchen from garden or farm to prepare *all* meals and snacks for the week. Amounts allow for a discard of about 5 per cent of the *edible* food as plate waste, spoilage, etc.

[b] Fluid milk and beverage made from dry or evaporated milk. Cheese and ice cream may replace some milk. Count as equivalent to a quart of fluid milk: natural or processed Cheddar-type cheese, 6 oz.; cottage cheese, 2½ lb.; ice cream or ice milk, 1½ qt.; unflavored yogurt, 4 cups.

[c] Bacon and salt pork should not exceed ⅓ lb. for each 5 lb. of this group.

[d] Weight in terms of dry beans and peas, shelled nuts and peanut butter. Count 1 lb. of canned dry beans—pork and beans, kidney beans, etc.—as 0.33 lb.

[e] Includes coffee, tea, cocoa, soft drinks, punches, ades, leavenings and seasonings. The use of iodized salt is recommended.

[f] Cereal fortified with iron is recommended.

[g] For pregnant and nursing teenagers, 7 qt. is recommended.

*From: Consumer Food Economics Institute, Agricultural Research Service. U.S. Department of Agriculture, 1975.

Table 18–4 LOW COST FOOD PLAN*

Amounts of Food for a Week[a]

FAMILY MEMBER	MILK, CHEESE, ICE CREAM[b] (Qt.)	MEAT, POULTRY, FISH[c] (Lb.)	EGGS (No.)	DRY BEANS AND PEAS, NUTS[d] (Lb.)	DARK GREEN, DEEP YELLOW VEGETABLES (Lb.)	CITRUS FRUIT, TOMATOES (Lb.)	POTATOES (Lb.)	OTHER VEGETABLES, FRUIT (Lb.)	CEREAL (Lb.)	FLOUR (Lb.)	BREAD (Lb.)	OTHER BAKERY PRODUCTS (Lb.)	FATS, OILS (Lb.)	SUGAR, SWEETS (Lb.)	ACCESSORIES[e] (Lb.)
Child															
7 mo.–1 yr.	5.70	0.56	2.1	0.15	0.35	0.42	0.06	3.43	0.71[f]	0.02	0.06	0.05	0.05	0.18	0.06
1–2 yr.	3.57	1.26	3.6	0.16	0.23	1.01	0.60	2.88	0.99[f]	0.27	0.76	0.33	0.12	0.36	0.68
3–5 yr.	3.91	1.52	2.7	0.25	0.25	1.20	0.85	2.95	0.90	0.30	0.91	0.57	0.38	0.71	1.02
6–8 yr.	4.74	2.03	2.9	0.39	0.31	1.58	1.10	3.67	1.11	0.45	1.27	0.84	0.52	0.90	1.43
9–11 yr.	5.46	2.57	3.9	0.44	0.38	2.13	1.41	4.81	1.24	0.62	1.65	1.20	0.61	1.15	1.89
Male															
12–14 yr.	5.74	2.98	4.0	0.56	0.40	1.99	1.50	3.90	1.15	0.67	1.88	1.25	0.77	1.15	2.61
15–19 yr.	5.49	3.74	4.0	0.34	0.39	2.20	1.87	4.50	0.90	0.75	2.10	1.55	1.05	1.04	3.09
20–54 yr.	2.74	4.56	4.0	0.33	0.48	2.32	1.87	4.81	0.93	0.71	2.10	1.47	0.91	0.81	2.11
55 yr. and over	2.61	3.63	4.0	0.21	0.61	2.38	1.72	4.92	1.02	0.62	1.73	1.23	0.77	0.90	1.16
Female															
12–19 yr.	5.63	2.55	4.0	0.24	0.46	2.17	1.17	4.57	0.75	0.63	1.44	1.05	0.53	0.88	2.44
20–54 yr.	3.02	3.21	4.0	0.19	0.55	2.34	1.40	4.17	0.71	0.55	1.31	0.94	0.59	0.72	2.13
55 yr. and over	3.01	2.45	4.0	0.15	0.62	2.54	1.22	4.57	0.97	0.58	1.24	0.86	0.38	0.64	1.11
Pregnant	5.25	3.68	4.0	0.29	0.67	2.80	1.65	4.99	0.95	0.66	1.52	1.06	0.55	0.78	2.56
Nursing	5.25	4.16	4.0	0.26	0.66	2.99	1.67	5.33	0.78	0.61	1.55	1.16	0.76	0.91	2.70

[a] Amounts are for food as purchased or brought into the kitchen from garden or farm. Amounts allow for a discard of about one tenth of the *edible* food as plate waste, spoilage, etc. Amounts of foods are shown to two decimal places to allow for greater accuracy, especially in estimating rations for large groups of people and for long periods of time. For general use, amounts of food groups for a family may be rounded to the nearest tenth or quarter of a pound.

[b] Fluid milk and beverage made from dry or evaporated milk. Cheese and ice cream may replace some milk. Count as equivalent to a quart of fluid milk: natural or processed Cheddar-type cheese, 6 oz.; cottage cheese, 2½ lb.; ice cream, 1½ qt.; unflavored yogurt, 4 cups.

[c] Bacon and salt pork should not exceed ⅓ lb. for each 5 lb. of this group.

[d] Weight in terms of dry beans and peas, shelled nuts and peanut butter. Count 1 lb. of canned dry beans—pork and beans, kidney beans, etc.—as 0.33 lb.

[e] Includes coffee, tea, cocoa, punches, ades, soft drinks, leavenings and seasonings. The use of iodized salt is recommended.

[f] Cereal fortified with iron is recommended.

*From: Consumer Food Economics Institute, Agricultural Research Service, U.S. Department of Agriculture, 1974.

Table 18–5   MODERATE COST FOOD PLAN*

Amounts of Food for a Week[a]

FAMILY MEMBER	MILK, CHEESE, ICE CREAM[b] (Qt.)	MEAT, POULTRY, FISH[c] (Lb.)	EGGS (No.)	DRY BEANS AND PEAS, NUTS[d] (Lb.)	DARK GREEN, DEEP YELLOW VEGETABLES (Lb.)	CITRUS FRUIT, TOMATOES (Lb.)	POTATOES (Lb.)	OTHER VEGETABLES, FRUIT (Lb.)	CEREAL (Lb.)	FLOUR (Lb.)	BREAD (Lb.)	OTHER BAKERY PRODUCTS (Lb.)	FATS, OILS (Lb.)	SUGAR, SWEETS (Lb.)	ACCESSORIES[e] (Lb.)
Child															
7 mo.–1 yr.	6.46	0.80	2.2	0.13	0.41	0.49	0.06	3.98	0.64[f]	0.02	0.06	0.05	0.05	0.19	0.08
1–2 yr.	4.04	1.69	4.0	0.15	0.29	1.24	0.59	3.44	1.03[f]	0.26	0.81	0.33	0.12	0.28	0.79
3–5 yr.	4.74	1.88	3.0	0.22	0.30	1.46	0.85	3.51	0.74	0.27	0.82	0.73	0.41	0.81	1.42
6–8 yr.	5.79	2.60	3.3	0.34	0.37	1.94	1.17	4.39	0.84	0.39	1.14	1.11	0.56	1.03	1.97
9–11 yr.	6.68	3.31	4.0	0.38	0.45	2.61	1.40	5.76	1.03	0.51	1.47	1.51	0.66	1.31	2.63
Male															
12–14 yr.	7.02	3.77	4.0	0.48	0.48	2.44	1.52	4.66	0.94	0.56	1.69	1.54	0.85	1.34	3.65
15–19 yr.	6.65	4.65	4.0	0.29	0.47	2.73	2.00	5.45	0.80	0.67	1.98	1.82	1.05	1.15	4.41
20–54 yr.	3.38	5.73	4.0	0.29	0.59	2.92	1.94	5.93	0.76	0.65	1.97	1.65	0.95	0.96	2.95
55 yr. and over	2.97	4.64	4.0	0.19	0.70	2.91	1.69	5.88	0.89	0.53	1.58	1.45	0.87	1.05	1.50
Female															
12–19 yr.	6.22	3.32	4.0	0.24	0.53	2.62	1.21	5.38	0.68	0.56	1.34	1.22	0.56	0.97	3.36
20–54 yr.	3.35	4.12	4.0	0.19	0.62	2.84	1.35	4.94	0.54	0.49	1.28	1.08	0.65	0.81	2.89
55 yr. and over	3.35	3.21	4.0	0.14	0.72	3.09	1.17	5.50	0.81	0.52	1.20	0.98	0.45	0.73	1.39
Pregnant	5.44	4.57	4.0	0.25	0.91	3.52	1.60	6.13	0.73	0.83	1.77	1.28	0.46	0.85	3.50
Nursing	5.31	5.01	4.0	0.26	0.91	3.76	1.73	6.52	0.74	0.81	1.84	1.42	0.69	1.00	3.79

[a] Amounts are for food as purchased or brought into the kitchen from garden or farm. Amounts allow for a discard of about one sixth of the *edible* food as plate waste, spoilage, etc. Amounts of foods are shown to two decimal places to allow for greater accuracy, especially in estimating rations for large groups of people and for long periods of time. For general use, amounts of food groups for a family may be rounded to the nearest tenth or quarter of a pound.

[b] Fluid milk and beverage made from dry or evaporated milk. Cheese and ice cream may replace some milk. Count as equivalent to a quart of fluid milk: natural or processed Cheddar-type cheese, 6 oz.; cottage cheese, 2½ lb.; ice cream, 1½ qt.; unflavored yogurt, 4 cups.

[c] Bacon and salt pork should not exceed ⅓ lb. for each 5 lb. of this group.

[d] Weight in terms of dry beans and peas, shelled nuts and peanut butter. Count 1 lb. of canned dry beans—pork and beans, kidney beans, etc.—as 0.33 lb.

[e] Includes coffee, tea, cocoa, punches, ades, soft drinks, leavenings and seasonings. The use of iodized salt is recommended.

[f] Cereal fortified with iron is recommended.

*From: Consumer Food Economics Institute, Agricultural Research Service, U.S. Department of Agriculture, 1974.

Table 18–6 LIBERAL FOOD PLAN*

Amounts of Food for a Week[a]

FAMILY MEMBER	MILK, CHEESE, ICE CREAM[b] (Qt.)	MEAT, POULTRY, FISH[c] (Lb.)	EGGS (No.)	DRY BEANS AND PEAS, NUTS[d] (Lb.)	DARK GREEN, DEEP YELLOW VEGETABLES (Lb.)	CITRUS FRUIT, TOMATOES (Lb.)	POTATOES (Lb.)	OTHER VEGETABLES, FRUIT (Lb.)	CEREAL (Lb.)	FLOUR (Lb.)	BREAD (Lb.)	OTHER BAKERY PRODUCTS (Lb.)	FATS, OILS (Lb.)	SUGAR, SWEETS (Lb.)	ACCESSORIES[e] (Lb.)
Child															
7 mo.–1 yr.	6.94	0.97	2.3	0.14	0.43	0.60	0.06	4.71	0.64[f]	0.02	0.05	0.06	0.05	0.20	0.09
1–2 yr.	4.26	2.07	4.0	0.17	0.31	1.50	0.59	4.10	1.07[f]	0.28	0.82	0.35	0.13	0.27	0.95
3–5 yr.	5.08	2.35	3.1	0.23	0.32	1.77	0.85	4.18	0.76	0.27	0.79	0.78	0.45	0.85	1.74
6–8 yr.	6.25	3.18	3.4	0.36	0.40	2.35	1.18	5.21	0.85	0.39	1.08	1.23	0.60	1.08	2.41
9–11 yr.	7.21	4.04	4.0	0.39	0.48	3.15	1.41	6.83	1.04	0.51	1.39	1.67	0.71	1.38	3.21
Male															
12–14 yr.	7.57	4.57	4.0	0.50	0.51	2.94	1.52	5.52	0.95	0.56	1.60	1.71	0.92	1.40	4.47
15–19 yr.	7.18	5.59	4.0	0.31	0.50	3.29	2.01	6.45	0.84	0.69	1.92	2.05	1.07	1.20	5.36
20–54 yr.	3.64	6.83	4.0	0.32	0.62	3.51	1.95	6.99	0.79	0.66	1.91	1.86	0.95	1.00	3.54
55 yr. and over	3.24	5.54	4.0	0.19	0.76	3.52	1.68	6.97	0.89	0.54	1.49	1.57	0.94	1.09	1.82
Female															
12–19 yr.	6.72	3.97	4.0	0.25	0.56	3.15	1.21	6.34	0.71	0.59	1.31	1.35	0.54	0.98	4.09
20–54 yr.	3.62	4.86	4.0	0.20	0.66	3.41	1.35	5.81	0.56	0.51	1.24	1.22	0.66	0.84	3.47
55 yr. and over	3.65	3.79	4.0	0.15	0.76	3.71	1.14	6.42	0.74	0.54	1.17	1.12	0.48	0.77	1.66
Pregnant	5.91	5.43	4.0	0.26	0.96	4.22	1.57	7.17	0.70	0.87	1.70	1.45	0.46	0.87	4.20
Nursing	5.76	5.97	4.0	0.28	0.97	4.51	1.72	7.66	0.75	0.84	1.76	1.58	0.68	1.02	4.52

[a] Amounts are for food as purchased or brought into the kitchen from garden or farm. Amounts allow for a discard of about one fourth of the *edible* food as plate waste, spoilage, etc. Amounts of foods are shown to two decimal places to allow for greater accuracy, especially in estimating rations for large groups of people and for long periods of time. For general use, amounts of food groups for a family may be rounded to the nearest tenth or quarter of a pound.

[b] Fluid milk and beverage made from dry or evaporated milk. Cheese and ice cream may replace some milk. Count as equivalent to a quart of fluid milk: natural or processed Cheddar-type cheese, 6 oz.; cottage cheese, 2½ lb.; ice cream, 1½ qt.; unflavored yogurt, 4 cups.

[c] Bacon and salt pork should not exceed ⅓ lb. for each 5 lb. of this group.

[d] Weight in terms of dry beans and peas, shelled nuts and peanut butter. Count 1 lb. of canned dry beans—pork and beans, kidney beans, etc.—as 0.33 lb.

[e] Includes coffee, tea, cocoa, punches, ades, soft drinks, leavenings and seasonings. The use of iodized salt is recommended.

[f] Cereal fortified with iron is recommended.

*From: Consumer Food Economics Institute, Agricultural Research Service, U.S. Department of Agriculture, 1974.

Table 18–7   COST OF FOOD AT HOME ESTIMATED FOR FOOD PLANS AT FOUR COST LEVELS[*a, b]

SEX-AGE GROUPS	COST FOR 1 WEEK				COST FOR 1 MONTH			
	Thrifty Plan[c]	Low Cost Plan	Moderate Cost Plan	Liberal Plan	Thrifty Plan[c]	Low Cost Plan	Moderate Cost Plan	Liberal Plan
FAMILIES								
Family of two[d]								
20–54 yr.	$23.10	$30.40	$38.20	$45.80	$100.00	$131.60	$165.10	$198.20
55 yr. and over	20.80	27.20	33.70	40.30	90.10	117.70	145.80	174.50
Family of four								
Couple, 20–54 yr. and children								
1–2 and 3–5 yr.	32.70	42.50	53.10	63.70	141.40	183.90	229.80	275.70
6–8 and 9–11 yr.	39.30	51.20	64.30	77.20	169.90	221.70	278.40	334.20
INDIVIDUALS[e]								
Child								
7 mo.–1 yr.	4.70	5.80	7.10	8.40	20.40	25.20	30.80	36.50
1–2 yr.	5.30	6.80	8.40	10.00	22.90	29.40	36.30	43.20
3–5 yr.	6.40	8.10	10.00	12.10	27.60	34.90	43.40	52.30
6–8 yr.	8.10	10.50	13.10	15.80	35.00	45.40	57.00	68.40
9–11 yr.	10.20	13.10	16.50	19.80	44.00	56.70	71.30	85.60
Male								
12–14 yr.	10.80	13.90	17.40	20.90	46.90	60.10	75.40	90.40
15–19 yr.	11.90	15.30	19.20	23.20	51.50	66.40	83.30	100.30
20–54 yr.	11.50	15.20	19.20	23.10	49.90	65.70	83.10	100.20
55 yr. and over	10.30	13.40	16.70	20.10	44.50	58.20	72.40	87.20
Female								
12–19 yr.	9.70	12.50	15.50	18.50	42.10	54.10	67.00	80.20
20–54 yr.	9.50	12.40	15.50	18.50	41.00	53.90	67.00	80.00
55 yr. and over	8.60	11.30	13.90	16.50	37.40	48.80	60.10	71.40
Pregnant	11.90	15.40	18.90	22.50	51.70	66.60	82.10	97.60
Nursing	12.60	16.30	20.30	24.10	54.70	70.50	87.80	104.50

[a] U.S. Average. March 1977.

[b] Assumes that food for all meals and snacks is purchased at the store and prepared at home. Estimates for each plan were computed from quantities of foods published in the Winter 1976 (Thrifty plan) and Winter 1975 (Low Cost, Moderate Cost and Liberal plans) issues of *Family Economics Review*. The costs of the food plans were first estimated using prices paid in 1965–66 by households from USDA's Household Food Consumption Survey with food costs at four selected levels. These prices are updated by use of "Estimated Retail Food Prices by Cities" released monthly by the Bureau of Labor Statistics.

[c] Coupon allotment in the Food Stamp Program based on this food plan.

[d] Ten per cent added for family size adjustment. See footnote *e*.

[e] The costs given are for individuals in four-person families. For individuals in other size families, the following adjustments are suggested: one-person, add 20 per cent; two-person, add 10 per cent; three-person, add 5 per cent; five- or six-person, subtract 5 per cent; seven- or more person, subtract 10 per cent.

*From: Family Economics Review, Consumer and Food Economics Institute, Agricultural Research Service, U.S. Department of Agriculture, Spring, 1977.

Table 18–8   FOOD PLANS THAT FAMILIES OF DIFFERENT SIZES AND INCOMES CAN USUALLY AFFORD*[a]

INCOME (BEFORE TAXES)	ONE-PERSON FAMILIES	TWO-PERSON FAMILIES	THREE-PERSON FAMILIES	FOUR-PERSON FAMILIES	FIVE-PERSON FAMILIES	SIX-PERSON FAMILIES
$2500 to $5000	Thrifty or Low Cost	Thrifty or Low Cost	Thrifty[b]	Thrifty[b]	Thrifty[b]	Thrifty[b]
$5000 to $10,000	Moderate Cost	Low Cost or Moderate Cost	Thrifty or Low Cost	Thrifty or Low Cost	Thrifty[b] or Low Cost	Thrifty[b]
$10,000 to $15,000	Liberal	Moderate Cost	Low Cost or Moderate Cost	Low Cost	Low Cost	Thrifty or Low Cost
$15,000 to $20,000	Liberal	Liberal	Moderate Cost	Low Cost or Moderate Cost	Low Cost	Low Cost
$20,000 to $30,000	Liberal	Liberal	Liberal	Moderate Cost	Moderate Cost	Low Cost or Moderate Cost
$30,000 or more	Liberal	Liberal	Liberal	Moderate Cost or Liberal	Moderate Cost or Liberal	Moderate Cost or Liberal

[a]Based on costs for the food plans estimated for winter 1976 and on data from the Consumer Expenditure Survey Series: Diary Data 1972 (BLS Report 448-1), updated to winter 1976.

[b]Many households of this size and income are eligible for assistance through the Food Stamp Program.

Note: The plan shown in the column corresponding to the number of persons in the family and opposite the family income before taxes costs about the amount a typical household of similar size and income spends for food. It is the plan a family of that size and income can usually afford.

*From: U.S. Department of Agriculture, Fall, 1976.

bake and cook can greatly lower the cost of meals. Ready-to-serve or partially prepared foods are proportionally expensive because the consumer is paying for the labor performed by the food manufacturer to save time for the consumer.

Cost Versus Adequacy

Foods in the plans provide for a nutritionally adequate diet that meets the RDA for *most* individuals, even though the thrifty and low cost plans contain less meat, poultry and fish than most families consume on the average. Since the proposal in 1973 to enrich bread with iron was not accepted, the thrifty plan, along with the three more expensive plans, is inadequate in iron for young children, teenage girls and women of childbearing age, when average selections are made. The plans provide about 6 mg. of iron per 1000 kcal., except if particularly iron-rich food choices are made. The plans, based on average food choices, meet only 80 per cent of the RDA for vitamin B_6 and magnesium. Since information on the content of vitamin E, folacin and zinc in foods is not adequate, the U.S.D.A. did not consider these nutrients when designing the food plans. Intakes for these nutrients may or may not meet the RDA.

Studies have shown that there is a relationship between income and an adequate diet. Education, or its lack, is as important as income in determining eating habits. In low income groups, some diets were good, while in high income groups some diets were poor. Education as to the foods that make up an adequate diet is essential. Studies of the food buying practices of urban low-income consumers indicate that they demonstrate considerable grocery shopping sophistication. The majority of these consumers purchase groceries at supermarkets. They tend to stretch the food budget by buying canned and dried milk, canned fruits and vegetables, breads, potatoes, rice and other cereals to substitute in part for meat, fresh milk, fruit and frozen foods.[9]

Food choices largely determine the cost of a diet and whether or not an individual's nutritional requirements will be met within the constraints of the food budget. For example, the cost of a calcium equivalent can range from $0.06 to $1.00, depending upon whether it comes from non-fat dry milk or from cream cheese. (See Table 18–9.) Table 18–10 gives the cost of 20 gm. of protein from various sources, and again the cost will vary depending upon the food chosen. Although the prices quoted are for 1976 and 1974, the relative differences among the foods are probably the

Table 18–9 COSTS OF MILK AND MILK PRODUCTS AS SOURCES OF CALCIUM*

MILK PRODUCT	MARKET UNIT	PORTION THAT PROVIDES AS MUCH CALCIUM AS 1 CUP WHOLE FLUID MILK	CALCIUM-EQUIVALENT PORTIONS PER MARKET UNIT	PRICE PER MARKET UNIT[a]	COST OF A CALCIUM-EQUIVALENT PORTION
Non-fat dry milk	38.4 oz. (makes 12 qt.)	⅓ cup dry (1 cup reconstituted)	48.0	$2.69	$0.06
Fresh skim milk	½ gal.	1 cup	8.0	0.69	0.09
Evaporated milk	large can (1⅔ cups)	½ cup	3.7	0.37	0.10
Whole fluid milk	½ gal.	1 cup	8.0	0.82	0.10
Cheese spread	2 lb.	1⅞ oz.	17.1	1.76	0.10
Buttermilk	1 qt.	1 cup	4.0	0.44	0.11
Grated Parmesan cheese	8 oz.	¾ oz. (2½ tbsp., packed)	10.7	1.44	0.14
Process American cheese	12 oz.	½ oz.	8.0	1.12	0.14
Natural Cheddar cheese	1 lb.	1⅓ oz.	12.0	1.70	0.14
Process American cheese	1 lb.	1½ oz.	10.7	1.58	0.15
Natural Swiss cheese	1 lb.	1¼ oz.	12.8	2.04	0.16
Cheese food	8 oz.	1⅞ oz.	4.3	0.78	0.18
Ice milk	½ gal.	1½ cups	5.3	0.99	0.19
Cheese spread	1 lb. jar	1⅞ oz.	8.5	1.66	0.20
Ice cream	½ gal.	1½ cups	5.3	1.09	0.21
Cheese spread	5 oz. jar	1⅞ oz.	2.7	0.57	0.22
Half-and-half	1 pt.	1⅛ cups	1.8	0.48	0.26
Plain yogurt	8 oz.	9½ oz. (1 cup)	0.8	0.24	0.30
Cottage cheese, creamed	2 lb.	10¾ oz. (1⅓ cups)	3.0	1.20	0.40
Sour cream	16 oz.	10 oz. (1¼ cups)	1.6	0.66	0.41
Fruit-flavored yogurt, 75% plain yogurt	8 oz.	12⅔ oz. (1⅓ cups)	0.6	0.29	0.49
Table cream	1 cup	1¼ cups	0.8	0.46	0.57
Natural blue cheese	4 oz.	3¼ oz.	1.2	0.85	0.71
Cream cheese	8 oz.	17 oz.	0.5	0.50	1.00

[a]Prices from three Washington, D.C. supermarkets, April 1976—store brand or least costly brand.
*From: Family Economics Review, Consumer and Food Economics Institute, Agricultural Research Service, U.S. Department of Agriculture, Summer 1976, p. 7.

Table 18–10   COST OF 20 GRAMS OF PROTEIN FROM SPECIFIED MEATS AND MEAT ALTERNATES*

FOOD	AMOUNT, READY-TO-EAT, TO GIVE 20 GRAMS PROTEIN[a]	MARKET UNIT	PART OF MARKET UNIT TO GIVE 20 GRAMS OF PROTEIN	PRICE PER MARKET UNIT[b]	COST OF 20 GRAMS OF PROTEIN
Peanut butter	4½ tbsp.	12 oz.	0.23	$0.58	$0.13
Bread, white enriched[c]	9 slices	1 lb.	0.51	0.34	0.17
Dry beans	1⅓ cups	1 lb.	0.24	0.78	0.19
Eggs, large	3	1 doz.	0.25	0.78	0.20
Chicken, ready-to-cook	3 oz.	1 lb.	0.37	0.56	0.21
Bean soup, canned	2½ cups	11½ oz.	0.96	0.22	0.21
Milk, whole, fluid[d]	2⅓ cups	½ gal.	0.29	0.80	0.23
Ground beef	3 oz.	1 lb.	0.24	1.01	0.25
Chicken breast halves	¾	1 lb.	0.25	0.98	0.25
Beef liver	2⅔ oz.	1 lb.	0.24	1.05	0.25
Tuna, canned	2½ oz., drained	6½ oz.	0.44	0.57	0.25
Turkey, ready-to-cook	2¼ oz.	1 lb.	0.35	0.76	0.27
Process American cheese	3 oz.	8 oz.	0.38	0.76	0.29
Cured ham	3⅓ oz.	1 lb.	0.29	1.09	0.31
Round beefsteak, bone in	2¼ oz., lean	1 lb.	0.22	1.79	0.39
Ocean perch fillet, frozen	3⅔ oz.	1 lb.	0.36	1.10	0.40
Frankfurters	3½	8 oz.	0.36	1.20	0.43
Chuck roast of beef, bone in	2½ oz., lean	1 lb.	0.35	1.25	0.44
Rump roast of beef, boned	2½ oz., lean	1 lb.	0.26	1.75	0.45
Pork chops, center	2⅓ oz.	1 lb.	0.35	1.50	0.52
Bologna	6 1-oz. slices	1 lb.	0.73	0.77	0.56
Bacon, sliced	10 slices	1 lb.	0.52	1.25	0.66
Porterhouse beefsteak	2⅓ oz., lean	1 lb.	0.34	2.06	0.69

[a]Approximately one third of the daily amount recommended for a man.

[b]Average retail prices in U.S. cities, April 1974. Bureau of Labor Statistics, U.S. Department of Labor.

[c]Bread and other grain products, such as pasta and rice, are frequently used with a small amount of meat, poultry, fish or cheese as main dishes in economy meals. In this way the high quality protein in meat and cheese enhances the lower quality of protein in cereal products.

[d]Although milk is not used to replace meat in meals, it is an economical source of good quality protein. Protein from non-fat dry milk costs less than half as much as from whole fluid milk.

*From: Chassy, J. P., and Nichols, J. B.: Food cost tables to help stretch your dollars. *In:* Shopper's Guide, 1974, Yearbook of Agriculture. Washington, D.C., U.S. Government Printing Office, 1974, p. 40.

same today, since food price increases are usually reflected equally in all foods.

MEAL PLANNING

Menus are usually planned several days in advance to be certain the essential nutrients and calories are included. These menus should be flexible, however, to make use of leftovers and to take advantage of special food buys.

There are many sources of help for planning attractive, appetizing and economical meals. Food editors of newspapers, magazines, radio and television programs regularly discuss plentiful foods and newer, more appetizing ways of serving them. Many food companies distribute leaflets and booklets containing tested recipes and other cooking information helpful for preparation and for teaching. Many official bulletins related to food and nutrition, meal plan-

ning, food preparation, budgets, buying, preservation and production are available from government agencies in most states, as well as from the United States Department of Agriculture, at a small cost or free of charge. Family Fare: a Guide to Good Nutrition, Home and Garden Bulletin Number 1, United States Department of Agriculture, is complete and easily understood. It can be used as a helpful guide for weekly shopping and family meal planning. The suggested food allowances are grouped to assure good nutrition for all members of the family. Additional planning guides are listed at the end of this chapter. Several community groups and colleges are beginning to offer courses in basic nutrition, food preparation and meal planning that are geared to the needs of the community.

Although wise planning of menus is the first step, the second step emphasizes careful selec-

tion of quality foods and the third is focused on good food preparation. Table 18–11 presents menus for one week based on the thrifty food plan.

Marketing List Made from Menus

After the menus are planned for the week, the foods included in the meals are listed. The list is checked against the foods on hand and a shopping list is written out. To facilitate shopping, foods are classified into 15 groups (see Tables 18–3 to 18–6). The amounts needed from each group for each family member are determined from one of the four food plans shown in Tables 18–3 to 18–6. The group totals should approximate the amounts of the foods required by the family for a week. Some adjustments may be needed at first to get the correct proportion of foods from each group into menus. With a little practice, however, these plans will prove easy to follow.

Regardless of the economic status of the family, these steps are followed in making a marketing list from the planned menus. The amount of the food budget determines only the selection of foods within the groups. Some types are less expensive than others.

ECONOMY HINTS

A limited food budget does not necessaily mean an inadequate diet. The budget can be stretched without sacrificing either variety or essential foods in the menu if the food choices are careful. The following hints for menu planning, marketing, storage and cooking are suggested when it is necessary to reduce costs. (See Figs. 18–10 and 18–11.)

Economy Hints for Menu Planning

1. Follow the papers for weekly market specials and seasonal, plentiful foods that are economical.
2. Plan menus a week in advance, with flexibility for leftovers and good buys.
3. In season, use foods that are plentiful and locally produced.
4. Use economical cuts and lower grades of meat. The food value is essentially the same as that of the higher priced cuts. For example, beef liver is much less expensive than calves' liver and is equal in nutritive value. Baby beef is less expensive than mature beef.
5. Use nutritious, low cost foods such as dried peas and beans frequently.
6. Use leftovers in appetizing combinations.
7. Use canned or frozen fruits and vegetables when fresh products are too expensive or out of season.
8. Poultry and fish are usually less expensive sources of protein than beef.
9. Combining incomplete proteins such as wheat, soybeans, rice, dried peas and seeds to make complete proteins is cheaper than buying meat, fish or poultry.
10. Eggs, skim milk and cheese are less expensive protein additions to a diet.
11. Bread is less expensive than rolls.

Economy Hints for Shopping

Armed with a carefully planned shopping list, you may save money in the following ways:

1. Shop in person and choose the most economical method, such as in the cash-and-carry chain stores or supermarkets. Shop at several stores if bargains are available.
2. Take advantage of sales and specials.
3. Buy foods in season and buy those that are plentiful.
4. Buy foods in bulk if sold under sanitary conditions. Join a food co-op and buy food in bulk with other families or individuals. This requires good pre-planning to avoid waste.
5. Buy foods in quantity if storage space is adequate and if they will be used before becoming stale.
6. Be familiar with brands and grades of foods. The less expensive standard brands or store brands are essentially the same in nutritive value as the more expensive, fancy grades and brands. Study the labels to become familiar with quality, size and weight.
7. Compare relative cost of different forms and packs of food (bulk, packaged, fresh, canned, frozen and dried).
8. Consider edible value of purchases. For example, a cheaper cut of meat with a high proportion of bone and fat may have so much waste it would be false economy. Wilted or decayed fruits or vegetables are usually a waste in both edible portion and nutritive value of vitamins.
9. When buying flour, get the "enriched," "restored," or whole grain for extra B vitamins and minerals. The cost is no more.
10. Buy the less expensive forms of food whenever possible. For example, evaporated, skim or dried skim milk is cheaper than fresh milk, satisfactory for cooking and can be used as a drink. Fortified margarine can be used in place of butter.
11. In choosing eggs, remember the color of the shell does not affect the food value or taste. Grade B eggs are usually cheaper than grade A and are just as nutritious.

Table 18–11   A WEEK'S MENUS BASED ON THE THRIFTY FOOD PLAN*

MEAL	SUNDAY	MONDAY	TUESDAY	WEDNESDAY	THURSDAY	FRIDAY	SATURDAY
Breakfast	Orange juice French toast Syrup Beverage	Orange juice Ready-to-eat cereal Doughnut Beverage	Peaches, sliced Grits Cinnamon toast Beverage	Orange juice Eggs Pan-fried potatoes Toast Beverage	Peaches, sliced Ready-to-eat cereal Toast Beverage	Apple juice Farina Toast Beverage	Apples, quartered Pancakes Syrup Beverage
Lunch	Beef pot roast Gravy Mashed potatoes Mixed vegetables Bread Ice milk Beverage	Grilled cheese sandwiches Macaroni salad Baked apples Beverage	Frankfurters Sauerkraut Bread Oatmeal cookies Beverage	Beef macaroni soup Saltine crackers Plums Beverage	Noodle soup Peanut butter and jelly sandwiches Carrot sticks Graham crackers Beverage	Frankfurter bean soup Saltine crackers Oatmeal cookies Beverage	Cheese sandwiches Gelatin (with apple juice and celery) Meringue pie Beverage
Dinner	Beans in tomato sauce Macaroni salad Pear halves Cornbread Gelatin Beverage	Beef stew with vegetables Cornbread Ice milk Beverage	Beef pie with vegetables Refrigerator biscuits Lettuce wedges with dressing Peanut butter cake Beverage	Fried chicken Rice Gravy Corn Bread Peanut butter cake Beverage	Beef patties Baked potatoes Stewed tomatoes Muffins Ice milk Beverage	Cheese rarebit on toast French-fried potatoes Collards Meringue pie Beverage	Spaghetti with meat sauce Tossed salad (lettuce, carrots, dressing) Bread sticks Ice milk Beverage
Snack	Doughnut	Bread and jelly sandwich	Cheese and saltine crackers	Doughnut	Peanut butter cake	Graham crackers	Ready-to-eat cereal

Note: Milk for everyone at least once daily and more often for children, teenagers and pregnant and nursing women. Spreads for bread and sugar for cereal, coffee and tea may be added, if desired.
*From: Consumer and Food Economics Institute, Agricultural Research Service, U.S. Department of Agriculture.

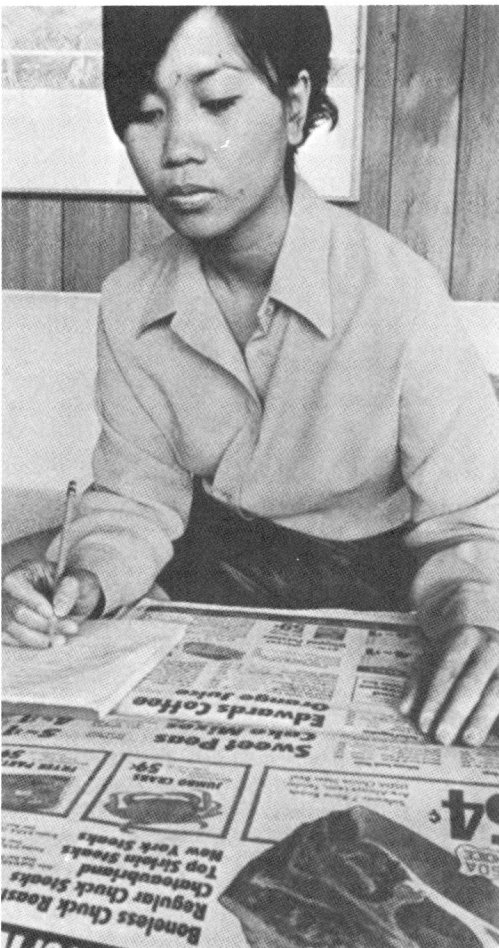

Figure 18–10 A listing of needed items, a week's menus and newspaper ads are useful in planning a shopping list. At grocery store, adjust plans to take advantage of specials. (Courtesy of: Ullrich, H. D.: Food Planning for Families at Three Different Cost Levels. Yearbook of Agriculture 1969, Food For Us All. Washington, D.C., U.S. Department of Agriculture, 1969, p. 280.)

If the difference in price between eggs of two different sizes is less than 9 cents per dozen, than it is cheaper to buy the larger eggs. If it is 9 cents or more, it is cheaper to buy the smaller eggs.

12. Home processing of foods (freezing and canning) is good economy when the foods are home-produced or purchased at the time the supply is plentiful.
13. Do not buy snack foods of low nutrient density. The price per pound will startle you, especially considering how little food value they contain.

Economy Hints for Storing Foods

No matter how good a buy, foods must be properly stored after their purchase to avoid loss of

vitamin values and to prevent spoilage or the result will be false economy.

1. Be sure there is adequate storage *space* for food.
2. All perishable foods need refrigeration, namely meat, eggs, fresh milk, cheese, butter, margarine and certain fruits and vegetables, such as salad greens and tomatoes.
3. Bread should be stored in a bread box that has a few holes for circulation of air. If kept in the refrigerator or freezer, it will stay fresh longer.
4. Store dried fruits in sealed containers in a cool place.
5. Store potatoes, root vegetables and cabbage in a dark, cool, dry place with good ventilation.
6. Keep frozen foods frozen until ready to use. Never refreeze after food has thawed.
7. Keep dry milk and cereals in covered containers in a cool, dry place.

Economy Hints for Cooking Foods

Much food value can be lost by improper cooking. Economy does not end with menu planning, buying and storage.

1. Use raw or cooked fruits and vegetables with the skin or peel very thinly. Much of the mineral and vitamin content is in the skin.
2. Save meat juice and drippings after the fat has been skimmed off to use in other cooking.

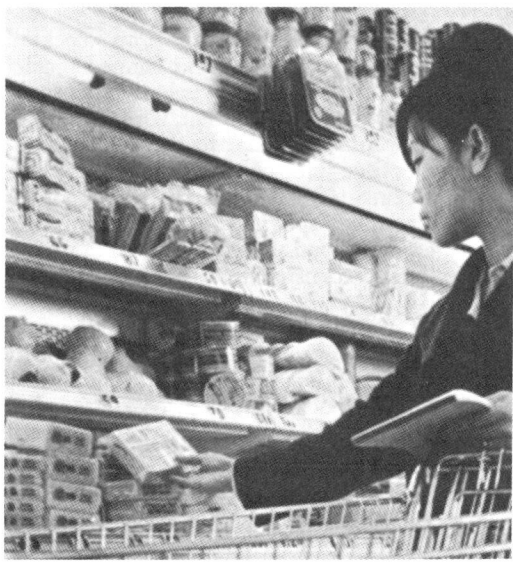

Figure 18–11 Choose package size that best suits family needs. Read labels for information on nutritive value, weight and price. Compare prices per serving. (Courtesy of: Ullrich, H. D.: Food Planning for Families at Three Different Cost Levels. Yearbook of Agriculture 1969, Food For Us All. Washington, D.C., U.S. Department of Agriculture, 1969, p. 283.)

3. Use leftover vegetable water in soups and sauces.
4. To retain the vitamins use as little liquid in cooking as possible and do not overcook. Steaming vegetables is the ideal method.
5. Use accurate measurements and tested recipes to eliminate failure.
6. In cooking, substitute fortified margarine for butter and inexpensive forms of milk for fresh milk.
7. Foods prepared in the home are usually less expensive than the ready-to-eat. Cereals, breads and rolls are examples.
8. Buying prepared foods in the delicatessen is an expensive practice.
9. Use bits of food in soups or in combination with other foods in casseroles and salads.
10. Use oven to best advantage by baking several foods at one time.
11. If space is available, disposing of food wastage in a compost pile will develop a source of fertilizer for next spring's garden.

FOOD ASSISTANCE PROGRAMS

U.S.D.A. Food Stamp Program

Through the Food Stamp Program, eligible low income households exchange an amount of money for an allotment of food stamps. Stamps may be used to purchase any foods except alcohol and certain imported items from retail stores at prevailing prices. Their purpose is to assist low income households to increase their food purchasing power and improve their diets. Effective in July 1977 a family of four with a maximum income of $570 per month after certain hardship deductions is eligible to buy $170 worth of food stamps each month. The cost of the stamps will vary from $146 for a family with this income to no cost if the monthly income is less than $30.

About 18 million people participate in the program, which is conducted under the auspices of the U.S.D.A. in almost all counties in the U.S. A program amendment passed in 1971 allows older people who are eligible for food stamps to use them for food prepared and delivered by private non-profit organizations such as the "Meals on Wheels" program.

U.S.D.A. Commodity Distribution Program

Some counties utilize U.S.D.A.'s Commodity Distribution Program for supplying food to institutions. It is no longer available to individuals. (See Table 18–12.)

Child Nutrition Programs

The School Lunch Program, started in 1946, presently serves 26 million school children. Many of these children receive reduced-price meals for which the schools are reimbursed by the federal government. (See Chapter 19.) The School Breakfast Program, started in the early 1970's, serves 2 million children. In this program, breakfast includes a serving of bread or cereal, milk and fruit or vegetables or full-strength fruit or vegetable juice. The Summer Food Program is provided for summer day camps and child care centers. See Table 18–12 for a summary of federal food assistance programs.

Some people doubt the effectiveness of federal food assistance programs, but local efforts at evaluation have shown some of these programs to be effective. One study of an urban black ghetto in South Memphis showed positive changes in the nutritional status of the children. After three years' participation in a U.S.D.A. supplemental food program for children up to 6 years of age, the food stamp program, a program providing iron-enriched formula for infants up to six months old and a free lunch program in day care centers, the children in the area showed statistically significant improvement in height and weight and reduction in the prevalence of anemia, low plasma vitamin A levels and low serum albumin levels. The improvement is a result of the increased availablity of higher quality food.[22]

FOOD TECHNOLOGY

During the past fifty years there has been tremendous progress in food technology. The ever-growing food industry markets food fresh, frozen, dried and canned, all especially processed for convenience to meet the public demands. The improved methods of food preservation through canning, freezing and freeze-drying, plus the growth of transportation systems, have made seasonal variation in food consumption less important. Trains, trucks, planes and barges are making longer but quicker trips from the farms and production centers to the cities. The increased use of certain fruits and vegetables is largely a result of these improvements. The improvements in the *production* of food have grown out of the improvement of agricultural methods. Insecticides, improved quality of seeds and an understanding of soil chemistry are some of the contributions of scientific agriculture. Better

Table 18–12 FEDERAL FOOD AND NUTRITION PROGRAMS

Administered by the Food and Nutrition Service, U.S. Department of Agriculture

PROGRAM	ELIGIBLE INDIVIDUALS OR GROUPS	YEAR STARTED	OBJECTIVES OF PROGRAM	COMPONENTS OF PROGRAM
Food Stamp Program	Needy families and individuals in participating counties (almost all counties).	1964	To supplement an individual's or a family's food-buying power.	Limited monthly allotment of food stamps at a reduced price, depending upon income. Stamps are used to pay for food.
Food Distribution Program	Supplemental food programs for mothers and infants. Elderly feeding programs. Schools and institutions.	1930's	To distribute surplus food to individuals and institutions to help agricultural support program.	Distribution of surplus food. Previously, to needy families, at present, only to eligible schools, institutions and persons in U.S. Trust territories.
Supplemental Food Program for Women, Infants and Children (WIC)	Pregnant and lactating women and infants and children up to five years of age who live in an approved project area and who are judged to be at nutritional risk because of inadequate nutrition or income.	1974	To improve the nutritional status of pregnant and lactating women and children up to five years of age in low income areas.	Cash grants to state health departments and comparable agencies who make available supplemental foods through participating health clinics. Health clinics provide specified nutritious food supplements or vouchers for these foods. Regular health exam of mother and child required.

Program	Participants	Year	Purpose	Support
National School Lunch Program	All children enrolled at participating schools, residential child care institutions, juvenile detention centers, orphanages and homes for the mentally retarded.	1946	To provide a nutritious Type A lunch (one that gives one third of the RDA for a child) at a reasonable cost to school children. To provide reduced-price lunches to needy eligible children.	Donated food to participating schools. Federal monetary support.
School Breakfast Program	All children enrolled in participating schools.	1973	To provide a nutritious breakfast at a low cost to children.	Donated food to participating schools. Federal monetary support.
Child Care Food Program	Preschool children in non-profit facilities such as day care centers, Head Start centers and family day care homes.	1968	To provide meal service for children in year-round day care centers and Head Start Programs.	Donated food to participating centers. Federal monetary support.
Non-Food Assistance Program	Schools participating in the National School Lunch or School Breakfast Programs.	1968	To help state educational agencies finance food service equipment to enable schools in low income areas to establish, expand or maintain food service programs.	Federal monetary support.
Special Milk Program	Schools, child care centers, settlement houses and summer camps.	1968	To reduce the cost of milk to children or provide it free to children who are also eligible for free meals.	Federal reimbursement to schools or centers for all or part of the cost of the milk served.
Summer Food Service Program for Children	Needy preschool and school-age children in non-profit recreation centers and summer camps and during vacations in areas with a continuous school calendar.	1968	To provide free lunches to children in summer programs.	Federal monetary contributions to cover the full cost of food service.

livestock, better quality of produce and better production are some of the contributions of genetics.

The easy-to-cook foods found in markets today were not widely available five years ago. It is predicted that the use of these "convenience" foods will increase. New names appear on lists of ingredients on packages. New items have different combinations of foods and some foods are synthesized to represent natural foods. Many contain preservatives of various kinds, to ensure better keeping qualities, and stabilizers and emulsifiers, to provide the desired texture and flavors. New equipment, processing methods, preservatives, packages and ways of getting foods to the stores have been developed. Technology has given us new varieties of foods that can be harvested more readily by machines. Special breeds of cattle and special types of feed have been selected that will give meat the desired qualities demanded by consumers. Farmers raise a breed of hogs with less fat, and young broilers come to the market cleaned and ready to cook. One farmer with a mechanized farm now can feed more than twice the number he did two decades ago.

New methods are used in processing foods. To keep foods from spoiling or ripening too fast the temperature and moisture and the oxygen and carbon dioxide content of the air are controlled. More ready-to-serve canned products ranging from soup to desserts are now on the market. New combinations of frozen foods are available: vegetables in cream sauce, entrées for one person or for a family, frozen egg noodles, canapés. In fact, almost every food prepared at home can also be bought frozen. The freeze-drying method of preservation will add more items that will keep without refrigeration and that can be reconstituted quickly. Newer items include imitation foods such as meatless meats, filled milk, imitation ice cream and imitation milk, whipped toppings and non-dairy coffee whiteners. These can be kept a long time without refrigeration. Packaging materials have been developed that will lengthen the shelf life of the product considerably.

The amount of work performed throughout our food supply system to make a variety of foods available all year and to save preparation time for the consumer makes that system very energy-intensive. To conserve non-renewable energy sources, Americans could do more of their own food preparation and individual food growing.

The marketing of new products relies on ad-vertising through the mass media, and this is another expense added to the cost of food. The cost of these new products in comparison with their homemade counterparts varies; most cost more, but a few cost less. The shopper must decide, and he or she is not always pleased with new convenience items. A recent consumer survey showed that one in five shoppers was rarely or never satisfied with such products, particularly with regard to their supposed healthfulness.[18]

The choice the shopper makes will depend upon the value placed on saving food preparation time. The development of new varieties of foods on the farm, new processes by the manufacturers and new ways to get the products to the market, to the family table and to eating places outside the home will affect the technology of the future. However, these activities are likely to be tempered by the increasing cost of petroleum and petroleum by-products such as plastic used in packaging.

The *distribution* of food is the effort to provide foods to meet the pressures and demands of population. When the population is concentrated in metropolitan areas, foods must be transported from various areas to provide canned goods, dairy products, fish, frozen foods, ingredients for bread and baked goods, meat, perishable fruits and vegetables, poultry products and staple supplies. Food production centers are usually located convenient to the sites of available foods.

THE PRODUCTION OF FOODS

The scientific advancements made in agriculture, animal husbandry, dairying and poultry raising have produced improvements in food quality. Hog cholera, tick fever of cattle and hookworm are some of the animal diseases that have been brought under control. As a result of our learning to control bacteria, milk pasteurization has been promoted along with improvements in the manufacture of butter and cheese. To bring about control of plant diseases, insecticides were introduced and the chemistry of the soil was investigated. Because the application of new technology resulted in greater efficiency, only 5 per cent of our population is now needed to produce food for the rest of us.

Scientific Agriculture

Agricultural science is a blend of many different areas. It includes a search for improve-

ment in technical skills, better breeds of livestock, higher-yielding, more disease-resistant pasture, better animal nutrition, improved control of pests, greater knowledge of marketing, storage, transportation, organization of the farm and farm machinery and careful management of expenditure. First, tests of many new techniques are made in the laboratory, then larger pilot tests are made in the field before farmers are encouraged to try the improved techniques. The findings of tests from different regions are classified and correlated and the results are organized for distribution. State experimental stations cooperate with the U.S. Department of Agriculture to put the research findings into practice. Grains, fruits, berries, vegetables and legumes now yield more quality produce per acre than during former years as a result of such testing.

Scientific Animal Husbandry and Poultry Raising

To bring about genetic improvement, the breeder selects animals carefully, then inbreeds and cross-breeds them to produce the desired qualities. The results are evident in the production of better milk and better meats.

Parasites often infest animals. For instance, arthropods live on the skins of animals, and worms and protozoa may be found inside the body of an animal. Control methods, which include sanitation, vaccination and treatment with drugs, have been used by veterinarians and farmers to fight an aggressive battle against animal plagues. Studies of animal nutrition have introduced new ideas in feeding to produce better quality livestock. Breeding by means of artificial insemination has been one of the greatest advancements in scientific animal husbandry during the past decade. To meet consumer demands, poultry breeds have been developed that furnish more white meat on breasts, and turkeys have been bred smaller to meet the needs of the smaller family.

Scientific Dairying

The improved dairy starts with a better breed of cows and better diets and living conditions for them. These factors have dramatically increased their milk output. In 1950, the average U.S. cow produced 5314 lb. of milk. In 1974, the average cow produced 10,291 lb. of milk.[25]

Because the greatest money value of whole milk is in the butterfat, emphasis is placed on the fat content of milk. Thus we see surplus whole milk converted into products such as butter, whole-milk cheese, evaporated and sweetened condensed milk and dried whole milk. From the production of butter, cheese, cream and ice cream there are by-products of skim milk, buttermilk and whey. Some of the skim milk is converted into cottage cheese, flavored milk drinks and cultured buttermilk, and some, in concentrated form, is used in ice cream, bread and other food products.

THE MARKETING AND DISTRIBUTION OF FOODS

Part of the increased cost of food has been a result of the increased cost of marketing. About 7 to 10 per cent of the retail cost of food goes into packaging. For some items this cost is slight, but for others it may equal the cost of the food itself. The public demands packages that are easy to handle and store, plus built-in-conveniences such as premixed foods and heat-and-serve dinners, all of which increase food costs. A large portion of marketing expenditure goes into the development of new products, most of which fail to sell. An average of 5000 new food products are introduced each year and 4500 of these fail. However, the number of food and non-food products on our grocery shelves is steadily increasing, so that the average store that carried 7200 items in 1965 carried 11,600 different items in 1975.

WORLD FOOD PRODUCTION

Sixty per cent of the world population lives in developing countries where there is great need for more and better food. Many countries will continue to have critical food problems for some time, in spite of large surpluses in countries such as the United States. It is not practical or advisable for the regions with abundant and efficient production to supply indefinitely the countries that have low production. With shortages developing everywhere, wealthy countries that are unable to meet their own food needs will buy the surplus food of productive nations, leaving those countries that have neither wealth nor adequate production unable to obtain food. The people of these countries must be educated to produce their own food supply. The World Health Organization of the United Nations is taking measures to increase the food supply in these countries through scientific agriculture. Cultivation projects, such as irrigation and flood control works, drainage projects and leveling of land for rice

fields, require time and an abundance of manual labor. In Asia, for example, where rice is the chief crop, mechanized agriculture on a large scale is impractical because of the topography of the countries. In countries such as India, China and Pakistan, which contain about 40 per cent of the world's population, soil erosion is a serious problem. (See Figures 18–12 and 18–13.)

Agricultural progress requires the adaptation and application of scientific agricultural practices to the local situation, as well as the use of fertilizer. However, production of adequate food supply in the needy areas also requires better food storage and food distribu-tion facilities. If even half of the world's food storage losses could be prevented, enough calories would be saved to satisfy the needs of 500 million people.[3] In a scientifically ignorant, tradition-bound population progress is necessarily slow. Death rates are declining in these areas despite widespread malnutrition and, consequently, the population is growing, but the supply of food is not keeping pace. A World Food Survey made by the United Nations Food and Agriculture Organization showed that intakes of animal protein ranged from 8 gm. per person per day in the Far East and 14 gm. in the Near East to 62 gm. in Oceania and 66 gm. in North America.[7]

Figure 18–12

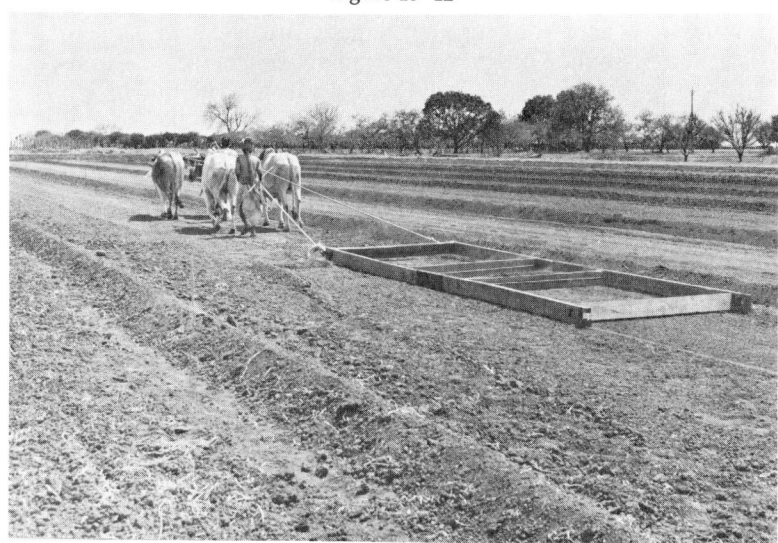

Figure 18–13

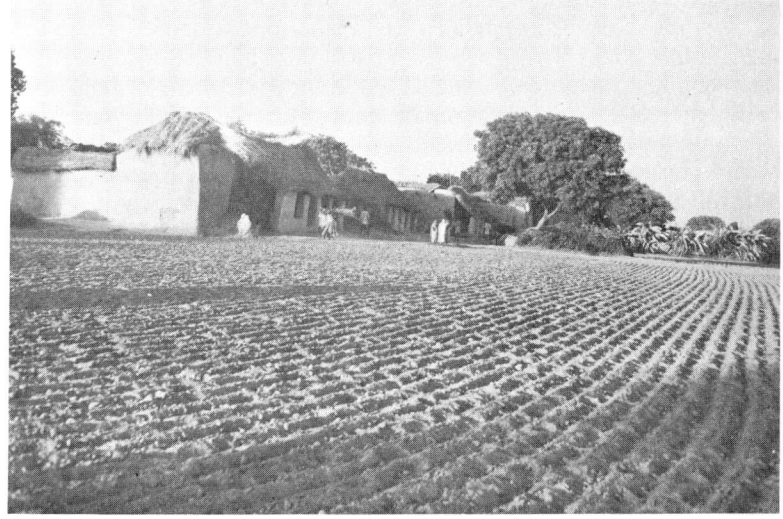

Figure 18–12   Using wooden floats to smooth the land in Central India. (Courtesy of the Agency for International Development (AID), India.)

Figure 18–13   Graded contour furrows for efficient irrigation and drainage in Etawon area, India. (Courtesy of AID, India.)

In the 1960's, because of the magnitude of the world food problem in contrast to the effectiveness of U.S. food production, the U.S. government, through research grants, encouraged U.S. food manufacturers to develop low-cost, nutritious foods for use in poor developing countries. The effort was doomed from the start because of low profit, high product costs, inadequate distribution systems in the host countries, lack of nutrition awareness by the intended consumers and mutual distrust between the host country and the U.S. firms. Very few of these efforts were successful in providing nutritious, low-cost foods at prices that the target group, the very poor, could afford. The local governments were not willing to subsidize the projects. A noted food economist, Alan Berg, predicts that until there is government financial support for such efforts, it is unlikely that the consumer food industry will be able to make a major contribution toward improving nutrition among the people of poor countries. "Problems are many, but the major impediment is the inability to reconcile the demand for corporate profit with a product low enough in cost to reach the needy in large numbers."[4] If improvement of the people's nutrition is the goal, then the governments have to be willing to provide support in the form of taxes and duties, loans, grants, guarantees and licenses. With this kind of support, the government could also regulate the food industry and prevent counterproductive activities such as the encouragement of early cessation of breast feeding in preference for commercial infant formula.[4]

THE PROCESSING AND PRESERVATION OF FOOD

The increasing complexity of present-day civilization makes the use of preserved foods necessary so that they can be carried long distances safely. The nutritive value of foods now receives careful consideration and should be improved whenever possible and desirable from the point of view of health safety. In evaluating food processing from a nutritional standpoint, the effects of the various processing methods on nutrition must be weighed against the advantage of increased food availability.

Like all living organisms, yeasts, molds and bacteria cannot survive and flourish unless the environmental conditions are favorable. Unfavorable conditions are extreme heat or cold, deprivation of water and sometimes of oxygen,

excess acidity in the medium in which they are suspended and the presence of certain chemicals. Treatment of food in one or more of these ways is the basis of food preservation. The method used to preserve a food product will vary with the type of food and the conditions under which it will be transported or stored.

Heat

Heat is a valuable defense against the growth of bacteria, but its effectiveness will depend upon the length of time it is used and the temperature maintained.

Boiling. Boiling (212°F. or 100°C.) will kill bacteria if the heat is maintained for a sufficient length of time to penetrate the food completely, but spores of the bacteria, such as those of the botulinus or of molds, may not be destroyed.

Pressure Cooker. A pressure cooker, which permits a temperature above boiling (240°F. or about 116°C.), will kill the very resistant bacteria and molds. It is a popular and safe method for preserving food in the home. The recipes and directions that accompany a pressure cooker give the recommended pressure and length of time for cooking specific foods.

Baking and Roasting. These are cooking methods that use temperatures up to 500°F. (260°C.). Standard cookbooks give the recommended times and temperatures for cooking meats, fish, poultry and all baked foods.

Canning. Commercially canned foods are considered safe from botulinus toxin; however, there have been isolated cases in which this was not so. The canning methods generally recommended for home canning or processing are the *boiling water bath* for fruits and tomatoes and the *steam-pressure* cooker for meats and all vegetables (low-acid foods) except tomatoes. In the boiling water bath a temperature of no higher than 212°F. (100°C.) is reached. This is considered adequate for canning fruits and tomatoes but not for other vegetables or for meats, because these require the higher temperatures of the pressure cooker to kill spores of bacteria.

To be sure of receiving maximum nutritional value from all methods of canning, only the freshest and best quality foods should be used. But freshness and safety are not synonymous. Safe canning means first that foods must be made free of bacteria that might cause fermentation. If such bacteria are not destroyed, their presence becomes obvious, for the molds, color changes, acids and gases they cause are easily seen, tasted or smelled; such products should, of course, be discarded at once.

Other methods of canning sometimes used include the so-called *open-kettle* method and *oven* canning. These are *not recommended*. In the open-kettle method, cooking of the food probably destroys the organism that causes spoilage of fruits and tomatoes, but yeasts, molds and bacteria may come in contact with food while it is being transferred from the kettle to the jar. In addition, there may not be enough heat present to produce a tight seal. If this method is used in canning fruits and tomatoes, the precaution of boiling the product for 10 minutes before serving should definitely be taken. The open-kettle method is not satisfactory for other vegetables or for meats.

Oven canning is influenced by so many variables that it cannot be recommended as a safe method of preservation for any food. One important reason is that when jars seal during processing in the oven, steam builds up inside the jars and can cause an explosion. Oven canning has resulted in some serious accidents.

Those interested in further information on canning should refer to the excellent national and state government bulletins, as well as state college and university extension service bulletins published on this subject.

Nutritive Value.   Some loss of nutritive value occurs in the process of canning or other heat processing of foods, but losses are not so great as supposed in the past. In general, there is some loss of vitamin A and vitamin E. There is some loss of ascorbic acid and thiamin. Meat, particularly, has been shown to lose considerable thiamin content. Riboflavin and niacin are fairly stable when exposed to heat. Because of better-controlled conditions, commercial canning will show less loss of nutrients than home methods.

Cold

Modern refrigeration is particularly effective in preventing the growth of dangerous numbers of bacteria. Most outbreaks of food poisoning have been caused by serving perishable foods that have been allowed to stand at room temperature after contamination.

Cold Storage.   Nearly every home has some form of cold storage, such as a refrigerator, for storing perishable foods and thus limiting the growth of organisms and food decay. Commercial firms preserve foods such as meat, eggs, fruit and vegetables for long periods of time in cold rooms.

Freezing.   Commercially frozen foods have been on the market for many years. However,

only comparatively recently have foods been successfully frozen in the home. Freezing takes from one third to one half the time and labor needed for canning. Besides fruits, vegetables and meats, a variety of baked goods, such as cookies, cakes, pies, bread and rolls, may be prepared ahead of time and stored in the freezer. Single-portion frozen food items are now available, which are of practical value to the individual living alone. Individual vegetables are frozen separately instead of being frozen in a solid block; thus, it is possible to remove and use only the desired amount. The development of frozen foods and concentrates has greatly influenced today's eating habits and nutrition.

For those interested in further information on freezing foods, the national and state government bulletins, as well as the state college and university extension service publications, are suggested.

Nutritive Value.   Frozen foods compare favorably in vitamin content with fresh foods, with the exception of vitamin E, some of which is lost in freezing. For other vitamins the only loss is in the blanching process, when approximately 10 per cent of the water-soluble vitamins are lost. In good commercial practice, crops are harvested at their prime and are frozen within three to four hours after harvesting. Fruits are packed under a sugar syrup with ascorbic acid added to retard oxidation and loss of color. Poultry are killed, bled, dressed and chilled, then frozen before any spoilage resulting from microbial action can occur. Not all the microorganisms are killed in freezing, and it is recommended that thorough cooking or reheating of frozen foods always be practiced.

Drying or Dehydration

The oldest method of food preservation is the removal of water from foods, or *drying*. This method has been greatly improved during the last 20 years and is used for meats, fish, milk, fruits, legumes, potatoes, cereals, soups, beverages and numerous cake, bread and dessert mixes. Microorganisms cannot grow in the absence of water. The process of drying does not cause a major loss of vitamins, but when stored dried foods are exposed to air, losses of vitamins A, C and E may occur from reaction with oxygen. If sulfur dioxide is used in the process of drying, as in the case of dried apricots, the ascorbic acid is protected, but the thiamin suffers. Eggs and milk, especially skim milk, are successful dried products. Foods that

contain fat become rancid by oxidation if kept too long. Dehydrated foods were used extensively during the world wars, since they take a minimum of space for shipping and storing. Today there is a resurgence in their use by the thousands of Americans who are "returning to nature" and discovering the pleasures of camping. The package mixes of cakes, cookies, quick breads and puddings are popular and used extensively. Potatoes are dried and packaged for preparation in various ways, such as mashed, scalloped, baked and fried. They save time in preparation and require fewer ingredients. Instant coffee, instant fruit juices, instant sauces and instant soups are also widely used. Substitutes for cream in coffee, which contain vegetable fat rather than butter fat, are available and quite economical.

Freeze-Drying. One of the newer processes in food preservation involves freezing a food and then placing it in a special drying chamber. Freeze-dried products retain their shape, color, fresh taste, texture and appearance, require no refrigeration until reconstituted and can be made ready to eat in a few seconds or minutes. Among products available are shrimp, crab meat, chicken, several of the red meats, eggs, vegetables and coffee.

Dehydrofreezing. Dehydrofreezing is a process that is just the opposite of freeze-drying. Here the food is first partially dehydrated and *then* frozen. Not all the moisture is removed and the products must be kept in frozen storage until reconstituted. Mashed potatoes processed by this method are an excellent product.

Nutritive Value. The nutrient content of a dehydrated food reflects the effect of the specific preparatory treatment and process used by the manufacturer, the growth conditions and the harvesting methods. The products, in general, compare favorably with canned foods and, in the case of very low temperature dried foods, with frozen and fresh foods.

Chemical Preservatives

The public is often concerned by the word "chemical," not realizing that all food is chemical in nature. The practice of adding chemicals to food for preservation is a very old one that probably began when humans first learned to preserve meat by putting salt on it. Sugar, salt, vinegar and spices are common preservatives used in the home. For centuries jellies, jams, preserves, pickles, sauerkraut, smoked hams and bacon have been made both commercially and at home. Today, preservatives are added to food in order to (1) inhibit microbial growth, (2) prevent oxidation or rancidity, (3) retain color, (4) maintain nutrients and (5) retain flavor. Government regulations limit the amount and kind of chemicals used. For example, benzoic acid or sodium benzoate may be used up to a concentration of 0.2 per cent if the foods treated with it are labeled. For a thorough discussion of food preservatives and additives, the reader is referred to reference 27.

FOOD ADDITIVES

Food additives come either from natural sources or from chemicals made in the laboratory. An extensive listing of additives and the level of their use in foods was made by Church and Church.[6] Lecithin is an example of an additive from a natural source. It comes from soybeans and from corn. It is used primarily as an antioxidant and an emulsifier. Additives synthesized in the laboratory are often the same as those found in food. For example, vitamins and minerals added to foods are identical to the vitamins and minerals found naturally in food.

Various chemicals are added during the production, processing and storage of almost everything we eat. By definition, a *chemical additive* is "a chemical or a mixture of chemicals of known or reproducible composition used in addition to the basic foodstuff in the production, processing, or storage of a food and is present in the food as purchased. A chemical additive may be either nutritive or non-nutritive and its presence in the food may be either intentional or incidental."[15] They improve the nutritional value, appearance, texture and flavor of food. Some additives retard rancidity and spoilage. Without additives in food, it would be nearly impossible to provide urban communities in America with sufficient untainted food daily.

An intentional additive is a chemical added by the processor to carry out a number of functions. In contrast, incidental or non-intentional additives, such as pesticide residue, detergent or substances from the packaging material, get into food accidentally during its production, processing or storage and are really food contaminants. Specified amounts of these incidental additives are allowed in certain foods. More than 2000 substances are used as direct additives. The essential purposes of an intentional additive in food must be (a) to improve the

Table 18–13   FUNCTIONS AND USES OF COMMON FOOD ADDITIVES*

FUNCTIONS	ADDITIVES USED	EXAMPLES OF FOODS IN WHICH ADDITIVES ARE USED
To improve nutritional value of certain foods.	Thiamin, riboflavin, niacin, iron, vitamin A, vitamin D, ascorbic acid, potassium iodide.	Wheat, flour, bread, rolls, biscuits, breakfast cereals, macaroni and noodle products, cornmeal, margarine, milk, iodized salt.
To maintain appearance, palatability and wholesomeness in certain foods (delaying undesirable changes in food caused by oxidation or microbial growth; preventing food spoilage caused by molds, bacteria, yeast).	Propionic acid, calcium and sodium salts of propionic acid, ascorbic acid, butylated hydroxyanisole (BHA) butylated hydroxytoluene (BHT), propylene glycol.	Bread, pie filling, cake mixes, potato chips, crackers, cheese, syrup, fruit juices, frozen and dried fruits, margarine, shortenings, lard.
To enhance flavor of certain foods.	Spices (cloves, ginger, cinnamon, etc.), citrus oils, amyl acetate, carvone, benzaldehyde, monosodium glutamate, vanilla.	Spice cake, gingerbread, ice cream, candy, carbonated beverages, fruit-flavored gelatins, toppings, sausage.
To give characteristic color to certain foods.	Annotto, carotene, cochineal, chlorophyll.	Baking goods, candy, carbonated beverages, cheese, ice cream, jams, jellies, oranges.
To maintain desired consistency in foods (emulsifiers and stabilizers).	Lecithin, mono- and diglycerides, gum arabic, carboxymethyl cellulose, carrageenan.	Bakery products, cake mixes, salad dressings, frozen desserts, ice cream, chocolate milk, candy, beer.
To control acidity or alkalinity in certain foods (leavening and neutralizing agents).	Potassium acid tartrate, tartaric acid, sodium bicarbonate, lactic acid, citric acid, adipic acid, fumaric acid.	Cakes, cookies, biscuits, crackers, waffles, muffins, butter, process cheese, cheese spreads, chocolates, carbonated beverages, confectionery.
To serve as maturing and bleaching agents.	Chlorine dioxide, chlorine, potassium bromate and iodate.	Wheat flour (to make it white), certain cheeses.
To help retain moisture (humectants), prevent caking or act as curing agents.	Glycerin, magnesium carbonate, sodium nitrate, calcium phosphate.	Coconut, marshmallows, table salt, garlic and onion powder, frankfurters, sausages, dietetic foods.

*Adapted from: Food Additives—Every Day Facts. Manufacturing Chemists Association, 1825 Connecticut Ave. N.W., Washington, D.C., 20009.

nutritive value, (b) to increase acceptability of the food item to the consumer through better physical appearance, flavor, color and texture, (c) to facilitate production and keep foods fresher for longer periods and (d) to lower cost. The functions of additives are numerous. A few of the commonly used additives, their uses and some of the foods in which they are used are shown in Table 18–13. New food products such as convenience foods require more additives than conventionally cooked foods, largely because of the conditions under which they are processed. They require additives to make up for partial loss of flavor, color and texture. Because these foods are not eaten immediately after they are prepared, they need special preservatives, antioxidants and other additives to maintain their freshness and desired physical properties over long periods of time. The public is interested in more sophisticated, flavorful, exotic and ethnic foods. Foods are shipped greater distances and stored for greater lengths of time. These foods require additives to prevent or retard food deterioration.

Much progress has been made in the removal of non-intentional additives from food by FDA inspectors (Fig. 18–14).

There has been considerable public concern about the safety of foods in relation to the number and kinds of chemicals that enter the food supply. The big problem that concerns chemists is the long-term effect on the body as a result of frequent exposure to these chemicals. Several years of feeding tests on different kinds

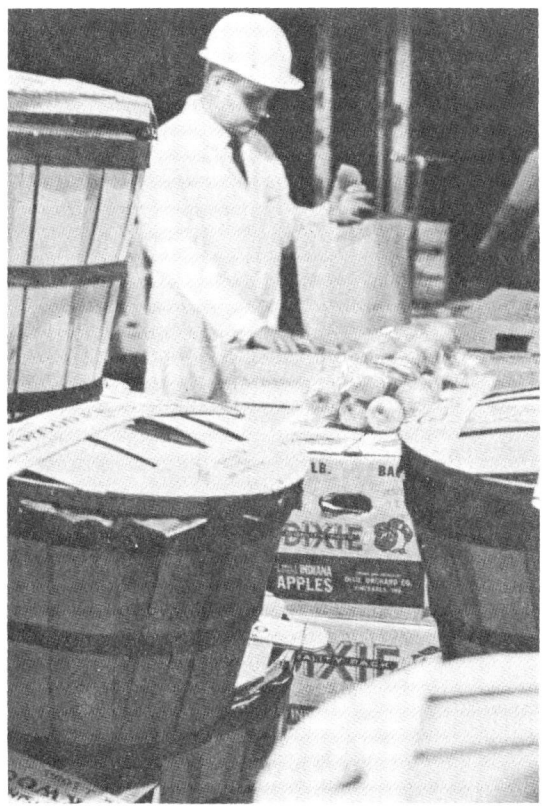

Figure 18–14 Samples of fresh foods are collected from the 800 carloads passing daily through Chicago's South Water Market. Inspector selects apples to be analyzed for pesticide residues. (From: FDA Papers, July–August 1970, p. 12.)

of animals are required to appraise these chronic aftereffects (Fig. 18–15). In 1950, this led to an investigation of the use of chemicals in foods by the Delaney committee, appointed by the U.S. House of Representatives. This committee reported that about 200 substances used as food additives were judged by experts to be *generally recognized as safe (GRAS)* under the conditions of current practice. Twenty years later the list had grown to approximately 600 items. About half of these are natural flavorings and spices or constituents of natural foods, which when added to other foods become "additives." Vitamins, minerals and other dietary supplements are another large group. Other agents such as preservatives, buffers, emulsifiers, stabilizers and antioxidants are included in the GRAS list. *Non-GRAS additives*, or *regulated additives*, are regulated more strictly than GRAS additives and require proof of their safety and usefulness. Their use is limited to allowable amounts (tolerances) in specific foods. Out of consideration for the public concern and because of the postwar release of a large number of new materials used in crop production or food processing, the Food and Nutrition Board of the National Research Council established the Food Protection Committee in 1950. This committee serves as a fact-finding and advisory body for government and industry on the use of chemicals in food. (See Additives Legislation, page 402.)

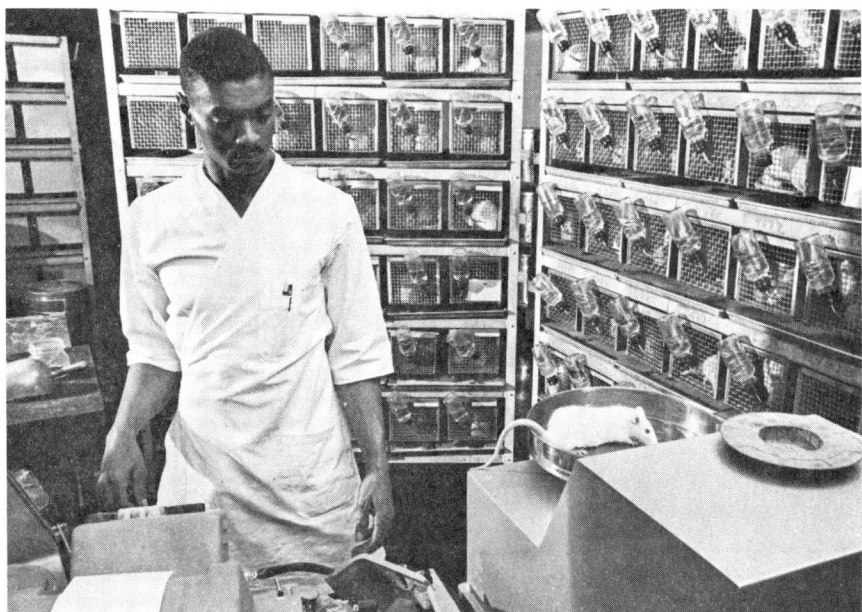

Figure 18–15   Technician records growth rate of rat in long-term food additive toxicity test. (Photo courtesy of the U.S. Food and Drug Administration.)

ADDITION OF NUTRIENTS TO FOODS

Enriched, Restored and Fortified Foods

The words *enriched, restored* and *fortified* are frequently confused. *Enriched* applies to flour, bread, degerminated corn meal and corn grits, and standards have been established as to how much of the food values can be added. Iron, niacin and thiamin are returned in about the same amounts as are lost in milling white flour from the whole grain, while riboflavin is added in larger amounts than found in whole wheat, and calcium and vitamin D may be added.

In *restored* foods the manufacturer puts back the nutrients lost in the processing. It is a voluntary move and not compulsory.

In *fortified* foods, the manufacturer adds nutrients that were not present in the food originally. For example, margarine is fortified with vitamin A and milk with vitamin D.

The 1953 joint report of the Food and Nutrition Board and the American Medical Association Council on Food and Nutrition approved the enrichment of flour, bread, degerminated corn meal and corn grits with thiamin, riboflavin and niacin.[1, 2] It also approved the nutritive improvement of whole grain corn meal and white rice, the retention or restoration of thiamin, niacin and iron in processed food cereals and the addition of vitamin D to milk (400 I.U. per qt.), vitamin A to margarine (15,000 I.U. per lb.), to bring it up to the average vitamin A content of butter, and iodine to table salt (1 part sodium or potassium iodide to 5000 parts salt).

Definite limits had to be set for the addition of nutrients to food products in order to protect the public from combinations that are irrational or even harmful. Most states have based their laws on the recommendations of the Food and Nutrition Board and the Council on Food and Nutrition. There is evidence that the recommended policies have benefited the public and have encouraged sound nutritional practices.

A well-controlled enrichment or fortification program can be an effective and inexpensive method of improving the intake of certain nutrients by a population. (See Table 18–14.) For example, it costs only $0.0004 to fortify a quart of milk with Vitamins A and D. See Chapter 3, Carbohydrates, and Chapter 40, Choosing Food for Nutrition and Health, for additional information on enriched, restored and fortified bread, flour and cereals.

"Organic" and Natural Foods

Although the words *organic* and *natural* are commonly used today in reference to food, the terms are frequently misunderstood. More unfortunate is the fact that there are no standards for the foods described in this way. Usually, the words refer to food growing and processing methods, but some people believe, erroneously, that such foods are "without chemicals." All substances are combinations of chemicals, some very complex. The only thing that makes one group organic is that its molecules contain carbon. All food is organic because it all comes from plant and animal sources, which contain carbon. Only a very few manmade foods could be considered inorganic.

More accurately, *organic* should refer to the

Table 18–14 COSTS AND SOURCES OF SELECTED VITAMINS AND MINERALS*

NUTRIENT	SOURCES	COST PER YEAR TO SUPPLY A 5 YEAR OLD'S TOTAL NEED[a]
Vitamin A	Cod liver oil	$ 3.08
	Raw carrots	0.48
	Butter	28.14
	Synthetic fortifier	0.02
	Mass dose	0.02
Vitamin D	Cod liver oil	4.94
	Fish	32.17[b]
	Synthetic fortifier	0.01
Thiamin (B₁)	Shelled peanuts	24.17
	Dried beans	8.67
	Whole wheat flour	26.73
	Synthetic fortifier	0.01
Riboflavin (B₂)	Non-fat dry milk	30.54
	Eggs	18.40
	Whole wheat flour	99.28
	Synthetic fortifier	0.01
Niacin	Chicken	34.55
	Whole wheat flour	43.44
	Dried beans	33.02
	Synthetic fortifier	0.02
Calcium	Fresh milk	30.78
	Dried beans	22.28
	Spinach	29.74
	Micronutrient fortifier[c]	0.08
Iron	Liver	16.85
	Dried beans	10.53
	Spinach	11.21
	Micronutrient fortifier[d]	0.13

[a]Ingredient cost only; does not include cost of carrier.
[b]Varies with type of fish.
[c]Calcium phosphate.
[d]Ferrous sulfate.
*From: Berg, A.: The Nutrition Factor. Washington, D.C., The Brookings Institution, 1973, p. 114.

process by which a food is grown. Unfortunately, there is no official definition for *organically grown,* but this one is useful: It is "food that has not been subjected to pesticides or artificial fertilizers and that has been grown in soil whose humus content has been increased by the addition of organic matter." To go one step further, *organically processed* food is organically grown food that, in its processing, has not been treated with preservatives, hormones, antibiotics or synthetic additives of any kind.[23]

Organic material or humus contains the same chemicals as commercial fertilizers—nitrogen, phosphorus, potassium, sulfur, magnesium and other minerals—except that in the organic material they are in complex combinations with carbon, hydrogen and usually oxygen. Commercial fertilizers contain the same chemicals in simpler forms and not always in combination with carbon. They are not any more artificial than the chemicals found in humus. In order for plants to use the chemicals in organic material, it must first be broken down by soil microorganisms, which convert them to simpler inorganic forms that can be used by the plants.

There is no scientific evidence that food grown organically or animals raised on organically grown food have higher nutritive values than those grown by other methods. Because organically grown food cannot be mass-produced, it is almost always more expensive. See Table 18–15 for a price comparison.

At present there are no federal regulations governing the production of organically grown food, although federal standards have been proposed. The only control that does exist is in the labeling of such foods. If the label says "no preservatives, no synthetic additives," then the food must not contain any of those substances. The lack of regulations distresses ethical producers and handlers of organically grown foods and allows unethical dealers to charge outrageous prices for foods grown in the regular way.

Natural foods are "those in the same form as they were harvested. They come from their place of growth to the consumer without having any alterations or treatments. They are unprocessed. Natural foods may or may not be grown organically."[23]

CITY, STATE AND FEDERAL CONTROL OF FOOD QUALITY

Most cities have food handling laws that apply to workers in the kitchens of institutions, hotels, clubs, hospitals, restaurants and food manufacturing plants. The workers are inspected by a doctor for the presence of any communicable disease or other illness that might contaminate foods.

State laws pertaining to food handlers and processors vary. When foods are sold to or distributed in another state, federal laws are enforced because this constitutes interstate commerce.

The Wiley Act or "pure food and drug law" of 1906 was the first effective food legislation: "An Act for preventing the manufacture, sale or transportation of adulterated or misbranded or poisonous or deleterious foods, drugs, medicines and liquors, and for regulating the traffic therein, and for other purposes."

Several amendments to the law were made and three were retained, although the Wiley Act was repealed when the 1938 Federal Food, Drug and Cosmetic Act was enacted by the 75th Congress. The Weight and Measure Amendment of 1913 clarified the rules about stating the quantity of the contents of packaged foods, and the Kenyon amendment of 1919 extended the rules to cover packaged meats. In 1923 the Butter Standard Amendment set the minimum milk fat content of butter at 80 per cent.

The McNary–Napes Amendment passed in 1930 authorized the Secretary of Agriculture to establish minimum standards for the quality, condition and amounts of food in containers, which were required to be met by all canned foods except meat products and milk. Products that did not comply with the standard were required to be labeled to show that they were below U.S. standard. While such food was probably entirely wholesome, this required statement served to identify the quality of the product for the consumer.

The Sea Food Inspection Amendment of 1935 authorized the Secretary of Agriculture "to provide government inspection of the packing of any sea food which might enter into interstate commerce for those packers desiring such inspection service."

The Meat Inspection Act of 1907 required that "all meat and meat food products in interstate commerce be prepared under the supervision of the U.S. Department of Agriculture."

In 1957 a law similar to the Meat Inspection Act was passed requiring inspection of dressed poultry and poultry products. The Production and Marketing Administration of the U.S. Department of Agriculture also offers a grading service to determine the quality of canned

Table 18–15   COST OF SELECTED FOODS ADVERTISED AS "ORGANIC" COMPARED WITH COSTS OF SIMILAR FOODS NOT LABELED "ORGANIC"*[a, b]

FOODS	REGULAR FOOD PRICE	ORGANIC FOOD PRICE AS A PERCENTAGE OF REGULAR FOOD PRICE	
	Supermarket	*Store No. 1[c]*	*Store No. 2[c]*
PROCESSED FOODS			
Canned fruits and vegetables, juices and preserves			
Apple juice (qt.)	$0.45	198%	182%
Apple sauce (lb.)	0.29	276	—
Peach preserves (lb.)	0.87	151	—
Pickles (qt.)	1.00	150	150
Tomatoes (lb.)	0.23	326	296
Dried fruits and vegetables (lb.)			
Lentils, hulled	0.37	338	100
Raisins	0.78	—	89
Flour, cereals, pastas and bread (lb.)			
Cornmeal, yellow	0.26	154	115
Granola	0.69	—	132
Grits	0.37	214	116
Oats, rolled (not quick-cooking)	0.52	—	56
Wheat cereal	0.49	82	61
Whole wheat bread	0.55	—	144
Whole wheat flour	0.22	205	177
Other			
Honey (lb.)	0.94	120	115
Peanut butter (lb.)	0.79	—	170
Vinegar, cider (qt.)	0.53	202	306
UNPROCESSED FOODS			
Meat and poultry			
Ground beef, regular (lb.)	0.75	313	—
Chicken:			
Fryer, whole (lb.)	0.65	254	—
Fryer, cut-up (lb.)	0.69	304	—
Breast with rib (lb.)	0.89	235	—

[a]Washington, D.C., February 1976.

[b]If a variety of brands or package sizes was available, the price of the best buy was chosen.

[c]Store No. 1 is a large natural food store that sells food, vitamins, cosmetics and literature. Store No. 2 is a natural—almost completely organic—food store owned cooperatively by the workers. Many foods are purchased in bulk. Some are repackaged at the store in smaller containers; some are sold in the customer's own container.

*From: Family Economics Review, Consumer and Food Economics Institute, U.S. Department of Agriculture, Summer 1976, pp. 10–11.

fruits and vegetables. Labeling of food products, food adulteration and food poisoning is also regulated by the 1938 Food, Drug and Cosmetic Act.

Standards of Identity

The Food and Drug Administration, an agency of the Department of Health, Education and Welfare, has the responsibility of enforcing the Food, Drug and Cosmetic Act, thereby carrying out the purpose of Congress to ensure that foods are safe, pure, and wholesome; are made or processed under sanitary conditions; and are honestly labeled and packaged. It carries on research and public education. *Food standard regulations* governing the definitions and standards of identity for foods, standards of quality and standards of container filling and labeling are established to promote honesty and fair dealing in the interest of the consumer. Standards of identity have been established for a number of common foods such as jellies, jams, mayonnaise, salad dressing, catsup, cheese, macaroni and noodles. The ingredients are not listed if these foods are prepared according to a fixed standard. These standards may be obtained from the FDA

Table 18–15   COST OF SELECTED FOODS ADVERTISED AS "ORGANIC" COMPARED WITH COSTS OF SIMILAR FOODS NOT LABELED "ORGANIC" (*Continued*)

FOODS	REGULAR FOOD PRICE	ORGANIC FOOD PRICE AS A PERCENTAGE OF REGULAR FOOD PRICE	
	Supermarket	*Store No. 1*[c]	*Store No. 2*[c]
UNPROCESSED FOODS			
Meat and poultry			
Leg (lb.)	0.79	265	—
Livers (lb.)	1.19	176	—
Eggs (doz.)	0.79	165	—
Fresh fruits and vegetables (lb.)			
Apples	0.33	173	142
Grapefruit	0.17	288	124
Oranges	0.18	228	117
Tangerines	0.21	186	143
Broccoli	0.55	125	129
Brussels sprouts	1.26	66	67
Cabbage, green	0.10	550	430
Cabbage, red	0.33	179	152
Carrots	0.23	183	152
Celery, pascal	0.44	148	109
Cucumbers	0.53	160	160
Garlic	2.45	90	65
Green beans	0.59	151	180
Green pepper	0.53	236	200
Greens (collards, kale)	0.39	144	233
Lettuce, head	0.39	164	144
Lettuce, romaine	0.49	131	129
Mushrooms	0.69	326	261
Onions	0.23	343	343
Potatoes, white	0.33	179	142
Spinach	1.10	95	82
Squash, summer	0.59	169	114
Tomatoes	0.52	208	138

without charge. Minimum standards of quality have been established for properties such as tenderness, color and freedom from defects. Standards of fill ensure that no air, water or space is sold as food and that the container fits the food. Standards for enrichment of foods are set. The product labeled "enriched" or "fortified" must contain the exact specified amount of added nutrients.

Nutritional Labeling

The 1973 Nutritional Labeling Act requires all canned and packaged foods to carry labels giving the nutrient content as a percentage of the U.S. Recommended Daily Allowances. The amounts of five vitamins and two minerals present in the package or can must be given (Table 10–9). See Chapter 10 for ways to use nutritional labeling in planning adequate meals.

Pesticide Legislation

In 1954, the Miller Pesticide Chemicals Amendment to the Federal Food, Drug and Cosmetic Act was passed to establish tolerances (that is, acceptable or relatively harmless levels) for pesticide chemical residues on raw agriculture commodities (fruits and vegetables). Under this amendment, the applicant must demonstrate the "usefulness" of a pesticide to the satisfaction of the U.S. Department of Agriculture and its "safety" (tolerance, or exemptions from tolerance) to the Food and Drug Administration. The regulations cover 26 pesticides, ranging from the virtually harmless to some of the most potent poisons known. Each pesticide is listed with the amount of tolerance (based upon results of animal tests that the pesticide manufacturer is required to submit) and the food crops on which it will be used.

Although other methods of pest control, such as the development of pest-resistant crops, the importing of insect predators and the breeding of sterile male insects, are being developed and used, it would be impossible to maintain the present U.S. level of food production without the use of chemicals.

Additives Legislation

In September 1958, a bill was signed into law requiring the safety of chemicals used in processing food to be proved by industry before being sold for use in foods. It became fully effective for all new chemicals in 1959. Up to this time, it was necessary for the government to prove a chemical unsafe after a food item containing it was already on the market and then bring court action to stop it from being sold.

Under the Delaney clause of the 1958 Food Additive Amendment, a food additive must be tested for safety on animals by the manufacturer or promoter and the results submitted to the Food and Drug Administration (FDA). If a food additive is found to produce cancer when ingested in any amount by test animals of any species, its use is prohibited. The statutes led to the banning of cyclamates in 1969 and may lead to the banning of saccharin in 1979. The safety requirements for an additive apply both to substances added directly to foods, including animal feeds, and to substances likely to contaminate food as a result of some incidental use in food processing. If the FDA is satisfied that no harm will result from the use of a proposed additive, it will issue a regulation specifying the amount that may be used and any other conditions of use. The Delaney clause is an extremely controversial one. Some feel it should be upheld and strengthened; others believe it is too inflexible for judging food additives fairly.

The use of any additive that tends to deceive the customer or otherwise result in adulteration or misbranding within the meaning of the Federal Food, Drug and Cosmetic Act is forbidden by law.

In 1960, the Color Additive Amendment was passed. It requires manufacturers to prove that their color additives are safe, and authorizes the FDA to establish and enforce tolerances for the use of color additives in foods, drugs and cosmetics. An estimated 18,000 firms use color additives in their products.

The "truth in packaging" law was enacted in 1966 and took effect in 1967. It requires fuller information and more prominent labels on packaged foods. Four basic regulations have been specified.[16]

1. A statement of the food's identity must appear on the principal display panel in bold type.
2. The name and address of the manufacturer, packer and distributor must be conspicuously stated.
3. A statement of the net contents must appear in concise standard measure. No qualifying terms such as "giant quart" or "jumbo pound" may appear.
4. A statement listing ingredients, when required, must appear in type of legible size on a single panel of the label. The common names of the ingredients must appear in decreasing order of predominance.

The regulations include proposals for special diet foods, with particular reference to vitamin and mineral supplementation and low-calorie foods. Guidelines for the nutritional quality of foods such as main dishes, snack foods, staples important in the diets of ethnic groups known to be malnourished, foods such as meat analogues, dairy products and fruits are under study by the National Research Council Food and Nutrition Board.

In 1969, when cyclamates (previously on the GRAS list) were found to be unsafe and were banned, the FDA was directed by the President to review all GRAS substances. The extensive reevaluation of every substance on that list is still under way. Our new knowledge about the effects of monosodium glutamate, red dye No. 2 and saccharin is a reflection of this new work by the FDA.

A survey of the substances generally recognized as safe was conducted in 1970 by the Food Protection Committee of the National Academy of Sciences, to establish the nucleus of a new GRAS list or its equivalent. This committee also compiled a list of appropriate and inappropriate uses of food additives. (See Table 18–16.) In evaluating the safety of a food additive, the hazards of its use must be balanced against the consequences if it is not used. Then a risk-to-benefit ratio can be determined.

Drugs and Additives in Livestock Feeds

Most commercial feeds currently contain some type of medication added to control animal diseases, increase yield of meat per pound of feed, shorten the period of feeding prior to

marketing or improve the texture and tenderness of meat.

The FDA has excluded certain antibiotics from use in food animals because of the possibility that, as the microorganisms in animals become resistant to these antibiotics, their resistance could be transferred to microorganisms that infect people. The result might be infections in humans that would resist treatment by antibiotics.

Drugs that leave any residue in meat, milk, eggs or other human food products must be proved safe before they can be marketed, just as additives in animal feed and human food must be. The federal agencies responsible for inspection of meat and poultry products also prevent the slaughter and processing of food animals that have been improperly fed with medicated foods. State and local officials cooperate with FDA inspectors in enforcing the feed additives safety rules.

Diethystilbestrol (DES), an estrogenic compound used to promote growth in steers, has been banned from animal feeds and injections that prepare beef for market because residues were found in the liver and other meat from treated animals.

FOOD POISONING

Food poisoning may be caused by different agents: bacteria, poisonous chemicals and foods that are intrinsically poisonous, such as

Table 18–16 APPROPRIATE AND INAPPROPRIATE USES OF FOOD ADDITIVES*[a]

INAPPROPRIATE USES
1. To disguise faulty or inferior processes.
2. To conceal damaged, spoiled or inferior goods.
3. To deceive customers.
4. To gain some functional property at the expense of nutritional quality.
5. To substitute for economical, well-recognized good manufacturing processes and practices.
6. To use in amounts in excess of the minimum required to achieve the intended effect(s).

APPROPRIATE USES
1. To improve or maintain nutritional value.
2. To enhance quality.
3. To reduce waste.
4. To enhance consumer acceptance.
5. To improve keeping quality.
6. To make the food more readily available.
7. To facilitate food preparation.

*From: Packard, V. S.: Processed Foods and the Consumer: Additives, Labeling, Standards and Nutrition. Minneapolis, University of Minnesota Press, 1976, p. 58.
[a]As compiled by the Food Protection Committee, National Academy of Sciences, 1970.

certain mushrooms and mussels. Most food poisoning is caused by bacteria. The general public often speaks of any food poisoning as synonymous with *ptomaine poisoning.* True ptomaines are formed only in the latter stages of food decomposition, and such foods are so obviously decayed that people would not eat them. Hence, ptomaine poisoning is extremely rare.

BACTERIAL FOOD POISONING

The distinctive feature of an outbreak of food poisoning is the sudden illness of several individuals following ingestion of a common meal. Usually a particular item of food served at the meal is the source of the poisoning. The victim suffers any one or all of the following symptoms: diarrhea, cramps, nausea, vomiting and fever. The symptoms may or may not be severe enough to require treatment. In the absence of specific diagnosis, the conditions may be grouped under the general heading of *gastroenteritis.*

The U.S. Public Health Service reported over 23,000 cases of microbial food poisoning in 1970. Since most food-related illnesses are probably not reported, however, the estimates of such illnesses range from 2 to 10 million cases per year.

Staphylococcal and Salmonella Food Poisoning. Physicians now distinguish two main subgroups of food poisoning: (1) *enterotoxic,* usually induced by a poison secreted by *staphylococci* and (2) *infectious,* induced by invasions of *Salmonella, Shigella, streptococci* and other organisms.

It is estimated that at least three fourths of reported gastroenteritis outbreaks are caused by staphylococcal enterotoxins. *Salmonella* infections appear to be the next most common cause, followed by *Shigella* infections.

The human carrier is the most common vector of both staphylococci and Salmonella. Approximately 25 of every 10,000 people are *Salmonella* carriers. It is estimated that the nation may suffer as many as one million enterotoxic cases a year without counting the vast number of mild, subclinical, undiagnosed and, therefore, unreported cases.

STAPHYLOCOCCAL POISONING. Staphylococcal food poisoning is caused by a toxin formed by *Staphylococcus* bacteria in the food before ingestion. Unfortunately, the enterotoxin is relatively heat-stable. The staphylococci multiply rapidly in certain foods at room temperature. These organisms hiber-

nate when refrigerated and are revitalized when exposed again to room temperature. A wide variety of foods have been implicated, but the usual vehicles for the enterotoxin are ham, poultry and cream- and custard-filled baked products.

Prevention. Since staphylococci are abundant in nature and are commonly present in the secretions of the nose and throat and in purulent lesions of the skin, it is impossible to exclude them from foods exposed to air. There is no perceptible change in flavor to warn someone eating the offending food. The best controls are cleanliness, elimination of flies, adequate refrigeration of all perishable foods and education of food handlers. *Staphylococcus* can be killed by heating foods to boiling temperature, but if toxins have developed before heating *they may not* be destroyed by boiling.

SALMONELLA POISONING. An increase in reports of *Salmonella* food-borne infections has been noted. The principal sources of human salmonellosis are livestock and domestic animals. The organisms have been found in animal feeds, in food processing places, among people who prepare and handle food and in other situations in which their presence invites the spread of disease. The natural habitat of *Salmonella* is the gastrointestinal tract of animal and human hosts. Salmonellosis is thus primarily an excremental disease transmitted by the fecal–oral route. The cycle of infection usually involves the transfer (direct or indirect) of viable salmonellae from one host to another and finally to humans, with food and water the most frequently implicated agents. Although salmonellosis may occur at any age, the highest incidence and most severe forms are observed in infants under one year of age and in aging persons. The foods most often implicated are poultry, prepared meats, desiccated coconut, cake mixes, custard-filled bakery products that are lightly cooked and subject to much handling, milk, milk products and eggs.

Prevention. Heat and refrigeration are the main tools to combat germ growth. The dangerous food temperatures at which germs thrive are between 40 and 120°F. (4 to 49°C.). To ensure destruction of *Salmonella* in food, the temperature must be raised throughout the food to an appropriately high degree for a sufficiently long time, such as 140°F. (60°C.) for 20 minutes or 149°F. (65°C.) for 3 minutes. Refrigeration does not kill the bacteria but will prevent their multiplication. See simple basic rules on this page.

Botulism. *Botulism* is the most serious form of food poisoning; the average mortality rate is about 68 per cent. The *Clostridium botulinum*, which tends to be found most often in non-acid canned foods, may or may not give an indication of its presence. Botulinum spores may remain resistant to a temperature of 212°F. (100° C.) despite several hours of processing. Subsequently, they can produce a deadly toxin in the canned product. This toxin can be destroyed by boiling canned foods for 10 to 15 minutes before serving.

Because of improved commercial canning and preserving practices, botulism now occurs relatively infrequently in the United States; however, some commercial cases have been reported. Outbreaks of botulism usually are caused by the consumption of home-canned vegetables or other foods that are inadequately cooked or preserved. *C. botulinum* is divided into types A, B, C, D and E on the basis of the type of toxin produced. In the past, the majority of outbreaks were found to be caused by type A and less frequently to type B botulism. However, the more recent outbreaks of botulism have caused grave concern. In 1963 fatalities occurred from canned tuna in Michigan and from prepared whitefish originating in the Great Lakes region. Three cases of botulism from home-canned gefilte fish were reported in 1969. The canned fish were prepared from Great Lakes whitefish that were first cooked and then stored in a sealed jar in a refrigerator for seven weeks. The fish were eaten cold. All of these outbreaks appeared to have been caused by the type E toxin, which had not previously been common in this country. Botulism organisms occur in garden and farm soil, in vegetables, in silt and in aquatic life. It appears that new and more stringent public health regulations relating to commercial processing are indicated to decrease the risk of botulism poisoning from processed foods.

Prevention of Bacterial Food Poisoning

Some simple basic rules to follow are:
1. Always wash hands before preparing a meal.
2. Never touch food with infected hands. Pimples, boils, paronychia and infected scratches teem with bacteria, especially staphylococci. These microorganisms multiply rapidly in certain foods such as custards, potato salad and cream-filled

pastries when exposed to room temperature. If there is a lesion on a finger, it should be kept well-covered or gloves should be worn while preparing meals and handling food.

3. Infections in the nose and throat increase the chances of contamination unless a mask is worn while handling food.
4. Keep perishables in the refrigerator until ready for use. This is essential for chopped and processed meats, custards, pastries, cream and similar products.
5. Wash uncooked fruits and vegetables thoroughly.
6. Cook meats thoroughly.
7. Inspect all leftovers and discard if signs of spoilage exist, such as changes in color or foul odor.
8. Inspect prepared foods for insect and rodent contamination.
9. Never eat partially spoiled foods.
10. Destroy cans that bulge. The same applies if the contents bubble out when the can is opened. Botulism may be present even though there are no changes in taste or smell.
11. Leftovers and food cooked for later use should be refrigerated immediately and not held until food reaches room temperature.

FOOD-BORNE AND WATER-BORNE DISEASES AND THEIR PREVENTION

Milk and water have long been known as carriers of disease, and we now know that other foods and food utensils may also be carriers. Food, water and utensils can be contaminated with bacteria, parasites or poisons. Food-borne diseases include brucellosis, tuberculosis, typhoid fever, paratyphoid, scarlet fever, diphtheria, tularemia, salmonellosis, septic sore throat, hepatitis and a variety of other disorders. Trichinae, tapeworms and other parasites and botulin, staphylococcal enterotoxin and other toxins can also contaminate the food supply. The possibilities of utensil-borne disease are increased by the fact that the bacterial count on spoons, glasses and cups in many restaurants is relatively high.

Despite the progress that has been made, food-borne illness continues to be a major public health problem. To reduce the incidence of such illness the basic principles of food protection must be applied.

Trichinosis. Uncooked or partially cooked meat is a serious cause of infection and disease, one example of which is *trichinosis.* It is suggested that up to 6 per cent of the hogs that are fed uncooked garbage in this country are infested with trichinous worm cysts. Fortunately, very few hogs are still fed in this manner. Trichinae are microscopic worms whose larvae burrow their way from the intestine into the muscles and mesenteric organs of swine and humans. The parasites are carried only if the host has eaten the uncooked flesh of an infested animal. When humans eat infected pork, they in turn become hosts to trichinae. Other animals such as bears also carry trichinae. One of the most unusual reported cases of trichinosis is that of three Swedish explorers who, on an expedition to the North Pole in 1897, shot and ate polar bears. They contracted trichinosis from infected bear meat, as was confirmed 33 years later when their frozen bodies and meat stores were found.[12]

PREVENTION. To prevent infection, pork should be *thoroughly cooked;* that is, large thick cuts should be cooked at least 30 minutes to the pound or until the internal meat is white. Thorough cooking is necessary for fresh, cured or smoked pork, for pork products such as sausages and frankfurters and also for hamburgers if they contain pork. As gauged by a meat thermometer, tenderized picnic shoulders should be heated to an internal temperature of 170°F. (78°C.), cured hams to 160°F. (71°C.) and fresh pork to 185°F. (85°C.). Freezing pork for 20 days at a temperature of 5°F. (minus 15°C.) or at minus 0.4°F. (minus 19°C.) for 24 hours is another way of killing trichinae. Tenderized hams with the stamp "Federally Inspected and Passed" have been processed to kill parasites and can be eaten safely with less cooking. From the standpoint of public health, trichinosis can be eliminated almost entirely if garbage is cooked before it is fed to hogs. (See Fig. 18–16.) It is reported that 40 per cent of infected swine get the disease from eating commerical raw garbage. Many cities dispose of their garbage by selling or giving it away for hog feed. However, cooking garbage intended for feed is now required by law in most states.

Tularemia. Although tick bites are considered the most common means of transmitting tularemia, infected rabbit meat is also a factor.

PREVENTION. Rabbits should never be handled with bare hands and rabbit meat must be *thoroughly cooked.*

Tapeworms. In certain lake regions fish are hosts to tapeworms, which can be transmitted

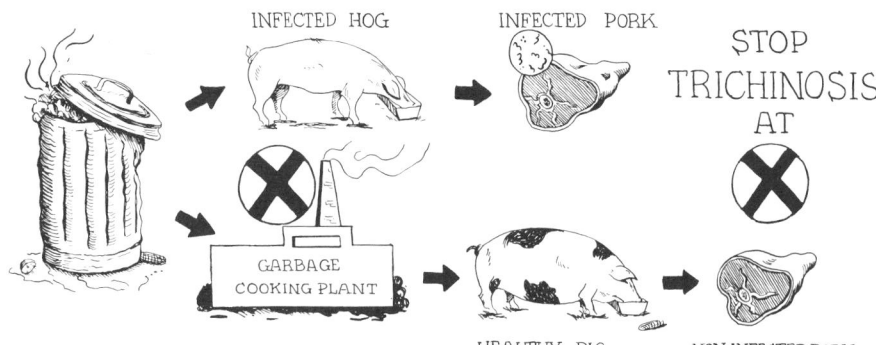

Figure 18–16 Cooking the garbage that is fed to hogs will help to eliminate trichinosis. (Adapted from: Publication No. 84, U.S. Public Health Service, 1951.)

to humans who eat them. As a rule, infection occurs when a person tastes chopped fish when seasoning it for cooking.

PREVENTION. Infected fish are not safe to eat unless they have been frozen or thoroughly cooked. If infected, they produce in the host a blood condition resembling pernicious anemia.

Diseases from Shellfish. In 1924 an outbreak of typhoid fever was reported and traced to oysters taken from contaminated waters off Long Island, New York. In 1964 and 1969 outbreaks of infectious hepatitis were associated with eating raw clams. As a result, the Public Health Service has developed a program to strengthen sanitary regulations for shellfish producers. Contaminated waters are restricted, and plants are inspected periodically.

Shellfish sanitation experts have become concerned with the apparent ability of shellfish to concentrate radioactive material, insecticides or other chemicals from the environment. Steps have been taken to solve this prob-

lem. The entire shellfish control program is one of interlocking and joint cooperation by industry, the states and the Public Health Service to assure that only safe shellfish are sold in the market. (See Fig. 18–17.)

Tuberculosis. Through the inspection of animals and the pasteurization of milk, the Public Health Service and state legislation have almost completely eliminated bovine tuberculosis.

Food Sanitation

Sanitation in the home and in restaurants, soda fountains, bars and similar places is essential to prevent the spread of food-borne diseases. The Public Health Service plays a large part in establishing sanitation programs for all public food handling and food processing establishments.

Following is a summary of Public Health Service activities related to food-borne diseases.

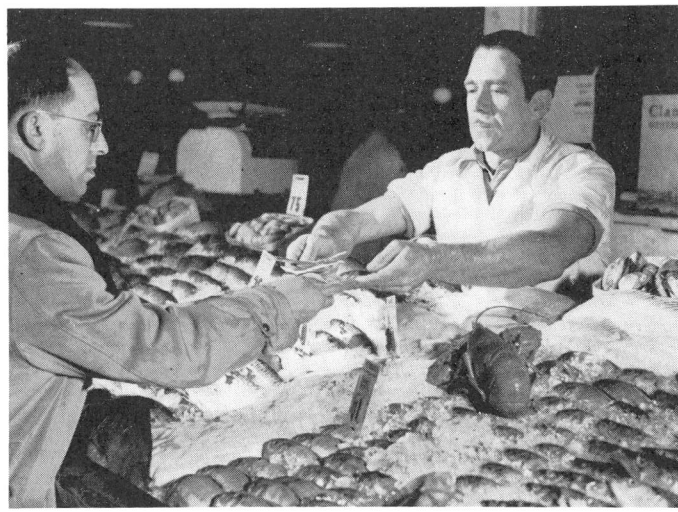

Figure 18–17 From shucker to consumer, the handling of shellfish must be sanitary. (From: Publication No. 84, U.S. Public Health Service, 1951.)

"The Public Health Service engages in the following activities to protect the nation from food-borne, including milk-borne, disease:

1. Develops and revises standards.
2. Promotes state and local programs based upon uniform standards and operations.
3. Advises and consults with state and industry officials on technical and administrative problems relating to sanitation of milk, shellfish and other foods.
4. Encourages the training of food handlers and food sanitarians.
5. Certifies state ratings of milk and shellfish shipped interstate.
6. Prepares educational materials to train sanitarians and food handlers.
7. Evaluates state and local programs upon request of state and local officials.
8. Consults with industry representatives on design and construction of food handling equipment and participates in joint industry–government development of equipment standards.
9. Inspects food handling facilities and practices in federal prisons, national parks, in Indian Service installations and on interstate carriers serving food to the public.
10. Conducts and advises on food sanitation and related research.
11. Compiles and publishes annual summaries of outbreaks of disease traced to food.
12. Serves on national and international bodies concerned with food sanitation.

"Food has both a positive and negative effect on health. On the positive side, there are the complex and imperfectly understood effects of food on long life, vigor, mental alertness and resistance to disease. On the negative side, there are hazards from swallowing food-borne organisms or poisons. Hazards may result from individual idiosyncrasies of the food or the person fed, but many are peculiarly a product of the environment: of polluted water, of careless handling, of contamination by insect vectors and of improper processing. To the extent that it is possible to do so, the Public Health Service seeks to provide assistance in eliminating these hazards."

FOOD POISONS OF NATURAL ORIGIN

Some of the poisons most dangerous to man are of natural origin, coming from plants, seeds, roots and animals. Certain varieties of mushrooms containing alkaloids are poisonous and extremely common in all parts of the United States. Dermatitis from handling pascal celery has been reported among farm workers. Rhubarb leaves contain considerable oxalic acid, cause illness and should not be used. The green part of sprouting white potatoes contains sufficient solanine (a narcotic alkaloid) to produce illness or even death. Ingestion of the fava bean or the inhalation of pollen causes a severe form of hemolytic anemia in susceptible individuals. Many wild plants are poisonous.

Clams and mussels found in the Pacific along the coast from California to Alaska may contain a poisonous alkaloid similar to strychnine. During the summer they feed on plankton, a marine organism, which infects the fish. Poisoning incurred by eating fresh, unspoiled fish of species not ordinarily poisonous was reported in 1957[29] in the South Pacific, the Philippines, Hawaii and the West Indies.

Swordfish was reported in 1970 to contain a sufficient amount of mercury to be toxic to humans. It seems that these fish, along with tuna and others, accumulate mercury because its level in sea water is high as a result of natural erosion and the action of rivers carrying mercury to the ocean and also as a result of modern industrial activities. Fish also accumulate selenium, which protects against the toxicity of methyl mercury. In the tragic incident of mercury poisoning from fish in Minamata Bay, Japan, the mercury level in the bay from industrial waste was so high that the amount of selenium in the water was not enough to protect against the effects of methyl mercury, and the humans who consumed the affected fish died.[21]

Only one fish, the puffer, is regarded as inherently poisonous. Puffers have a gland containing the neurotoxin tetraodontoxin. Death ensues from the poison soon after ingestion. Some fish are poisonous some of the time in some parts of the world. To list a few examples, herring is toxic in Cuba and Tahiti from May to October; many species of the fish native to New Hebrides waters are most toxic from April to July; and yet some of these are poisonous at all times at one location and harmless 20 miles away. This is a real public health problem, since with the increased use of freezing to preserve foods and the increased transporting of frozen foods, fish poisoning may appear in parts of the world where it was unknown before.

PESTICIDES

Pesticides have played an important role in agriculture's phenomenal success and are ex-

pected to continue to be the chief deterrent against pests that menace food production. A disadvantage in their use is their poisonous nature, which gives rise to harmful residues. The effects of pesticides on other organisms in the environment and the amounts of residues on agricultural produce have been the subject of much debate and controversy. The current system for regulating residues on food is based on the "tolerance principle," which assumes that, while all pesticide chemicals can be poisonous at high levels, there are low levels at which injury does not occur. There is evidence that, in general, adherence to tolerances by food producers is good.

The Food and Drug Administration made determinations on market basket samples for residues of 20 chlorinated hydrocarbons, including DDT, and for organic phosphate-type insecticides. Most of the samples were reported to contain no residues or mere traces of chlorinated hydrocarbons; a few contained amounts measurable by extremely sensitive techniques; and only a few traces of organic phosphate residues were found. However, because of its lasting effects on the environment, DDT was banned in 1972 and can now be used only in very limited ways. The acceptable daily intake levels of pesticide residues were established by the World Health Organization and the Food and Agricultural Organization of the United Nations and were revised in 1971.[28]

A weakness in the current system of regulating residues is that the FDA regulations apply only to products in interstate commerce. Individual state programs are needed to fill the gap left in the federal regulations. The search for compounds of lower mammalian toxicity is meeting with encouraging results, and similar progress is expected in finding substitutes for broad-spectrum insecticides, such as selective crop breeding for pest resistance and the control of insects through biological means. The system currently employed in regulating the agricultural use of pesticides is directed chiefly to the problem of residues on agricultural products.

It is well recognized that traces of pesticides retained on fruits, vegetables and forage material may be ingested either directly by humans or by edible animals that are in turn consumed by humans. The chlorinated hydrocarbon pesticides are more likely than others to be of biologic significance in a food chain because of their relative stability and their solubility and persistence in animal fat.

Before the ban on DDT, chemical analysis disclosed minute traces of that pesticide in every food. Fatty dishes and foods cooked in fat contained more of it because DDT is soluble in oil, grease and fat. When fed to animals and humans, it is stored in their fatty tissues. The more it is absorbed the greater the amount that is stored, until a saturation point is reached, but nothing adverse happens. Evidence shows that DDT is changed into another chemical, which leaves the body via the kidneys.

Persons sensitive to DDT may develop dermatitis, bleeding tendencies or destruction of blood cells. Acute, uncomplicated DDT poisoning is a recognized condition, but so far no deaths from it have been reported. Fatalities have been reported after swallowing the compound with other products, but in each instance one of the other products has proved to be responsible.

To investigate the nature and extent of the storage of chlorinated pesticides in human fat, Hoffman and colleagues[20] analyzed fat specimens obtained at autopsy from 282 persons who had died of various diseases. The data obtained confirmed earlier conclusions that, for any chronic intake level of DDT, equilibrium between intake of DDT and excretion of the sum of its metabolic derivatives is eventually achieved, after which the concentration of total DDT in the fat tends to remain constant. The most significant finding of the analysis is that the results indicate no progression of storage of DDT in the general population since 1951, when the first studies were made. Also, the intake of lindane, dieldrin and other pesticides is so low or the rate of excretion is so rapid that the levels of these pesticides in human fat are either insignificant when measurable or not even measurable by the most sensitive methods now available. We need to intensify our national effort to understand and weigh the long-term effects of pesticides on health and the total environment. It is very important that anyone who uses a pesticide understand its purpose and properties.

RADIOACTIVITY IN FOODS

Atomic energy has assumed an important role in our civilization, and the problem of fallout contamination of foods has been discussed frequently. Comar[10] reported that there is no indication for a change in our dietary habits or food technology as a result of fallout contamination. This has been confirmed. However, broadscale research on the problem of

radioactivity in foods and its implications is continuing for future public welfare.

Strontium-90, a dangerous element of radioactive fallout, is absorbed by the body in much the same ways that calcium is, and if a significant amount were to find its way into the food supply, a serious health problem would result. Like calcium it concentrates in bone, and the irradiation of bone tissue may cause cancer or leukemia. Calcium appears to reduce the amount of radioactive strontium-90 that may be deposited in the body. The relationship of the amount of strontium-90 to the amount of calcium is referred to as the strontium-to-calcium ratio. Plants take up strontium-90 along with their necessary calcium. Animals eat the plants and human beings eat both plants and animal products such as milk, meat and eggs.

Although there is a high concentration of strontium-90 in milk compared with other foods, milk is also high in calcium. Since both strontium-90 and calcium concentrate in bone tissue, a reduction of calcium in the diet by lowering milk intake may cause the bones to take up more strontium from other sources such as vegetables. Experiments under the joint auspices of the Public Health Service, the Department of Agriculture and the Atomic Energy Commission showed that strontium-90 can be removed from milk. Other ways to reduce radioactive material in foods are agricultural practices that lessen fodder and crop contamination and a change in cattle feeding practices. At present, cows in the United States do not take in enough strontium-90 to make milk dangerous.

In a survey made by the U.S. Public Health Service, a slight increase in the average daily intake of strontium-90 during 1962 was observed at 21 boarding schools and institutions throughout the country. The strontium-90 intake ranged from 9 to 46 picocuries (pc.) per day; the average was 25 pc. per day. The 1961 average was 19 pc. per day. These averages are well below those that the Federal Radiation Council's radiation guide lists as acceptable health risks. Two hundred picocuries per day is listed as compatible with the orderly development of nuclear industry in the United States. The guidelines are not intended to be limits for safe radiation levels, but are meant to indicate when detailed evaluation of possible exposure risks is needed and when it is necessary to consider taking protective action. A warning system is in operation in the United States so that, should radiation levels exceed the guidelines and standards that have been established, the public will be informed.

PROBLEMS AND SUGGESTED TOPICS FOR DISCUSSION

1. Explain food poisoning. How can 't be prevented?
2. What are the main types of bacterial food poisoning and how can they be prevented?
3. List four food poisons of natural origin.
4. List the food-borne diseases and explain how each can be controlled.
5. Describe four methods of preventing food spoilage.
6. What are the possible dangers of the use of pesticides on fruits and vegetables?
7. What methods of food preservation retain the most nutritive value? List the advantages and disadvantages of (a) canned foods, (b) frozen foods, (c) dehydrated foods, (d) freeze-dried foods, (e) dehydrofrozen foods.
8. Report on nutrition and health programs in your community.
9. Discuss the purpose of and the legislation pertaining to food additives. List seven classes of food additives and give an example of each. Read the labels on ten canned or packaged foods and list the additives in each. What purpose does each of the listed additives serve?
10. What is the role of the nurse in the health of society?
11. Discuss the public health hazards of antibiotics in the milk supply. To what purpose are antibiotics used in food preservation?
12. Keep a record of your food expenditures for two weeks. Are there ways to reduce your food expenses?
13. Think about your food buying, storage and preparation practices. Are there ways in which the energy required could be reduced or replaced with a renewable energy source such as human energy?

PLANNING GUIDES

Better Health Care for People with Low Incomes. Washington, D.C., U.S. Department of Health, Education and Welfare, Bureau of Family Services, 1966.

Family Fare: A Guide to Good Nutrition. Home and Garden Bulletin No. 1. Washington, D.C., Consumer and Food Economics Research Division, Agricultural Research Service, U.S. Department of Agriculture, 1970.

Family Food Buying. A Guide for Calculating Amounts to Buy and Comparing Costs. Home Economics Research Report No. 37. Washington, D.C., Agricultural Research Service, U.S. Department of Agriculture, 1973.

CITED REFERENCES

1. The Addition of Specific Nutrients to Foods. Public Health Report No. 69, March, 1954, p. 275.
2. American Medical Association Council on Foods and Nutrition: A statement of general policy concerning the addition of specific nutrients to foods. JAMA 154:145, 1954.
3. Berg, A.: The Nutrition Factor. Washington, D.C., The Brookings Institution, 1973, p. 70.
4. Berg, A.: Problems and promise of private industry. In: The Nutrition Factor. Washington, D.C., The Brookings Institution, 1973, pp. 143–159.

5. Center for Disease Control: Ten–State Nutrition Survey, 1968–70. DHEW Publ. No. (HSM) 72–8130–34. Washington, D.C., Health Services and Mental Health Administration, U.S. Department of Health, Education, and Welfare, 1972.

6. Church, C. F., and Church, H. N.: Food Values of Portions Commonly Used, 12th ed. Philadelphia, J. B. Lippincott Co., 1975, pp. 156–78.

7. Clark, F.: A scorecard on how we Americans are eating. In Food for Us All, 1969 Yearbook of Agriculture. Washington, D.C., U.S. Department of Agriculture, 1969.

8. CNI Weekly Report, 7(19):8, May 12, 1977 (Community Nutrition Institute).

9. Coltrin, D. M., and Bradfield, R. B.: Food buying practices of urban low-income consumers—A review. J. Nutr. Educ., 1:16, 1970.

10. Comar, C. L.: Radioactivity in foods. JAMA, 171:1221, 1959.

11. Consumption of Foods in the United States 1909–1952. Supplements for 1956. Agricultural Handbook No. 62. Washington, D.C., U.S. Government Printing Office, 1957.

12. Dangers of eating bear meat (editorial). JAMA, 220:274, 1972.

13. Fincher, L. J., and Rauschert, M. E.: Diets of men, women and children in the United States. Washington, D.C., Nutrition Program News, U.S. Department of Agriculture, September–October 1969.

14. Food and Nutrition Board: Recommended Dietary Allowances, 8th ed. Washington, D.C., National Research Council, National Academy of Sciences, 1974.

15. Food Protection Committee: Principles and Procedures for Evaluating the Safety of Intentional Chemical Additives in Foods. Washington, D.C., National Research Council, 1957.

16. Friedelson, I.: Fair packaging: Synopsis of food packaging and labeling regulations. FDA Papers, 1:21, 1967.

17. Gallo, A.: Marketing Developments, National Food Situation. Washington, D.C., Economic Research Service Publication No. 159, U.S. Department of Agriculture, 1977, p. 23.

18. Handy, C. R., and Pfaff, M.: Consumer Satisfaction with Food Products and Marketing Services. Agricultural Economics Report No. 281. Washington, D.C., Economic Research Service, U.S. Department of Agriculture, 1975.

19. Health and Nutrition Examination Survey, 1971–74. Rockville, Maryland, National Center for Health Statistics, Health Resources Administration, Public Health Service.

20. Hoffman, W.S., et al.: Pesticide storage in human fat tissue. JAMA, 188:819, 1964.

21. Jukes, T. H.: Mecury in fish. JAMA, 233:1001, 1975.

22. Kafatos, A. G., and Zee, P.: Nutritional benefits from federal food assistance. A survey of preschool black children from low-income families in Memphis. Am. J. Dis. Child., 131:265, 1977.

23. Leverton, R. M.: Organic, inorganic: What they mean. In: Shopper's Guide, 1974 Yearbook of Agriculture. Washington, D.C., U.S. Government Printing Office, 1974, p. 70.

24. Lowenstein, F. W.: Preliminary clinical and anthropometric findings from the first health and nutrition examination survey. Am. J. Clin. Nutr., 29:918, 1976.

25. Niedermeier, R. P., Bohstedt, G., and Baumann, C. A.: Move over, milky way—Our cows are stars too.

In: That We May Eat, 1975 Yearbook of Agriculture, Washington, D.C., U.S. Government Printing Office, 1975, p. 144.

26. Owen, G. M., et al.: A study of nutritional status of preschool children in the United States, 1968–70. Pediatrics, 53:597, 1974.

27. Packard, V. S., Jr.: Processed Foods and the Consumer: Additives, Labeling, Standards and Nutrition. Minneapolis, University of Minnesota Press, 1976.

28. Pesticide Residues in Food. Report of the 1971 Joint FAO/WHO Meeting. WHO Technical Report No. 502. Geneva, World Health Organization, 1972.

29. Poisonous fish (editorial). JAMA, 162:118, 1957.

ADDITIONAL REFERENCES

Adelson, S. F.: Changes in diets of households 1955–65. Implications for nutrition education. Washington, D.C., U.S. Department of Agriculture, Nutrition Program News, May–June 1968.

Agar, E. A., and Dolman, C. E.: Type E botulism. JAMA, 187:538, 1964.

Agriculture, Volume III: Science, Technology and Development. U.S. papers prepared for the U.N. Conference on the Application of Science and Technology for the Benefit of the Less Developed Areas. Washington, D.C., U.S. Government Printing Office, 1962.

Anderson, L., and Browe, J. H.: Nutrition and Family Health Service. Philadelphia, W. B. Saunders Company, 1960.

Beacham, L. M.: Food standards. FDA Papers, 1:4, 1967.

Bond, R. G., and Stauffer, L. D.: Food sanitation and/or the infectious process. J. Am. Diet. Assoc., 31:993, 1955.

Brooke, M. M.: Epidemiology of amebiasis in the U.S. JAMA, 188:519, 1964.

Burr, H. K., and Elliott, R. P.: Quality and safety in frozen foods. JAMA, 174:1178, 1960.

Cannon, P. R.: Why we have a safe and wholesome food supply. Am. J. Public Health, 53:626, 1963.

Characteristics of Food Stamp Households, September 1975. Washington, D.C., Food Stamp Division, Food and Nutrition Service, F.N.S. Publication No. 160, 1976.

Coon, J. M.: Protecting our internal environment. Nutrition Today, 5:14, 1970.

Darby, W. J.: Food additives in animal production. National Live Stock and Meat Board. Food and Nutrition News, 33(No. 1), 1961.

Duggan, R. E., and Dawson, K.: Pesticides: a report on residues in food. FDA Papers, 1:4, 1967.

Dunning, G. M.: Radioactivity in the diet. J. Am. Diet. Assoc., 42:17, 1963.

Eadie, G. A., et al.: Type E botulism. JAMA, 187:496, 1964.

Echols, B. E., and Arena, J. M.: Food additives and pesticides in foods. Pediatr. Clin. North Am., 24:175, 1977.

Editorial: Salmonella control. JAMA, 189:691, 1964.

Editorial: The most deadly poison. JAMA, 187:530, 1964.

Egan, M.C.: Federal nutrition support programs for children. Pediatr. Clin. North Am., 24:229, 1977.

Family Economics Review: Washington, D.C., Consumer and Food Economics Research division, U.S. Department of Agriculture.

Food Protection Committee, Food and Nutrition Board:

Chemicals used in food processing. Washington, D.C., National Research Council, Publication No. 1274, 1965; An evaluation of public health hazards from microbiological contamination of foods. Publication No. 1195, 1964.

Friedman, L.: Safety of food additives. FDA Papers, *4*:4, 1970.

Hussemann, D. L.: Food-borne disease—A continuing problem. J. Am. Diet. Assoc., *31*:253, 1955.

Institute of Food Technologists: The effects of food processing on nutritional values. Nutr. Rev., *33*:123, 1975.

Ireland, L. M.: Low-income Life Styles. Washington, D.C., U.S. Department of Health, Education and Welfare, Publication No. 14, 1967.

Jukes, T. H.: Antibiotics in meat production. JAMA, *232*:292, 1975.

Kupchik, G. L.: Environmental health in the ghetto. Am. J. Public Health, *59*:220, 1969.

Larrick, G. P.: The role of the Food and Drug Administration in nutrition. Am. J. Clin. Nutr., *8*:377, 1960.

Lindsay, D. R.: Food safety. FDA Papers, *4*:4, 1970.

Monge, B., and Throssell, D.: Good nutrition on a low income. Am. J. Nurs., *60*:1290, 1960.

Moore, M. L.: When families must eat more for less. Nurs. Outlook, *14*:66, 1966.

Most, H.: Trichinellosis in the United States. JAMA, *193*:871, 1965.

Owen, G., and Lippman, G.: Nutritional status of infants and young children, U.S.A. Pediatr. Clin. North Am., *24*:211, 1977.

Patterson, M. L., and Marble, B.: Dietetic foods. Am. J. Clin. Nutr., *16*:440, 1965.

Piper, G. M.: Nutrition in coordinated home care programs. J. Am. Diet. Assoc., *39*:198, 1961.

Protecting Our Food, 1966 Yearbook of Agriculture. Washington, D.C., U.S. Department of Agriculture, 1966.

Report: Analysis of pesticide residues. FDA Papers, *1*:17, 1967.

Report by the Council on Foods and Nutrition: General policy on addition of specific nutrients to foods. JAMA, *178*:1024, 1961.

Report by the Council on Foods and Nutrition: Safe use of chemicals in foods. JAMA, *178*:749, 1961.

Review: Freezer storage and vitamin stability in beef. Nutr. Rev., *23*:18, 1965.

Review: Radionuclides in American diets. Nutr. Rev., *21*:105, 1963.

Sanders, H. J.: Food additives. Chemical and Engineering News, October 10, 1966, p. 100.

Senate Select Committee on Nutrition and Human Needs, 90th Congress. Part B: The National Nutrition Survey. Washington, D.C., U.S. Government Printing Office.

Senate Select Committee on Nutrition and Human Needs: Food Price Changes and Nutritional Status, 1973–74, Part I. Washington, D.C., U.S. Government Printing Office, 1974.

Smillie, W. G., and Kilborne, E. D.: Preventive Medicine and Public Health, 3rd ed. New York, The Macmillan Company, 1963.

Smith, E. H.: Problems in the safe and effective use of pesticides in agriculture. Nutr. Rev., *22*:193, 1964.

Stare, F. J., Myers, M. L., and McCann, M. B.: Nutrition education via the public press. J. Am. Diet. Assoc., *39*:124, 1961.

Stoll, N., and Miyauchi, D.: Acceptability of irradiated fish and shellfish. J. Am. Diet. Assoc., *46*:111, 1965.

Tschirley, F. H.: Pesticides. Relation to environment quality. JAMA, *224*:1157, 1973.

Vaughn, R. H., and Stewart, G. F: Antibiotics as food preservatives. JAMA, *174*:162, 1960.

Walsh, H. E.: The changing nature of public health. J. Am. Diet. Assoc., *46*:93, 1965.

Welch, H.: Problem of antibiotics in foods. JAMA, *170*:2093, 1959.

Werrin, M., and Krondich, D.: Salmonella control in hospitals. Am. J. Nurs., *66*:528, 1966.

White, P. L.: National nutrition survey. JAMA, *223*:1272, 1973.

Chapter 19

TEACHING NUTRITION

Nutrition has rapidly become a complicated, highly specialized science, with every indication that it will become more so. To interpret the findings of nutrition research into practical working knowledge is a tremendous undertaking and a challenge. However, until this knowledge is applied, the teaching and learning processes are not fully effective. The nutritional needs and interests of the individual or group should determine the appropriate educational programs. Active participation by the individual or group in a problem-solving approach to nutrition is essential to making the subject interesting and personal. Group proj-

ects, such as one for weight control, may be one way to arouse and sustain interest and to motivate people to improve their eating habits.

TEACHING NUTRITION AROUND THE WORLD

Interpreting nutrition to all people of the world calls for high specialization and concentrated effort. As was pointed out in Chapter 1, the combined efforts of FAO, WHO and UNESCO are directed toward setting up stations and nutrition education programs in all parts of the world to foster better diets and, as a result, better health (Fig. 19–1). Scientific knowledge in the field of nutrition is increasing so rapidly that it is difficult to keep abreast of it, yet there is a great lag between the discoveries of research and their practical application.

Food is generally plentiful in the United States. The average citizen can buy more calories than he can consume. However, intelligent application of knowledge about food and nutrition is needed to prevent malnutrition and chronic disorders and to rehabilitate people whose disabilities result from poor nutritional status. Educational efforts directed toward developing programs that stimulate desirable food habits and modify poor ones are needed.

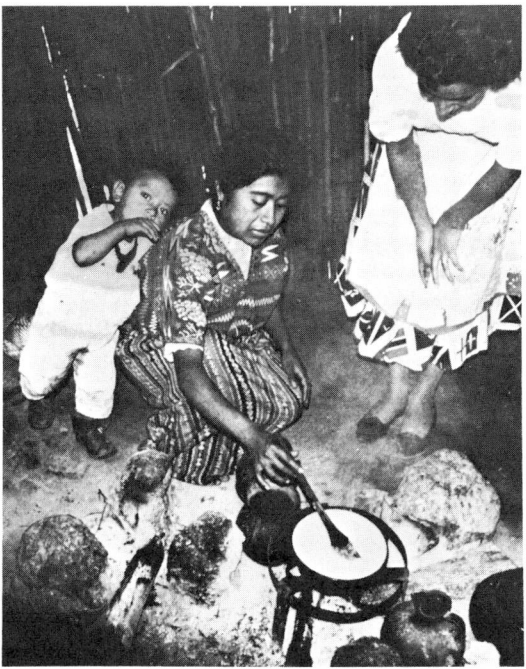

Figure 19–1 Guatemalan mother learns to prepare nourishing meals for her family with help of a nutritionist from the Institute of Nutrition of Central America and Panama (INCAP). (Courtesy of UNICEF. Photo by Bernard Cole.)

Food has a basic meaning in every culture and to every individual. (See Chapter 17, Geographic and Cultural Dietary Variations.) One must understand this in order to plan and execute sound nutritional education approaches. Changes in cultural food patterns take place only when people are involved and convinced that the proposed changes will further the attainment of some goal. The World Health Organization has recognized this factor and is sending cultural anthropologists into the field to assist in learning and understanding the role of food in particular societies, the attitude toward food and toward changes in food habits. The ways people are motivated to improve or change food habits are many and varied. Any improvement of nutritional status can be attained only through a nutrition education program suitable to the needs of the group or individual.

NUTRITION EDUCATION

All people, regardless of their level of education, social or economic status or geographic location, need nutrition education. Humans have no instinct nor do they inherit knowledge that will guide them to choose those foods that meet the nutritional needs of the body. Each generation learns which foods to select and why and how different foods affect health.

The function of nutrition education is to make it possible for everyone to learn and to use nutrition information through individual responsibility and action. The greatest job in nutrition education is to look at problems through the eyes of the people who need to learn. Educators are concerned with helping people understand how to select foods to meet nutrient and energy needs. Individuals who evaluate knowledge and are motivated to apply it will implement the changes necessary to improve their dietary habits. There are many people, however, who may not realize their need to change.

Concepts summarizing all the nutrition knowledge applicable to food for health were developed by a subcommittee of the Interagency Committee on Nutrition Education in 1964, and in simple terms, as represented here, reflect the research findings that constitute the knowledge of nutrition needed for wise food selection.

1. Nutrition is the food a person eats and how the body uses it. A person eats food to live, to grow, to keep healthy and well and to get energy for work and play.

2. Food is made up of different nutrients needed for growth and health. Some of these nutrients and how they work in the body are well understood; others are little understood and perhaps even unknown. All nutrients needed by the body are available through food. Eating many kinds and combinations of food can lead to a well-balanced diet. No food by itself has all the nutrients needed for full growth and health. Each nutrient has specific uses in the body. Most do their best work in the body when teamed with other nutrients.

3. All persons throughout their lives need the same nutrients in varying amounts. The amounts of nutrients needed are influenced by age, sex, size, activity and state of health. Suggestions for the kinds and amounts of food needed are made by scientists.

4. The way food is handled influences the amount of nutrients in it, its safety, appearance and taste. Handling includes everything that happens to food while it is being grown, processed, stored and prepared for eating.

These basic concepts do not imply that nutrition is eating what you don't like because it is good for you. There is a need for a variety of foods; there is an interdependence between the nutrients and the foods that supply them; and the best source of the nutrients is food. A useful tool for obtaining these nutrients is the daily food guide (basic food groups). The daily allowances (Recommended Dietary Allowances) are the quantitative amounts of nutrients needed by healthy people differing in age, sex, size and activity. The directions for the selection, care and preparation of foods based on research combine procedures that ensure safety, maximize eating quality and minimize loss of nutritive value.[6]

The effectiveness of nutrition education reflects the degree to which provision is made for the application of basic learning principles. Any change in the behavior of people depends upon the emphasis placed on the individual as a member of a family unit. The person must be helped to determine or clarify his or her goals and to become personally involved in attaining them. Fleming[3] lists the following factors that are important in the teaching–learning process.

1. Learning takes place more readily when *emphasis is placed on the individual.* Each individual is unique, with a different hereditary, social and home background.

The aims and motivations of individuals differ and must be recognized. Individuals should participate in the planning of ways to accomplish their goals.

2. Learning tends to occur as *emphasis is placed on the learner's perception of the tasks to be accomplished.* The individual's perception of the task often differs from that of the teacher. The leader facilitates learning through creating an opportunity for the fulfillment of important tasks.

3. Learning is facilitated as *emphasis is placed on human factors.* As emphasis is given to the feelings, anxieties, concerns, questions and problems of the learner, a setting is created for growth. Feelings of belonging and of security are basic to maximum learning and permissive leadership fosters learning.

4. Learning is facilitated as *the learner is involved in an active way.* Learning is an active process and teachers should help students clarify goals and plan, experience, try out, manipulate and explore ideas. As learners assume responsibility, their growth is extended.

5. Learning is facilitated as *emphasis is placed on the wise use of materials and resources.* The use of a variety of appropriate materials contributes to the effectiveness of learning. The teacher is but one resource; there are many people, places and things in the local environment that will, if carefully used, contribute to the learning operation.

Briefly, when helping people to improve their nutritional habits, it is important to begin with the person's interest and point of view rather than with the teacher's knowledge of nutrition. Begin with present dietary practices and modify these only as much as necessary to achieve good nutrition. When the approach is centered on people rather than on the diet the teaching is more effective. Food habits are ingrained, and it is not human nature to make sudden changes. Pick up the good points in each individual's diet and build from what he or she is already used to eating rather than change the entire food pattern.

PATTERN FOR APPLICATION OF DIETARY ALLOWANCES

In nutrition interpretation, one must be able to take the scientific facts resulting from research and put them into terms that are under-

standable and can be applied to everyday habits.

The Bureau of Human Nutrition and Home Economics of the U.S. Department of Agriculture[7] interpreted the Recommended Daily Dietary Allowances into the "Basic Seven" food groups. Although this was first published as far back as World War II, it is still sound and an excellent aid in teaching nutrition and evaluating dietary patterns.

In response to many requests for a simpler grouping of foods to use in nutrition education programs, the Institute of Home Economics of the U.S. Department of Agriculture[9] interpreted the Recommended Daily Dietary Allowances (see Chapter 10) as falling into four groups. These four food groups form the foun-

dation of an adequate diet. The number of servings in each are suggested in Figure 19–2 and in Table 10–4. These foods are rich sources of the essential food elements and are called the "protective foods." More of these foods and additional foods such as butter, margarine, oil, sugar and desserts that supply calories and added nutrients will be used as needed to round out meals for growth, activity and desirable weight. By following such a pattern it is not difficult to plan meals to meet the body's needs for nutrients. Meal planning is discussed in Chapter 10.

The choice of teaching devices depends upon the needs of the group or individual. Cultural and regional factors, seasonal differences in food supplies and variations in nutritive

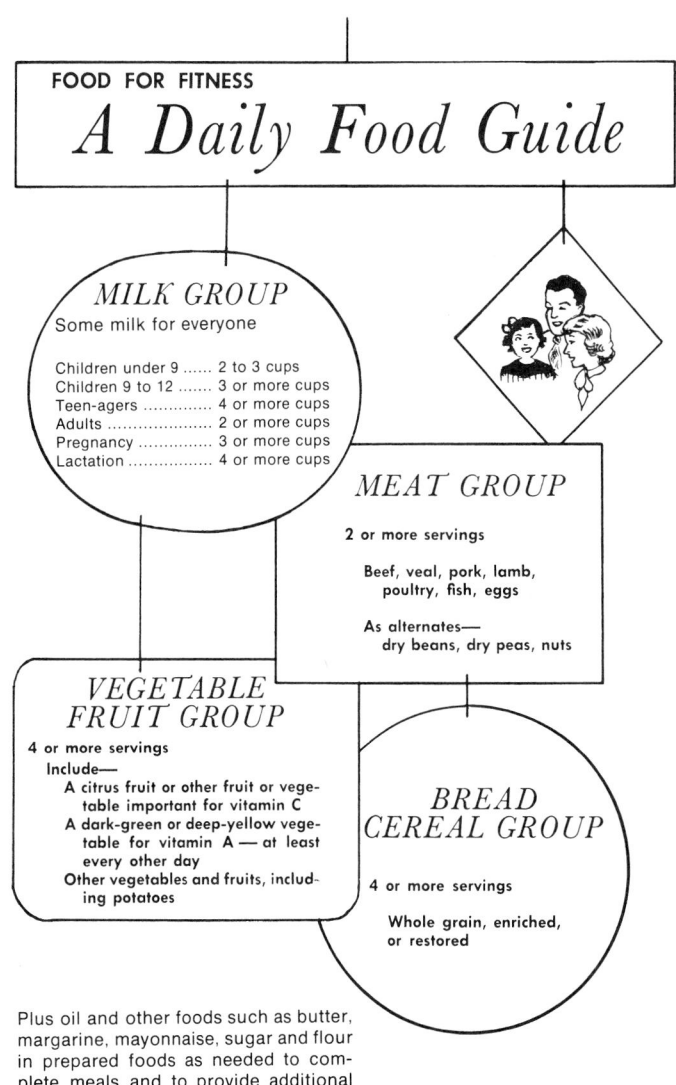

Figure 19–2 The "Basic Four Food Groups" dietary pattern. (Modified from: Leaflet No. 424, Institute of Home Economics, U.S. Department of Agriculture, Washington, D.C.)

needs and economic resources determine the choice to make and procedure to use. Daily food intakes must meet the body's nutritional needs. These nutrients and their relation to body needs and health have been discussed in preceding chapters.

THE DIETARY HISTORY

Any desired dietary change for an individual (or group) begins with the person's customary food intake and food habits. An evaluation of present habits indicates to the teacher and the learner where changes are needed to improve nutrition. This approach helps the person to identify areas in which changes should be made and provides an opportunity to make his or her own evaluations.

In a hospital or clinic situation, the nurse or dietitian-nutritionist has access to personal information about the individual, much of which is related to food intake and food habits. Age, sex, occupation, marital status, ethnic group, economic status, present weight, pertinent laboratory findings, diagnosis (determined or probable) and physician's dietary order are a matter of record.

The interviewer asks the patient to recall the usual foods eaten on a typical day. A notation is made while the person is supplying the information, or the person may write it himself. In this way, both the counselor and the patient can be looking at and thinking objectively about the dietary pattern while it is recorded, as shown in the following example:

10:00 A.M.:	coffee
	doughnut
Noon meal:	sandwich
	cheese
	egg
	hamburger
	Coke
Evening meal:	meat, fish, chicken
	potatoes or grits
	vegetables
	bread
	cake
	Jello
Late evening:	crackers
	cookies
	Coke

The counselor may also ask the patient to keep a food record or diary (Chapter 11) in which he or she records all foods eaten. This can be brought to the next session with the counselor. Besides providing invaluable insight into the eating behavior of the patient, it also provides the counselor with an idea about the patient's commitment to changing his or her eating habits.

The nurse or nutritionist accepts the patient's dietary pattern and proceeds to analyze the intake for serving sizes and added condiments such as cream in coffee and butter on bread. The nurse also determines the place and time food is eaten, who prepares the food, the number for whom the food is prepared or the number in the family, the kinds of meat, vegetables and desserts eaten, the kinds and amounts of food eaten between meals or for snacks and the time of day they are eaten. If the weekend pattern differs from that of the typical day, notation of the differences is made. The dietary history is discussed more fully in Chapter 11, Assessment of Nutritional Status.

The person becomes involved in giving information and is usually interested in knowing how his or her diet rates. The nurse or nutritionist evaluates the adequacy of the food pattern, points out the positive practices and designates the areas that are in need of improvement. In the example given, milk, vegetables and fruit seem to be the foods that the nutrition counselor would try to stimulate the person to think about. When given an opportunity the person usually suggests which foods and how much of them he or she is willing to include on a daily basis. The counselor may need to explore further with the person the ways to implement dietary changes. Together the counselor and patient formulate an acceptable dietary pattern.

This illustrates briefly a practical method for the nurse or nutritionist to use to obtain the dietary pattern of an individual and utilize it to improve nutrition. When evaluating the dietary intake, some interviewers may prefer to score the person's dietary pattern or have the person do it himself. An example of a score card is shown in Table 19–1. From this exercise the patient can learn where the low scores in the diet occur. Further discussion relating to the kind of meals, time of meals and other pertinent information is needed to help improve the dietary pattern and food habits.

A brief statement of the interviewer's evaluation of the patient's diet and how the problem was handled or resolved should be recorded in the patient's chart. The patient might be referred to the dietitian or nutritionist for further instruction as indicated.

Obviously these methods serve only to determine the individual's present dietary pattern and to show the teacher and learner what the

Table 19–1   FOOD SELECTION SCORE CARD

Score your diet for each day and determine your average score for the week. If your final score is between 85 and 100, your food selection standard has been good. A score of from 75 to 85 indicates a fair standard. A score below 75 indicates a low standard.

MAXIMUM SCORE FOR EACH FOOD GROUP	CREDITS	COLUMNS FOR DAILY CHECK						
20	Milk Group: Milk (including foods prepared with milk as cheese and ice cream). Adults: 1 glass, 10; 1½ glasses, 15; 2 glasses, 20. Children: 1 glass, 5; 1½ glasses, 10; 2 glasses, 15; 4 glasses, 20.							
35	Vegetable and Fruit Group: Vegetables: 1 serving, 5; 2 servings, 10; 3 servings, 15. Potatoes may be included as one of the above servings. If dark green or deep yellow vegetable is included, extra credit, 5. Fruits: 1 serving, 5; 2 servings, 10. If citrus fruit or raw vegetables or canned tomatoes are included, extra credit, 5.							
15	Bread and Cereal Group: Bread: dark whole grain, enriched or restored. Cereals: dark whole grain, enriched or restored. 2 servings of either, 10; 4 servings of either, 15.							
25	Meat Group: Eggs, meat, cheese, fish, poultry, dry peas, dry beans and nuts. 1 serving of any one of above, 10. 1 serving of any two above, 20. If liver (beef, lamb, pork or calf's) or kidney is used, extra credit, 5.							
5	Water (total liquid including coffee, tea or other beverage): Adults: 6 glasses, 2½; 8 glasses, 5. Children: 4 glasses, 2; 6 glasses, 5.							
100	Final Score							

needs are and where to place the emphasis to obtain better nutrition. Detailed forms and specific procedures are available and are well documented for use in nutritional surveys of populations and in research activities in which an accurate record of the nutrients ingested is required. See Chapter 11.

TEACHING TECHNIQUES

There is no one way or method to teach nutrition. The method must be adapted to the individual or group needs. Telling, informing, going over a list and showing are not effective ways of learning. The problem-solving approach is effective because it involves the learner. People are interested in what change means to them. The teaching–learning process may occur at the bedside or, if the patient is ambulatory, in the environment of a nutrition clinic or a classroom or possibly in the home. In any situation, the atmosphere should be as free of distractions and interruptions as possible. (See Fig. 19–3).

Obtaining a patient's dietary pattern requires a personal approach, respect and consideration for the person. Through use of words, action and attitude the individual can be made aware of the interviewer's concern about resolving the dietary problem. Rapport is achieved when the person develops confidence in the interviewer. By allowing an individual to talk about what food means to him, the interviewer can

get an idea of how to begin the dietary evaluation. The person responds with interest to the request, "Tell me which foods you regularly eat" and usually proceeds (but sometimes hesitates) to give the necessary information. Eating habits are very personal and many people may hesitate to discuss them, especially if for some reason they feel the habits are "bad" or if they are embarrassed by them. The interviewer listens without judging and begins the evaluation when the person is ready. Using the given dietary pattern (p. 415), the interviewer would review briefly the positive aspects of the person's diet and follow with "I did not hear you mention milk." Following the person's explanation or rationalization, the question "How could you use milk?" might bring further suggestions and give the interviewer some idea of what and how other suggestions could be offered. It could open a discussion about the nutrients in milk that are beneficial for the person. The use of vegetables could be approached in a similar manner. Thus the individual would have some part in planning the changes needed to improve his diet. A person is more likely to try and adopt a diet he or she had a part in revising.

Not all patients will change their behavior. They may show signs of being aware of and interested in a change and may appear to understand the changes recommended but may not necessarily be motivated to do so. The decision to adopt the changes is an individual matter. One thing is certain—it is the learner who must go through the process and adopt the change.

"Timing" and patient readiness to learn are exceedingly important. There may be days when no learning can take place and other days when the patient is ready and eager to learn. Effective points can be put across through conversation rather than lecturing, possibly through conversation during a meal. Sharing facts about nutrition with patients help them to feel important, an essential part of the feeling of well-being (Fig. 19–4). The patient may be ready to talk about what he or she likes to eat and what foods would make a good meal. This is an opening to look at the patient's present dietary pattern. It serves as the basis for teaching both normal and therapeutic nutrition. In both instances, all essential nutrients and calories for energy are needed by the individual. The therapeutic regimens are modifications of the normal diet, depending upon the characteristics of the therapy given for the disease.

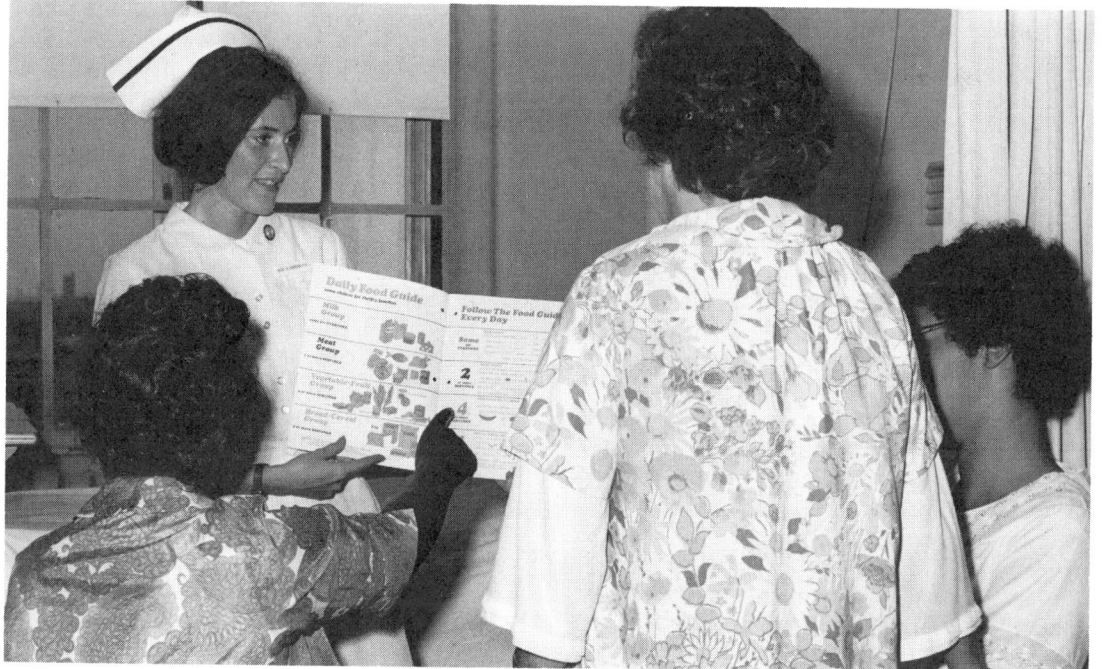

Figure 19–3 Some of the best opportunities for teaching occur during discussion with small groups of patients. Here the nurse is discussing the selection of well-balanced meals. (Courtesy of Graduate Hospital of the University of Pennsylvania. Photo by Paul Axler.)

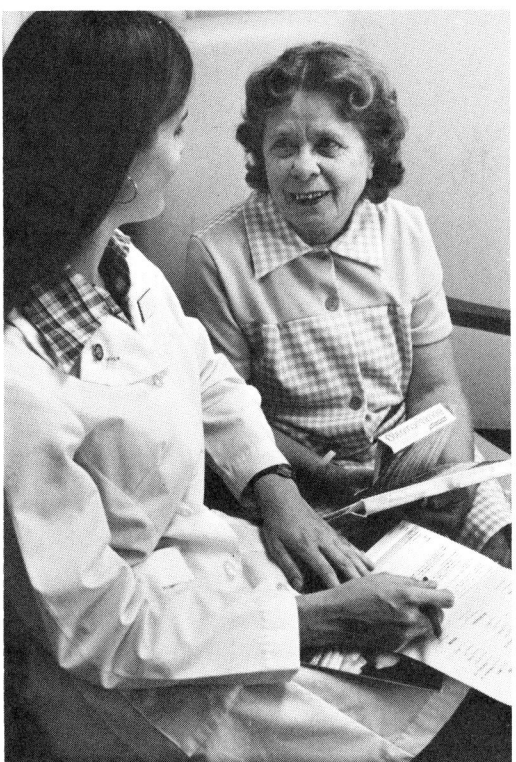

Figure 19–4   Dietitian and patient discussing dietary changes. (Photograph courtesy of Nutrition Department, Lutheran General Hospital, Park Ridge, Ill.)

If necessary changes must be made in the person's diet, he or she should be given a written copy of the plan discussed, especially if there are many changes in the customary pattern. With a normal, non-therapeutic diet, often the person can write the dietary program that he or she plans to adopt and be given appropriate supplementary visual aids. It is more meaningful when the nurse or dietitian-nutritionist approves the plan. If the person's dietary management is related to a therapeutic condition, he or she should have a written copy of the plan that he or she helped develop along with appropriate supplementary materials. More than one opportunity should be granted a person to discuss such an important topic as the changes required in the dietary pattern. Learning and the beginning of change should take place before the day of discharge from the hospital.

Follow-up sessions to answer questions or to adjust the pattern to meet changing needs are necessary. Circumstances (economic, social, psychological, seasonal) alter conditions, and adjustments in the dietary pattern may be needed. Change in eating behavior does not come after a few counseling sessions but takes quite a while and requires conscientious effort on the part of the patient and continual support from the nutrition counselor. Frequent contact by phone or mail may also be necessary to answer questions and handle problems.

Giving people a standardized printed diet sheet and expecting them to follow it exactly is an unrealistic and unsound practice. A person tends to choose foods from the list that conform to the customary pattern and discard other recommendations for dietary treatment. If such a practice prevails, the patient should be given an opportunity to indicate the pattern he or she will choose and then this pattern should be evaluated. It is important that the person and interviewer tailor the plan of therapy to fit the individual's needs and lifestyle.

In most cases, the patient will be unable to make at one time all the dietary changes necessary to follow a new diet. The changes should be made in steps, and as the changes become comfortable, more can be added.

Nurses have many opportunities to teach sound nutrition facts and dietary practices while giving bedside care, during the bath and when the trays are served at mealtime. Other opportunities are available in discussions with groups of patients who are on similar modified diets and with groups of patients on "general" or "regular" diets. The role of the nurse as a member of the team teaching nutrition is a vital one. Nursing includes meeting the nutritional needs of patients, and meeting these needs on an individual basis is vital to complete patient care.

NUTRITION CLINIC

Nutrition clinics in the outpatient departments of hospitals provide educational programs. Physicians refer to the clinic those patients who need nutrition counseling for specific conditions in which dietary management is an important part of therapy. Nurses, social workers and dental hygienists also refer people to the clinic for counseling.

The nutritionist begins by taking a careful dietary history. The counseling follows in the same way as has been explained. The dietary history, the nutritional care plan for the patient and progress notes are recorded in the patient's record, thus sharing and promoting continuity of care. Food models, leaflets, posters and other visual aids are widely used to help people learn about nutrition and how to plan an adequate diet for themselves. Frequently, the

nutritionist will use food models to help the patient visualize the size of the serving of food under discussion. Exhibits of actual foods or models, posters and films are used in the waiting rooms of clinics to stimulate interest in nutrition facts and to provide an opportunity to learn about foods in general. Sometimes cooking classes are conducted to introduce a discussion on food and nutrition. The focus of the discussion group could be on weight control, vegetarianism, saturated fat, the relationship of hypertension and sodium intake, sugar as a cause of dental caries, food economics or some other concern of the group.

PRENATAL AND POSTPARTUM CLINIC

In the prenatal clinic the teaching centers around the nutritional needs of mother and fetus during pregnancy. The diet during pregnancy is a normal one for the individual mother, with additional nutrients required during the second half to provide for the needs of the fetus. (See Chapter 13.) Counseling begins with the patient's dietary pattern and focuses on the areas needing improvement. The time spent in going over the standardized diet sheets frequently distributed in clinics could be used more appropriately to study the individual's dietary practices to see where changes are necessary.

During the postpartum period there are many opportunities for teaching. Weight control, adequate diet and eating habits, breast feeding and infant feeding are areas to be considered. This is the time to emphasize good nutrition and eating habits for the entire family, including the new baby. It is a time to review the dietary problems manifested during pregnancy and to stress the importance of good nutritional status prior to conception.

WELL BABY CLINIC

The mother in the well baby clinic is concerned with the progress of her child and is ready to learn about the foods her child should have. She is eager to discuss the problems she encounters. These are important clues to observe and incorporate in a plan of teaching. The mother is the "gatekeeper" in Kurt Lewin's "channel theory" of why people eat what they do. She determines largely what and how food comes to the table and, as a mother, is likely to modify and change food habits in the desired direction.

PRESCHOOL NUTRITION PROGRAMS

The Head Start Nutrition and Food Program administered in Child Development Centers under the auspices of the Office of Economic Opportunity brings children and food together in a good emotional and physical environment. The emphasis is "to establish sound nutritional practices by providing food to program participants as well as educating families in the selection and preparation of food in the home." Children attending the Center are given food at snack time and at lunch, and in some instances breakfast is served.

Parents participate actively in the program by developing policies and working in the Centers. There are many opportunities to interview and counsel parents, to feed the children and to train staff and health aides in developing sound attitudes toward nutrition and good sound practices. The program draws heavily on the skills of nutrition, health, education, psychology, social work and recreation professionals. Non-professionals play an important role in working with the children and parents. In Figure 19–5, the health aides are shown in a training session where they gain knowledge and skill in nutrition education.

SCHOOL LUNCH PROGRAMS

A type of food service is available to public school children in the United States and is provided by local school districts or subsidized by the National School Lunch Act. If the child is fed inadequately at home, the school lunch program offers an opportunity to provide at least one sufficiently nutritious meal five days a week and to teach facts about food. The school nurse can play an active role in the nutrition education program of the school system. The nurse is in a position to know which areas of nutrition education need emphasis through findings of physical and dental examinations, discussions on health, office visits of students and contact with parents.

The child may carry a packed lunch from home and supplement it with a hot beverage, hot dish or soup at school, or the entire meal may be prepared and served as part of the school lunch program. The National School Lunch Program encourages schoolchildren to eat more nutritious lunches. It carries out the National School Lunch Act of 1946, which authorized federal aid to school lunch programs in the form of a state grant-in-aid program, providing both for cash and food assistance. The

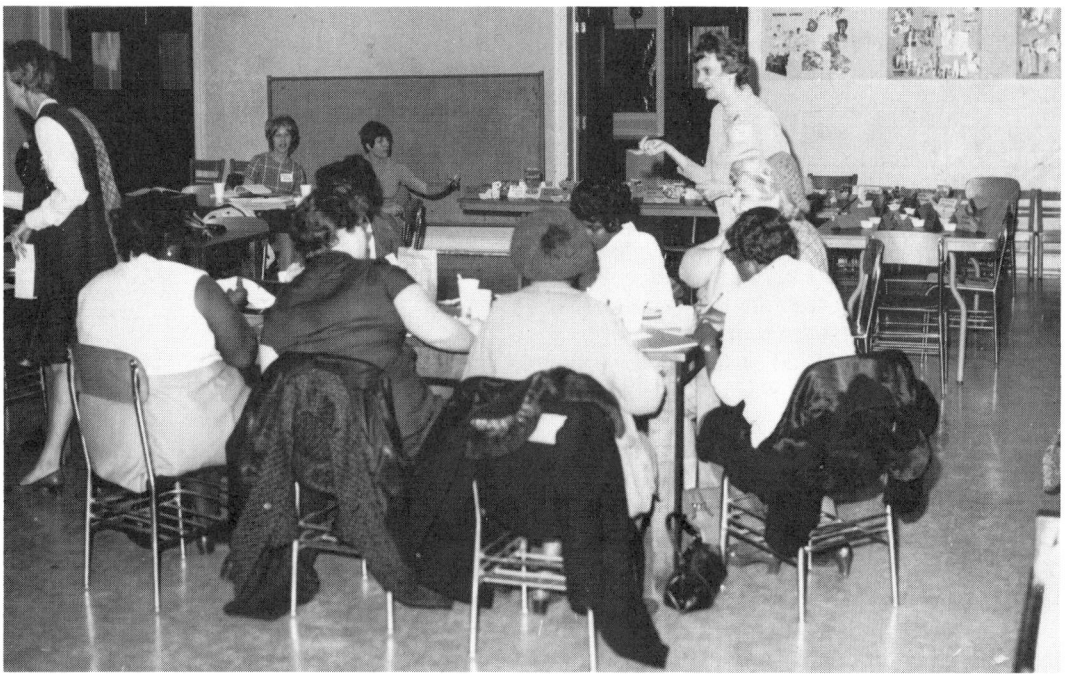

Figure 19–5 Health aides gain interest and skills in nutrition as they set their own goals and learn by doing at a training session coordinated by Maryland State Department of Health nutritionists. (Photo courtesy of Division of Nutrition, Maryland State Department of Health.)

federal government has subsidized many school lunch programs that provide nourishment for children at an economical cost or at no cost for those who cannot afford to pay. Surplus food commodities have been allotted to the school lunch programs of participating schools and technical assistance has been provided. Major responsibility for program operations rests with the state and local governments. Applications for subsidy must come from the school district. The standards set by the Department of Agriculture are expressed in terms of the food groups that make up a well-balanced lunch, called the "Type A" lunch. (See Fig. 19–6).

The "Type A" Lunch

In order to be eligible for reimbursement under the National School Lunch Program, schools must serve lunches that contain as a minimum:[8]

1. One half pint of fluid whole milk as a beverage.
2. Two ounces (edible portion as served) of lean meat, poultry, or fish; or two ounces of cheese; or one egg; or one half cup of cooked dry beans or peas; or four table- spoons of peanut butter or an equivalent quantity of any combination of these foods. To be counted in meeting this requirement, these foods must be served either in a main dish or in a main dish and one other menu item.
3. Three fourths of a cup of two or more vegetables or fruits or both. Full-strength vegetable or fruit juice may be counted to meet not more than one fourth cup of this requirement. An ascorbic acid–rich food should be served daily and a vitamin A–rich food at least twice a week. Several sources of iron should be included each day.
4. One serving of whole-grain or enriched bread or muffins, cornbread, biscuits or rolls made of enriched or whole-grain flour.
5. Two teaspoons butter or fortified margarine used as a spread, as a seasoning or in food preparation.
6. Other foods to round out meals and supply energy.

Part of the cost of milk to schools, non-profit child care centers, Head Start programs and summer camps is subsidized under the Special Milk Program of the U.S. Department of Agriculture. (See Chapter 18.)

If these foods are included in the lunch, in general, one third of the daily dietary needs of children aged 10 to 12 years or about one fourth of their total nutritive needs for the week will be met. Larger portions are served to older children.

The idea of serving lunches to schoolchildren is not new to this century. As early as 1849 France operated some school lunch programs and was one of the first countries to provide school lunches on a national scale. In 1904 the English Parliament authorized the installation of facilities for preparing and serving food as part of standard school equipment. The first record of an organized school feeding program in the United States was in 1853, when the Children's Aid Society of New York opened a vocational school for poor children and served meals to them. The program has grown, and today serving food in school has become a generally accepted part of the American school system; yet there are many schools without food preparation units. More work is needed to provide all children with the opportunity to obtain an adequate lunch at school.

Some of the objectives of the school lunch program are the provision of (1) nutritious food in sufficient quantities, (2) time to enjoy the lunch, (3) a pleasant eating place and (4) improvement of food habits of the child and, indirectly, of the parents and family.

The school lunch program offers an opportunity for children to participate in the planning of menus and to learn about the nutrients in foods as they relate to good nutrition and the building of healthy bodies. Various aspects of nutrition can attract interest in class discussions in social studies, mathematics, biology, English, art and science. Field trips to local plants, markets and farms are ways to utilize community resources. The school lunchroom should be the laboratory in which the principles learned in the classroom are put into action. A useful tool for teaching older children about nutrition is the *Food For Youth Study Guide*.[4]

The school lunch program is potentially

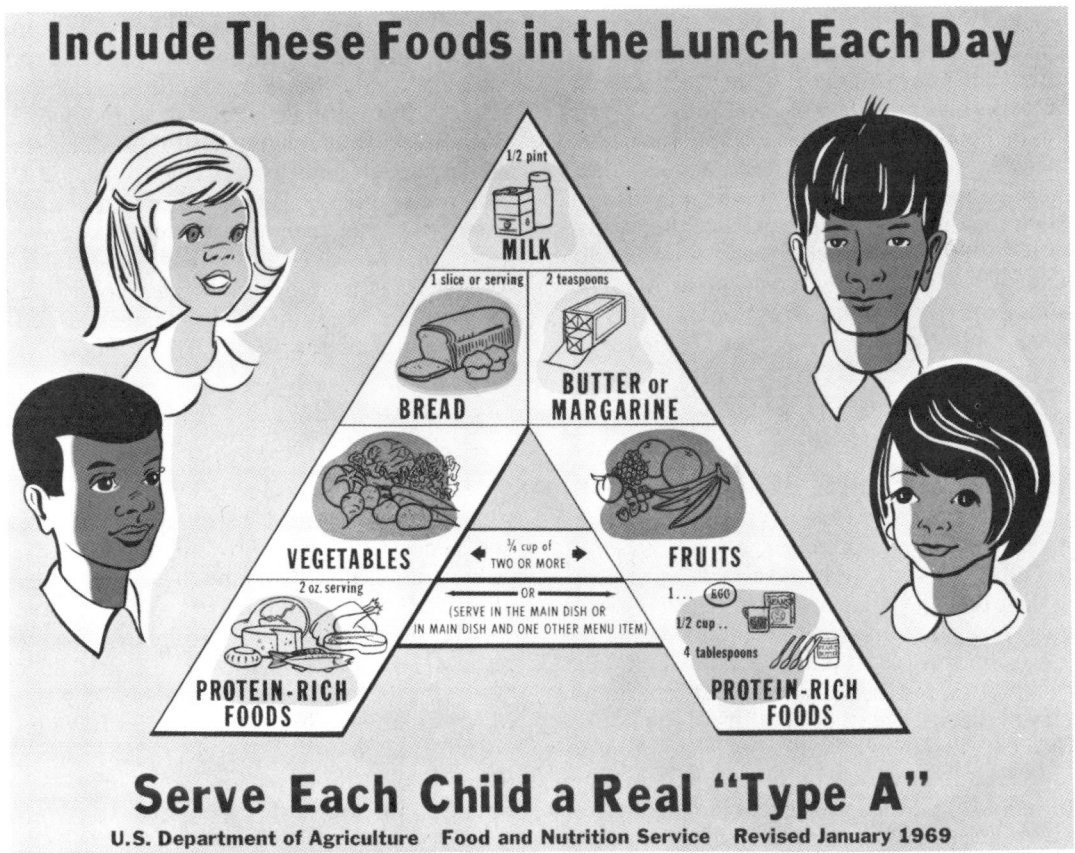

Figure 19–6 The National School Lunch Program's plan for a well-balanced lunch expressed as the "Type A" lunch. (Courtesy of the U.S. Dept of Agriculture, Agricultural Marketing Service.)

one of the best ways to promote better health and reinforce good nutritional habits, but the widespread availability of confections and carbonated beverages in vending machines on school premises may tempt children to spend lunch money for them and may lead to poor food habits. The high energy value and constant availability of such "junk" foods are likely to affect children's appetites for regular meals. In addition, the nutritional yield of these foods is greatly inferior to that of milk, fruit and other basic foods. The Council on Foods and Nutrition of the American Medical Association[1] opposed the sale and distribution of these foods in school lunchrooms.

EXPANDED FOOD AND NUTRITION EDUCATION PROGRAM (EFNEP)

This program, started in 1968, encourages nutrition education and is funded through the U.S. Department of Agriculture and administered through the Cooperative Extension Service. Reflecting a unique approach to nutrition education, the program's objective is to train community nutrition aides from low income areas to teach nutrition to others in the community and thus to improve the dietary intake and eventually the nutritional status of community members. The aides visit people in their homes or work with groups in the community. The advantage of this type of educational effort is that the nutrition aides, who are themselves members of the community and thus familiar with it, are in a better position to influence eating patterns than a professional who is unfamiliar with the area.

THE CONSUMER'S NUTRITION KNOWLEDGE

From a recent survey of 1400 households, the Economic Research Service of the U.S. Department of Agriculture reports that about one half of the surveyed households were altering their diets because of health problems or to avoid potential ones. Households changing diets reported an avoidance of sweets and snacks, fried foods, fatty red meat, ice cream and soft drinks. Nearly two fifths of the households checked labels for health-relevant information. Larger households, higher income households and those whose homemakers had more schooling were more likely than others to introduce preventive diet changes.[5]

The FDA Consumer Nutrition Knowledge

Survey revealed that nine out of 10 people who were the principal grocery shoppers for their households felt that they had no problems providing a nutritious diet for their families. Yet when asked to define a nutritous diet most were unable to do so. Shoppers under the age of 34 were most confident of their nutrition knowledge, while those over 50 years of age were least confident. Twenty per cent of those scoring low on a nutrition knowledge test felt that they knew a great deal about nutrition. About 50 per cent of those scoring well on a nutrition knowledge test were aware of their knowledge, while 40 per cent felt they knew little or nothing about nutrition.[2]

From these studies it appears that consumers are aware of the relationship between health and nutrition and are attempting to make dietary changes to improve health, but they seem to need more information about the basic principles of nutrition.

NUTRITION IN THE HEALTH EDUCATION CURRICULUM

A dynamic nutrition education program that begins in early childhood and continues through the elementary and secondary schools can help young children to acquire positive attitudes toward food. It can also help older children to assume responsibility for their own food selection and prepare them for adult and parental responsibility. As future citizens in a democracy, children must develop acceptable nutritional practices and a sense of social consciousness to enable them to participate intelligently in the adoption of public policy affecting the nutrition of people.*

TEACHING AIDS

Charts, posters, pictures, pamphlets and slides help a great deal in teaching patients and some excellent ones are available. Practical and accurate graphic presentation is particularly useful if there are language differences to overcome. Copies of the food pattern shown in Figure 19–2 are available from the U.S. Department of Agriculture at small cost. This can be used as a guide for individuals or groups. Many commercial food companies have good posters and colorful materials that are adapted from reliable sources. These, of course, should be used with discretion in reference to advertis-

---

*White House Conference on Food, Nutrition and Health, 1969.

ing. At the end of this chapter is a list of sources of health education material on nutrition, available free or at small cost. Wax or paper food models are also good visual aids, especially for demonstration of serving size. Even standard household measures—a cup or a tablespoon— are good visual aids. If you don't have any visual aids, make some!

PROBLEMS AND SUGGESTED TOPICS FOR DISCUSSION

1. Obtain a dietary history from a patient. Score the diet using Table 19–1.
2. How would you go about teaching a patient who is eating a "general diet"?
3. Keep a personal record of food consumed during a three day period. Compare it with the basic food groups.
4. Visit the nutrition clinic and the well baby and pre-natal clinics in your hospital or medical center and report observations.
5. Prepare a teaching aid, either individually or in group work, that will be useful in teaching patients nutrition facts.
6. What is meant by the "Type A" school lunch? Plan a week's menus for packed lunches for a boy aged 11 years to carry from home. How does it compare with the lunch served at school?
7. What are the objections to the sale of confections and carbonated beverages on school premises?
8. List reasons for providing a good school lunch. In what way can a school nurse aid in bringing about the improvement of food habits of schoolchildren.?

CITED REFERENCES

1. Council on Foods and Nutrition: Confections and carbonated beverages in schools. JAMA, *180*:1118, 1962.
2. FDA Consumer Nutrition Knowledge Survey, Report II, 1975. DHEW Publication No. (FDA) 76–2059. Washington, D.C., Division of Consumer Studies, Office of Nutrition and Consumer Sciences, Food and Drug Administration, 1976.
3. Fleming, R. S.: Principles of Learning. Proceedings of Nutrition Education Conference, April 1 to 3, 1957. USDA Publication No. 745. Washington, D.C., U.S. Department of Agriculture, p. 17.
4. Food for Youth Study Guide. USDA Publication No. FNS–140. Washington, D.C., U.S. Department of Agriculture, 1975.
5. Jones, J. L.: Are health concerns changing the American diet? National Food Situation, No. 159, March 1977, p. 27. (Published by Economic Research Service, U.S. Department of Agriculture.)
6. Leverton, R. M.: Development of Basic Nutrition Concepts for Use in Nutrition Education. Proceedings of Nutrition Education Conference, February 20 to 22, 1967. USDA Publication No. 1075. Washington, D.C. U.S. Department of Agriculture.
7. National Food Guide. USDA Leaflet No. 288. Washington, D.C., U.S. Department of Agriculture, 1957.
8. National School Lunch Program. USDA Bulletin PA–19. Washington, D.C. U.S. Department of Agriculture, 1959.
9. Page, L., and Phipard, E. F.: Essentials of An Adequate Diet . . . Facts for Nutrition Programs. Home Economics Research Report No. 3. Washington, D.C., Agricultural Research Service, U.S. Department of Agriculture, 1957.

SOURCES OF NUTRITION AND HEALTH EDUCATION MATERIAL

American Can Company, Home Economics Section, 100 Park Avenue, New York, New York, 10017.
American Dietetic Association, 430 North Michigan Avenue, Chicago, Illinois, 60611.
American Institute of Baking, 400 East Ontario Street, Chicago, Illinois, 60611.
Borden Company, 350 Madison Avenue, New York, New York, 10017.
California Fruit Growers Exchange, Educational Department, Los Angeles, California.
Campbell Soup Company, 375 Memorial Avenue, Camden, New Jersey, 08101.
Cereal Institute, Inc., 135 South LaSalle Street, Chicago, Illinois, 60603.
Evaporated Milk Association, 228 North LaSalle Street, Chicago, Illinois, 60601.
General Foods Corporation, 250 Park Avenue, New York, New York, 10017
General Mills, Inc., Dept. of Nutrition, 9200 Wayzata Blvd., Minneapolis, Minnesota, 55426.
Gerber Products, Department of Nutrition, Fremont, Michigan, 49412.
H. J. Heinz Company, P. O. Box 5, Pittsburgh, Pennsylvania, 15230.
Institute of American Poultry, 110 North Franklin Street, Chicago, Illinois, 60606.
Merck and Company, Rahway, New Jersey, 07065.
Metropolitan Life Insurance Company, 1 Madison Avenue, New York, New York, 10010.
National Dairy Council, 111 North Canal Street, Chicago, Illinois, 60606.
National Live Stock and Meat Board, 36 South Wabash Avenue, Chicago, Illinois, 60603.
National Research Council, 2101 Constitution Avenue, N.W., Washington, D.C., 20037.
Office of Child Development, Department of Health, Education and Welfare, Washington, D.C. 20203.
Pet Milk Company, Home Economics Department, St. Louis, Missouri.
Poultry and Egg National Board, 250 West 57th Street, New York, New York, 10019.
U.S. Department of Agriculture, Institute of Home Economics, Washington, D.C., 20251.
Wheat Flour Institute, 309 West Jackson Boulevard, Chicago, Illinois, 60606.

ADDITIONAL REFERENCES

Aldrich, C. K.: Prescribing a diet is not enough. J. Am. Diet. Assoc., *33*:785, 1957.
Babcock, C.: Attitudes and the use of food. J. Am. Diet. Assoc., *38*:546, 1961.
Beeuwkes, A. M.: Teaching nutrition—Progress and problems. J. Am. Diet. Assoc., *35*:797, 1959.
Bergevin, P.: Telling vs. teaching—Learning by participation. J. Am. Diet. Assoc., *33*:781, 1957.
Blackburn, M. L.: Who turns the child "off" to nutrition? J. Nutr. Educ., *2*:45, 1970.

Burke, B. S.: The dietary history as a tool in research. J. Am. Diet. Assoc., *23*:1041, 1947.

Cassel, J.: Social and cultural implications of food and food habits. Am. J. Public Health, *47*:732, 1957.

Craig, D. G.: Guiding the change process in people. J. Am. Diet. Assoc., *58*:22, 1971.

Davis, A. J.: The skills of communication. Am. J. Nurs., *63*:66, 1963.

Gifft, H. H., Washbon, M. B., and Harrison, G. G.: Nutrition, Behavior and Change. Englewood Cliffs, New Jersey, Prentice–Hall, Inc., 1972.

Ginther, J. R.: Educational diagnosis of patients. J. Am. Diet. Assoc., *59*:560, 1971.

Hearings Before the Select Committee on Nutrition and Human Needs of the United States Senate. Part 2, National School Lunch Program. Washington, D.C., March 23, 1970.

Hill, M. M.: A conceptual approach to nutrition education. J. Am. Diet. Assoc., *49*:20, 1966.

Homemakers' Food and Nutrition Knowledge, Practices and Opinions. Home Economics Research Report No. 39. Washington, D.C., Agricultural Research Service, U.S. Department of Agriculture, 1975.

Kintzer, F. C.: Approaches to teaching adults. J. Am. Diet. Assoc., *50*:475, 1967.

Knudson, A. L., and Newton, M. E.: Behavioral factors in nutrition education. J. Am. Diet. Assoc., *37*:222 and 226, 1960.

Lewin, K.: Forces behind food habits and methods of change. Washington, D.C., Committee on Food Habits. National Research Council, 1943.

Mann, G. V.: Nutrition education—U.S.A. Food and Nutrition News, *41*:November, 1969. (Published by National Live Stock and Meat Board, Chicago.)

Morris, E.: How does a nurse teach nutrition to patients? Am. J. Nurs., *60*:67, 1960.

Myers, M. L.: The ambulatory clinic in community and public health nutrition. J. Am. Diet. Assoc., *59*:48, 1971.

Neihoff, A.: Changing food habits. J. Nutr. Educ., *1*:10, 1969.

Niemeyer, K. A.: Nutrition education is behavioral change. J. Nutr. Educ., *3*:No. 1, 1971.

Nutrition . . . Food for Thought. Is the Consumer Getting the Message? A. C. Nielson Company, 1976.

Pattison, M., Barbour, H., and Eppright, E.: Teaching Nutrition. Ames, Iowa, Iowa State College Press, 1963.

Proceedings of Nutrition Education Conference, April 1 to 3, 1957. Washington, D.C. U.S. Department of Agriculture, Miscel. Pub. No. 745, 1957.

Proceedings of Nutrition Education Conference, January 29 to 31, 1962. Washington, D.C., U.S. Department of Agriculture, Miscel. Publ. No. 913, 1962.

Proceedings of Nutrition Education Conference, February 20–22, 1967. Washington, D.C., U.S. Department of Agriculture, Miscel. Pub. No. 1075, 1967.

Review: The effects of a balanced lunch program on the growth and nutritional status of school children. Nutr. Rev., *23*:35, 1965.

Roth, A.: The teenage clinic. J. Am. Diet. Assoc., *36*:27, 1960.

Schild, D. T.: Make your own visual aids! J. Am. Diet. Assoc., *37*:581, 1960.

Sipple, H. L.: Problems and progress in nutrition education. J. Am. Diet. Assoc., *59*:19, 1971.

Sliepcevich, E. M., and Creswell, W. H.: A conceptual approach to health education: complications for nutritive education. Am. J. Public Health, *58*:684, 1968.

Vargas, J. S.: Teaching is changing behavior. J. Am. Diet. Assoc., *58*:512, 1971.

Vaughn, M. E.: An agency nutritionist looks at home health care under Medicare. J. Am. Diet. Assoc., *51*:146, 1967.

Young, C. M.: Teaching the patient means reaching the patient. J. Am. Diet. Assoc., *33*:42, 1957.

Young, C. M.: The interview itself. J. Am. Diet. Assoc. *35*:677, 1959.

Young, C. M.: Interviewing the patient. Am. J. Clin. Nutr., *8*:523, 1960.

Zifferblatt, S. M., and Wilbur, C. S.: Dietary counseling: Some realistic expectations and guidelines. J. Am. Diet. Assoc., *70*:591, 1977.

Part Two

DIET THERAPY AND NUTRITIONAL CARE IN DISEASE

This section of the book deals with the role of nutrition in the prevention and treatment of disease. All the therapeutic diets are modifications of the normal adequate diet pattern based on the Recommended Dietary Allowances as suggested by the Food and Nutrition Board of the National Research Council, with amounts of nutrients adjusted to cover the additional requirements created by disease or injury. Space does not permit the inclusion of all diets in use for each disease. Only those diets most generally accepted are outlined here.

DEVELOPMENT OF DIET THERAPY

Nursing and medicine have always been concerned with the feeding of the sick. From the time of the Egyptian medical era, a relationship has been recognized between food and disease, and some form of diet therapy has been practiced. Celsus emphasized the role of foods in preventive medicine about 25 B.C., when he wrote: ". . . we come to those which nourish, namely food and drink. Now these are of general assistance not only in disease of all kinds but in preserving health as well." In 1671 Nicolai Venette recognized the efficacy of using vegetables and fresh fruits as antiscorbutics; and Bachstrom's writings in 1734 demonstrate that he recognized scurvy as a deficiency disease. As early as 1843, Jonathan Pereira, a member of the Royal College of Physicians in London, published a book in collaboration with Dr. Charles A. Lee of New York based on experimental

work in the feeding of "paupers, lunatics, criminals, children and the sick in metropolitan institutions." In 1854 during the Crimean War, Florence Nightingale and her staff, located at Scutari, were as devoted to the problems of feeding the sick and wounded as they were to other phases of nursing. Florence Nightingale is historically recorded as the founder of dietetics as well as of nursing. Between 1854 and 1865 there seems to have been a lull in the study of dietetics until after the Civil War. History appears to repeat itself in that it takes the increased demands of war to further the interest and study of foods and nutrition. In the early 1870's, Dr. F. W. Pacy, Fellow of the Royal College of Physicians, London, began a treatise on food and dietetics. It is recorded that in his lectures he emphasized that the correct feeding of the well and sick should be of deep concern. He stated, "Ill management of food kills off the weak and ruins the middling." Thus, the role of nutrient requirements in disease and the necessity of supplying certain essential nutrients as a preventive to disease were recognized by the earliest physicians.

Others became interested and approached and treated the subject from various angles. Cooking schools were founded in the East (New York, Boston and Philadelphia). In the 1880's, graduates from these schools began taking positions as instructors in foods and cookery in nurses' training schools, to teach the nurses how to prepare foods for the sick. The next step was a diet kitchen supervised by a graduate from a cooking school. Progress continued and has reached our present-day system of dietitians in charge of food service in the hospital. It has been a long journey, one in which the nurse played a major role. The nurse continues to function as a vital and necessary member of the team in feeding the sick. She sees more of the patient than anyone else, and when the food is served, she should be able to observe, encourage and guide the learning process intelligently. With the cooperation of everyone—nurse, doctor, dietitian and patient—effective management of the patient's dietary needs and provision of complete nutritional care will be achieved.

UNIT FIVE

PRINCIPLES OF NUTRITIONAL CARE

Chapter 20

THE NUTRITIONAL CARE PROCESS

THE CHANGING PICTURE OF NUTRITIONAL DISEASE

Scientific progress is changing the picture of nutritional disease in America. In the early 1900's frank deficiency diseases—pellagra, beriberi, scurvy and rickets—were endemic. Today fully developed cases are rare or at least uncommon. In fact, in 1955 the United States Public Health Service discontinued reporting the occurrence of pellagra and other deficiency diseases. Today, the majority of cases of pellagra, beriberi, xerophthalmia and protein–calorie malnutrition are the result of special conditioning circumstances, e.g., the existence of a primary disease that produces secondary nutritional deficiency disease. Nevertheless, sporadic cases do occur and could be diagnosed incorrectly if these diseases are not borne in mind.

Reasons for the changing face of nutritional disease include advances in research, steady improvement of general economic status, fortification and enrichment of foods and education of the public. Along with these advancements there has been rapid and wide-reaching technological progress in the food industry itself.

However, while certain nutritional diseases are largely disappearing in America, there is a steady increase in the recognition of new nutrition-related disorders, most of which fall into one of four categories: (1) lack or imbalance of nutrients (disorders of magnesium deficiency, vitamin E deficiency anemia); (2) in-

born errors of metabolism (phenylketonuria); (3) iatrogenic diseases (caused by medications and treatments affecting the intestinal flora, the appetite or the absorption, utilization and excretion of nutrients) and (4) overnutrition (obesity, diabetes mellitus, toxicity, imbalances, atherosclerosis).

Definite relationships exist between diet and wound healing, stress, burns, gastrointestinal diseases, infectious diseases, diseases of the liver, diseases of the heart and circulatory system, diseases of the bone, cancer and possibly mental disorders. The relationship between nutrition and disease and the nutritional care needed with certain diseases will be described in subsequent chapters.

THE NUTRITIONAL CARE PROCESS

In the course of a lifetime a person's nutritional status and nutritional needs will change. They will reflect the individual's environment and his or her phase in the life cycle. Because an individual is changing, the health care, including the nutritional care, must also be dynamic. Nutritional care is the *process* of meeting a person's changing nutritional needs. The type of care depends on the presence of disease or potential disease, on the environment and on the state of growth and development of the individual. The *nutritional care process* is the assessment of the individual's nutritional status, the identification of nutritional needs or

427

problems, the planning of objectives of nutritional care to meet these needs, the implementation of nutritional activities, including education, necessary to meet the objectives and the evaluation of the nutritional care.

For a healthy person, nutritional care may mean only assessment of nutritional status, identification of adequate nutritional health without problems and encouragement to continue the good work. A healthy person usually requires nutritional care in the form of education regarding eating habits that will help to prevent disease and maintain the present good health. (See Chapter 19, Teaching Nutrition.)

Nutritional care for the ill or hospitalized patient is more complex. It means far more than simply providing the hospitalized person with a tray of food three times each day. It should include the monitoring of food intake and, when intake is inadequate, should also include taking action through counseling the patient, providing emotional support and encouragement, or initiating a tube feeding, an elemental diet, parenteral nutrition, or protein, calorie or vitamin and mineral supplementation. (See Chapter 35.) It is obvious that thorough nutritional care requires the attention and contributions of many professionals, particularly those of the nurse, clinical dietitian and physician.

One of the reasons for the frequency of malnutrition in our hospitals today is that no one health professional or group has taken complete responsibility for the nutritional care of the patient. This has happened in many phases of health care, and nutrition is no exception. Since nutritional care involves so many disciplines, one way to improve it is to have a group of professionals take responsibility for the care and its outcome. Several institutions are developing nutritional support teams composed of physicians, dietitians, nurses, surgeons, pharmacists and physical therapists, who can capitalize on each other's expertise and be responsible for the patient's nutritional care. They work with the primary care providers to ensure that the proper nutritional care is carried out.[6] For provision of effective nutritional care by all of these health professionals, a *nutritional care plan* or written documentation of the nutritional care process is a necessity. It allows for proper communication and the interaction necessary for complete nutritional care.

THE NUTRITIONAL CARE PLAN

The nutritional care plan consists of a nutritional assessment, the identification of nutri-

tional problems, the setting of objectives of nutritional care, nutritional intervention activities (including education) and evaluation of the nutritional care.

Assessment

Collection of the data needed for assessment of nutritional status is discussed thoroughly in Chapter 11, Assessment of Nutritional Status. In summary, this data base includes anthropometric, biochemical, clinical, dietary and psychosocial information that is pertinent to the nutritional status of the patient. (See Table 20–1.)

From the data base an assessment of nutritional status is made and any problems or needs are identified. The relative importance of these problems should also be evaluated so that they can be given levels of priority. Each problem is then numbered and future notes taken about this problem are identified by the same number. This facilitates record keeping and allows a quick review of the care being provided for one nutritional problem. It is desirable that the nutritional problems, as the dietitian-nutritionist, nurse or physician perceives them, will be given the same priority by the patient, but frequently this is not the case.

The following is an example of a nutritional assessment and the identification of nutritional problems:

Patient: Ms. Anderson—20 years old, white, female. From the health record, laboratory data, anthropometric measurements and nutritional history, the following information serves as the data base:

Laboratory data:	Elevated fasting blood sugar. Ketosis. Hypoglycemia.
Anthropometric data:	Underweight; below-normal triceps skinfold thickness.
Dietary data:	Caloric intake below energy needs: 10-lb. weight loss in past year. Meals three times per day; coffee frequently.
Medical history:	Diagnosed one year ago as having juvenile-onset diabetes. Was given little instruction about diet and complains of hypoglycemia.

Nutritional Assessment: Ms. A., although diagnosed one year ago as having diabetes, is not in good control of her condition and does not completely understand her diet. She has been consuming fewer calories than she requires and does not follow a regular dietary pattern. Ms. A.'s *nutritional problem* can be stated as juvenile-onset diabetes mellitus in poor control. However, her nutritional

Table 20–1 ASSESSMENT OF NUTRITIONAL STATUS—THE DATA BASE IN THE NUTRITIONAL CARE PROCESS

This data base includes all information—anthropometric, biochemical, clinical, nutritional-dietary and psychosocial—that is pertinent to the nutritional status, problems and care of the patient. It includes the following information:*

ANTHROPOMETRIC
Weight, height and weight changes. Growth parameters (in infants, children, adolescents): chest circumference, head circumference; (in pregnant women): weight gain.
Skinfold thickness: triceps, scapular, abdominal, and so on.
Arm circumference and muscle circumference.
Skeletal radiographic information.

BIOCHEMICAL
Blood, serum, plasma measurements.
Urinary measurements.
Tissue assays or biopsies.

CLINICAL EXAMINATION
Findings indicative of nutritional status.
Findings indicative of disease that may affect nutritional status.
Pertinent medical history.

NUTRITIONAL HISTORY
Dietary intake.
24-hour recall.
Food frequency questionnaire.
Nutrition-related information.
Use of vitamin and mineral supplementation.
Allergies, food intolerances.
Nutrition knowledge.
Physical activity.

PSYCHOSOCIAL INFORMATION
Cooking and eating atmosphere.
Attitudes toward food and eating.
Number of persons in household.
Economic factors.
Food buying and cooking facilities.
Pertinent social history.
Ethnic background.

*See Chapter 11 for a complete discussion.

problem could be stated more specifically as three problems: (1) hypoglycemic episodes related to poor control of diabetes mellitus, (2) weight loss and (3) little knowledge of proper dietary management.

The identification of nutritional problems evolves naturally from a thorough nutritional assessment, which should include all present and potential problems. Identification of the potential problems brings attention to those that might be prevented from developing by taking immediate action.

Objectives for Nutritional Care

After the identification of nutritional problems, the next step is to formulate a plan for dealing with each of them, with the greatest attention being paid to the problems of highest priority. If the nutrition information is not complete, the first objective would be to collect more of it. For example, one objective might be to find out when Ms. A.'s hypoglycemic attacks occur.

The objectives should be patient-centered, which means that they should be stated in terms that show what the patient will achieve if the objective is met. For example, the objective would be: "Ms. A. will be able to select a 2000 kcal. diet from the hospital menu after three days of instruction," rather than "I will teach Ms. A. how to select a 1500 kcal. diet from the hospital menu," which is not patient-centered. Stated in the latter way, the objective identifies what needs to be done but does not make the nurse, clinical dietitian or even Ms. A. responsible for Ms. A.'s learning. One session in which the dietitian does all the talking and Ms. A. does all the listening but learns little would meet the objective but not the patient's needs.

In addition, the objectives should be realistic and should take into consideration the educational level of the patient and the economic and social resources of the patient and his family.

The objectives should be stated in *quantifiable* terms. In order to know if objectives have been met, they must be stated in measurable ways. The plan or objective of care made

for each problem should carry the same number in notations in the medical record as the problem it is designed to deal with. Returning to our example, the objectives for each of the three nutritional problems identified for Ms. A. might be the following:

Problem No. 1—Hypoglycemic episodes.

Objectives: (1) The nutrition counselor will find out when the hypoglycemic attacks occur, (2) Ms. A. will demonstrate an understanding of hypoglycemia through a verbal explanation of why it happens, what the body needs when it does happen and how to prevent it and (3) Ms. A. will modify her diet in order to avoid hypoglycemia.

Problem No. 2—Weight loss.

Objective: Ms. A. will stop losing weight and will demonstrate this by check-ups at three months, six months, nine months and one year.

Problem No. 3—Lack of knowledge about proper diet to control her diabetes.

Objective: Ms. A. will understand the principles of her modified diet by being able to select the proper foods from the hospital menu to meet her dietary requirements.

Implementation of Nutritional Care

This part of the nutritional care process includes all of those activities or interventions that will enable the patient to meet the objectives already defined. Such activities include the diet prescription, nutritional counseling and education, provision of food and necessary nutritional supplements (if the patient is hospitalized), vitamin and mineral medication or activities such as public aid advice and food stamp counseling that will help the patient to meet his nutritional needs economically. The diet prescription will be discussed on page 433; nutrition counseling and education are discussed in Chapter 19; and food assistance programs are discussed in Chapter 18.

For each objective there are specific interventions or actions that are numbered to correlate with the objective they are designed to meet. The nutritional interventions should be complete and *specific* and should include the "what, where, when and how" of the activity. Nothing should be vague or left open to question. With complete and specific interventions outlined and documented, the entire health team (including the patient) will know what is being done, especially at those times when the primary care providers are not available. No one can be with a patient for 24 hours every day. Information about the treatment and progress of a patient should be accessible to the health team from a central record. Referring again to Ms. A., the nutritional interventions for each objective might be stated as follows:

Objective No. 1: Ms. A. will modify her diet in order to avoid afternoon hypoglycemia.

Intervention: No. 1–1. Carbohydrate will be distributed throughout the day as follows: breakfast (8:00 A.M.): 80 gm.; lunch (noon): 85 gm.; afternoon snack: 30 gm. and dinner (6:30 P.M.): 85 gm.

Objective No. 2: Ms. A. will stop losing weight.

Intervention: No. 2–1. Caloric intake will be increased to 2000 kcal. per day using the following diet: 280 gm. of carbohydrate, 43 gm. of protein and 80 gm. of fat.

Objective No. 3: Ms. A. will understand the principles of her modified diet and will be able to select the proper foods from the hospital menu.

Intervention: No. 3–1. Teach Ms. A. how to select a 2000 kcal. diet from the hospital menu by giving her the opportunity on February 7, 8 and 9 at 10:30 A.M. to select (with supervision and discussion) a 2000 kcal. diet from the hospital menu.

Evaluation of Nutritional Care

The last step is evaluation of the nutritional care provided. This step makes the nutritional care plan dynamic and responsive to the patient's needs. If the objectives have been written in measurable behavioral terms, the evaluation becomes very easy, since present behavior is being measured against behavior already defined. For example: "Ms. A. was not able to select a 2000 kcal. diet after three days of instruction because she does not understand the food exchange system." A revision in the care plan at this point might include the following: "Ms. A. will attend classes for diabetics during the week of February 14 to 18 in order to learn the concept of a food exchange."

Another aspect of this last step is the evaluation of the extent to which the patient's nutritional requirements are being met. This can be done by using the *nutritional index*.[2] The nutritional index quantifies the extent to which the patient's *actual intake* of a nutrient meets the recommended or *desirable intake* defined for that patient. The nutritional index (NI) can be used to evaluate the adequacy of the calorie, protein, vitamin or mineral intake of the patient. Nutrients of special importance in the pa-

tient's diet should be evaluated using this method. To calculate the nutritional index:

$$\text{Nutritional Index (NI)} = \frac{\text{Actual Intake of Nutrient} - \text{Desirable Intake}}{\text{Desirable Intake}} \times 100$$

If the actual daily intake exceeds the desirable intake, the nutritional index is stated as a positive percentage. If actual intake equals desirable intake, the index is stated as +1 per cent to avoid an index of zero. If the actual intake is less than the desirable intake, then the nutritional index is stated as a negative percentage. Obviously, the goal of nutritional care is to meet the nutritional requirements of the patient and thus to have as many days as possible with a positive nutritional index. Having several days with a negative nutritional index means that the objectives of the nutritional care are not being met and that the care should be evaluated and changed.

Example: Mr. M., who was burned in a fire, requires 60 kcal. per kg. of body weight per day. His daily intake per kg. for one week was: Monday, 30 kcal.; Tuesday, 20 kcal.; Wednesday, 30 kcal.; Thursday, 36 kcal.; Friday, 40 kcal.; Saturday, 45 kcal. and Sunday, 60 kcal. The nutritional index for Monday would be calculated as follows:

$$\text{NI} = \frac{30 \text{ kcal./kg.} - 60 \text{ kcal./kg.}}{60 \text{ kcal./kg.}} \times 100$$

$$\text{NI} = \frac{-30 \text{ kcal./kg.}}{60 \text{ kcal./kg.}} \times 100$$

$$\text{NI} = -0.5 \times 100 = -50\%$$

For the entire week the nutritional indexes are: Monday, −50 per cent; Tuesday, −66 per cent; Wednesday, −50 per cent; Thursday, −40 per cent; Friday, −33 per cent; Saturday, −25 per cent and Sunday +1 per cent. The average nutritional index for the week is −37.7 per cent.

On the seventh day Mr. M. finally achieved a positive nutritional index. During the week, Mr. M.'s average was 38 per cent below his desirable intake. The goal now would be to achieve equally high positive nutritional indexes to offset the days with negative indexes. At the least, the indexes should remain positive. If they do not, nutritional care should be modified, and parenteral nutrition (Chapter 35) may be necessary. The same kind of evaluation can be made for protein intake, vitamin C intake or the intake of any other nutrient. The NI for each nutrient can be plotted on a graph to provide a visual as well as a percentage evaluation of the patient's actual nutrient intake compared with the desirable intake.

As the evaluation reveals that objectives are not being met or that new needs have arisen, the process begins again with reassessment, identification of new needs, setting of objectives and so on. Table 20–2 summarizes the nutritional care process, including the criteria necessary for each step.

THE NUTRITIONAL CARE RECORD

The nutritional care process, as applied to a patient either in a hospital or an outpatient setting, must be documented in the health record. Documentation of the nutritional care plan has the following advantages:

1. It helps the patient to understand his nutritional care and to know that he will have to be an active participant.
2. It helps ensure that nutritional care will be relevant, complete and effective by providing a record that identifies the problems and sets criteria for evaluating the care.
3. It allows the entire health team to understand the rationale for nutritional care and the means by which it will be provided.
4. It allows the entire health team to participate in the nutritional care and to reinforce the patient's education whenever there is an opportunity.

Fortunately, much of the information needed for nutritional care is already collected by various health professionals: dietitian-nutritionists, physicians, nurses and social workers. For example, a physician will ask about gastrointestinal disturbances and a nurse usually will weigh and measure the patient and ask about any food allergies. Social workers frequently ask about the amount of money available for food and about the patient's living conditions. But this information needs to be organized and recorded in one place as part of the nutritional care record, so that it can be used to make a nutritional assessment and formulate a picture of nutritional needs. The nutritional care record ensures that all aspects of nutritional care are noted in one place as part of the total health record.

A detailed nutritional care record may be kept by the clinical dietitian, but if this is the case, the information it contains should be summarized periodically in the permanent health record (Fig. 20–1). This detailed infor-

Table 20–2   THE NUTRITIONAL CARE PROCESS

STEPS	COMPONENTS	FACTORS TO CONSIDER
1. *Assessment of Nutritional Status* 　　Collect information (data base). 　　Identify problems.	Dietary history. Biochemical data. Clinical examination findings. Medical history. Anthropometric data. Psychosocial data.	The information should be accurate, pertinent to the patient and appropriately interpreted. The problems should be numbered the same as those in the medical record, given priority ratings in the order of their importance, related to assessment data and should include present and potential problems.
2. *Planning of Nutritional Care* 　　Set objectives.	Additional information needed. Available resources. Educational level of patient and family. Modification of dietary intake. Supplementation of nutrient intake. Measures to enable patient to meet nutritional requirements. Treatment of medical problems affecting nutritional status.	Objectives should be patient-centered, stated in behavioral terms, realistic, measurable, designated as short- or long-term and numbered according to problem that they are designed to deal with.
3. *Implementation of Nutritional Care* 　　Determine nutritional interventions.	Modification of intake as required to make it acceptable to the patient. Teaching patient and family about the nutritional care plan. Provision of necessary nutritional supplements in acceptable form. Resolution of health problems. Enrollment of the patient in food assistance programs if necessary.	Interventions should be numbered according to the problem and objective, individualized for each patient and specific in describing what, how, why, when and where.
4. *Evaluation of Nutritional Care*	Monitoring of food and fluid intake; evaluation of intake for adequacy in meeting patient's nutritional needs. Assessment of nutritional knowledge as reflected in behavioral change. Monitoring of biochemical data related to nutritional status. Monitoring of anthropometric data. Monitoring of clinical condition.	Evaluation should include a comparison between observed behavior and expected behavior, a determination of the effectiveness of intervention in meeting objectives, an explanation of the effectiveness or ineffectiveness of intervention and suggestions for revision of the care plan based on evaluation.

mation is especially important for hospital care audits, professional standards review committees and other efforts to maintain quality health care. See Figure 20–2 for an example of a nutritional care record.

Parts of the nutritional care record may be incorporated into the nursing care plan, which is a detailed record kept by the nurse and periodically summarized for inclusion in the medical record.

NUTRITIONAL INTERVENTION—DIET MODIFICATION

ADEQUATE NORMAL DIET AS A BASIS FOR THERAPEUTIC DIETS

All therapeutic diets are modifications of the normal or adequate diet pattern. The hospital's general diets and the individual's normal diet are the basis for therapeutic diets. Regardless of the type prescribed, the aim or purpose of the diet is to supply needed nutrients to the body. Before discussing any therapeutic diets, either general or specific, the adequate normal diet will be reviewed. (Also review Chapter 10.)

There are many ways to plan a diet that will be nutritious and adequate. To be certain that the dietary allowances are fulfilled, the safest procedure is to include certain specified amounts of foods in the daily diet. The Basic Food Groups (Table 10–4) will serve as guides when planning adequate therapeutic diets, taking into consideration the adjustments and changes necessary to meet the abnormal conditions.

For the normal healthy adult the foundation of an adequate diet provides approximately 63

gm. of protein and 1200 kcal. (See Table 10–4.) To provide heat and energy and to produce or maintain normal weight, more of the foods listed or other foods are added. Eating these additional foods will also raise the amounts of required nutrients taken in.

In evaluating the foundation of an adequate diet, the amount of protein allowed is adequate but not excessive. The fruits and vegetables recommended provide bulk to avoid feelings of hunger and residue to prevent constipation. Mineral salts and vitamins are furnished by the foods. Iodized salt is recommended unless its use is contraindicated. Since every food is needed in the specified amount, any item omitted should be replaced by another food of equal value.

The Recommended Dietary Allowances developed by the Food and Nutrition Board of the National Research Council (Table 10–1) have been used extensively as a guide for good dietary planning in hospitals, institutions, school feeding programs, the Armed Forces and in normal everyday living. The foundation of an adequate diet, which has already been described, is patterned after the recommended allowances. There are many combinations of foods that will provide the recommended nutrient allowances. When normal or therapeutic diets are planned, the best use can be made of the allowances by using foods that are available in the locality and that are particularly suited to the nationality and specific income level of the individual, with amounts adjusted to cover the needs caused by illness.

The normal diet is not rigid. It is a flexible plan that supplies the body with all the nutrients needed in the *normal* processes of metabolism. Each nutrient must be supplied in sufficient amounts and with relation to each other so the diet will be both adequate and correctly balanced.

Balanced Diet. A diet that supplies all the nutrients needed for good health in the right amounts with the right relationships to each other is what nutritionists call a *balanced diet.* Balance can be attained by eating a large variety of protective foods. These include the Basic Food Groups or the foundation of an adequate diet, described here and in Chapter 10.

Normal Diet. A *normal diet* is an adequate diet that furnishes the body with all the nutrients necessary for the growth and repair of tissues and the normal functioning of the organs. *Normal* is a relative term, and what can be considered "normal" depends to some extent upon the individual. The body's requirements are very definite. It needs protein for building and repairing body tissue, carbohydrate and fat for providing heat and energy and minerals for making bones and teeth, maintaining the proper reaction of the body fluids and regulating the body processes. Vitamins, indispensable in regulating the body functions, and water, essential to every cell, are included in the adequate normal diet. For optimum health the body must have food that supplies the nutrients in correct amounts and proportions.

Standardization. The term *diet standardization* is not readily accepted by people who have been accustomed to the freedom of selection. It sounds perilously like regimentation and it is apt to produce a feeling of physical and spiritual limitation among those whom it affects. Diets should not be standardized even though the basic requirements have been established. Allowing selection from a wide variety of foods shows recognition of individual likes and dislikes.

THE DIET PRESCRIPTION

Modifications of the normal diet pattern are indicated for a number of diseases. The following are some general principles of dietary man-

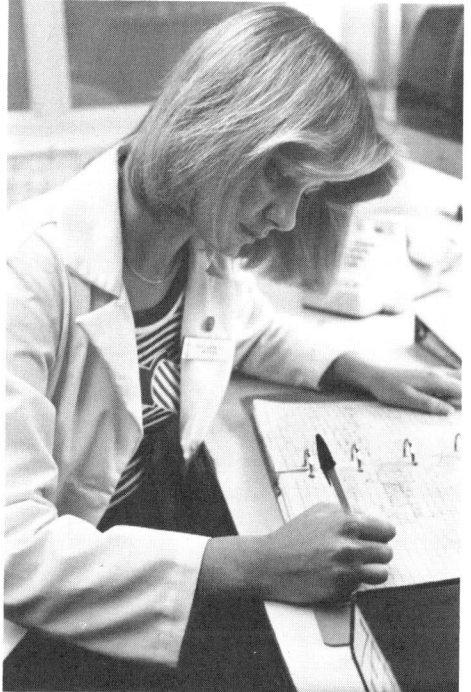

Figure 20–1 Dietitian documenting nutritional care. (Courtesy of Ms. Sheila Henderson, R. D., and the nutrition staff of Lutheran General Hospital, Park Ridge, Ill.)

NUTRITIONAL CARE RECORD

Dr. _____ Rm. No. _____

Address _____
and
Phone No. _____

Age _____ Sex _____

Problem List

Nutritional Care Flow Sheet: Weights, Lab Values, I&O& Dates									
Date									
Wgt.									
N/kcal. ratio									
Intake–tray pro./kcal.									
Intake–Supps. pro./kcal.									
Intake–P. Vein pro./kcal.									
Intake–C. Vein pro./kcal.									
Urine cc./24 hr.									
Stools Avg./24 hr.									

NUTRITIONAL CARE PLAN

Basal Energy Expenditure: _____ kcal.
Anabolic Req.: _____ kcal. _____ gm. pro. _____ gm. N
Maintenance Req.: _____ kcal. _____ gm. pro. _____ gm. N

Diet Calculation _____ kcal.
CHO =   Pro =   Fat =   Na$^+$ =

Time					
Milk					
Meat					
Bread					
Fruit					
Fat					
Veg.					
Misc. CHO					
Total P F C	P F C	PFC	PFC	PFC	PFC

EVALUATION OF NUTRITIONAL CARE—
PROGRESS NOTES

Date

RECOMMENDATIONS FOR FOLLOW-UP

NUTRITIONAL CARE RECORD (*Continued*)

ASSESSMENT—Data Base

Diet HX _____ Date 24 Hr. Recall	Medications/Vits. & Mins./Supplements
	<table><tr><td></td><td>Date</td><td></td><td>Date</td><td></td></tr></table>
	Medical HX and Clinical Findings
Allergies: Use of sugar: _____ salt: _____ Use of alcohol: _____ none _____ occas. _____ oz. _____ often Fluid intake _____	Social HX

Feeding and G.I. Habits
   Consistency of food:
   Appetite:
   Bowel habits:
   Recent chngs. in eating habits:
   Recent wgt. chngs.:
   Dental condition:
	Activities
	   Occup.: _____ hr./wk.
	   Exercise _____

	Anthropometry
	   Skinfold thickness: Arm circumf.: % Body fat:
	   Arm muscle circumf.:
	   Frame type: S M L IBW: Surface area:

Evaluation of Intake
   P _____ Cal. _____ _____ _____
   F _____ _____ _____ _____
   C _____ _____ _____ _____
	Patient's
	Hgt: Wgt: Wgt. goal: Usual wgt:

Figure 20–2   Nutritional care record records assessment data, the nutritional care plan, intervention strategies and monitoring and evaluation data.

agement and nutritional care for a specific disease:

1. The therapeutic diet should vary from the individual's normal diet as little as possible, unless the normal diet is inadequate.

2. The diet should meet the body's requirements for essential nutrients as generously as the disease condition permits.

3. The diet regimen should recognize and take into account the patient's food intake habits and food preferences, his economic status and religious practices and any environmental factors that have bearing on the diet, such as where the meals are eaten and who prepares them. (See Fig. 20–3.)

The diet prescription in nutrition serves the same purpose as the drug prescription in medicine. It designates the type, amount, frequency and route of food ingestion just as the drug prescription identifies the drug name, dosage, frequency and route of administration. The diet prescription includes the daily caloric

requirements based on the individual's desirable weight and normal activity plus the amounts and forms of needed protein, fat, carbohydrate, minerals, vitamins and other substances such as fluid and fiber. The Recommended Dietary Allowances for different age groups may be used as a *guide* only, since variations or deviations from the average are not considered in the RDA. In the food prescription the individual variations are taken into account. The construction of the diet prescription will be discussed in detail.

Calorie Allowance to Meet Energy Requirement

It is quite possible to estimate roughly the calories required by a normal person. Nature supplies a very good checking device, the appetite, and in most normally active people it regulates the weight with surprising accuracy. However, the appetite cannot always be

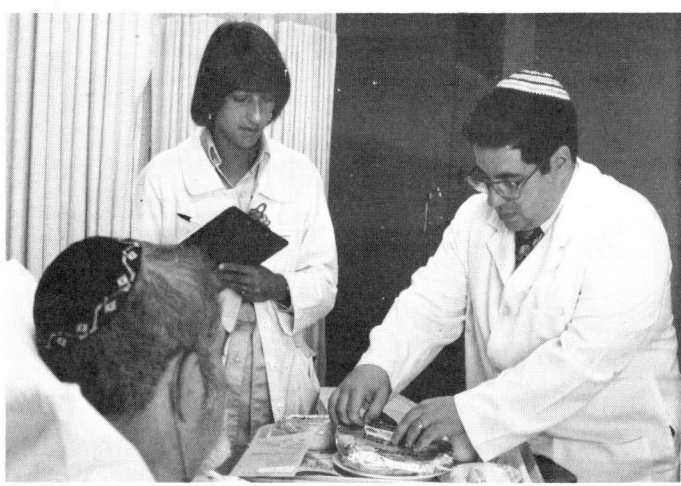

Figure 20–3 Rabbi blessing a kosher meal. (Courtesy of Ms. Sheila Henderson, R.D., and the nutrition staff of Lutheran General Hospital, Park Ridge, Ill.)

trusted or depended upon in disease and in obesity.

The average adult afebrile patient at bed rest with minor injury or illness can maintain caloric balance by an intake of about 1600 kcal. per day. Severe injury or illness may increase the needs from 2500 to 4000 kcal. per day. An individual who was severely depleted before the illness or injury may require an intake of 3500 kcal. or more. Other situations requiring increased calories will be discussed in the forthcoming chapters. It should be mentioned that the caloric requirement must be considered in relation to the need for other nutrients. In diseases or injuries in which there is a tendency to lose protein, the administration of 50 to 100 per cent more calories than the calculated requirement has, at times, made it possible to maintain protein equilibrium. For ambulatory patients, the factors for determining calorie requirements are their levels of activity and the appropriateness of their present weights.

For practical purposes, the energy requirement of an individual may be determined by either (1) calculating the number of kcal. per kilogram per day or (2) calculating the per cent increase over basal demands. To make the determinations, the desirable weight based on sex, age, height and body build (frame) is used. (See Chapter 2, Energy.) The desirable weight for an individual may be obtained from Appendix Tables 14 to 17. The daily caloric allowances are determined according to the activity of the individual. (See Table 20–3.) Restlessness of a bed patient may increase the requirement 10 to 20 per cent. Fever increases calorie requirements 10 per cent for each degree Celsius above normal temperature. Desirable weight is used instead of actual weight in determining a patient's requirements because the present weight of the individual may be abnormal as a result of undernutrition or obesity. Synonyms for desirable weight are *ideal, standard, normal, average* and *expected* weight. The abbreviation IBW, for ideal body weight, is often used.

The determination of the energy requirement of an individual is illustrated in the following example.

Example: Let's suppose that the patient referred to earlier in this chapter (Ms. A.) is a 20 year old student who has a height of 162.5 cm. (5 ft., 5 in.) and medium body build. According to Appendix Table 15 she has a desirable weight of 53.6 kg. (118 lb.). Her activity level is light, which, according to Table 20–3, shows that she requires 35 to 40 kcal. per kg. per day. Thus, her average calorie allowance would be 53.6 multiplied by 35 to 40 or 1876 to 2144 (average 2010) kcal. per day.

The energy requirement could also be calculated by determining the percentage increase over the basal calorie requirement. By consulting the third column in Table 20–3, one finds that there would be a 40 to 60 per cent increase over the student's basal demands. Energy requirements calculated for the same student using this method would be as follows:

53.6 kg. × 25 kcal./kg./day = 1340 kcal. = basal requirement.

To this add 40 to 60 per cent for activity:

1340 + 536 to 804 = 1876 to 2144 kcal./day

Rapid Calorie Requirement Calculations. Food specialists in the USDA worked out a formula for calculating a person's daily energy requirement rapidly. The desirable weight in pounds is multiplied by 21 for a man and by

18 for a woman. The result is the approximate number of calories used daily by a moderately active adult. For very active individuals, 25 per cent more calories are required; for a sedentary individual, 25 per cent less.

Example: Using the same subject as above, the calories used daily would be:

118 lb. × 18 = 2124 kcal.

Protein Allowance

After calculating the daily calorie allowance, the protein fraction of the diet is determined. At least one third of the adult protein fraction should consist of animal or complete protein, which contains the essential amino acids. Vegetable proteins are termed incomplete because they do not contain all the essential amino acids. (See Chapter 5, Proteins.)

Protein is essential to life. The recommended daily allowance based on the utilization value of 70 per cent for food proteins is 0.8 gm. of protein per kg. of body weight for adults (54 gm. and 46 gm. for the reference man and woman, respectively). The RDA is usually considered adequate for previously well-nourished individuals who are ambulatory patients or who require only brief periods of hospitalization. The minimum protein for nitrogen equilibrium ranges from approximately 25 to 40 gm., depending upon the quality of protein ingested. The bed patient who requires more than 10 days' hospitalization, the patient losing protein (from burns, exudates, ascites or renal disease) and the patient not forming sufficient protein (hepatic disease) will require an increase. Currently, the trend is to use a liberal protein allowance rather than limit the fraction. Therefore, optimum rather than adequate protein levels are recommended.

Severe depletion of body protein can lead to prolonged convalescence, poor wound healing, an increase in complications after surgery, anemia and increased susceptibility to infections, as well as other complications.

The protein foods of high biological value are usually the most expensive diet items. Thus, there is often a tendency among individuals in the low income groups to consume less animal protein than the recommended amount. If the income is limited, less expensive proteins such as cheese, canned evaporated or powdered milk, beans and legumes are used, since most animal proteins (meat, eggs, fresh milk and poultry) are frequently more expensive. See Table 18–10 for the cost of various servings of protein.

Cultural customs, individuaal food habits and the supply of foods available are additional factors that influence the protein intake.

The determination of the protein fraction of an individual's diet is illustrated in the following example.

Example: Using the same 20 year old female student previously mentioned, the protein allowance would be:

53.6 × 0.8 = 43 gm. of protein per day

Fat and Carbohydrate Allowances

Following the calculation of the protein fraction, the remainder of the calories in the diet are determined and are assigned to fat and carbo-

Table 20–3   RECOMMENDED CALORIE ALLOWANCES FOR ENERGY REQUIREMENTS

	ADULT[a]			CHILD[b]	
Activity	*Kcal./ Kg./Day*	*Increase Over Basal Calories (%)*		*Age*	*Kcal./ Kg./Day*
			Both sexes:		
Basal or standard	25		1–2		100–95
Minimal (bed rest)	27.5	10	3–5		95–80
Very light (typist)	30–35	20–40	6–9		80–75
Light (medical student, teacher, nurse)	35–40	40–60	10–13		75–60
			Girls:		
Moderate (homemaker, metal worker)	40–45	60–80	14–15		50–45
Hard (carpenter, housemaid at hard work)	45–50	80–100	16–17		45–40
Severe (farmer, laundress at hard work)	50–70	100–180	18–19		40–35
			Boys:		
Very severe (miner, lumberman)	75	200	14–17		65–60
			18–19		55–50

[a]Based on desirable weight.
[b]Based on age.

Table 20–4   SUGGESTED PROTEIN, FAT AND CARBOHYDRATE ALLOWANCES

AGE OR CONDITION	PROTEINS (*Gm./Kg.*)	FATS (*Gm./Kg.*)	CARBOHYDRATES (*Gm./Kg.*)
Under 1 year	2.0–2.2	2–3	6–10
1–3	1.8	2–3	6–10
4–6	1.5	2–3	6–10
7–10	1.2	2–3	6–10
11–18	0.9–1.0	2–3	6–10
Adult	0.8	1–2	4–6
Pregnancy	+30	1–2	4–6
Lactation	+20	1–2	4–6

hydrate. What is the correct or optimum proportion of fat to carbohydrate to meet the requirements of the body under various conditions? Exact data on this ratio are scarce. Economic factors dictate the diets of much of the population, and they select a high percentage of the cheaper carbohydrates. The present recommendation for Americans is to increase the carbohydrate content of the diet so that it provides 50 to 60 per cent of the calories.

Present knowledge of nutrition emphasizes the possible harmfulness of too much fat. The American Heart Association and the Senate Select Committee on Nutrition and Human Needs recommend that 30 to 35 per cent of total calories in the diet come from fat.[5] A suggested distribution of proteins, fats and carbohydrates in the diet is shown in Table 20–4. (Review Chapter 3, Carbohydrates, and Chapter 4, Lipids.)

The average daily food intake of an individual without dietary restrictions amounts to about 60 to 90 gm. of protein, 90 to 120 gm. of fat and 300 to 400 gm. of carbohydrate. This proportion may have to be varied to meet the needs caused by certain diseases, and this will be discussed later.

A rapid, satisfactory clinical method for calculating the constituents of a food prescription consists of dividing the total calorie allowance into approximately 10 to 15 per cent protein, 25 to 35 per cent fat and 50 to 65 per cent carbohydrate.

Example: Continuing with the same 20 year old female student used in the examples for calorie and protein allowances, the fat and carbohydrate needs are calculated.

Protein intake already determined: 43 gm.
4 kcal./gm. × 43 gm. protein = 172 kcal. or 8 per cent of kcal. from protein.

Fats make up 25 to 35 per cent of kcal., in this case 35 per cent.

Total kcal. requirement (2010) × 0.35 = 703 kcal. from fat.

$$\frac{703 \text{ kcal.}}{9 \text{ kcal./gm. fat}} = 78 \text{ gm. of fat}$$

$$= 1.5 \text{ gm. fat/kg.}$$

(Note: fats in the diet average 1 to 2 gm. per kg. IBW, depending on energy needs.)

Carbohydrates make up remainder of kcal.: 57 per cent in this case.

Total kcal. requirement (2010) × 0.57 = 1146 kcal. from carbohydrate.

$$\frac{1146 \text{ kcal.}}{4 \text{ kcal./gm. CHO}} = 286 \text{ gm. of carbohydrate}$$

$$= 5.3 \text{ gm. CHO/kg.}$$

(Note: carbohydrates in the diet usually average 4 to 6 gm. per kg. IBW.)

Minerals and Vitamins

In addition to total calorie, protein, fat and carbohydrate allowances, the diet must satisfy the requirements for the essential minerals and vitamins. All of the foods included in the basic plan were selected particularly because of their essential mineral and vitamin contributions.

Minerals. The requirements for sulfur, phosphorus and potassium, which are laid down with nitrogen in the formation of tissue protoplasm, are increased in certain conditions such as starvation, injury, burns and diabetic acidosis. The efficiency of a high-protein diet may be decreased if these minerals are not supplied in sufficient amounts. In acute conditions, sodium and chloride are also of special concern. The Recommended Dietary Allowances (Table 10–1) are considered adequate for

the other minerals in acute or semiacute situations, but in long-term hospitalization or rehabilitation, calcium, iron, iodine and zinc are of major importance.

The amount of iron in the average American diet is believed to be about 6 mg. per 1000 kcal. For the adult male 10 mg. daily is recommended. The adult female in the childbearing years needs 18 mg. according to the RDA revised in 1974. A supplement of iron or iron-fortified foods is indicated.

In severe sodium-restricted diets the iodine content may be below the requirements of approximately 1 μg. per kg. These will be considered in subsequent chapters with the various diseases.

The RDA for zinc is 15 mg. per day but may be higher in patients with malabsorption syndromes. Zinc sulfate therapy has been shown to improve wound healing. (See Chapter 34, Nutritional Care for Patients with Surgery, Burns or Trauma; and review Chapter 7, Minerals.)

Vitamins. Vitamin requirements under stress situations have not been completely determined, although we know more about them now than before. Vitamin requirements during specific disease states or when using particular medications will be discussed in subsequent chapters.

Sometimes up to ten times the normal Recommended Dietary Allowances will be necessary. However, in many instances these large intakes are probably not indicated, and in the case of vitamins A and D they may be harmful. Since accurate metabolic studies of vitamin requirements during and after disease and injury are lacking, the requirements must be approximated. In arriving at suggested allowances, Pollack and Halpern consider the following factors: (1) requirements for normal individuals, (2) the nature of the disease or injury, (3) the known capacity of the body to store certain vitamins, (4) known losses through the skin, urine or intestinal tract produced by various phenomena and (5) the interrelations of nutrient requirements.[4] (Review Chapter 8, Vitamins.)

THIAMIN. Evidence indicates that a person's thiamin requirement is related to body weight and the caloric content of the diet. (See p. 164.) The requirement is further influenced by the amount of carbohydrate in the diet, since the enzymes containing thiamin are involved in carbohydrate metabolism. A liberal allowance of thiamin is advisable when patients are recieving glucose intravenously. There is no evidence that in minor injuries or illness the thiamin requirements are greatly increased above normal. However, in severely injured and diseased individuals the thiamin allowance may be increased to about 5 mg. daily. When a definite depletion exists, as is possible in chronic alcoholism, 10 to 25 mg. of thiamin per day may be indicated for the first week to ten days, followed by a maintenance dose of 5 mg. daily until convalescence is well along.

Thiamin deficiency is sometimes precipitated during the refeeding of starved persons. The increased calorie and carbohydrate intake sharply increases the body demands for this vitamin. When oral antibiotics are administered, thiamin requirements, as well as requirements for the other B-complex vitamins, may be increased as a result of the drugs[2] interference with the biosynthesis of thiamin. The excessive use of antacids may cause an alkaline destruction of thiamin before it is absorbed from the gastrointestinal tract.

Example: Continuing with the same 20 year old female student, the thiamin allowance would be: 0.5 mg. per 1000 kcal. per day or 1.0 mg. per 2000 kcal. diet per day.

RIBOFLAVIN. The allowances recommended by the Food and Nutrition Board of the National Research Council are based on calorie intake and body size. Riboflavin requirements in disease have not been clearly defined. Minor illnesses and injuries should not alter the requirement if food consumption is normal. However, after a severe injury, illness or burn the requirements may be increased five to ten times over what is normal.

Example: Continuing with the same 20 year old female student, the riboflavin allowance would be: 0.6 mg. per 1000 kcal. per day or 1.2 mg. per 2000 kcal. diet per day.

NIACIN. Niacin requirements in health and disease are related to the intake of tryptophan-containing protein. The amino acid tryptophan can serve as a precursor of niacin. Like thiamin, it plays an important role in intermediary carbohydrate metabolism. The current RDA of 6.6 mg. per 1000 kcal. per day is based on calorie intake and expressed as niacin equivalents, including dietary sources of the preformed vitamin and the precursor tryptophan. (See p. 167.)

Little is known concerning the metabolism and requirement for niacin in stress situations. It has been suggested that, following severe injury, infection and burns, the metabolism of niacin is altered in a manner similar to that of other members of the B-complex. During the

acute phase of the disease or injury and also in the early period of convalescence, at least 50 to 100 mg. of niacinamide has been recommended. In cases of previous depletion or deficiency, niacinamide in amounts up to 500 mg. per day is administered during the first seven to ten days or longer.

Example: Continuing with the same 20 year old female student, the niacin allowance would be: 6.6 mg. per 1000 kcal. per day or 13.2 mg. niacin equivalent per 2000 kcal. diet per day.

PANTOTHENIC ACID AND VITAMIN B_6 (PYRIDOXINE). It is generally believed that the amount of pantothenic acid needed is 5 to 10 mg. (10 times the thiamin requirement). A 2000 kcal. diet will provide about 10 mg. Authorities recommend that this vitamin and pyridoxine be included in the dietary supplements of individuals who have undergone nutritional depletion or who are forced to subsist on processed foods for any length of time.

There is no evidence to indicate that the requirements for these two substances are related to calories. A specific relationship exists between vitamin B_6 and the metabolism of tryptophan; the requirement for vitamin B_6 increases with the protein in the diet. (See p. 170.) The Food and Nutrition Board of the National Research Council recommended an intake of 2 mg. per day, which they believed would be adequate for the metabolism of 100 gm. of protein.

FOLIC ACID AND VITAMIN B_{12}. During certain stress situations, the hematopoietic system may be depressed. Both vitamin B_{12} and folic acid have some relation to normal hematopoiesis. Folacin is used in the treatment of nutritional megaloblastic anemia caused by folate deficiency. The amount needed is influenced by body size and metabolic rate. The RDA for adults has been set at 0.4 mg.

Many pregnant women manifest a folacin deficiency in the last trimester. Stressful conditons such as hemolytic anemia, leukemia, Hodgkin's disease, carcinomatosis, hyperthyroidism and malabsorption syndromes as well as the consumption of alcohol also increase the requirement for folacin.

Folacin does not relieve the neurological symptoms of pernicious anemia. If absorption is normal, a dietary intake of 3 μg. per day of vitamin B_{12} is required to meet the needs of adults. Pernicious anemia patients will respond to as little as 0.1 μg. by intramuscular injection or 5 to 15 μg. taken orally with the intrinsic factor. A diet of 15 μg. will gradually replenish body stores. A B_{12} deficiency can precipitate a folic acid deficiency because of the "folate trap." (See page 614.)

ASCORBIC ACID. Ascorbic acid requirements in stress are reported to be abnormally high. This is most likely caused by increased utilization, not necessarily by a pre-existing deficiency. However, opinions differ fairly widely regarding normal and therapeutic requirements for vitamin C. The Committee on Therapeutic Nutrition recommends as much as 1 to 2 gm. daily during acute stages of stress, and 300 mg. thereafter. Patients with burns, excessive trauma and fractures of the long bones probably require 1 gm. of ascorbic acid daily during the acute phase and 300 mg. thereafter until convalescence is established. Seventy to 100 mg. daily is then believed to be adequate. Under moderate stress circumstances, about 300 mg. daily is advised.

VITAMIN A. There is no evidence to date of an *increased* need for fat-soluble vitamin A for short-term illnesses *except* in hepatic disease where storage or availability of the vitamin may be less than normal. However, the normal requirement of 4000 to 5000 I.U. (800 to 1000 R.E.) should always be ensured.

VITAMIN D. There have been no studies to indicate that acute febrile bacterial diseases, surgical procedures and burns in any way alter the metabolism of vitamin D in adults. For fracture cases, however, because of the role of vitamin D in calcium and phosphorus metabolism, 400 I.U. of vitamin D should be ensured. Renal disease alters vitamin D metabolism (see Chapter 30), thus making large doses of the vitamin or small doses of the analog of the active form (1α -OHD_3) necessary. In malabsorption syndromes vitamin D is frequently not absorbed.

VITAMIN E. Therapeutic use of vitamin E has been under study in the treatment of a large number of conditions. It is known to be a useful treatment for hemolytic anemia of neonates. Some evidence supports its use among women who have had repeated spontaneous abortions. Some types of ulcers have responded to vitamin E therapy. Claims have been made for its effectiveness in treating complications of menopause, muscular dystrophy, diabetes, male infertility and heart disease, but evidence is lacking to support these claims. Those conditions that interfere with the absorption of fat (biliary tract diseases, pancreatic insufficiency, cystic fibrosis and ingestion of mineral oil) also interfere with the absorption of vitamin E. The

vitamin E requirement is increased when the intake of polyunsaturated fat is increased and in severe protein deficiency conditions.

VITAMIN K.   It is believed that vitamin K requirements are fulfilled by any mixed diet, except in certain stress conditions that may interfere with the absorption or metabolism of the vitamin and result in a deficiency. Oral administration of streptomycin greatly reduces the synthesis of vitamin K by intestinal organisms and other antibiotics may have similar effects. It is therefore suggested that vitamin K always be given when antibiotics or sulfonamides are given orally.

Fluids

Water, although not considered a food, is an indispensable nutrient and plays an important role in the proper functioning of the human body. It is always listed with foods.

Optimum convalescence demands normal tissue hydration. A normal healthy adult at rest and not sweating needs 1800 to 2500 ml. of water daily to provide for urinary secretion and to replace losses from insensible perspiration. Additional fluids must be added to replace water lost by excessive sweating, vomiting, diarrhea, tube drainage or other conditions in which there is increased water loss. (See Chapter 9, Water and Electrolytes.) If sufficient water is not obtained through fluid intake and food (Fig. 20–4), it must be supplied parenterally.

The sample in Table 20–5 shows how a completed food prescription for a normal adult, as described in the preceding pages, looks when finally assembled.

MODIFICATIONS OF THE NORMAL DIET

The normal diet may be modified and thereby become a specific therapeutic diet. The

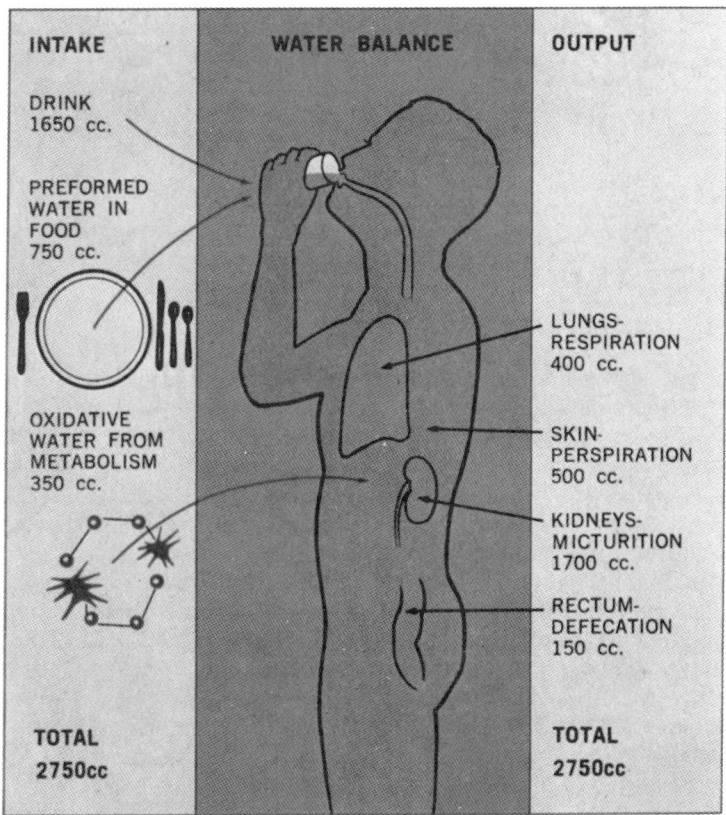

Figure 20–4   Humans maintain the osmotic pressure of body fluids at optimum level by adjusting water intake and output. Most of the amount needed is supplied by the liquid itself. Some is drawn from the moisture in food and the remainder is manufactured by the body itself. The importance of this "water of oxidation" varies according to species: the kangaroo rat, for example, drinks no water at all. His water need, proportionately the same as a human's, is met by the moisture in his diet and by what he manufactures himself. (From: Nutrition Today, 5:22, 1970.)

Table 20–5   CONSTRUCTION OF DAILY DIET PRESCRIPTION FOR A NORMAL ADULT

STANDARD ALLOWANCES		DIET PRESCRIPTION
Desirable Weight for:		53.6 kg. (118 lb.)
Sex		Female
Age		20 yr.
Height		162.5 cm. (5 ft., 5 in.)
Protein Allowance		
0.8 gm./kg. ideal body weight (IBW) or approximately 10 to 20% of total calories.		53.6 × 0.8 = 43 gm. protein.
Fat and Carbohydrate Allowances		
Fats average 1 to 2 gm./kg. IBW or approximately 25 to 35% of total calories.		53.6 × 1.5 = 80 gm. fat.
Carbohydrates average 4 to 6 gm./kg. IBW or approximately 50% of total calories.		53.6 × 5.2 = 280 gm. carbohydrate.
Energy or Calorie Allowance		
Activity: light.		
Calories required per kg. IBW per day: 35 to 40 kcal.		53.6 × 35 to 40 = 1876 to 2144 kcal. (2010 avg.)
Calories from Food Constituents		
Protein = 4 kcal./gm.		43 × 4 = 172 kcal.
Fat = 9 kcal./gm.		80 × 9 = 720 kcal.
Carbohydrate = 4 kcal./gm.		280 × 4 = 1120 kcal.
		2012 kcal.
Mineral Allowances		
Calcium:	0.8 gm./day.	Calcium: 0.8 gm./day.
Iodine:	100 μg./day.	Iodine: 100 μg./day.
Iron:	18 mg./day.	Iron: 18 mg./day.
Phosphorus:	0.8 gm./day.	Phosphorus: 0.8 gm./day.
Magnesium:	300 mg./day.	Magnesium: 300 mg./day.
Zinc:	15 mg./day.	Zinc: 15 mg./day.
Vitamin Allowances		
Vitamin A:	4000 I.U. (800 R.E.)/day.	Vitamin A: 4000 I.U. (800 R.E.)/day.
Thiamin:	0.5 mg./1000 kcal./day.	Thiamin: 1.0 mg./day.
Riboflavin:	0.6 mg./1000 kcal./day.	Riboflavin: 1.2 mg./day.
Niacin equiv.:	6.6 mg./1000 kcal./day.	Niacin equiv.: 13.2 mg./day.
Folacin:	400 μg./day.	Folacin: 400 μg./day.
Vitamin B_6:	2.0 mg./day.	Vitamin B_6: 2.0 mg./day.
Vitamin B_{12}:	3.0 μg./day.	Vitamin B_{12}: 3.0 μg./day.
Ascorbic acid:	45 mg./day.	Ascorbic acid: 45 mg./day.
Vitamin D:	400 I.U./day.	Vitamin D: 400 I.U./day.
Vitamin E:	12 I.U./day.	Vitamin E: 12 I.U./day.

substitutions and modifications are made to help compensate for the dysfunction of the affected body part, to meet the specific needs induced by a disease or to prevent a disease from developing or worsening.

Therapeutic diets may be classified as qualitative and quantitative modifications of the normal diet. The qualitative diet is an adequate diet adjusted according to the type of food allowed. The quantitative diet is calculated with an increase or decrease in the amount of the food constituents. To illustrate: gastrointestinal diets are qualitative while a diabetic diet is quantitative.

The adjustment in diet may take any of the following forms:

1. Change in consistency of foods. Examples: liquid diet, soft diet, low fiber diet, high fiber diet.
2. Increase or decrease in energy value of diet. Examples: reduction diet, high calorie diet.
3. Increase or decrease in type of foods. Examples: sodium-restricted diet, lactose-free diet.
4. Omission of specific foods. Example: allergy diet.
5. Adjustment in the ratio and balance of food constituents: proteins, fats and carbohydrates. Examples: diabetic diet, ketogenic diet, high protein diet, low fat diet.
6. Rearrangement of the number and frequency of meals. Example: gastric ulcer diet.

Some of the modifications may overlap in individual diets. For example, a patient may be on a diabetic diet but because of acute indigestion or poor teeth he may also require a soft diet.

Diets must be flexible in order to be practical and usable. Therefore, it is impossible to divide diets into separate and distinct categories. The recommended dietary allowances for food constituents established for normal body requirements are considered, with amounts of nutrients adjusted to cover the needs created by disease or injury, when modifications in the diet are indicated.

THE PRINCIPAL SOURCES OF FOOD CONSTITUENTS

To be familiar with the various foods included in a diet, it is necessary to know their analysis. For that reason, Table 20–6 was planned as an aid in learning the contents of various foods. Knowing the nutrients contained in different foods is essential for correctly evaluating therapeutic diets. Chapter 10 on an adequate diet may also be helpful. A more complete analysis of the nutrient content of foods can be found in Appendix Table 1.

NUTRITIONAL CARE FOR THE HOSPITALIZED PATIENT

Food served in any institution is not like that to which patients are accustomed, and the food served in hospitals is no exception. Patients come from all cultures and economic groups, and they bring their food habits with them.

Table 20–6 THE PRINCIPAL SOURCES OF THE VARIOUS FOOD CONSTITUENTS*

Daggers on the chart below give a rough idea of how servings from groups of familiar foods contribute toward dietary needs—the more daggers, the better the food as a source of the nutrient. The percentages given below the chart are based on the National Research Council's recommended dietary allowances for a young, moderately active man. Some foods within a group have more of a nutrient, some less; but in a varied diet, which is common in this country, a group is likely to average as shown.

KIND OF FOOD	SIZE OF SERVING (READY-TO-EAT)	PROTEIN	CALCIUM	IRON	VIT. A	THIAMIN	RIBOFLAVIN	NIACIN	VIT. C	KCAL.
Milk	1 cup	†	††††		†	†	††			165
Cheese, process Cheddar	1 oz.	†	†††		†		†			105
Meat, poultry, fish	4 oz.	††		††	†	†	†	††		195
Eggs	1 large	†		†	†		†			80
Dry beans and peas, nuts	¾ cup cooked	††	†	†††		†	†	†		170
Whole grain or enriched products	2 slices	†	†	†		†	†	†		120
Citrus fruits	½ cup								†††††	50
Other fruits	½ cup			†	†				†	60
Tomatoes, tomato juice	½ cup			†	†††			†	†††	25
Dark green and deep yellow vegetables (except sweet potatoes)	½ cup		†	†	†††††		†		††††	40
Sweet potatoes	1 medium		†	†	†††††	†	†	†	†††	170
Light green vegetables[b]	½ cup		†	†	†				††	35
Potatoes	1 medium			†		†		†	†††	90
Other vegetables	½ cup			†					†	40
Butter, margarine	1 tbsp.				†					100
Other fats	2 tbsp.									220
Sugar, all kinds	2 tsp.									35
Molasses, syrups	2 tbsp.			††						110

†††††More than 50 per cent of daily need. †††About 30 per cent of daily need.
††††About 40 per cent of daily need. ††About 20 per cent of daily need.
†About 10 per cent of daily need.

[a]Foods supplying thiamin, riboflavin and niacin are good sources of other members of the B vitamin group.
[b]Includes asparagus, green snap beans, peas, green lima beans, green cabbage, brussels sprouts, green lettuce.
*From: Family Fare: Food Management and Recipes. Home and Garden Bulletin No. 1. Washington, D.C., U.S. Department of Agriculture, 1960.

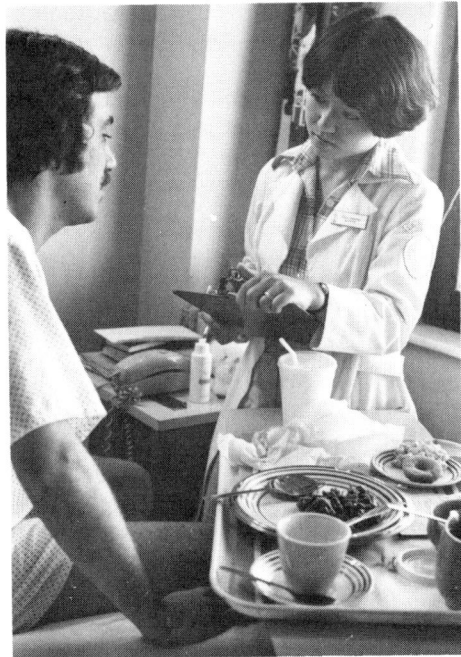

Figure 20–5 Clinical dietitian talking with a patient. (Courtesy of Ms. Sheila Henderson, R.D., and the nutrition staff of Lutheran General Hospital, Park Ridge, Ill.)

Illness with its stress and anxiety affects appetite, taste, the digestion and utilization of foods and the personalities of individuals. The kind of diet is suitable for the person's nutritional needs is prescribed by his physician or recommended by the clinical dietitian. (See Fig. 20–5.) An important aspect of the therapeutic measures instituted for the hospitalized person is the nutritional care.

Food service to patients requires imagination and ingenuity in planning for a variety of foods familiar to them. The appearance of the food on the tray—its color, texture, composition and temperature—is important to most people. Seasonings and flavorings are often restricted and this usually adds to the eating problems encountered in giving care.

NUTRITIONAL ADEQUACY OF HOSPITAL DIETS

All hospitals and institutions engaged in feeding the sick have some specific, basic, routine diets designed for uniformity and convenience of service. These standard diets are based on the foundation of an adequate diet pattern (Chapter 10, Table 10–4), which is formulated from the Recommended Daily Dietary Allowances, as already outlined and discussed in this chapter.

The nutritional requirements for the hospitalized patient should be determined after assessment of:

1. The nutritional status of the individual.

2. The individual's history of recent surgery, medication, radiation therapy, chemotherapy or other medical treatments.

3. The amount and types of nutrients being lost from the body.

4. The effect of the present disease and of the medical and surgical therapy on the individual's ingestion, absorption, utilization and excretion of nutrients.

5. The anticipated duration of the stress, disease or injury and the proposed medical and surgical therapy.

Unfortunately, too many of the therapeutic diets outlined in hospital manuals do not supply the nutrients necessary for maintaining good nutrition during the acute phase of an illness, and insufficient attention is given to the extra requirements needed for the convalescent and rehabilitative phases of medical care. The Recommended Dietary Allowances are intended for healthy, active people and are not adequate for many sick and injured individuals. A normally adequate diet may be inadequate for an individual suffering from prolonged physical or emotional stress or receiving medical therapy. These conditions may interfere with the utilization of food and bring about a nutritional deficiency. Standard hospital diets must attempt to fulfill the increased metabolic demands created by stress or illness. The interpretation of the standard diets for the individual patient must be a liberal one, since we unfortunately do not know the exact nutritional requirements of patients who have various diseases.

Standard Diets

The types of standard diets are usually referred to as *general, light, soft* and *liquid*. These diets are used routinely for patients not requiring a therapeutic diet, depending upon their food tolerance and physical condition. It is important for the nurse to be familiar with the principles and contents of the various diets, since they serve as a foundation for the diversified therapeutic diets.

Food Intake

An important observation for the nurse to make is that the food *served* does not necessarily represent the food *intake* of the patient. In a hospital food intake study conducted by one of

the authors (unpublished data), a week's survey of the patients who were served general diets showed a daily variation in patients' intake of between 1900 and 3200 kcal., with the average patient's intake approximately 2570 kcal. When the patients in semiprivate rooms selected food from a menu of approximately 2500 to 3000 kcal., about 25 per cent of the bread, butter and vegetables and 37 per cent of the salads were not eaten. The ward patients on a nonselective general diet of approximately the same number of calories left between 5 and 10 per cent of the food uneaten.

In another hospital food intake study[1] it was observed that patients eating from trays appeared to consume diets of higher nutritive value than did ambulatory patients eating in a dining room. However, possible food consumption outside of regular meals was not observed or known. The *average* figures showed a food intake approximating the Recommended Dietary Allowances for the healthy subject, but *individual* records indicated that the food selection and consumption of some patients would not provide sufficient nutrients to meet the standard. Most noticeable was the low intake of fruits and vegetables by some patients, which resulted in a large number whose intakes were below recommendations for ascorbic acid and vitamin A.

One of the ways to prevent iatrogenic malnutrition in our hospitals is to observe and record the patient's intake frequently and as accurately as possible. In a few hospitals, the nutrient content of each person's recorded food intake can be determined by using a specially programmed computer; in others the dietitian can manually calculate the composition of the food intake.

Regardless of the type of diet prescribed for a patient, it is important to check both the food served and the food left on the tray in order to obtain an accurate indication of the patient's calorie and nutrition intake. This is very important and should not be overlooked.

THE GENERAL OR ADEQUATE NORMAL DIET

In some hospitals the general diet is also known as the "regular," "full" or "house" diet. The general diet is a basic adequate normal diet of approximately 2000 to 2500 kcal. and contains 60 to 80 gm. of protein, 80 to 100 gm. of fat and 200 to 300 gm. of carbohydrate. All the protective foods outlined in the foundation of an adequate diet pattern, which includes the basic four food groups (meat, milk, eggs, citrus fruits, vegetables, whole grain or enriched breads and cereals) are included. Additional foods or more of the same food, such as butter or fortified margarine, desserts, salad dressing, crackers and sugar, are added to increase calories and to make the diet more palatable. There are no particular food restrictions. However, foods that may cause digestive disturbances, such as cooked cabbage and fried pork, are used with discretion. A few hospitals are instituting the prudent diet of the American Heart Association, which is low in saturated fat and cholesterol, as the general diet. (See Chapter 28.)

An example of an average general diet is shown in Table 20–7. In most hospitals the general diet may be selected by the patient from a menu of nutritious foods. This allows the patient to select foods that he or she likes, yet controls the adequacy of the diet to some extent.

THE SOFT OR LIGHT DIET

The soft or light diet (Table 20–8) is used as a transition diet. It is an adequate diet that is moderately low in cellulose and connective tissue. Fried foods are omitted. The soft diet is planned for conditions in which mechanical ease in eating, digestion or both is desired. It is also a diet low in residue. It is good for patients who have few or no teeth or ill-fitting dental plates.

The average composition of the soft diet is 1800 to 2000 kcal. However, the calories as well as the protein, fat and carbohydrate allowances are adjustable according to the individual's needs, based on activity, height, weight, sex, age and any specific demands caused by disease.

The current trend in diet planning fosters liberal interpretation of the soft diet, particularly with regard to vegetables. Vegetable purées are notoriously unpopular and patients often refuse to eat them. To prove the point one large hospital[3] omitted vegetable purées from the soft diet in favor of cooked low-fiber vegetables. The result was a more palatable diet and happier patients, who benefited from eating vegetables that previously they had refused.

The hospitals following the trend of more liberal diet interpretation and planning serve fine whole-grain or enriched bread and cereals on soft diets.

Foods Included
Milk: Milk beverage, buttermilk, cream.

Table 20–7 GENERAL OR ADEQUATE NORMAL DIET

MEAL PLAN	SAMPLE MENU	SERVINGS GRAMS	SERVINGS HOUSEHOLD MEASURE
	Breakfast		
Fruit	Fresh grapefruit	100	1 half (no skin)
Cereal	Cooked oatmeal (cooked weight)	118	½ cup
Egg	Soft cooked egg	50	1
Bread	Whole wheat toast	23	1 slice
Butter	Butter or fortified margarine	7	1 pat
Milk	Milk	244	1 cup
Cream	Cream	60	2 oz.
Sugar	Sugar	15	3 tsp.
Coffee	Coffee	200	2 coffee cups
	Lunch		
Soup	Beef broth with rice	125	½ cup
Crackers	Saltines	8	2
Entrée	Macaroni and cheese	110	½ cup
Vegetable	Cooked asparagus	96	6 spears
Salad	Tomato and watercress	100	1 serving
Salad dressing	French dressing	15	1 tbsp.
Bread	Whole wheat roll	30	1 average-size
Butter	Butter or fortified margarine	7	1 pat
Milk	Milk	244	1 glass
Fruit	Stewed royal Anne cherries	100	10 cherries with juice
	Dinner		
Meat	London broil	85	3 oz.
Potato	Stuffed baked potato	150	1 medium
Vegetable	Savory green beans	75	½ cup
Bread	Rye bread	23	1 slice
Butter	Butter or fortified margarine	7	1 pat
Dessert	Strawberry ice cream	62	1 average scoop (3½ oz. or ½ cup)
Milk	Milk	244	1 glass

Eggs: Soft or hard cooked, poached, scrambled.

Meat, fish, poultry: Prepared by boiling, broiling or roasting—ground beef, lamb, veal; liver; fish; poultry without skin; bacon.

Cheese: Cottage, pot and cream cheese; other cheeses may be used for flavoring in cooking, such as American or Cheddar of a mild variety.

Breads: Plain or toasted fine whole wheat, rye without seeds, enriched white; white crackers.

Cereals: Enriched, refined or finely ground.

Cereal products: Macaroni, spaghetti, noodles, rice.

Fats: Butter, oil, fortified margarine.

Vegetables: Cooked vegetables of low fiber—asparagus, beets, carrots, green beans, young peas, potatoes, spinach and squash—boiled or steamed, mashed, creamed, baked, or escalloped; vegetable purées; vegetable juices; lettuce and tomato salad. (Some hospitals do not serve any whole vegetables on the soft diet.)

Fruits: Cooked without skin or seeds; cooked fruit purées; fruit juices and ripe banana.

Soups: Clear soup broths, strained vegetables and strained cream soups.

Desserts: Plain puddings, cakes, cookies and frozen desserts prepared without nuts.

Beverages: All liquids.

Foods Omitted. Salads, raw fruits with the exception of bananas and fruit juices, coarse vegetables, coarse breads and cereals, rich pastries and nuts are not included in this diet.

LIQUID DIETS

Liquid diets are commonly ordered for patients with conditions requiring easily digested and easily consumed nourishment that is free

from mechanical irritants and irritating condiments or that has minimal residue. Patients who have chewing or swallowing difficulties or dental wiring may also require a liquid diet. The two varieties of liquid diets are the full liquid diet and the clear or restricted liquid diet.

Full Liquid Diet

The full liquid diet (Table 20–9) uses all foods that are liquid at room or body temperature. For example, ice cream is considered a liquid.

The diet, if properly designed and *consumed,* may be considered adequate for maintenance requirements, except with regard to fiber. The average composition of the diet is approximately 1300 to 1500 kcal., 45 gm. of protein, 65 gm. of fat and 150 gm. of carbohydrate. By careful planning, the diet can be increased in protein and caloric value to approach the normal diet or even a high-calorie diet. Increasing the protein and calories in a liquid diet is necessary when a patient must

remain on such a diet for an indefinite period. Protein and vitamin supplements (Table 35–5) can be added to the liquids to increase the protein and vitamin intake.

Full liquid diets can be planned to meet the needs of a patient with diabetes, renal disease or any other disorder. For the lactose-intolerant patient this is more difficult because the diet is usually based on milk as the protein source. A lactose-free product such as Ensure (Ross Laboratories) may be necessary. A fluid restriction might also make the full liquid diet inadequate because only a limited amount of it will be consumed. In this situation the liquids used should be very nutritious and highly concentrated.

Foods Included
Milk: Milk and milk beverages, cream.
Soups: Clear broth, strained cream soups, strained vegetable soups.
Cereals: Cereal gruel.
Fruits: Strained fruit juices.
Vegetables: Strained vegetable juice and vegetable water.

Table 20–8   SOFT OR LIGHT DIET

		SERVINGS	
MEAL PLAN	SAMPLE MENU	GRAMS	HOUSEHOLD MEASURE
Breakfast			
Fruit	Orange juice	124	½ glass
Cereal	Cooked farina (cooked weight)	119	½ cup
Egg	Poached egg on toast	50	1
Bread	Toasted bread (enriched)	23	1 slice
Butter	Butter or fortified margarine	7	1 pat
Cream	Cream	60	2 oz.
Milk	Milk	244	1 cup
Sugar	Sugar	15	3 tsp.
Coffee	Coffee	200	2 coffee cups
Lunch			
Soup	Tomato consommé	120	½ cup
Entrée	Baked macaroni and cheese	110	½ cup
Vegetables	Cooked asparagus tips or purée	96	6 spears
Bread	Light rye bread	23	1 slice
Butter	Butter or fortified margarine	7	1 pat
Fruit	Applesauce	127	½ cup
Milk	Milk	244	1 glass
Dinner			
Meat	Sliced chicken	85	3 oz.
Potato	Mashed potato	98	½ cup
Vegetable	Buttered spinach purée	90	½ cup
Bread	Light rye bread	23	1 slice
Butter	Butter or fortified margarine	7	1 pat
Dessert	Chocolate ice cream	62	1 average scoop (3½ oz. or ½ cup)
Milk	Milk	244	1 glass

Beverages: Tea, coffee, carbonated beverages, eggnog, malted milk beverages.

Desserts: Plain gelatin dessert, ice cream without seeds or nuts, ices, sherbet, milk-rennet pudding, soft custard.

Sweets: Sugar.

Fats: Butter, fortified margarine, oil.

Because this diet is inadequate in fiber, constipation may result from its prolonged use.

Clear or Restricted Liquid Diet

The clear or restricted liquid diet (Table 20–10) is frequently ordered for postoperative patients to furnish nourishment prior to the return of gastrointestinal function. It is an *inadequate* diet composed chiefly of water and carbohydrates; therefore, it is used a *very short time.* The average clear or restricted liquid diet contains 400 to 500 kcal., 5 to 10 gm. of protein, no fat and 100 to 120 gm. of carbohydrate.

The liquid is served at frequent intervals to supply the tissues with fluid and to relieve thirst. As the name indicates, the diet consists of clear liquids such as tea, broth, carbonated beverages, strained fruit juice and gelatin (liquid at body temperature). Milk and liquids prepared with milk are omitted, as are fats. Some patients' stomachs become distended and very uncomfortable if given fruit juice, especially orange juice. Fruit juices that do not agree with the patient are omitted from the diet. Carbonated beverages, especially ginger ale, seem to be tolerated by the majority of the patients. As usual, the diet is planned with due consideration to the patient's food preferences.

Foods Included

Fruits: Strained fruit juices and fruitades.

Soups: Clear soup broths.

Beverages: Tea, coffee (decaffeinated), carbonated beverages.

Desserts: Plain gelatin, plain fruit ice made with strained fruit juices.

Sweets: Sugar, lactose

Table 20–9   FULL LIQUID DIET*

MEAL PLAN	SAMPLE MENU	SERVINGS Grams	SERVINGS Household Measure
	Breakfast		
Fruit	Strained orange juice	124	½ cup
Cereal	Cooked thin farina gruel (cooked weight)	120	½ cup
Cream	Cream	60	2 oz.
Sugar	Sugar	15	3 tsp.
Coffee	Coffee	200	2 coffee cups
	10:00 A.M.		
Milk beverage	Milk	244	1 glass
	Lunch		
Soup	Tomato consommé	120	½ cup
Fruit juice	Grape juice	254	1 cup
Dessert	Vanilla ice cream	62	1 average scoop (3½ oz. or ½ cup)
	3:00 P.M.		
Milk beverage	Vanilla malted milk	270	1 cup
	Dinner		
Soup	Strained cream of pea soup	122	½ cup
Dessert	Raspberry gelatin	60	¼ cup
Beverage	Tea	200	2 teacups
Sugar	Sugar	10	2 tsp.
	8:00 P.M.		
Milk beverage	Eggnog	233	1 cup

*To increase the calories for the daily diet, add sugar, cream, butter or fortified margarine whenever possible.

Table 20–10 CLEAR OR RESTRICTED LIQUID DIET

| | | SERVINGS | |
MEAL PLAN	SAMPLE MENU	Grams	Household Measure
	Breakfast		
Fruit juice	Orange juice (strained)	124	½ cup
Beverage	Coffee (decaffeinated)	200	2 coffee cups
Sugar	Sugar	10	2 tsp.
	10:00 A.M.		
Fruitade	Lemonade	240	1 cup
	Lunch		
Soup	Consommé	120	½ cup
Fruit juice	Grapefruit juice (strained)	123	½ glass
Tea	Tea	200	2 teacups
Sugar	Sugar	10	2 tsp.
	3:00 P.M.		
Carbonated beverage	Ginger ale	230	1 cup
	Dinner		
Soup	Chicken broth	125	½ cup
Gelatin	Raspberry gelatin	60	¼ cup
Tea	Tea	200	2 teacups
Sugar	Sugar	10	2 tsp.
	8:00 P.M.		
Fruit juice	Orange juice (strained)	248	1 cup

See Table 20–11 for a summary of all these diets.

PSYCHOLOGICAL FACTORS IN FEEDING THE SICK PERSON

Throughout the text an effort has been made to bring out the psychological factors in feeding the sick. It is suggested that the part of Chapter 1 dealing with the care and feeding of patients be reviewed at this point.

The three daily meals and between-meal nourishments are often highlights of the day and are looked forward to by the patient, so the nurse should attempt to make mealtime a pleasant experience. A comfortable temperature in a room free of drafts, a comfortable eating position in bed or on a chair located away from unpleasant sights and pleasant conversation or music encourage good food intake. Most patients prefer to wash their hands and faces before eating and to eat from a table that is free of other objects.

The arrangement of the tray should reflect thoughtfulness and consideration of the patient's needs and wishes. The china, glassware and silver on the tray should be in a convenient location and within the patient's reach. Independence should be encouraged in patients who require assistance in eating. The nurse can accomplish this by having patients specify the sequence of foods to be eaten and by having them participate in eating, even if only by holding their bread.

A *patient's attitude* toward his illness and hospitalization frequently is reflected in the rejection of meals or the prescribed diet. Other reasons for poor acceptance of hospital meals may be unfamiliar foods and eating schedule and improper food temperatures. By giving patients an opportunity to express themselves and by accepting their attitudes, the nurse can help patients overcome their feelings and improve their acceptance of the hospital food. Food acceptance is also improved when selection of menus by the patients themselves is encouraged and when patients are given an explanation of why a particular diet has been prescribed. Problems with food acceptance that the nurse cannot handle should be communicated to the clinical dietitian.

If the nurse will take the time to encourage

Table 20–11 SUMMARY OF BASIC HOSPITAL DIETS

FOOD	GENERAL OR ADEQUATE NORMAL DIET	SOFT OR LIGHT DIET	FULL LIQUID DIET	CLEAR LIQUID DIET
Milk, cream, buttermilk	Included.	Included.	Included.	Not included.
Eggs	Raw and cooked.	Included.	In beverages.	Not included.
Cheese	All varieties.	Cottage, pot, cream, mild American, Cheddar.	Not allowed.	Not included.
Fats	All kinds.	Butter, fortified margarine, oil, mayonnaise and French dressing.	Butter, fortified margarine, oil.	Not included.
Meat, fish, poultry	All included.	Ground and tender beef, lamb, veal; liver, bacon, fish, poultry.	Not allowed.	Not included.
Vegetables	All included.	Cooked vegetables of low fiber; lettuce and tomato salad; potatoes boiled, mashed, baked, creamed, scalloped; vegetable juices.	Vegetable juices, vegetable purée used in soups.	Vegetable water.
Fruits	All included.	Fruit juices, ripe bananas, cooked fruit without skin or seeds.	Fruit juices, fruitades.	Strained fruit juices, fruitades.
Breads	All varieties.	Fine whole grain, rye without seeds, enriched white, refined crackers.	Not allowed.	Not included.
Cereals	All varieties.	Refined; finely ground.	Cooked gruel.	Not included.
Cereal products	All varieties.	Cooked macaroni, spaghetti, noodles, rice.	Not allowed.	Not included.
Soups	All varieties.	Clear broth, consommé, strained cream and vegetable soups.	Clear broth, consommé; strained vegetable and cream soups.	Clear broth and consommé.
Beverages	All kinds.	All kinds.	Tea, decaffeinated coffee; carbonated beverages; eggnog.	Tea, decaffeinated coffee; carbonated beverages.
Desserts	All kinds.	Plain puddings, simple cakes and cookies; frozen desserts without nuts; custard, gelatin, milk-rennet pudding.	Plain gelatin dessert, ice cream without nuts and seeds; ices. sherbets, milk-rennet pudding, soft custard.	Plain gelatin desserts and ices.

patients and show interest in their food, the result will often be most rewarding. Patients' acceptance of their diet is closely related to the nurse's attitude toward it. It is no more necessary to convince patients that they *like* their diets than it is to convince them that they *like* unpalatable medication. There is every need, however, to approach the patients and win their confidence so that they will accept the diet. The nurse who is convinced that the diet contributes to the restoration of her patients' health will communicate this conviction to them by her actions, her facial expressions and her conversation. Patients who understand that the diet contributes to the success of their medical or surgical therapy will usually accept it more willingly. In this capacity the nurse serves as an interpreter of the therapeutic diet.

When patients must adhere to a therapeutic dietary program indefinitely, the nurse may

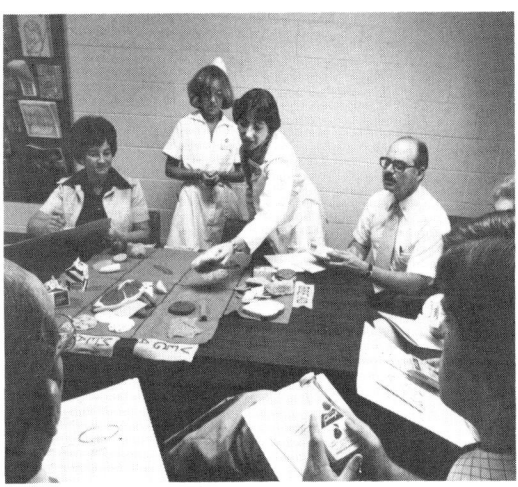

Figure 20–6 Dietitian and nurse teaching a group of patients about diet. (Courtesy of Ms. Sheila Henderson, R. D., and the nutrition staff of Lutheran General Hospital, Park Ridge, Ill.)

need to confer with the dietitian, the social worker or the community health nurse. She may want to bring the members of the health team together to help patients resolve their nutritional problems. In this role the nurse is a coordinator.

During the course of nursing care the nurse comes in contact with many individuals who do not require a therapeutic dietary program. Informal opportunities for discussing nutrition principles with all patients are often available, especially with those individuals receiving regular diets. Frequently, and usually most effectively, the nurse and dietitian can combine their skills to teach groups of patients normal nutriton or dietary modification for a disorder from which all of the patients suffer. Classes on the diet for coronary artery disease, diabetes and hypertension have been developed. (See Fig. 20–6.)

PROBLEMS AND SUGGESTED TOPICS FOR DISCUSSION

1. What dietary adjustments necessary for the sick are frequently overlooked?
2. What is meant by routine house diets and what purpose do they serve? What are their (a) advantages and (b) disadvantages or limitations?
3. Compare diets served in the hospital where you are located with those outlined in this chapter. If there are any differences between the diets, justify the discrepancy.
4. Plan a full liquid diet for a 46 year old female patient requiring 2000 kcalories. Check with recommended allowances for adequacy.
5. List the foods usually allowed on a clear liquid diet. How adequate is a clear liquid diet? Why is it not necessary that the diet meet requirements for nutritional adequacy?
6. Discuss the conditions (diagnosis of patient and hospital management) for which it is advantageous to use the soft diet.
7. Discuss the advantages and disadvantages of the current trend for more liberal treatment and management of various diet plans.
8. List the psychological factors to be considered when feeding the sick. How can the nurse help?
9. Design a nutritional care plan for a patient, including assessment, objectives, nutritional interventions and evaluation. What criteria will you use to evaluate the nutritional care? Did the patient meet the objectives?

CITED REFERENCES

1. Ahart, H. E.: Assessing food intake of hospital patients. J. Am. Diet. Assoc., 40:114, 1962.
2. Ghadimi, H. (ed.): Total Parenteral Nutrition: Premises and Promises. New York, John Wiley and Sons, 1975, p. 190.
3. Krause, M. V.: Some modern concepts concerning hospital diets. J. Am. Diet. Assoc., 20:610, 1944.
4. Pollack, H., and Halpern, S. L.: Therapeutic Nutrition. Publication No. 234. Washington, D.C., National Research Council, 1952.
5. Select Committee on Nutrition and Human Needs of the U. S. Senate: Dietary Goals for the United States. Washington, D.C., U. S. Government Printing Office, 1977.
6. Wade, J. E.: Role of a clinical dietitian specialist on a nutrition support service. J. Am. Diet. Assoc., 70:185, 1977.

ADDITIONAL REFERENCES

American Hospital Association: Recording Nutritional Information in Medical Records. American Hospital Association, 840 N. Lake Shore Dr., Chicago, Illinois, 60611, 1976.
Babcock, C. G.: Problems in sustaining the nutritional care of patients. J. Am. Diet. Assoc., 28:222, 1952.
Babcock, C. G.: Comments on human interrelations. J. Am. Diet. Assoc., 33:871, 1957.
Bean, W. B.: The clinician interrogates nutrition. Am. J. Clin. Nutr., 13:263, 1963.
Cooper, L. F.: Florence Nightingale's contribution to dietetics. J. Am. Diet. Assoc., 30:121, 1954.
Cousins, N.: Anatomy of an illness (as perceived by the patient). N. Engl. J. Med., 295:1458, 1976.
Davis, J., and Hodges, R. E.: A "new" approach to diet therapy. Dietetic Currents, 1(5), 1974. (Published by Ross Laboratories, Columbus, Ohio.)
English, O. S.: Psychosomatic medicine and dietetics. J. Am. Diet. Assoc., 27:721, 1951.
Food and Nutrition Board, National Research Council: Recommended Dietary Allowances, 8th ed. Washington, D.C., National Academy of Sciences, 1974.
Goodhart, R. S., and Shils, M. E. (eds.): Modern Nutrition in Health and Disease, 5th ed. Philadelphia, Lea & Febiger, 1973.
Goodhue, P. J., Collins, M. E., and Baumgarten, S.: Continuing nutritional care for the discharged patient. Dietetic Currents, 3(1), 1976.
Hegsted, D. M.: Nutritional requirements in disease. J. Am. Diet. Assoc., 56:303, 1970.
Hodges, R. E.: The effect of stress on ascorbic acid metabolism in man. Nutrition Today, 5:11, 1970.
Jolliffe, N., and Krehl, W. A.: Principles of nutrition therapy. In: Jolliffe, N., Clinical Nutrition, 2nd ed. New York, Harper and Bros., 1962.
Kocher, R. E.: Monitoring nutritional care of the long-term patient. J. Am. Diet. Assoc., 67:45, 1975.
Mayo Clinic: Mayo Clinic Diet Manual, 4th ed. Philadelphia, W. B. Saunders Co., 1971.
Moore, H. B.: Psychologic facts and dietary fancies. J. Am. Diet. Assoc., 28:789, 1952.
Selye, H.: On just being sick. Nutrition Today, 5:2, 1970.
Turner, D.: Handbook of Diet Therapy, 5th ed. Chicago, University of Chicago Press, 1970.
Youmans, J. B.: The changing face of nutritional disease in America. JAMA, 189:672, 1964.

Chapter 21

THE INTERACTIONS BETWEEN DRUGS, NUTRIENTS AND NUTRITIONAL STATUS

In a period in the development of medical care when most diseases are chronic ones requiring long-term management and drug therapy, it is essential to be aware of the effects of drugs administered over long periods of time. One of the factors that deserves attention is the interaction between drugs and the nutritional status of an individual, which was previously little appreciated and is still poorly understood. Both the side effects and the therapeutic effects of a drug can affect a person's nutrient intake, metabolism and requirements and ultimately, his nutritional status. Just as important, food and the nutrients in it can affect the action of a drug by altering its absorption, metabolism and excretion. When administering a drug, it is important to note its action and side effects in terms of nutritional implications. Some drugs have been reported as inducing actual clinical deficiency states in humans; others have caused decreased serum levels of certain nutrients; while still others have caused nutritional changes in animals only, and we have no evidence about their nutritional effects in humans.

Drug-induced malnutrition is most likely to develop in those patients receiving long-term drug therapy who take medication for the control of a chronic disease for many years.

When studying nutrient and drug interrelationships, it is important to remember that clinical nutritional deficiency states are usually the result of a *combination of factors*. A nutritional deficiency is more likely to occur in those patients who have a marginal nutritional status before the drug is prescribed. If the nutritional status and the present intake are good, the patient is not as likely to become nutritionally

deficient. Patients who have a catabolic disease, weight losses of 10 per cent or more of their ideal body weight, poor dietary intakes (alcoholics, for example), chronic disease of the gastrointestinal tract or increased nutritional requirements as a result of recent major surgery or infection are more likely to be put into nutritional jeopardy by the use of certain drugs. If patients in these categories are then placed on long-term drug therapy, it becomes especially important to assess their dietary intakes and nutritional status and, if necessary, to institute preventive or rehabilitative measures such as providing additional food or vitamin and mineral supplements along with the drug therapy. An increased requirement for nutrients can usually be met by supplementation. (See Table 21–1.)

It is useful to categorize the interactions of drugs and nutrients into (1) those by which drugs affect the body's intake, absorption, metabolism and requirements for nutrients and (2) those by which nutrients or foods affect the absorption, metabolism, action and excretion of drugs.

THE EFFECTS OF DRUGS ON NUTRIENT INTAKE, ABSORPTION, METABOLISM AND REQUIREMENTS

The effects of drugs on nutritional status can also be classified into various types of actions: (1) alteration of food intake, (2) alteration of nutrient absorption, (3) alteration of nutrient metabolism and utilization and (4) alteration of nutrient excretion. See Table 21–2 for a summary of these actions.

Table 21–1 NUTRIENTS SIGNIFICANTLY AFFECTED BY DRUGS

NUTRIENT	DRUG ACTION	DRUGS
Vitamin B_6	Function as vitamin B_6 antagonists or increase the turnover of B_6 in the body.	Isonicotinic acid hydrazide, cycloserine and other antituberculous drugs. Hydralazine. Penicillamine. L-Dopa. Oral contraceptives. Alcohol.
Folic Acid	Function as folic acid antagonists; affect the absorption of folic acid or increase the turnover or loss of folate from the body.	Para-aminosalicylic acid. Methotrexate. Pyrimethamine. Isonicotinic acid hydrazide. Anticonvulsants. Triamterene. Trimethoprim. Oral contraceptives. Cycloserine. Salicylazosulfapyridine (Azulfidine). Aspirin. Pentamidine. Alcohol.
Vitamin B_{12}	Affect the absorption of vitamin B_{12}.	Neomycin. Biguanides. Para-aminosalicylic acid. Cholestyramine. Potassium chloride. Alcohol.
Niacin	By antagonizing Vitamin B_6, cause depletion, because vitamin B_6 is a necessary coenzyme in the synthesis of niacin from tryptophan.	Isonicotinic acid hydrazide. 6-Mercaptopurine. 5-Fluorouracil.
Riboflavin	Decreases riboflavin absorption by increasing G.I. motility.	Thyroxine.
	Displaces riboflavin from plasma binding site and causes hyperexcretion of riboflavin.	Boric acid.
Thiamin	Impairs absorption of thiamin or impairs the formation of the coenzyme form of the vitamin.	Alcohol.
	Increase requirements.	Digitalis alkaloids.
Ascorbic Acid	Decrease the absorption or stimulate the metabolism of the vitamin.	Oral contraceptives.
	Deplete the tissues of the vitamin.	Aspirin. Alcohol. Anorectic agents. Anticonvulsants. Tetracycline.
	Depletes adrenal ascorbic acid.	ACTH.
Vitamin A	Acts as a solvent for carotene and vitamin A and thus prevents absorption.	Mineral oil.
	Decrease absorption by damage to mucosa; inhibition of pancreatic lipase and inactivation of bile salts.	Cholestyramine. Neomycin. Alcohol. Colchicine (affects carotene).

Table continued on the following page

Table 21–1   NUTRIENTS SIGNIFICANTLY AFFECTED BY DRUGS (*Continued*)

NUTRIENT	DRUG ACTION	DRUGS
Vitamin D	Affect absorption or metabolism of vitamin D.	Cholestyramine. Laxatives. Antacids. Mineral oil. Phenolphthalein.
	Accelerate the degradation of $25\text{-}OHD_3$.	Anticonvulsants. Glutethimide.
	Block the production of $1,25\text{-}OH_2D_3$ in the kidney.	Diphosphonates. Corticosteroids.
Vitamin E	Diminishes the carrier lipoprotein for vitamin E.	Clofibrate.
Vitamin K	Decrease synthesis of vitamin K_2 by intestinal bacteria, but no effect on vitamin status unless vitamin K intake is inadequate.	Tetracyclines and other broad-spectrum antibiotics.
	Decrease absorption of vitamin K.	Mineral oil. Neomycin. Cholestyramine.
	Cause vitamin K deficiency.	Coumarin anticoagulants. Aspirin and other salicylates.
Iron	Depresses iron absorption.	Bicarbonate.
	Increases iron absorption.	Isonicotinic acid hydrazide.
	Impairs the uptake of iron into protoporphyrin; capable of causing sideroblastic anemia.	Cholestyramine.
Zinc	Cause excessive urinary excretion of zinc.	Alcohol. D-Penicillamine. Corticosteroids. Estrogen component of oral contraceptives. Chlorthalidone. Thiazides. Furosemide.
Magnesium	Increase urinary excretion of magnesium.	Chlorothiazide. Hydrochlorothiazide. Ethacrynic acid. Ammonium chloride. Mercurial diuretics. Alcohol.
	Drug-induced steatorrhea causes formation of magnesium soaps and excessive fecal excretion of magnesium.	
Calcium	Cause malabsorption of calcium.	Prednisone and other glucocorticoids. Phenobarbital. Phenytoin. Primidone. Glutethimide. Diphosphonates. Phenolphthalein. Neomycin.
	Cause excessive urinary excretion of calcium.	Furosemide. Ethacrynic acid. Triamterene. Alcohol.
	Increase intestinal absorption of calcium.	Combination oral contraceptives.

Table 21–1 NUTRIENTS SIGNIFICANTLY AFFECTED BY DRUGS (*Continued*)

NUTRIENT	DRUG ACTION	DRUGS
Protein	Cause malabsorption of protein.	Neomycin.
	Inhibit protein synthesis.	Actinomycin D. Corticosteroids.
Fat	Cause malabsorption of fat.	Neomycin. Colchicine. Cholestyramine. Para-aminosalicylic acid.
Carbohydrate	Cause malabsorption of lactose.	Neomycin. Colchicine.
	Causes malabsorption of sucrose.	Neomycin.
Sodium and Potassium	Increase fecal excretion.	Neomycin. Colchicine.
Phosphate	Increase fecal excretion.	Aluminum hydroxide antacids.

DRUGS THAT AFFECT THE INTAKE OF FOOD AND NUTRIENTS

Drugs can affect the intake of food and nutrients either through a side effect accompanying their required action or as the reason for their administration. An example that immediately comes to mind is the anorectic agents used to *diminish appetite* and thus the quantity of food consumed. These are used most often to aid in weight reduction. Because most of these agents are amphetamines and act on the central nervous system (CNS) to depress the appetite, they have several side effects, among which is hyperactivity. The individual usually develops a tolerance to the drug's appetite-depressive effect after about 10 days, and consequently the use of such drugs for weight reduction should be only for a short term.

These same drugs are used to control behavioral difficulties in hyperactive children. Paradoxically, in hyperactive children the amphetamine dextroamphetamine and the structurally related compound methylphenidate have a calming effect. However, their use has been shown to cause growth retardation in children who take them for several months or longer.[23] When the medication is discontinued during the summer, a child grows faster than normal and experiences some "catch-up" growth.[24] Dextroamphetamine (Dexedrine) seems to have a greater growth-retarding effect than methylphenidate (Ritalin). Possibly this

growth retardation is a result of the decreased food intake associated with the drug-induced appetite depression. Lucas and Sells studied two hyperactive boys and found reduced nutritional intakes on those days when the boys were taking drugs.[16] These reductions were enough to have caused the depressed growth in these children, and their findings suggest that some children may never develop a tolerance to the appetite-depressing effects of amphetamines. For ways to plan meals around the drug therapy and thus to increase the caloric intake of these children, see the Lucas reference.[16]

Some of the tranquilizing drugs such as chlorpromazine and lithium carbonate can lead to an increase in body weight. It is thought that these agents cause an increase in appetite sec-

Table 21–2 EFFECTS OF DRUG ACTION ON NUTRITIONAL STATUS

Alteration of food intake.
    Changes in appetite.
    Changes in sense of taste and smell.
    Nausea and vomiting.
Alteration of nutrient absorption.
    Luminal Effects
        Changes in gastrointestinal motility.
        Changes in bile acid activity.
        Formation of drug–nutrient complexes.
    Mucosal Effects
        Inactivation of absorptive enzyme systems.
        Damage to gastrointestinal mucosal cells.
Alteration of nutrient metabolism and utilization.
Alteration of nutrient excretion.

ondary to their alteration of mental status or effect on the CNS. This effect is non-specific, but patients taking these drugs who have a weight gain should be evaluated and possibly the drug dosage should be reduced. Numerous other drugs decrease the appetite as a side effect of their action, and this should always be appreciated when they are administered. Information on the side effects of a particular drug usually states whether the appetite is affected.

Another side effect of drugs that affects the intake of food is *taste alteration*. Drugs can cause abnormal taste sensation (dysgeusia) or reduced acuity of the taste sensation (hypogeusia) or may leave an unpleasant aftertaste. Griseofulvin (an antifungal agent), D-penicillamine (a copper-chelating agent), clofibrate (an agent used to bind cholesterol in the gastrointestinal tract), 5-fluorouracil (a cancer chemotherapeutic agent) and some tranquilizers decrease or alter taste. Furthermore, they seem to have a systemic effect not related to the concomitant ingestion of food. Table 21–3 lists some drugs and their effects on the taste sensation. Radiotherapy given to treat carcinoma of the tongue, tonsils or nasopharynx also reduces taste acuity by damaging the salivary glands and taste organs. When taking these drugs or receiving radiotherapy, patients should be informed of the possible alteration of taste, and every effort should be made to season their food well. Patients should be encouraged to eat well during periods when they are not receiving drugs or radiation therapy. (See Chapter 36, Nutrition, Diet and Cancer.)

Zinc deficiency also causes hypogeusia and dysgeusia. Because of extended periods of inadequate nutritional intake or inadequate mineral supplementation, patients may become zinc-deficient and complain of taste changes. In this case, zinc supplements, usually in the form of zinc sulfate, are administered.

Other drugs that affect food intake are those that cause nausea and vomiting as a side effect of their action. Many of the drugs used in the chemotherapy of cancer have this effect. (See Table 36–2.)

Some drugs may cause a craving or unusual desire for certain foods. For instance, patients taking diuretics may crave salt in their food because of the increased excretion of sodium, and will increase their sodium intake unless counseled about ways to avoid it.[13]

DRUGS THAT AFFECT THE ABSORPTION OF NUTRIENTS

Because most drugs and most nutrients are absorbed in the small intestine, it is not surprising that drugs affect nutrient absorption and vice versa. It is unfortunate that so little is known about these effects. The interaction of food and drugs with the mechanical, secretory, digestive, absorptive and excretory functions of the gastrointestinal tract is complicated and depends on the drug dosage, type and amount of food, timing and the presence of disease.

In general, drugs can cause malabsorption by (1) exerting an effect in the intestinal lumen or (2) impairing the absorptive ability of the

Table 21–3 EFFECTS OF MEDICATIONS ON TASTE SENSITIVITY*

DRUG	EFFECT
Amphetamines	Decreased sweet sensitivity in some; differs with individuals. Increased bitter sensitivity.
Anesthetics	
Cocaine	Decreased sensitivity, especially sweet and bitter.
Eucaine	Decreased bitter and sweet sensitivity.
Amydricaine	Decreased bitter and sweet sensitivity.
Amylocaine	With high intake, loss of salt detection, decreased bitter sensitivity.
Isococaine and tropacocaine	Decreased sweet sensitivity.
Benzocaine	Increased sour sensitivity.
Amethocaine	Increased bitter sensitivity. Decreased sweet sensitivity.
Lidocaine	Decreased salt and sweet sensitivity.
Acetyl sulfosalicylic acid	Decreased sensitivity.
Clofibrate	Decreased sensitivity.
Dinitrophenol	Loss of salt taste; general hypogeusia.
D-Penicillamine	General decrease in sensitivity.
5-Fluorouracil	Some alterations in bitter and sour sensitivity. Increased sweet sensitivity.
Griseofulvin	Decreased sensitivity.
Insulin	With prolonged use, decreased sweet and salt sensitivity.
Lithium carbonate	Strange, unpleasant taste.
Phenindione	Decreased sensitivity.
Phenytoin	Decreased sensitivity.
Oxyfedrine	Decreased sensitivity.
Anti-thyroid agents	
Methimazole	Decreased sensitivity.
Methylthiouracil	Decreased sensitivity.

*Adapted from: Carson, J. A. S., and Gormican, A.: Disease-medication relationships in altered taste sensitivity. J. Am. Diet. Assoc., 68:550, 1976.

gastrointestinal mucosa. These effects can be limited and specific for a particular nutrient, or they can be general, resulting in a more severe malabsorption.

Luminal Effects

Drugs can *affect the transit time* of food and nutrients in the gut and reduce nutrient absorption. Cathartic agents such as podophyllin, jalap and colocynth may reduce gastrointestinal transit time. Calcium and potassium losses along with steatorrhea have been reported after using these agents.[4] Bisacodyl, oxyphenisatin and phenolphthalein, commonly used as laxatives, can decrease the absorption of glucose.[8]

A number of drugs *affect bile acid activity* and thus the absorption of fat, fat-soluble vitamins (A, D and K), carotene and other micellar components such as cholesterol. By sequestering bile acids through a binding effect, these drugs inhibit the intraluminal phase of fat digestion and absorption, and steatorrhea results. Drugs that have this action are cholestyramine, clofibrate, colestipol and neomycin. Cholestyramine, clofibrate and colestipol are usually given for the purpose of reducing cholesterol absorption and thus blood cholesterol, while neomycin is an antibiotic used to reduce the gut flora. Malabsorption has been reported in the form of vitamin K deficiency and hypoprothrombinemia.[6] Osteomalacia that responded to vitamin D therapy has also been reported;[9] however, the osteomalacia in this case was in a woman who also had a bile salt diarrhea, so that a deficiency of bile salts may have also contributed to the vitamin deficiency. Fat-soluble vitamins and possibly calcium should be given to patients taking cholestyramine.[15]

The status of fat-soluble vitamins in patients receiving these drugs should be monitored with periodic determinations of serum carotene for vitamin A status, of serum calcium, serum phosphorus and alkaline phosphatase for vitamin D evaluation, of serum alpha-tocopherol for vitamin E status and of prothrombin time to assess vitamin K status. Night blindness, osteomalacia, hemolysis of red blood cells when exposed to H_2O_2 and easy bruising are clinical signs that may reflect a deficiency of one or more of these fat-soluble vitamins. (See Chapter 12.)

Another drug that *prevents the absorption of* the fat-soluble vitamins is mineral oil, frequently used as a laxative.[3] Of course, excessive use of this oil is more likely to cause a deficiency than occasional use. The vitamins

become dispersed in oil, with the result that they are not absorbed but excreted in the feces. Mineral oil may also impair micelle formation in the gastrointestinal lumen.

Finally, a drug may affect the environment of the gastrointestinal lumen and prevent the absorption of a nutrient. Antacids change the pH of the stomach and if used extensively and frequently can significantly reduce the absorption of iron, which requires an acidic gastric environment in order to be changed from the ferric to the absorbable ferrous form. The absorption of iron is reduced in an alkaline environment.

Mucosal Effects

Those drugs with the greatest effect on nutrient absorption are those that *damage the intestinal mucosa*. Such drugs destroy the structure of the villi and microvilli, which results in an inhibition of the brush border enzymes and intestinal transport systems needed for optimal nutrient absorption. The result is general or specific malabsorption of varying degrees. The irritating cathartics already mentioned may have this effect and thus cause a mild steatorrhea. This often happens with chronic laxative abuse.

Neomycin is known to cause histological changes in the gut mucosa within six hours of administration and results in diminished absorption of sucrose and xylose.[10, 12] This action of neomycin is in addition to its bile acid binding activity, which has already been discussed. Increased excretion of protein, sodium, potassium and calcium also occurs. Neomycin illustrates malabsorption by three mechanisms: (1) mucosal damage, (2) precipitation of bile salts and (3) inhibition of pancreatic lipase. Mucosal damage probably has the greatest effect on nutrient absorption.

One drug that *affects the intestinal transport mechanisms* of the mucosa is colchicine, an anti-inflammatory agent used in the treatment of gout. Patients taking colchicine have reduced serum cholesterol levels, increased fecal excretion of bile acids, sodium, potassium, fat and protein and impaired absorption of vitamin B_{12}. Although the drug causes some change in the intestinal mucosa, this does not seem to be enough to account for the extensive reduction in absorption. The malabsorptive effect of colchicine may be a result of changes in the mucosal transport systems.[19]

Para-aminosalicylic acid (PAS) seems to work in a similar manner to reduce the absorption of vitamin B_{12}. It does not appear to inter-

Table 21–4   PRIMARY INTESTINAL ABSORPTIVE DEFECTS INDUCED BY DRUGS*

DRUG	USE	MALABSORPTIVE OR FECAL NUTRIENT LOSS	MECHANISM
Mineral oil	Laxative.	Carotene, vitamins A, D, K.	Physical barrier. Nutrients dissolve in mineral oil and are lost. Micelle formation ↓.
Phenolphthalein	Laxative.	Vitamin D, Ca.	Intestinal hurry. K depletion. Loss of structural integrity.
Neomycin	Antibiotic to "sterilize" gut.	Fat, nitrogen, Na, K, Ca, Fe, lactose, sucrose, vitamin B_{12}.	Structural defect. Pancreatic lipase ↓. Binding of bile acids (salts).
Cholestyramine	Hypocholesterolemic agent. Bile acid sequestrant.	Fat, vitamins A, K, B_{12}, D, Fe.	Binding of bile acids (salts) and nutrients, e.g. Fe.
Potassium chloride	Potassium repletion.	Vitamin B_{12}.	Ileal pH ↓.
Colchicine	Anti-inflammatory agent in gout.	Fat, carotene, Na, K, vitamin B_{12}, lactose.	Mitotic arrest. Structural defect. Enzyme damage.
Biguanides: Metformin Phenformin	Hypoglycemic agents (in diabetes).	Vitamin B_{12}.	Competitive inhibition of B_{12} absorption.
Para-aminosalicylic acid	Antituberculosis agent.	Fat, folate, vitamin B_{12}.	Mucosal block in B_{12} uptake.
Salicylazosulfapyridine (Azulfidine)	Anti-inflammatory agent in ulcerative colitis and regional enteritis.	Folate.	Mucosal block in folate uptake.

*From: Roe, D. A.: Drug-induced Nutritional Deficiencies. Westport, Conn., Avi Publishing Co., 1976, p. 130.

fere with the production of intrinsic factor or with its binding to vitamin B_{12} but rather with the uptake and transport of the vitamin across the mucosal wall.[26]

It has also been postulated that the biguanides phenformin and metformin cause a malabsorption of sugar from the gastrointestinal tract by blocking a mucosal enzyme and thus the transport of sugar across the mucosa into the blood stream. This is the reason for their use in the treatment of hyperglycemia. See Table 21–4 for a summary of the primary intestinal absorptive defects induced by drugs.

DRUGS THAT AFFECT THE METABOLISM AND EXCRETION OF NUTRIENTS

Antivitamins

Drugs that *interfere with the action of a vitamin with its enzymes* can be antimetabolites, antivitamins or enzyme inducers. Anti-

vitamins and antimetabolites, with structures similar to those of the real vitamins and metabolites, can block enzymatic reactions. The enzymes take up the antivitamin or antimetabolite instead of the actual vitamin or metabolite. Cancer chemotherapeutic agents work on this principle. The antivitamins are taken up by the most rapidly growing cells in the body, the cancer cells, which die or malfunction when the antivitamin does not function like the real vitamin. Common antivitamins are the folate antagonists methotrexate and pyrimethamine. Methotrexate is used to treat leukemia, choriocarcinoma and psoriasis that is resistant to other forms of therapy. Pyrimethamine is used in the treatment of chloroquine-resistant malaria and ocular toxoplasmosis. These drugs act as folic acid analogs and are bound to the dihydrofolate reductase enzyme instead of folic acid. Folic acid is then unable to bind with the enzyme and is put out of the metabolic system and excreted. Without the real folic acid, deoxyribonucleic acid

(DNA) synthesis, which depends on the presence of folic acid, is inhibited, cell replication stops and the cell dies. In addition, the folic acid deficiency can cause macrocytic anemia. (See Chapter 12, Nutritional Deficiency Diseases.)

Clinical rickets and osteomalacia in patients receiving long-term anticonvulsant therapy are due to increased induction of hepatic enzymes, which interfere with the metabolism of vitamin D_3 to 25-OHD$_3$ so that there is a smaller amount of active vitamin D available.[17] In addition, the 25-OHD$_3$ form of the vitamin may be inactivated. It is usually recommended that patients taking anticonvulsants receive a vitamin D supplement and possibly a folate supplement. From 8000 to 10,000 I.U. of vitamin D has been recommended weekly, especially for blacks, patients with limited sun exposure and patients with limited activity.[7] See p. 659 for further discussion of anticonvulsants.

A drug may also affect the metabolism of a nutrient by *forming a complex* with it, making it unavailable for use by the body. Isonicotinic acid hydrazide (INH) functions in this manner. This drug, used in the long-term treatment of tuberculosis, forms a complex with pyridoxine (vitamin B_6) with the result that the pyridoxine is excreted in the urine and is not used by the body. Urinary levels of vitamin B_6 breakdown products are then above normal and indicate a biochemical vitamin B_6 deficiency. Other drugs that function as vitamin B_6 antagonists are hydralazine, penicillamine, L-dopa, cycloserine, pyrazinamide and ethionamide. Clinical signs of vitamin B_6 deficiency are, in order of appearance, seborrheic dermatitis, glossitis, stomatitis, cheilosis, conjunctivitis and later, severe sensory neuritis. Cycloserine and pyrazinamide (other antituberculous drugs) when given in conjunction with INH will cause a sideroblastic anemia that is not seen when INH is given alone. A dose of 50 mg. of vitamin B_6 daily will protect against vitamin B_6 deficiency when the patient is taking one of these drugs.

Excretion of Nutrients

Drugs act to increase the excretion of a nutrient by *displacing the vitamin from its binding site on a plasma protein*. If unbound to a protein, the vitamin will be filtered through the kidneys and excreted.[20] Aspirin may alter the transport of folate by competing for sites on the serum proteins that transport folate, and thus folate is excreted.[2]

D-penicillamine, used to treat heavy metal poisoning (such as lead poisoning), Wilson's disease, cystinuria or rheumatoid arthritis, besides chelating with the intended metal such as lead or copper, may also *chelate with other metals* and increase their excretion in the urine. D-penicillamine increases the excretion of zinc through formation of a zinc-penicillamine chelate.[18] In the reported cases, the patient's absorption of zinc from food offset the excessive loss of that mineral, so that a balance was maintained. However, an ill patient who is not eating could not maintain that balance. EDTA (ethylenediaminotetraacetate) administered intravenously to treat lead poisoning may also cause excessive urinary excretion of zinc.[5]

Drugs can also increase the excretion of a nutrient by *decreasing its reabsorption by the kidneys*. Oral diuretics such as furosemide, ethacrynic acid and triamterene can produce significant hypercalciuria by reducing reabsorption of calcium from the convoluted tubule in the kidney. Because of this, furosemide has also been utilized as a temporary measure to control symptoms of hypercalcemia. Diuretics may also affect the status of magnesium and zinc in the body by increasing renal excretion of these minerals.[27] See Table 21–5 for a synopsis of the nutritional implications of the use of selected drugs.

SUMMARY OF SOME OF THE ACTIONS OF THE COMMON DRUGS

Anticonvulsants

The anticonvulsants phenytoin, phenobarbital and primidone are capable of inducing a biochemical or clinical folate deficiency state or a vitamin D deficiency manifested by the development of rickets or osteomalacia. The prevalence of megaloblastic anemia in people who take anticonvulsants ranges from 0.15 to 0.75 per cent.[21] It is thought by some that these drugs interfere with the conversion of folic acid to 5-methyltetrahydrofolate, the active form of folic acid. Others feel that these drugs, particularly phenytoin, impair the absorption of folate from food by inhibiting intestinal conjugase, which is necessary for breaking down the polyglutamates of folic acid in food to the monoglutamate form that can be absorbed. Vitamin B_{12} levels, although usually unaffected by the use of anticonvulsants, may fall if folic acid is given to remedy low serum folate levels. The increased hematopoiesis increases the

Table 21–5   EFFECTS OF SOME DRUGS ON NUTRITIONAL STATUS*

DRUG	MECHANISM	NUTRITIONAL IMPLICATION
Analgesics		
Alcohol	Toxic effect on intestinal mucosa. Impairs pancreatic enzyme secretion.	Decreased absorption of thiamin, folic acid, vitamin B_{12}. Increased urinary excretion of magnesium and zinc.
Aspirin (salicylates)	Block uptake of vitamin C by platelets.	Decreased serum folate. Increased urinary excretion of vitamin C.
Colchicine	Decreases activity of intestinal disaccharidases. Damages G.I. mucosa by blocking mucosal cell replication.	Decreased absorption of vitamin B_{12}, fat, carotene, sodium, potassium, lactose, xylose, protein. Decreased serum cholesterol, carotene and vitamin B_{12}.
Amphetamines Dextroamphetamine Methylphenidate	Decrease appetite.	Decreased caloric intake and possibly reduced growth.
Antacids Aluminum hydroxide	Decreases absorption of phosphate.	Phosphate depletion.
Others	Basic environment inactivates thiamin.	Inadequate amount of thiamin.
Anticonvulsants Phenobarbital Phenytoin Primidone	Increase turnover of vitamin D, may block hydroxylation of vitamin D.	Decreased serum levels of folate, vitamin B_{12}, pyridoxine, 25-hydroxyvitamin D_3 and calcium. Possible osteomalacia.
Barbiturates	Accelerate inactivation of vitamin D.	Decreased absorption of thiamin. Increased urinary excretion of vitamin C. Decreased serum vitamin B_{12}.
Antidepressants Lithium carbonate	May increase appetite.	Possible weight gain.
Antivitamins Methotrexate Pyrimethamine	Inhibits dihydrofolate reductase. Causes gastrointestinal mucosal injury.	Malabsorption of vitamin B_{12}, folate, fat and xylose. Weight loss, diarrhea, nausea, anorexia, vomiting, gingivitis, stomatitis.
Antimicrobials Chloramphenicol	Decreases protein synthesis by blocking mRNA–ribosome bond.	Possibly increased need for riboflavin, pyridoxine and vitamin B_{12}. Possible peripheral neuritis, optic neuropathy.
Penicillin	Carries potassium with it into urine.	Hypokalemia.
Tetracyclines	Chelate divalent ions. May decrease synthesis of mucosal iron-carrier protein.	Decreased absorption of calcium, iron, magnesium, xylose, amino acids and fat. Increased urinary excretion of vitamin C, riboflavin, nitrogen, folic acid and niacin. Decreased synthesis of vitamin K by intestinal bacteria.
Neomycin	Decreases activity of disaccharidases. Causes mucosal injury. Precipitates bile acids and disrupts micelle formation.	Decreased absorption of fat, carbohydrate, protein, fat-soluble vitamins, vitamin B_{12}, calcium, iron.

*From: March, D. C.: Handbook: Interactions of Selected Drugs with Nutritional Status in Man. Chicago, American Dietetic Association, 1976.

Table 21–5 EFFECTS OF SOME DRUGS ON NUTRITIONAL STATUS (*Continued*)

DRUG	MECHANISM	NUTRITIONAL IMPLICATION
Antitubercular Agents		
Para-aminosalicylic acid	Affects mucosal transport mechanism.	Decreased absorption of vitamin B_{12}, iron, folate, fat and xylose. Possible peripheral neuritis. Decreased intestinal mucosal disaccharidases.
Isonicotinic acid hydrazide (INH)	Structurally related to pyridoxine and niacin.	Increased urinary excretion of pyridoxine. Causes pyridoxine depletion. Can cause polyneuropathy, megaloblastic anemia. Causes niacin depletion.
Cycloserine	Acts as a pyridoxine antagonist.	Decreased protein synthesis. May decrease absorption of calcium and magnesium. May decrease serum folate, vitamin B_{12} and pyridoxine.
Cathartics	Can cause intestinal hyperperistalsis. May irritate intestine.	Can cause steatorrhea. Can increase intestinal calcium and potassium loss. Decreased glucose absorption.
Chelating Agents Penicillamine	Chelates with pyridoxine. Chelates with zinc and copper.	Increased urinary excretion of pyridoxine, zinc and copper. Can cause pyridoxine depletion.
Corticosteroids	Stimulate protein catabolism. Depress protein synthesis.	Decreased absorption of calcium and phosphorus. Increased urinary excretion of vitamin C, calcium, potassium, zinc and nitrogen. Decreased serum zinc. Increased blood glucose, serum triglycerides, serum cholesterol.
Diuretics Furosemide		Increased excretion of calcium, magnesium and potassium. Decreased serum magnesium and potassium. Decreased carbohydrate tolerance.
Mercurials		Increased urinary excretion of thiamin, magnesium, calcium and potassium. Possibly induced magnesium depletion and bone resorption.
Thiazides	May increase intestinal calcium absorption or increase bone resorption.	Increased urinary excretion of potassium, magnesium, zinc and riboflavin. Decreased carbohydrate tolerance. Possible potassium and magnesium depletion.
Triamterene	Competitive inhibition of dihydrofolate reductase; reduces activation of folic acid.	Decreased serum folate, serum vitamin B_{12}. Possibly increased calcium excretion.

Table continued on the following page

Table 21–5   EFFECTS OF SOME DRUGS ON NUTRITIONAL STATUS (*Continued*)

DRUG	MECHANISM	NUTRITIONAL IMPLICATION
Hypocholesterolemics Cholestyramine	Binds bile salts and disrupts micelles. Binds intrinsic factor at ileal pH.	Decreased absorption of cholesterol, vitamins A, D, K and B_{12}, folate, fat, medium-chain triglycerides (MCT), glucose, xylose, carotene, iron. Decreased calcium absorption. Decreased serum calcium and vitamin B_{12}. Increased urinary calcium.
Clofibrate	May decrease activity of intestinal disaccharidases.	Decreased taste acuity, unpleasant aftertaste. Decreased absorption of carotene, glucose, iron, MCT, vitamin B_{12}.
Hypotensive Agents Hydralazine	Inactivates pyridoxine. May chelate trace metals.	Increased excretion of pyridoxine; pyridoxine depletion. Possible peripheral neuritis.
Laxatives Mineral oil	Dissolves fat-soluble vitamins.	Decreased absorption of carotene, vitamins A, D, E and K, calcium and phosphate.
L-Dopa (levodopa)	Pyridoxine involved in metabolism of L-Dopa. Antagonizes pyridoxine.	Possible polyneuropathy related to pyridoxine depletion. Increased need for ascorbic acid and pyridoxine. Decreased absorption of tryptophan and other amino acids. Increased urinary excretion of sodium and potassium.
Oral Contraceptives	May increase catabolism, decrease absorption or alter tissue uptake of vitamin C. May inhibit folate conjugase. May increase transport proteins for vitamin A. Estrogens increase the rate of conversion of tryptophan to niacin.	Altered tryptophan metabolism. Decreased serum vitamin C levels. Possibly decreased serum vitamin B_{12}, folate, pyridoxine, riboflavin, magnesium and zinc. Increased hemoglobin, hematocrit, serum levels of vitamins A and E, total lipids, triglycerides, iron, total iron-binding capacity (TIBC) and plasma copper. Possible polyneuropathy, peripheral neuritis and megaloblastic anemia.
Sedative-Hypnotics Glutethimide	Possibly increases inactivation of 25-hydroxy vitamin D_3.	Increased vitamin D turnover. Increased bone resorption.
Sulfonamides Salicylazosulfapyridine (Azulfidine)		Decreased absorption of folate. Decreased serum folate and serum iron.
Other sulfonamides		Decreased sources of folate, vitamin K, B vitamins from intestinal bacterial synthesis.
Tranquilizers Chlorpromazine	Can reduce physical activity.	Possible weight gain.

body's need for vitamin B_{12}. Serum B_{12} should always be watched when the patient taking anticonvulsant therapy is also being given folate treatment.[22] The action of anticonvulsants in causing vitamin D deficiency was discussed earlier.

Oral Contraceptives

Oral contraceptives have many effects on nutrition, some of which are clinically important. Oral contraceptives increase plasma triglyceride levels, elevate blood glucose slightly and increase nitrogen retention.[14] Plasma levels of vitamins A and E are increased and levels of magnesium, zinc, riboflavin, ascorbic acid, folacin and vitamins B_{12} and B_6 are decreased. The fact that these changes are not found in all women illustrates that some women are more sensitive to the effects of oral contraceptive agents (OCAs) than others. Dietary intake probably influences the development of a biochemical deficiency.

Vitamin B_6 metabolism is affected so that there is an increased excretion of tryptophan metabolites after a tryptophan loading test. Thus, the requirement for vitamin B_6 is increased. Another result is a decrease in the brain amine serotonin and its metabolite 5-hydroxyindoleacetic acid (5-HIAA). This decrease could cause the depression sometimes seen in women who have biochemical signs of vitamin B_6 deficiency. In these women, depression was relieved when vitamin B_6 was given. Such women should probably take a vitamin B_6 supplement of 20 to 40 mg. daily.[1] Vitamin B_6 is probably not routinely necessary for all women taking contraceptives.

Some women who take oral contraceptives develop biochemical signs of folate deficiency; that is, lowered serum folate and lowered red cell folate with increased excretion of formiminoglutamic acid (FIGLU), a urinary metabolite of folic acid. Whether folate deficiency develops while a woman is taking oral contraceptives depends largely on her intake of folate and use of folate supplements. One theory postulates that oral contraceptives interfere with the deconjugation of polyglutamic acid to the monoglutamate form that is necessary for folic acid absorption from the gastrointestinal tract.[25]

Changes in plasma levels of minerals are likely a result of the redistribution of the minerals within the body rather than of excessive excretion or impaired absorption of the minerals.

THE EFFECT OF NUTRIENTS AND NUTRITIONAL STATUS ON THE ABSORPTION AND METABOLISM OF DRUGS

Drug metabolism may be altered in states of nutritional deficiency, since the activity of the hepatic microsomal enzyme drug-metabolizing system is influenced by the intake of protein, carbohydrate, lipid, riboflavin, ascorbic acid, magnesium and zinc. For example, manipulation of the diet from a normal one to a high-protein, low-carbohydrate diet resulted in a 35 to 40 per cent reduction in the plasma half-lives of antipyrine and theophylline.[11] Manipulation of major components of the diet could be of particular clinical significance in some situations, such as a protein increase for weight reduction or postoperative therapy using only intravenous glucose.

Other factors that influence the metabolism of drugs are the rate of intestinal absorption and delivery of the drug to the liver; the presence of other disease, including malnutrition; liver function; and the concomitant administration of other drugs that can either increase or decrease the metabolism of the first drug.

An example of an interaction between a drug and a food constituent is seen with the monoamine oxidase inhibitors (MAOIs) (used to treat depression) and the tyramine content of food. These drugs, particularly phenelzine and tranylcypromine, block monoamine oxidase activity, and thus tyramine is not deaminated in the liver but is allowed to reach the circulation. The tyramine causes the release of norepinephrine, which induces a hypertensive crisis through sympathetic overstimulation. The patient gets an occipital headache and a severe increase in blood pressure. Foods such as cheeses and wine, which contain tyramine, should be avoided by patients taking MAOIs. (See Table 21–6.)

The absorption of many drugs from the gastrointestinal tract is affected by the presence of food and nutrients in the lumen. Generally, drugs are absorbed more slowly when they are taken with food, and thus the total absorption may be reduced, usually because of delayed gastric emptying and dilution. By reducing the absorption of a drug, food reduces its therapeutic dosage. The drug may never reach effective levels in the blood, or the slow absorption may act as a sustained release, prolonging the effects of the drug.

These actions can be clinically significant. Changes in gastrointestinal acidity generally

Table 21-6   TYRAMINE CONTENT OF VARIOUS FOODS*

FOOD	TYRAMINE CONTENT (mcg./gm. or mcg./ml.)
Cheeses	
Camembert	86
Stilton	466
Brie	180
Emmentaler	225
N.Y. State Cheddar	1416
Gruyère	516
Processed American	50
Cream	ND[a]
Cottage	ND
Yeast	ND
Yogurt	ND
Beer	
Brand A	1.8
Brand B	2.3
Brand C	4.4
Wine	
Sherry	3.6
Sauterne	0.4
Riesling	0.6
Chianti	25.4
Port	ND

[a]ND = not detected.

*From: Horwitz, D., et al.: Monoamine oxidase inhibitors, tyramine and cheese. JAMA, *188*:1108, 1964.

affect the rate of absorption of a drug rather than the total amount of drug absorbed.

The rate of gastric emptying, influenced by the type of meal or food ingested, can influence the absorption of a drug. For example, drugs such as L-dopa and penicillin G are metabolized or degraded in the stomach, so that situations of delayed gastric emptying would cause increased destruction of these drugs and a smaller effective dosage. On the other hand, delayed gastric emptying in the case of nitrofurantoin, a broad-spectrum antibacterial agent, would increase the time the product is in the stomach, allowing a greater portion of the drug to be dissolved by the gastric juice before it entered the duodenum where the absorption would be maximal. Food in this case would increase the effective dosage of a drug.

Certain nutrients can affect the absorption of drugs. Foods of dairy origin, which contain large amounts of calcium, inhibit the absorption of tetracycline because calcium forms a complex with the drug that prevents its absorption from the gastrointestinal tract. Tetracycline derivatives should probably be given without milk or milk products.

Another example of a food constituent affecting the absorption of a drug is the effect of a high-fat meal on the absorption of griseofulvin. A large intake of fats increases the absorption of griseofulvin, which is highly lipid-soluble. It may be that the fat stimulates the secretion of bile, which enhances the solubility of the drug by making it more water-soluble. See Table 21-7 for a summary of those mechanisms that can interfere with drug therapy.

Table 21-7   MECHANISMS BY WHICH FOOD INTERFERES WITH DRUG THERAPY*

Alteration of absorption of orally administered drugs by affecting:
   G.I. transit time and motility.
   G.I. secretions and pH.
   osmolality of G.I. tract.
   ionization of drug.
   stability of drug.
   solubility of drug.
   complexing of drug with a dietary component.
Alteration of drug's distribution.
Alteration of drug's metabolism.
Alteration of drug's excretion.
Exertion of antagonistic pharmacological response by active substance in food.

*Adapted from: Hethcox, J. M., and Stanaszek, W. F.: Interactions of drugs and diet. Hospital Pharmacy, *9*(10): 373, 1974.

PROBLEMS AND SUGGESTED TOPICS FOR DISCUSSION

1. Evaluate one of your patients for possible nutritional problems resulting from his or her drug therapy. What are your recommendations for nutritional care?
2. Why are drugs more likely to induce nutritional deficiency in chronically ill, debilitated patients? What can be done to prevent this?
3. Evaluate a patient with a malabsorption syndrome (sprue, regional enteritis or small bowel resection, for example). Is he or she taking any medication? How is the absorption of medication changed? Evaluate the patient's nutritional status. What nutritional care would you recommend?
4. Evaluate a patient receiving a cancer chemotherapeutic agent.
   a. Is he or she suffering from oral or gastrointestinal side effects of the therapy? What are these side effects?
   b. Is the nutritional intake adequate? Is there any weight loss? If so, why?
   c. What would you recommend for nutritional care?
   d. How would you help the patient make any necessary changes in diet?

CITED REFERENCES

1. Adams, P. W., et al.: Effect of pyridoxine hydrochloride (vitamin B_6) upon depression associated with oral contraceptives. Lancet, *1*:897, 1973.

2. Alter, H. J., Zvaifler, M. J., and Rath, C. E.: Interrelationship of rheumatoid arthritis, folic acid and aspirin. Blood, 38:405, 1971.
3. Burrows, M. T., and Farr, W. K.: The action of mineral oil per os on the organism. Proc. Soc. Exper. Biol. Med., 24:719, 1927.
4. Faloon, W. W.: Drug production of intestinal malabsorption. N.Y. State J. Med., 70:2189, 1970.
5. Fell, G. S., et al.: Urinary zinc levels as an indication of muscle catabolism. Lancet, 1:280, 1973.
6. Gross, L., and Brotman, M.: Hypoprothrombinemia and hemorrhage associated with cholestyramine therapy. Ann. Intern. Med., 72:95, 1970.
7. Hahn, T. J., et al.: Serum 25-hydroxycalciferol levels and bone mass in children on chronic anticonvulsant therapy. N. Engl. J. Med., 292:550, 1975.
8. Hart, S. L., and McColl, I.: The effect of the laxative oxyphenisatin on the intestinal absorption of glucose in rat and man. Br. J. Pharmacol., 32:683, 1968.
9. Heaton, K. W., Lever, J. V., and Barnard, D.: Osteomalacia associated with cholestyramine therapy for postileectomy diarrhea. Gastroenterology, 62:642, 1972.
10. Jacobsen, E. D., Prior, J. T., and Faloon, W. W.: Malabsorption syndrome induced by neomycin: Morphologic alterations in the jejunal mucosa. J. Lab. Clin. Med., 56:245, 1960.
11. Kappas, A., et al.: Influence of dietary protein and carbohydrate on antipyrine and theophylline metabolism in man. Clin. Pharmacol. Ther., 20:643, 1976.
12. Keusch, G. T., Troncale, E. J., and Plant, A. G.: Neomycin-induced malabsorption in a tropical population. Gastroenterology, 58:197, 1970.
13. Langford, H. G.: Rationale for diets modified in sodium and potassium. Paper presented at the 57th Annual Meeting of the American Dietetic Association, Philadelphia, 1974.
14. Lecocq, F. R., Bradley, E. M., and Goldzieher, J. W.: Metabolic balance studies with norethynodrel and chlormadinone acetate. Am. J. Obstet. Gynecol., 99:374, 1967.
15. Longstreth, G. F., and Newcomer, A. D.: Drug-induced malabsorption. Mayo Clin. Proc., 50:284, 1975.
16. Lucas, B., and Sells, C. J.: Nutrient intake and stimulant drugs in hyperactive children. J. Am. Diet. Assoc., 70:373, 1977.
17. Matheson, R. T., et al.: Absorption and biotransformation of cholecalciferol in drug-induced osteomalacia. J. Clin. Pharmacol., 16:426, 1976.
18. McCall, J. T., et al.: Comparative metabolism of copper and zinc in patients with Wilson's disease (hepatolenticular degeneration). Am. J. Med. Sci., 254:13, 1967.
19. Roe, D. A.: Drug-induced nutritional deficiencies. Westport, Connecticut, Avi Publishing Co., 1976, p. 135.
20. Roe, D. A.: Drug-induced Nutritional Deficiencies, p. 150.
21. Roe, D. A.: Drug-induced Nutritional Deficiencies, p. 211.
22. Roe, D. A.: Drug-induced Nutritional Deficiencies, p. 217.
23. Safer, D., Allan, R., and Barr, E.: Depression of growth in hyperactive children on stimulant drugs. N. Engl. J. Med., 287:217, 1972.
24. Safer, D. J., Allan, R. P., and Barr, E.: Growth rebound after termination of stimulant drugs. J. Pediatr., 86:113, 1975.
25. Streiff, R. R.: Folate deficiency and oral contraceptives. JAMA, 214:105, 1970.
26. Toskes, P. P., and Deren, J. J.: Selective inhibition of vitamin B_{12} absorption by para-aminosalicylic acid. Gastroenterology, 62:1232, 1972.
27. Wester, P. O.: Zinc during diuretic treatment. Lancet, 1:578, 1975.

ADDITIONAL REFERENCES

Carson, J. A. S., and Gormican, A.: Disease–medication relationships in altered taste sensitivity. J. Am. Diet. Assoc., 68:550, 1976.
Carson, J. A. S., and Gormican, A.: Taste acuity and food attitudes of selected patients with cancer. J. Am. Diet. Assoc., 70:361, 1977.
Clinical nutrition: Folic acid absorption, anticonvulsant and contraceptive therapy. Nutr. Rev., 32:39, 1974.
Cummings, J. H., et al.: Laxative-induced diarrhea: A continuing clinical problem. Br. Med. J., 1:537, 1974.
Faloon, W. W. (ed.): Symposium: Drug–nutrient relationships. Am. J. Clin. Nutr., 26:103, 1973.
Goodman, L. S., and Gilman, A. (eds.): The Pharmacological Basis of Therapeutics, 5th ed. New York, Macmillan Publishing Company, 1975.
Hahn, T. J.: Bone complications of anticonvulsants. Drugs, 12:201, 1976.
Hartshorn, E. A.: Food and drug interactions. J. Am. Diet. Assoc., 70:15, 1977.
Hethcox, J. M., and Stanaszek, W. F.: Interactions of drugs and diet. Hospital Pharmacy, 9(10):373, 1974.
Malnutrition and drug metabolism in man. Nutr. Rev., 34:237, 1976.
March, D. C.: Handbook: Interactions of Selected Drugs with Nutritional Status in Man. Chicago, American Dietetic Association, 1976.
Pierpaoli, P. G.: Drug therapy and diet. Drug Intell. Clin. Pharm., 6:89, 1972.
Symposium: Oral contraceptives and nutrients. Am. J. Clin. Nutr., 28:371, 1975.
Theuer, R. C.: Effect of oral contraceptive agents on vitamin and mineral needs: A review. J. Reprod. Med., 8:13, 1972.
Visconti, J. A.: Drug–food interaction. In: Nutrition in Disease. Columbus, Ohio, Ross Laboratories, 1977.
Wynn, V.: Vitamins and oral contraceptive-use. Lancet, 1:561, 1975.

UNIT SIX

DISEASES OF THE GASTROINTESTINAL SYSTEM

Chapter 22

NUTRITIONAL CARE FOR PATIENTS WITH ESOPHAGEAL AND GASTRIC DISEASES

Gastrointestinal diseases can be classified as (1) organic and (2) reflex or functional. The latter are the more common. An *organic* disease of the stomach is one in which a definite pathological change has taken place in the structural tissues. Peptic ulcer and cancer are examples. A *reflex* or *functional* disorder of the stomach is a disturbance, either sensory, motor, absorptive or secretory in origin, for which no lesion or other pathological cause can be found. Functional disorders have, in addition, a hard-to-define emotional and psychological component. As we learn more about gastrointestinal disorders, it becomes harder to separate them into organic and functional categories. For example, a "functional" disorder such as ulcerative colitis has characteristic pathological manifestations; and an "organic" disorder such as peptic ulcer is caused by excessive gastric acidity, a functional aspect. It appears that most gastrointestinal diseases have both organic and functional components.

A gastrointestinal disorder, whether it is the patient's primary disease or the gastrointestinal manifestation of a systemic disease, is a potential threat to the individual's nutritional status. The objectives of the nutritional care are not only to alleviate the gastrointestinal

symptoms but also to maintain good nutritional status.

The first objective requires application of knowledge about how various foods may affect the gastrointestinal tract and aggravate the present pathological condition. The second objective, maintenance of good nutritional status, requires an understanding of the way in which the gastrointestinal disorder impairs the individual's ability to consume, absorb and utilize nutrients. It is important to recognize the *nutrient limitations* of the therapeutic diet modifications, especially when the patient must change usual dietary intake patterns and is suffering from anorexia, nausea, vomiting, constipation or diarrhea.

NUTRITIONAL ASSESSMENT

The assessment of nutritional status, especially the dietary history, is crucial in the nutritional care of a patient with a gastrointestinal disorder. Besides being the basis for setting the nutritional care objectives (see Chapter 20), the assessment has special significance in gastrointestinal disease. First the dietary history can reveal eating patterns or changes that reflect symptoms characteristic of a disorder. For

466

Table 22–1   DIETARY HISTORY INFORMATION THAT CAN GIVE CLUES TO
GASTROINTESTINAL DISEASE

SYMPTOM	POSSIBLE DISORDER
Ingestion of solid food causes distress but liquids do not.	Esophageal stricture or tumor.
Difficulty in swallowing; food sticks in throat.	Esophageal spasm; achalasia.
Epigastric pain when eating.	Gastric ulcer.
Pain 2–5 hours after a meal, relieved upon eating.	Duodenal ulcer.
Abdominal pain several hours after a fatty meal.	Pancreatic or biliary tract disease.
Cramps, distention and flatulence several hours after drinking milk.	Lactose intolerance probably due to lactase deficiency.
Heartburn after a fatty meal.	Hiatal hernia; achalasia; esophageal motility problem.

example, the patient who complains of pain four to five hours after a fatty meal gives a clue of possible gallbladder disease. Consider esophageal disease when the patient gives a history of difficulty in swallowing dry foods such as bread or toast. Table 22–1 presents more clues to be gained from the dietary history.

Second, the nutritional status assessment can forewarn the nurse or nutritionist about potential nutritional problems. Gastrointestinal disease will probably worsen borderline nutritional status, and measures should be taken to prevent this.

Third, a nutritional assessment taken after the patient has started a therapeutic regimen can tell how the patient is coping with the disease and its treatment. Because eating problems are individual, because eating can be painful and because food and the gastrointestinal reactions related to it are fraught with mystery and misconception, patients may follow very restricted and inadequate diets. The nurse, nutritionist or physician should know how the patient is eating at home, where the patient must care for himself and try to comply with the medical regimen. If the diet is inadequate, the nutritionist can give advice and encouragement for necessary changes.

DISEASES OF THE ESOPHAGUS

In normal swallowing, the muscles of the pharynx, upper esophagus and upper esophageal sphincter are smoothly coordinated with the muscles of the lower esophagus and lower esophageal sphincter.* The entire esophagus functions as one tissue during swallowing. The bolus of food is voluntarily moved

*Although these muscles are referred to as "sphincters" they are really no different from the rest of the esophagus; however, physiologically they remain constricted and closed, unlike the rest of the esophagus.

from the mouth to the pharynx. The upper sphincter relaxes, the food moves into the esophagus, and the lower esophageal sphincter (LES) relaxes to receive the food bolus. Peristaltic waves move the bolus down the esophagus and into the stomach. (See Fig. 22–1.) For a more complete discussion of the physiology of the esophagus the student is referred to other texts.[8, 9]

Disorders of the esophagus are due to obstruction, inflammation or derangement of the swallowing mechanism. Although all esophageal disorders are potential deterrents to the person's ability to consume food, only those common disorders for which nutritional care is indicated will be discussed here.

ACHALASIA (ESOPHAGEAL DYSSYNERGIA)

Achalasia, also called *esophageal dyssynergia* or *cardiospasm*, is a disorder of lower esophageal motility. Decreased numbers of ganglion cells in Auerback's plexus cause impaired cholinergic innervation of the esophageal musculature. The result is failure of the LES to relax and open during swallowing. Consequently, patients complain of *dysphagia*, or difficulty in swallowing, and describe the sensation of food sticking in the esophagus under the sternum. Dysphagia, which can be mild and infrequent, becomes severe and painful as the achalasia worsens. During eating, the esophagus fills with food and fluid until either the pressure forces the esophageal sphincter to open and allow small amounts of food to enter the stomach, or the person is forced to vomit up the food. Extreme dilatation of the esophagus develops, while the LES opening narrows. When the patient finally seeks help, he or she is usually eating very little because of the physical and social discomfort involved and has usually lost weight.

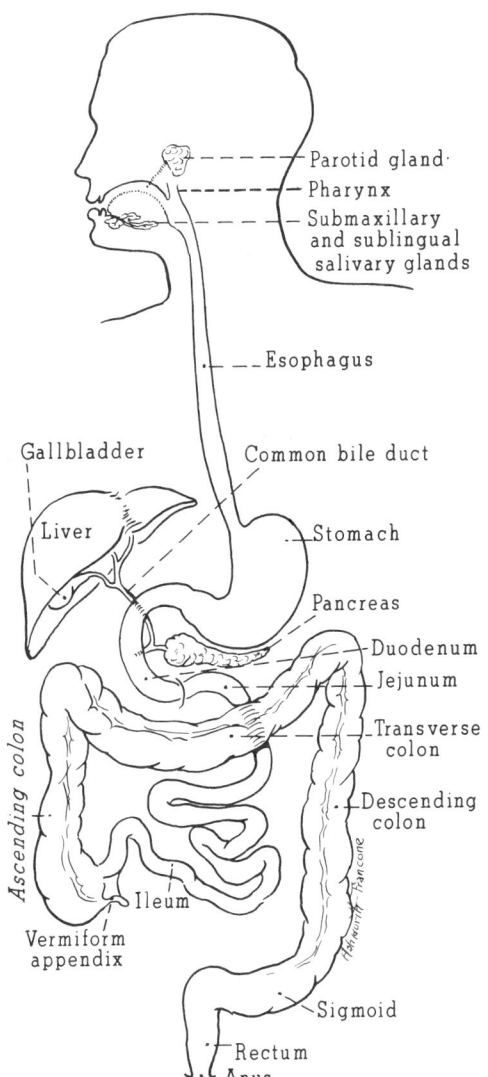

Figure 22–1 The digestive system and its associated structures. (From: Jacob, S. W., and Francone, C. A.: Structure and Function in Man, 4th ed. Philadelphia, W. B. Saunders Co., 1978.)

Treatment

Treatment of achalasia is the forceful dilatation of the LES with small inflatable bags. In this way, dysphagia can be relieved for years and perhaps permanently; however, esophageal motility is not restored. Surgery is often required, although this pneumatic dilatation may be performed first in order to rehabilitate the patient nutritionally prior to surgery. After dilatation or surgery the esophagus, now permanently open, functions by means of gravity and oropharyngeal pressure.

Until the LES can be opened, the use of liquid foods and fluids with meals will facilitate swallowing and maintain the patient's nutritional intake. If this does not work, feeding by means of a nasogastric tube, jejunostomy, gastrostomy or intravenous line is necessary. (See Cahpter 34, Nutritional Care for Patients with Surgery, Burns or Trauma.)

Permanent opening of the LES through dilatation or surgery alleviates dysphagia, but it also allows reflux of the gastric contents into the esophagus. The gastroesophageal reflux is highly acidic and causes inflammation of the esophagus or *esophagitis*.

ESOPHAGITIS

Esophagitis usually occurs in the lower esophagus as a result of the irritating effect of acidic gastric reflux on the esophageal mucosa. The common symptom is *heartburn*, a burning epigastric substernal pain. In the rare situation when esophagitis appears in the upper esophagus, it is usually a consequence of iron deficiency (Plummer-Vinson syndrome.) Iron deficiency causes atropic changes in the esophageal mucosa that make it vulnerable to the minor trauma from food.

The gastroesophageal reflux that causes lower esophagitis occurs because the LES pressure is lower than normal so that the LES does not close as it should between swallows. The LES pressure is controlled by many factors, some of which are the gastrointestinal hormones. Gastrin increases LES pressure and secretin and cholecystokinin decrease LES pressure. Low LES pressure may be caused by gastrin deficiency.[3] When lower esophagitis is chronic, an inflammatory stricture and eventually dysphagia can develop.

Nutritional Care

The objectives of nutritional care for esophagitis are (1) to prevent irritation of the inflamed esophageal mucosa in the acute phase, (2) to prevent esophageal reflux and (3) to decrease the irritating capacity or acidity of the gastric juice.

In the acute phase, the patient may want a liquid diet, which is less abrasive to the esophagus. Orange juice and tomato products can be irritating because of their acidity, and omission of these from the diet can be helpful.

Certain foods affect gastrointestinal hormone release and LES pressure:

1. Protein meals stimulate gastrin release and *increase* LES pressure.

2. Fatty meals cause release of cholecystokinin from the small intestine, which *decreases* LES pressure.

3. Chocolate, which contains caffeine and theobromine, *decreases* LES pressure.

4. Coffee, which contains caffeine, *decreases* esophageal pressure and stimulates gastric acid secretion.

5. Alcohol *decreases* LES pressure.

6. Cigarette smoking (nicotine) *decreases* LES pressure.

7. Peppermint and spearmint oils, such as might be found in liqueurs, *decrease* LES pressure.

Those foods and other factors that decrease LES pressure should be restricted or omitted from the diet.

To decrease the irritating capacity or acidity of the gastric juice, the patient is advised to take antacids and Gaviscon. Gaviscon is a mixture of aluminum hydroxide and alginic acid that floats on top of the gastric acid pool. It prevents the movement of gastric acid into the esophagus.

Other helpful suggestions are for the patient to sleep on a bed that has its upper portion raised 4 to 6 inches and to lose weight if overweight. See Table 22–2 for a summary of the nutritional care for esophagitis.

Bethanechol, a cholinergic drug, increases LES pressure and may be prescribed if the esophagitis does not respond to other measures. Esophagitis that does not respond after three to six months of medical therapy should be treated surgically.

HIATAL HERNIA

Hiatal hernia is an outpouching of a portion of the stomach into the chest through the esophageal hiatus of the diaphragm. Depending on the form of the outpouching, a hiatal hernia may be *paraesophageal* or *sliding,* in which part of the stomach but not the esophagus herniates through the diaphragm into the thorax, or it can be *gastroesophageal,* in which the lower esophagus and part of the stomach protrude through the diaphragm into the thorax. The major symptoms of either type of hernia are reflux of gastric contents into the esophagus and esophagitis. (See Fig. 22–2.)

Treatment

Treatment aims to reduce gastroesophageal reflux, so the nutritional care is similar to that

Table 22–2 NUTRITIONAL CARE FOR PATIENTS WITH ESOPHAGITIS

The patient with esophagitis should:
1. Avoid those foods that he knows will cause heartburn.
2. Eat small, frequent meals to prevent stomach distention and resulting gastric acid secretion.
3. Eat high-protein meals, which stimulate gastrin secretion and increase lower esophageal sphincter pressure.
4. Avoid high-fat meals and decrease fat in the diet. Fat decreases lower esophageal pressure.
5. Avoid chocolate, alcohol and caffeine-containing beverages such as coffee, tea and cola drinks.
6. Avoid lying down, bending over or straining immediately after eating.
7. Avoid eating within two to three hours of going to bed.
8. Avoid tight-fitting clothing, especially after a meal.
9. Lose weight if he is overweight.

given for esophagitis. Again, surgical repair is indicated if the esophageal distress is resistant to medical therapy.

DISEASES OF THE STOMACH

INDIGESTION

Indigestion or dyspepsia is an indefinite term frequently used to describe any discomfort occurring from a disorder of the digestive tract. The core of the trouble may be in the stomach, or it may be a reflex symptom of the derangement of some other organ, such as the colon, or of gallbladder disease, renal calculi, chronic appendicitis or diabetes. Indigestion as a manifestation of psychoneurosis is frequently encountered. The association between emotional and gastrointestinal disturbances is so frequent that the relationship cannot be denied. Many people complain of a "nervous stomach," which they attribute to the eating of certain foods. Besides psychic disturbance, other avoidable causes of indigestion are rapid eating, poor mastication, overindulgence in rich foods and a poor diet.

Nutritional Care

Before dietary treatment begins, the cause of indigestion must be determined. The symptoms may be a warning of a more serious illness. A therapeutic diet for simple indigestion is seldom necessary. A well-balanced diet plus correct eating habits are usually sufficient. Treating the cause, whether it is a mental or a physical one, is the important factor. Emphasis

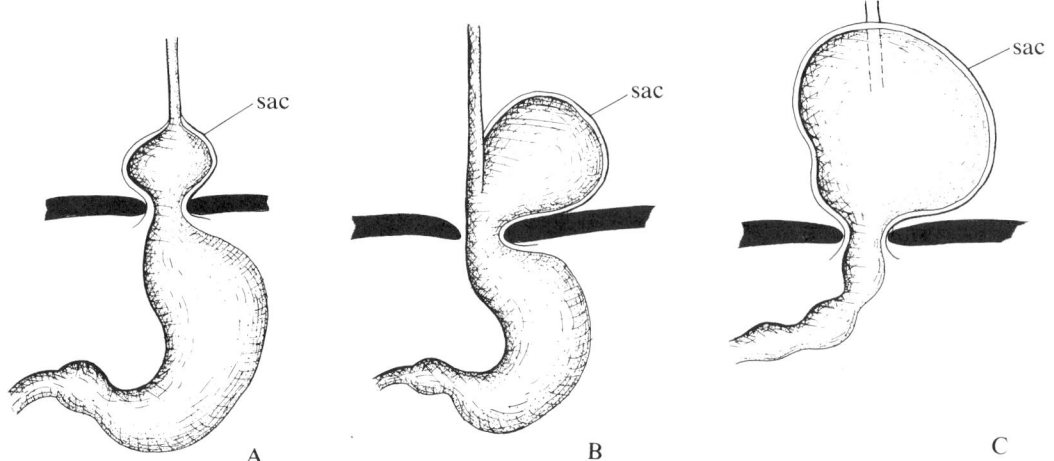

Figure 22–2   Sketches of various types of hernias. *A*, bell (or sliding) hernia; *B*, paraesophageal hernia; *C*, massive (or gastroesophageal) hernia. (From: Hagarty, G.: A classification of esophageal hiatus hernia with special reference to sliding hernia. Am. J. Roentgenol., *84*:1056, 1960.)

should be placed on the improvement of the patient's customary dietary and eating habits.

HYPOCHLORHYDRIA

Hypochlorhydria is a condition is which the gastric juice secreted by the stomach glands contains a diminished amount of hydrochloric acid, although some free hydrochloric acid is present. As a result, proteins are not digested properly in the stomach, carbohydrates ferment very readily and the gastric mucosa becomes hypersensitive. The lack of sufficient hydrochloric acid in the gastric juices lowers resistance to bacterial action, both fermentative and putrefactive. Diarrhea is a common symptom. Disturbances may occur anywhere along the digestive tract.

To avoid confusion, two other conditions similar to hypochlorhydria deserve mention. *Achlorhydria* is a condition in which free hydrochloric acid is not found, but combined acid is present. *Achylia gastrica* is a condition in which neither free nor combined acid is present.

These conditions often accompany other diseases such as pernicious anemia, sprue, carcinoma, diabetes, nephritis and chronic gastritis. They commonly occur after irradiation of the stomach in the treatment of cancer or gastric ulcer, when parietal cells are destroyed.

Nutritional Care

Every precaution should be taken to prevent the introduction of bacteria into the digestive tract and to avoid foods that will favor their development. Milk, one of the chief offenders, must be selected carefully or treated to keep the bacterial count low. A low-fiber diet is advised, as fibrous foods have a tendency to delay the emptying of the stomach and thus favor bacterial activity. The minimal fiber diet (p. 490 and Table 23–4) is especially recommended when diarrhea is present. In cases of severe diarrhea it may be advisable to boil the drinking water.

Because fats inhibit the secretion of hydrochloric acid and retard the emptying of the stomach, the amount in the diet should be restricted to a minimum, about 70 to 90 gm. Fried foods and rich desserts should be avoided. Iced and very cold beverages and foods are contraindicated.

Because broth and clear soups stimulate gastric secretion, they may be included in the diet. Carbohydrates in the form of starch are less likely to ferment, so they are preferred to the sugar type of carbohydrates. Cooked fruits and vegetables (or fruits and vegetables of low fiber content) are recommended.

ACUTE GASTRITIS

Acute gastritis is an inflammation of the gastric mucosa, sudden and sometimes violent in onset, but the term is often applied to any stomach discomfort. Attacks very often follow dietary indiscretions such as overeating, the eating of specific foods to which the individual is sensitive, eating too fast or eating when overtired or emotionally upset. Too much alcohol,

tobacco and highly seasoned foods may also be contributing factors.

The possible ingestion of certain toxic substances, such as spoiled food (which might contain staphylococcal toxin) or drugs such as salicylates and ammonium chloride, can be another factor. The toxin of an infectious disease or of germs from the teeth, tonsils or sinuses may also bring on an attack of gastritis.

The initial treatment is to get rid of the offending substance as soon as possible. It may be necessary to empty the stomach by induced vomiting, lavage or both. Irrigation of the colon and the administration of a laxative may also be of value in hastening the cleansing process.

Nutritional Care

To allow the stomach to rest and heal, food is usually withheld for 24 to 48 hours. Since it can stimulate gastric acid secretion, even the water taken by mouth is restricted, with the exception of cracked ice, which may be held in the mouth to relieve thirst. Fluids are given intravenously.

Following the fast period, low-fiber liquid foods are added as tolerated. (See the description of the full liquid diet, p. 447 and Table 20–9.) Milk is usually a good food to start the diet. Small amounts of milk toast, cereal and cream soups are fed at intervals of 30 to 45 minutes. Stimulating broths and highly seasoned foods should be avoided. The amount of food and the number of feedings are increased according to the patient's tolerance until he or she is eating a full regular diet. The nurse or dietitian should discuss the patient's customary dietary pattern, eating habits and any changes needed with the patient himself.

CHRONIC GASTRITIS

The cause of chronic gastritis is not known. The attacks follow the same type of conditions described for acute gastritis. Chronic gastritis often precedes the development of organic gastric lesions such as cancer and ulcer. It may be due to an antral defect that closely resembles these diseases. It may also be related indirectly to diseases such as tuberculosis, myocardial failure and nephritis. The same dietary indiscretions listed for acute gastritis seem to be frequent causes of the chronic variety. The stomach seems to be a long-suffering organ, willing and capable of accepting neglect, abuse and ill treatment. But there comes a time—sooner in some, later in others—

when the stomach rebels. Chief among the manifestations of this rebellion is pain, which may be mild at times but severe and cutting at intervals.

Endoscopy

There is a simple way to ascertain the true state of affairs. A gastroscope can be passed down the esophagus into the stomach, and the appearance of the stomach mucosa can be viewed, studied and even photographed. Erosions, ulcerations, changes in the blood vessels, and destruction of surface cells can be seen. These can then be correlated with chemical, histological and clinical findings to help make a diagnosis.

Nutritional Care

Because the conception of chronic gastritis is vague, the nutritional care must follow general principles. The diet should be adequate in calories and nutrients and soft in consistency. The patient should eat at regular intervals and chew the food well. Highly seasoned foods are not usually tolerated well. Excess amounts of liquids with meals tend to cause discomfort. The same principle for ulcer care, that is, reduction of gastric acidity, is followed for gastritis. (See Table 22–3.) Frequent small meals interspersed with antacid therapy are the mainstay of treatment. (See Table 22–4.) Most important is to determine the cause of the discomfort and then to prescribe individualized treatment.

Chronic gastritis can result in atrophy and loss of stomach oxyntic cells. This results in a loss of gastric secretion and possible vitamin B_{12} malabsorption because of a lack of intrinsic factor. Vitamin B_{12} status should always be assessed in these patients. (See Chapter 11, Assessment of Nutritional Status.)

GASTRIC AND DUODENAL ULCERS

An eroded lesion in the gastric mucosa or intestinal mucosa (duodenum) is termed an *ulcer*. The location of the ulcer determines its nomenclature. That is, if the ulcer is located in the stomach, it is a *gastric ulcer;* if it is located in the duodenum, it is called a *duodenal ulcer* (see Fig. 22–3). Often both types are grouped together under the general term *peptic ulcer*. Since the treatment for both types is essentially the same, the nutritional care for them will be

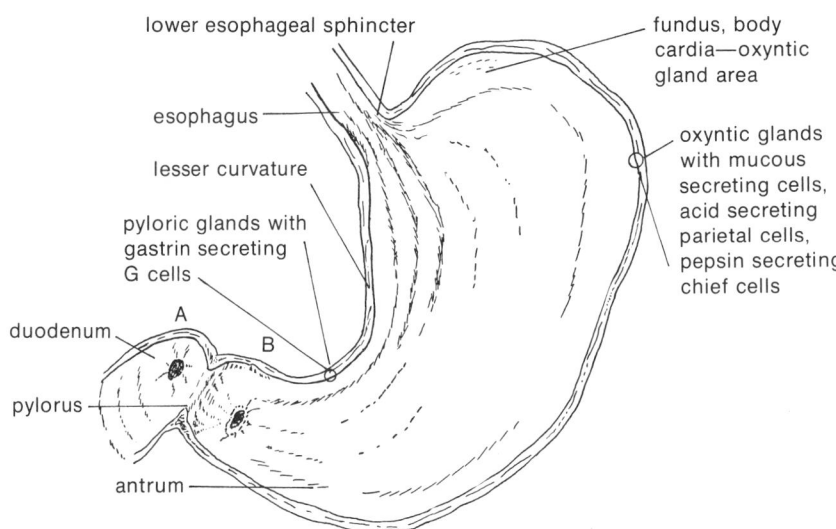

Figure 22–3 Diagram showing stomach and duodenum with eroded lesions. *A,* duodenal ulcer; *B,* gastric ulcer.

considered together. Duodenal ulcers are much more common than gastric ulcers, and both kinds occur in the male more frequently than in the female, usually in people who are naturally tense, hard-working and hard-worrying.

It is reported that approximately 10 per cent of our population is or has been afflicted with gastric or duodenal ulcers. Sometimes during routine x-ray examination ulcer scars are found, although the individual never knew that the disorder existed. This would seem to indicate that healing sometimes takes place spontaneously. Ulcers tend to recur in 75 to 80 per cent of patients. The disease appears to run a course that lasts about 15 years.[6]

During the years 1960 to 1972, there was a 50 per cent decrease in the incidence of duodenal ulcer that cannot be explained until we know more about the pathogenesis of peptic ulcer disease.[14] However, the frequency of duodenal ulcer seems to be increasing among U.S. females, possibly as a result of the fact that more American women are now pursuing aggressive careers.

Pathogenesis of Ulcer Disease

An acidic gastrointestinal environment is believed to be the principle cause of peptic ulcer disease. Normally, the mucosa of the stomach is protected from the strongly acidic digestive juices by the mucus secreted by glands from the lower esophagus to the upper duodenum. The duodenum is also protected by the pancreatic secretions, which contain large quantities of

sodium bicarbonate that neutralize the hydrochloric acid in the gastric juice. In the alkaline environment, pepsin is inactivated and cannot digest the duodenal mucosa.

The reasons why the gastric or duodenal acidity gets too high and why the mucosa loses its resistance to normal gastric acidity are not clear, but many theories have been suggested.

Duodenal Ulcer. Most duodenal ulcers occur within 3 cm. of the pylorus, at a point where the gastric acidity is high. The following have been observed in patients with duodenal ulcer and may help to explain the pathogenesis of the disease:[11, 21]

1. Increased capacity to secrete acid in response to gastrin because of a greater number of parietal cells (acid-secreting cells). Maximal acid secretion has been found to be twice that of persons without duodenal ulcer disease.
2. Increased sensitivity of parietal cells to gastrin.
3. Hypersecretion of gastrin in response to meals.
4. Decreased ability to inhibit gastrin release when the acidity of the gastric contents drops too low.
5. Increased nocturnal gastric acid secretion.
6. Rapid entry of acidified chyme into the duodenum; it cannot be neutralized rapidly enough.

All of these abnormal functions result in an increased acid load to the duodenum and the development of a duodenal ulcer.

Gastric Ulcer. Most gastric ulcers are found

in the antrum of the stomach. Their pathogenesis seems to be different from that of the duodenal ulcer. The following are possible pathological processes:

1. Gastritis or inflammation of the antrum or pyloric gland area tends to occur with gastric ulcer and may be a "pre-ulcer" condition.
2. Chronic backward diffusion of H^+ ions after the normal gastric mucosal barrier is disrupted results in gross mucosal damage. The mucosal damage leads to release of pepsin in large quantities, which contributes to further mucosal damage.
3. A disturbance in antroduodenal motility can cause bile acids from the duodenum to reflux back into the stomach, where they break the mucosal barrier and cause gastritis. The damaged mucosa then becomes susceptible to peptic ulceration. Other agents that break the barrier are salicylates and alcohol.

Although chronic ulcer usually follows a typical course and produces characteristic symptoms, occasionally the symptoms are either non-existent or indefinite, and hemorrhage or perforation may be the first sign of the illness. Ulcers can perforate into the peritoneal cavity or penetrate into an adjacent organ (usually the pancreas), and they may erode an artery and result in massive hemorrhage.

Predisposing Factors

Faulty dietary habits, excessive smoking, excessive aspirin ingestion and *excessive drinking of coffee and cola drinks* are associated with an increased risk of developing an ulcer.[7] Rushing through meals, improper selection of food and irregular mealtimes are poor nutrition and eating habits that set the stage for ulcer development.

Heredity has been mentioned as a possible factor in the development of ulcers. It has been observed that patients with type O blood have ulcers more often than do persons with other blood types.

Physical stress can cause ulcers. Therefore, inadequate sleep and rest or disease or trauma may be predisposing factors in their development.

Emotional conflicts, psychological stress, nervous strain or *psychic trauma* cause a disturbance of the nerves that control the blood supply to the lining of the stomach and the duodenum, thus weakening the lining and

making it susceptible to attack by the gastric juices. Excessive stimulation of the vagus by impulses originating in the cerebrum increases gastric acid secretion.

Protective factors in unrefined foods may help to prevent ulcer disease. Based on epidemiological studies in populations that eat unrefined diets, some investigators feel that factors present in fiber can protect the gastrointestinal epithelium from ulcer disease through a buffering activity.[20]

Treatment

The objectives of treatment are relief of pain, healing of the ulcer, reduction of the tendency to recurrence and maintenance of good nutritional status. Unfortunately, there is no cure for peptic ulcer disease, and the ulcers do tend to recur.

Medical Therapy. The accepted medical treatment at present for peptic ulcer is based on the fact that these ulcers do not exist in the absence of hydrochloric acid. Accordingly, therapy is directed toward the neutralization of acids and the reduction of acid secretion by the stomach. By elevating the pH of the gastric contents, the proteolytic activity of pepsin and the damaging effect of acid are reduced. In addition, therapy aims to preserve the resistance of the epithelium to the destructive action of gastric juice. With these objectives, therapy consists of taking antacids and anticholinergics, modifying the diet and avoiding stressful situations.

REST. Because resistance must be kept at a high level, physical and mental rest are important. If the ulcer is moderately advanced, bed rest either at home or in the hospital may be advocated for a period of one to three weeks. An equal period of convalescence is prescribed, particularly for the working person, who should stay away from disturbing office situations. In mild cases the patient can usually continue his regular routine work activities while following the diet and taking medication. If the atmosphere and surroundings at home or at work are unpleasant and cause emotional upsets, the patient may be advised to consider a complete change.

ANTACIDS. Antacids have long been clinically effective in reducing the pain from duodenal ulcer, and it was always thought that relief was due to a reduction in gastric acidity. This is questionable now in the light of evidence showing that pain relief in duodenal ulcer patients was the same whether they were given

an antacid or a placebo that looked and tasted like chalky white antacid but had no buffering capacity.[18] This does not exclude the use of antacids but suggests that factors other than acid neutralization are important in the relief of ulcer pain. The degree to which a patient responds to antacids depends on the individual, the extent of the parietal cell mass, the rate at which the antacid is emptied from the stomach and the gastric acid response to eating. Antacids vary in their ability to neutralize acid, and this should be considered when prescribing the amount to be used.

The preferred antacid is aluminum hydroxide-based, because it has good acid-neutralizing ability and is not absorbed by the body. Antacids containing calcium, such as calcium carbonate preparations, are less desirable. Calcium stimulates gastrin secretion, which increases gastric acid secretion. Magnesium frequently is added to antacid mixtures to prevent constipation. However, aluminum hydroxide binds phosphorus in the gut and prevents its absorption, which could result in a lowered serum phosphate level.

Antacids should be taken one hour after eating. Taken this way they have a longer buffering effect, about three to four hours. More antacid is usually required for the patient with duodenal ulcer than for the patient with gastric ulcer, because the duodenal ulcer patient usually has hypersecretion of acid.

ANTICHOLINERGICS AND OTHER DRUGS. Anticholinergics decrease gastric acid secretion and gastric motility. They inhibit vagal stimulation of acid-secreting parietal cells, vagal-stimulated release of gastrin and gastric motility. They are generally given during the active phase of ulcer disease. During inactive phases they may be taken only at night, since during sleep basal gastric acid secretion increases. Unfortunately, they have side effects such as mouth dryness, blurred vision and retention of urine.

Other drugs such as cimetidine (a histamine antagonist or H_2 receptor antagonist), which block the stimulatory action of histamine on acid-secreting parietal cells; prostaglandins; and certain gastrointestinal hormones are also used at times in ulcer therapy.

Nutritional Care. Like the other measures, nutritional care aims to reduce the secretion of stomach acid, to neutralize it, to maintain the resistance of gastrointestinal epithelial tissue to the acid and to restore the patient's nutritional status. There is little disagreement about these objectives of nutritional care, but controversy does exist regarding the dietary modifications needed to meet these objectives. As is usually the case, the controversy exists because of the ignorance regarding what happens to an individual food item in the gut, its effect on the alimentary tube and the explanation of symptoms that might follow its ingestion. Many of the diets used are a result of deep-rooted practice, without true scientific justification.

It is known that sight, smell and taste, water and practically anything else taken into the stomach stimulate gastric secretions to a greater or lesser degree. Neither those foods that are chemically, mechanically or thermally irritating to the mucosa nor those believed to be soothing have been determined. Although the chemical composition and physical properties of foods before ingestion are available, correlations between the nature of a food and its gastrointestinal effects in most cases are unknown.

When trying to reduce gastric acidity, it is important to consider both the immediate and delayed effects of foods and even of antacids. Antacids and food act as buffers, so their immediate effect is a lowering of gastric acidity. However, when the acidity gets too low, a feedback mechanism in the stomach stimulates it to begin secreting acid again.

FOOD ACIDITY. The effect of acidic foods on gastric acidity must be evaluated. The pH of foods ranges from about 2 in lime juice to 8 in egg whites and graham crackers. Most foods have a pH of between 5 and 7. The pH of both orange juice and grapefruit juice is 3.2 to 3.6, which is considerably less than the normal gastric acid pH of about 1.6. Theoretically (on the basis of their immediate acidity), acid fruit juices are contraindicated only for patients who have oral or esophageal lesions and possibly for patients with gastric lesions, particularly if the stomach is achlorhydric. Otherwise, the pH of a food before it is ingested has little therapeutic importance. Diluting fruit juices with water affects the pH very little.

FOODS THAT CAUSE GAS. In thinking about foods that give them distress, many ulcer patients will mention several that cause them to belch and have gas. The lack of knowledge about intestinal gas and the many factors influencing its production make it unwise to classify foods on the basis of their gas-forming properties. Data on the laxative properties of foods are very sparse. It is not known which foods do or can have laxative properties or on what part of the intestines they act or how they

Table 22–3   FACTORS THAT AFFECT GASTRIC
                      ACIDITY

INCREASE GASTRIC ACIDITY
Cephalic phase of digestion
   Thought, taste and smell of food, chewing and
   swallowing initiate vagal stimulation of parietal
   cells in fundic mucosa to secrete gastric acid.
Gastric phase of digestion
   Effect of food in stomach:
      Distention of fundus stimulates parietal cells to
      produce acid.
      Increased alkalinity of antrum causes release of
      gastrin.
      Distention of antrum causes release of gastrin,
      which stimulates gastric acid secretion.
      Substances in food and digestive products can in-
      crease acidity:
         alcohol
         caffeine
         polypeptides and amino acids (products of
         protein digestion).

DECREASE GASTRIC ACIDITY
Gastric phase of digestion
   Acidification of antrum reduces gastrin release and
   thus gastric acid secretion.
   Food, especially protein, has an initial buffering
   effect.
Intestinal phase of digestion
   Fat, acid and hyperosmolarity in the small intestine stimulate release of one or more gastrointestinal hormones which inhibit gastric acid
   secretion.

function. Flatulence is discussed further in Chapter 23, Nutritional Care for Patients with Intestinal Disease.

FACTORS THAT DAMAGE GASTROINTESTI-NAL MUCOSA.   Usually the stomach is protected by its epithelium, and the duodenum is protected by the thick alkaline mucoid secretions of Brunner's glands. All foods and environmental factors known to cause epithelial irritation and possible breakdown should be avoided, but we have only very limited knowledge in this area. Alcohol is known to damage the gastric mucosa, however. Black pepper, chili powder, cloves, nutmeg and mustard seed have been thought to cause a slight reddening of the mucosa. Black pepper has been shown to be an irritant causing a specific and localized hyperemia, whereas other spices are apparently innocuous in this respect.[16] Salicylates and some other drugs can cause damage to gastric mucosa.

FOODS THAT STIMULATE GASTRIC ACID SECRETION.   Caffeine and alcohol are known to stimulate gastric juices when consumed by themselves and should be avoided by ulcer patients. Cigarette smoking may increase gastric acid secretion and gastric motility or may impair neutralization of gastric acid by inhibiting pancreatic bicarbonate secretion, but this has not been proved.[2, 17] Garlic, paprika, horseradish, mustard and other spices have been shown to increase gastric secretion, but only when they were used alone and in fairly large amounts.[4] Many more studies show that nonspicy diets are no more effective in reducing ulcer pain or in aiding ulcer healing than are regular diets. (See Table 22–3.)

Pepsin secretion in response to the intake of different foods tends to parallel gastric acid secretion. The production of mucus in response to various foods is not known. Secretory or motor activity increases the vascularity of gastric mucosa.

**Diet and Eating Pattern
Recommendations**

Frequent and regular meals and antacid therapy are more important than the type of food ingested. It is important to eat small meals frequently (every two hours or so) so that the buffering action of food will be present in the stomach and yet the stomach will not be distended with a large meal, which enhances gastric acid secretion.

Protein foods have a dual role related to gastric content and secretions. They act as a buffer, but their buffering action is only temporary. As the protein digestion products (amino acids and polypeptides) reach the antrum, they stimulate the secretion of gastrin and thus the secretion of gastric acid.

Fat inhibits gastric secretion. However, there are no experimental observations to verify that the dairy fats traditionally recommended to the ulcer patient are any more effective in depressing gastric secretions than are animal fats or fried foods.

Whether or not a food will be tolerated by an ulcer patient is best determined by trying it. Intelligent individuals will probably avoid any food that they know from experience causes indigestion, pain or other digestive symptoms. Doll and associates[5] observed 121 patients with peptic ulcer who received a controlled dietary regimen and reported that a conventional bland diet does not increase the healing rate. Lennard-Jones and Babouris reported no difference in the gastric acidity of 12 duodenal ulcer patients whether they received a "free choice" diet or a traditional ulcer diet.[13] Todd[19] found no proof that the avoidance of certain foods customarily considered irritating is beneficial, unless these foods cause immediate

Table 22–4 PRINCIPLES OF NUTRITIONAL CARE FOR PEPTIC ULCER DISEASE— THE LIBERAL DIETARY REGIMEN

The patient with peptic ulcer disease should:
1. Eat frequently—at least every three hours.
2. Eat small meals to avoid stomach distention.
3. Avoid drinking coffee, tea, cola and other caffeine-containing beverages and alcohol.
4. Cut down on or quit smoking cigarettes.
5. Avoid using large amounts of aspirin or other drugs known to damage the stomach lining.
6. Avoid using excessive amounts of pepper in cooking or on food.
7. Avoid those foods or drinks that cause discomfort.
8. Eat meals in as relaxed an atmosphere as possible.

distress. He believes that the therapeutic ulcer diet has no proven virtue other than that it diminishes stomach acid. Roth's[15] study indicated that a rigid dietary regimen is difficult for the patient. He reported that the majority of patients given the traditional ulcer diet did not understand the regimen and were apt to be more restrictive than necessary.

The Liberal Approach. In 1971, the American Dietetic Association stated that nutritional care for the patient with ulcer disease should be liberalized considerably, based on information showing that the bland diet has had no significant effect on the healing of ulcers.[1] The Liberal Dietary Regimen as outlined in Table 22–4 is recommended. Table 22–5 lists recommended foods and amounts and also those foods that *may* cause distress. These should be discussed with the patient, and those that do not cause distress should be allowed in the diet. Table 22–6 gives a sample menu.

Counseling the Patient. The application of the liberal concept centers around the person rather than the diet and around normal nutritional needs rather than a special regimen. Regularity and frequency of meals and moderation in eating habits are important in the long-term care. An understanding, common-sense approach to the dietary treatment, which considers the patient as a whole person and not just the ulcer, will provide the essential nutritional needs and acid-reducing features that are therapeutic to the individual. Using such an approach, the nurse might ask, for example, what changes should the patient make in the present dietary pattern to provide the necessary calories and nutrients? What changes must be made in eating habits? How will the patient implement the changes? What changes must he or she make in lifestyle? Who can help in making these changes?

Traditional Ulcer Diet. Although it is not recommended in this text, the traditional treatment remains widely used and for that reason is presented here.

Unlike the foods used in the liberal approach, foods included in the conventional ulcer diet are soft in consistency, with a minimum amount of fiber. All foods believed to stimulate gastric secretion and gastric motility are omitted.

Milk. In 1915 Sippy introduced a progressive regimen. Milk (or milk and cream) is the basis of the diet and is conventionally used for its acid-buffering capacity. It is now questionable whether milk should be used to such a large extent in the diet for the ulcer patient. In a study of five patients with duodenal ulcer and five patients without gastrointestinal disease, it was shown that milk (whole, low-fat or skim) significantly increased gastric acid secretion in all patients, and that this stimulatory effect lasted for at least three hours. The fat content of the milk had no effect on the gastric acid secretion.[10] Second, in other patients who received hourly drinks of milk and cream, gastric contents were more acidic (pH 1.3) than in patients who received only three meals per day. In those patients who received only meals, the gastric pH was greater than 2.0 for 90 to 120 minutes.[12] Third, calcium, of which milk is a rich source, is known to increase gastric acid secretion by stimulating gastrin release. It may be that ulcer pain that occurs two to four hours after a meal is due to milk ingestion with that meal. Fourth, whole milk and whole milk products contribute saturated fat to the diet. The milk-based diet predisposes patients who follow it to atherosclerosis and myocardial infarction because of the high content of saturated fats. The neutralizing effects of cream, whole milk and skim milk are identical, and the delayed emptying time of the stomach produced through the use of cream can generally be duplicated by prescribing anticholinergic drugs, so that the use of fat-containing milk products is not necessary.

Other Foods. Enriched, refined or finely ground whole-grain cereals are included early in the diet. Eggs are usually added to the diet during the same period as bread and cereal. Fruits and vegetables are cooked to soften fiber. Chicken, fish and meat are withheld until the convalescent stage is approached. Meat extracts (broth, soups and gravies), tea, coffee, cocoa, concentrated chocolate, alcohol, condiments and spices are avoided because they tend to stimulate gastric activity. Fried foods

are traditionally excluded. Although sweets in concentrated form are thought to be somewhat irritating, custard, simple puddings, gelatin desserts and vanilla ice cream are well tolerated and may be added to the diet near the beginning of the treatment.

FEEDING INTERVALS.   Small meals or feedings are served at intervals of one, two or three hours, depending upon the acuteness of the patient's condition.

AMOUNT OF FOOD.   It is customary to start the diet treatment with 3- to 4-oz. feedings of milk or milk and cream at intervals of one to two hours. Nonabsorbable antacid is given for ap-

proximately one week. When additional food is allowed, small feedings (12 to 20 oz.) of soft-fiber foods are added to or substituted for some of the milk or milk and cream feedings, and the number of feedings is increased until a total of six are served. The next stage consists of low-fiber foods divided into six small meals or into three meals with milk served in between. The foods allowed in each stage are outlined in the following section. The physician prescribes the diet treatment best suited to meet the patient's condition. Surgical patients who have had gastric resections usually can tolerate small amounts of food fed regularly. Medical patients

Table 22-5   LIBERAL DIET FOR PEPTIC ULCER*

FOOD GROUPS	FOODS RECOMMENDED	FOODS THAT MAY CAUSE DISTRESS
Milk and Milk Products (2 or more cups daily)	All milk and milk drinks	None
Vegetables (2 or more servings daily)	All vegetable juices All raw or cooked vegetables	None
Fruits (2 or more servings daily)	All fruit juices All raw, cooked or dried fruits	None
Breads and Cereals (4 or more servings daily)	Whole-grain or enriched breads and cereals	None
Potatoes or Substitutes	Potatoes Enriched rice, barley, noodles, spaghetti, macaroni and other pastas	Any of these items fried, including snack foods such as potato chips and other snack chips
Meats or Substitutes (6 or more oz. daily)	All meats, poultry, fish and shellfish Eggs Crisp bacon Cheese Dried peas and beans Smooth peanut butter Soybeans and other meat substitutes	Any of these items fried or very highly seasoned Chunky peanut butter
Fats	Butter or fortified margarine Mild salad dressings such as mayonnaise, French or vinegar and oil All fats and oils	Highly seasoned salad dressings
Soups	Mildly seasoned meat stock and cream soups	Highly seasoned soups
Sweets and Desserts	All sweets and desserts except those listed to avoid	All sweets and desserts containing nuts or coconut Fried pastries such as doughnuts
Beverages	Decaffeinated coffee, cocoa, fruit drinks, 99% caffeine-free cola and other carbonated beverages, except other cola drinks	Coffee, tea, alcohol and cola drinks
Miscellaneous	Iodized salt, flavorings Mildly flavored gravies and sauces Herbs, spices, mustard, ketchup and vinegar in moderation, *if tolerated*	Strongly flavored seasonings and condiments such as garlic, pepper, barbeque sauce, chili sauce, chili pepper, horseradish Popcorn, nuts, coconut

*From: Chicago Dietetic Association, Inc.: Manual of Clinical Dietetics. Downers Grove, Ill., Johnson Printers, 1975, pp. III-23-25.

Table 22–6 SAMPLE MENU FROM THE LIBERAL DIET PLAN FOR ULCER PATIENTS*

BREAKFAST	LUNCH	DINNER
½ cup orange juice 1 poached egg or egg substitute 2 slices bacon or bacon substitute 1 slice toast 1 tsp. butter or margarine 1 tbsp. jelly 1 cup decaffeinated coffee 1 oz. cream or non-dairy creamer 2 tsp. sugar	2 oz. beef patty on bun Sliced tomato and lettuce French dressing ½ cup sherbet 4 oz. milk (whole or low-fat)	2 oz. broiled chicken ½ cup mashed potatoes ½ cup peas ½ cup fruited Jello salad 1 tsp. butter or margarine 1 cup decaffeinated coffee 1 oz. cream or non-dairy creamer 2 tsp. sugar

MIDMORNING SNACK	MIDAFTERNOON SNACK	BEDTIME SNACK
½ cup oatmeal 4 oz. milk (whole or low-fat) 2 tsp. sugar ½ cup peaches	2 slices bread 1 oz. American cheese 1 tsp. butter or margarine 4 oz. milk (whole or low-fat) Fresh apple	½ cup custard 2 sugar cookies ½ cup apricots 4 oz. milk (whole or low-fat)

APPROXIMATE NUTRITIVE VALUE OF SAMPLE MENU

Protein	100 gm.	Riboflavin	2.377 mg.
Fat	110 gm.	Thiamin	1.497 mg.
Carbohydrate	320 gm.	Calcium	1309 mg.
Calories	2670	Phosphorus	1701 mg.
Vitamin A	9199 I.U.	Iron	12.7 mg.
Vitamin C	132 mg.	Sodium	3124 mg.
Niacin	18.5 mg.eq.	Potassium	3030 mg.

*From: Chicago Dietetic Association, Inc.: Manual of Clinical Dietetics. Downers Grove, Illinois, Johnson Printers, 1975, pp. III-23–25.

who are ambulatory seem to get along well on the schedule of three meals plus milk served midmorning, midafternoon and at bedtime.

STAGES OF PEPTIC ULCER DIET THERAPY. Following are typical stages in the traditional nutritional care given for peptic ulcer.

First Stage. For the patient with an active, acute peptic ulcer, 3 to 4 oz. of milk or milk and cream (half-and-half or one third cream and two thirds milk) are served at intervals of one to two hours from 7:00 A.M. through 9:00 or 10:00 P.M. (and during the night if the patient is awake) until pain disappears, or for about one week. When whole milk alone is ordered, with 15 hourly 4-oz. feedings the diet contains approximately 68 gm. protein, 68 gm. fat, 90 gm. carbohydrate and 1245 kcal. When milk and cream (half-and-half) is prescribed, the diet contains approximately 60 gm. protein, 210 gm. fat, 83 gm. carbohydrate and 2460 kcal. Sometimes pain may not disappear entirely even after three or four days on this feeding schedule. These patients will usually react favorably to a continuous intragastric drip of the same milk and cream mixture for a few days.

Second Stage. As pain disappears, small feedings of soft-fiber foods are added to or replace some of the milk or milk and cream feedings. The initial feedings of 3 to 4 oz. served at frequent and regular intervals throughout the waking hours are gradually increased in size, and the interval between feedings is lengthened until the patient is established on a schedule of six feedings daily. Thorough mastication of all foods to promote mixing with saliva in preparation for gastric digestion is important.

Foods are selected from among the following:

Milk toast
Egg: poached or soft-cooked
Cereal: enriched Cream of Wheat, farina, boiled rice or oatmeal
Strained cream soup
Toasted enriched white bread and butter or margarine
White crackers and butter or margarine
Dessert: rennet-milk pudding, custard, gelatin dessert, vanilla ice cream, bread pudding, tapioca pudding, plain sugar cookies

Stages one and two are outlined in Table 22–7.

Third Stage: Six-feeding Restricted Bland Diet. Small feedings (12 to 20 oz.) are given

Table 22–7 FIRST AND SECOND STAGES OF TRADITIONAL DIETARY MANAGEMENT FOR PEPTIC ULCER

		8 A.M.	10 A.M.	12 NOON	3 P.M.	6 P.M.
First Stage 3 to 4 oz. milk or milk and cream (half-and-half) served every 1 to 2 hours on the hour, 7 A.M. through 9 P.M. and during the night if necessary.						
Second Stage Supplementary feedings added as tolerated (6 to 8 oz.)	1 feeding	Farina with cream and sugar				Baked custard
	2 feedings	Boiled rice with cream and sugar				
	3 feedings	Farina with cream and sugar		Milk toast		Gelatin and cream
	4 feedings	Oatmeal with cream and sugar	Poached egg on toast	Cream soup with soda crackers		Vanilla ice cream with sugar cookies
	5 feedings	Cream of Wheat with cream and sugar	Soft-cooked egg with 1 slice toast	Boiled rice with cream and sugar	Bread pudding with cream	Cream soup with croutons

Table 22–8   SIX FEEDING RESTRICTED BLAND DIET*

FOOD GROUPS	FOODS RECOMMENDED	FOODS WHICH MAY CAUSE DISTRESS
Milk and Milk Products (2 or more cups daily)	All milk and milk drinks	None
Vegetables (2 or more servings daily)	All vegetable juices Cooked vegetables as tolerated Salads made from allowed foods	Raw vegetables, dried peas and beans, corn Gas-forming vegetables such as broccoli, Brussels sprouts, cabbage, onions, cauliflower, cucumber, green pepper, rutabagas, turnips and sauerkraut
Fruits (2 or more servings daily)	All fruit juices Cooked or canned fruit Avocado and banana Grapefruit and orange sections without membrane	All other fresh and dried fruit Berries and figs
Breads and Cereals (4 or more servings daily)	Enriched breads and cereals	Very coarse cereals such as bran Seeds in or on breads, rolls and crackers Bread and bread products made with nuts or dried fruit Any fried breads
Potatoes or Substitutes	Potatoes Enriched rice, barley, noodles, spaghetti, macaroni and other pastas	Potato chips, fried potatoes, fried rice, wild rice
Meats or Substitutes (6 or more ounces daily)	All lean, tender meats, poultry, fish and shellfish Eggs; crisp bacon; lean ham Mild cheeses Smooth peanut butter Soybean and other meat substitutes	Highly seasoned, cured or smoked meats, poultry or fish, such as corned beef, luncheon meats, frankfurters and other sausages, sardines, anchovies and strong-flavored cheeses Chunky peanut butter
Fats	Butter or fortified margarine Mayonnaise All fats and oils	Salad dressings
Soups	Mildly seasoned meat stock and cream soups made with allowed foods	All other soups
Sweets and Desserts	Sugar, syrup, honey, jelly, seedless jam, hard candies, plain chocolate candies, molasses, marshmallows Cakes, cookies, pies, puddings, custard, ice cream, sherbet and Jello made from allowed foods	All sweets and desserts containing nuts, coconut or fruit that is not allowed Fried pastries such as doughnuts
Beverages	Decaffeinated coffee, cocoa, fruit drinks, 99% caffeine-free cola and other carbonated beverages, except other cola drinks.	Coffee, tea, alcohol and all cola drinks
Miscellaneous	Iodized salt, flavorings Mildly flavored gravies and sauces Mild herbs and spices	Strongly flavored seasonings and condiments such as ketchup, pepper, barbeque sauce, chili sauce, chili pepper, horseradish, garlic, mustard, vinegar Olives, pickles, popcorn, nuts and coconut

*From: Chicago Dietetic Association, Inc.: Manual of Clinical Dietetics, Downers Grove, Ill., Johnson Printers, 1975, pp. III-20–22.

Table 22–9 SAMPLE MENU FROM THE SIX FEEDING RESTRICTED BLAND DIET*

BREAKFAST	LUNCH	DINNER
½ cup orange juice	2 oz. beef patty	2 oz. broiled chicken
1 poached egg or egg substitute	½ cup rice	½ cup mashed potatoes
1 slice toast	½ cup spinach	½ cup peas
1 tsp. butter or margarine	1 slice bread	1 tsp. butter or margarine
1 cup decaffeinated coffee	1 tsp. butter or margarine	1 cup decaffeinated coffee
1 oz. cream or non-dairy creamer	4 oz. milk (whole or low-fat)	1 oz. cream or non-dairy creamer
2 tsp. sugar		2 tsp. sugar

MIDMORNING SNACK	MIDAFTERNOON SNACK	BEDTIME SNACK
½ cup oatmeal	6 oz. vegetable soup	½ cup cottage cheese
8 oz. milk (whole or low-fat)	½ cup sherbet	½ cup apricots
2 tsp. sugar	2 sugar cookies	2 saltine crackers
½ cup peaches	1 cup decaffeinated coffee	4 oz. milk (whole or low-fat)
	1 oz. cream or non-dairy creamer	
	2 tsp. sugar	

APPROXIMATE NUTRITIVE VALUE OF SAMPLE MENU

Protein	95 gm.	Riboflavin	1.985 mg.
Fat	85 gm.	Thiamin	1.467 mg.
Carbohydrate	280 gm.	Calcium	1028 mg.
Calories	2265	Phosphorus	1466 mg.
Vitamin A	16,354 I.U.	Iron	14.3 mg.
Vitamin C	124 mg.	Sodium	3047 mg.
Niacin	20 mg.eq.	Potassium	3015 mg.

*From: Chicago Dietetic Association, Inc.: Manual of Clinical Dietetics. Downers Grove, Illinois, Johnson Printers, 1975, pp. III-20–22.

six times a day. Fried foods, most raw fruits and vegetables, caffeine, alcohol, coarse breads and cereals, highly seasoned foods and any other foods known to cause the patient discomfort are omitted. See Table 22–8 for foods included in this diet and Table 22–9 for a sample menu. The diet contains approximately 100 gm. of protein, 90 gm. of fat, 280 gm. of carbohydrate and 2300 kcal. If fewer calories or a reduction of serum lipids is desired, cream may be omitted from the diet, or the amount of cream may be reduced or replaced by whole or skim milk.

POSSIBLE NUTRITIONAL INADEQUACIES. Over a long period, the large amount of alkali administered to the peptic ulcer patient may lead to alkalosis. Calorie and protein deficiencies frequently accompany ulcers, especially during the initial treatment, and interfere with the healing of the lesions. Avitaminosis, particularly of vitamin C, may develop unless vitamin supplements or specific vitamin-rich foods are added to the diet. Before accurate information about vitamins was available, it was not unusual to see ulcer patients in the hospital who had typical symptoms of ascorbic acid deficiency, such as areas of bluish skin (weakened capillary walls that may lead to hemorrhages) and bleeding gums. When signs of avitaminosis are detected today they may be attributed to neglect, carelessness, lack of knowledge or insufficient income for an adequate diet.

Secondary anemia may develop in the ulcer patient during treatment with antacids. Iron absorption depends upon an acid medium; thus, neutralization of gastric acids interferes with iron absorption (see p. 131). Possible blood loss from an unhealed ulcer can result in an iron deficiency.

Patients receiving restricted ulcer diets need careful supervision. Whenever there is doubt about the adequacy of the diet, protein, vitamin and iron supplements should be added. Radiographs show that complete healing takes from 14 to 100 days, with an average of 40. This is why medical treatment is sometimes continued for six to seven weeks before changes are made in the medication and diet.

Bleeding Ulcers

Dietary Treatment. Whether it is advisable to prescribe food for a patient who has a bleed-

ing ulcer remains controversial. The conservative method of dietary treatment withholds all food by mouth for a period of 24 to 72 hours after hemorrhage has stopped. Glucose is given intravenously. When food is allowed orally, milk and cream are offered at hourly intervals. Feedings are added as tolerated.

Surgery

Peptic ulcer is primarily a medical disease, but surgery is advised when the ulcer is complicated by hemorrhage, perforation, obstruction or intractability or when the patient is unable to follow the medical regimen. For a review of surgical procedures for peptic ulcer, see the Cooperman reference at the end of this chapter. The nutritional implications of vagotomy, antrectomy and gastric resection are covered in Chapter 34. After the ulcer has been removed, the patient should be informed that permanent dietary discretion and lifestyle changes are essential, since an operation is not a cure-all. Recurrences of ulcers are common following both medical and surgical treatment.

CARCINOMA OF THE STOMACH

The etiology of carcinoma of the stomach is unknown and is believed by some authorities to include a number of causes rather than a single cause. (See Chapter 36, Nutrition, Diet and Cancer.) Symptoms are so slow to manifest themselves and the growth of the tumor is so rapid that frequently carcinoma of the stomach is overlooked until it is too late for an effective cure. Because it is a disease of middle age, any unusually prolonged gastric discomfort appearing at this stage in life should be investigated, even though it seems slight. Loss of appetite, loss of strength and loss of weight frequently precede other symptoms. Extreme hypochromic anemia is associated with cancer of any part of the alimentary tract. Achylia gastrica or achlorhydria has been shown to exist for years preceding the onset of gastric carcinoma. However, in some cases increased secretory activity is evident, especially when cancer develops on the site of an old gastric ulcer.

Periodic physical examinations or check-ups are encouraged for middle-aged people. X-ray examinations and gastroscopy aid in making a very early diagnosis, so that surgical treatment is more likely to be successful. Speculation as to the role of diet in the etiology of cancer of the stomach has been growing. Chapter 36 deals with this subject more fully.

Nutritional Care

The dietary regimen for carcinoma of the stomach is determined somewhat by the location of the cancer, the nature of the functional disturbance and the stage of the development of the disease. The patient with advanced, non-operable cancer should receive a diet adjusted to provide comfort. Any food preferences, unless definitely harmful, are granted, and living should be made as bearable as possible. In the later stages of the disease the patient may tolerate only a liquid diet, and it may be necessary to resort to parenteral administration of fluids or to transfusions. As long as other therapeutic procedures such as surgery, radiation therapy or chemotherapy are being performed, the nutritional support for the patient should be equally aggressive. (See Chapter 36.)

Anorexia is almost always present in patients who have stomach cancer, from the early stages throughout the entire course of the disease. Patients who are encouraged to select their own menus and who suggest foods that are appealing to them usually ingest more than when they are not involved in the selection or when they are forced to eat.

When gastric secretion is depressed or lacking, the diet discussed for *hypochlorhydria* is used; when gastric secretion is increased, the diet outlined for liberal ulcer therapy is used.

After an operation, the diet outlined for gastric surgery (Chapter 34) is prescribed.

PROBLEMS AND SUGGESTED TOPICS FOR DISCUSSION

1. Interview a patient with dysphagia due to achalasia. Obtain a dietary history and assess his or her nutritional intake. With the patient, plan the nutritional care and submit a written care plan.
2. What are the principles of dietary treatment for peptic ulcer? List a food to illustrate each principle.
3. Compare the medical dietary treatment for ulcers used in your hospital with the dietary treatment outlined in this chapter.
4. Study the eating habits of three ulcer patients of different nationalities who are in the hospital. Check for adequacy.
5. Obtain the diet history of a patient with peptic ulcer admitted to the hospital. Follow up the prescribed treatment and plan the necessary nutritional care with the patient. If possible, follow the patient's progress in the outpatient clinic. Check the diet for adequacy.
6. Obtain a dietary history from a patient who complains of

indigestion. How adequate is his or her dietary pattern? Indicate where improvement is needed. How will he or she implement the changes?

7. How would a patient suffering with hypochlorhydria modify his or her dietary and eating habits?

8. What is the rationale for liberal peptic ulcer diet therapy?

CITED REFERENCES

1. American Dietetic Association: Position paper on bland diet in the treatment of chronic duodenal ulcer disease. J. Am. Diet. Assoc., 59:244, 1971.

2. Boden, G., et al.: Effect of nicotine on serum secretin and exocrine pancreatic secretion. Am. J. Dig. Dis., 21:974, 1976.

3. Castell, D. O.: The lower esophageal sphincter: Physiologic and clinical aspects. Ann. Intern. Med., 83:390, 1975.

4. Demling, L., and Koch, H.: Condiments. Acta Hepatogastroenterol., 21:377, 1974.

5. Doll, R., Friedlander, P., and Pygott, F.: Dietetic treatment of peptic ulcer. Lancet, 1:5, 1956.

6. Fry, J.: Peptic ulcer: A profile. Br. Med. J., 2:809, 1964.

7. Grossman, M. I., et al.: A new look at peptic ulcer. Ann. Intern. Med., 84:57, 1976.

8. Guyton, A. C.: Textbook of Medical Physiology, 5th ed. Philadelphia, W. B. Saunders Co., 1976, pp. 850–866.

9. Hightower, N. C.: Applied anatomy and physiology of the esophagus. In: Bockus, H. L.: Gastroenterology, vol. 1, 3rd ed. Philadelphia, W. B. Saunders Co., 1974.

10. Ippoliti, A. F., Maxwell, V., and Isenberg, J. I.: The effect of various forms of milk on gastric acid secretion. Ann. Intern. Med., 84:286, 1976.

11. Isenberg, J. I., et al.: Increased sensitivity to stimulation of acid secretion by pentagastrin in duodenal ulcer. J. Clin. Invest., 55:330, 1975.

12. Kirsner, J. B., and Palmer, W. L.: Effect of various antacids on the hydrogen ion concentration of the gastric contents. Am. J. Dig. Dis., 7:85, 1940.

13. Lennard-Jones, J. E., and Babouris, N.: Effect of different foods on the acidity of the gastric contents in patients with duodenal ulcer. Gut, 6:113, 1965.

14. Mendeloff, A. I.: What has been happening to duodenal ulcer? Gastroenterology, 67:1020, 1974.

15. Roth, H. P., and Caron, H. S.: Patients' misconceptions about their peptic ulcer diets: Potential obstacles to cooperation. J. Chronic Dis., 20:5, 1967.

16. Schneider, M. A., De Luca, V., Jr., and Gray, S. J.: Effect of spice ingestion on stomach. Am. J. Gastroenterol., 26:722, 1956.

17. Solomon, T. E., and Jacobson, D. E.: Cigarette smoking and duodenal ulcer disease. N. Engl. J. Med., 286:1212, 1972.

18. Sturdevant, R. A. L., et al.: Antacid and placebo produced similar pain relief in duodenal ulcer patients. Gastroenterology, 72:1, 1977.

19. Todd, J. W.: Treatment of peptic ulcer. Lancet, 1:113, 1952.

20. Tovey, F.: Duodenal ulcer and diet. In: Burkitt, D. P., and Trowell, H. C. (eds.): Refined Carbohydrate Foods and Disease: Some Implications of Dietary Fiber. London, Academic Press, 1975.

21. Walsh, J. H., Richardson, C. T., and Fordtran, J. S.:

pH dependence of acid secretion and gastrin release in normal and ulcer subjects. J. Clin. Invest., 55:462, 1975.

ADDITIONAL REFERENCES

Atkinson, M.: Dysphagia. Br. Med. J., 1:91, 1977.

Brown, M., et al.: Personality factors in duodenal ulcer. Psychosom. Med., 12:1, Jan.–Feb., 1950.

Brunner, L. S.: What to do (and what to teach your patient) about peptic ulcer. Nursing' 76, 6:27, 1976.

Buchman, E., et al.: Unrestricted diet in the treatment of duodenal ulcer. Gastroenterology, 56:1016, 1969.

Castell, D. O.: Diet and the lower esophageal sphincter. Am. J. Clin. Nutr., 28:1296, 1975.

Cooperman, A. M. (ed.): Peptic ulcer disease. Surg. Clin. North Am., 56(6), 1976.

Foltz, E. L.: Neurophysiological mechanisms in production of gastrointestinal ulcers. JAMA, 187:413, 1964.

Friedman, G. D., Siegelaub, A. B., and Seltzer, C. C.: Cigarettes, alcohol, coffee and peptic ulcer. N. Engl. J. Med., 290:469, 1974.

Hartroft, W. S.: The incidence of coronary artery disease in patients treated with the Sippy diet. Am. J. Clin. Nutr., 15:205, 1964.

Kirsner, J. B.: Facts and fallacies of current medical therapy for uncomplicated duodenal ulcer. JAMA, 187:423, 1964.

Kramer, P., and Caso, E. K.: Is the rationale for gastrointestinal diet therapy sound? J. Am. Diet. Assoc., 42:505, 1963.

Laureta, H. C., et al.: An appraisal of the management of peptic ulcer including comparative studies of the value of a polyunsaturated fat nutritional preparation in the management of gastric hypersecretion. Am. J. Clin. Nutr., 15:211, 1964.

McMillan, D. E., and Freeman, R. B.: The milk alkali syndrome. A study of the acute disorder with comments on the development of the chronic condition. Medicine, 44:485, 1965.

Moeller, H. C.: Conventional dietary treatment of peptic ulcer. Am. J. Clin. Nutr., 15:194, 1964.

Morson, B. C.: Precancerous lesions of upper gastrointestinal tract. JAMA, 179:311, 1962.

Odell, A. C.: Ulcer dietotherapy: Past and present. J. Am. Diet. Assoc., 58:447, 1971.

Rubin, H.: The Ulcer Diet Cook Book. New York, M. Evans and Company, Inc., 1963.

Sandweiss, D. J.: The Sippy treatment for peptic ulcer: Fifty years later. Am. J. Dig. Dis., 6:929, 1961.

Sippy, B. W.: Gastric and duodenal ulcers: Medical cure by an efficient removal of gastric juice erosion. JAMA, 64:1625, 1915.

Snorf, L. D.: Emotional factors in gastrointestinal disorders. JAMA, 162:857, 1956.

State, D.: Gastrointestinal hormones in the production of peptic ulcer. JAMA, 187:410, 1964.

Symposium: Clinical management of peptic ulcer. Am. J. Clin. Nutr., 15:191 and 235, 1964.

Thorn, G. W., et al.: Harrison's Principles of Internal Medicine, 8th ed., New York, McGraw-Hill Book Co., 1977.

Weinstein, L., et al.: Diet as related to gastrointestinal function. JAMA, 176:935, 1961.

Wirts, C. W., et al.: Effect of tea on gastric secretions and motility. JAMA, 155:725, 1954.

Chapter 23

NUTRITIONAL CARE FOR PATIENTS WITH INTESTINAL DISEASE

PHYSIOLOGY AND FUNCTIONS OF THE INTESTINES

The absorption of food is practically completed in the small bowel. Food is emptied from the stomach into the duodenum where the breaking-down process continues. Secretions from the intestine, the pancreas and the liver have prepared the gastric contents for absorption, which for the most part takes place in the upper half of the small intestine. The only nutrients that are absorbed in the distal small intestine (the terminal ileum) are fats and vitamin B_{12}.

The large intestine or colon takes up considerable space in the abdomen. It is about 1.5 meters long and starts with the cecum, the segment from which the appendix projects. From the lower right side of the abdomen, the colon extends upward (ascending), crosses (transverse) underneath the liver and stomach to the spleen and turns downward (descending) on the left side. It is connected with the rectum by a small section called the sigmoid. (See Fig. 23–1.)

The main functions of the colon are (1) the absorption of water and (2) the transfer of feces from the ascending colon to the descending colon, then via the rectum to the exterior. This latter function is accomplished mainly by periodic, relatively frequent intervals of progressive mass peristalsis. The sigmoid sphincter prevents the passage of fecal material into the rectum until the urge to defecate is felt. Normal rectal sensibility is needed for the desire for evacuation, and regularity of habit and ample roughage are prime requisites for proper functioning of the colon.

The mechansim of the entire alimentary tract is controlled by the nervous and endocrine systems. When an individual becomes tense or overfatigued, the colon may go into a single spasm or series of spasms. The constriction may be associated with alternating constipation and diarrhea.

This brief review has been presented as a guide to better understanding of the various diseases in the intestinal region and their dietary treatment. A review of Chapter 6 is recommended. Figure 6–9, illustrating the sites of normal absorption of nutrients from the small bowel, will be helpful when studying intestinal disease and the nutritional care necessary for treating it.

Since many intestinal disorders appear to be functional ones, that is, involving motility, absorption and secretion problems in the absence of recognizable pathological conditions, it seems probable that diet is related to both the exacerbation and remission of these diseases. However, this area of study is largely unex-

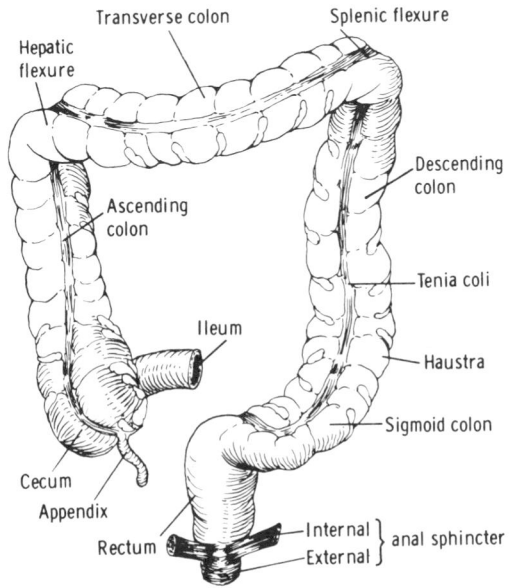

Figure 23–1 The human colon. (From: Ganong, W. F.: Medical Physiology, 6th ed. Los Altos, California, Lange Medical Publications, 1973, p. 375.)

plored, and there is only limited evidence to incriminate certain foods in some individuals. In these cases, elimination of individual foods may be beneficial. Distress after ingestion would seem to incriminate that particular food. Although there are some general principles to follow, *nutritional care for all patients with diseases of the intestines must be individualized*. The principles presented here are only *guidelines*.

FLATULENCE

Because human gas production has not been studied extensively, it is not well understood. Almost all intestinal gas is composed of five gases: N_2, O_2, CO_2, H_2 and CH_4 (methane). The normal individual usually excretes less than 100 ml. of gas per hour. If this amount is exceeded, he or she usually complains of "excessive gas."

The causes of excessive gas are (1) *aerophagia* (the swallowing of air while eating or drinking), (2) increased intestinal motility (decreased intestinal transit time) and (3) excessive bacterial fermentation of bowel contents.

An analysis of rectal gas can give a clue to the reason for excessive flatulence. Excessive amounts of H_2 and CO_2, which are not present in the atmosphere in large quantities, indicate excessive bacterial fermentation and point to malabsorption of a fermentable substrate such as lactose. High N_2 and O_2 concentrations in the flatus result from aerophagia. Methane is produced by only one third of the population. However, a person's flatus is rarely analyzed for its composition. If it were, suggestions and methods for nutritional care to minimize gas production would be more effective.

Patients with "too much gas" frequently do not have more gas than other people, but may have problems with gastrointestinal motility. Normally, gas is reabsorbed through the colonic wall as the feces move down to the rectum. If colonic motility is increased for any reason, less gas can be reabsorbed. If colonic motility is disordered so that gas cannot pass through to the rectum, the result is eructation, pain and distention, and the patient will complain of "too much gas."

Nutritional Care

Nutritional care begins with cautioning the patient to eat slowly, chew with the mouth closed and avoid gulping food. Lactose may be the offending agent if the person has a lactose

intolerance, in which case a lactose-free diet should be prescribed. (See page 500.) To determine whether lactose is the gas-causing agent, the patient should omit all milk and milk sugar-containing products (such as ice cream, puddings and custards) from the diet for a trial period and observe whether there is a beneficial effect.

The following fruits and vegetables could *possibly* be gas-forming. Trial periods of omitting them and observing the results can determine which of them affect individual patients.

VEGETABLES

Beans, kidney	Onions
Beans, lima	Peas, split or black-eyed
Beans, navy	Peppers, green
Broccoli	Pimentos
Brussels sprouts	Radishes
Cabbage	Rutabagas
Cauliflower	Sauerkraut
Corn	Scallions
Cucumbers	Shallots
Kohlrabi	Soybeans
Leeks	Turnips
Lentils	

FRUIT

Apples (raw)	Cantaloupe
Avocados	Honeydew melon
	Watermelon

CONSTIPATION

Definition

Constipation may be defined as a retention of the feces in the colon beyond the normal emptying time. It is a condition of stasis in the large intestine. Under normal conditions, the residue of food eaten one morning will reach the large bowel (but not the rectum) the following morning. Defecation takes place normally 24 to 72 hours or longer after the intake of food. The type of diet eaten is believed to influence to some degree the length of time before defecation takes place. A diet high in fiber content resists enzymatic digestion or absorbs liquids in its passage along the intestinal tract and thereby produces bulk, a stimulant to defecation. The opposite is true of a diet low in fiber. Burkitt found that the transit time for food through the gut was approximately 30 to 40 hours for people in rural communities of Africa who had high fiber intakes and 70 to 100 hours for people eating the British diet. The daily stool size was less for people who ate the low-fiber British diet—150 gm. compared with 400 gm. for those eating the African diet.[4]

Many people believe it is necessary to have a daily bowel movement, become disturbed when this does not occur and purge themselves with laxatives and cathartics. For comfort and

health, most people should have a daily bowel movement; however, there are individuals who require an evacuation only every second or third day, and sometimes the intervals may be longer. At the extreme is the reported case of a young man who did not defecate at all for 368 days.[7]

Etiology

The causes of constipation are numerous and varied. The strain and speed of modern life and the resulting poor habits of hygiene are contributing factors. Repeated lack of response to the urge for defecation, failure to establish a regular time for defecation, lack of exercise (which causes a loss of tone in the intestinal musculature), the use of cathartics for long periods of time, nervous strain and worry are the most common causes. Hypothyroidism, dehydration and certain medications such as those containing iron, aluminum or calcium compounds can cause constipation. Inadequate diet or improper food habits could be the cause. Insufficient fiber in the diet may cause constipation because there is little residue reaching the colon, and stool bulk is needed to promote normal peristalsis. Lack of thiamin and insufficient intake of water can also cause constipation.

Chronic constipation may result from an organic disorder such as a physical defect, obstruction or constriction associated with a debilitating disease or may be functional in origin, as occurs in old age. There are three types of constipation generally recognized: (1) atonic, (2) spastic or irritable colon syndrome and (3) obstructive.

ATONIC CONSTIPATION

Atonic constipation is sometimes called "lazy bowel" constipation because of the loss of rectal sensibility; the rectum is full of feces but the urge to defecate is lacking. The peristaltic waves that are normally strong become weak, and fecal matter moves slowly and accumulates. This type of constipation is often observed in older people, whose body processes are slowing down. It also occurs in obesity, accompanying fevers, following operations and during pregnancy. Inadequate diet, irregular meals, insufficient intake of liquids and failure to respond to the urge to defecate are the most frequent causes of atonic constipation.

Treatment

The treatment is to develop regularity of habit through a bowel training program and the establishment of good health habits: regular meals, adequate diet providing ample fiber, regular time for elimination, rest, relaxation, adequate intake of fluids and exercise.

Nutritional Care

The adequate normal diet is used for patients with atonic constipation. It includes enough bulk (vegetables, fruit and whole-grain cereal products) so that the fiber residue left in the bowel after digestion will encourage the movement of the intestinal contents and stimulate periodic evacuation. Approximately 800 gm. of fruits and vegetables is needed to produce a daily normal bowel movement. Raw and cooked fruits and vegetables, cereals including their skins and bran will provide the fiber. Eight hundred gm. of fruits and vegetables is equal to about four pieces of fresh fruit and a large salad. See page 41 for a definition of fiber. Table 23–1 gives the fiber content of some foods.

Prunes and prune juice have been found to stimulate intestinal motility by pharmacological means. The laxative substance found in prunes is *dihydroxyphenyl isatin*. Other foods may have this same ability; but data on pharmacological laxative properties of food are very limited.

Because water is absorbed by the colon, the habitual intake of 8 to 10 glasses of fluid daily is necessary. If the fluid intake is less than this, constipation is likely to result. Some people believe milk to be constipating. Usually the cause for the constipation will be found in other factors.

Bran, the most concentrated source of food fiber, should be used in moderation. Excessive amounts given right away may irritate a sensitive alimentary tract, and large quantities may cause flatulence, loose stools or intestinal blockage. The large amount of phytates in bran may reduce absorption of calcium, magnesium, iron and zinc. However, bran should be included gradually in the diet in breakfast cereals and bran muffins or added to stews and baked goods.

The typical high-fiber diet suggested for use in average cases of atonic constipation is an adequate normal diet with an increase in the amount of whole-grain cereal products, fruits and vegetables (Table 23–2).

Table 23–1 FIBER CONTENT OF SOME FOODS*

FOOD	GM. CRUDE FIBER	
	per 100 gm.	*per half cup*
Bran flakes (100% bran)	7.8	2.2
Bran flakes (40% bran)	3.6	1.0
Raisin Bran	3.0	0.8
Puffed wheat	2.0	0.6
Shredded wheat	2.3	0.6
Sunflower seeds (kernels)	3.8	1.1
Sesame seeds	6.3	1.8
Pumpkin seeds (kernels)	1.9	0.5
English walnuts	2.1	1.2
Peanuts, with skins	2.7	2.7
Almonds, with skins	2.6	2.2
Pecans	2.3	1.3
Peanut butter (2 Tblsp.)	1.9	0.7
Whole-grain bread (1 slice)	0.9	0.4
Bran muffin	1.8	0.7
Fresh fruit with skin (1 average)	1.5	1.5
Fresh fruit without skin (1 serving)	1.0	1.0
Raw vegetables	1.1	1.1
Cooked vegetables	1.3	1.3

*From: Watt, B. K., and Merrill, A. L.: Composition of Foods. Agriculture Handbook No. 8. Washington, D.C., U.S. Department of Agriculture, 1963.

Laxatives

There are several types of laxatives; bulk-increasing agents, stool softeners, chemical stimulants and saline cathartics.

Cellulose and hemicellulose derivatives are common bulk-increasing agents. Taken in large amounts, they have been shown to decrease the absorption of nitrogen and fat. The excessive use of mineral oil can affect nutritional status by interfering with the absorption of the fat-soluble vitamins A, D, K and carotene. (See Chapter 21.)

IRRITABLE BOWEL SYNDROME OR SPASTIC COLON

The irritable bowel syndrome or spastic constipation (also known as *spastic colitis, spastic colon* or *mucous colitis*) is a common disorder of unknown cause that does not appear to be characterized by any organic abnormality. It is the result of overstimulation of the intestinal nerve endings that causes irregular contractions of the bowel. There is excessive or in-coordinated sigmoidal motility and loss of rectal sensibility, which can cause either rapid transit through the bowel or constipation. It is accompanied by abdominal pain and sometimes by nausea, constipation or diarrhea, which may alternate. Mucus may be found in the stool. Because of the spasms, the mass moves irregularly along the intestinal tract. Attacks are frequently associated with an emotional upset or a prolonged period of stress. Contributing causes vary and include the excessive use of cathartics, laxatives and tobacco, drinking too much tea, coffee or alcohol, stress or emotional disturbance, previous gastrointestinal illness, antibiotic therapy, enteric infections and lack of regularity in sleep, rest, fluid intake and evacuation. Patients complain of heartburn, distention, flatulence, a full feeling and mild or severe cramping pain.

Treatment

A therapeutic regimen must include helping the patient to cope with stressful situations and to relieve pent-up emotions. Good habits of personal hygiene must be established, with adequate time allowed for a bowel movement.

Nutritional Care

Persons suffering from spastic constipation are frequently underweight, tense and upset. Because of past experience they are afraid to eat and fearful of additional pain. The aim of the nutritional therapy is to relieve the condition, nourish the patient and bring the patient's weight back to normal.

The normal diet is recommended, with emphasis on high-fiber foods that will add bulk to

Table 23–2   HIGH-FIBER DIET*

FRUIT		VEGETABLES		CEREAL
3–5 servings daily		*4 servings daily*		*1 serving daily*
[a]Apples	Grapefruit	Asparagus	Okra	Oatmeal
[a]Apricots	[a]Peaches	Broccoli	Onions	Shredded wheat
Bananas	[a]Pears	Brussels sprouts	Parsnips	Whole-wheat cereal
Berries	Pineapple	Carrots	Peas (all varieties)	Bran cereal
Cherries	[a]Plums	Cabbage	Peppers	Puffed wheat
Figs	Prunes	Cauliflower	Potatoes (white,	Brown rice
Oranges	Dried fruit	Celery	sweet)	Bran (include 2 tblsp. daily)
		Corn	Radishes	
		Eggplant	Rhubarb	
		Endive	Sauerkraut	
		Kohlrabi	Spinach	
		Lettuce	Squash	
		Greens (all varieties)	Tomatoes	
		Green Beans	Turnips	
		Lima Beans	Watercress	
		All other beans		
		Mushrooms		

SOUPS	PROTEIN		BREAD
As desired	*3 servings daily*		*3–5 servings daily*
Hearty varieties such as vegetable, mine-	Beef	Pork	100% whole-wheat bread
strone, chowder, bean, chili	Veal	Bacon	Cracked wheat bread
	Lamb	Eggs	Rye bread
	Fish	Chicken	Buckwheat bread
	Ham	Peanut butter	Corn bread made with
	Turkey	(crunchy)	course-ground meal

DESSERTS	MISCELLANEOUS	FATS
As desired		*As desired*
Ices and sherbets	Sunflower seeds	Butter
Fruit (fresh, frozen, canned)	Pumpkin seeds	Margarine
Fruit whips	Popcorn	Cream
	Nuts	Salad oil
		Salad dressing

BEVERAGES	AVOID
6–8 glasses daily	Highly refined cereals:
Water	white rice
Milk (2–3 cups)	cream of wheat
Fruit juice	farina
Cocoa	white bread
Tea	pastries
Coffee	pies
	cakes
	macaroni
	spaghetti
	noodles
	Ice cream

*From: Department of Food and Nutrition Services, Shands Teaching Hospital and Clinics, University of Florida, Gainesville, Florida, 1975.

[a]Unpeeled.

the stool and may relieve the constricting pressure and promote normal bowel motility. An increase in dietary fiber is not the cure-all for irritable bowel syndrome that many people believe it to be. A study of patients who were given either high-bran or regular biscuits daily found no difference in the relief of their symptoms.[16] The beneficial effect of bran for some people may be a psychological one or a placebo effect.

OBSTRUCTIVE CONSTIPATION

In obstructive constipation, an obstruction or closure hinders the passage of intestinal residue. The obstruction may be complete or partial. Adhesions, cancer, a tumor or an impaction usually causes the obstruction. Surgical treatment is frequently indicated.

Nutritional Care

Bowel residue is minimized to a degree that depends on the size of the obstruction. If the obstruction is very extensive, a full liquid diet may be necessary. In such cases the liquids should provide ample nutrients. (See page 447.) Chemically defined or elemental diets, which leave no residue but provide concentrated nutrition, may be the best choice, depending on the extent of debilitation of the patient. See page 707 for a discussion of elemental diet formulas. Sometimes it may be more desirable to administer foods and fluids parenterally (See Chapter 35). Regardless of the type of diet, attention should be directed toward insuring that the patient receives sufficient calories, protein, electrolytes, vitamins and fluids.

The dietary regimen following intestinal resections and colostomy will be discussed in Chapter 34.

HEMORRHOIDS

Hemorrhoids are ruptured blood vessels located around the anal sphincter. They may be either external or internal and may or may not cause pain and discomfort (Fig. 23–2). It is important for the patient with hemorrhoids not to become constipated, because the pressure from the dry, hard feces often causes bleeding and severe pain. Surgery usually is advised if the hemorrhoids become progressively worse. Some of the causes of hemorrhoids are constipation, pregnancy and the prolonged and continued use of cathartics or enemas. Sometimes they appear without apparent cause.

Nutritional Care

Diet is not used as a treatment for the condition but to provide comfort for the patient and possibly to prevent the development of more hemorrhoids. The high-fiber diet shown in Table 23–2 plus 8 to 10 glasses of water or liquids per day is recommended to avoid constipation and reduce straining at defecation. Those foods known by the patient to be irritating to the perianal area (such as highly seasoned foods) should be avoided. A discussion with the patient of a normal diet and regular eating and elimination habits is indicated. In the acute phase of hemorrhoid flare-up, the patient may require a low residue, low-fiber diet (see Table 23–4). Gradual return to the high-fiber diet should be the objective.

DIARRHEA

Diarrhea, which is a symptom and not a disease, is the occurrence of frequent liquid stools. The passage of food through the intestines is abnormally rapid and impairs complete digestion and absorption. The fecal matter passes through the colon so quickly that there is no chance for the fluid to be absorbed. Because of this, fluid replacements are necessary. Diarrhea is the direct opposite of constipation, in which the fecal matter remains dormant and becomes hard and dry.

Classification

Diarrhea is classified as both *functional* and *organic* in origin. The functional type is less severe than the organic and may occur in any normal person whose intestines are exposed to an irritant or who is faced with a stressful situa-

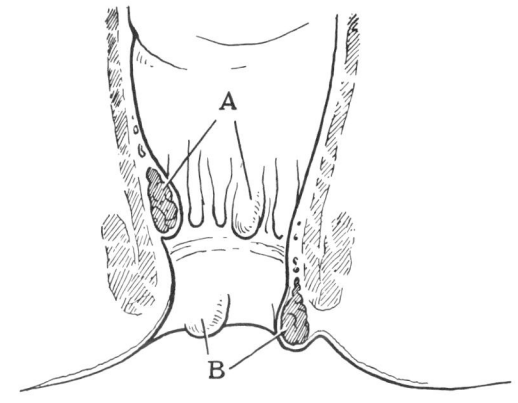

Figure 23–2 Hemorrhoids. *A,* internal hemorrhoids; *B,* external hemorrhoids.

tion. In organic diarrhea there is a demonstrable lesion of the intestinal mucosa, which is not present in functional diarrhea. However, as we learn more about intestinal disease, it becomes more difficult to classify a case of diarrhea as exclusively functional or organic.

Etiology

There are many causes of diarrhea. Some of the major causes of *functional diarrhea* are overeating or eating the wrong foods, putrefaction in the intestinal tract, fermentation caused by incomplete digestion, the habitual use of cathartics, nervous irritability or endocrine disturbance. During periods of stress, strain or excitement, children and adults may have diarrhea. In children, fright may cause diarrhea. One of the most obstinate varieties of diarrhea is exhibited during hysteria. During hot weather diarrhea occurs frequently. Food poisoning is a common culprit. The bacteria produce toxins in the food, which are irritating to the gastrointestinal tract. (See Chapter 18.)

Caffeine consumption in amounts of 75 to 300 mg. per day (the amount in one to two cups of coffee) may cause functional diarrhea in some people. In these doses, caffeine increases intestinal secretion, which may account for the diarrhea.[18] Patients should be questioned about their caffeine consumption, and a trial period of decreased intake may be effective. Table 23–3 gives the caffeine content of some beverages.

Organic diarrhea may be caused by external poison, such as food poisoning, or by parasite invasion, and it may accompany certain diseases such as tuberculosis, amebic dysentery, typhoid fever, viral hepatitis, chronic ulcerative colitis, regional ileitis and enteritis. It may be caused by enzyme deficiencies that result in impaired digestion and absorption of carbohydrates.

Nutritional Care

For all types of diarrhea the dietary treatment is similar. The aim of the medical treatment is to remove the cause. The diet generally adopted is one that will leave very little residue in the intestinal tract. The low-fiber diet is presented in Table 23–4.

In the beginning of the dietary treatment for severe diarrhea, a fast of 24 to 48 hours is often prescribed to provide rest for the gastrointestinal tract. The nature and severity of the diarrhea determine the duration of the rest.

Acute diarrhea is most dangerous in infants and small children, who can easily become dehydrated from the large fluid losses. In these cases parenteral administration of fluids and electrolytes is usually necessary.

Besides bowel rest, the nutritional care for adults usually includes replacement of lost fluids and electrolytes by increasing the oral intake of liquids, sodium and potassium. Fruit juices and bouillon are examples of fluids high in potassium. (See Appendix Table 9 for more foods high in sodium and potassium.) After about 48 hours, simple foods such as broth, gruel, dry toast and tea are given. Return to the normal diet is guided by the patient's condition and tolerance for food.

Pectin has value in the treatment of diarrhea. Scraped raw apple or liberal amounts of applesauce may be given every two to four hours, as tolerated, for their pectin content.

Losses of electrolytes, especially of potassium and sodium, should be corrected early with saline solutions that have potassium added. Glucose, ascorbic acid and the B vitamins are added to minimize protein and vitamin depletion. If the parenteral feeding must be continued for longer than 72 hours, amino acids in a 3 per cent solution may be added to prevent further protein catabolism. In the event that the diarrhea continues and cannot be diagnosed or treated, total intravenous hyperalimentation may be necessary, especially if exploratory surgery is anticipated. (See Chapter 35.)

When the diarrhea stops and the patient begins to tolerate food, the amounts given should be increased gradually as the patient can accept

Table 23–3   CAFFEINE CONTENT OF BEVERAGES*

BEVERAGE	CAFFEINE[a] (mg./200 ml.)
Prepared coffee[b]	66–150
Tea	70–150
Cola drinks	20–26
Decaffeinated coffee	1.8–6
Cocoa	0.25–345

*From: Handbook of Nutrition Care, 5th ed. St. Louis, Mo., Barnes Hospital, 1975, p. 163.

[a] It is obvious that there is a wide range of figures represented in the literature. Part of this variance is due to the fact that the caffeine content of beverages is based on the amount of water, the method of brewing, and the blend of coffee or tea used. Since caffeine is water soluble, the longer the exposure to hot water, the greater will be the extraction of caffeine.

[b] Coffee prepared by the drip or vacuum method has less caffeine than percolated coffee.

Table 23–4   MINIMAL-FIBER DIET*

FOOD GROUP	FOODS ALLOWED	FOODS NOT ALLOWED
Potatoes and Substitues	Potatoes without skin; rice, pasta	Kasha
Breads and Cereals	Enriched white bread or rolls made from finely milled flour; graham crackers, saltines, refined cereals, croutons; bread sticks without seeds; bread crumbs, rusks, matzoth, bagels, pancakes, waffles, biscuits, cornbread, French toast	All-Bran, cracked wheat bread and rolls, bran flakes, shredded wheat, Wheat Chex, Grape Nuts Flakes, Pettijohns, barley
Fruit	Strained fruit juices	All fruits
Fats	Any fat	None
Combination Dishes	Those made with rice or pasta and meat, cheese or fish	Any made with vegetables, fruits or other foods not allowed
Snacks	Plain crackers without seeds or cracked grain, potato chips, pretzels, corn chips (note: because of the nature of these foods, patients may not want them)	Any made from foods not allowed
Beverages		
Milk	Any	None
Milk-free Beverages	Any	None
Available Supplements	Any	None
Soups	Any creamed or broth-based soups without vegetables	Soups with vegetables
Animal Protein		
Meat	Any	None
Poultry	Any	None
Fish	Any	None
Non-meat Protein		
Dairy Products	Any cheese	None
	Yogurt made without fruit or seeds	Yogurt with seeds or fruit
	Any eggs	
Other Sources	Meat extenders	Dried beans, peas, nuts, seeds, lentils, chunky peanut butter
Vegetables	None	All vegetables
Desserts and sweets	Any without seeds or fruit	Any made with cracked wheat, seeds or fruit
Miscellaneous	Salt, spices, herbs, sugar substitute, meat tenderizers, MSG, mustard, catsup, soy sauce, Worcestershire sauce, brewer's yeast, extracts, flavorings, food coloring, vinegar, Tabasco sauce, baking powder, baking soda, cornstarch, horseradish, gravy without vegetables	Pickles, relishes, olives, gravy with vegetables such as onions

*From: Handbook of Nutrition Care, 5th ed. St. Louis, Mo., Barnes Hospital, 1975, pp. 74–75.

them. The foods given should be low in fiber and concentrated in protein and calories.

To achieve the high protein and calorie level, protein concentrates such as dry skim milk powder can be added to milk beverages, desserts and creamed dishes, and suitable carbohydrates such as glucose can be added to beverages. See Table 35–5 for some high-calorie, high-protein liquid supplements. Furthermore, increased intake of cereals, custards, simple puddings and jelly will increase the protein and calorie level, and butter, margarine and cream can be added to foods as tolerated. In the beginning, only vegetable and fruit juices will be included, then creamed vegetable soup and, finally, selected whole cooked foods. Diet changes are always guided by the patient's condition and toleration for foods. The return

to the normal diet is gradual. High calorie and protein intakes may be required for several months to correct protein deficiencies.

If the diarrhea becomes chronic, it may be associated with a number of nutritional deficiencies. Except for certain types of neurogenic diarrhea, impaired absorption resulting from abnormal anatomical changes or from mucosal alterations of the small bowel is a common feature in most nutritional complications of diarrhea.

Besides impaired absorption there is a heavy loss of electrolytes, vitamins, minerals and protein, which will have to be replaced. Potassium is probably the most important electrolyte lost, reflecting tissue depletion rather than specific changes in the circulating plasma levels. The loss of potassium alters bowel motility, encourages anorexia and can introduce a cycle of bowel distress. Loss of iron from gastrointestinal bleeding may be severe enough to cause anemia. Protein is poorly digested and absorbed. If antibiotic therapy is used, intestinal synthesis of some of the B vitamins is impaired. Deficiencies of folic acid, vitamin B_{12} and niacin have been reported.

In diseases with chronic diarrhea, low fiber diets may have to be used initially. To avoid great loss of body weight and tissue protein it may be necessary to provide up to 4000 kcal. and 150 gm. of protein daily for several months.

After the diarrhea begins to lessen, adding more fiber to the diet may be effective. A larger stool bulk helps to restore normal bowel motility. Large quantities of fluid (2 to 3 qt. daily) are required in an attempt to replace body fluids lost in the stools.

STEATORRHEA

Steatorrhea is a diarrhea characterized by an excess of fat in the stool and is a symptom of malabsorption. It is generally indicative of serious organic disease. The excessive amount of exogenous fat in the stool may result from (1) failure of proper digestion, such as in pancreatitis (Chapter 24), and following gastric resection (Chapter 34), (2) bile salt deficiency, such as in diseases of the liver and biliary tract system, blind loop syndrome or ileal resection (Chapter 34), (3) failure of normal absorption due to mucosal damage, such as occurs in nontropical sprue and regional enteritis, after gastrointestinal radiation therapy or resection of over half of the intestine and (4) decreased fat re-esterification and decreased chylomicron formation and transport, as seen in abetalipo-

proteinemia and intestinal lymphangiectasia. (See Table 23–5).

Normally, the fecal fat amounts to about 4 per cent of ingested fat or 2 to 5 gm. daily, but when there are defects in absorption or digestion, fat from food appears in the stool in amounts as high as 60 gm. daily. Occasionally, the fecal fat level may be high in a normal person after ingestion of large amounts of dietary fat.

Nutritional Care

Since steatorrhea is a symptom and not a disease, the underlying disorder must be determined and treated. Weight loss is always present, so patients require an increased caloric intake. Dietary protein should be high, with carbohydrates and fats added as tolerated to meet individual needs. Multiple vitamin and mineral deficiencies are common, making supplemental vitamin therapy necessary, with special emphasis on fat-soluble vitamins, calcium, zinc, magnesium and iron. Foods high in these vitamins and minerals are recommended, plus medication as necessary. Hematopoietic factors, such as vitamin B_{12} and folic acid, should be included when macrocytic anemia is present. (See Chapter 29.) Potassium should be increased in the diet and, in some cases, is required as medication in the form of KCl syrup or powder.

Medium-Chain Triglycerides. Inadequate caloric intake resulting from faulty digestion and absorption of fat may be alleviated by the use of medium-chain triglycerides in the diet. Medium-chain triglycerides (MCT) are hydrolyzed more rapidly than the longer-chain fats for a given lipase concentration and can rely on the small amount of intestinal lipase rather than on pancreatic lipase. The products of MCT hydrolysis are easily dispersed and absorbed without the presence of bile acids. Resynthesis of free fatty acids into triglycerides within the mucosal cell is not necessary with these fatty acids. Following absorption, the short- and medium-chain fatty acids enter the portal venous blood and are transported to the liver directly, without being resynthesized into triglycerides. Besides being more easily absorbed, MCT have also been found to be more rapidly absorbed, approximately as fast as glucose. MCT are available in oil and dry powder preparations, which supply protein, carbohydrate, minerals and vitamins as well. The infant formula Pregestimil and the elemental diet Flexical (both by Mead Johnson) contain MCT

Table 23–5 EXAMPLES OF DISEASES MANIFESTING STEATORRHEA FROM POSSIBLE DEFECTS IN FAT ABSORPTION*

POSSIBLE DEFECT	REPRESENTATIVE DISEASE	DEGREE OF STEATORRHEA
Decreased lipolysis	Chronic pancreatitis	Severe
	Pancreatic carcinoma	Severe
	Cystic fibrosis	Moderate
Decreased micellar solubilization	Extrahepatic or intrahepatic biliary obstruction	Mild
	Intestinal stasis (blind-loop syndrome)	Mild
	Ileal resection	Mild to moderate
	Drugs, e.g., cholestyramine	Mild
Decreased mucosal uptake	Gluten enteropathy	Moderate
	Tropical sprue	Mild
	Nongranulomatous jejunitis	Moderate
	Whipple's disease	Moderate
	Amyloidosis	Mild
	Extensive intestinal resection	Severe
	Lymphoma	Moderate
Decreased re-esterification	Small bowel ischemia (?)	Mild to moderate
Decreased chylomicron formation	Abetalipoproteinemia	Mild
Decreased chylomicron transport in lymph	Intestinal lymphangiectasia	Moderate
	Retroperitoneal fibrosis or malignancy	Moderate

*Adapted from: Westergaard, H., and Dietschy, J. M.: Normal mechanisms of fat absorption and derangements induced by various gastrointestinal diseases. Med. Clin. North Am., *58*:1413, 1974.

oil. Medium-chain triglycerides are used as a source of calories for the patient with steatorrhea and not as a primary form of therapy, unless the steatorrhea cannot be treated in any other way.

Because these triglycerides are not very palatable, most patients cannot tolerate more than 50 gm. per day, which supplies about 400 kcal.

INFLAMMATORY DISEASES OF THE BOWEL

DIVERTICULAR DISEASE

Diverticula are herniations of the colonic wall. It was thought in the past that aging and fatty degeneration of the colon were responsible for the development of *diverticulosis*. But now that it is possible to measure intraluminal pressure in the colon, it is thought that the outpouchings result from segmentation of the colon and the resulting high intracolonic pressures.[11] (See Fig. 23–3.)

The diverticula may occur anywhere along the intestinal tract but are most frequently observed in the colon. The accumulation of fecal matter in these pockets often results in infection and inflammation and sometimes causes ulceration or even perforation. This is *diverticulitis*. Surgery is sometimes advised, especially if perforation occurs. Approximately 10 to 15 per cent of patients with diverticulosis develop diverticulitis.

Nutritional Care

The reason why segmentation and high intracolonic pressures occur has not been definitely elucidated, but a most plausible theory gaining acceptance is that of Burkitt, Painter and their colleagues. They theorize that the decreased stool size resulting from decreased fiber intake is responsible for the development of diverticular disease. This argues against the traditional diet therapy. Because undigested fragments of fiber were frequently found near perforated diverticula that required surgery, physicians and surgeons felt that roughage aggravated the condition and prescribed low-roughage diets. Now it appears that a fiber-deficient diet favors the development of diverticulosis.

Painter reported that his patients who had diverticulosis defecated easier, had less pain and less distention when the dietary fiber was increased. The swiftly passed soft stool sub-

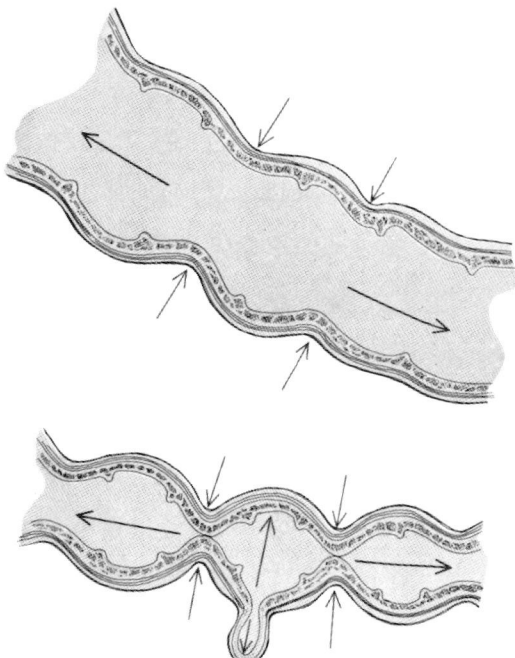

Figure 23-3 Mechanism by which low-fiber, low-bulk diets might generate diverticula is shown schematically. Where colon contents are bulky (top) muscular contractions exert pressure longitudinally. If lumen is smaller (bottom), contractions can produce occlusion and exert pressure against colon wall, which may produce a diverticular "blowout."

jects the sigmoid to less strain and does not favor the development of diverticula (Fig. 23-3). After treating 70 patients who had diverticulosis by giving them unprocessed bran, all-bran cereal and whole-meal bread, Painter found that 2 tsp. of bran three times per day (the equivalent of 2 to 3 gm. of fiber) relieved the symptoms of the disease for most patients.[12] Table 23-1 gives the crude fiber content* of some foods. Table 23-2 lists a variety of foods that provide a high-fiber diet.

Patients with diverticular disease being taught about the new diet may require extensive encouragement, because the high-fiber approach is probably the complete opposite of all previous advice the patient has received.

REGIONAL ENTERITIS (CROHN'S DISEASE)

Enteritis is an inflammation or irritation of the bowel of varying degree. Regional enteritis or Crohn's disease is chronic inflammation

---

*See Chapter 3 for the difference between crude fiber and dietary fiber.

with a granulomatous response that may occur in any part of the gastrointestinal tract. It most commonly affects all layers of the intestinal wall of the ileum and colon. The bowel wall thickens and the intestinal lumen becomes narrowed.

Crohn's disease may take a benign course and eventually disappear, or it may become severe, with complications such as intestinal obstruction or fistula formation. When confined to the colon, Crohn's disease has a patchy distribution and thus is more likely to be successfully managed through surgical removal of the diseased sections. However, when found in the small intestine Crohn's disease is diffuse and continues to spread and damage the intestine even after surgical resection. The patient who has Crohn's disease in the small intestine will probably have many problems and require a number of surgical resections in attempting to control the disease.

The disease occurs most often between the ages of 15 and 35, both sexes are equally affected, and it is two to three times more common among Jews than among non-Jews. The cause of the disease is unknown, but current theories include genetic, infectious and immunological factors. The patient typically complains of fatigue, variable weight loss, right lower quadrant pain or cramping and diarrhea.

Treatment

Emotional support is especially important, since the disease is chronic with unknown etiology and variable prognosis. The patient, usually a young person, frequently is resentful about this physical weakness in the most productive period of his or her life.

Most important during acute periods are maintenance of fluid and electrolyte balances and administration of an antidiarrheal agent. Sometimes salicylazosulfapyridine is given to suppress bowel activity. Corticosteroids are given in severe cases that do not respond to other measures. Surgical removal of the diseased portion of the ileum or colon is indicated in cases of recurrent, complicated regional enteritis.

Nutritional Care

The diet should be low in residue, high in caloric value, liberal in animal proteins and rich in vitamins and minerals (see Table 23-4). In regional enteritis with malabsorption steatorrhea, there usually is improvement when fats are restricted to 25 per cent of

calories (about 50 gm.) per day; sometimes severe restriction (to 10 per cent of calories) is necessary. Improvement may result from the use of medium-chain triglycerides. Ideally, fat in the stool should be less than 10 gm. daily.

Elemental diet formulas (see Chapter 35) or total parenteral nutrition may be necessary if the patient cannot absorb nutrients or if food exacerbates the diarrhea.

Patients with regional enteritis seem to have lower serum and leukocyte vitamin C levels than do normal individuals.[8] This could be a result of the low-fiber diets that these patients usually follow, which are low in vitamin C, or it could be due to an increased need for vitamin C as a result of this disease. Since it has also been found that patients who developed fistulas (a common complication of regional enteritis) also had ileal tissue and blood ascorbate levels lower than patients without fistulas, it has been postulated that fistulas might form more easily in patients who have a depressed vitamin C content. Possibly the defect occurs in the collagen formation process which requires vitamin C.[8] Increased intake of vitamin C (at least 500 mg. per day) is indicated until the levels of the vitamin improve.

ULCERATIVE COLITIS

Ulcerative colitis is a chronic inflammation and ulceration of the mucosa of the large intestine. (See Fig. 23–4.) The etiology is unknown, although a number of theories have been offered by medical authorities. The four most common theories are: (1) it is of infectious origin, (2) it is an autoimmune disorder, (3) it is an allergic condition and (4) it is a result of psychogenic disturbances. That individuals who develop the disease are frequently depressed, irritable and emotionally unstable is a common observation. A combination of causal factors probably is involved.

The general characteristics of ulcerative colitis are rectal bleeding, diarrhea accompanied by pain and spasm, fever, ulcerative lesions in the mucosa of the large intestine, nutritional edema, negative nitrogen balance, avitaminosis, dehydration, electrolyte imbalance, anorexia and malnutrition. Anemia may be present as a result of blood loss. The disease usually occurs in young people (under age 40 to 50), though no age is exempt. Chronic ulcerative colitis has a striking tendency to exacerbation and remission. Unlike Crohn's disease, which can affect both the small and large intestines, ulcerative colitis affects only the colon.

Elimination test diets are sometimes employed for diagnosis when a food allergy is suspected (see Chapter 31). Milk, eggs, oranges, wheat, spinach and tomatoes are the foods most frequently found to be the cause of the allergy. Rider and Moeller[13] obtained good clinical results by removing foods from the diet that produced a hypersensitivity reaction when injected intramucosally. Others have reported dramatic results after withholding milk from the diet.[10]

If medical treatment fails to produce results, surgery may be advised. Surgery is required for 20 to 30 per cent of patients with chronic ulcerative colitis. Because this disease is so nutritionally debilitating, the patient should always receive nutritional support and rehabilitation prior to surgery.

Nutritional Care

The frequent stools characteristic of the disease tend to limit the absorption of nutrients in the diet. Unless the dietary treatment receives special attention, evidence of multiple nutritional deficiencies invariably appears. Nutritional care is an important part of the therapy, and the diet should consist of adequate nutrients that are not disturbing to the patient's physiological condition. Severe dietary restrictions not only cause nutritional deficiencies but also add to the problems most individuals with this ailment exhibit. The importance of restoring normal nutrition in patients with ulcerative colitis cannot be overemphasized; in some cases this alone may initiate improvement. A daily intake of 2500 to 3500 kcal. in-

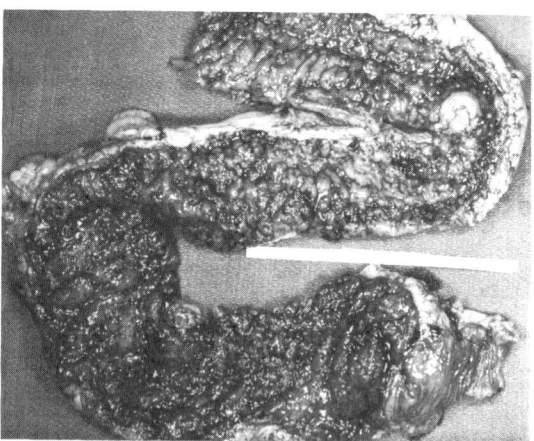

Figure 23–4 The mucosal lining of the colon in ulcerative colitis is greatly disturbed. (From: Sabiston, D. C. (ed.): Davis-Christopher Textbook of Surgery, 11th ed. Philadelphia, W. B. Saunders Co., 1977, p. 1117.)

cluding 125 to 150 gm. of protein, is recommended. High-protein, high-calorie diets are discussed in Chapters 34 and 35.

The foods included in the diet are selected from those listed in the minimal-fiber diet (Table 23–4) and should provide large amounts of vitamins and minerals. Vitamin and mineral supplements are recommended.

"Fiber," "Roughage" and "Residue" Diets. There is confusion and misunderstanding about the definitions of the terms *low residue, low fiber* and *low roughage* when applied to diets. The word *residue* is mistakenly used to describe two different characteristics: (1) the indigestible content of a food, i.e., the dietary fiber and (2) the increased fecal output from a food, regardless of whether any portion of the food remained after chemical digestion.

All foods have some residue. Even if no food is eaten, there is residue in the intestinal tract from the normal body metabolism and processes of life. Milk and fats seem to increase the bulk of stools, although they are actually low in fiber content. Milk, while reported and considered by many to be a high-residue food, should be classified as medium-residue on the basis of fecal studies. Thus, while a food might be high-residue because of its fiber content, it does not necessarily follow that a low-fiber food is also low-residue.

In general, foods can be listed in order of increasing fecal output as follows: protein < fat < milk < digestible carbohydrate < carbohydrate with non-digestible material. To have minimal gut residue would mean unrealistic dietary restriction. The term *low residue* will only be used in reference to elemental diet formulas. (See Table 35–7C.) These are composed of substances that are almost completely absorbed.

MINIMAL-FIBER DIET. The minimal-fiber diet (Table 23–4) follows the normal diet pattern, with modifications in consistency. Turner[17] defines it as "a diet which contains a minimum of indigestible carbohydrates and no tough connective tissue."

For purposes of this text, diets composed of whole foods of which little remains in the colon after digestion will be referred to as *minimal-* or *low-fiber* diets. A diet containing large amounts of food substances that resist digestion is a high-fiber diet.

Frequent small feedings are advised and are usually more acceptable to the individual than the customary three meals a day. The frequent small feedings are more beneficial, permitting better absorption of the nutrients in the diet.

The nurse can be of great help by giving encouragement and understanding to these patients, who are frequently described as dependent, immature, obsessive and hostile. These individuals are often highly vulnerable to the ordinary events of life. An understanding of their emotional difficulties is indispensable to the effective treatment of ulcerative colitis. Attention to the attractive service of food, cheerful surroundings, efforts to inspire confidence and encouragement to eat the diet prescribed are of primary importance to effective total therapy. The nurse has an opportunity to study the patient's eating habits and to assist in making the changes or improvements that are indicated in his or her customary diet. Emphasis on the patient's needs is more apt to bring a change in eating habits than sessions on the diet that stress do's and don't's. As with all patients who have intestinal diseases, the dietary regimen should be individualized.

GASTROINTESTINAL ALLERGY

A group of disorders termed *eosinophilic gastroenteritis* are chronic relapsing conditions that often exist for long periods without symptoms. They occur in the stomach or small bowel and are characterized by clinical symptoms of abdominal pain, belching, bloating, distention, flatus and diarrhea. Pathologically, there is tissue edema and infiltration of the intestinal wall with eosinophils. These disorders are thought to be allergic reactions and seem to be more common in men. The allergy most frequently involves food, but can also be a reaction to a drug, an insect sting or an inhaled antigen such as grass pollen.

Treatment consists of eliminating those items known to cause exacerbation. The most difficult step is to identify the allergens. In determining the source of a food allergy, the elimination diets discussed in Chapter 31 are used.

MALABSORPTION SYNDROMES

There are a number of disorders that interfere with adequate intestinal absorption of essential food elements. Among those discussed elsewhere in this text are celiac disease (Chapter 39), pancreatitis (really maldigestion, Chapter 24) and short bowel syndrome (Chapter 34). Other causes of malabsorption are the toxic influences of some drugs, (Chapter 21), gastrointestinal parasites or malignancies. (See Table 23–6.)

Table 23–6 SOME DISEASES AND CONDITIONS ASSOCIATED WITH MALABSORPTION

Inadequate Digestion
    Pancreatic insufficiency
    Gastric acid hypersecretion
    Gastric resection
Altered Bile Salt Metabolism with Impaired Micelle Formation
    Hepatobiliary disease
    Interrupted enterohepatic circulation of bile salts
    Bacterial overgrowth
    Drugs that precipitate bile salts
Abnormalities of Mucosal Cell Transport
    Biochemical or genetic abnormalities
        Disaccharidase deficiency
        Monosaccharide malabsorption
        Specific disorders of amino acid malabsorption
        Abetalipoproteinemia
        Vitamin B_{12} malabsorption
        Non-tropical sprue (gluten-sensitive enteropathy)
    Inflammatory or infiltrative disorders
        Regional enteritis
        Ulcerative colitis
        Amyloidosis
        Scleroderma
        Tropical sprue
        Gastrointestinal allergy
        Infectious enteritis
        Whipple's disease
        Intestinal lymphoma
        Radiation enteritis
        Drug-induced enteritis
    Endocrine and metabolic disorders
    Inadequate absorptive surface after surgery
Abnormalities of Intestinal Lymphatics and Vascular System
    Intestinal lymphangiectasia
    Mesenteric vascular insufficiency
    Chronic congestive heart failure

SPRUE

Sprue is a disease of unknown etiology believed by many to be a nutritional deficiency disorder. There is atrophy of the villi in the proximal small intestine, which is less severe in tropical sprue than in celiac sprue. While *steatorrhea* is the outstanding characteristic of the disease, impaired absorption caused by biochemical or organic disease of the bowel affects the absorption of all nutrients. A form of *anemia*, generally of the macrocytic type, is present. The onset of symptoms usually is very gradual, covering a period of months or years. The patient has *loss of appetite* and consequent *loss of weight* and emaciation. *Osteomalacia* and impaired vitamin D and calcium absorption resulting in *hypocalcemia* may occur. Other symptoms include easy bruising or abnormal bleeding as a result of hypothrombinemia (vitamin K deficiency); peripheral edema caused by hypoalbuminemia;

neuropathy; glossitis; stomatitis (from B-vitamin deficiencies) and skin changes from carotene or vitamin A deficiencies. (See Table 23–7.)

Incidence

Although found in all parts of the United States and Europe (non-tropical), sprue is more common in the Southern states and the tropics (tropical); women are affected more frequently than men; and the age group in which it usually occurs is from 20 to 40 years.

Nutritional Care

Since there is a difference in response to treatment between tropical and non-tropical sprue, they will be considered separately.

Tropical Sprue. Folic acid deficiency is believed to be the primary cause of tropical sprue. Dramatically favorable results have been obtained in patients having tropical sprue with megaloblastic anemia, who were treated with an adequate diet, vitamin B_{12} and folic acid. Tropical sprue may also be caused by infection since antibiotic treatment has had some success.

The diet should be high in protein (120 gm. or more), including liver and lean meat, and low in carbohydrates and fats. Carbohydrates are limited to those available from simple sugars, low-starch vegetables, fruits and fruit juices because of faulty absorption. Fats are usually restricted to those that are easily digested and absorbed. Medium-chain triglycerides may be used. Folic acid supplementation, frequently as much as 5 to 10 mg. daily, is necessary. Vitamin supplements, especially of vitamin

Table 23–7 LABORATORY ABNORMALITIES FOUND IN THE MALABSORPTION SYNDROME*

Macrocytic, hyperchromic, hypochromic or normochromic anemia (B_{12} and folic acid deficiency)
Microcytic, hypochromic anemia (iron and protein deficiency)
Hypocholesterolemia
Low prothrombin
Low serum calcium
Low serum phosphorus
Low serum potassium
Low serum albumin
Elevated alkaline phosphatase

*From: Ross, J. R., and Moore, V. A.: Axioms of malabsorption. Hospital Medicine, *11*:98, 1975.

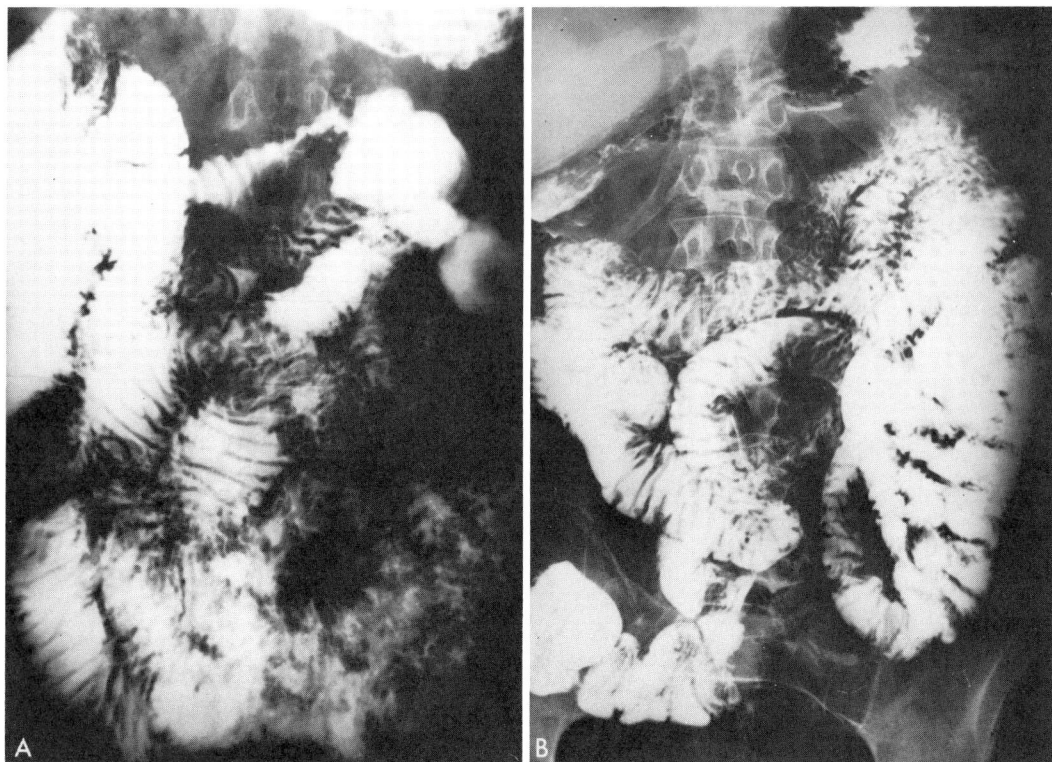

Figure 23–5   Barium contrast studies from a patient with celiac sprue. Before treatment *(A)*, there is significant dilatation of some of the loops of small bowel, as well as marked distortion and coarsening of the mucosal pattern. After six weeks of maintenance on a gluten-free diet *(B)*, there is a significant reduction in the dilatation and improvement in the mucosal pattern, although it has not yet returned to normal. (From: Sleisenger, M. H., and Fordtran, J. S.: Gastrointestinal Disease, Philadelphia, W. B. Saunders Co., 1973, p. 877.)

B-complex, calcium and iron should also be given.

In the beginning of the treatment, only those foods that can be tolerated by the patient are offered. However, the response to folic acid is usually dramatic, and gradually a more liberal food allowance can be given.

Gluten-sensitive Enteropathy (Non-tropical Sprue). Current evidence indicates that non-tropical sprue is adult celiac disease. One theory explains the disease as being due to an abnormal (either defective or deficient) enzyme in the mucosal cell that fails to digest a toxic peptide contained in the gliadin fraction of gluten (the protein in wheat). Other theories state that the reaction to gluten is a defect in immunity or a defect in the mucosal cell membrane that allows gluten to act as a cytotoxic agent.

Apparently, the intestinal epithelium of patients who have this disease cannot tolerate the glutamine-rich polypeptide contained in gluten, and so this polypeptide acts as a cytotoxin. It interferes with the normal maturation of the intestinal epithelium, thus injuring the

mucosa and causing the pathological changes.[1] The villi of the intestinal mucosa become atrophied and flattened, so that the absorptive surface is decreased and the cells of the villi become deficient in the disaccharidases needed for digestion and in the carriers needed for the transport of nutrients into the blood stream. (See Fig. 23–5.) The result is a malabsorption of lipid, carbohydrate, protein, iron, magnesium, zinc and vitamins, especially the fat-soluble ones.

The anemia seen in these patients is commonly associated with folic acid deficiency, which appears to be caused by unknown interferences with the absorption of this vitamin. Therapy for non-tropical sprue is complicated by the impairment of absorption of multiple nutrients from foods. Therefore, vitamin B_{12} or folic acid administered orally may not relieve the symptoms, and intramuscular administration may be necessary.

The treatment includes correcting the nutritional malfunction of the small bowel and thus the deficiency states. Removal of gluten

from the diet results in the histological appearance of the intestinal mucosa returning to normal (Fig. 23–5).

GLUTEN-FREE DIET. A specific diet that omits the glutamine-bound fraction (glutenin and gliadin) of protein is the treatment of choice for non-tropical sprue. In this diet wheat, rye, barley and oats are excluded, since they all contain large amounts of this protein fraction, which becomes the toxic substance. This means that all bakery products and packaged foods must be scrutinized before they are used. Labels must be read carefully. (See Table 23–8 for the recommended diet.) Additional recipes

may be found in the Sheedy reference listed at the end of this chapter. Cereal products that can be used as substitutes are corn flour, cornmeal, potato flour, rice flour, soybean flour and wheat-starch flour (gliadin-free). (See Table 23–9.) During the first few weeks of gluten restriction, the diet should be supplemented with vitamins and minerals in order to cure deficiencies and replenish nutrient stores.

Bayless and associates[2] report on six patients with adult celiac disease who followed the gluten-free diet for 15 months and improved clinically and biochemically, with the histological appearance of their intestinal mucosae be-

Table 23–8   WHEAT-, RYE-, BARLEY- AND OAT-FREE DIET[*a]

FOODS ALLOWED		FOODS OMITTED	
Milk	2 glasses or more (more for children); flavored if desired.	Meats, fish and poultry	Meat patties and meat, fish or chicken loaf made with bread or bread crumbs; croquettes; breaded meats, fish or chicken; chili con carne and other canned meat dishes; cold cuts, unless guaranteed pure meat; bread stuffings.
Eggs	1 or 2 a day.		
Meat, fish and poultry	2 medium servings daily (not breaded, creamed or served with thickened gravy; no bread dressings; otherwise, prepared as desired).		
Cheese	As desired.	Gravies, sauces	All gravies or cream sauces thickened with wheat flour.
Bread	Made from rice, corn, soybean and gluten-free wheat flour only.	Bread	All bread, rolls, crackers, cake and cookies made from wheat or rye; Ry-Krisp; muffins, biscuits, waffles; pancake flour and other prepared mixes; rusks; zwieback; pretzels; any products containing oatmeal, barley or buckwheat; breaded foods; bread crumbs.
Cereals	Corn flakes, corn meal, hominy, rice, Rice Krispies, Puffed Rice, precooked rice cereals.		
Fats	Butter and other fats as desired (note restrictions under *Foods Omitted*).		
Vegetables, potatoes	As desired, except creamed; include 2 servings green or yellow vegetables and at least 1 raw vegetable daily (the last may be omitted for very young children); rice may be substituted occasionally for potatoes.	Cereals and cereal products	All wheat and rye cereals; wheat germ; barley; oatmeal; buckwheat; kasha; noodles, macaroni, spaghetti; dumplings.
		Fats	Commercial salad dressings, except pure mayonnaise (read labels).
Fruits	As desired; 3 servings daily; include citrus fruit once a day.	Vegetables	Any prepared with cream sauce or breaded.
Soups	All clear and vegetable soups; cream soups thickened with cream, cornstarch, or potato flour only.	Soups	All canned soups, except clear broth; all cream soups, unless thickened with cream, cornstarch or potato flour.
Desserts	Any of the following: gelatin, fruit gelatin, ice or sherbet; homemade ice cream; custard; Junket; rice pudding; cornstarch pudding (homemade); or blancmange, if thickened with cornstarch.	Desserts	Cakes, cookies, pastry; commercial ice cream and ice cream cones; prepared mixes; puddings; all homemade puddings thickened with wheat flour.
Beverages	Milk, fruit juices, ginger ale, cocoa (read label to see that no wheat flour has been added to cocoa or cocoa syrup); for adults, add: coffee (made from ground coffee), tea, carbonated beverages.	Beverages	Postum, malted milk, Ovaltine (read labels on instant coffees to see that no wheat flour has been added); for adults: beer, ale.
Sweets	Sugar, white or brown; molasses; jellies and jams; honey; corn syrup.	Sweets	Commercial candies containing cereal products (read label).

WARNING: *Read labels on all packaged and prepared foods.*

*From: Sleisenger, M. H., et al.: Treatment of non-tropical sprue. J. Am. Diet. Assoc., *33*:1138, 1957.

[a]This diet is free from cereal proteins, except those found in rice and corn. It is adequate for normal nutrition. The diet for the adult contains approximately 90 gm. of protein, 90 gm. of fat, 200 gm. of carbohydrate and 2000 kcal. A high-calorie wheat-, rye-, barley- and oat-free diet may be ordered, if desired. (All quantities listed are for adults. For children, the amount of milk should be increased and size of servings of other foods decreased according to the age of the child.)

Table 23–9 SUGGESTIONS FOR
SUBSTITUTIONS FOR WHEAT FLOUR IN
RECIPES*

One cup of wheat flour may be substituted in standard recipes by the following:

  1 cup corn flour
  ¾ cup coarse cornmeal
  1 scant cup fine cornmeal
  ⅝ cup potato flour
  ⅞ cup rice flour

There are some problems in the use of substitutes for wheat flour. The following suggestions will improve the eating quality of the final product:

1. Rice flour and cornmeal tend to have a grainy texture. A smoother texture may be obtained by mixing the rice flour or cornmeal with the liquid called for in the recipe, bringing this mixture to a boil and then cooling before adding to the other ingredients.
2. Soy flour must always be used in combination with another flour, not as the only flour in a recipe.
3. When using other than wheat flour in baking, longer and slower baking is required. This is particularly necessary when the product is made without milk and eggs.
4. When using coarse meals and flours in place of wheat flour, the amount of leavening must be increased. For each cup of coarse flour, use 2½ tsp. of baking powder.
5. Substitutes for wheat flour do not make a satisfactory yeast bread.
6. Muffins or biscuits, when made with other than wheat flour, are of better texture if baked in small sizes.
7. Dryness is a common characteristic of cakes made with flours other than wheat. Moisture may be preserved by (a) frosting or (b) storing in closed containers.

*From: Ohlson, M. A.: Experimental and Therapeutic Dietetics, 2nd ed. Minneapolis, Burgess Publishing Co., 1972, pp. 142–43.

coming virtually normal. Ruffin[15] reports follow-up observations on 10 patients with celiac sprue who were treated exclusively with the gluten-free diet for 10 years. Both the immediate and prolonged effects have been clinically satisfactory. Any relapses were due to dietary indiscretions and promptly subsided when gluten was removed from the diet.

Drugs

Adrenocortical steroids have been observed to facilitate intestinal absorption in the acute stage of the disease in most patients. However, intestinal biopsies taken from these individuals continue to show marked abnormalities despite the improvement of symptoms.

GASTROINTESTINAL ENZYME DEFICIENCIES

Intestinal enzyme deficiency states involve deficiencies of the brush border disac-charidases, which hydrolyze disaccharides at the mucosal cell membrane and allow the absorption of monosaccharides. (See Table 3–2.) Deficiencies or low levels of these enzymes can result in malabsorption of the carbohydrates.

There are three types of disaccharidase deficiencies: (1) rare congenital defects, such as sucrase-isomaltase or lactase deficiencies seen in the newborn, (2) generalized forms that are secondary to diseases such as regional enteritis or celiac sprue, which damage the intestinal epithelium (these are discussed in relation to the diseases that cause them) and (3) an adult form of lactase deficiency, which usually appears after childhood but can appear as early as two years of age.

ADULT LACTASE DEFICIENCY

Low lactase activity in adults is a common disorder and can result in an intolerance to lactose, the sugar in milk. It is more prevalent among blacks, Asians, Orientals and South Americans than among Caucasians. In fact, most populations except for Northern European Caucasians have high incidences of adult lactose intolerance. It has been estimated that there are 30 million people in the U.S. who cannot absorb lactose, including 2 million elementary school children.[3]

Unable to be hydrolyzed into galactose and glucose, lactose is not absorbed but remains in the gut and acts osmotically to draw water into the intestines. (See Fig. 23–6.) In addition, bacteria ferment the undigested lactose and generate lactic acid and other organic acids, carbon dioxide and hydrogen gas. The result is bloating, flatulence, cramps and diarrhea. It is presumed that the person with lactase deficiency can utilize the protein, fat, vitamins and minerals in milk.

Lactase deficiency is diagnosed from a history of gastrointestinal symptoms that occur after milk ingestion, from a breath or hydrogen test, an abnormal lactose tolerance test or biopsy of the intestinal mucosa. For a lactose tolerance test, the patient takes an oral dose of lactose (1.5 to 2 gm. per kg. of body weight or up to 50 gm. in an adult—the equivalent of the amount of lactose in 1 qt. of milk) after an overnight fast. Measurements are made of the blood glucose at specified times afterward. For the breath test, the amount of H_2 produced by the bacteria acting on lactose and then released into the gut is measured in the breath. In the lactose-intolerant person, gastrointestinal symptoms will appear after administration of

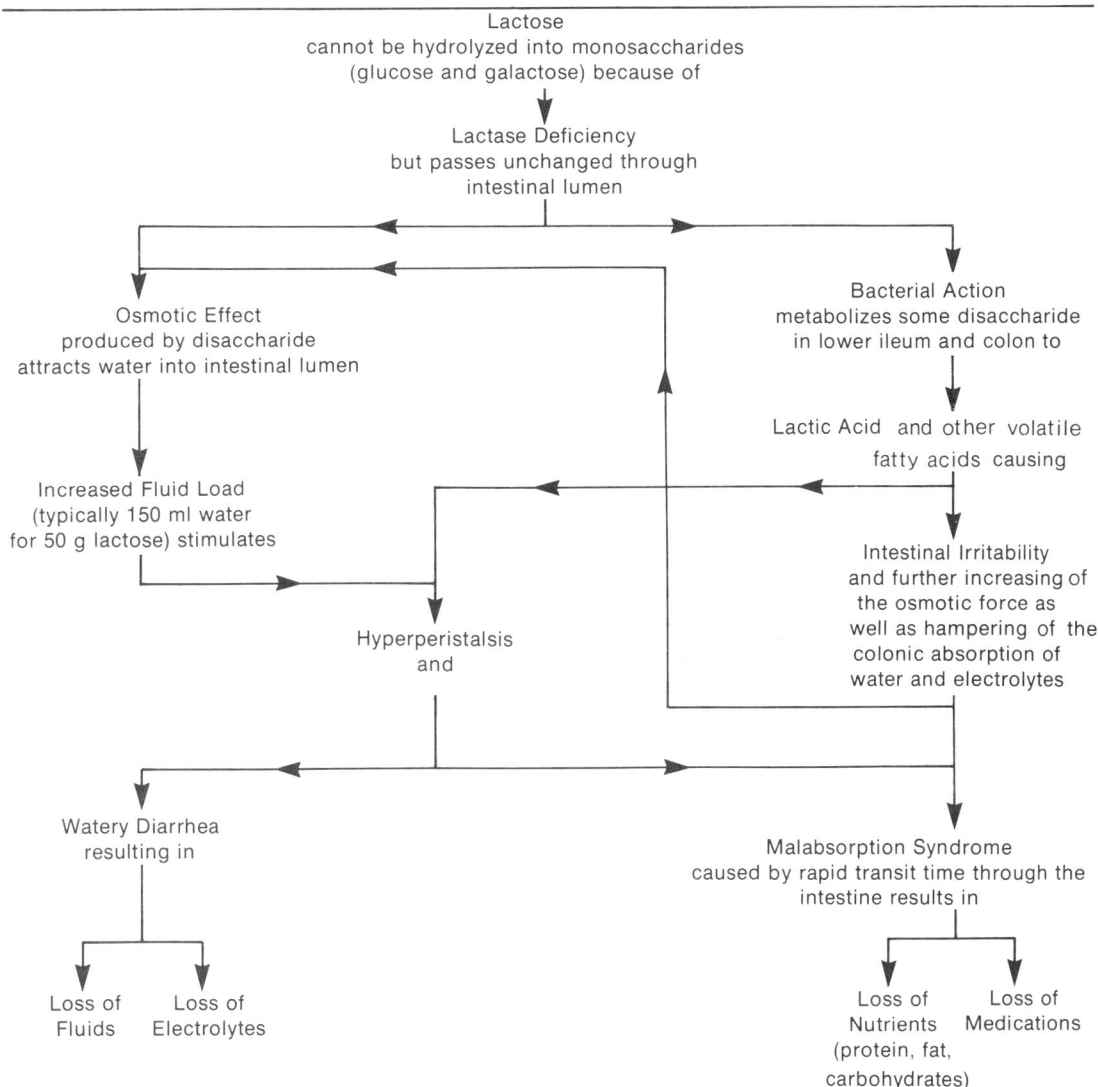

Lactose
cannot be hydrolyzed into monosaccharides
(glucose and galactose) because of

Lactase Deficiency
but passes unchanged through
intestinal lumen

Osmotic Effect
produced by disaccharide
attracts water into intestinal lumen

Bacterial Action
metabolizes some disaccharide
in lower ileum and colon to

Lactic Acid and other volatile
fatty acids causing

Increased Fluid Load
(typically 150 ml water
for 50 g lactose) stimulates

Intestinal Irritability
and further increasing of
the osmotic force as
well as hampering of the
colonic absorption of
water and electrolytes

Hyperperistalsis
and

Watery Diarrhea
resulting in

Malabsorption Syndrome
caused by rapid transit time through the
intestine results in

Loss of   Loss of
Fluids   Electrolytes

Loss of   Loss of
Nutrients   Medications
(protein, fat,
carbohydrates)

Figure 23–6 Pathogenesis and clinical implications of lactose intolerance. (From: Ensure Plus. Columbus, Ohio, Ross Laboratories, 1977, p. 11.)

the lactose, and blood glucose will increase less than 25 mg. per 100 ml. of serum above the fasting level. Although some patients will appear abnormal when tested, they will have no history of intolerance to milk. This raises the question of whether the blood glucose level is truly an indicator of lactose intolerance. Such patients appear able to tolerate the small amount of milk in their diets but cannot accommodate the large test load of 50 gm. when it is given undiluted and on an empty stomach.

Nutritional Care

With the omission of milk and lactose-containing foods, the symptoms of lactose intolerance are alleviated. Cheese contains very minute amounts of lactose, but most patients can tolerate it. The amount of lactose in creamed cottage cheese varies widely, since lactose is an optional ingredient added to the creaming mixture.[5] Yogurt contains lactose but for some unknown reason is tolerated by some patients.[6] For others it may have to be omitted. Ice cream and other milk dishes, cooked or uncooked, contain lactose and should be avoided or restricted. See Table 39–13 for a lactose-free (galactose-free) diet. If after strict adherence to a lactose-free diet the symptoms do not disappear, then lactose intolerance is probably not the reason for the gastrointestinal symptoms, and another cause should be sought.

Although studies have shown that the amount of the enzyme sucrase in the body can be increased by feeding fructose (which is part of sucrose), feeding studies using lactose could not induce the production of more lactase. Lactase production seems to be under genetic control.

The production of those enzymes that can be induced in the body by feeding the specific sugar has tremendous therapeutic implications. It seems to take two to five days before sucrase activity is seen, which is the same length of time the intestinal epithelium needs to renew itself or that a crypt cell needs to move up the villus to the tip, where it would function with the new enzyme.[14]

BLIND LOOP SYNDROME

This is a disorder characterized by intestinal stasis and bacterial overgrowth that results from obstructive disease, stricture, fistula formation or surgical repair of the intestine (see Chapter 34). Because stasis favors their growth, the bacteria undergo a population explosion. Bacteria unconjugate bile salts, which besides being cytotoxic in the unconjugated form are also less effective as micelle formers. With reduced micelle formation, steatorrhea secondary to the bowel stasis results. There is also malabsorption of vitamin B_{12} because the bacteria use the vitamin for their own growth. Treatment is directed toward removal of the blind loop or control of the bacterial growth with antibiotics.

PROTEIN-LOSING ENTEROPATHY

Protein-losing enteropathy, a secondary disorder to many diseases, is a condition of excessive gastrointestinal loss of protein and can occur anywhere along the G.I. tract. Four mechanisms have been proposed to explain this abnormal loss of protein into the gut:[9]

1. Because of an inflamed or ulcerated mucosa, plasma proteins may pass into the G.I. lumen (regional enteritis, ulcerative colitis).

2. Disordered mucosal cell structure may permit plasma protein loss (non-tropical sprue).

3. Increased lymphatic pressure causes increased movement of plasma proteins into the lumen through spaces between mucosal cells in the epithelium.

4. Dilated lymph vessels in the intestinal mucosa rupture and discharge their protein-rich contents into the lumen (idiopathic intestinal lymphangiectasia).

A normal person will catabolize 5 to 10 per cent of the intravascular albumin pool daily, but the person with protein-losing enteropathy will catabolize 50 to 60 per cent.

Nutritional Care

Treatment aims to relieve the underlying disorder and to supply large amounts of calories and protein (150 gm. or more daily) to offset the protein loss. This is done with a high-protein diet and protein supplements, with a defined-formula diet that is high in protein, such as High-Nitrogen Vivonex, or with total parenteral nutrition. It is very important to maintain nutritional status in these patients so that they will respond to the medical treatment and endure the diagnostic tests.

PROBLEMS AND SUGGESTED TOPICS FOR DISCUSSION

1. Describe the physiology and functions of the intestines.
2. Classify foods into low- and high-fiber types.
3. Differentiate between the low-fiber and low-residue diets. List the foods that are good sources of cellulose. Why does cellulose form residue? What is the difference between residue and roughage?
4. When is a low-fiber diet used? A high-fiber diet?
5. Plan a high-protein, high-calorie, low-fiber diet for a patient with regional enteritis. The patient is a 40 year old male, 20 pounds overweight, who works in a factory and carries his lunch.
6. Plan menus for a two-week period for a patient with (a) ulcerative colitis and (b) atonic constipation. The patient is a 25 year old female who lives alone, clerks in a store and eats lunch and dinner in a restaurant. Check the menus for adequacy.
7. What are the principles of a diet for chronic diarrhea? Differentiate between diarrhea and steatorrhea.
8. Interview a patient with ulcerative colitis and find out which foods bother him or her. Is the patient afraid to eat certain foods? Is his or her diet adequate? What changes would you recommend?
9. What are the general principles of nutritional care for a patient with a malabsorption syndrome?
10. Do a nutritional assessment of a patient with gluten-sensitive enteropathy.

CITED REFERENCES

1. Baker, H., Frank, O., and Sobotka, H.: Mechanisms of folic acid deficiency in nontropical sprue. JAMA, 187:119, 1964.
2. Bayless, T. M., Yardley, J. H., and Hendrix, T. R.: Adult celiac disease: Treatment with gluten-free diet. Arch. Intern. Med., 111:83, 1963.
3. Bedine, M. S., and Bayless, T. M.: Intolerance of small amounts of lactose by individuals with low lactase levels. Gastroenterology, 65:735, 1973.
4. Burkitt, D. P., Walker, A. R. P., and Painter, N. S.:

Effect of dietary fiber on stools and transit-times, and its role in causation of disease. Lancet, *2*:1408, 1972.

5. Feeley, R. M., Criner, P. E., and Slover, H. T.: Major fatty acids and proximate composition of dairy products. J. Am. Diet. Assoc., *66*:140, 1975.

6. Gallagher, C. R., Molleson, A. L., and Caldwell, J. H.: Lactose intolerance and fermented dairy products. J. Am. Diet. Assoc., *65*:418, 1974.

7. Geib, D. and Jones, J. D.: Unprecedented case of constipation. JAMA, *38*:1304, 1902.

8. Gerson, C. D.: Ascorbic acid deficiency in clinical disease including regional enteritis. Ann. N.Y. Acad. Sci., *258*:483, 1975.

9. Greenberger, N. J., and Isselbacher, K. J.: Disorders of absorption. In: Thorn, G. W., et al. (eds.), Harrison's Principles of Internal Medicine, 8th ed. New York, Mc Graw-Hill Book Co., 1977, p. 1535.

10. Idiopathic ulcerative colitis and milk. Nutr. Rev., *22*:262, 1964.

11. Painter, N. S.: Diverticular disease of the colon—A disease caused by fiber deficiency. Plant Foods for Man, *1*(1):67, 1973.

12. Painter, N. S., Alameida, A. Z., and Colebourne, K. W.: Unprocessed bran in treatment of diverticular disease of the colon. Br. Med. J., *1*:137, 1972.

13. Rider, J. A., and Moeller, H. C.: Hypersensitivity factors in ulcerative colitis. JAMA, *183*:545, 1963.

14. Rosensweig, N. S.: Diet and intestinal enzyme adaptation: Implications for gastrointestinal disorders. Am. J. Clin. Nutr., *28*:648, 1975.

15. Ruffin, J. M., et al.: Gluten-free diet for nontropical sprue: Immediate and prolonged effects. JAMA, *188*:42, 1964.

16. Søltoft, J., et al.: A double-blind trial of the effect of wheat bran on symptoms of irritable bowel syndrome. Lancet, *1*:270, 1976.

17. Turner, D.: Handbook of Diet Therapy, 5th ed. Chicago, University of Chicago Press, 1970.

18. Wald, A., Back, C., and Bayless, T. M.: Effect of caffeine on the human small intestine. Gastroenterology, *71*:738, 1976.

ADDITIONAL REFERENCES

Ament, M. E.: Inflammatory disease of the colon: Ulcerative colitis and Crohn's colitis. J. Pediatr., *86*:322, 1975.

Burkitt, D. P., and Trowell, H. C. (eds.): Refined Carbohydrate Foods and Disease: Some Implications of Dietary Fiber. New York, Academic Press, 1975.

Cummings, J. H.: Progress report—Dietary fiber. Gut, *14*:69, 1973.

Debry, G., and Drouin, P.: Diet in functional disorders of the colon. Prog. Food Nutr. Sci., *2*:1, 1976.

Elsborg, L., and Bastrup-Madsen, P.: Folic acid absorption in various gastrointestinal disorders. Scand. J. Gastroenterol., *11*:333, 1976.

Farmer, R. G.: The protean manifestations of Crohn's disease. Postgrad. Med., *57*:129, 1975.

Goldstein, F.: Diet and colonic disease. J. Am. Diet. Assoc., *60*:499, 1972.

Hosoi, K., Alvarez, W. C., and Mann, F. C.: Intestinal absorption: A search for the low residue diet. Arch. Intern. Med., *41*:112, 1928.

Idea Exchange: Fiber in the diet. J. Am. Diet. Assoc., *66*:50, 1975.

Jeffries, G. H., Weser, E., and Sleisenger, M. H.: Malabsorption. Gastroenterology, *56*:777, 1969.

Katz, A. J., and Falchuk, Z. M.: Current concepts in gluten sensitive enteropathy (celiac sprue). Pediatr. Clin. North Am., *22*:767, 1975.

Kaufmann, M.: Answers to questions on gastrointestinal allergy. Hospital Medicine, *11*:61, 1975.

Kramer, P.: The meaning of high and low residue diets. Gastroenterology, *47*:649, 1964.

The lactose tolerance test and milk consumption. Nutr. Rev., *34*:302, 1976.

Levitt, M. D., et al.: Studies of a flatulent patient. N. Engl. J. Med., *295*:260, 1976.

McCarthy, C. F.: Nutritional defects in patients with malabsorption. Proc. Nutr. Soc., *35*:37, 1976.

Mendeloff, A. I.: Dietary fiber. Nutr. Rev., *33*:321, 1975. The role of lactose in the diet. Dairy Council Digest, *45*(5) 1975 (Published by the National Dairy Council, Chicago).

Senior, J. R. (ed.): Medium Chain Triglycerides. Philadelphia, University of Pennsylvania Press, 1968.

Sheedy, C. M., and Keifetz, N.: Cooking for Your Celiac Child: Dietary Management in Malabsorption Disorders. New York, Dial Press, Inc., 1969.

Simoons, F. T., Johnson, J. D., and Kretchmer, N.: Perspective on milk during drinking and malabsorption of lactose. Pediatrics, *59*:98, 1977.

Sleisenger, M. H., and Fordtran, J. S. (eds.): Gastrointestinal Disease: Pathophysiology, Diagnosis, Management, 2nd ed. Philadelphia, W. B. Saunders Co., 1978.

Thompson, W. G.: Constipation and catharsis. Can. Med. Assoc. J., *114*:927, 1976.

Trowell, H.: Definition of dietary fiber and hypotheses that it is a protective factor in certain diseases. Am. J. Clin. Nutr., *29*:417, 1976.

Zamcheck, N., and Broitman, S. A.: Nutrition in diseases of the intestines. In: Goodhart, R. S., and Shils, M. E. (eds.), Modern Nutrition in Health and Disease, 5th ed. Philadelphia, Lea and Febiger, 1973.

Chapter 24

NUTRITIONAL CARE FOR PATIENTS WITH DISEASES OF THE LIVER, EXOCRINE PANCREAS AND BILIARY SYSTEM

PHYSIOLOGY AND FUNCTIONS OF THE LIVER

In the metabolism of food, the liver is one of the most important of the body organs (see Fig. 24–1). It is the largest glandular organ of the body, contributing between 2.5 and 3 per cent of the body weight.

The liver also has the greatest number of and most varied functions of any organ in the body. Most of the end products of the digestion of food are transported directly to the liver. Compounds that it manufactures or stores are sent to other parts of the body as needed. Poisons

that enter the body through food or that are produced in other parts of the body are detoxified in the liver. Since the liver has many functions in the metabolism of all major nutrients, a brief summary of its role in the metabolic process follows.

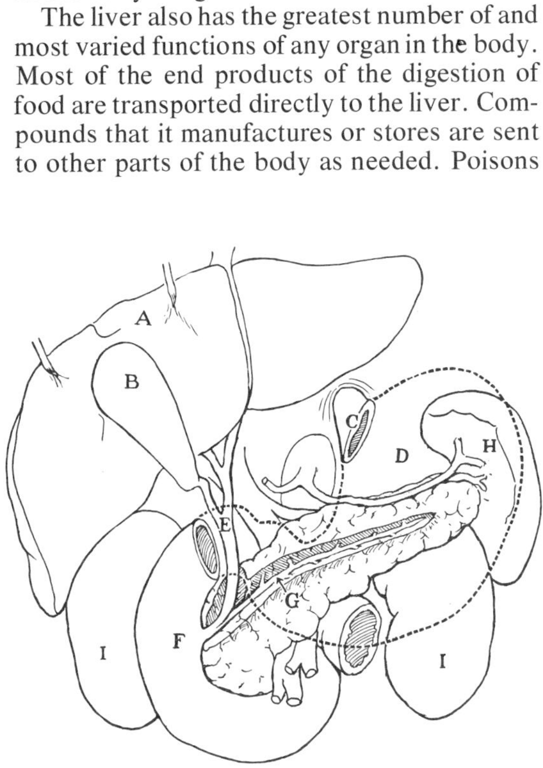

Carbohydrate Metabolism

The hepatic cells serve as a storehouse for glycogen, which is formed in the liver from the glucose, fructose and galactose received from the portal circulation (glycogenesis). When glucose is needed by the body, glycogen is converted to glucose (glycogenolysis) and returned to the blood stream. When glucose concentration in the blood begins to fall below normal, conversion of protein and fat to glucose (gluconeogenesis) occurs in the liver, after which it is sent to the blood stream to maintain normal blood glucose level.

Figure 24–1 Schematic drawing showing relationship of organs of the upper abdomen. *A*, liver (retracted upward); *B*, gallbladder; *C*, esophageal opening of stomach; *D*, stomach (shown in dotted outline); *E*, common bile duct; *F*, duodenum; *G*, pancreas and pancreatic duct; *H*, spleen; *I*, kidneys.

Fat Metabolism

The liver synthesizes fat from fatty acids, deaminized amino acids (keto acids) and carbohydrates. It synthesizes cholesterol and converts about 80 per cent of it into bile salts; the remainder is transported in the form of lipoproteins in the blood. Triglycerides are synthesized from fatty acids, as are phospholipids. Both are incorporated into lipoproteins for transport to the adipose tissue, where they are stored. Oxidation of fatty acids to acetoacetic acid and then to acetyl-CoA occurs in the liver. Acetyl-CoA in turn can enter the Krebs cycle and be oxidized to liberate energy. About 60 per cent of all initial oxidation of fatty acids in the body takes place in the liver.

Protein Metabolism

In the metabolism of proteins, deamination of the amino acids must take place in the liver cells before they can be used for energy or converted to carbohydrate and fats. Keto acids and ammonia are also formed from this deamination process. Conversion of amino acids into other amino acids (non-essential) occurs in the liver through several stages of *transamination.* They are released from the liver to maintain normal blood levels of each amino acid. Other important chemical compounds (such as purines and pyrimidines) are synthesized from amino acids through transamination. The formation of urea by the liver removes ammonia, which is excreted. The carbon residues are converted into fatty acids or glucose for energy or storage. Most of the plasma proteins (albumin, globulin, fibrinogen, prothrombin and heparin) are synthesized by the hepatic cells. A reserve of these proteins is maintained in the liver to replenish serum proteins as needed.

Minerals and Vitamins

The greatest portion of the body's iron is stored in the liver in the form of ferritin until needed by the body. Copper is also stored in the liver and is necessary for the production of hemoglobin. Iron is an integral part of hemoglobin, and vitamin B_{12} (also stored in the liver) brings about the maturation and release of red blood cells in the bone marrow. The iron from discarded red blood cells is recovered and stored by the liver.

All the fat-soluble vitamins are present in the liver. Considerable amounts of vitamins A, D and K are stored there. The liver converts carotene into vitamin A, vitamin K into prothrombin and vitamin D into an active form (25-OH-vitamin D_3). It also stores appreciable amounts of ascorbic acid and the B-complex vitamins.

DISEASES OF THE LIVER RELATED TO DIET

The type of diet used in treating diseases of the liver is related directly to the liver's functions. An understanding of its role in the metabolic process is necessary to determine the character of the diet for any hepatic disturbance. An organ that performs so many varied activities will manifest many types of pathological conditions. Fortunately, the liver has great powers of reserve and compensation and responds to treatment even under adverse conditions.

Objectives of Nutritional Care

The important role of diet in the treatment of liver is recognized and clinical improvement observed as the result of appropriate nutritional care. The objectives of nutritional care are: (1) to maintain or improve the patient's nutritional status through the provision of adequate calories and nutrients and (2) to enable the damaged organ to function as easily and efficiently as possible. These two principles of nutritional care apply for all hepatic disturbances.

Liver Function Tests.   During the course of liver disease, liver function can change drastically, and the nutritional care must be adjusted according to the deteriorating or improving liver function. Liver function tests listed in Table 24–1 provide clues to changing liver function. For instance, a person's serum albumin level reflects his or her protein nutriture. Decreased serum albumin levels show that the liver is unable to synthesize protein or that not enough protein is being provided in the diet. Elevated levels of serum ammonia show that the liver cannot synthesize urea from ammonia in the blood, and that too much ammonia is entering the blood stream from the action of colonic bacteria on protein in the gut. Bacterial enzymes deaminate the amino acids in the gut, thus forming ammonia, which is absorbed through the intestinal mucosa. Intestinal bleeding also contributes protein to the gut and thus to ammonia formation.

VIRAL HEPATITIS

Hepatitis is an inflammation of the liver caused by a virus, toxins, obstruction, parasites or drugs (chloroform, carbon tetrachloride). Viral hepatitis is caused by two different types of viruses, called type A and type B. (There may possibly be a third virus, type C.) Hepatitis caused by the type A virus is called *hepatitis A* or *infectious hepatitis.* This disease, common among children and young adults, is mildly contagious and readily transmitted through contaminated drinking water, food or sewage. In the acute phase there are symptoms of nausea, vomiting, anorexia, fever, headache, weight loss, fatigue and abdominal discomfort.

The symptoms of *serum hepatitis* or type B viral hepatitis are similar to those of infectious

Table 24–1   COMMON LIVER FUNCTION TESTS*

DIAGNOSTIC TEST	FUNCTION EVALUATED
Van den Bergh Icterus index Urine bilirubin Urobilinogen Fecal urobilinogen	Formation and excretion of bile
Total protein Albumin Globulin Fibrinogen Thymol turbidity Cephalin flocculation	Protein metabolism and formation of albumin, globulin, fibrinogen
Prothrombin time	Production of prothrombin
Urea Uric acid Ammonia	Formation of urea and uric acids and removal of ammonia

Glucose tolerance
Galactose tolerance
	Carbohydrate metabolism
	    Gluconeogenesis
	    Glycogenesis
	    Glycogenolysis

Serum phospholipids, triglycerides Cholesterol (total or ester) Ketone	Lipid metabolism Synthesis of cholesterol Formation of ketone bodies
Bromsulphalein (BSP) Hippuric acid	Detoxification Excretion of substances withdrawn from the blood Conjugation, oxidation or reduction
Serum glutamic-oxaloacetic transaminase (SGOT) Serum glutamic-pyruvic transaminase (SGPT) Lactic dehydrogenase (LDH) Alkaline phosphatase Leucine aminopeptidase (LAP) 5′-Nucleotidase Cholinesterase	Enzyme production

*From: Given, B. A., and Simmons, S. J.: Gastroenterology in Clinical Nursing, 2nd ed. St. Louis, C. V. Mosby Co., 1975, p. 273.

hepatitis but are usually more severe. This disease can be transmitted through transfusions of blood or serum from a person who is a carrier of the virus or through improperly sterilized medical instruments, dental drills, tattooing needles or any other skin-puncturing instrument that has come in contact with contaminated blood. Less commonly, it can also be transmitted by other than the parenteral route, which makes its specific cause more obscure. In 5 to 10 per cent of cases, acute serum hepatitis can develop into chronic active hepatitis. This rarely happens after infectious hepatitis. Some people may be carriers of the hepatitis B antigen (HB$_s$Ag) while remaining asymptomatic. These people are the most dangerous to the health of the community.

Nutritional Care

The nutritional care is the same for both forms of hepatitis. Since there is no proven medication to counteract viral hepatitis, every attempt is made to spare the liver. Complete bed rest is essential. In severe cases that are accompanied by vomiting, a 5 to 10 per cent solution of glucose is administered intravenously, and protein hydrolysates or amino acids (3.5 per cent solution) are added if prolonged parenteral feeding is indicated, or protein-containing solutions such as concentrated human plasma and albumin may be used. Concentrated liquid formulas administered orally or by tube feeding provide essential nutrients and sufficient calories and should be given until the person is able to consume an adequate

diet. The same type of diet as outlined for cirrhosis of the liver is prescribed. (See page 509.) The diet should supply 3000 kcal. or more and be high in carbohydrate (300 to 400 gm.) and protein (100 to 150 gm.). It is usually supplemented with B vitamins (especially thiamin and B_{12}), vitamin K and ascorbic acid. At one time it was believed that fat in the diet should be low to prevent fatty deposits in the liver, but the various studies have shown no adequate rationale for fat restriction. Alcohol is forbidden, however.

While most attacks are not serious, they may be severe in older people. If liver damage is extensive in older patients, fatty infiltration of the liver may occur, and hepatic coma may develop. In cases of impending hepatic coma, a maintenance quantity of protein is prescribed. (See page 510.)

PRECAUTIONS AGAINST CONTAMINATION. Disposable dishes, utensils, cups and trays should be used when serving food to the patient who has viral hepatitis of *either the A or B type*. The paper or plastic service and all uneaten food should be disposed of in the patient's room, not in the central dishwashing area of the hospital. Nurses or family members who feed the patient should take all precautions to avoid contracting the disease.

CIRRHOSIS

Cirrhosis is the most serious or final stage of liver injury and degeneration. The normal liver tissue is gradually destroyed and inactive fibrous connective tissue replaces the liver cells, following fatty degeneration of long standing. (See Fig. 24–2.) An intermediate stage called *alcoholic hepatitis* may develop, in which some liver cells die and cause necrotic inflammation. In contrast to the enlarged fatty liver, the cirrhotic liver is contracted and has lost most of its function. Once the dense vascular and fibrous

bands have formed, scarring is reported to be permanent.

Etiology

Alcohol. Chronic alcoholism is the most common cause of cirrhosis. The alcohol-induced liver injury is due to the constant presence of alcohol itself and the metabolic derangements it causes, rather than to the malnutrition commonly associated with alcoholism.[8] Alcohol causes disordered liver metabolism because of its conversion to acetaldehyde and the excessive production of hydrogen that results from this reaction. See Figure 24–3 for the metabolic and toxic effects of alcohol. Fatty liver commonly occurs even after acute alcohol ingestion.

Not all alcoholics go on to develop alcoholic hepatitis and cirrhosis. Whether they do depends on the duration and amount of their alcohol intake and on undefined genetic and possibly immunological factors. An adequate diet does not protect against the development of fatty liver, alcoholic hepatitis or cirrhosis in the alcoholic.

Studies by Lieber[7] indicate that an intake of 11 to 12 oz. of 86 proof whiskey per day can lead to the development of fatty liver in humans, regardless of the maintenance of an adequate diet. When rats were fed this amount of alcohol, a fatty liver could be produced within two to six weeks, even though a well-balanced and controlled dietary intake was maintained.

MALNUTRITION. The chronic alcoholic with liver disease is usually also malnourished, which can aggravate the liver disease. He or she is malnourished for several reasons. First, alcohol replaces food in the diet. It is possible for humans to obtain their maintenance energy needs from the calories in the alcohol consumed, but they will be malnourished because

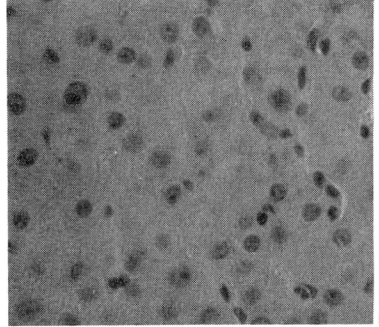

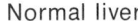

Figure 24–2 Fatty changes in the liver. (From: Halpern, S. L.: Nutrition and chronic disease. Reprinted from Health News, monthly publication of the New York State Department of Health, September, 1955.)

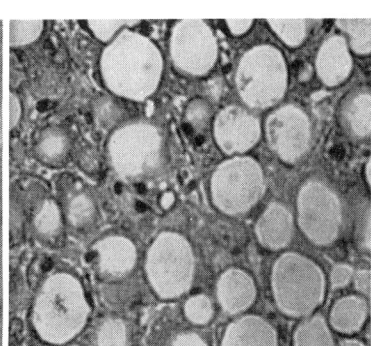

Normal liver   Fatty infiltration of liver

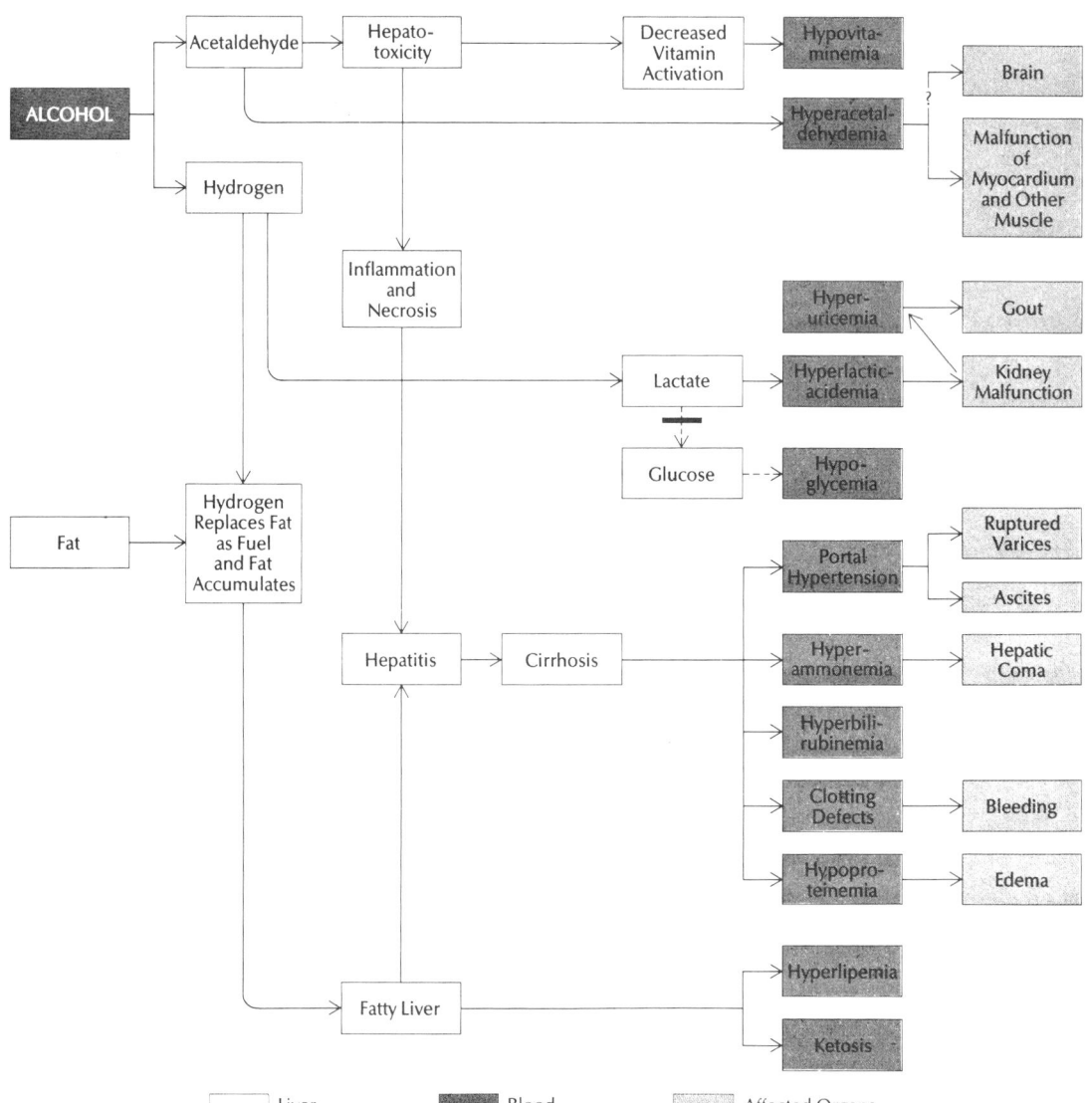

Figure 24–3 Complications of excessive alcohol consumption stem largely from excess hydrogen and from acetaldehyde. Hydrogen produces fatty liver and hyperlipemia, high blood lactic acid and low blood sugar. The accumulation of fat, the effect of acetaldehyde on liver cells and other factors as yet unknown lead to alcoholic hepatitis. The next step is cirrhosis. The consequent impairment of liver function disturbs blood chemistry, notably causing a high ammonia level which can lead to coma and death. Cirrhosis also distorts liver structure, inhibiting blood flow. High pressure in vessels supplying the liver may cause ruptured varices and accumulation of fluid in the abdominal cavity. There are individual differences in response to alcohol; in particular, not all heavy drinkers develop hepatitis and cirrhosis. (From: Lieber, C. S.: The metabolism of alcohol. Sci. Am., *234*:33, 1976. Copyright © 1976 by Scientific American, Inc. All rights reserved.)

of an inadequate intake of nutrients. Alcohol is a notable source of empty calories, since 20 oz. of 86 proof liquor provides 1500 kcal., or about one half to two thirds of the daily caloric requirement, but it contains no protein, vitamins or minerals.

Second, alcohol causes inflammation of the stomach, pancreas and intestine and interferes with the normal processes of digestion and absorption, resulting in malabsorption of nutrients and a secondary malnutrition. The absorption of thiamin, vitamin B_{12}, folic acid and ascorbic acid is depressed.

Third, alcohol and its conversion product acetaldehyde can interfere with the activation of vitamins by liver cells. For example, low serum levels of 25-OH-vitamin D_3, an active form of vitamin D produced by the liver, have

been reported in cirrhotic patients. Vitamin B_6 cannot be converted to its metabolically active form by a diseased liver.

Fourth, alcohol increases the body's requirements for B vitamins, which are needed to metabolize alcohol. It also increases the requirement for magnesium, a mineral excreted after alcohol consumption, so that magnesium deficiency is common among alcoholics.

Fifth, the malnutrition–alcoholism relationship is a vicious circle, because malnutrition seems to potentiate the destructive effects of alcohol on the liver and also causes gastrointestinal changes that contribute to the malabsorption problem and the continuing poor nutritional status already provoked by the alcohol. Folate deficiency and, to a lesser extent, protein deficiency seem to be be most responsible for the malabsorption caused by malnutrition.[1]

These five reasons combined with social and economic factors lead to a malnourished chronic alcoholic. He or she will frequently exhibit signs of clinical deficiency, such as cardiac changes from thiamin deficiency or macrocytic anemia from folate deficiency (see Chapter 12).

Other Causes. Cirrhosis may also be caused by various toxic and infectious agents that cause destruction of the liver cells, as is seen in viral hepatitis, which ultimately leads to fibrosis of the liver.

Nutritional Care

Malnutrition should be corrected, but this is usually difficult because of social and economic factors. Nutritional care for the cirrhotic patient should include a diet that is high in calories, high in carbohydrates and high in protein (1.5 to 2.0 gm. per kg. body weight), with moderate fats and an abundance of vitamins, especially the B complex. This diet is designed to prevent further degeneration of the liver cells and to regenerate the tissue that has not been too seriously damaged.

Calories. Since there is often extreme weight loss, a high-calorie diet with at least 45 to 50 kcal. per kg. desired body weight per day is indicated to rehabilitate the cirrhotic patient.

High Carbohydrate. Increased carbohydrate in the diet for patients with liver disease is well tolerated and seems to have a definite therapeutic value. The carbohydrate content of the diet protects and supports hepatic function. Three hundred to 400 gm. is recommended to spare the available protein and to aid in re-

covery. Liquids and solid foods such as fruit juices with sugar or lactose added, hard candies, jelly, honey, bread, cereals, potatoes, vegetables and fruits or a concentrated-formula supplement are given by mouth as soon as is feasible.

High Protein. A liberal protein intake offers protection in cirrhosis of the liver and is essential for the repair of hepatic cells and the formation of cholic (or cholalic) and other bile acids. A daily intake of 1.5 to 2.0 gm. per kg. of desired body weight or 100 to 150 gm. per day (p. 510) is usually adequate. A cause for *exception to the high protein intake is hepatic coma* (p. 510). Both the quality and quantity of protein are important. It should be of high biological value and rich in the lipotropic factors methionine and choline, which mobilize liver fat and thus counteract fatty infiltration and degeneration of the parenchyma. Meat, fish, poultry, eggs, milk, skim milk powder and cottage cheese are good sources of proteins to include in the diet prescribed for cirrhosis.

CONCENTRATED ORAL AND PARENTERAL PROTEIN. If a patient is too ill to eat or has a poor appetite and cannot consume the large quantity of protein food he or she needs, concentrated protein may be included, such as calcium caseinate, dried milk, soybean flour, dried yeast or Promix. See Table 35–5 for high-calorie and high-protein nutritional supplements. Tube feeding may be necessary but is contraindicated for patients who have esophageal varices. Intravenous administration of amino acids, carbohydrates and water-soluble vitamins may be prescribed if the oral consumption is inadequate.

High Vitamins. A therapeutic vitamin preparation that is a good source of the vitamin B complex, especially folic acid, should be given. All of the vitamins should be supplied in abundance to fortify the liver against stress and to repair damage already done. Vitamin K should be prescribed if evidence of hypoprothrombinemia exists.

Moderate Fat. The lowering of dietary fat to 25 per cent of total calories has been shown to reduce the amount of fatty deposition in the liver when alcohol is being consumed. Substitution of medium-chain triglycerides (MCT) for normal longer-chain dietary fats also resulted in a reduced accumulation of fat in the liver. Whether these measures hasten the recovery from alcoholic fatty liver after the patient has stopped drinking is not known.

On the other hand, food is more palatable and easier to prepare when moderate amounts

of fat are allowed. In addition, the inclusion of fats increases calories. From 70 to 100 gm. of fat, or about 25 to 30 per cent of total calories, is recommended along with the use of MCT oil in salad dressings and spreads.

Steatorrhea is found in about 50 per cent of cirrhotic patients, whether they are alcoholics or not. This malabsorption of fat appears to have several causes, which vary among patients: cirrhosis-associated pancreatic insufficiency, decreased amounts of bile salts, administration of neomycin and, possibly, lymphatic hypertension.

Fluids and Sodium. One of the complications of advanced cirrhosis is the development of edema and *ascites* (the accumulation of fluid in the abdominal cavity). The ascites is due to (1) hypoalbuminemia, (2) high portal pressure from obstruction by the damaged liver and (3) renal sodium retention from secondary hyperaldosteronism. To reduce the fluid accumulation, sodium and fluids are restricted according to the individual's needs (1000 to 1500 ml. of fluid per day). Sodium is restricted to between 250 mg. and 1000 mg. per day (10 to 43 mEq.), depending upon the rate of diuresis and the tolerance of the patient. Diuretics are also given. Since potassium is also lost by the cirrhotic patient, a potassium-sparing diuretic is used.

Dried low-sodium milk products are recommended to help provide the necessary protein and calories in this diet, since eggs, meat and milk are relatively high in sodium. Therefore, when sodium is restricted these protein foods, as well as table salt, will have to be limited. (See sodium-restricted diets in Chapter 28.)

Patients should be weighed and their abdomens palpated daily to check for fluid retention. As diuresis progresses there will be weight loss, until the patient is "dry." Then there should be a steady, slow gain in weight as the nutritional status improves, if the patient was underweight.

Diet
FOODS TO INCLUDE DAILY

Milk: 1 pt. of milk; 2 oz. cream, 20%

Eggs: 2 poached, hard- or soft-cooked.

Meat, fish, poultry: 6 oz. of lean or moderately fat meat, fish or poultry.

Cheese: Pot or uncreamed cottage cheese, as desired.

Bread: 6 slices whole-grain or enriched white bread.

Cereals: 1 serving enriched or whole-grain cereal.

Cereal products: Macaroni, spaghetti, noodles and rice as alternates for potatoes.

Fats: 3 pats of butter or fortified margarine.

Vegetables: 4 to 5 servings, including 1 to 2 servings potato or equivalent, 1 serving green leafy or yellow vegetable, 1 to 2 servings other vegetables.

Fruits: Fresh and canned fruits as tolerated; at least 1 serving of citrus fruit daily; 2 servings of other fresh fruits or sweetened canned fruit.

Soups: Clear soups.

Desserts: Cake, pie, gelatin, sherbets, ice cream and ices as desired.

Beverages: Tea, coffee, Postum, carbonated beverages, fruit juices.

Sweets: Sugar, lactose, jelly, honey and syrup (at least 9 tblsp. daily).

FOODS OMITTED

Foods known to cause discomfort, salty foods if sodium is restricted, excessively fatty foods and alcohol.

Problems in Feeding. Great care should be taken to have the patient select food attractive to him whenever possible. This cannot be overemphasized, since food for these patients is the most important single therapeutic measure. The appetite is almost always poor, and much difficulty is frequently encountered in maintaining nutritional intake. The division of meals into six to eight small feedings per day is usually more inviting than three large meals. Patients tend to experience nausea at the end of the day, so the major part of the caloric intake should be given in the morning. The patient's understanding of the importance of the nutritional therapy helps him to ingest the food he selected. Guidance from the nurse or dietitian in assisting the person to make the right choices is helpful. Appetite tends to improve as the patient eats more. Establishing a regular eating pattern often alleviates the problem.

HEPATIC COMA (PORTAL-SYSTEMIC ENCEPHALOPATHY)

In patients having severely impaired liver function, particularly those having advanced cirrhosis or vascular shunts between the portal and caval venous systems, hepatic encephalopathy is a common occurrence. Signs of encephalopathy or impending hepatic coma include confusion, apathy, personality changes, muscle contractions and spasticity.

Hyperammonemia. An elevated level of serum ammonia is one cause of portal-systemic

encephalopathy but not the only one. Ammonia gains access to the general circulation, raising the blood ammonia and causing intoxication of the central nervous system. Following ingestion of protein or an episode of bleeding into the gastrointestinal tract, intestinal bacteria act on the protein to produce ammonia, which passes through the intestinal wall into the blood stream. The liver is unable to convert ammonia to non-toxic urea, and ammonia accumulates in the blood stream. The accumulation of blood in the gastrointestinal tract has the same effect as the ingestion of a high-protein meal because of the very high protein content of blood.

Neurotransmitters. Another approach in exploring the etiology of hepatic encephalopathy involves the neurotransmitters in the brain and those amino acids that are their precursors. Abnormally high levels of certain amino acids lead to abnormally high levels of neurotransmitters that produce encephalopathy.[4] If the protein given orally or by infusion to patients with impaired liver function could be low in the amino acids that are precursors of neurotransmitters, then encephalopathy could be avoided. When such amino acid mixtures were given intravenously to patients who had hepatic dysfunction, there was a reduction in encephalopathy.[5] However, the application of this principle to whole foods is unrealistic.

Nutritional Care

While generous quantities of protein are essential in the treatment of liver diseases, they must be avoided in impending hepatic coma. When signs and symptoms of ammonia intoxication are manifested (such as the "flapping" tremor of the hands when extended in front of the chest), the dietary intake of protein must be markedly reduced to about 30 gm. (0.5 gm. per kg. body weight) per day or even eliminated completely. With improvement, the dietary protein is gradually increased until a normal or high protein intake is tolerated, but the patient must always be watched for signs of impending coma, and serum ammonia should be monitored. Protein intake as low as 30 to 40 gm. daily (using protein of high biological value) will permit nitrogen balance in an otherwise adequate diet supplying adequate calories.

Ammonia Content of Foods. Some foods are

A diet of 30 to 40 grams of protein for the day consists of the following:

Meat, fish or poultry (2 to 3 oz.)	14–21 gm. of protein
Milk (8 oz.)	8 gm. of protein
Bread and cereals (3 servings)	6 gm. of protein
Vegetables (2 to 3 servings)	4 gm. of protein
Non-protein foods: enough to supply calories needed (sugar, jelly, fruit, oil, salt-free butter)	0
Vitamin and mineral supplements	0
Total	32–39 gm. of protein

See Chapter 30 for further discussion of low-protein diets.

more potent in causing hyperammonemia than others because they contain substantial amounts of pre-formed ammonia along with protein. Eliminating these foods could help patients with hyperammonemia. Table 24–2 gives the ammonia content of 64 foods as well as their nitrogen or protein content (nitrogen × 6.25 = protein). Those foods that raise the serum ammonia the most in cirrhotic patients are: several varieties of cheese, chicken, buttermilk, gelatin, hamburger, ham, potatoes, onions, peanut butter and salami.[10]

Other foods have an ammoniogenic effect because they contain large amounts of certain amino acids* that are deaminated in the patient's tissues and produce ammonia, which then enters the blood stream. One can speculate that, if amino acid precursors (alpha ketoacids) were given to the patient, perhaps they would combine with the excess ammonia to make amino acids and thus use up the excess ammonia.[3] These newly formed amino acids would also improve the nutritional status of the patient.

Other methods of reducing blood ammonia are the oral administration of neomycin to destroy gut flora and the use of lactulose, a nondigestible carbohydrate that induces diarrhea and so removes the intestinal contents. Lactulose may also reduce colonic absorption of ammonia by lowering the luminal pH.

*glycine, serine, threonine, glutamine, histidine, lysine and asparagine

Table 24–2   AMMONIA (NH₃) CONTENT OF FOODS*

FOOD	N (gm./100 gm. Wet Weight)	NH₃-N (% Total N)	FOOD	N (gm./100 gm. Wet Weight)	NH₃-N (% Total N)
American cheese[a]	3.712	2.19	Half milk/half cream	0.512	2.27
Apples	0.032	3.36	Ham[b]	2.704	0.58
Bacon	4.864	0.33	Hoap cheese[b]	3.520	1.75
Banana	0.176	0.00	Hot dog	2.000	0.32
Beer	0.048	1.62	Idaho potatoes[b]	0.416	2.33
Beer cheese[b]	3.760	2.44	Lemon juice (frozen)	0.080	2.90
Bread	0.320	0.94	Lettuce	0.144	0.55
Breakfast cereal (Rice Krispies)	0.944	0.00	Lima beans	1.344	0.21
			Margarine	0.096	21.96
Brewer's yeast	6.208	0.35	Mayonnaise	0.176	23.33
Broccoli	0.496	1.26	Milk	0.560	0.35
Brussels sprouts	0.512	2.15	Mushrooms	0.304	2.18
Buttermilk[a]	0.576	2.75	Mustard	0.352	1.00
Cabbage	0.208	0.82	Onions[b]	0.240	11.20
Carrots	0.176	0.81	Orange juice (frozen)	0.112	3.16
Catsup	0.320	11.00	Peaches	0.064	3.78
Cauliflower	0.302	1.41	Peanut butter[b]	4.448	1.10
Celery	0.144	0.00	Pears	0.112	2.67
Cheddar cheese[a]	4.000	2.76	Pecans	1.472	0.48
Chicken[b]	3.808	0.45	Pickle relish	0.080	10.84
Corn	0.560	0.25	Potato chips	0.848	2.83
Cucumbers	0.144	3.27	Radishes	0.160	2.77
Domestic blue cheese[a]	3.440	4.00	Raisins	0.400	2.37
Egg white	0.744	0.05	Rice	0.320	0.04
Egg yolk	2.560	0.16	Salami[a]	2.800	3.97
French dressing	0.096	14.00	Spanish olives	0.224	4.16
Grapefruit	0.800	2.07	Spinach	0.480	0.20
Grapes	0.208	4.20	Squash	0.192	4.28
Grape wine	0.016	11.20	String beans	0.160	0.46
Gelatin[a]	13.696	0.25	Sweet potatoes	0.288	0.61
Green peas	1.008	0.60	Tilsit cheese[b]	4.000	1.38
Grits (corn)	0.192	0.00	Tomatoes	0.176	2.09
Ground beef (hamburger)[a]	3.872	0.26	Turnip greens	0.400	0.73

[a] and [b]These foods are exceptionally high in NH₃-N or ammonia. Foods marked with *a* are higher than foods marked with *b*.

*From: Rudman, D., et al.: Ammonia content of food. Am. J. Clin. Nutr., 26:487, 1973.

If the patient remains neurologically clear after about a week on the low-protein diet, protein intake should be increased by 10 to 15 gm. intervals each week until a level of 1 gm. per kg. of body weight per day (65 to 85 gm.) or higher is reached. If encephalopathy develops, the dietary protein must again be reduced.

PHYSIOLOGY AND FUNCTION OF THE GALLBLADDER

The gallbladder, shaped like a pear with the large end pointing upward (Fig. 24–1), is attached to the right side of the undersurface of the liver. Variations in shape and position are not unusual. Diseases of the biliary tract and gallbladder are closely associated with liver disorders.

Function

The main task of the gallbladder is to store the bile secreted by the liver. The bile is composed of bile salts and acids, color pigments, lipids, mucin and water, and after secretion from the liver it is concentrated in the gallbladder. During the concentration process water and electrolytes are reabsorbed by the gallbladder mucosa. Other constituents, particularly the bile salts, and lipid substances such as cholesterol are not reabsorbed. They become highly concentrated in the gallbladder bile. Approximately one quart of bile is produced daily.

Bile assists in the digestion and absorption of fats and in the absorption of fat-soluble vitamins A, D, E and K and the minerals iron and calcium. It is necessary for the formation of micelles, the form in which fat, cholesterol and

fat-soluble vitamins are absorbed. In addition it has a slightly laxative action and is believed to retard fermentation.

The rate of secretion of bile is directly related to the type of food digested. Fatty foods excite the secretory activity of the gallbladder. A high percentage of the bile salts that pass into the intestines is reabsorbed in the terminal ileum, enters the portal vein and returns to the liver to be secreted again into bile. This *enterohepatic circulation* of bile salts maintains the bile salt pool. The bile is a carrier of waste products such as bile pigments, which are finally excreted with the feces and account for the feces' normal brown color.

The gallbladder is ordinarily full and relaxed between meals, with the sphincter of Oddi closed. During the course of digestion, food fat or fatty acids reach the duodenum and stimulate the production of the hormone *cholecystokinin* in the intestinal mucosa. When brought to the gallbladder by the blood stream, this hormone causes the gallbladder to contract and the sphincter of Oddi to relax, thus releasing the concentrated bile into the duodenum via the common duct. (See Fig. 24–4.)

DISEASES OF THE GALLBLADDER

Women are victims of gallbladder disease more frequently than men are. It is a disease that occurs most often in obese women over 40 years of age. The common diseases of the biliary tract are biliary dyskinesia, cholecystitis (acute and chronic) and gallstones.

BILIARY DYSKINESIA

Biliary dyskinesia produces vague abdominal complaints. The sphincter of Oddi, which controls the opening and closing of the bile duct into the duodenum, does not open properly and can go into spasm. Bile then builds up in the gallbladder, causing increased pressure. This spasm of the sphincter of Oddi can exist even after cholecystectomy.

CHOLECYSTITIS

Inflammation of the gallbladder is known as *cholecystitis*. Cholecystitis due to gallbladder infection is fairly common. Bacteria may stray from any part of the body, such as the tonsils, teeth, sinuses or even the appendix, and travel via the blood stream to the gallbladder. Other elements influencing abnormal functioning include overweight, preg-

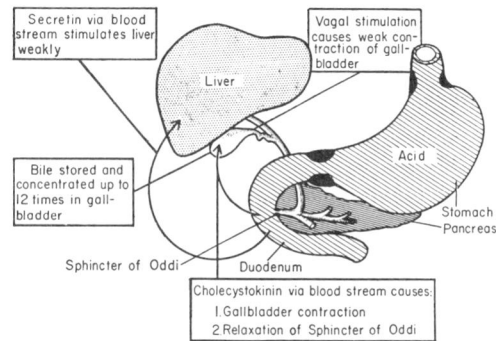

Figure 24–4 Mechanisms of liver secretions and gallbladder emptying. (From: Guyton, A. C.: Textbook of Medical Physiology. 5th ed. Philadelphia, W. B. Saunders Company, 1976.)

nancy, constipation, constricting clothes, improper diet and digestive upsets. The walls of the gallbladder become red and swollen, and sometimes pus collects, which causes distention. During such episodes, the patient is aware of pain in the region of the gallbladder, accompanied by nausea, vomiting, flatulence and soreness in the upper right side of the abdomen. Jaundice may appear.

Jaundice, a symptom of various diseases of the biliary tract, is a discoloration of tissues and body fluids by bile pigment. Much of the pigment that gives the bile its greenish color is derived from the breakdown of red corpuscles. Should the biliary tract become obstructed by a stone or by inflammation so that bile is no longer able to reach the intestine, the coloring matter undergoes changes and returns to the circulation as bilirubin. This overflow of bile into the general circulation as bilirubin causes the yellow pigmentation of the skin and discoloration of the eyes that are typical of jaundice. Jaundice may be either *obstructive*, the result of a complete or partial obstruction caused by stones, tumor or inflammation within the common bile duct or duodenum (Fig. 24–1), or *hepatocellular*, which means it is caused by a liver disease or injury.

GALLSTONES

The formation of gallstones without infection of the gallbladder is called *cholelithiasis*. *Choledocholithiasis* develops when stones slip into the common bile duct, producing obstruction and cramps. The existence of stones may cause no symptoms and the patient may be unaware of their presence until this happens. In choledocholithiasis the passage of bile into the duodenum is interrupted

and jaundice develops. Absorption of fat and fat-soluble vitamins is impaired, and stools become light-colored because they contain no bile pigments. If not corrected, the backup of bile can cause liver damage, biliary cirrhosis or pancreatitis. In most cases, however, the stones remain stationary and the symptoms are similar to chronic inflammation. If the gallbladder and stones are removed by surgery, the majority of patients are cured completely.

Gallstones are composed of *cholesterol* crystals or of bile salt and pigment, or both. Most stones are found to contain a high percentage of cholesterol. Therefore, the stones are probably caused by stagnation of the bile, with the formation of calculi, a change in the colloidal state of the bile and an increase in the percentage of cholesterol in the bile. However, there is no evidence to suggest that a low-cholesterol diet will lower bile cholesterol.

Nutritional Care

Because fats stimulate gallbladder secretion and sphincter of Oddi action, they should be avoided by the patient with a gallbladder problem. The patient learns through experience that he is more comfortable if he eats plain, simple foods and avoids rich pastries, nuts and chocolate and fatty, fried and gas-forming foods. Condiments and highly seasoned foods may cause distention and increase peristalsis, which ultimately results in irritation to the gallbladder. However, *the disturbance varies with the individual patient* and the dietary management should be individualized.

Acute Attack. An acute attack almost always occurs in connection with an obstruction. When it does occur, the gallbladder should be kept as inactive as possible. All visible fat in the diet is omitted. An all-liquid diet of 2 to 3 liters per day and parenteral supplementation may be required. The protein (30 to 40 gm.) is supplied by skim milk, and carbohydrate (200 to 300 gm.) is obtained from sweetened fruit juices, fruit nectars and gelatin. As soon as tolerated, limited amounts of fat and solid food are added.

The patient is advised to adhere to a low-fat (about 50 gm. of fat) diet until it is known whether surgical removal of the gallbladder is indicated. A combination of foods to provide 50 gm. of fat is as follows:

Lean meat, fish or poultry (3 oz.)	15 gm. of fat
Egg (1)	5 gm. of fat
Butter, margarine or oil (2 tblsp.)	30 gm. of fat
Total	50 gm. of fat

Skim milk, low-fat cottage cheese, cereals, breads, vegetables, fruits, ices, jello and puddings made with skim milk are used. Sweets are taken in amounts that will supply adequate calories. A regimen free of fat would restrict the protein foods to skim milk, cream-free cottage cheese and egg whites only, with no meat, margarine or butter. No fat of any kind would be allowed in cooking or otherwise added to food.

Chronic Condition. For the dietary treatment of patients with chronic cholecystitis it is desirable to keep the diet *low in fat* (about 25 per cent of total calories). Too strict limitation, however, is undesirable, since fat in the intestines is important for some gallbladder drainage of the biliary tract. Many patients with cholecystitis or gallstones are overweight. Attention should be given to weight reduction.

The *protein* allowance is kept at the normal requirement and the carbohydrate allowance is normal, decreased or increased to maintain the patient's weight at the desired level. Increasing the amount of *carbohydrate* serves as a therapeutic measure in cases complicated by jaundice.

Individuals differ considerably as to the foods that are "gas-forming" or cause them discomfort. It is best to discuss this with the patient, who can then eliminate those foods that bother him. A survey of patients hospitalized with gallbladder disease failed to show any greater incidence of specific food intolerances than among patients without gastrointestinal disorders.[6]

The Low-fat Diet. The low-fat diet contains approximately 80 gm. of protein, 50 gm. of fats, 275 gm. of carbohydrates and 1870 kcalories. If the patient is overweight, calories can be reduced by eliminating sweets such as jelly, sugar and gelatin. If further reduction of fat is indicated, butter and margarine are eliminated.

FOODS LIMITED
Milk, skim milk: 2 cups (1 pt.) daily.
Eggs: 1 poached, hard- or soft-cooked, daily.
Meats, fish or poultry: 3 oz. of meat, fish or poultry, lean and free from all visible fat and from skin of chicken, daily.
Fats: 2 pats (4 level tsp.) of butter, fortified margarine or oil daily.
FOODS INCLUDED
Cheese: Pot cheese or uncreamed cottage cheese.
Breads: Whole-grain or enriched white preferred.
Cereals: Whole-grain preferred, except the very coarse varieties.

Cereal products: Macaroni, spaghetti, noodles, rice.

Vegetables: As tolerated (to include 1 serving green leafy or yellow vegetable daily).

Fruits: As tolerated (to include at least 1 serving citrus fruit daily). Fruit juices.

Soups: Clear soups with fat removed or soups made with skim milk.

Desserts: Angel food cake, gelatin desserts with fruits as tolerated, sherbets and ices.

Beverages: Tea, coffee, Postum, carbonated beverages.

Sweets: Sugar, jelly, honey, hard candy and syrup.

FOODS OMITTED

Meats, fish or poultry: Fat of meat, skin of chicken, bacon, scrapple, cold cuts, sausages, fatty fish (mackerel), duck, goose, fish canned in oil.

Fats: All fat except allowed butter or fortified margarine and oil.

Desserts: Except those included.

Miscellaneous: Chocolate, peanut butter, cream, nuts, pastries, fried foods, highly seasoned foods, pickled foods and pickles, rich gravies and cream sauces.

VITAMIN SUPPLEMENTATION. Because fat and therefore the fat-soluble vitamins are poorly absorbed, administration of water-soluble forms of vitamins A, D, E and K may be necessary. Vitamin K plays an important role in controlling bleeding in individuals afflicted with certain types of jaundice. When given parenterally or orally with bile salts, vitamin K can be transported to the liver where it helps to produce prothrombin, which is necessary for blood clotting.

Postoperative Cholecystectomy Diet. If the patient has the gallbladder removed surgically, it is still advisable to continue the low-fat diet regimen for several months following the operation to permit the inflammation to subside. When the gallbladder is removed, the bile is stored in the large common duct connecting the liver and small intestine. The tube stretches to perform its new function.

Chenodeoxycholic Acid and Lecithin. These two substances are being used in the conservative management of cholelithiasis. Chenodeoxycholic acid (CDCA), a normal constituent of human bile, will dissolve gallstones in most patients when given in a daily dose, but this therapy may be necessary for 6 to 30 months. It appears the CDCA reduces hepatic cholesterol synthesis and thus the biliary concentration of cholesterol. There are mild side effects such as abdominal discomfort and diarrhea that can be controlled by modification of dosage but, more important, the long-term effects of CDCA on hepatic function are not known.[2]

Lecithin, another natural bile component, also dissolves gallstones and it too is being used with good results.

PHYSIOLOGY AND FUNCTION OF THE PANCREAS

The pancreas is located deep in the upper abdomen, behind the stomach (Fig. 24–1). Some of its cells manufacture insulin (endocrine function) and others secrete powerful enzymes that aid in the digestion of protein, fats and carbohydrates in the intestine (exocrine function). This *exocrine* function, known to be under the control of gastrointestinal hormones (see Table 6–1), may also be controlled by the endocrine function of the pancreas.[9] The duct leading from the pancreas joins a common tube through which both bile and pancreatic juices drain into the duodenum.

PANCREATITIS

Pancreatitis is an inflammation of the pancreas characterized by edema, cellular exudate and fat necrosis. It can be mild and self-limiting or severe, with necrosis of pancreatic tissue, and can be acute or chronic, with pancreatic destruction so extensive that exocrine or endocrine pancreatic function is lost and steatorrhea or diabetes results.

The symptoms of pancreatitis can range from those of a mild upset stomach to severe abdominal pain, edema and shock, and death may result.

Etiology and Pathogenesis

The precise mechanisms that cause pancreatitis and pancreatic destruction are unknown, but the following are associated with and perhaps are causes of pancreatitis: chronic alcoholism, biliary tract disease, ingestion of certain drugs, trauma and hypercalcemia.

One theory states that an obstruction to the flow of pancreatic juice develops, either from a malfunctioning sphincter of Oddi, a stone in the common duct or a protein plug in a pancreatic ductule. The pancreatic juices then back up into the pancreas. Somehow, these pancreatic enzymes become activated, possibly by backed-up bile, and they move out of the ductules and into the pancreatic parenchyma, where they begin to digest the organ itself. In severe cases the enzymes move out of the

Table 24–3   SOME TESTS OF PANCREATIC
FUNCTION

TEST	SIGNIFICANCE
Secretin Stimulation Test	Measures pancreatic secretion, particularly bicarbonate, in response to secretin stimulation
Glucose Tolerance Test	Assesses endocrine function of pancreas by measuring insulin response to a glucose load
72-Hour Stool Fat Test	Assesses exocrine function of pancreas by measuring fat absorption, which reflects pancreatic lipase secretion

pancreas and begin to digest surrounding fat tissue. When this happens, serum calcium falls to a dangerously low level, which is a bad prognostic sign. It may be that serum calcium falls because of "soap" formation by the calcium and the fatty acids created by fat necrosis. Serum amylase and lipase, two pancreatic enzymes, move from the inflamed pancreas into the lymphatic system and the blood stream, leading to elevated serum amylase and lipase levels, which are characteristic of pancreatic disease.

A common cause of pancreatitis is alcoholism. Presumably alcohol causes duodenitis and edema of the papilla of Vater, where the common bile duct opens into the duodenum. This condition obstructs pancreatic and bile flow, which back up into the pancreas. The backed-up bile appears to activate the pancreatic enzymes so that they begin their destruction. It is also possible that alcohol has a direct cytotoxic effect on the pancreas by causing excessive precipitation of protein in the pancreatic ductules, which blocks the release of pancreatic juice.

Some tests for monitoring pancreatic function are given in Table 24–3.

Nutritional Care

The liberation and activation of the potent pancreatic digestive enzymes are brought about by a strong stimulus such as food or alcohol. In addition, fatty foods excite the secretory activity of bile. Thus, the dietary treatment of pancreatitis must be adjusted to consist of foods that will not stimulate these systems into action.

During severe acute attacks of pancreatitis, all oral feeding is withheld, and a nasogastric tube frequently is used to remove all gastric acid. After 24 to 48 hours the patient may be given a clear liquid diet to see how he tolerates it. One of the biggest mistakes made in treating these patients is to start them eating again too soon. A nutritious clear liquid diet can be made by giving the patient a defined formula diet consisting of amino acids, glucose and a small amount of fat. This diet is "predigested" and will not stimulate pancreatic secretions. Total parenteral nutrition may be necessary in prolonged severe pancreatitis. Chapter 35 discusses these feedings in greater detail.

In less severe attacks, easily digested, non-stimulating foods that are very low in fat (25 to 30 gm.), with increased carbohydrate and protein, should be given. Foods are better tolerated if divided into six small meals rather than the usual three. The low-fat diet described on page 514 can be used.

Chronic pancreatitis ensues when inflammation fails to subside or recurs at intervals. The patient almost always presents feeding problems because food provokes nausea and vomiting, which make it difficult to maintain good nutritional status. To complicate matters, the pancreas does not secrete a sufficient amount of enzymes, and maldigestion and malabsorption result. Steatorrhea is a common occurrence. *Pancreatin,* a pancreatic enzyme replacement, may be administered orally after each meal to facilitate digestion of carbohydrate, protein and fats. Since pancreatic bicarbonate secretion will frequently be defective, antacids should also be given to maintain the optimum pH level for enzyme activity. Effort should be made to cater to the patient's tolerances and preferences insofar as the diet prescription permits. In the interval phase, the low-fat diet may be used. Alcohol is prohibited, since it acts as an intestinal irritant and encourages recurrences.

In chronic cases with extensive pancreatic destruction, the insulin-secreting capacity of the pancreas decreases and glucose intolerance develops. Treatment with insulin and nutritional care similar to that used for a patient with diabetes mellitus is then required. (See Chapter 25.)

Malabsorption of vitamin B_{12} has been observed in some patients with pancreatic insufficiency, so for these patients vitamin B_{12} status should be assessed, and the vitamin should be given parenterally if needed.

ZOLLINGER-ELLISON SYNDROME

A gastrin-secreting tumor or gastrinoma of the pancreas is the cause of this disease. The high serum levels of gastrin cause hypersecretion of gastric acid and the development of duodenal ulcers in 95 per cent of cases. The nutritional care is the same as that for a duodenal ulcer (Chapter 22); however, the preferred treatment is surgical removal of the tumor.

PROBLEMS AND SUGGESTED TOPICS FOR DISCUSSION

1. List the various functions of the liver and then determine the relationship of each function to the metabolism of food.
2. Take a dietary history of a patient with cirrhosis of the liver. Identify the areas of his diet that need improving. How will the patient implement the changes?
3. Under what conditions does hepatic coma appear? Why is a low-protein diet used?
4. Adjust the diet in problem 2 to limit sodium to 250 mg. When would such a diet be required in cirrhosis of the liver?
5. Plan a diet containing 30 gm. protein for a patient with hepatic coma. The patient is a 40 year old male requiring 2600 kcal. Why is it important to maintain adequate calorie intake?
6. Obtain the dietary history of a patient with gallbladder disease. What adjustments need to be made to restrict the diet to 40 gm. of fat? Adjust the protein and carbohydrate to meet the individual's caloric needs. Why does a patient with gallbladder disease experience pain on the ingestion of fat?
7. What is the rationale for using a high-protein diet in treating viral hepatitis?
8. What are the principles of diet for chronic pancreatitis? Plan a diet and meal pattern for a patient with chronic pancreatitis who is 50 years old and requires 2300 kcal.
9. Explain why a chemically defined diet or "predigested diet" is useful in the nutritional care of a patient with pancreatitis.

CITED REFERENCES

1. Baraona, E., and Lindenbaum, J.: Metabolic effects of alcohol on the intestine. In: Lieber, C. S. (ed.): Metabolic Aspects of Alcoholism. Lancaster, England, MTP Press Ltd., 1977, p. 107.
2. Carey, M. C.: Editorial: Cheno and urso: What the goose and the bear have in common. N. Engl. J. Med., *293*:1255, 1975.
3. Close, J. H.: The use of amino acid precursors in nitrogen-accumulation diseases. N. Engl. J. Med., *290*:663, 1974.
4. Fischer, J. E., and Baldessarini, R. J.: False neurotransmitters and hepatic failure. Lancet, *2*:75, 1971.
5. Fisher, J. E., et al.: The effect of normalization of plasma amino acids on hepatic encephalopathy in man. Surgery, *80*:77, 1976.
6. Koch, J. F., and Donaldson, R. M.: A survey of food intolerances of hospitalized patients. N. Engl. J. Med., *271*:657, 1964.
7. Lieber, C. S.: The prolonged cocktail hour and liver disease. JAMA, *185*:419, 1963.
8. Lieber, C. S., and DeCarli, L. M.: Metabolic effects of alcohol on the liver. In: Lieber, C. S. (ed.): Metabolic Aspects of Alcoholism. Lancaster, England, MTP Press Ltd., 1977, p. 45.
9. Malaisse-Lagae, F., et al.: Exocrine pancreas: Evidence for topographic partition of secretory function. Science, *190*:795, 1975.
10. Rudman, D., et al.: Ammonia content of food. Am. J. Clin. Nutr., *26*:487, 1973.

ADDITIONAL REFERENCES

Baraona, E., et al.: Alcoholic hepatomegaly: Accumulation of protein in the liver. Science, *190*:794, 1975.

Council report on dietary fat regulation. Nutr. Rev., *21*:36, 1963.

Dreiling, D. A.: New hypotheses on pancreatitis. Warren-Teed G. I. Tract, *5*(4):4, 1975. (Published by Warren-Teed Pharmaceuticals, Inc., Columbus, OH)

Fischer, J. E.: Amino acid infusion in hepatic encephalopathy. Dietetic Currents, *3*(2), 1976. (Published by Ross Laboratories, Columbus, OH)

Guyton, A. C.: Textbook of Medical Physiology, 5th ed. Philadelphia, W. B. Saunders Company, 1976.

Hepner, G. W., Roginsky, M., and Moo, H. F.: Abnormal vitamin D metabolism in patients with cirrhosis. Am. J. Dig. Dis., *21*:527, 1976.

Herbert, V., Zalusky, R., and Davidson, C. S.: Correlation of folate deficiency with alcoholism and associated macrocytosis, anemia, and liver disease. Ann. Intern. Med., *58*:977, 1963.

Kater, R. M. H., et al.: Relationship of serum tocopherol to beta-lipoprotein concentrations in liver diseases. Am. J. Clin. Nutr., *23*:913, 1970.

Leevy, C. M., Thompson, A., and Baker, H.: Vitamins and liver injury. Am. J. Clin. Nutr., *23*:493, 1970.

Maddrey, W. C., et al.: Effects of keto analogues of essential amino acids in portal-systemic encephalopathy. Gastroenterology, *71*:190, 1976.

Soeters, P. B., and Fischer, J. E.: Insulin, glucagon, amino acid imbalance and hepatic encephalopathy. Lancet, *2*:880, 1976.

Symposium on nutrition and liver injury, Pts. I and II. Am. J. Clin. Nutr., *23*:445–507; 579–656, 1970.

Toskes, P. P., et al.: Vitamin B_{12} malabsorption in chronic pancreatic insufficiency. N. Engl. J. Med., *284*:627, 1971.

Tuzhilin, S. A., et al.: The treatment of patients with gallstones by lecithin. Am. J. Gastroenterol, *65*:231, 1976.

Nutrition and Alcoholism

Alcohol, gastritis, and nutrient absorption. Nutr. Rev., *35*:8, 1977.

Davidson, C. S.: Cirrhosis in alcoholics: Protein nutrition and hepatic coma. JAMA, *160*:390, 1956.

Iber, F. L.: In alcoholism the liver sets the pace. Nutr. Today, *6*:2, 1971.

Isselbacher, K. J.: Metabolic and hepatic effects of alcohol. N. Engl. J. Med., *296*:612, 1977.

Lieber, C. S.: The metabolism of alcohol. Sci. Am., *234*:25, 1976.

Williamson, D., and Turl, M.: Nutrition in the treatment of the alcoholic. Dietetic Currents, *2*(1), 1975. (Published by Ross Laboratories, Columbus, OH)

UNIT SEVEN

DISEASES OF METABOLISM AND THE ENDOCRINE GLANDS

Chapter 25

NUTRITIONAL CARE FOR PATIENTS WITH DISORDERS OF THE ENDOCRINE PANCREAS: DIABETES MELLITUS AND HYPOGLYCEMIA

DIABETES MELLITUS

Diabetes mellitus is generally considered to be an inborn error of metabolism in which the body is unable to utilize sugars completely. Manifestations may appear in youth, referred to as *juvenile-onset* type (ketosis-prone), or in later life, as *maturity-onset* type (ketosis-resistant). The main differences between these two types of diabetes are that juvenile-onset diabetes begins abruptly, manifests severe symptoms immediately and requires insulin to control, while the maturity-onset type develops insidiously, has milder symptoms and can frequently be controlled by diet alone. In some instances, diabetic clinical manifestations may remain latent even though the inherent pattern can be demonstrated by laboratory methods. The clinical syndrome is characterized by (1) an impaired ability to metabolize carbohydrates, (2) an increased concentration of glucose in the circulating blood (hyperglycemia) and (3) the excretion of varying amounts of glucose in the urine (glycosuria). The etiological development of diabetes mellitus is unknown, but it is fairly well established that the entire endocrine system is involved, particularly the pancreas. (See Figure 25–1.)

Hormonal Relationships. The beta cells in the islands of Langerhans of the pancreas secrete the hormone *insulin,* and the adjacent alpha cells secrete the hormone *glucagon.* Both are important in controlling the blood glucose level. These two hormones have opposite effects on blood sugar concentration: Insulin lowers and glucagon raises blood glucose. In diabetes mellitus, insulin is absent, deficient or ineffective, and this partially accounts for the metabolic derangement. However, glucagon is present in excessive amounts in diabetes and may account partially for the hyperglycemia of the disease. Insufficient insulin results in decreased removal of glucose from the blood, and excess glucagon causes the liver to release excess glucose into the blood stream. However, it has been documented that suppression of insulin does not result in hyperglycemia if glucagon is also suppressed. Conversely, hyperglucagonemia does not result in hyperglycemia if

518

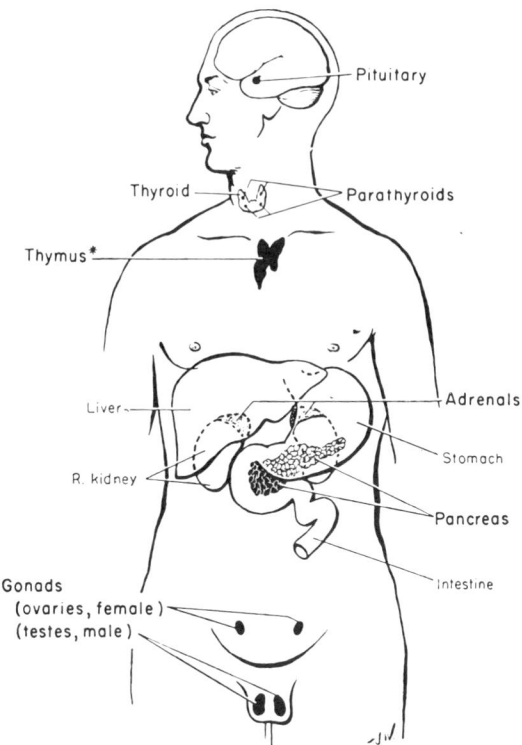

Figure 25–1   Location of principal endocrine glands. *The thymus is present only up to puberty. (From: Brooks: Basic Facts of General Chemistry. Philadelphia, W. B. Saunders Company, 1956.)

insulin is also present in sufficient amounts.[18] Insulin and glucagon exist in a delicate balance: High concentrations of insulin should stimulate glucagon release, and low concentrations should suppress glucagon release. In diabetes the coordination of insulin and glucagon secretion is lacking, and glucagon levels become high in relation to insulin levels (I:G ratio); thus, hyperglycemia increases.[22] See page 46 for further discussion of insulin and glucagon.

In the early 70's another hormone, *somatostatin,* attracted the interest of diabetologists. Among other activities, this hormone inhibits the release of both insulin and glucagon in humans. It also inhibits the release of growth hormone, increased levels of which have been seen in uncontrolled diabetes and which is suspected in the development of diabetic microangiopathy.[10, 11]

Etiology

Any serious disturbance of the pancreas that interferes with the production and balance of insulin and glucagon predisposes a person to

have clinical manifestations of diabetes. There are several factors to consider.

Genetic Factor. Heredity is involved in the development of diabetes or of its metabolic variations that lead to vascular complications, but its role is poorly understood. Although since the work of Pincus and White in 1933 the mode of transmission has been thought to be Mendelian autosomal recessive, subsequent genetic studies have brought this into question. It is now supposed that the diabetic predisposition is due to a number of genetic characteristics (upon which environment has an influence) that result in the final clinical presentation. The presentation may be chemical diabetes without symptoms of overt diabetes. It has also been postulated that there is a genetic difference between childhood diabetes and that which develops in an adult.[19]

Viral Factor. Because it is known that some viruses replicate in the pancreas, viral infection is being studied as a possible factor in the etiology of diabetes. Several viruses, including mumps, hepatitis, rubella, coxsackie and influenza are being investigated. There is strong epidemiological evidence to suggest a connection with juvenile-onset or insulin-dependent diabetes. It is thought that the susceptibility to pancreatic damage (and thus deficient insulin production) resulting from viral infection has a genetic link.[12]

Obesity. The onset of diabetes in adulthood is usually associated with overweight. With every 20 per cent increase in body weight, the chance of becoming diabetic doubles. Hyperinsulinism is also seen, and it is thought that insulin resistance develops from an increase in adipose tissue mass. It has been reported[3] that the insulin receptor located on the surface of the adipose cell in the obese person is different from the receptor in the non-obese person. The insulin is not able to attach to the receptor in the obese person and so cannot exert its effect. This may account for the hyperinsulinism and increased incidence of diabetes in the obese.

Stress. The ramifications of stress in the development of diabetes are poorly understood. Infectious diseases such as influenza, pneumonia and scarlet fever, accidents or trauma or the physiological stress of pregnancy may precipitate symptoms of diabetes. These situations decrease glucose tolerance in the diabetic. Diseases of the liver, gallbladder, thyroid, pituitary and pancreas are frequently associated with diabetes. Mental stress may aggravate the disease by causing the release of catecholamines, which decrease glucose toler-

ance and promote mobilization of fatty acids and possible ketoacidosis.

Trace Minerals. It has been observed that diabetics excrete increased amounts of *zinc* in their urine and that their plasma leukocyte and erythrocyte zinc levels are reduced. Glucose tolerance is lowered in zinc-deficient rats, and zinc has been shown to enhance the action of insulin in promoting uptake of glucose by adipose tissue.[16] It is not known whether reduced zinc levels are a causative factor in diabetes development or a consequence of the metabolic defect.

Another trace element possibly involved in diabetes mellitus and glucose intolerance is *chromium.* In fact, a sensitive indicator of chromium deficiency in rats is glucose intolerance. A "glucose tolerance factor" has been identified as a natural form of chromium. This factor seems to potentiate the action of insulin, and long-term oral supplementation with chromium was found to improve glucose tolerance in some diabetic persons, probably in those with a chronic low-chromium state.[8, 9]

Progression of the Disease

Diabetes can be thought of as beginning at conception with a genetic tendency. The time between conception and the development of overt diabetes varies from months to years, depending upon environmental factors. The progression of the disease is shown in Table 25-1.

Incidence. The reported incidence of diabetes is increasing by about 6 per cent per year.[5] It is impossible to evaluate the reason, although

greater food consumption, reduction in physical exercise, greater incidence of obesity, improved methods of diagnosis, increased longevity, reproduction by known diabetics and concentrated efforts of the medical profession to seek out diabetic individuals undoubtedly contribute. The American Diabetes Association has established that one out of four Americans may be a carrier of diabetes. It is diagnosed in all ages. One in 2500 juveniles under age 15 has overt diabetes. The younger the individual in whom clinical symptoms appear, the more serious the condition. (Diabetes in children is discussed in Chapter 38.) In about two thirds of diabetics the condition manifests itself after 40 years of age.

The lack of clinical symptoms is indicated dramatically by the fact that 78 per cent of the selectees in World War II who were found to have diabetes did not know they had it. Approximately one person in twenty has diabetes or is a potential diabetic. According to various estimates the prevalence of diabetes is 5 per cent of the population.

Diagnostic Tests. To make a definite diagnosis of diabetes mellitus certain laboratory tests are used.

URINE. The urine is tested for total volume, specific gravity, glucose and fatty acids. Although glucose in the urine does not necessarily mean diabetes mellitus, with the exception of mere traces it may be indicative of the disease. Tests are available in which the concentration of glucose in the urine is read colorimetrically: (1) by indicator paper (Tes-Tape), (2) by paper stick (Clinistix) or (3) by adding a tablet to urine (Clinitest).

Table 25–1 METABOLIC AND VASCULAR CHANGES IN VARIOUS STAGES OF DIABETES*

| DIABETIC STAGE | CARBOHYDRATE TOLERANCE | | | INSULIN-LIKE ACTIVITY AND SYNALBUMIN ANTAGONIST[a] | VASCULAR CHANGES[b] |
	FASTING BLOOD SUGAR	GLUCOSE TOLERANCE	CORTISONE-GLUCOSE TOLERANCE		
Prediabetes	Normal	Normal	Normal	May be increased	+
Subclinical	Normal	Normal (abnormal during pregnancy, infection, emotional stress, and physical trauma)	Abnormal	Increased	+
Latent	Normal or increased	Abnormal	Test not necessary	Increased	+ +
Overt	Increased	Test not necessary	Test not necessary	Increased	+ + +

*From: Waife, S. O. (ed.): Diabetes Mellitus, 7th ed. Indianapolis, Lilly Research Laboratories, Eli Lilly & Company, 1970, p. 9.

[a]Test used for screening large numbers of people.

[b]+ = degree of vascular change present.

Ketonuria, the presence of fatty acids (ketone bodies) in the urine, indicates the incomplete oxidation of fats. This is considered a serious condition and requires immediate adjustment of diet and insulin.

BLOOD. Fasting blood sugar (FBS) is elevated in all but the mildest cases of diabetes; the normal blood glucose level is 70 to 100 mg. per 100 ml. The oral *glucose tolerance test* indicates the ability of the patient to utilize a specific amount of glucose calculated at the rate of 1 gm. per kg. of body weight. (Glucose flavored with lemon, or Glucola is commonly used.)

A blood sugar estimate is made before the glucose preparation is served and again ½ hour, 1 hour, 2 hours, and 3 hours after the glucose preparation has been taken. Figure 25–2 illustrates the difference in the glucose tolerance curves of a normal person (*A*) and two diabetics (*B, C*). The intravenous glucose tolerance test, the insulin tolerance test, the cortisone- and prednisone-glucose tolerance tests and the oral and intravenous tolbutamide tolerance tests are also used in the diagnosis of diabetes.

Symptoms. When symptoms are present, they usually include *increased thirst (polydipsia), increased urination (polyuria), increased appetite (polyphagia),* failing strength and loss of weight. Pruritus vulvae, skin infection or irritation and visual disturbances are frequently present. Excessive urinary output and the failure to balance it by fluid intake causes dehydration and electrolyte imbalance. Inability of tissues to heal and degenerative changes occur, especially in advanced cases. Acidosis or ketosis is a symptom of the accumulation of fatty acids in the blood. The failing strength and loss of weight result from starvation, because the body is unable to utilize food. Glycosuria is not necessarily diagnostic of diabetes mellitus, because it may have another cause, such as emotional upset, overeating, pregnancy, hyperthyroidism or malfunction of the kidneys.

There are four other carbohydrates that may appear in the urine without creating any suspicion of the disease: pentose, galactose, fructose and lactose. Glucose is the specific sign in the urine of the diabetic.

Physiological Disturbances. In order to understand the controls for maintaining normal blood glucose levels and the impairment of these controls in diabetes, intermediary metabolism should be reviewed (Chapter 6) as well as carbohydrate, lipid and protein metabolism (Chapters 3, 4 and 5).

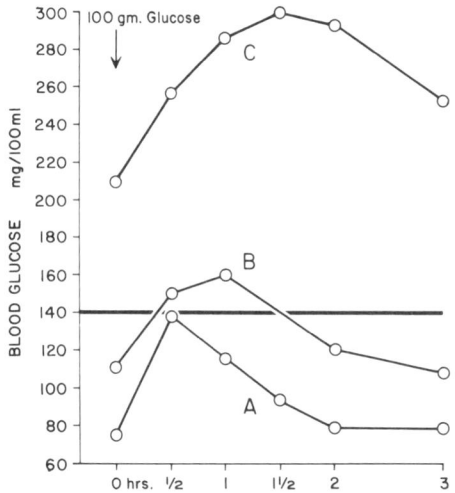

Figure 25–2 Glucose tolerance curves. *A* depicts a normal glycemic response of an adult to the oral administration of 100 gm. of glucose. The rise is rapid but the peak does not exceed 150 mg./100 ml., and the mild degree of hyperglycemia has subsided by 1½ hours. In *B* the fasting blood glucose value is slightly above normal but the peak at 1 hour exceeds 140 and the 2-hour value exceeds the upper border of normal (100 mg./100 ml.), as seen in mild diabetes. *C* depicts the fasting hyperglycemia with values far exceeding 140 mg. at 1½, 2 and 3 hours, as seen in uncontrolled diabetes, which is identifiable by finding glycosuria and a hyperglycemia *without resorting to a glucose tolerance test.* Glycosuria usually occurs when the blood sugar level is maintained for varying periods above 140 mg./ml., as indicated by the heavy black line. (From: Duncan, G. G. (ed.): Diseases of Metabolism, 5th ed. Philadelphia, W. B. Saunders Co., 1964.)

Glucose from dietary carbohydrate, protein and fat and from liver glycogen (glycogenolysis) maintains blood glucose levels. Normally glucose combines with a carrier substance in the cell membrane and is transported to the inside of the membrane, where it is released to the interior of the cell in most tissues of the body. An exception to this is the brain, in which glucose transport is more dependent on diffusion through the blood-brain barrier than through the cell membrane. Insulin affects the rate of glucose movement through the membrane of cells.

Glucose is handled normally by the body in different ways: (1) it may be utilized for energy at once (cell oxidation), (2) it may be converted to glycogen for storage in the liver (glycogenesis), (3) it may be converted to fat for storage in adipose tissue (lipogenesis) or (4) it may be converted to muscle glycogen (see Chapter 3). Non-diabetics dispose of the glucose in these ways as rapidly as it enters the blood stream. This rapid disposition prevents

the concentration of blood glucose from rising above the threshold established by the kidneys. The diabetic, however, with little or no insulin activity, has lost the ability to perform these functions completely, because the glucose cannot cross the cell membrane and be oxidized through the glycolytic pathway in the cell to supply energy, and it cannot be converted or stored. Hyperglycemia and glycosuria follow.

The normal renal threshold for glucose averages 160 to 180 mg. per 100 ml. of blood. The non-diabetic may, however, have a normally low threshold. If so, glucose may be excreted from the kidneys, but this does not mean that he has diabetes. Whether the person has a low or high renal threshold is determined by the glucose tolerance test.

Fatty acid synthesis decreases and fatty oxidation increases in diabetes. When the glycogen stores are depleted, fatty acids are used for energy through acetyl-CoA and the citric acid cycle. When the acetyl-CoA cannot be used fast enough it is converted into the ketone bodies beta-hydroxybutyric acid and acetoacetic acid, which accumulate rapidly in the blood. They combine with basic ions and are excreted in the urine. Acetone is excreted by the lungs and gives a "fruity" odor to the breath. Acidosis develops when the basic ions are depleted; diabetic coma then ensues and, if not treated, death occurs.

In the absence of insulin, free fatty acids, triglycerides, cholesterol and phospholipids increase in the blood. These high concentrations have been suggested as factors in the development of arteriosclerosis in people with diabetes.

Protein synthesis is affected by insulin, since it promotes the transport of amino acids through the cell membrane in much the same carrier transport system that transports glucose. Normally the total quantity of protein stored in the tissues of the body is increased by insulin.

In diabetes there is an increase in protein breakdown. Amino acids are deaminized, and the non-nitrogenous part of the molecule forms glucose and fatty acids. This leads to an increase of glucose and incompletely oxidized fatty acids in the blood and an increased excretion of nitrogen and potassium in the urine.

It has been noted previously that glucose in the body is derived from other food sources besides carbohydrate in the diet. It should be remembered that carbohydrates are estimated to yield approximately 100 per cent, proteins 58 per cent and fats 10 per cent of their weight as available glucose in the body.

MANAGEMENT OF DIABETES

Hormonal

Insulin. The diabetic frequently has to resort to commercial insulin preparations; he must inject a fixed amount of the hormone into his body each day. Because the amount of the daily injection is fixed and constant, he cannot have the same freedom in the intake of food as the non-diabetic. A balance must be maintained between the insulin and the glucose received from food.

Commercial Insulin. Insulin is a protein extracted from the pancreas of animals and is packaged in crystalline form. In 1964, the synthesis of insulin was completed—another step forward in scientific achievement. A *standardized unit of insulin* provides for the use of 1.5 to 3.0 gm. of glucose.

There are three general types of commercial insulin: (1) the quick-acting regular crystalline or unmodified insulin, (2) the slow-acting protamine zinc insulin and (3) the intermediate insulin. The types and characteristics of the insulins available in the United States are summarized in Table 25-2. The diabetic's response to the insulin determines the kind and amount that the physician will prescribe.

Administration of Insulin. The insulin preparations currently available require parenteral administration because the digestive juices would digest insulin, which is a protein.

The type, dosage and frequency of insulin administration is individualized for the patient, depending upon his stage of growth, physical state, activity and psychological stability. It may be a single dose or a mixture of insulins in one injection or a regimen of two or three injections during a 24-hour period.

Injections of insulin must be continued during the period when the pancreas is unable to function adequately. Very often improvement occurs, in which event the amount of insulin is either reduced or omitted. For example, an obese person who requires insulin at first may, after sufficient weight loss, be able to control his diabetes by diet alone or by diet plus one of the oral hypoglycemic agents. The *severity* and the *nature* of the diabetes determine whether insulin must be continued. See page 764 for a discussion of the decrease in insulin requirements commonly found following initiation of insulin therapy in juvenile diabetics.

Table 25-2   TYPES AND CHARACTERISTICS OF INSULIN AVAILABLE IN THE UNITED STATES*

TYPE OF INSULIN	APPEAR-ANCE	ACTION	DURATION (Hours)	ZINC CONTENT (mg./100 Units)	BUFFER	PROTEIN Type	mg./100 Units
Regular Crystalline	Clear	Rapid	5–7	0.016–0.04	None	None	–
Semilente®	Turbid	Rapid	12–16	0.2 –0.25	Acetate	None	–
Globin	Clear	Intermediate	18–24	0.25 –0.35	None	Globin	3.8
NPH	Turbid	Intermediate	24–28	0.016–0.04	Phosphate	Protamine	0.5
Lente®	Turbid	Intermediate	24–28	0.2 –0.25	Acetate	None	–
Protamine Zinc	Turbid	Prolonged	36+	0.2 –0.25	Phosphate	Protamine	1.25
Ultralente®	Turbid	Prolonged	36+	0.2 –0.25	Acetate	None	–

*From: Waife, S. O. (ed.): Diabetes Mellitus, 7th ed. Indianapolis, Lilly Research Laboratories, Eli Lilly & Company, 1970, p. 41.

Another situation is the *Somogyi phenomenon,* in which there is deterioration of diabetic control in the face of increasing dosages of insulin. The person becomes overinsulinized, as is frequently seen in children when attempts are made to eliminate glucosuria completely. This should be suspected in a child receiving more than 1.5 units of insulin per kg. body weight per day. The insulin dosage should be slowly reduced or split into two injections.

Insulin is best injected where the skin is loose, in a pocket between the fat and muscle. The sites of injection should be frequently changed or rotated (see Fig. 25–3). Because the nurse most often has the responsibility of teaching the use and administration of the insulin to a patient, she should become very familiar with the technique used in her institution. Other procedures are given in diabetic manuals. Frequently in the areas where insulin is injected there will be atrophy or hypertrophy of the adipose tissue. Unfortunately, the cause of this condition is not well understood, but rotating injection sites may help to prevent it.

INSULIN RESISTANCE. In some cases antibodies to injected insulin can develop. An immune reaction occurs, and the insulin becomes ineffective. Depending on the degree of resistance, insulin dosages are greatly increased, sometimes up to several hundred units per day. It is then necessary to switch to another type of insulin (from pork to beef, for instance). More common causes of insulin resistance are physiological stresses such as pregnancy, infection, an endocrine disorder or obesity.

INSULIN ALLERGY. Insulin allergies develop in the form of an allergy to the insulin being used (especially to pork insulins) or to the

alcohol used for cleansing or sterilization. Treatment involves changing the type of cleansing solution or insulin. A purer insulin called "single peak insulin" (a description of the protein's electrophoretic pattern) has been developed. This type is 99 per cent insulin, compared with the old U.S.P. variety, which was 92 per cent insulin. It has less extraneous protein and thus fewer allergic properties. An even purer insulin, "single component insulin," is being developed and should be available soon.

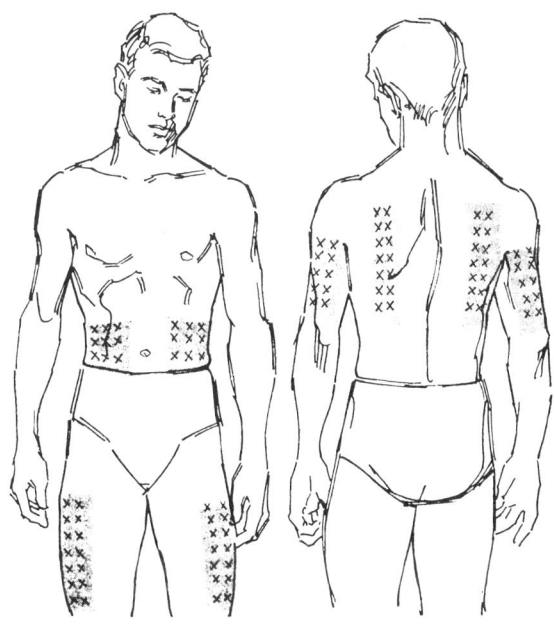

Figure 25–3 Sites for insulin injection. (From: Luckman, J., and Sorensen, K. C.: Medical-Surgical Nursing. Philadelphia, W. B. Saunders Co., 1974, p. 1329.)

Special care is required in the handling, storage and administration of insulin. Insulin, regardless of the source, is sold in a standard potency, U-100 (100 units per cc.). Made from pork or beef insulin, it has varying levels of impurities that may be responsible for insulin allergy. "Single peak" insulin is the purest form.

Glucagon. Glucagon, usually in excess in diabetics, may be used to increase blood glucose in the case of a hypoglycemic attack.

Somatostatin. The rationale for using somatostatin in addition to insulin is that somatostatin lowers blood glucagon levels. In fact, in studies of insulin-dependent diabetics done by Gerich and his colleagues, it was found that insulin and somatostatin together resulted in lower blood glucagon levels after a meal and lower blood glucose levels than when insulin alone was used.[7]

Because glucagon seems to be a key in the development of ketoacidosis, it is postulated by Gerich that somatostatin may be more effective than insulin in the treatment of ketoacidosis, since it can reduce the level of blood glucagon more effectively.

At present, there are several problems with the use of somatostatin: (1) it can be given only by infusion rather than injection because of its short half-life, (2) it may be inappropriate for children because it also inhibits the release of growth hormone and (3) it has been shown by some researchers to exert a transient effect on the aggregation of platelets.

Oral Hypoglycemic Agents

There are two types of hypoglycemic agents, the sulfonylurea and phenethylbiguanide compounds. The *sulfonylurea* compounds lower the blood sugar level and reduce glycosuria in certain diabetic patients. Current results indicate that these drugs act by *stimulating the pancreatic beta cells to secrete endogenous insulin.* These compounds are effective only in diabetics who have beta cells that can respond to the stimulus. The insulin then appears to exert its main effect in the liver by promoting a decrease in the output of glucose from the liver glycogen into the blood stream. Results to date have generally not been satisfactory in young diabetics or in treating such complications as infection, surgery or acidosis, but a lowering of blood glucose has been reported in mild or moderately severe and stable diabetics of the older age group who have a residual insulin

supply (require less than 20 units daily) and in whom onset took place after age 40. The current available hypoglycemic compounds are shown in Table 25-3.

The *phenethylbiguanide, phenformin* (DBI), has been reported to have hypoglycemic activity when used alone or in combination with sulfonylurea in treating mild cases, the elderly and the obese. In addition, when used as a supplement to insulin in certain young diabetics, it has made possible a significant reduction in the insulin dosage. The mode and site of action of the biguanides are different from those of the sulfonylureas, since they seem to *stimulate glucose utilization by the tissues.*

In 1961, the University Group Diabetes Program (UGDP), a prospective clinical trial, was begun to determine the efficacy of sulfonylureas and biguanides in preventing the vascular complications of diabetes. In 12 University Centers, over one thousand patients with insulin-independent diabetes were studied. After eight years of research, the group stated that both tolbutamide and phenformin were found to be less effective than diet alone or diet plus insulin in preventing cardiovascular complications of diabetes. Although these findings were endorsed by the FDA, the AMA and the American Diabetes Association, they are controversial. The general use of oral hypoglycemics has decreased in favor of insulin, but there is still some use of the oral hypoglycemics, particularly in cases that cannot be controlled by diet and for which it is impossible to give insulin.

Table 25-3 AVAILABLE ORAL HYPOGLYCEMIC COMPOUNDS*

COMPOUNDS	MAXIMUM RECOMMENDED DAILY DOSE *(gm.)*	DURATION OF ACTION *(Hours)*
Sulfonylureas		
Tolbutamide (Orinase)	2–3	6–12
Acetohexamide (Dymelor)	1.5	12–24
Chlorpropamide (Diabinese)	0.5	up to 60
Tolazamide (Tolinase)	0.75	12–24

*From: Waife, S. O. (ed.): Diabetes Mellitus, 7th ed. Indianapolis, Lilly Research Laboratories, Eli Lilly & Company, 1970, p. 125.

Artificial Pancreas

Research continues for a device capable of monitoring blood glucose and delivering insulin into the blood stream when necessary. There would be enough insulin within the device to keep the person supplied for an extended period. Problems of miniaturization and replacement and of rejection by the body still remain to be solved.

Urine Testing

Urine glucose and acetone concentrations are the best measurements of the adequacy of diabetes management. Urine specimens should be checked four times daily: before breakfast, lunch, dinner and bedtime. Ideally, the specimens should be *double-voided,* which means emptying the bladder and then testing the urine voided half an hour later. The insulin dosage or food intake is then adjusted depending upon the presence or absence of glucosuria or ketonuria.

Nutritional Care

The diet of a diabetic is a normal diet which consists of sufficient calories for activity and the maintenance of ideal weight and is adequate in carbohydrate, protein, fat, minerals and vitamins. The dietary treatment of diabetes consists essentially of reducing and systematizing the intake of carbohydrate in order to place as little strain as possible on the impaired blood glucose–regulating mechanism. Treatment with exogenous insulin more or less restores the regulating mechanism, and dietary management currently being prescribed for diabetics corresponds closely in composition and quantity to that deemed optimal for healthy non-diabetic persons of similar age.

The role of the diet in diabetes is (1) to provide sufficient calories to maintain ideal body weight, (2) to adjust food ingestion to the available insulin, allowing only small amounts or no glucose to spill into the urine and permitting the blood sugar to rise slightly above normal, (3) to prevent acidosis and shock and (4) to furnish an adequate diet for good health and normal activity. For a large percentage of maturity-onset diabetics, it is possible to control blood sugar by diet alone. Though the secretion of insulin is diminished, there is enough to take care of dietary needs. Other diabetic patients need specific food restrictions plus the administration of insulin or an oral hypoglycemic agent.

Clinical Control. The methods by which adequate control of diabetes may be accomplished have been the subject of much study and debate. On the one hand, the patient may be treated by permitting him to eat what he likes so long as he is free from clinical symptoms, maintains or gains weight (as necessary) and is free from ketosis and hypoglycemia. This is known as clinical control. Insulin dosage under these circumstances must be adjusted frequently. Continuous glycosuria and hyperglycemia are permitted as long as the patient maintains his normal weight and shows no ketone bodies in the urine. Concentrated sweets such as sugar, candy, syrup, jelly and sweet desserts are omitted or limited.

Chemical Control. In contrast, many physicians use a measured diet and insulin, when indicated, that is regulated to control the blood sugar within normal limits and to keep the urine free or nearly free of sugar. By this means an adequate intake of calories, protein, minerals and vitamins is assured, while the amount of carbohydrates and calories is limited. With this type of regulation, a constant insulin requirement is more readily established, and normoglycemia may be maintained for long periods. This is known as chemical control.

The question arises as to whether it is true that the meticulous control gained by using the regulated diet with nearly perfect insulin balance will minimize the incidence of complications throughout the years. The group advocating a liberal diet feels that glycosuria is not incompatible with well-being and intimates that vascular damage is perhaps inevitable and not delayed by strict regimen. Many years of study and observation are needed for the complete answer. However, the weight of evidence suggests that the microvascular complications of diabetes are decreased by reduction and control of blood glucose concentration.[4]

Caloric Allowance. The same procedure used to plan the normal diet is followed when computing a diet prescription for a diabetic patient. First, the caloric allowance is determined, based on the patient's height, weight, age, sex and occupation or activity. Details for calculating a diet have already been given (Chapter 20). Most authorities consider it advisable to keep the weight of the diabetic slightly below average (about 10 per cent). However, at the lower equilibrium the individual is sometimes incapable of a full, active, healthy life and will fatigue easily, have decreased resistance to infection and suffer mental apathy and depression. This must always be watched for, and the diet should be adjusted to supply sufficient energy for full activity. En-

ergy requirements can be calculated in the following way:

1. To determine the basal calories expended for 24 hours, the patient's ideal weight in pounds is multiplied by 10 or in kilograms by 4.5.
2. If the person is young, tall, and male, 100 to 200 calories are added to the basal calorie requirement.
3. If the person is elderly, short and female, 100 to 200 calories are subtracted from the basal calorie requirement.
4. Light activity requires 30 per cent added to the calculated basal calories. Greater activity requires an addition of 50 to 75 per cent of the calculated basal calories.

Chapter 2 gives other methods for calculating energy requirement.

Protein Allowance.   Next, the protein allowance is determined, which is essentially the same as that for the normal individual and may vary from 0.8 to 1.5 gm. of protein per kg. of desirable body weight or 0.4 to 0.7 gm. per lb.

Untreated or poorly regulated diabetics excrete large quantities of nitrogen in the urine, the result of the increase in the conversion of proteins to carbohydrates. Because of this a large protein deficit may occur. It is advisable to allow 1.5 gm. of protein during the beginning few weeks of the treatment to correct this deficit. Later in the course of treatment, 0.8 gm. per kg. of desirable body weight or a minimum of 65 gm. of protein daily may be sufficient for an adult. However, current practice is to prescribe from 80 to 100 gm., because there is less available glucose in protein, and the metabolism to glucose is slower. Reserve protein is needed during episodes of ketosis, whether very mild or severe.

Carbohydrate Allowance.   The carbohydrate allowance is the next determination of the diet. The estimation is guided by the patient's blood sugar, urinalysis and available insulin. Carbohydrates provide 45 to 50 per cent of the total calories in the diet of most Americans. In diabetics this percentage should remain the same, with the avoidance of highly concentrated sugars. An amount less than 100 gm. is inadvisable, since a low level frequently leads to ketosis. An amount over 300 gm. may overtax the metabolic capacity of the diabetic.

Fat Allowance.   To balance the caloric requirement, the remaining calories in the diet are supplied by fats. It is recommended that fat be restricted to between 30 and 35 per cent of calories and contain mostly polyunsaturated fatty acids as a preventive measure against atherosclerosis.

Minerals and Vitamins.   Vitamin and mineral requirements of patients with well-controlled diabetes do not differ significantly from those of normal subjects. There is no necessity for mineral and vitamin supplements when the diet is adequate and the glycosuria is controlled.

Weighed Versus Measured Diets.   Dietary control is highly desirable, though strict arithmetical standards do not seem warranted. With the exception of rare cases, it is no longer considered necessary to weigh the food on a gram scale. Measured amounts of foods using the available and familiar household measures of teaspoon, tablespoon and measuring cup will suffice.

Meal Planning with Exchange Lists.   In 1950 the American Diabetes Association, working jointly with the U.S. Public Health Service and the American Dietetic Association, published a simplified, widely used method of calculating a diabetic diet and planning the diabetic's meals. An effort was made to reclassify and standardize food values and reduce the complexity of diabetic diets. This material has been revised, and the present booklet, "Exchange Lists for Meal Planning," is available at small cost for use in planning menus.[6]

The Diet.   The present dietary pattern of the patient is evaluated for the presence of the protective food groups, which are the same as for a non-diabetic. Appropriate dietary practices are noted and become the foundation for planning the revised pattern with the patient. It should include high-quality protein foods such as meat and milk, vegetables, fruits, whole-grain or enriched cereals and breads and fortified margarine.

After the calories, protein, fat and carbohydrate requirements have been determined, foods to meet these requirements are outlined, using the dietary history information obtained.

The foods to meet the carbohydrate allowance are determined before the protein and fat requirements are considered. The analysis of some carbohydrate foods shows that they contain fat and protein. (See Table 25–4.) For example, using the Exchange List, 8 oz. of skim milk contains 12 gm. carbohydrate, 8 gm. protein and a trace of fat. A slice of bread from list 4 contains 15 gm. of carbohydrate and 2 gm. of protein.

The protein foods (meats, eggs, cheese) are identified. Most of the protein foods contain a percentage of fats. For example, 3 oz. of a lean meat such as boiled ham contains 21 gm. protein and 9 gm. fat.

The fat allowance is the last adjustment

Table 25–4 COMPOSITION OF FOOD EXCHANGE GROUPS

EXCHANGE GROUP	WEIGHT (gm.)	APPROX. MEASURE		COMPOSITION FOR 1 EXCHANGE OR 1 SERVING[a]	CALORIES
List 1	240	1 cup		Milk (C, 12 gm.; P, 8 gm.; F, trace)	80
List 2	100	½ cup		Vegetables (C, 5 gm.; P, 2 gm.)	25
List 3	varies	varies		Fruit (C, 10 gm.)	40
List 4	25 (varies)	1 slice	Other	Bread exchanges (C, 15 gm.; P, 2 gm.)	70
List 5	30 (varies)	1 oz.	items	Meat exchanges (P, 7 gm.; F, 3 gm.)	55
List 6	5 (varies)	1 tsp.	vary	Fat exchanges (F, 5 gm.)	45

[a]C = carbohydrate, P = protein, F = fat.

made in the diet. Because butter, fortified margarine, oil and mayonnaise are considered pure fats, their inclusion or exclusion from the diet can be easily and simply adjusted to meet the fat requirement.

In the simplified method of calculating the diabetic diet, *food exchanges are basic*. The principal foods allowed the diabetic are classified into six groups, determined by the composition of the food. Each group contains similar kinds and amounts of food according to the nutritional value of carbohydrate, protein and fat. The groups are shown in Table 25–5. See Table 25–6 for an example of a diabetic diet plan.

Meal Planning

The need for insulin is the determining factor that decides how the foods of the diet should be distributed among meals. Also, the *kind* of insulin employed by the patient affects the meal planning. Some convenient methods for distributing the required foods into meals will be discussed.

Using No Insulin. When no insulin is prescribed, the daily carbohydrate allowance usually is divided equally among three meals, with one third each at breakfast, lunch and dinner. In some patients the blood sugar is higher in the morning, and for these individuals a smaller amount of carbohydrate is given then, for example, one fifth at breakfast, two fifths at lunch and two fifths at dinner.

Using Regular (Crystalline) Insulin. When regular, quick-acting (crystalline) insulin before each meal is employed, the carbohydrate allowance is divided equally into three meals, following the same proportions suggested when using no insulin. Regular insulin alone is little used today except for diabetics undergoing surgery or those with ketoacidosis. Frequently, it is used in children in conjunction with a slower-acting insulin to give a more balanced level of blood sugar.

Using Prolonged-acting Insulin. Protamine zinc insulin, for example, has a prolonged activity of approximately 24 hours. When arranging meal schedules to synchronize with insulin injections, Pollack and Dolger[14] originally demonstrated how important it is that the maximum availability of glucose from foods should coincide with the maximum availability of insulin. Thus, when protamine zinc insulin is administered, an evening feeding (bedtime) is usually required to prevent hypoglycemia during the night or early morning. For a correct distribution of *carbohydrate*, the amount planned for the bedtime feeding is deducted from the total daily carbohydrate allowance, and the remaining carbohydrate is then divided into the three daily meals as follows: one fifth at breakfast, two fifths at lunch, two fifths at dinner, with 25 to 30 gm at bedtime (when indicated), deducted from the total carbohydrate allowance before division into meals.

Using Regular and Protamine Zinc Insulin. When regular insulin and protamine zinc insulin are employed together, the daily carbohydrate allowance is frequently divided into three meals following these proportions: breakfast, two fifths, lunch, one fifth, dinner, two fifths.

The larger proportion of carbohydrate served at breakfast will synchronize with the regular insulin availability if it is injected before breakfast.

Using Intermediate-acting Insulins. The intermediate-acting insulins have an action that is intermediate in duration and intensity. When an insulin of intermediate action (globin zinc insulin, NPH or Lente) is given before breakfast, a late afternoon nourishment (3:30 to 4:00 P.M.) is frequently required to counteract any hypoglycemic tendency at this time. This is particularly characteristic of globin. A bedtime feeding often is unnecessary when intermediate insulin preparations are used. The carbohydrate allowance may be divided as follows: breakfast, one sixth, lunch, two sixths, afternoon snack, one sixth, dinner, two sixths.

Text continued on page 532

Table 25–5   DIABETIC EXCHANGE LISTS*

*List 1—Milk Exchanges (Includes **Non-fat,** Low-fat and Whole Milk)*

This list shows the kinds and amounts of milk or milk products to use for one Milk Exchange. Those that appear in **bold type** are **non-fat.** Low-fat and whole milk contain saturated fat. One Exchange of milk contains 12 grams of carbohydrate, 8 grams of protein, a trace of fat and 80 calories.

TYPE	AMOUNT
Non-Fat Fortified Milk	
Skim or non-fat milk	1 cup
Powdered (non-fat dry, before adding liquid)	⅓ cup
Canned, evaporated skim milk	½ cup
Buttermilk made from skim milk	1 cup
Yogurt made from skim milk (plain, unflavored)	1 cup
Low-Fat Fortified Milk	
1% fat fortified milk	1 cup
(omit ½ Fat Exchange)	
2% fat fortified milk	1 cup
(omit 1 Fat Exchange)	
Yogurt made from 2% fortified milk (plain, unflavored)	1 cup
(omit 1 Fat Exchange)	
Whole Milk (omit 2 Fat Exchanges)	
Whole milk	1 cup
Canned, evaporated whole milk	½ cup
Buttermilk made from whole milk	1 cup
Yogurt made from whole milk (plain, unflavored)	1 cup

List 2—Vegetable Exchanges

This list shows the kinds of vegetables to use for one Vegetable Exchange. One Exchange is ½ cup. One Exchange of vegetables contains about 5 grams of carbohydrate, 2 grams of protein and 25 calories. All vegetables listed are non-fat.

Asparagus	Greens:
Bean sprouts	Mustard
Beets	Spinach
Broccoli	Turnip
Brussels sprouts	Mushrooms
Cabbage	Okra
Carrots	Onions
Cauliflower	Rhubarb
Celery	Rutabaga
Cucumbers	Sauerkraut
Eggplant	String beans, green or yellow
Green pepper	Summer squash
Greens:	Tomatoes
Beet	Tomato juice
Chard	Turnips
Collards	Vegetable juice cocktail
Dandelion	Zucchini
Kale	

The following raw vegetables may be used as desired:

Chicory	Lettuce
Chinese cabbage	Parsley
Endive	Radishes
Escarole	Watercress

Starchy vegetables are found in the Bread Exchange list.

*From: Exchange Lists for Meal Planning. American Diabetes Association, Inc., 1 West 48th Street, New York, New York, 10020; and American Dietetic Association, 430 N. Michigan Avenue, Chicago, Illinois, 60611, 1976.

Table 25–5   DIABETIC EXCHANGE LISTS *(Continued)*

List 3—Fruit Exchanges

This list shows the kinds and amounts of fruits to use for one Fruit Exchange. One Exchange of fruit contains 10 grams of carbohydrate and 40 calories. All fruits listed are non-fat.

FRUIT	AMOUNT	FRUIT	AMOUNT
Apple	1 small	Mango	½ small
Apple juice	⅓ cup	Melon	
Applesauce (unsweetened)	½ cup	Cantaloupe	¼ small
Apricots, fresh	2 medium	Honeydew	⅛ medium
Apricots, dried	4 halves	Watermelon	1 cup
Banana	½ small	Nectarine	1 small
Berries		Orange	1 small
Blackberries	½ cup	Orange juice	½ cup
Blueberries	½ cup	Papaya	¾ cup
Raspberries	½ cup	Peach	1 medium
Strawberries	¾ cup	Pear	1 small
Cherries	10 large	Persimmon, native	1 medium
Cider	⅓ cup	Pineapple	½ cup
Dates	2	Pineapple juice	⅓ cup
Figs, fresh	1	Plums	2 medium
Figs, dried	1	Prunes	2 medium
Grapefruit	½	Prune juice	¼ cup
Grapefruit juice	½ cup	Raisins	2 tablespoons
Grapes	12	Tangerine	1 medium
Grape juice	¼ cup		

Cranberries may be used as desired if no sugar is added.

List 4—Bread Exchanges (Includes Bread, Cereal and Starchy Vegetables)

This list shows the kinds and amounts of breads, cereals, starchy vegetables and prepared foods to use for one Bread Exchange. Those that appear in **bold type** are **low-fat.** One Exchange of bread contains 15 grams of carbohydrate, 2 grams of protein and 70 calories.

FOOD	AMOUNT	FOOD	AMOUNT
Bread		**Starchy Vegetables**	
White (including French and Italian)	1 slice	**Corn**	⅓ cup
Whole wheat	1 slice	**Corn on cob**	1 small
Rye or pumpernickel	1 slice	**Lima beans**	½ cup
Raisin	1 slice	**Parsnips**	⅔ cup
Bagel, small	½	**Peas, green (canned or frozen)**	½ cup
English muffin, small	½	**Potato, white**	1 small
Plain roll, bread	1	**Potato (mashed)**	½ cup
Frankfurter roll	½	**Pumpkin**	¾ cup
Hamburger bun	½	**Winter squash, acorn or butternut**	½ cup
Dried bread crumbs	3 tbsp.	**Yam or sweet potato**	¼ cup
Tortilla, 6″	1		
		Prepared Foods	
Cereal		Biscuit, 2″ dia.	1
Bran flakes	½ cup	(omit 1 Fat Exchange)	
Other ready-to-eat unsweetened		Corn bread, 2″ × 2″ × 1″	1
cereal	¾ cup	(omit 1 Fat Exchange)	
Puffed cereal (unfrosted)	1 cup	Corn muffin, 2″ dia.	1
Cereal (cooked)	½ cup	(omit 1 Fat Exchange)	
Grits (cooked)	½ cup	Crackers, round butter type	5
Rice or barley (cooked)	½ cup	(omit 1 Fat Exchange)	
Pasta (cooked)		Muffin, plain small	1
Spaghetti, noodles, macaroni	½ cup	(omit 1 Fat Exchange)	
Popcorn (popped, no fat added)	3 cups	Potatoes, french fried, length 2″ to 3½″	8
Cornmeal (dry)	2 tbsp.	(omit 1 Fat Exchange)	
Flour	2½ tbsp.	Potato or corn chips	15
Wheat germ	¼ cup	(omit 2 Fat Exchanges)	

Table continued on the following page

Table 25–5   DIABETIC EXCHANGE LISTS *(Continued)*

List 4—Bread Exchanges (Includes Bread, Cereal and Starchy Vegetables) (Continued)

This list shows the kinds and amounts of breads, cereals, starchy vegetables and prepared foods to use for one Bread Exchange. Those that appear in **bold type** are **low-fat.** One Exchange of bread contains 15 grams of carbohydrate, 2 grams of protein and 70 calories.

FOOD	AMOUNT	FOOD	AMOUNT
		Pancake, 5″ × ½″	1
Crackers		(omit 1 Fat Exchange)	
Arrowroot	3	Waffle, 5″ × ½″	1
Graham, 2½″ sq.	2	(omit 1 Fat Exchange)	
Matzoth, 4″ × 6″	½		
Oyster	20		
Pretzels, 3⅛″ long × ⅛″ dia.	25		
Rye wafers, 2″ × 3½″	3		
Saltines	6		
Soda, 2½″ sq.	4		
Dried Beans, Peas and Lentils			
Beans, peas, lentils (dried and cooked)	½ cup		
Baked beans, no pork (canned)	¼ cup		

List 5—Meat Exchanges (a) Lean Meat

This list shows the kinds and amounts of lean meat and other protein-rich foods to use for one low-fat meat exchange. One Exchange of lean meat (1 oz.) contains 7 grams of protein, 3 grams of fat and 55 calories. To plan a diet low in saturated fat, select only those exchanges that appear in **bold type.**

	TYPE	AMOUNT
Beef:	**Baby beef (very lean), chipped beef, chuck, flank steak, tenderloin, plate ribs, plate skirt steak, round (bottom, top), all cuts rump, spare ribs, tripe**	1 oz.
Lamb:	**Leg, rib, sirloin, loin (roast and chops), shank, shoulder**	1 oz.
Pork:	**Leg (whole rump, center shank), ham, smoked (center slices)**	1 oz.
Veal:	**Leg, loin, rib, shank, shoulder, cutlets**	1 oz.
Poultry:	**Meat without skin of chicken, turkey, cornish hen, guinea hen, pheasant**	1 oz.
Fish:	**Any fresh or frozen**	1 oz.
	Canned salmon, tuna, mackerel, crab and lobster	¼ cup
	Clams, oysters, scallops, shrimp	5 or 1 oz.
	Sardines (drained)	3
Cheeses containing less than 5% butterfat		1 oz.
Cottage cheese, dry and 2% butterfat		¼ cup
Dried beans and peas (omit 1 Bread Exchange)		½ cup

Meat Exchanges (b) Medium-Fat Meat

This list shows the kinds and amounts of medium-fat meat and other protein-rich foods to use for one medium-fat meat exchange. For each Exchange of medium-fat meat omit ½ Fat Exchange.

	TYPE	AMOUNT
Beef:	Ground (15% fat), corned beef (canned), rib eye, round (ground commercial)	1 oz.
Pork:	Loin (all cuts tenderloin), shoulder arm (picnic), shoulder blade, Boston butt, Canadian bacon, boiled ham	
Liver, heart, kidney and sweetbreads (these are high in cholesterol)		1 oz.
Cottage cheese, creamed		¼ cup
Cheese:	Mozzarella, ricotta, farmer's cheese, Neufchatel,	1 oz.
	Parmesan	3 tbsp.
Egg (high in cholesterol)		1
Peanut butter (omit 2 additional Fat Exchanges)		2 tbsp.

Table 25–5 DIABETIC EXCHANGE LISTS (*Continued*)

List 5—Meat Exchanges (c) High-Fat Meat

This list shows the kinds and amounts of high-fat meat and other protein-rich foods to use for one high-fat meat exchange. For each Exchange of high-fat meat omit 1 Fat Exchange.

TYPE	AMOUNT
Beef: Brisket, corned beef (brisket), ground beef (more than 20% fat), hamburger (commercial), chuck (ground commercial), roasts (rib), steaks (club and rib)	1 oz.
Lamb: Breast	1 oz.
Pork: Spare ribs, loin (back ribs), pork (ground), country style ham, deviled ham	1 oz.
Veal: Breast	1 oz.
Poultry: Capon, duck (domestic), goose	1 oz.
Cheese: Cheddar types	1 oz.
Cold cuts	4½″ × ⅛″ slice
Frankfurter	1 small

List 6—Fat Exchanges

This list shows the kinds and amounts of fat-containing foods to use for one Fat Exchange. To plan a diet low in saturated fat select only those Exchanges that appear in **bold type.** They are **polyunsaturated.** One Exchange of fat contains 5 grams of fat and 45 calories.

FOOD	AMOUNT
Margarine, soft, tub or stick†	1 tsp.
Avocado (4″ in diameter)††	⅛
Oil: corn, cottonseed, safflower, soy, sunflower	1 tsp.
Oil, olive††	1 tsp.
Oil, peanut††	1 tsp.
Olives††	5 small
Almonds††	10 whole
Pecans††	2 large whole
Peanuts††	
Spanish	20 whole
Virginia	10 whole
Walnuts	6 small
Nuts, other††	6 small
Margarine, regular stick	1 tsp.
Butter	1 tsp.
Bacon fat	1 tsp.
Bacon, crisp	1 strip
Cream, light	2 tbsp.
Cream, sour	2 tbsp.
Cream, heavy	1 tbsp.
Cream cheese	1 tbsp.
French dressing†††	1 tbsp.
Italian dressing†††	1 tbsp.
Lard	1 tsp.
Mayonnaise†††	1 tsp.
Salad dressing, mayonnaise type†††	2 tsp.
Salt pork	¾ inch cube

†Made with corn, cottonseed, safflower, soy or sunflower oil only
††Fat content is primarily monounsaturated
†††If made with corn, cottonseed, safflower, soy or sunflower oil can be used on fat modified diet

Table continued on the following page

Table 25–5   DIABETIC EXCHANGE LISTS *(Continued)*

List 7—Beverages, Seasonings, Condiments and Foods Allowed as Desired

The following may be used as desired, unless the physician finds a special reason to limit them. The foods listed have no appreciable carbohydrate, protein or fat content if used in ordinary amounts.

Coffee	Rennet tablets	Garlic	Parsley seasoning
Tea	Celery seasoning	Lemon	Pepper
Clear broth	Cinnamon	Mint	Saccharin, Sucaryl and other non-caloric sweeteners
Bouillon, without fat		Mustard	Vinegar
Gelatin, unsweetened		Nutmeg	Pickles (sour or unsweetened dill)
		Onion seasoning	

If a midafternoon feeding is not given, the carbohydrate deducted from breakfast is added to the noon meal. With NPH and Lente insulins, the division of carbohydrate is frequently apportioned as described for protamine zinc insulin.

Protein Allowance Divided into Meals.   There are some authorities who like to divide the *protein* allowance of the diet among the meals in a manner similar to that described for carbohydrate. Because of the present trend of liberalizing the diabetic diet, however, a more liberal procedure is to subdivide only the *carbohy-*

drate allowance. However, it should be remembered that an adequate meal contains a complete protein.

Pollack and Dolger[14] established that it is advisable to include about one half of the proteins in the evening and bedtime meals if protamine zinc insulin is used, thereby allowing a continuous flow of glucose during the night. The other half is divided to include one sixth for breakfast and one third at noon. They state: "When the patient consumes one half to two thirds of the daily protein allowance (meat) at supper time, it is rare to find nocturnal hypo-

Table 25–6   EXAMPLE OF A METHOD FOR PLANNING A DIABETIC DIET

Diet prescription: Calories, 2100; C, 250 gm.; P, 85 gm.; F, 85 gm.
Approximate % of calories: C = 49%, P = 16%, F = 35%

		TOTAL DAY'S FOOD			
FOOD	AMOUNT	LIST	C *(gm.)*	P *(gm.)*	F *(gm.)*
Milk, skim	2 cups	1	24	16	
Vegetables	3 servings	2	15	6	
Fruits	6 exchanges	3	60		
			99 (total)		
Bread exchanges	10	4	150	20	
				42 (total)	
Meat exchanges	3	5a		21	9
	2	5b		14	11
	1	5c		7	8
					28 (total)
Fat exchanges	11	6			55
		Totals:	249	84	83

The number of servings of bread, meat and fat exchanges required to complete the diet prescription were determined in the following way:

1. Subtract the carbohydrate grams (99) furnished by the milk, vegetables and fruit from the grams of carbohydrate prescribed (250); divide the result by 15, which is the amount of grams of carbohydrate in one bread exchange (List 4).
   250 − 99 = 151; 151 ÷ 15 = 10 bread exchanges
2. The protein grams in a diet are adjusted by the addition of one or more meat exchanges (List 5).
   85 − 42 = 43; 43 ÷ 7 = 6 meat exchanges
3. The fat grams in a diet are adjusted by the addition of one or more fat exchanges (List 6).
   85 − 28 = 57; 57 ÷ 5 = 11 fat exchanges

glycemic episodes, the reason for this being that about one half of the protein consumed is converted into available carbohydrate. This conversion is slow. . . . The slow rise in blood sugar concentration, and the absence of any tendency to rapid fluctuations after the ingestion of meat, establishes its usefulness without question.''[14]

When using insulin of intermediate action, protein in the night meal or feeding also helps to prevent early morning hypoglycemia.

Special Diabetic Foods. Contrary to popular belief, the purchase or preparation of special diabetic foods is not necessary. The diabetic patient can and should eat the same variety of foods as the rest of the family, with the exception of sugar and foods prepared with sugar. Canned and frozen fruits present the greatest problem because of the syrup in which they are prepared. However, water-packed fruits, both canned and frozen, are quite widely available and are becoming more equitable in price. As a diabetic person becomes less accustomed to sugar, sweetened foods are no longer enticing. Presenting the diet in terms of exchanges with meal patterns makes it much easier for the diabetic patient to select foods available at home or in a restaurant to fit into his personally prescribed plan. Every patient should know the food equivalents to encourage variety in the selection of foods.

The diabetic diets in Tables 25–7 and 25–8 are examples of (1) a diabetic diet for a patient using regular insulin or no insulin and (2) a diabetic diet for a patient using protamine zinc insulin or an intermediate-acting insulin.

SUGAR SUBSTITUTES. To replace sugar and sweetness in the diet for the diabetic, non-nutritive sweeteners have been developed. The oldest of these sweeteners is saccharin, which at present is the only sweetener available for household use. In early 1977 the FDA proposed banning the use of this sweetener in foods because Canadian studies reported the development of bladder tumors in rats that were fed large doses of saccharin. However, it is still available as a non-prescription drug.

Cyclamate, a popular, good-tasting sweetener, was banned in 1971. Because of the controversy about saccharin and cyclamates, new sweeteners are being used or being developed. *Maltitol* from maltose is 90 per cent as sweet as sucrose, and claims have been made that it is not absorbed by the body and therefore could be used as a non-nutritive sweetener. Another product being developed is *aspartame*, which has not yet been approved by the FDA.

Xylitol, the alcohol of xylose, is as sweet as sucrose and is also used as a sweetener in the diets of diabetics. Like sorbitol and mannitol (see Chapter 3), this sugar can be taken by diabetics because it is absorbed less quickly than sucrose. However, these sugars are eventually absorbed and therefore must be considered in the diet calculation. It is best to prescribe natural foods but if an artificial sweetener is necessary, then saccharin, if available, is preferable, since it has no nutritive value and does not need to be counted in the diet.

Food Values. The composition and classification of the most frequently served foods will be found in Appendix Tables 1 and 2. The classifications of fruits and vegetables according to their carbohydrate content are offered in Appendix Table 12. These tables may be useful if a system other than the method described in this text using exchange lists is employed. The exchange lists have been emphasized because of their wide use and greater simplicity.

However, other systems have certain merits that probably warrant their continued use. For example, some clinicians and educators use fewer groupings of food, combining fruits and some vegetables into one group, including milk with the meat group and other vegetables on the free food list, or other simplifications. With these or similar modifications, the system used might consist of five exchange or serving groups: (1) free foods, (2) protein foods, (3) low-carbohydrate foods, (4) high-carbohydrate foods and (5) foods consisting mostly of fats and oils.[13, 15] The most effective systems for teaching are those adapted by the nurse or dietitian to the learning abilities of the diabetic person.

The total value of the ingredients makes up the nutrient value of any prepared dish. For example, when a custard is analyzed for its nutrient value, the ingredients of the custard are listed, namely milk or cream, sweetening, egg, and flavoring. The nutrient value of the custard is the total of the nutrients.

DIABETES IN PREGNANCY AND CHILDHOOD

The diet of the pregnant diabetic woman was discussed in Chapter 13. The diabetic child's diet will be discussed in Chapter 38.

DIABETES IN THE ELDERLY

Glucose tolerance declines with age, so that a large number of elderly patients seem to have diabetes. For this reason several authorities

Table 25–7   AN EXAMPLE OF MEAL PLANNING FOR AN ADULT USING REGULAR
INSULIN OR NO INSULIN

Diet Prescription: Calories, 2140; protein, 110 gm.; fat, 100 gm.; carbohydrate, 200 gm.
The carbohydrates are divided approximately as follows: breakfast, one-third, 67 gm.; lunch, one-third, 67 gm.; dinner, one-third, 69 gm.

FOOD	AMOUNT	LIST	C *(gm.)*	P *(gm.)*	F *(gm.)*
		TOTAL DAY'S FOOD			
Milk, whole	1 pt.	1	24	16	20
Vegetables	2 servings	2	10	4	
Fruits	3 servings	3	30		
Bread exchanges	9 servings	4	135	18	
Meat exchanges (medium-fat)	10 servings	5b		70	55
Fat exchanges	5 servings	6			25
		(total)	199	108	100

SAMPLE MEAL PLAN

		LIST
Breakfast:	Fruit, 1 serving	3
	Bread exchanges: 3 servings	4
	Eggs: 2 or 2 other meat exchanges	5
	Milk: 1 glass (8 oz.)	1
	Butter: 1 level tsp., or 1 other fat exchange	6
	Tea or coffee, as desired	
Lunch:	Meat exchanges: 2 servings	5
	Bread exchanges: 3 servings	4
	Butter: 2 tsp., or 2 other fat exchanges	6
	Vegetables: 1 serving	2
	Fruit: 1 serving	3
	Milk: ½ glass (4 oz.)	1
Dinner:	Meat exchanges: 6 servings	5
	Vegetables: 1 serving	2
	Bread exchanges: 3 servings	4
	Butter: 2 level tsp., or 2 other fat exchanges	6
	Fruit: 1 serving	3
	Milk: ½ glass (4 oz.)	1
	Tea or coffee, as desired	

SAMPLE MENU

Breakfast:	Orange juice	½ cup
	Poached egg on toast	2 2 slices
	Butter	1 tsp.
	Cornflakes	¾ cup
	Milk, whole	6 oz.
	Coffee	As desired
	Evaporated milk	1 oz.
Lunch:	Sandwich:	
	Ham	2 oz.
	Rye bread	2 slices
	Butter	2 tsp.
	Lettuce and tomato salad	
	Apple	1 small
	Graham crackers	2
	Milk, whole	4 oz.
Dinner:	Rib eye steak	6 oz.
	Browned potato	2 (2 in. in diameter)
	Green peas	½ cup
	Muffin	1 (2 in. in diameter)
	Butter	2 tsp.
	Honeydew melon	⅛ (7 in. in diameter)
	Milk, whole	4 oz.
	Tea with lemon	

Table 25–8 AN EXAMPLE OF MEAL PLANNING FOR AN ADULT USING PROTAMINE ZINC INSULIN OR AN INTERMEDIATE-ACTING INSULIN

Diet Prescription: Calories, 2100; proteins, 85 gm., carbohydrates, 250 gm. The carbohydrates and proteins are divided approximately:

MEAL	CARBOHYDRATES *(gm.)*	PROTEINS *(gm.)*
Breakfast	$^1/_5$ 37	$^1/_6$ 17
Lunch	$^2/_5$ 85	$^1/_3$ 24
Dinner	$^2/_5$ 90	$^1/_2$ 43 (including bedtime)
Bedtime feeding	37 (subtracted from total carbohydrates)	

The total day's food is calculated in Table 25–6.

	SAMPLE MENU PLAN	LIST
Breakfast:	Fruit: 1 serving	3
	Bread: 1 serving	4
	Fat: 2 level tsp. or 2 other fat exchanges	6
	Eggs: 1 or other meat exchange (Meat "a" exchange + ½ fat)	5
	Milk (non-fat): 1 glass (8 oz.)	1
	Coffee or tea, as desired	
Lunch:	Meat "a" exchanges: 2 servings	5
	Vegetables: 1 serving	2
	Bread exchanges: 4 servings	4
	Fat: 3 level tsp. or 3 other fat exchanges	6
	Fruit: 2 servings	3
	Tea or coffee, as desired	
Dinner:	Meat "b" exchanges: 2 servings	5
	Vegetables: 2 servings	2
	Bread exchanges: 4 servings	4
	Fat: 4 level tsp. or 4 other fat exchanges	6
	Fruit: 2 servings	3
	Tea or coffee, as desired	
Bedtime: *	Bread exchanges: 1 serving	4
	Fruit: 1 serving	3
	Meat "c" exchanges: 1 serving	5
	Milk (non-fat): 1 glass (8 oz.)	1
	Fat: 2 level tsp. or 2 other fat exchanges	6

*If an intermediate-acting insulin is used, the bedtime feeding may be given in the afternoon (3:30–4:30 P.M.).

	SAMPLE MENU	
Breakfast:	Banana	½ small
	Egg	1 soft boiled
	Toast	1 slice
	Margarine	2 tsp.
	Milk, skim	1 glass (8 oz.)
	Coffee or tea	As desired
Lunch:	Meat balls	2 oz.
	Boiled spaghetti	1½ cup
	Mixed green salad with olive oil and vinegar	2 tsp.
	Blueberries	1 cup
	Plain sponge cake	1½ in. cube
	Margarine	1 tsp.
	Tea or coffee, as desired	
Dinner:	Tomato juice	4 oz.
	Broiled liver	2 oz.
	Crisp bacon	1 slice
	Baked potato, large	1
	Carrots	½ cup
	Whole wheat bread	1 slice
	Margarine	3 tsp.
	Applesauce, without sugar	1 cup
	Graham crackers	2
	Tea or coffee, as desired	
Bedtime:	Bread	1 slice
	Cheese, cheddar	1 oz.
	Mayonnaise	1 tsp.
	Grapes	12
	Milk	1 glass (8 oz.)

argue that different glucose tolerance standards should be used in diagnosing true cases of maturity-onset diabetes in the elderly. Since the relationship between blood glucose control and the development of the debilitating vascular complications of diabetes is still unclear, how to care for the elderly patient becomes questionable.

The long-term effects of oral hypoglycemic agents have already been discussed, and the use of insulin can mark the end of independence for an elderly patient and force him or her into accepting outside supervision or chronic institutionalization. Insulin injections can be hazardous for the nearly blind, forgetful, frightened and unconfident elderly patient. Hypoglycemia is always a danger because the elderly patient may neglect to eat or may give himself a second injection, forgetting that he had already injected himself.

Before treating diabetes, it should be clear to what extent the person is afflicted by it. Foot care education is extremely important in all cases, and dietary control of blood glucose levels should be tried first, before other measures. This change itself may be difficult for the patient and will require a great deal of time and empathy on the part of the clinician.

DIABETES AND SURGERY

If the diabetic patient's condition has been kept under control, he may undergo needed surgery without any unusual risk. When the surgery is an emergency, preoperative preparation is impossible. In emergency surgery cases, the regulation of insulin, intravenous fluids and glucose is begun during the actual operation and carried on after its completion. Frequent urinalyses and necessary insulin injections for a sugar-free urine are carried out.

In elective surgery, it is advisable to plan a preoperative program for the patient, following the same principles suggested for the non-diabetic. To prevent dehydration, large amounts of fluids are administered by mouth or parenterally, especially the day preceding the operation. Additional carbohydrates are prescribed to allow an adequate storage of glycogen, and sufficient insulin is given to enable the patient to oxidize the carbohydrates, thereby guarding against acidosis. Food is permitted until 4 or more hours prior to the operation and resumed as soon as possible postoperatively. The degree of severity of the surgery will help to guide the preoperative and postoperative diet treatment.

To maintain fluid and electrolyte balance, abundant amounts of saline fluids are administered parenterally immediately after the operation. Glucose is usually given in the fluid, with adequate injections of insulin to metabolize the glucose.

Food in liquid form is usually the first type of food permitted orally. After minor surgery, the patient may be given his usual diet immediately. The diet advances in a procedure similar to that described for the non-diabetic. If fruit juices cause gas and bring discomfort to the patient, ginger ale or glucose solution is prescribed. The blood sugar determination and urinalysis govern the amount and type of insulin injections.

DIABETIC DIETS IN EMERGENCIES

Illness

During an illness insulin should still be taken, although caloric intake should be decreased by about 20 per cent, because insulin requirements usually increase during febrile illness. Glucagon levels also increase, which puts the diabetic out of control. The person should be watched for the development of ketoacidosis and treated with insulin accordingly.

Sometimes a diabetic patient may become too ill to eat the foods prescribed. When such a condition occurs, a soft or liquid diet is indicated. It is most important that the calculated carbohydrate allowance be consumed daily even on a limited-calorie diet. If necessary, the protein and fat allowances may be sacrificed and the amounts limited to coincide with the comfort of the patient. (See Table 25-9.)

The advantages of the soft or liquid diet are

Table 25-9   CARBOHYDRATE CONTENT OF SOME FOODS

FOOD	CARBOHYDRATE CONTENT (gm./240 c.c.)
Whole milk	12
Orange juice	24
Coke	20
Ginger ale	21
Other soft drinks	25
Sugar	5/tsp.
Candy bar	22/oz.
Honey	16/tbsp.

that the foods included are easily ingested and digested and contain a limited amount of bulk.

Here are some suggested adjustments that may be made to the prescribed diabetic diet:

1. Fruit juices and ginger ale may be served instead of whole fruits.

2. Cooked cereal may be diluted with the milk allowance in the diet to make a soft gruel, which is usually tolerated by a sick person.

3. Soft cooked cereal may be substituted for the potato or bread included in the diet.

4. Some of the bread and milk allowance can be served as milk toast.

5. Eggs or cottage cheese or both may be substituted for the meat allowed in the diet. Use the eggs for an eggnog or custard and blend with the milk allowed in the diet.

6. The cooked vegetables may be puréed and then diluted with some of the milk allowance in the diet to make a vegetable-milk soup.

Consult the lists of food substitutions and equivalents for diabetics, which will suggest further possibilities.

Diabetic Coma

Uncontrolled diabetes can lead to ketosis followed by ketoacidosis and coma. (See Fig. 25–4.) This *ketoacidosis* occurs when there is an *insulin lack* either through deliberate or unavoidable omission of prescribed insulin injections, an infection or a surgical operation. The increase of glucose in the blood and urine in a controlled diabetic indicates that the patient's metabolism demands additional insulin. If this urgent need is not recognized and the insulin supplied immediately, the patient may go into a diabetic coma.

Ketoacidosis does not usually appear in maturity-onset diabetics because, even though there is not enough effective insulin for proper glucose uptake by the tissues, enough still exists to inhibit excessive fat mobilization and development of ketonemia. For this reason, another less common diabetic coma is seen in adults with maturity-onset diabetes—the *nonketotic hyperosmolar coma*. It has an insidious onset and is frequently seen in adults

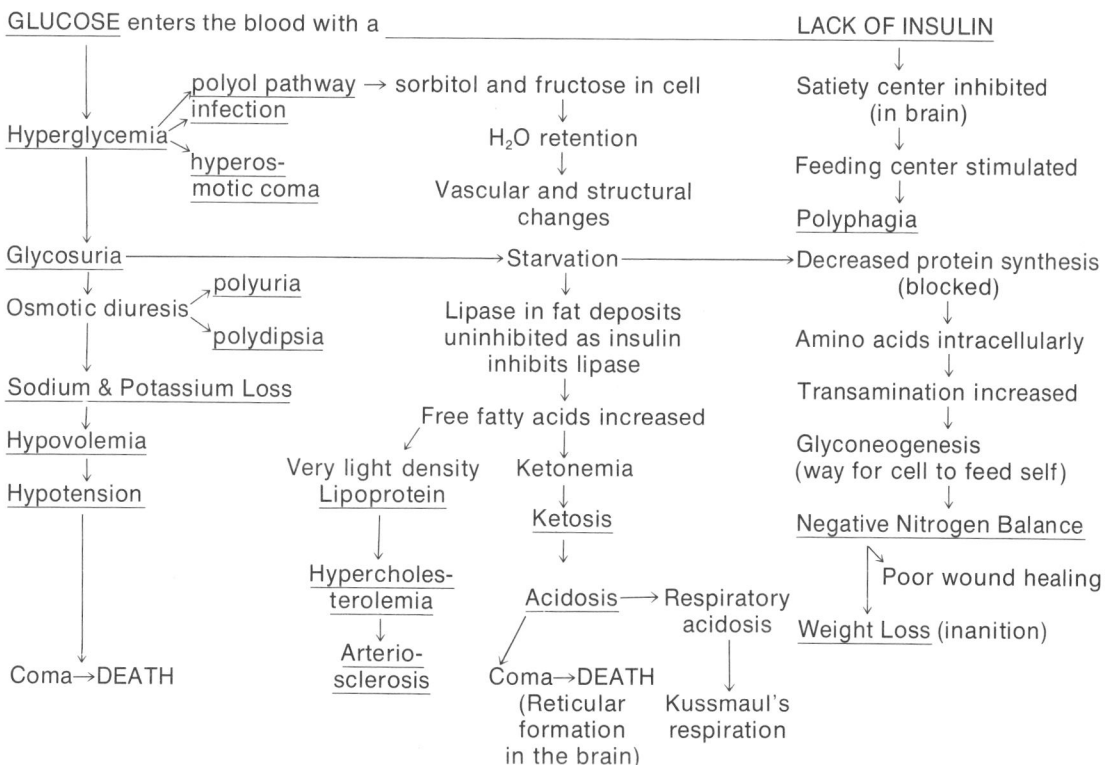

Figure 25–4 Pathophysiology of diabetes mellitus.

with undiagnosed or mild diabetes who experience a precipitating stress, such as acute pancreatitis, myocardial infarction, septicemia or gastroenteritis. The resulting hyperglycemia, 600 to 3000 mg. per 100 ml., leads to a hyperosmolarity and osmotic diuresis. The inevitable consequence is severe dehydration and hypovolemia, leading to compromised renal blood flow and thromboembolic complications and eventually to cerebral dehydration and coma.

A last form of diabetic coma occurs from *lactic acidosis,* but the reason for its association with diabetes is obscure. It is characterized by even greater acidosis and compensatory deep breathing than seen in ketoacidosis. Both hyperosmolar coma and lactic acidosis are variants of ketoacidosis from the point of view of therapy as well as pathophysiology.

The warning symptoms of coma are: thirst and dry mouth, flushed face, progressive drowsiness, nausea, vomiting, abdominal pain, cold and dry skin, characteristic acid breath (ketoacidosis), difficult breathing, headache, dizziness, pain in back and legs and extreme weakness. When one of the symptoms occurs, it may not indicate anything seriously wrong, but when several or all of the symptoms appear, it is cause for alarm. The urine will contain large amounts of sugar.

Treatment. Coma caused by ketoacidosis, hyperglycemic hyperosmolarity or lactic acidosis may prove fatal if not treated promptly and efficiently. Speed in treatment is essential.

The treatment consists of (1) insulin, (2) electrolytes and (3) fluids. Usually regular insulin is given intravenously at least every six hours or by continuous infusion. In severe ketoacidosis, fluid and electrolyte replacement usually requires the intravenous route and consists of normal saline solution and sometimes bicarbonate. As hyperglycemia and glycosuria diminish, 5 per cent glucose is added. If there is no nausea or vomiting, oral replacement may be attempted using salty broth with supplementary water and tea. Later, carbohydrates such as fruit juice (orange juice), ginger ale and skim milk are added. Sufficient sugar must be present for metabolism: about 5 to 8 gm. per kg. of body weight during the first 24 hours, either by mouth or by vein. Intravenous administration should be maintained until oral intake is assured, since one cannot rely on the patient to eat or drink when necessary. The hypoglycemia that could result from the administration of insulin is very dangerous, and the damage could be irreparable. Potassium is

given after 4 to 6 hours, preferably monitored by electrocardiogram; urinary output must be adequate. For the next few days it is desirable to supplement the diet with a B-complex vitamin, because B-complex intake may have been inadequate.

Insulin Reaction (Hypoglycemia)

Insulin reactions occasionally experienced by diabetics result from the sudden decline of the percentage of glucose in the blood—*hypoglycemia.* The early symptoms are usually sweating, impatience, double vision, hunger, pallor, trembling, palpitation, headache, faintness and an "all gone" feeling. Although fleeting, these reactions can be relieved by the immediate consumption of an easily digested carbohydrate such as fruit juice, Life Savers or sugar.

An insulin reaction from regular insulin is rapid and requires immediate recognition and treatment; with a slow-acting insulin the onset is more gradual. When the reaction occurs from protamine zinc insulin, it may be necessary to repeat for several hours the administration of the rapidly absorbed carbohydrate plus a more slowly absorbed food such as crackers and milk. Some diabetologists prefer giving a more slowly digested and absorbed carbohydrate, such as bread, combined with a rapidly digested carbohydrate, such as jam, for a reaction from protamine zinc insulin. When severe reactions result in unconsciousness, the patient receives glucose intravenously or by stomach tube. Assuming that the insulin is given before breakfast, reactions from regular unmodified insulin often occur before lunch (between 3 and 6 hours after injection); reactions from intermediate-acting insulins (globin, NPH, Lente) are apt to occur in the afternoon before the evening meal; and reactions from protamine zinc insulin occur later. Reactions may be caused by an unusual amount of exercise, a delay in eating, the omission of a meal or of the prescribed amount of food, by an error in the administration of an excessive amount of insulin or by a decreased need for insulin.

A more serious type of insulin reaction is one that develops slowly and results from an excessive and continuous overdosage of insulin. The result is not only a lowering of blood sugar but also a depletion of glycogen reserves. Central nervous system involvement finally results, and gastric stasis often is present. In this case the use of oral glucose is futile, and the patient should be given intravenous glucose or gluca-

gon immediately, followed by oral glucose after the person responds to intravenous treatment.

If reactions occur too frequently, the insulin dose should be adjusted to prevent permanent brain damage. Patients taking insulin are advised to carry lump sugar or Life Savers for such emergencies, and to avoid dangerous delays, diabetics should carry cards of identification. More than one staggering diabetic afflicted with an insulin reaction has been shunned as being intoxicated.

Glucagon produced in the alpha cells of the islands of Langerhans may be used in the treatment of hypoglycemic reactions. Subcutaneous injection of 1 or 2 mg. is used. Glucagon stimulates glycogenolysis in the liver, and glucose is released rapidly into the blood stream.

COMPLICATIONS OF DIABETES MELLITUS

Diets for control of diabetes should be designed not merely to avoid signs and symptoms but also to minimize the development of complications. The modern treatment of the diabetic patient has as its primary goal the prevention of vascular degenerative complications. Evidence is accumulating that early control of diabetes can postpone and minimize the onset of such complications as retinopathy, neuropathy, severe atherosclerosis and renal vascular disease.

Degenerative Vascular Complications. The increased life span of the diabetic made possible by improved control of the disease has brought a steady increase in the incidence of vascular complications in these patients. The vascular disease is of two types: arteriosclerosis and microangiopathy. The relationship between diabetes and the vascular diseases is not clear, but it is known that they frequently appear together. *Atherosclerosis* is not specific to diabetes, but it generally develops at an earlier age in diabetics than in non-diabetics and is the major cause of death in patients with maturity-onset diabetes.

Microangiopathy, unique to diabetes, is characterized by a thickening of the capillary basement membrane and accounts for most of the deaths in juvenile-onset diabetics. It has been stated by Siperstein[20] that microangiopathy is seen before clinical symptoms of diabetes and thus is independent of the hyperglycemia and metabolic changes of that disease. This has been the rationale for liberal control of the diabetic patient. Evidence is accumulating, however, that refutes this idea and supports the hypothesis of R. G. Spiro:

The metabolic hypothesis holds that diabetic microangiopathy is a true consequence or "complication" of insulin deficiency. Either the lack of insulin itself or secondary phenomena such as hyperglycemia and/or somatotropin elevation would be responsible for capillary alterations.[21]

There is still no agreed-upon answer to the question of which comes first: the small vessel disease or the metabolic disorder.

To explain the vascular changes and the relationship to hyperglycemia, some diabetologists refer to the *polyol pathway* of glucose metabolism. This insulin-dependent pathway functions in the lens of the eye, in some nerve cells, in the aorta and in capillary tissue of the diabetic with hyperglycemia.[17] Via this pathway, sorbitol and fructose accumulate within the cell, causing an increase in osmotic pressure. In the eye this results in a movement of water into the lens and a disruption of the lens fibers, allowing cataracts to form. A similar process takes place in the aorta and capillaries. Areas of disruption become necrotic and fill with cholesterol, and atherosclerotic plaques develop.

A second possible fate for the excess glucose in the cell is its use for the over-production of saccharide-rich basement membrane and eventual thickening of the membrane—microangiopathy.[21] The diabetic patient should learn about how the disease can affect his circulatory system. Besides involving the eyes, the vascular complications can affect the kidneys (*nephropathy, Kimmelstiel-Wilson syndrome*) and lead to renal failure; the heart and coronary arteries, causing impairment of physical activities; and the limbs (*dermopathy*), which are frequently the site of mild to extreme degeneration of the arteries, resulting in gangrene of one or both legs. Wounds heal slowly, especially in the feet, so the diabetic should take reasonable precautions. *Neuropathy,* or deterioration of nervous tissue, can also develop in the diabetic.

For the diabetic patient with atherosclerosis, a reduction of dietary cholesterol to 200 mg. and moderate reduction of total fat to between 30 and 35 per cent of total calories, with a polyunsaturated to saturated fat ratio of 2:1, is recommended. See dietary management of hyperlipoproteinemia (Chapter 28).

Infections. The diabetic is highly susceptible to infection. Uncontrolled diabetes favors uncontrollable infections. The nurse must be aware of this and be alert to any signs. Usually

an infection will destroy the glucose-insulin homeostasis and put the diabetic "out of control."

Underweight. The diabetic should determine his ideal weight, and try to reach it or maintain it. Overzealous insulin therapy will result in a weight gain as the resulting hypoglycemia triggers an appetite response and increased food consumption. In addition, the diabetic under treatment is not losing as many calories through glucosuria.

Uncontrolled diabetics will often lose weight, especially during the onset of the disease, because of the body's inability to utilize glucose. The underweight condition is more prevalent in diabetic children than in adults. Children have the additional physiological stress of body growth and development. (See Chapter 38 for discussion of diabetes mellitus in children.)

Education of the Patient

Every person with diabetes should know how to calculate and plan his own diet. The patient or a member of his family should be given an opportunity to learn how to do it. If for any reason this is not possible, he should be involved in the planning of a program that he can reasonably follow. Changes in eating habits and dietary pattern are not easily attained, and frequent adjustments are necessary until an acceptable pattern evolves. It is important that the nurse and dietitian recognize when the patient is *ready to learn* about his disease and the management of it. Frequently, when a person realizes that he has diabetes, learning about appropriate diet is the least important focus of his attention. He is likely to be much more concerned about giving himself an insulin injection, and the education regarding his diet may have to wait until a more appropriate time.

The first step in the teaching-learning process is to begin with the patient's customary dietary patterns and eating habits and retain as many of them as possible. (See Chapter 19.) The more familiar he becomes with food values the better he is able to meet changing situations. Timing and spacing of meals, so important in the treatment, should be planned with the person to conform to his lifestyle. The diet and the insulin dosage must be adjusted to the person and not vice versa.

At each follow-up visit to the clinic, hospital or doctor's office, the interview should begin with a determination of the dietary pattern the patient is now following. If there has been a change in weight or abnormal blood and urine tests, or both, the well-informed diabetic usually knows the reason. Many times he needs assistance in adjusting to life's changing conditions.

Standardized diet sheets are seldom applicable to the person's needs. Distributing the sheets and going over them with the person requires little preparation and could be done by a clerk. It is the role of the professional interviewer (dietitian, nurse, physician) to involve the diabetic person in planning his own program. The time thus spent will be rewarding to all concerned.

Most people resist changes in diet. Furthermore, they resist being different from other people. The nurse can help to develop a healthy mental attitude in the patient. Her daily association with the patient at mealtime, during the administering of insulin and during the bath offers an opportunity to help him accept his handicaps. Teaching aids to demonstrate the importance of substituting foods equal in caloric, protein, carbohydrate, fat, mineral and vitamin content should be used. An understanding of the function of foods, the relationship of the diet to health and the purpose of insulin administration, body care and the testing of urine for sugar content will abolish fear.

The diabetic patient requires skillful care and thoughtful guidance to help him gain confidence. The cooperation of the physician, dietitian, nurse and patient is important. If there is failure in the control of the diabetic condition, it may be attributed to the patient's ignorance of the complications and consequences. To the diabetic patient, "knowledge is freedom."

Programs for patients with diabetes are available throughout the United States, sponsored by various health agencies, dietetic associations, hospitals and clinics. The aim is to give practical and continuing education, guidance and support to the diabetic and his family.

The bimonthly magazine published for diabetics by the American Diabetes Association and the paper published by the Association of American Diabetic Educators contain helpful information about the disease, diets and recipes based on the Exchange Lists, plus interesting and pertinent stories.

HYPOGLYCEMIA

Hypoglycemia is not a disease but a symptom of a derangement in carbohydrate metabolism. As mentioned, hypoglycemia may occur in the diabetic person (from not eating or from too much insulin) but may also be caused by other disorders. It is usually defined as a

blood glucose level below 50 mg. per 100 ml. A person may or may not have any symptoms when his blood sugar is this low. Andreasen and Maraspini report a case of symptomless hypoglycemia in which the fasting blood glucose level was 7 mg. per 100 ml.[2] The symptoms of sweating, weakness, hunger, tachycardia and "inward trembling" are produced by a compensatory increase in epinephrine secretion as the body attempts to increase hepatic glycogenolysis to offset the falling blood glucose level. Other non-specific symptoms are headache, blurred vision, mental confusion, incoherent speech, bizarre behavior or convulsions, which usually result from a slow and severe decline in blood sugar.

Basically, hypoglycemia is of two types: that which is present in the fasting state (organic hypoglycemia) and that which is present in the "fed" state. Fasting hypoglycemia is characterized by the development of hypoglycemic symptoms 8 or more hours after a meal. Although fasting hypoglycemia is rare in occurrence, there are several possible causes, some of which are: hypersecretion of insulin due to an insulinoma (tumor of the pancreatic islet beta cells), other endocrine tumors, an endocrine deficiency, overadministration of insulin or sulfonylureas, liver damage or starvation. The treatment for this type of hypoglycemia is to remove the tumor, correct the underlying medical problem or treat the symptoms with diazoxide, which decreases secretion of insulin and elevates blood glucose.

Hypoglycemia in the "fed" state, or reactive hypoglycemia, is caused by intake of food, especially of carbohydrates, in sensitive individuals. Such individuals are those with certain inherited metabolic disorders, gastrojejunostomy dumping syndrome (see Chapter 34) or functional hypoglycemia, a poorly understood disorder.

Functional hypoglycemia, although not rare, has recently been diagnosed in situations where it is not supported by biochemical evidence such as an abnormal glucose tolerance test or a low blood glucose level. Because the symptoms are non-specific and the disease has been popularized in the lay literature, people complaining of periodic tremulousness or weakness are misdiagnosed or led to believe that reactive hypoglycemia is the problem when there may be other emotional or psychological factors involved.[23] With reactive or functional hypoglycemia, the patient usually experiences symptoms within 2 to 4 hours after eating. This peculiar timing is attributed to the rapid absorption of sugar into the circulation even though the carbohydrates are ingested along with the other nutrients. If tests were made at this stage, a marked elevation of the blood sugar would be noted. When the rise in blood sugar occurs, the pancreas is signaled to produce sufficient insulin to utilize the excessive amount. In the healthy person, the pancreas furnishes the correct quantity of insulin, and the blood sugar falls to the normal level. In reactive hypoglycemia, as demonstrated by a 5-hour oral glucose tolerance test (GTT), the initial rise in blood glucose is normal but there is an oversecretion of insulin, which causes the blood glucose to fall to below-normal levels 2 to 4 hours after eating. A reactive hypoglycemia indicative of the early stage of diabetes is characterized by a delay in secretion of insulin, which causes blood sugar to remain high longer and then to fall to hypoglycemic levels several hours after eating. (See Fig. 25–5.)

In summary, the work-up for the patient complaining of hypoglycemia symptoms should include a dietary history to determine the content of the diet and timing of symptoms, a 5-hour glucose tolerance test and a 72-hour fast if the GTT is normal.

Nutritional Care

Surgery to remove the pancreatic tumor is the preferred treatment when a tumor is established definitely as the cause. Some patients refuse to have an operation, and others, with mild symptoms, may prefer to try medical regimens, including diet. The basic principles of the diet treatment for hypoglycemia are focused upon the quick utilization of carbohydrates, which stimulate the islet cells of the pancreas to secrete insulin and draw glucose from the blood. Because the glucose available after the absorption and metabolism of fats and proteins is released into the blood stream evenly and more slowly, causing less stimulation of insulin secretion, a diet rich in proteins and fats and moderate in carbohydrates is recommended.

The diet for hypoglycemia is calculated in a procedure similar to that used to plan the diabetic diet, and the Exchange Lists (Table 25–5) can be used. A diet divided into five or six meals, with a protein in each meal in order to provide a less rapidly available source of glucose, helps maintain blood glucose at a normal level.

The calories for the diet are based upon the patient's normal requirements, and this procedure has been discussed previously. When the total calories are known, the amounts of pro-

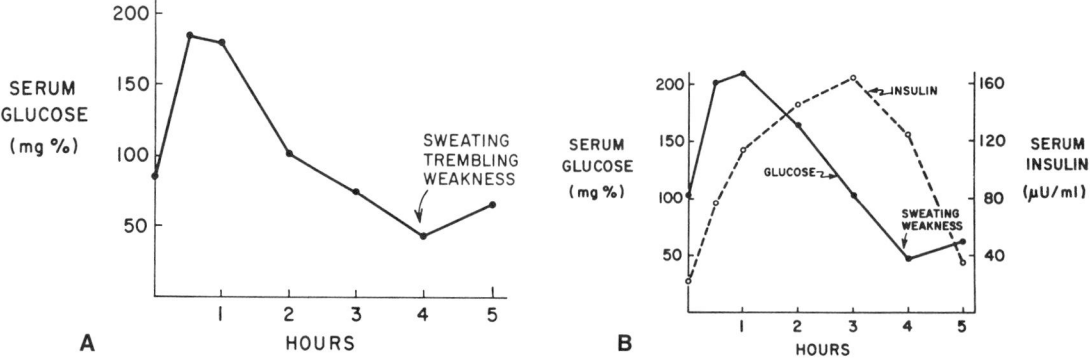

Figure 25–5 (A) Oral glucose tolerance test shows typical reactive hypoglycemia 4 hours after ingestion of glucose. (B) Oral glucose tolerance test shows reactive hypoglycemia in a patient with diabetes mellitus of maturity onset. Note that the blood glucose remains higher longer and then falls precipitously. (From: Crofford, O. B., and Graber, A. L.: Symptomatic hypoglycemia in adults: A protocol for clinical and laboratory evaluation. South. Med. J., 66:74, 1973.)

teins and carbohydrates are determined. A high protein content of 70 to 130 gm. (15 to 20 per cent of calories) is average; and a moderate carbohydrate content of 40 to 45 per cent of calories is the usual range.[1] After deducting these two requirements, the balance of the calories is allotted to fats. Caution must be exercised to prevent the development of any dietary inadequacies. Calcium and riboflavin levels may be very low because of the limited amount of milk permissible on a moderate carbohydrate diet. In such cases it is often advisable to prescribe the necessary calcium and riboflavin by medication as a supplement to the diet.

Since concentrated sweets are rapidly digested and absorbed and stimulate insulin production, sugar, sweetened desserts, jelly, jams, honey, syrups, candy, sweetened fruits, fruits high in carbohydrates and soft drinks are omitted. Fruits, vegetables, breads, cereals and potatoes should make up the carbohydrate in the diet.

Alcohol should be omitted or restricted to one drink per day, since alcohol can potentiate hypoglycemia by blocking gluconeogenesis. Caffeine should also be omitted because it affects blood glucose levels.

PROBLEMS AND SUGGESTED TOPICS FOR DISCUSSION

1. What is diabetes mellitus? Give the possible contributing factors. What tests are used to diagnose the disease?
2. List the symptoms of an untreated diabetic. How can they be controlled?
3. What is the purpose of insulin? Describe the different kinds and point out how they differ.
4. Describe the oral hypoglycemic agents and explain their use in the treatment of diabetes mellitus.

5. Describe diabetic acidosis or ketosis. What is the cause and treatment?
6. What is an insulin reaction? How is it treated?
7. What percentage of *each*—carbohydrate, protein and fat—is possibly metabolized as glucose in the body?
8. Interview a patient with diabetes and show how his present dietary pattern can be modified for diabetic management.
9. Plan the menu guide with the patient, using the Exchange Lists.
10. Check the planned menus for nutritional adequacy.
11. Compare the differences and similarities of chemical regulation and clinical regulation of diabetes mellitus.
12. Study the diabetic diets used in your institution and analyze the characteristics.
13. (a) Calculate a diet for a patient with reactive hypoglycemia containing daily: 180 gm. carbohydrate, 100 gm. protein and 80 gm. fat.
    (b) Determine the total calories.
    (c) Plan a meal pattern.

MANUALS, COOKBOOKS AND SOURCES OF INFORMATION FOR PATIENTS WITH DIABETES

A.D.A. Forecast (published bimonthly) and the A.D.A. Exchange Lists for Meal Planning. American Diabetes Association, Inc., 1 West 48th Street, New York, New York, 10020.

Behrman, Sister M.: A Cookbook for Diabetics. New York, American Diabetes Association, Inc., 1959.

Danowski, T. S.: Diabetes as a Way of Life. New York, Coward-McCann, 1964.

Donahoe, V.: Diabetic Cooking Made Easy. Minneapolis, Burgess Publishing Co., 1976.

Fischer, A. E., and Horstmann, D. L.: A Handbook for the Young Diabetic, 4th ed., New York, Intercontinental Medical Book Corp., 1972.

Gormican, A.: Controlling Diabetes with Diet. Springfield, Illinois, Charles C Thomas, 1971.

Joslin, E. P.: A Diabetic Manual. Philadelphia, Lea & Febiger, 1959.

MacRae, N.: How to Have Your Cake and Eat It Too! Anchorage, Alaska, Alaska Northwest Publishing Co., 1975.

Pollack, H., and Krause, M. V.: Your Diabetes, A Manual for the Patient. New York, Harper and Brothers, 1951.

Rogers, F. L., et al.: Your Diabetes and How to Live with It. Lincoln, Neb., University of Nebraska Press, 1961.

Rosenthal, H., and Rosenthal, J.: Diabetic Care in Pictures, 4th ed. Philadelphia, J. B. Lippincott Company, 1969.

CITED REFERENCES

1. Anderson, J. W., and Herman, R. H.: Effects of carbohydrate restriction on glucose tolerance of normal men and reactive hypoglycemic patients. Am. J. Clin. Nutr., 28:748, 1975.
2. Andreasen, A. T., and Maraspini, C.: Symptomless hypoglycemia. S. Afr. Med. J., 50:1339, 1976.
3. Arker, J. A., Gordon, P., and Roth, J.: Defect in insulin binding to receptors in obese man: Amelioration with calorie restriction. J. Clin. Invest., 55:166, 1975.
4. Cahill, G. F., Etzwiler, D. D., and Freinkel, N.: Control and diabetes. N. Engl. J. Med., 294:1004, 1976.
5. Crofford, O.: Report of the National Commission on Diabetes to the Congress of the United States (DHEW Publication No. NIH 76–1018). Washington, D.C., U.S. Government Printing Office, 1975.
6. Exchange Lists for Meal Planning. American Diabetes Association, Inc., and American Dietetic Association, 1976.
7. Gerich, J. E., et al.: Prevention of human diabetic ketoacidosis by somatostatin: Evidence for an essential role of glucagon. N. Engl. J. Med., 292:985, 1975.
8. Glinsmann, W. H., and Mertz, W.: Effect of trivalent chromium on glucose tolerance. Metabolism, 15:510, 1966.
9. Levine, R. A., Streeten, D. H. P., and Doisy, R. J.: Effects of oral chromium supplementation on glucose tolerance of elderly human subjects. Metabolism, 17:114, 1968.
10. Lundbaek, K., et al.: Diabetes, diabetic angiopathy and growth hormone. Lancet, 2:131, 1970.
11. Lundbaek, K., et al.: The pathogenesis of diabetic angiopathy and growth hormone. Dan. Med. Bull., 18:1, 1971.
12. Maugh, T. H.: Diabetes III: New hormones promise more effective therapy. Science, 188:920, 1975.
13. Miller, G.: Diet and diabetes—A new approach to planning meals. Minn. Med., 55:167, 1972.
14. Pollack, H., and Dolger, H.: Advantages of prozinsulin (protamine zinc insulin) therapy: Dietary suggestions and notes on the management of cases. Ann. Intern. Med., 12:2019, 1939.
15. Power, L.: New approaches to the old problem of diabetes education. J. Nutr. Educ., 5:230, 1973.
16. Quarterman, J., and Florence, E.: Glucose tolerance and plasma levels of FFA and insulin in zinc-deficient rats. Br. J. Nutr., 28:75, 1972.
17. Rosio, E. A., Morrison, A. D., and Winegrad, A. J.: Demonstration of polyol pathway activity in an isolated capillary preparation. Diabetes, 21:330, 1972.
18. Sherwin, R. S., et al.: Glucagon and glucose regulation in normal and diabetic subjects. N. Engl. J. Med., 294:455, 1976.
19. Simpson, N. E.: Heritabilities of liability to diabetes when sex and age of onset are considered. Ann. Hum. Genet., 32:283, 1969.
20. Siperstein, M. D., Unger, R. H., and Madison, L. L.: Studies of muscle capillary basement membrane in normal subjects, diabetic and prediabetic subjects. J. Clin. Invest., 47:1973, 1968.

21. Spiro, R. G.: Search for a biochemical basis of diabetic microangiopathy. Diabetologia, 12:1, 1976.
22. Unger, R. H.: Glucagon and blood sugar. N. Engl. J. Med., 294:1239, 1976.
23. Yager, J., and Young, R. T.: Non-hypoglycemia is an epidemic condition. N. Engl. J. Med., 291:907, 1974.

ADDITIONAL REFERENCES

Bondy, P. K., and Felig, P.: Disorders of carbohydrate metabolism. In: Bondy, P. K., and Rosenberg, L. E. (eds.): Duncan's Diseases of Metabolism, 7th ed. Philadelphia, W. B. Saunders Co., 1974, pp. 246–309.

Cohn, C.: Meal-eating, nibbling and body metabolism. J. Am. Diet. Assoc., 38:433, 1961.

Conn, J. W., and Pek, S.: On spontaneous hypoglycemia. Current Concepts. Kalamazoo, Michigan, The Upjohn Company, 1970.

Danowski, T. S. (ed.): Diabetes Mellitus, Diagnosis and Treatment. New York, American Diabetes Association, 1964.

Joslin, E. P.: A renaissance of the control of diabetes. JAMA, 156:1584, 1954.

Joslin, E. P., et al.: The Treatment of Diabetes Mellitus, 11th ed. Philadelphia, Lea & Febiger, 1969.

Kaufman, M.: Programmed instruction materials on diabetes. J. Am. Diet. Assoc., 46:36, 1965.

Karam, J. H., Grodsky, G. M., and Forsham, P. H.: Excessive insulin response to glucose in obese subjects as measured by immunochemical assay. Diabetes, 12:197, 1963.

Martin, D. B.: Insulin resistance: New insights. N. Engl. J. Med., 294:778, 1976

Maugh, T. M.: Diabetes: Epidemiology suggests a viral connection. Science, 188:347, 1975.

Maugh, T. M.: Diabetes II: Model systems indicate viruses a cause. Science, 188:436, 1975.

Pincus, G., and White, P.: On the inheritance of diabetes mellitus. Am. J. Med. Sci., 186:1, 1933.

Pollack, H.: Dietary management of diabetes mellitus. Am. J. Med., 25:708, 1958.

Pollack, H.: Fat content of the diabetic diet. Diabetes, 9:145, 1960.

Shagan, B. P.: Diabetes in the elderly patient. Med. Clin. North Am., 60:1191, 1976.

Singer, D. L., and Hurvitz, D.: Long-term experience with sulfonylureas and placebo. N. Engl. J. Med., 227:450, 1967.

Skillman, T. G., and Tzagournis, M.: Diabetes Mellitus. Kalamazoo, Michigan, The Upjohn Co., 1973.

Stone, D. B.: A rational approach to diet and diabetes. J. Am. Diet. Assoc., 46:30, 1965.

Tani, G. S., and Hankin, J. H.: A self-learning unit for patients with diabetes. J. Am. Diet. Assoc., 58:331, 1971.

Waiffe, S. O. (ed.): Diabetes Mellitus, 7th ed. Indianapolis, Lilly Research Laboratories, Eli Lilly Company, 1970.

Williams, F. F., et al.: Dietary errors made at home by patients with diabetes. J. Am. Diet. Assoc., 51:19, 1967.

Williams, T. F., et al.: The clinical picture of diabetic control studied in four settings. Am. J. Public Health, 57:441, 1967.

Wilson, J. L., et al.: Controlled versus free diet management of diabetes. JAMA, 147:1526, 1951.

Wolf, S., and Berle, B. B. (eds.): Dilemmas in diabetes. Adv. Exp. Med. Biol., vol. 65. New York, Plenum Press, 1975.

Wood, F. C., and Bierman, E. L.: New concepts in diabetic dietetics. Nutrition Today, 7:4, 1972.

Chapter 26

NUTRITIONAL CARE FOR PATIENTS WITH DISEASES OF THE ADRENAL CORTEX AND THYROID GLAND AND OTHER DISEASES OF METABOLISM

The adrenal cortex and thyroid gland are very potent endocrine glands, and the consequences of their functioning abnormally are extensive. This malfunctioning can affect metabolism and cause nutritional imbalances, loss of body weight control and much discomfort. Fortunately, hormonal replacement therapy is very effective and usually restores the patient to productive and comfortable living. Nutritional care is important to help maintain metabolic balance during the acute phase of the disease and to rehabilitate the patient nutritionally after the hormonal treatment has started.

ADRENAL CORTEX INSUFFICIENCY

Addison's disease is a rare metabolic disorder in which there is an insufficiency of the hormones of the adrenal cortex, either because of an infection such as tuberculosis, a tumor, spontaneous atrophy or atrophy following removal of the pituitary gland in the treatment of cancer (hypophysectomy). The adrenals, two small glands of vital importance, are deeply imbedded in the back tissues near the kidneys. (See Fig. 25–1.) They consist chiefly of two parts. The central portion (medulla) contains cells originating from nerve structures that secrete *epinephrine* and *norepinephrine*. The outer shell (cortex) secretes *aldosterone*, a *mineralocorticoid* that controls water and electrolyte balance; the *glucocorticoids* cortisol (hydrocortisone) and cortisone, which function in gluconeogenesis; and the *androgenic hor-*

mones, which stimulate protein synthesis and the formation of sex hormones.

Mineralocorticoid Deficiency. In Addison's disease the lack of aldosterone decreases sodium reabsorption and allows the excretion of sodium ions, chloride ions and water in the urine in excessive quantities. A greatly decreased extracellular fluid volume results; acidosis develops because of the failure of hydrogen ions to be excreted in exchange for sodium reabsorption; potassium retention is increased and serum potassium rises sharply; blood volume falls and cardiac output decreases. A crisis develops in a few days.

Glucocorticoid Deficiency. In Addison's disease the lack of cortisol secretion makes it impossible for the person to maintain normal blood glucose levels between meals because he cannot synthesize sufficient amounts of glucose by gluconeogenesis. Rapid glycogen depletion occurs and *hypoglycemia* follows. Severe hypoglycemia may be experienced by a person without food for 10 or more hours. Mobilization of fats and protein from tissues is reduced, and many other metabolic functions are depressed. Most people with Addison's disease have a *melanin pigmentation of the skin* of a deep tan or bronze. The cause is believed to be an excessive secretion of melanocyte-stimulating hormone (MSH) by the pituitary to exert an inhibiting effect when the adrenal steroids are lacking. These patients frequently experience abdominal discomfort, diarrhea, nausea, vomiting, anorexia and weight loss. The prognosis for Addison's disease was grave, but modern therapy has improved the outlook.

Treatment

Hormonal. Supplying the missing adrenal cortex hormones to the patient has proved advantageous. Cortisone, cortisol, prednisone or hydroxycortisone is given to meet glucocorticoid needs, and fluorocortisol or desoxycorticosterone is given to meet mineralocorticoid needs. Hormone therapy has enabled the person with adrenocortical insufficiency to lead a normal life, provided the proper medication is taken faithfully.

Nutritional. Hormone replacement therapy causes the release of serum potassium and the retention of salt and water, with the sodium and potassium reaching or approaching a normal concentration level. However, 4 to 6 gm. of additional salt daily is often advised to spare the need for hormones and thus reduce the expense of the treatment. In a few cases, sodium chloride therapy alone is sufficient to relieve the symptoms for years. If electrolyte balance is not thus achieved, then active cortical extracts or aldosterone is given.

Because of the tendency to hypoglycemia and the extreme weakness experienced by patients with Addison's disease, frequent feedings of an adequate diet, high in protein and moderate in carbohydrate—similar to that described under hypoglycemia (Chapter 25)—may be necessary. The individual with Addison's disease must understand the symptoms of hypoglycemia and carry crackers and a protein food (such as cheese) with him to control attacks if they occur frequently. He should have a fairly substantial meal at bedtime in order to prevent an early morning hypoglycemic reaction.

Because the sufferer is frequently dehydrated, a generous intake of fluids is required. Vitamins, particularly ascorbic acid and those of the B-complex that function as components of metabolic enzymes, should be given in liberal amounts to provide for the increased metabolism. A concentrated vitamin supplement may be prescribed. Foods rich in potassium (Appendix Table 9) should be included, along with a potassium supplement, since hormonal therapy tends to cause potassium depletion.

Anorexia is often a symptom of untreated chronic adrenocortical insufficiency, and many such patients will have lost weight. A return to normal weight through dietary management may need to be included in the treatment. See Chapter 27 on underweight.

Prior to the introduction of desoxycorticosterone, dietary treatment consisted of a diet low in potassium and high in sodium, in an attempt to correct the faulty mineral metabolism. Such a diet is difficult to prepare and is not very acceptable to the patient. With present therapy it is not necessary.

ADRENOCORTICOTROPIC HORMONE THERAPY

The steroids of the adrenal cortex and the adrenocorticotropic hormone of the anterior pituitary gland (ACTH), which stimulates the adrenal cortex, are used for the treatment of a variety of disorders. The effect of their long-term usage on metabolism is important to note here.

Therapeutic doses of cortisone may produce hypokalemia, and hypochloremic alkalosis may result. Potassium is provided by an adequate intake of fruits, fruit juices, vegetables, whole-grain cereals, meat and broth.

Protein Metabolism. The administration of a large amount of cortisone may result in a negative nitrogen balance and wasting of muscle tissue. An equilibrium may be maintained with a diet sufficient in calories, high in protein (at least 1 gm. per kg. per day) and liberal in carbohydrate to exert the maximum protein-sparing effect.

Lipid Metabolism. Cortisol increases total body fat, but the mechanisms by which the lipid metabolic changes take place are still unclear. Fat deposition occurs in the face ("moon face"), supraclavicular areas ("buffalo hump") and over the lower cervical vertebrae of the trunk. This can be disconcerting to patients and must be explained to them. Little can be done to prevent this other than regulating the hormonal medication.

Carbohydrate Metabolism. Cortisone therapy stimulates gluconeogenesis. Insensitivity to insulin is manifested, so diabetics taking cortisone require additional insulin. Previously unrecognized latent diabetes often is unmasked in these patients and may become clinical diabetes requiring insulin.

Ascorbic Acid. Considerable amounts of ascorbic acid are present in adrenal tissue. ACTH depletes the adrenal tissue of this vitamin. A supplement of ascorbic acid may be necessary with ACTH therapy.

Other Manifestations. Adrenocortical steroid therapy increases hydrochloric acid secretion. Peptic ulceration may develop and if not treated may result in hemorrhage. Frequent feedings are indicated, along with the use of antacids.

Dietary Management. A diet adequate in calories, high in protein (100 gm.), moderate in carbohydrate (200 to 300 gm., with avoidance of concentrated sugar) and moderate in sodium (2 to 3 gm.) plus an ascorbic acid supplement may be indicated when ACTH therapy is given over an extended period of time.

HYPERTHYROIDISM (EXOPHTHALMIC GOITER, THYROTOXICOSIS, BASEDOW'S DISEASE OR GRAVES' DISEASE)

Hyperthyroidism is a condition in which the thyroid gland is overactive, with a consequent increase in the rate of metabolism. It is thought to be an *autoimmune disorder;* and is much more common in women. Disorder of carbohydrate metabolism (with abnormal blood sugar curves and increased glucose metabolism), increased protein metabolism, calcium imbalance, disorder of creatine metabolism and depressed serum cholesterol are frequently present. There are also changes in the liver and destruction of the muscle tissue. The condition is also referred to as exophthalmic goiter, thyrotoxicosis, Basedow's disease or Graves' disease. In many cases, a partial thyroidectomy is performed. However, even following a successful operation, many symptoms remain. Therefore, the medical treatment is of paramount importance. (See Fig. 26–1.)

Treatment

Medical. Treatment for hyperthyroidism includes one of the following therapies, with the choice depending on the patient's age and extent of disease: (1) administration of antithyroid drugs such as propylthiouracil or methimazole, (2) surgery or (3) radioiodine therapy.

Nutritional. Since in hyperthyroidism all the metabolic processes in the body are accelerated, a high calorie diet is indicated to prevent the destruction of body tissue and a rapid loss of weight.

CALORIES. The increase of calories over normal allowances should be in accordance with the elevation of the metabolic rate. In mild cases the increase may be from 15 to 25 per cent above the normal allowance, while in severe cases an increase of 50 to 75 per cent is re-

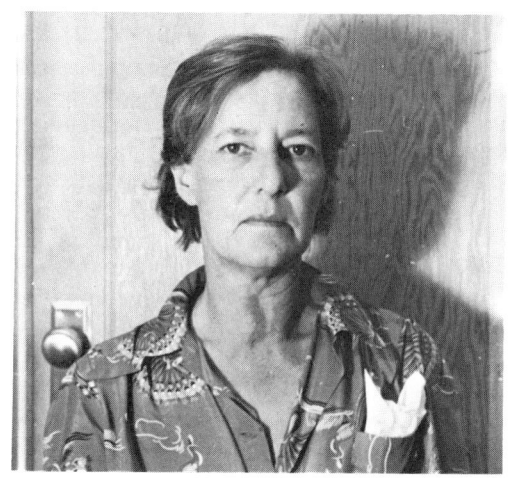

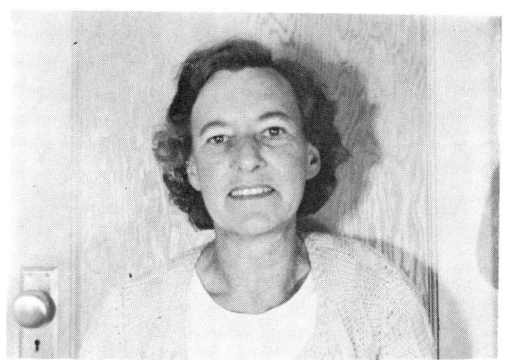

Figure 26–1 Before and after 2½ months of treatment for severe hyperthyroidism (without exophthalmos). An antithyroid drug was administered. Patient was later treated with I^{131} and made a complete recovery despite a stormy course. Note weight loss, enlarged thyroid (goiter) and tense expression before treatment. (Courtesy of Dr. R. H. Hoffman.)

quired. A diet containing 4500 to 5000 kcal. or more is frequently prescribed and consumed, since these patients exhibit a ravenous appetite.

PROTEIN. Hyperthyroidism is characterized by *negative nitrogen balance* and a decrease in muscle mass. Therefore, the protein allowance should be liberal—sufficient to meet the increased need for nitrogen. By supplying sufficient calories through carbohydrates and fats, an allowance of 100 gm. of protein will usually be adequate to maintain nitrogen balance.

CARBOHYDRATE. Carbohydrate intake should be increased to compensate for the disturbance in carbohydrate metabolism and to supply an excellent source of easily assimilated food energy. The increase in carbohydrates will spare the proteins in the diet.

MINERALS AND VITAMINS. The diet should be abundant in all essential food nutrients. Supplements, especially B vitamins, should be a regular part of any diet program to meet the greatly increased demand. The high-calorie diet discussed and outlined in Chapter 27 can be used as a basic diet.

IODINE. Iodine administration plays a significant role in the treatment of Graves' disease. Iodine is an essential component of the thyroid hormone *thyroxine,* the active principle of the thyroid gland. In hyperthyroidism, administration of iodine in large doses (as potassium iodide) will increase the storage of thyroid hormone and prevent its release. Consequently its effects on hyperthyroidism are striking, even if only temporary. It is normally used only for a short period of time in conjunction with antithyroid drugs and before surgery or other therapy.

STIMULANTS. The stimulating effect of tea, coffee, tobacco and alcohol is limited or avoided, as indicated or ordered by the physician.

PSYCHOLOGY OF FEEDING. The psychological aspect of hyperthyroidism is important and should be considered seriously in the dietetic treatment of the condition. When the person is *involved in planning* the dietary regimen, successful adoption of the prescribed amount of food is apt to occur. Physical rest and peace of mind are essential in the successful treatment of these patients.

Diagnostic Test Diet. The *low creatine-creatinine* diet is used sometimes as a test diet for cases of hyperthyroidism and diseases of the muscles. The purpose of the diet is to aid in determining the creatine content of the patient's urine. After lowering the creatine and creatinine in the diet, the measurement of urinary excretion of creatine becomes more helpful as a diagnostic tool. Excretion of creatine in the urine will be above normal in hyperthyroidism.

All meats, meat products, fish, poultry, cranberries, plums, prunes and gelatin are omitted from the regular diet for the day before the 24-hour urine collection. This same diet may be prescribed as a therapeutic diet when indicated.

HYPOTHYROIDISM (MYXEDEMA OR GULL'S DISEASE)

Hypothyroidism is an endocrine condition characterized by the deficient activity and less-ened secretion of *thyroxine* or *triiodothyronine,* or both, which are the thyroid gland hormones. In adults, the medical term for the advanced stage of this difficulty is *myxedema.* In women it is frequently caused by *Hashimoto's thyroiditis.* Often, it develops after treatment for hyperthyroidism. A similar disorder in children, termed *cretinism* or infantile myxedema, develops in fetal life or early infancy if the mother has severe hypothyroidism. (See Fig. 38–7.) It will be discussed in Chapter 38.

In myxedema (Gull's disease), the thyroid undergoes a slow, progressive, specific type of atrophy. The cause is unknown. Symptoms may develop slowly and proceed unrecognized.

Because of the lowered basal metabolic rate (ranging from 15 per cent to 30 per cent, or more), there is rapid increase in weight, elevated blood cholesterol value, cold intolerance, dry skin and lethargy. See Table 26–1 for a list of symptoms. Myxedema is more frequent in the female than the male. (See Fig. 26–2.)

Treatment

Treatment consists of the administration of *thyroid extract,* preferably by mouth, and regulation of the diet. Because most of the patients suffering with myxedema are overweight, a low-calorie diet is indicated. The calories should be reduced in accordance with the low metabolic rate and the degree of overweight. This, combined with the administration of thyroid hormone, should result in a return to normal weight. Principles of calorie reduction are described in Chapter 27.

Because hypothyroidism causes decreased peristalsis, which results in constipation, nu-

Table 26–1 CLINICAL FEATURES OF HYPOTHYROIDISM

Physical and mental slowness; drowsiness
Dry skin and hair
Decreased hearing acuity
Slow thick speech
Decreased appetite
Intolerance to cold
Constipation
Menorrhagia and sterility in menstruating women
Paresthesia of hands and feet
Muscular aching and cramping

All or most of these symptoms and signs may be present in patients with severe hypothyroidism, but only a few are noted in patients with early or mild hypothyroidism.

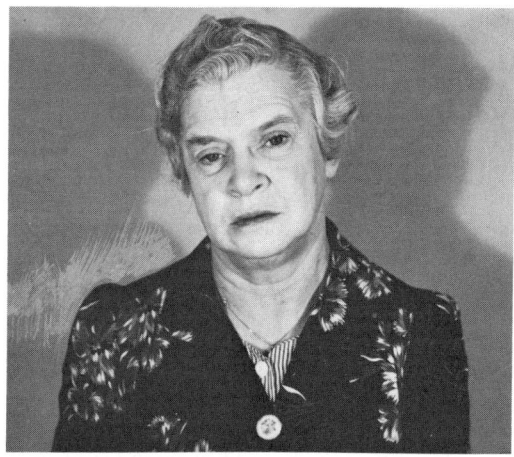

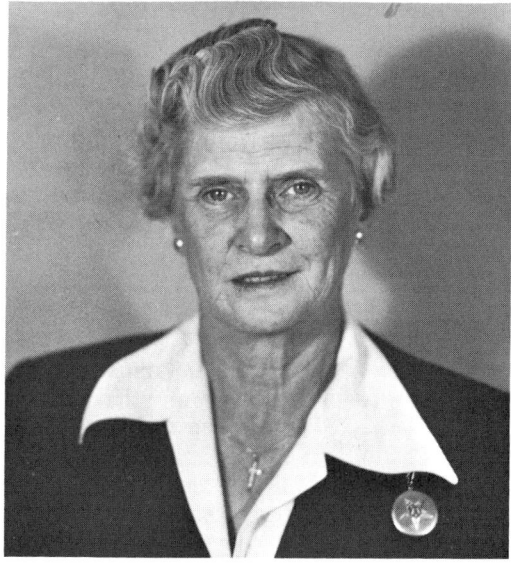

Figure 26–2 Above, severe case of myxedema prior to therapy. Below, same case following adequate thyroid therapy. (Courtesy of Arnold S. Jackson, M.D., Jackson Clinic, Madison, Wisconsin, and JAMA, *165*:122, 1957.)

tritional care during rehabilitation should include serving high-fiber, natural laxative foods such as bran, prunes or apples and encouraging the patient to drink 6 to 8 glasses of water per day. See Table 23–2 for a high fiber diet.

TETANY (SPASMOPHILIA)

Tetany is a condition caused by abnormal calcium metabolism and manifested by *convulsions, cramps* or *muscle twitching*. It is commonly classified as (1) hypocalcemic tetany, the result of parathyroid hypofunction, and (2) alkalosis, the result of vomiting or the ingestion of alkaline salts.

Hypocalcemic tetany (low blood calcium),

most frequently observed in children, is usually associated with rickets, acute infections and gastrointestinal disease. In adults it occurs as a result of injury to the parathyroids during a thyroidectomy, pregnancy, severe gastrointestinal disease, pancreatitis, osteomalacia, kidney disease or hypermagnesemia. A deficiency in the intake or absorption of vitamin D or calcium may also cause the disease.

Nutritional Care

A normal adequate diet, emphasizing the foods rich in calcium and vitamin D, is prescribed, particularly when the blood calcium is low (hypocalcemic tetany). (See Table 7–2 and Appendix Table 7 for foods high in calcium content.) Milk and cheese are excellent sources of calcium, and at least 1 to 1½ qt. of milk should be included in the daily diet. In addition to foods rich in calcium, medicinal calcium is also given, because it is difficult to get large doses of calcium through food alone. Vitamin D is given to promote the absorption and utilization of calcium. Vitamin D–enriched milk is an excellent source of calcium and vitamin D. However, vitamin D intoxication (hypercalcemia) must be watched for. In patients with hypocalcemia due to hypoparathyroidism, supplementation with magnesium may improve the response to vitamin D and calcium.[2]

Tetany occurring from *alkalosis* is treated by administering large doses of an acid-producing salt or hydrochloric acid.

HYPERCALCEMIA

Like hypocalcemia, *hypercalcemia* is a symptom of many disorders: various bone diseases, including carcinoma of the bone, hyperthyroidism, overconsumption of antacids and milk in ulcer therapy (milk-alkali syndrome) or hyperparathyroidism. Some of the symptoms of hypercalcemia (defined as serum calcium levels higher than 5.8 mEq. per liter) and the resulting *hypophosphatemia* (as serum calcium levels increase, serum phosphorus levels decrease) are osteoporosis, kidney stones, nausea, anorexia, constipation, lethargy, and irritability.

Treatment

Hypercalcemia is treated by caring for the underlying disorder. However, in the event that this must be delayed, the following medical therapy is usual.

Fluids. A high fluid intake is encouraged to prevent formation of calcium-containing renal stones.

Sodium. Sodium (usually infused intravenously) promotes renal clearance and excretion of calcium.

Acid-ash Diet. This diet acidifies urine and prevents calcium stone formation. (See Chapter 30.) Prune juice and cranberry juice, for example, result in an acidic urine.

Phosphate. Phosphate promotes deposition of calcium into the skeleton and is used as intravenous therapy in hypercalcemia. Complications of intravenous therapy are metastatic calcification and acute renal failure. They appear less commonly with oral phosphate therapy; however, diarrhea is a common problem with oral therapy.

GOUT

Gout is one of the oldest diseases recorded in medical history. Even Hippocrates mentioned gout in his writings. It is a disorder of purine metabolism, in which an *excess of uric acid* appears in the blood, and the sodium urates are deposited as *tophi* in the small joints and the surrounding tissues; their most common site in chronic gout is the helix of the ear (Fig. 26–3). For some unknown reason, individuals with gout have trouble eliminating uric acid, an end product of *purine* metabolism formed in the breakdown of *nucleoproteins,* chiefly those of animal origin. The normal person eliminates 700 mg. of uric acid daily via the kidneys. The body maintains a reserve pool of at least 1000 mg. in solution in body fluids. In gout, not only is there overproduction of uric acid, so that the amount in the pool increases from 3 to 15 times normal, but excretion is decreased.

Characteristics

The disease resembles arthritis. Sudden pain in the big toe, with the pain continuing up the leg, is characteristic of the disease.

Gout usually occurs after the age of 35 and is characterized by specific heritable metabolic defects. The ailment manifests itself in attacks, which in the beginning may last but a few days and then disappear for a period of months. With the advancement of the disease, the symptoms occur more frequently and are more prolonged. Trivial injury or unaccustomed exertion may encourage the episodes, and questions arise as to whether the attacks are related to excessive eating, drinking and exercise. There are indi-

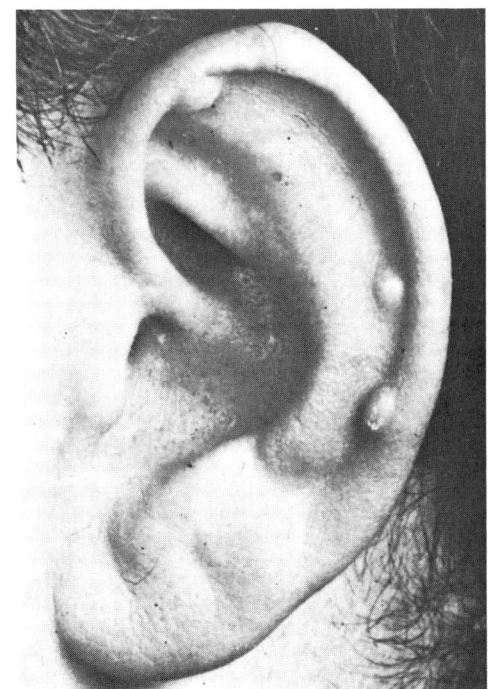

Figure 26–3 Tophi on the ear of a patient who had had gout for many years. (Courtesy of Dr. John H. Talbott. From: Seminar Report, Merck, Sharp and Dohme, Div. of Merck and Co., Inc., Fall 1956.)

vidual food allergies that will bring on an acute attack regardless of the purine content of these foods. Occasionally, the disturbance is a sequel to an operation. Obesity is usually associated with a gouty condition.

Nutritional Care

The emphasis that should be placed on purine restriction in the diet is debatable. Drugs have largely replaced the need for rigid restriction of purine in the diet of patients with gout. From a practical point of view, it is almost impossible to plan a diet devoid of purine, since all foods have some traces of *nucleoprotein* from which purines are derived. However, a number of foods are almost purine-free (Table 26–2). Robinson[3] points out that *exogenous* sources of uric acid can be decreased by a diet eliminating foods high in preformed purine; however, the *endogenous* formation of uric acid is apparently influenced very little by dietary regulation. Purines are synthesized in the body from simple metabolites, which are constantly available from dietary carbohydrate, fat and protein as well as from endogenous purine breakdown. Thus, it is unlikely that avoidance

Table 26–2   FOODS GROUPED ACCORDING
TO PURINE CONTENT

GROUP 1: HIGH PURINE CONTENT
(100 to 1000 mg. of purine nitrogen per 100 gm. of food)

Anchovies	Mackerel
Bouillon	Meat extracts
Brains	Mincemeat
Broth	Mussels
Consommé	Partridge
Goose	Roe
Gravy	Sardines
Heart	Scallops
Herring	Sweetbreads
Kidney	Yeast, baker's and
Liver	brewer's

Foods in this list should be omitted from the diet of patients who have gout (acute and remission stages).

GROUP 2: MODERATE PURINE CONTENT
(9 to 100 mg. of purine nitrogen per 100 gm. of food)

Meat and Fish	
(except those in Group 1):	*Vegetables*
Fish	Asparagus
Poultry	Beans, shell
Meat	Lentils
Shellfish	Mushrooms
	Peas
	Spinach

One serving (2 to 3 oz.) of meat, fish or fowl or 1 serving (½ cup) vegetable from this group is allowed each day or five days a week (depending upon condition) during remissions.

GROUP 3: NEGLIGIBLE PURINE CONTENT

Bread, enriched white and crackers	Fruit
	Gelatin desserts
Butter or fortified margarine (in moderation)	Herbs
	Ice cream
Cake and cookies	Milk
Carbonated beverages	Macaroni products
Cereal beverage	Noodles
Cereals and cereal products (refined and enriched)	Nuts
	Oil
	Olives
Cheese	Pickles
Chocolate	Popcorn
Coffee	Puddings
Condiments	Relishes
Cornbread	Rennet desserts
Cream (in moderation)	Rice
Custard	Salt
Eggs	Sugar and sweets
Fats (in moderation)	Tea
	Vegetables (except those in Group 2)
	Vinegar
	White sauce

Foods included in this group may be used daily.

of foods high in purine content will significantly decrease the uric acid pool. However, since purine metabolism is disturbed, restriction of foods containing *nucleoproteins,* which give rise to purines, is indicated. Excessive use of *fats* should be avoided, since fats are believed to prevent the normal excretion of urates. *Protein* intake should be adequate but not excessive. The calories should be maintained with *carbohydrates,* which have a tendency to increase uric acid excretion.

Acute Stage.   Rigid restriction of foods containing purines is generally recommended in the acute stage of gout so as not to add exogenous purines to the existing high uric acid load. Usually a diet that is relatively high in carbohydrate, moderate in protein and low in fat is indicated. Fluids such as water and fruit juice (up to 3 liters per day) should be forced to assist the excretion of uric acid and to minimize the possibility of calculi formation. Sodium bicarbonate or trisodium citrate can also be given to alkalinize the urine and increase the solubility of uric acid in the urine. Patients with a sodium restriction would require a potassium salt of carbonate or citrate instead.

Interval Stage.   Dietary management during intervals between attacks is used, along with uricosuric drugs (such as probenecid), to achieve negative uric acid balance and control the urate deposits and serum uric acid level. The current dietary treatment for patients who are maintained on medication for gout is a normal adequate diet adjusted so that the patient achieves his or her ideal weight. The diet should be moderate in protein (60 to 70 gm.), increased in carbohydrate and relatively low in fat, and should exclude foods of high purine content such as liver, kidney, sweetbreads, meat extracts, smoked meat, anchovies, sardines and leguminous vegetables. In the majority of patients, further dietary restriction does not seem to be justified. However, in severe or advanced cases, a further restriction of purine intake and the limitation of protein to 50 to 75 gm. daily (in the form of plant and dairy protein products as much as possible) may be helpful. Protein intake is limited because it has been shown that endogenous uric acid biosynthesis may be accelerated in both normal and gouty patients by a high intake of protein. Most of the proteins in the therapeutic diet come from *cheese, eggs and milk, which are low in nucleoproteins.* Fluids should be adjusted to produce a normal urinary output (2000 ml.).

Alcohol.   It is now believed that mild or moderate use of alcohol by the patient with gout will not necessarily induce an acute attack. However, "lactic acid, which appears during the metabolism of ethanol, has a demonstrable effect on the metabolism of uric acid."[1] It results in the renal retention of urate.

Obesity.   It is advisable that the obese pa-

tient reduce and then maintain a body weight that is 10 to 15 per cent below the calculated normal weight. However, weight loss should not be drastic but should occur gradually over a period of several months. A sudden reduction of calories that results in a metabolic state comparable to fasting, with the development of ketonemia, is recognized as a precipitating factor of acute attacks. Weight reduction should be deferred until the serum uric acid concentration has been brought under control.

Low-purine Diet. Foods grouped according to purine content are listed in Table 26–2. The normal diet contains from 600 to 1000 mg. of purines daily. In cases of severe or advanced gout the purine content of the daily diet is restricted to approximately 100 to 150 mg. Fat is kept to 40 per cent of the caloric intake. The diet may be prescribed according to these groupings, allowing for considerable individualization among patients.

LOW-PURINE DIET
Foods Included Daily

Milk: 2 to 3 cups.
Cheese: 1 or 2 oz.
Eggs: 1 or 2.
Lean meat, fish or poultry: 2 to 3 oz.
†*Vegetables:* 4 servings including 1 serving potato, 1 to 2 servings green leafy or yellow variety, 1 serving other vegetable.
Fruit: as desired, including 1 serving citrus fruit.
Bread, cereals and cereal products (enriched): 4 to 6 servings or as desired.
Fat: 2 to 5 servings depending on calorie allowance (see fat exchange list, Table 25–5).
Omit all foods in Group 1, Table 26–2.
Omit for low-fat diets: Pastries, chocolate, nuts, olives, cream, ice cream, cream cheese, whole milk (use skim milk).

Use of Drugs

Most patients require continuous administration of a urate eliminant such as *probenecid* (Benemid) or *sulfinpyrazone*. They decrease the uric acid level in the blood by increasing the elimination of the acid through the kidneys. Another useful drug is *allopurinol,* which inhibits uric acid production. Both probenecid and sulfinpyrazone are frequently used with colchicine. *Colchicine* has proved helpful in re-

SAMPLE MENUS

Remission Stage

Breakfast
    Half grapefruit
    Cream of Wheat with milk and sugar
    Poached egg on toast
    Butter or fortified margarine if allowed
    Coffee with milk and sugar

Lunch or Supper
    Macaroni and cheese
    Lettuce and tomato salad
    Chocolate pudding
    Milk (whole or skim)

Dinner
    2–3 oz. roast beef or hamburger
    Baked potato
    Mashed yellow squash
    Enriched white bread, butter and jelly
    Fruit gelatin dessert and cookie
    Milk (whole or skim)
    Coffee or tea

Bedtime
    Milk or fruit juice

Acute Stage

Breakfast
    Orange juice
    Cream of Wheat with milk and sugar
    Poached egg on toast
    Coffee with milk and sugar

Lunch
    Macaroni and cheese
    Broiled tomato
    Chocolate pudding
    Milk (whole or skim)

Dinner
    Scrambled eggs or jelly omelet
    Baked potato
    Mashed yellow squash
    Enriched white bread and preserves
    Fruit gelatin dessert
    Milk (whole or skim)
    Coffee or tea

Bedtime
    Milk (whole or skim) or fruit juice

Fruit juice and carbonated beverages between meals

lieving the joint pains of gouty arthritis but has no effect on uric acid metabolism. It is of more value during the acute stage but may be needed during symptom-free periods as a preventive. The nutritional effects of long-term colchicine ingestion are discussed in Chapter 21. In some instances, ACTH (adrenocorticotropic hor-

---

*Omit during the acute phase.
†Omit vegetables in Group 2, Table 26–2 in acute phase.

mone) can be used during the acute stage. It is usually given as a single injection.

PROBLEMS AND SUGGESTED TOPICS FOR DISCUSSION

1. (a) Interview a patient with Addison's disease and obtain a diet history.
   (b) Plan with the patient a menu pattern that meets his requirements.
   (c) Check the menu for adequacy of calcium, protein, iron, vitamins and calories.
2. Interview a patient receiving ACTH therapy.
   (a) Note the fat distribution of the person.
   (b) Note whether the person requires insulin.
   (c) Ask if his appetite or diet has changed since beginning ACTH therapy.
3. (a) Interview a patient suffering with Graves' disease and obtain a list of his average daily food intake.
   (b) Has he had any weight changes?
   (c) Estimate the amount of proteins and calories in his daily intake.
   (d) Estimate the *normal* daily calorie and protein requirements for the patient and compare with the estimated intake.
   (e) Determine the patient's *present* daily calorie and protein requirements. What is the percentage of increase in calories over the normal requirements?
   (f) With the patient, plan a diet that will meet his psychological and physiological needs.
   (g) Check the nutritional adequacy of the menus, particularly for minerals and vitamins.
4. (a) Obtain the diet history of a patient suffering with myxedema.
   (b) Determine the patient's *normal* calorie requirements per day.
   (c) Estimate her average calorie intake for the day.
   (d) Determine her *present* daily calorie requirements; then compare with the calculations made for the present calorie intake and normal calorie requirements.
5. What is tetany and how may it be treated?
6. Read the chart of a patient with hypercalcemia.
   (a) Note the cause of the hypercalcemia.
   (b) What kind of therapy is the patient receiving?
7. Interview a chronic gouty patient in the interval stage.
   (a) What are his complaints?
   (b) How much does he weigh?
   (c) Obtain a diet history.
   (d) What recommendations would you make?

CITED REFERENCES

1. Editorial. Ethyl alcohol in the pathogenesis of gout. JAMA, *183*:203, 1963.
2. Potts, J. T., and Deftos, L. J.: Parathyroid hormone, calcitonin, vitamin D, bone and bone mineral metabolism. In: Bondy, P. K., and Rosenberg, L. E. (eds.): Duncan's Diseases of Metabolism, 7th ed. Philadelphia, W. B. Saunders Co., 1974, p. 1374.
3. Robinson, W. D.: Nutrition and joint diseases. JAMA, *166*:253, 1958.

ADDITIONAL REFERENCES

Astwood, E. B.: Management of thyroid disorders. JAMA, *186*:585, 1963.
Bondy, P. K.: The adrenal cortex. In: Bondy, P. K., and Rosenberg, L. E. (eds.): Duncan's Diseases of Metabolism, 7th ed. Philadelphia, W. B. Saunders Co., 1974, pp. 1125–32, 1140–51 and 1156–57.
Clifford, A. J., et al.: Effect of oral purines on serum and urinary uric acid of normal, hyperuricemic and gouty humans. J. Nutr., *106*:428, 1976.
Eisenstein, A. B., and Singh, S.: Hormonal control of nutrient metabolism. In: Goodhart, R. S., and Shils, M. E. (eds.): Modern Nutrition in Health and Disease. Philadelphia, Lea & Febiger, 1973, pp. 457–73.
Jackson, A. S.: Hypothyroidism. JAMA, *165*:121, 1957.
Krane, S. M.: Selected features of the clinical course of hypoparathyroidism. JAMA, *178*:472, 1961.
Kupperman, H. S., and Epstein, J. A.: Oral therapy of adrenal cortical hypofunction. JAMA, *159*:1447, 1955.
Maclachan, M. J., and Rodnan, G. P.: Effects of food, fast and alcohol on serum uric acid and acute attacks of gout. Am. J. Med., *42*:38, 1967.
McConahey, W. M.: Hypothyroidism. Hospital Medicine, *11*:98, 1975.
Murlin, J. R.: Historical background for the nutritional treatment of metabolic diseases. J. Am. Diet. Assoc., *24*:381, 1948.
Review. Relationship between thyroid hormone and vitamin B$_{12}$. Nutr. Rev., *19*:274, 1961.
Talbot, J. H., and Ricketts, A.: Gout and gouty arthritis. Am. J. Nursing, *59*:1405, 1959.
Watkins, E., et al.: Incidence and current management of post-thyroidectomy hypoparathyroidism. JAMA, *182*:140, 1962.

UNIT EIGHT

BALANCE AND IMBALANCE OF BODY WEIGHT

Chapter 27

NUTRITIONAL CARE IN CONDITIONS OF OVERWEIGHT AND UNDERWEIGHT

REGULATION OF ENERGY INTAKE AND BALANCE OF BODY WEIGHT

As mentioned in Chapter 2, the balance between energy intake and energy expenditure is very precise, as evidenced by the fact that most people maintain a body weight with remarkable tenacity. This can be frustrating to the many people who would like to lose weight, maintain a reduced weight or gain weight. How does this system of body weight regulation function in body weight balance? How is weight maintained when food availability or energy expenditure changes?

Because the economy of energy is extremely important to an animal for the maintenance of its life, it is not surprising that something so important as energy balance is under the influence of more than one mechanism or factor. The regulation of energy intake (eating) and expenditure (activity) is the result of the integration of many neural, chemical and hormonal influences. This integration takes place for the most part in the hypothalamus of the brain.

Definitions. Before going further in the discussion of energy balance, some frequently used terms should be defined. *Hunger* is the stimulus, usually unpleasant, that compels a person to seek food and to eat. It is associated with gastric sensations (tenseness, rumbling, a feeling of emptiness), sensations in the mouth and throat (salivation, dryness, emptiness) and, in extreme hunger, sensations in the head (headache, dizziness, faintness).[18] *Appetite,* on the other hand, is a not unpleasant response that causes a person to desire and anticipate food. An appetite can be specific for a certain kind of food. *Satiety* is the sensation accompanying the satisfaction of the desire for food that comes after eating. This is a much vaguer feeling than the opposite one of hunger and has far fewer sensations. Unlike hunger, which builds up slowly, satiety occurs rapidly. *Anorexia* is the absence of a desire for food in a situation when one would normally expect it or in the presence of a physiological need for food. Anorexia is abnormal.

The Hypothalamus in Hunger and Satiety

The hypothalamus is a portion of the brain about 5 to 6 cm. in size that lies at the base of the brain near the brain stem. It is in this small area that the primary regulator of eating activity is located. From studies using animals and

553

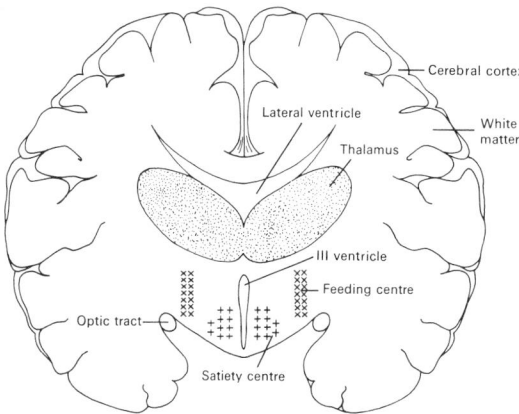

Figure 27–1 Cross-section of the brain indicating the feeding centers below the thalamus (hypothalamic area). (From: Davidson, S., Passmore, R., and Brock, J. F.: Human Nutrition and Dietetics, 6th ed. Baltimore, Williams & Wilkins Co., 1976.)

limited study of human beings, we can now identify the portions of the hypothalamus that are important in this regulation—the *ventromedial hypothalamus (VMH)* and the *lateral hypothalamus (LH)*. (See Figure 27–1.)

In working with the VMH in rats, investigators have found that when lesions are inflicted in this area, the rats become hyperphagic and overeat to the point of obesity. However, when lesions are applied only to the LH, the rats become anorexic and stop eating. From these observations we can now conclude that the VMH is a *"satiety center or system"* that, if destroyed, causes the rat to eat past the point of physiological need to the point of obesity. In contrast, the LH has come to be known as the *"feeding center or system,"* since it seems to be needed to stimulate the animal to eat. This lateral area is also thought to be involved with qualitative aspects of appetite such as taste as well as with thirst regulation. After observing the eating behavior of people who had some part of either the VMH or LH destroyed by an accident or a tumor, similar conclusions can be drawn for humans regarding the body's regulation of eating.

When stimulated, the VMH sends out satiety signals that inhibit the LH, or feeding center, when the organism has had enough to eat. It is believed at present that eating will continue until VMH signals turn off the desire to eat and that signals from the VMH travel through a fiber system to *inhibit LH feeding activity*. We eat because we are no longer satiated, not because we are hungry. The LH system controls feeding behavior, and the VMH regulates it.

satiety → satiety $\overset{+}{\rightarrow}$ VMH $\overset{+}{\rightarrow}$ LH $\overset{-}{\rightarrow}$ stop feeding
        signal

hunger → lack of $\overset{-}{\rightarrow}$ VMH $\overset{-}{\rightarrow}$ LH $\overset{+}{\rightarrow}$ start or continue feeding
        signal

What are the factors that stimulate the VMH so that it is activated to regulate the LH? What registers in the VMH as either hunger or satiety? Let's look first at sensory input.

Sensory Influences. In the study of hunger it was initially thought that a person felt hungry because of hunger contractions in the stomach. However, experience has shown that even when there is complete denervation of the upper gastrointestinal tract there is no interference with the normal maintenance of energy balance. Thus, gastrointestinal signals are not the only regulators but are probably modifiers. We know that there are both *stretch* and *chemoreceptors* in the oropharynx, stomach, liver and intestines that record the distension of the stomach and the presence of food after a meal and relay this information to the brain. This may be a cue for immediate satiety or *short-term regulation*. However, this regulation may not be completely accurate. To illustrate, men given an intake of liquid *before* the test meal reduced their intake of the meal somewhat but not quite enough. They ate more calories than they would have without the preload. The intakes were not isocaloric,[29] which shows that the short-term regulation does not have the precision that long-term weight balance would suggest.

Other sensory stimuli coming from the taste, smell and texture of food are relayed to the cortex of the brain, where they are interpreted on the basis of previous food experiences. They are then channeled through the hypothalamic system and may result in a VMH signal to stop or to continue eating. Interestingly, it has been observed that in experiments administering liquid food through a tube, hunger was not as well satisfied when the food went straight into the stomach as when an equal amount of the food was administered into the mouth. The oral factor seems to play a significant role in subjective satiation.[29] In addition, the person was less comfortable estimating the intake given through the intragastric tube than that given through the mouth tube, even though in neither case had he seen how much had been administered.

Further, *cortical* influences are apparent when we knowingly eat past satiation, such as at a special holiday or celebration. We pur-

posely ignore satiety signals and as a result of conscious effort (although often it doesn't require that much!) eat past the point of fullness. People can continue to eat when they derive pleasure from the sensation. The reverse may be true in unpleasant situations, such as arguments at the dinner table. In summary, many sensory factors, both learned and innate, contribute to feelings of hunger or satiety.

Metabolic Influences. It is postulated that metabolic mechanisms account for the medium-term and long-term control of energy intake and body weight. It is evident from the previous discussion that sensory factors are too variable and would not be able to maintain complete balance by themselves. Several theories of metabolic regulation have been proposed.

GLUCOSTATIC THEORY. This theory, developed by Jean Mayer, is the oldest of the chemical or metabolic mechanisms to be discussed and is useful in attempting to explain *medium-term control,* perhaps the day-to-day rather than the month-to-month or year-to-year control. It states that there are *glucoreceptors* in the VMH and LH and possibly in the liver that are sensitive to the *rate of glucose utilization.* The rate of utilization is measured as an *A/V ratio,* which compares the arterial (A) concentration of glucose with the venous (V) concentration. The higher the ratio, the greater the rate of tissue utilization of glucose. When the ratio is high, the glucoreceptor sends a signal to the VMH that is registered as satiety, and the VMH then sends a signal to the LH, inhibiting its stimulation of feeding behavior. When the ratio is low, the receptor sends a signal to the VMH that is registered as hunger, and the VMH stops sending signals to the LH. The LH, now uninhibited, signals the commencement of feeding behavior. Insulin concentration may also be involved in this system, since it is related to glucose concentration in the blood. (When the rate of glucose utilization is high, blood insulin also is high.) It may also have a direct effect on the brain, since the VMH, unlike the rest of the brain, has been found to be sensitive to insulin. Animals with VMH injury develop hyperinsulinism before they develop obesity. Perhaps the insulin, controlled by the VMH, plays a role in the metabolic changes.[4]

THERMOSTATIC THEORY. It has been observed that mammals make feeding adjustments in response to environmental temperature; that is, they eat more in the cold and less in the heat. This is thought to be due to the presence in the brain of a heat-responsive center (also in the hypothalamus) called the *preop-tic anterior hypothalamus (POAH).* Brobeck states that animals eat to keep warm and stop eating to prevent hyperthermia.[5] When this brain center is destroyed in rats, the animals are observed to overeat in the heat and undereat in the cold.

There may be a relationship between the POAH and the *specific dynamic action (SDA)* of food (see Chapter 2). After eating, the SDA of food causes an increase in metabolism with a resulting increase in heat production. This increase in heat may be registered in the POAH as a satiety signal, which then acts alone or relays this information to the VMH. Miller has shown that *thermogenesis* (heat production) following a meal can differ between obese and non-obese individuals. In persons of normal weight, overeating resulted in a 25 to 50 per cent increase in thermogenesis, which tends to dissipate the excess intake. The increase in thermogenesis observed in obese individuals who overeat was less marked.[19]

AMINOSTATIC THEORY. It has been found that rats will modify their intake to meet their protein requirements. Not only will they eat more of a diet with a lower percentage of protein, but they will also select diets that have balanced amino acid patterns (see Chapter 5). Amino acid–imbalanced diets will decrease the appetite in both animals and humans, as measured by decreased food intake.[11] This effect appears to be related to the plasma concentration of non-essential amino acids and the abnormality of the plasma amino acid pattern produced by the diet. It is possible that plasma amino acid patterns are perceived in the central nervous system.

Since many brain *neurotransmitters* are affected by the supply of amino acids in the blood stream and from the diet, and since many aspects of physiology and behavior are mediated through brain neurotransmitters, it is entirely possible that feeding behavior could also be so influenced.[15] Receptors in the hypothalamus are sensitive to the catecholamines dopamine and norepinephrine, which are neurotransmitters. The VMH has an alpha-noradrenergic excitatory system for feeding, and the LH has a beta-adrenergic system for satiety. The function of these systems is still controversial.[14]

LIPOSTATIC THEORY. This theory attempts to explain a mechanism of *long-term body weight regulation.* There is no significant relationship between food intake and energy expenditure on the same day, but there is significant correlation when subjects are observed for a period of weeks.[9] This theory, attempting to explain this phenomenon, is

based on the assumption that adipose tissue is a distinct anatomical organ. The body has a *"set point"* of adipose reserves or total caloric storage that is individual and that influences the body's intake and metabolism of energy. These caloric stores are "sensed" and regulated so that a constant body weight can be maintained by making changes in energy intake and possibly in absorption, metabolism and expenditures. For instance, when the VMH-lesioned animal referred to earlier overeats, it only does so to a certain point. At the new weight its intake decreases to maintain that weight. Its body determines a new, higher "set point" for adipose reserves, and the rat eats to maintain this higher level but does not continue to gain. When volunteers are force-fed and gain weight, they will stop eating or reduce their daily intake as soon as the force-feeding stops and will return to their normal weights.[27] It is this same principle of a "set point" of adipose or energy reserves that is thought to be active in migratory birds who overeat before flying south. In the late summer and fall they develop a higher "set point" that allows them to build up adipose reserves to provide the energy they will need for the long migration.

How does the body monitor these adipose reserves? *Plasma glycerol concentration* during basal lipolysis correlates with the size of the adipocyte in the adipose tissue. During lipolysis, or fat breakdown, triglyceride is metabolized to fatty acids, which can pass back into the fat cell, but glycerol, which cannot be reused, is released. Most of it is used for gluconeogenesis in the liver. The extent of the gluconeogenesis from glycerol may be registered in the VMH as a measure of adipose stores.[4]

Plasma free fatty acids released from adipose tissue stores may function as another marker of the triglyceride stores in adipose tissue. Plasma free fatty acids increase as the body is deprived of food.

Hormonal Factors. As already mentioned, *insulin* may act indirectly by affecting the rate of glucose utilization, which can be sensed by hypothalamic glucoreceptors, or it may act directly on the hypothalamus.

Glucagon reduces food intake, possibly in an indirect way through its effect of raising peripheral blood glucose levels.

Glucocorticoids in large doses will lead to obesity, and adrenalectomy without glucocorticoid replacement will lead to a decrease in food intake and weight loss.

Thyroid hormone enhances the catabolism

of fat, protein and carbohydrate, with increased lipolysis appearing first.

Growth hormone increases lean body mass and decreases adipose stores.

In short term regulation *CCK-PZ*, a gastrointestinal hormone released into the blood upon the presence of food in the G.I. tract, may also inhibit food intake by registering a satiety signal. There may even be other factors not yet known, possibly hormones.[7]

In summary, the system for energy balance control is flexible and redundant—good qualities for a system that is so important to life. (See Fig. 27–2.) However, the system can vary as a result of environmental and possibly of genetic factors and cause an imbalance: overweight or underweight.

OVERWEIGHT OR OBESITY

In the U.S., by far the most prevalent type of body weight imbalance is excess body weight or obesity. Obesity in the United States is recognized as a medical problem of growing concern. Society has created an abundant food supply while physical activity continues to diminish. Because overweight is definitely detrimental to health and tends to shorten life, it is a public health problem. It is estimated that approximately 30 per cent of the population in the United States is overweight as a result of imbalances between food calorie intake and calorie expenditure, although this depends on how overweight is defined.

Definition. Overweight or obesity is a condition of the body in which there is an excessive deposit of fat. The condition may be either slight (overweight) or gross (obese). A weight that is 10 per cent above the desirable weight in the normal individuals is considered *overweight* and a deviation of 20 per cent above this weight is indicative of *obesity. Morbid obesity* has been defined as 100 lb. (45.4 kg.) above ideal weight.

Social Deviance of Fatness. Unfortunately, almost every facet of our society—advertising, fashion, insurance, employment—stigmatizes the obese or overweight person. A society that is health-conscious and values self-denial labels the overweight as social deviants lacking self-restraint. The overweight person then learns a whole set of self-defeating and self-degrading social responses that serve to perpetuate the image of a social deviant. He or she feels that being fat is "bad" and enters a vi-

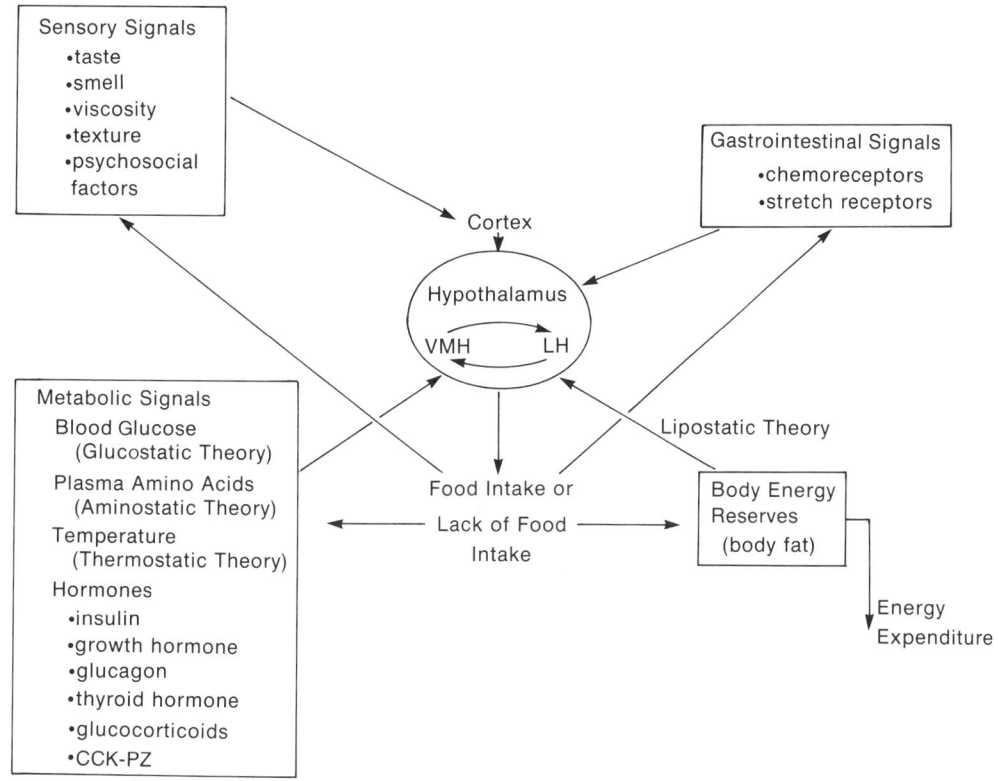

Figure 27-2 Summary of the regulation of energy intake.

cious cycle of low self-esteem, depression, overeating for consolation, increased fatness, social rejection and a further lowering of self-esteem.[10]

Weight reduction cannot be achieved until the person raises his self-image and stops punishing himself. As caring professionals it is important to help in this process and to avoid stigmatizing the overweight person. In fact, for some people it may be much healthier psychologically, emotionally and socially to maintain their present weight and learn to accept it than to struggle to reduce and have to cope with discomfort and guilt when they fail.

Think about how you view the obese individual. Who do you feel is obese? How do you feel when you gain weight? How would you respond to the obese individual who says, "I can't help it, I will always be fat."?

Classification. Obesity is generally accepted to be the result of excess caloric intake over energy output, and it may result from any combination of increased caloric intake or decreased energy expenditure. Obesity may be classified as (1) exogenous or (2) endogenous.

The *exogenous* or alimentary type develops through an excessive food intake and low activity level. *Endogenous* or constitutional obesity is the result of some metabolic or other physiological or psychological disorder.

Heredity. Heredity is believed to influence the endogenous or constitutional type of obesity. Genetic characteristics of heavy bone structure and muscle mass may cause the weight to vary from the "ideal" weight standards. The observations of Seltzer and Mayer[25] that, as a group, obese adolescent girls differ from the non-obese population in morphological features other than their greater adiposity, are of special significance. It would appear that there are constitutional factors operating in the predisposition to obesity. Many authorities do not recognize the endogenous type, believing that overindulgence in food is the basic cause of obesity.

Mayer states that a child has a 10 per cent chance of becoming obese if his parents are of normal weight, a 50 per cent chance if one parent is obese and an 80 per cent chance if both are obese. Generally, it is believed that children of obese parents gain weight because they eat the same foods and are exposed to the same eating habits as their parents, but there probably is a genetically controlled predisposition to the development of obesity as well.

Endocrine Factors. A glandular basis for obesity is uncommon. Obesity may involve a disturbance in the functioning of one or more of the ductless glands, either the thyroid or the pituitary, but usually an excessive food intake is a contributing factor. Endocrine factors may only facilitate the weight imbalance. Correction of the hormonal deficiency does not obviate the need for dietary restriction.

Activity. Overweight is more likely to develop in the inactive person for two reasons. First, the inactive person expends fewer calories each day, which must then be balanced by an intake of fewer calories each day. Second, it appears that energy intake and expenditure can only be balanced by the body when there is moderate activity. At a point of low activity there is, surprisingly, an *increase* in food intake and a gain in body weight. Mayer has observed this both in rats and humans (see Fig. 27–3).[17] This situation has been attributed to decreased glucose utilization due to the low level of activity. Unfortunately, this situation may exist frequently in a country such as ours, where the energy intake is abundant and the energy expenditure can be very low.

The widely accepted reasons for overeating and obesity are summarized as: (1) emotional, when compulsive eating becomes a compensation for emotional and psychological problems; (2) regulatory, when the brain's appetite control center is not functioning properly; and (3) cultural, when parents, family and friends overeat and children learn the same habit (see Fig. 27–4).

Danger of Overweight. Excessive overweight can become a menace to health. If the vitality and functioning of the body are to be kept at a maximum level of efficiency, a normal weight must be maintained.

Statistics show that obesity decreases life expectancy. Only 60 per cent of obese people reach the age of 60, compared with 90 per cent of slim persons. Thirty per cent of the obese reach the age of 70, while 50 per cent of the slim reach 70. The age of 80 is reached by only 10 per cent of the obese, compared with 30 per cent of the thin, a ratio of one to three.

Overweight is often a dangerous complication or the forerunner of another disease. As described in Chapter 25, individuals with a diabetic tendency or whose family history reveals the disease should strive to maintain a normal or slightly below-normal weight. These individuals are considered "potential diabetics" and must avoid obesity in an attempt to

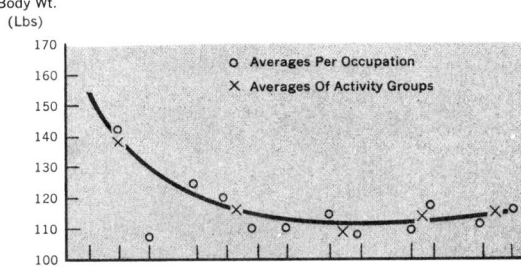

BODY WEIGHT AND CALORIC INTAKE AS A FUNCTION OF PHYSICAL ACTIVITY IN MAN

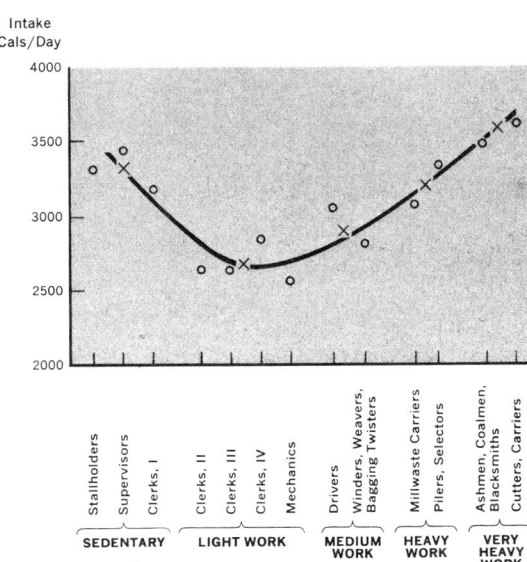

Figure 27–3 In a study done in West Bengal by J. Mayer, the voluntary food intake of 300 workers was studied. Note that the lowest voluntary food intake is seen in workers who engage in light regular activity. Sedentary workers eat more and are much fatter. Workers performing heavy work eat more but their weight is still light. (From: Mayer, J.: Why people get hungry. Nutr. Today, 1:2, 1966.)

prevent or delay the development of the disease. (See Fig. 27–5.)

Obesity encourages circulatory disorders, and patients with cardiovascular disease should maintain a body weight approximately 10 per cent below the computed normal weight to lessen the work of the heart and circulatory system. (See Chapter 28.) Arthritis, gout and nephritis are some of the other diseases in which it is necessary to maintain normal weight. Even without disease symptoms, the obese patient is advised to reduce for optimum health. Years ago a fat person was considered healthy, but present medical knowledge and longevity statistics have proved such beliefs

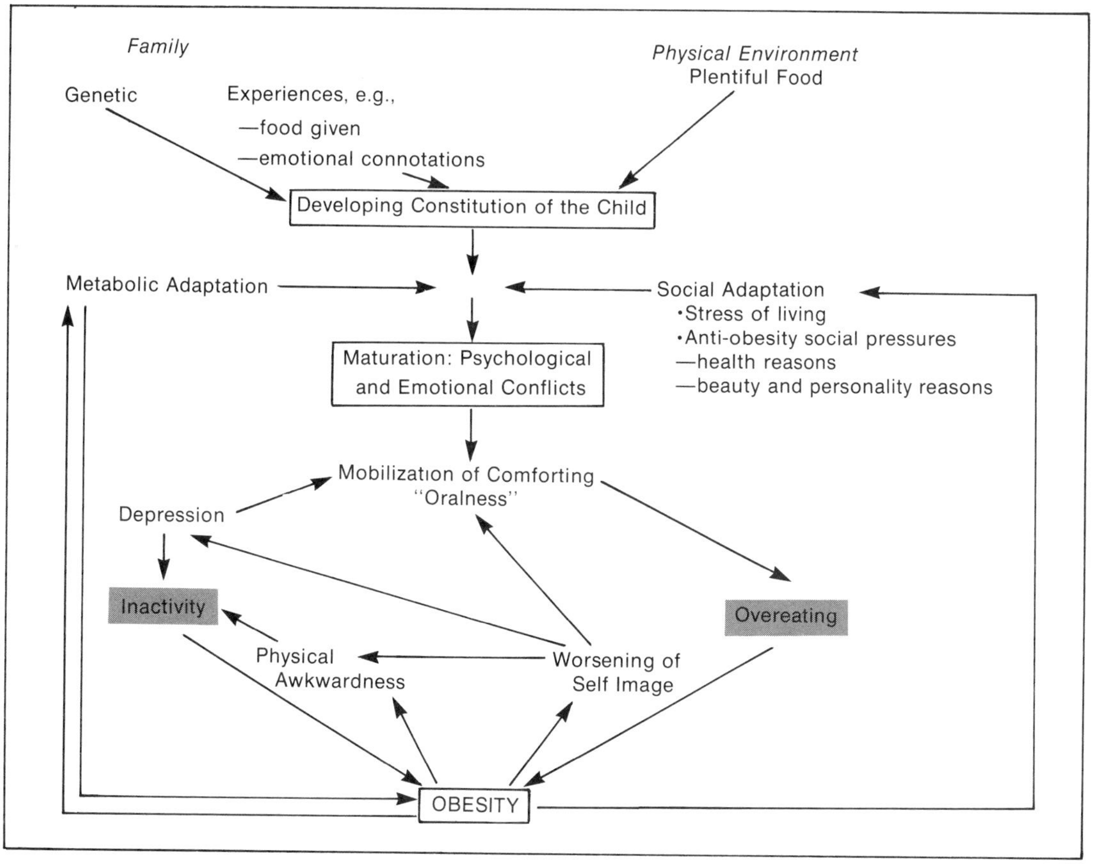

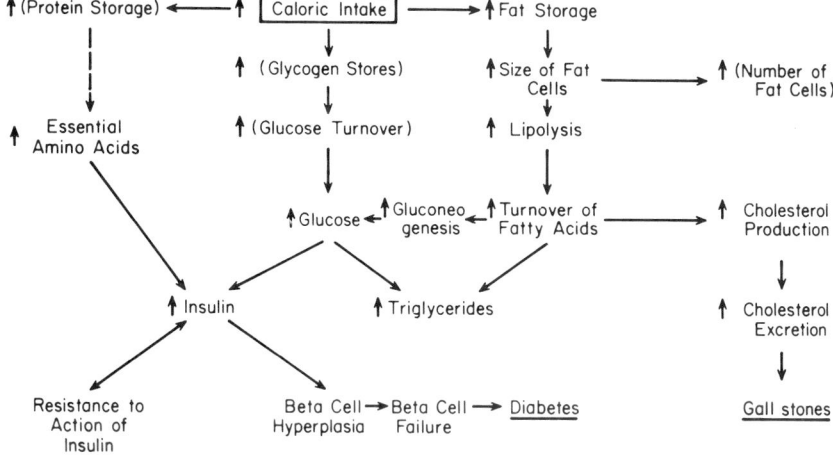

Figure 27–4 The complex network of psychological, emotional and social factors in obesity.

Figure 27–5 A schematic diagram for some of the metabolic consequences of ingesting excess calories. The parentheses and broken lines indicate uncertainty about the proposed metabolic changes. This diagram allows a formulation of the pathogenesis of gallstones and diabetes, two of the major diseases associated with obesity. (From: Bray, G. A.: The Obese Patient. Philadelphia, W. B. Saunders Co., 1976, p. 265.)

false. It is interesting to note that fashion has followed the path of medical knowledge.

Standards of Desirable Weight

A fixed set of desirable weight standards (i.e., weights associated with lowest mortality) based on height and bodily frame (small, medium or large) for women and men aged 25 and over was compiled by the Society of Actuaries (see Appendix Tables 14 and 15). These standards represent data gathered by 26 insurance companies between the years 1935 and 1953. Because of individual variations, the figures given as desirable or normal standards must be used only as a guide. Height-weight standards for children were discussed in Chapter 11. Chapter 2 outlines a rule of thumb for determining ideal body weight.

Body composition is also important in determining the desirable weight of an individual. One measure of variation in body composition is the thickness of subcutaneous fat tissue, determined by calipers. Appendix Table 19 gives the standards developed for triceps skinfold thickness measurements, and Figure 27–6 compares the triceps skinfold of an average-weight and an obese person. Figure 11–5 gives instructions for measuring skinfold thickness. Anthropometric measurements can be used to determine body contour and size of body frame; underwater body weight measures fat content of the body; x-ray shadows measure the fat surrounding organs; and radioactive potassium count measures body leanness.

Physiology of Obesity

Studies reported[12] indicate that human obesity is accompanied by a marked increase in adipose cell number. A decrease in cell size can be achieved by weight loss while cell number remains high. The increase in cell number may be greater when obesity has an early onset than when it begins later in life. It is not yet known whether the stimuli that increase adipose cell number are nutritional, endocrine, behavioral, genetic or some mixture of these.

Accompanying the greater number of fat cells seen in people who have been obese since childhood is the observation that, when these individuals reduce to a lower weight, they experience extreme hunger symptoms equivalent to those seen in starved non-obese people. Possibly the obese person feels hungry during or after reducing because of ever-present "starving" fat cells. Losing weight may not be normal for these people but may put them into a chronic, starvation-like state in which they are genuinely hungry.[21] In other words, their "set point" for body adipose stores may be higher than for normal-weight individuals, so that their bodies constantly try to maintain or regain the "set point" during periods of reduced caloric intake and weight reduction. The obese person has an energy balance but it is at a higher "set point" than normal. The overweight body is just as defensive of its "set point" as is the normal weight body. Further investigations of these theories may lead to a more rational approach to the prevention and treatment of human obesity than is available at present.

Intestinal length, found to be significantly greater in obese people as compared with non-obese subjects, may be another factor in the development of obesity or may be a result of obesity that helps to maintain the obese state. The increased absorptive surface may allow more rapid absorption of food and cause an earlier onset of hunger after eating.[1]

AVERAGE WEIGHT   OBESE

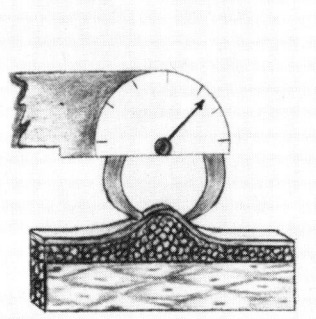
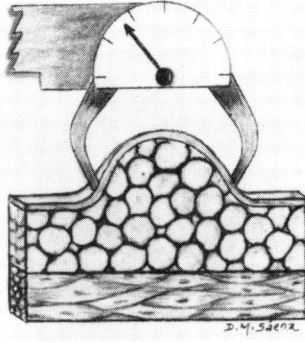

Figure 27–6 Skinfold calipers measure in mm. the thickness of the subcutaneous fat tissue. This gives a rough measurement of adiposity. (Diagram courtesy of Dr. Dorice Czajka-Narins.)

Psychosocial Aspects of Overeating and Obesity

Some overweight individuals eat to satisfy an inner need; gorging overcomes their emotional problems. "Overindulgence in food compensates and substitutes in significant measure for the disagreeable affective elements generated by the intrapsychic conflicts."[26] People who experience frustration, depression, worry, guilt, shame, hopelessness, isolation and unusual stress often seek compensations from eating. To the obese patient, food may represent love, security or satisfaction and provide a means of relieving an ever-present nervous tension. A compulsive pattern becomes established, and frequently the underlying causes are overshadowed by habit and addiction. It is not unusual for individuals to gain weight after giving up cigarette smoking. The gain in weight is actually due to the substitution of eating for smoking and is not related to any alteration in basic metabolic processes. It is common to see a weight change, either a gain or a loss, in people who are having a stressful or traumatic experience in their lives (e.g., divorce, family death, job change or geographic move). Through emotional and psychological factors, stress affects food intake and thus weight balance.

Once established, obesity is sometimes clung to as a defense against social contact. In other instances, the obese person may decide that excessive food and weight are a sign of wealth, prosperity or success in life, which is unrelated to the physiological sense of satiety.

Often there is a conflict between a desire to lose weight and the enjoyment of the attention gained through failing to cooperate with treatment. Usually the causes of obesity are many. An adequate explanation of the physiological and psychological factors influencing excessive appetite awaits further research.

TREATMENT

Dietary

Regardless of the type or cause of obesity, the overweight individual must curtail his food intake. The safest and best way for an individual to lose weight is to adopt a regimen that is adequate in the essential nutrients. During the course of losing weight, the reduction of calorie intake enables the body to deplete its adipose tissue stores.

Fad Diets. Periodically, new diets for weight reduction become popular. Some of these may be followed effectively for short periods, whereas others are nutritionally inadequate. A drastic reduction diet should be followed only with the consent or advice of a physician. In the overanxious desire to lose the pounds that were put on so easily by uncontrolled eating habits, different varieties of reducing diets have been followed indiscreetly. An endless number of low-calorie diets, with emphasis on first one and then another dietary component, with and without special medication, have been proposed, tried, abandoned and resurrected. It is not surprising that the reduction diet is often abused and ridiculed.

A diet that frequently reappears under various names is the no- or low-carbohydrate, high-protein, moderate- or high-fat diet. The diet is meant to put the dieter into a state of ketosis, which supposedly increases the rate of weight loss and may reduce hunger. In fact, followers of these diets do lose weight rapidly during the first week or 10 days because of fluid loss and usually because of calorie restriction. Although the diet does not state that calories are reduced, the average dieter cannot make up the calories normally present as carbohydrate by increasing protein and fat intake and thus naturally reduces calorie intake. The problem usually comes with the return to the normal diet, when the person often regains the lost weight.

Formula Diets. Formula diets for reducing weight come into vogue periodically. They are supplied by pharmaceutical, dairy and food companies and are in liquid, powder or solid (wafers, etc.) form. The recommended daily quantity supplies approximately 900 calories and consists of 20 per cent protein, 30 per cent fat and 50 per cent carbohydrate.

The use of the formula diets is simple, since they require no meal planning and no decisions. However, since weight reduction is usually a long-term procedure, the individual, through the process of change in behavior, strives to adopt better eating habits and an adequate dietary pattern. The change is best accomplished by building the diet around customary foods. Liquid formulas soon become monotonous and are often discarded in favor of another fad. The person will most likely return to previous dietary habits and regain the pounds lost.

Formula diets may be of value in the early treatment of obesity or for those individuals who watch the scales and use formulas occasionally to lose a few pounds, but they should be restricted to a limited period. On the long-term

basis, they may be useful as a substitute for one meal per day. They also have a limited use for patients with a serious medical disorder that requires immediate weight reduction, patients requiring surgery whose obesity poses a hazard or patients who have become discouraged after many futile attempts at dieting. The formula diets are not a panacea for overweight, and the best approach to excessive weight still is a combination of reduced calories and increased exercise, carefully balanced to meet the individual's nutritional needs in terms of his sociological, cultural, economic, physiological and psychological requirements.

Starvation or Fasting. Fasting is a severe treatment for obesity, with quick results that may or may not be lasting. Loss of 4 to 8 lb. in 24 hours in the early days of the fast are not rare. Some of this is water and sodium diuresis, which is usual during the first day or two. As the treatment progresses, the nitrogen loss tends to increase while the loss of salt and water decreases, but the rate of nitrogen excretion finally goes down, and the person maintains a slow, steady nitrogen loss.

Starvation treatment should be given in a hospital under strict medical supervision because severe complications may develop, such as gouty arthritis, normochromic or normocytic anemia and orthostatic hypotension. Individuals with a history of gout or cardiac, renal, cerebral or hepatic disorders are not suitable candidates for this strenuous treatment. Fasting is used chiefly for extremely obese individuals so that normal weight can be achieved in a reasonable length of time. The other advantage of fasting is that the person goes into ketosis, and the high levels of blood ketones can prevent feelings of hunger.

Vitamin supplements are given to meet the recommended allowances. Some physicians allow limited amounts of such low-calorie foods as lettuce, celery and tomatoes, plus black coffee and tea. Other regimens include protein intakes of 40 to 100 gm. (1.3 to 1.5 gm. per kg. ideal body weight) per day to replace muscle and visceral protein that is being metabolized, thus promoting the loss of adipose tissue only. This has been called a protein-sparing modified fast (PSMF).[2] Water intake is liberal (2 liters per day) to prevent dehydration. Normal exercise is encouraged. After the first week, when weight loss is rapid because of fluid loss, the fasting person will lose one third to one half lb. (0.1 to 0.2 kg.) per day, even with an intake of 100 gm. of protein per day.

How effective this method of reducing

weight will prove to be for large numbers of patients over a period of many years remains to be seen. One great difficulty is the need to change eating habits so that weight can be maintained at the new low level. Another point of concern involves lay people who might overextend the starvation period to achieve extra weight loss, thus provoking serious complications.

When a person begins eating after a prolonged fast, the intake should be gradually increased after starting with some carbohydrate-containing liquids. With refeeding there is usually a marked weight gain due to expansion of the fluid space, but a spontaneous diuresis will occur after 10 days to 3 weeks. The caloric intake should be low because the basal metabolic rate (BMR) has decreased during the fast, and the person requires fewer calories. After a while the BMR returns to normal.

The Calorie-restricted Diet Plan

CALORIES. Calorie restriction is a popular method of weight reduction. The number of calories is decreased to the point where excess calories are no longer deposited as fat in the tissues, and the body is forced to draw on some of its own fat stores to meet energy needs. When this stage is reached the individual will lose weight. This is true with any regimen when a reduction in calorie intake occurs. The caloric value of body fat is 3500 kcal. per pound. This is the figure on which weight loss depends. Thus, to lose one pound a week 500 fewer kcal. must be ingested each day.

The number of calories a person ingests can be estimated by determining his basal needs and adding the activity increment. The basal needs for an adult male are estimated to be 1 kcal. per kg. per hr. (see Chapter 2). The estimated activity needs are also listed in Chapter 2. For example, a man engaged in sedentary activity weighing 253 lb. (115 kg.) needs approximately 3000 to 3500 kcal. (12,500 to 14,600 kJ.) to maintain his weight.

$$115 \text{ kg. } (253 \text{ lb.}) \times 1 \times 24 = 2760$$
$$+ \quad \text{activity increment} = 225 \text{ to } 750$$
$$\overline{\text{Total kcal.} = 2985 \text{ to } 3510}$$

His desirable weight for his height and age is 165 lb. (75 kg.). To maintain this weight he needs approximately 2000 to 2200 kcal. (8360 to 9200 kJ.). The difference is 1000 kcal. (4200 kJ.). If he elects to reduce his present intake by 1000 kcal. per day (to lose 2 lb. or 0.9 kg. per week), it would take him about 297

days or approximately 10 months to lose 85 lb. (39 kg.). Looking at weight reduction only in terms of a decrease of a calculated number of calories tends to oversimplify the problems of obesity. Although the method of estimating calories is a good rule of thumb, there may be people who will not lose at the predicted rate. Bray reported a 15 per cent decrease in BMR in obese patients who were put on a severe caloric restriction of 450 kcal. per day.[3] There may be other physiological changes that help the obese person maintain his current weight even in the presence of caloric restriction.

If a person is currently consuming 4000 kcal. and his work includes a great deal of activity, then a reduction diet of 2000 to 3000 kcal. could be instituted at first and later reduced to the number of calories that will maintain weight loss.

PROTEIN. Protein in the diet is kept at the maximum amount permitted by the regimen. Frequently the protein ranges from 0.8 gm. to 1.5 gm. or more per kg. of ideal body weight. Animal protein foods such as eggs, milk and meats have high satiety value. In contrast, carbohydrate foods such as fruits and vegetables are emptied quickly from the stomach. A person gets hungry about two hours after ingestion of a meal composed largely of carbohydrate foods. From a socioeconomic viewpoint, however, a high-protein diet is not always practical.

CARBOHYDRATES AND FATS. After the protein allowance is determined, the remaining calories in the diet are divided between carbohydrates and fats.

The apparent superiority of low-calorie diets composed chiefly of protein and fat as compared with the usual protein-carbohydrate low-calorie diets has been reported.[32] Subjects maintain that fats eliminate the hunger and fatigue commonly experienced when fat is greatly limited. The efficacy of such diets has been attributed to the fact that no change in basal metabolic rate occurs on the low-calorie fat-protein diet. When the same number of calories is provided by a carbohydrate-protein diet, however, there appears to be a compensatory drop in the basal metabolic rate that apparently allows the body to adapt to the lowered calorie intake, preventing any significant weight loss.

Others disagree and feel that the relative composition of the diet in terms of protein, fat and carbohydrate and the timing of meals are of little long-range consequence. Weight loss occurs when there is a deficit of calories.[30]

MEAL FREQUENCY. Even though rats given infrequent access to food became heavier than rats allowed to nibble unrestrictedly, there is still controversy regarding the implications of these findings for weight maintenance or weight reduction in human beings. The evidence suggests that frequent small meals result in decreased lipogenesis, lowered blood cholesterol levels and improved glucose tolerance; however, the meaning of this for weight maintenance is still obscure.[31] After a period of several weeks for metabolic adaptation, some people may be able to lose weight on a regimen of many low-calorie meals even though they could not reduce on a regimen that contained the same number of kcal. in three or fewer meals per day.

MINERALS AND VITAMINS. The foods selected for the diet should supply an adequate amount of minerals and vitamins. If the diet has an extremely low caloric value (800 kcal.), vitamin and mineral supplements are necessary.

WATER BALANCE. When a person reduces his calorie intake drastically he may experience a large weight loss during the first week. This is due to loss of water.

However, during the period of weight reduction there may be a week or 10 days when a plateau is reached and no weight loss is experienced. The body reconstitutes the early large fluid loss. During this time the patient may lose large amounts of adipose body tissue before he shows a reduction in weight.

Because water weighs more than fat, the scales may show a gain in the patient's weight during the period of fluid retention. However, water intake is not restricted in the diet unless complications occur. In such cases, salt (sodium) is also restricted to allow the release of fluids from the tissues and to avoid thirst. Weight gain can be deceptive because of the water retention. After a period of no loss or a gain due to fluid balance, the patient will usually experience a sudden substantial weight reduction. It is very helpful if this is explained to patients, who often become discouraged.

FOODS TO INCLUDE. The calorie-restricted diet plan is basically the same as any well-balanced normal diet. To be certain that it meets the standards for adequate nutrition, the protective foods are included (Chapter 10 and Table 10–4). The lower the calorie intake, the more necessary it is to eat a diet of high quality. When the food intake is large, there is greater probability of obtaining all necessary nutrients. When the intake is low, food choices become

important. To increase satisfaction, sufficient bulk should be included. Amounts and kinds of the person's customary foods are adjusted for weight loss. A faulty diet program would result in the development of a nutritional deficiency.

Sample Low-calorie Diets. Examples of two low-calories diets are given in Tables 27–1 and 27–2. Both provide 1200 kcal. and 80 to 85 gm. of protein. The first is a low-fat (30 gm.), moderate-carbohydrate (150 gm.) diet for an adult. The second example for an adult has a

moderate fat (55 gm.) and low carbohydrate (100 gm.) content.

Caloric Value of Foods. The caloric value of foods varies within specific limits. Fats offer the highest caloric value. Protein and carbohydrates contain less than half as many calories as the same number of grams of fat. Butter, margarine, oil, bacon and mayonnaise are examples of foods that are primarily fat. Meats, eggs, milk and cheese are protein foods. Fruits and vegetables are composed chiefly of carbo-

Table 27–1　1200 KCAL. DIET FOR AN ADULT (HIGH PROTEIN, LOW FAT, MODERATE CARBOHYDRATE)

Diet Prescription: Kcal., 1200; protein, 85 gm.; fat, 30 gm.; carbohydrate, 150 gm. Calculation based on Food Exchange Lists, Chapter 25. All diets are calculated with a leeway of 3 to 5 gm. above or below the diet order.

FOOD	FOOD EXCHANGES (no.)	LIST[b]	CARBO-HYDRATE (gm.)	PROTEIN (gm.)	FAT (gm.)
Milk, skim	2	1	24	16	—
Vegetables	2	2	10	4	
Fruits	4	3	40		
Bread	5	4	75	10	
Meat,[a] lean	8	5		56	24
Fat	1	6			5
			Totals　149	86	29

SAMPLE MEAL PLAN

Breakfast — List
Fruit, 1 exchange — 3
Bread, 2 exchanges — 4
Meat, lean, 2 exchanges — 5
Milk, skim, 1 exchange — 1

Lunch or Supper
Vegetables, 1 exchange — 2
Bread, 2 exchanges — 4
Meat, lean, 3 exchanges — 5
Fruit, 1 exchange — 3
Milk, skim, 1 exchange — 1

Dinner or Supper
Meat, lean, 3 exchanges — 5
Vegetable, 1 exchange — 2
Bread, 1 exchange — 4
Fat, 1 exchange — 6
Fruit, 2 exchanges — 3

SAMPLE MENU

Breakfast	*Lunch*	*Dinner*
½ grapefruit (small)	5 small oysters with catsup and horseradish	Bouillon
½ cup plain cottage cheese	Sandwich:	1 parsley potato
2 slices whole-wheat toast	2 slices rye bread	(2 in. diameter)
1 glass (8 oz.) skim milk	2 oz. cold sliced tongue	3 oz. roast veal, lean
Coffee or tea as desired	2 stalks celery	½ cup peas and carrots
	1 carrot	1 tsp. mayonnaise
	1 peach (medium)	1 cup applesauce
	1 glass (8 oz.) skim	(unsweetened)
	buttermilk	Tea or coffee as desired

[a]Lean meat with visible fat removed is used, reducing the fat content from 5 to 3 gm. per Meat Exchange. Limit eggs to 1 per day and omit peanut butter.
[b]From Exchange lists, Table 25–5.

Table 27–2 1200 KCAL. DIET FOR AN ADULT (HIGH PROTEIN, MODERATE FAT, LOW CARBOHYDRATE)

Diet Prescription: *Kcal., 1200; protein, 85 gm.; fat, 50 gm.; carbohydrate, 100 gm. Calculation based on Food Exchange Lists, Chapter 25. All diets are calculated with a leeway of 3 to 5 gm. above or below the diet order.*

FOOD	FOOD EXCHANGES (no.)	LIST[b]	CARBO-HYDRATE (gm.)	PROTEIN (gm.)	FAT (gm.)
Milk, skim[a]	2	1	24	16	
Vegetables	3	2	15	6	
Fruit	3	3	30		
Bread	2	4	30	4	
Meat, lean	9	5		63	27
Fat	5	6			25
			Totals 99	89	52

SAMPLE MEAL PLAN

	List
Breakfast	
Fruit, 1 exchange	3
Bread, 1 exchange	4
Meat, 2 exchanges	5
Milk, skim, 1 cup (8 oz.)	1
Fat, 1 exchange	6
Coffee	
Lunch or Supper	
Meat, 3 exchanges	5
Vegetables, 1 exchange	2
Fat, 2 exchanges	6
Fruit, 1 exchange	3
Milk, skim, 1 cup (8 oz.)	1
Dinner	
Meat, 4 exchanges	5
Bread, 1 exchange	4
Vegetable, 2 exchanges	2
Fruit, 1 exchange	3
Fat, 2 exchanges	6
Tea or Coffee	

SAMPLE MENU

Breakfast	*Lunch*	*Dinner*
½ cup orange juice	3 oz. broiled halibut	4 oz. lean roast beef
2 eggs (omit 1 tsp. fat)	½ cup cooked turnip greens	½ cup cooked rice
1 slice whole-wheat toast	Dried prunes, 2	½ cup baked winter squash
8 oz. skim milk	2 tsp. butter	Mixed green salad
Coffee or tea as desired	1 glass (8 oz.) skim milk	with 1 tsp. oil and vinegar
		1 tsp. butter
		Strawberries (1 cup)
		Tea or coffee

[a] If whole milk is used, substitute 6 oz. lean meat with visible fat removed for 6 Meat Exchanges allowed.
[b] From Exchange lists, Table 25–5.

hydrates. Food values were discussed in Chapter 25 and may be found in Appendix Tables 1 and 2.

The calculation figures for the low-calorie diets in Tables 27–1 and 27–2 are based upon the Food Exchange Lists in Chapter 25. However, the nutritive value of specific foods varies. For example, apples vary from 12 to 35 per cent in their carbohydrate content, depending upon the kind and the conditions of growth.

In the nutritive analysis of an apple, most authorities list the average carbohydrate content as 15 per cent. The cited example is applicable to many foods. Some of the foods listed in the tables have been analyzed in the uncooked form, while in reality cooked foods are eaten. The method of cooking may reduce the caloric value as much as 50 per cent. Usually these variations may be discounted.

ALCOHOL. Alcohol is relatively high in

calorie content. One gm. of alcohol yields about 7 calories or 200 kcal. per oz.—almost as much as fat. In addition, sugar or some form of carbohydrate (such as Coke or ginger ale) is frequently added to alcoholic beverages, and they are often taken along with a snack (see Appendix Table 3).

A pint of beer (4 per cent alcohol) yields about 200 kcal.; a 4 oz. glass of wine (10 per cent alcohol) has about 75 kcal. and 1 oz. of distilled liquor, such as whiskey, brandy, gin or rum, yields from 75 to 80 kcal. See Table 2–1 for a method of calculating the caloric content of liquor.

One martini has about the same number of calories as 2½ slices of bread (a bread slice averages 60 to 75 kcal.). One whiskey highball has the same number of calories as 6 tsp. of sugar and an old fashioned contains the same number of calories as 6 tbsp. of cream. Add potato chips at the rate of 100 kcal. for 8 to 10 of them; or peanuts, around 50 kcal. for 10; or almonds at 100 kcal. to the dozen, and one has a very calorically expensive cocktail hour.

SNACK FOODS AND BEVERAGES. In Appendix Table 3 is a list of other foods and beverages commonly consumed between meals. This table is included for the purpose of showing how easy it is to add calories, especially "empty" calories, to a day's intake. A few snacks taken during the day can equal or exceed the entire day's calorie allowance.

FOODS ALLOWED AS DESIRED. Foods that have little or no caloric value and can be taken in unrestricted amounts by diabetic and obese patients, unless the diet order specifies to the contrary, are listed in Table 25–5.

ACTIVITY EQUIVALENTS OF FOOD CALORIES. The energy equivalents of various activities in relation to energy value of common foods are shown in Table 27–3.

Psychology of Weight Reduction. The overweight person first of all must be aware that he needs to lose weight. Many times attention to the need is given in the hospital or in the physician's office. In the hospital the patient is introduced to the regimen through the meals served to him. In the physician's office most likely he is given a diet list to follow.

It is of utmost importance to utilize the principles of learning in assisting patients with the dietary program to lose weight. The plan is individualized to his needs and in terms of how he perceives his task and is developed from the dietary history.

The person may be *aware* of his need to change but not interested in losing weight. One who is *interested* in losing weight is usually ready to learn how the task can be achieved. He *evaluates* possible solutions and becomes involved in planning his regimen. He then gives the plan a *trial*. Satisfaction may or may not occur and adjustments are necessary before complete satisfaction with the program and its adoption take place. These are the stages[6] that an individual undergoes to change former eating habits and dietary patterns. Some people do not progress beyond the awareness stage. They may "go on diets" but never become involved in a change of eating habits and dietary pattern.

Eating habits are acquired. The person who is overweight, regardless of age, in most instances has poor food habits. If the past food habits have caused overweight, then the patient must change eating habits and not just restrict calories for a limited period of time.

The overweight patient should be reminded that it took time to accumulate the excessive weight and that the effective changes occur gradually. He should understand the reasons for losing weight and become familiar with the role of food and food habits. Good habits acquired during weight reduction should be those that can be continued for an indefinite time. The best motivating force to reach and maintain desired weight is the possibility of improved health, appearance and efficiency. The person's motivation and ability to bring about change in food habits and avoid returning to former habits and obesity means success.

The process of re-education on the part of the individual is difficult. He has to make the necessary changes and adopt a pattern that he can reasonably follow. The greatest hurdle for the patient is to lose the first few of the accumulated pounds. The task seems quite hopeless if the excessive weight amounts to 70 to 80 or more pounds. Even for those individuals, the loss of 3 to 5 pounds will arouse enthusiasm and encourage them to continue to reach the goal.

The correction of obesity poses dual problems: (1) the balance between calorie intake and energy expenditure and (2) the dependence upon food for satisfaction. Attempts at weight reduction are futile if a large share of food—and satisfaction—is denied and there is no compensatory replacement. Attention to other activities (away from eating) helps some individuals. (See Table 32–3.)

Aids to Dietary Treatment. The essence of weight reduction is decreased caloric intake. Various indirect approaches have been popularized. These include administration of

Table 27-3 ENERGY EQUIVALENTS OF FOOD CALORIES EXPRESSED
IN MINUTES OF ACTIVITY*

FOOD	CALORIES	ACTIVITY				
		Walking[a] *(min.)*	*Riding Bicycle*[b] *(min.)*	*Swimming*[c] *(min.)*	*Running*[d] *(min.)*	*Reclining*[e] *(min.)*
Apple, large	101	19	12	9	5	78
Bacon, 2 strips	96	18	12	9	5	74
Banana, small	88	17	11	8	4	68
Beans, green, 1 c.	27	5	3	2	1	21
Beer, 1 glass	114	22	14	10	6	88
Bread and butter	78	15	10	7	4	60
Cake, 1/12, 2-layer	356	68	43	32	18	274
Carbonated beverage, 1 glass	106	20	13	9	5	82
Carrot, raw	42	8	5	4	2	32
Cereal, dry, 1/2 c., with milk and sugar	200	38	24	18	10	154
Cheese, cottage, 1 tbsp.	27	5	3	2	1	21
Cheese, Cheddar, 1 oz.	111	21	14	10	6	85
Chicken, fried, 1/2 breast	232	45	28	21	12	178
Chicken, TV dinner	542	104	66	48	28	417
Cookie, plain, 148/lb.	15	3	2	1	1	12
Cookie, chocolate chip	51	10	6	5	3	39
Doughnut	151	29	18	13	8	116
Egg, fried	110	21	13	10	6	85
Egg, boiled	77	15	9	7	4	59
French dressing, 1 tbsp.	59	11	7	5	3	45
Halibut steak, 1/4 lb.	205	39	25	18	11	158
Ham, 2 slices	167	32	20	15	9	128
Ice cream, 1/6 qt.	193	37	24	17	10	148
Ice cream soda	255	49	31	23	13	196
Ice milk, 1/6 qt.	144	28	18	13	7	111
Gelatin, with cream	117	23	14	10	6	90
Malted milk shake	502	97	61	45	26	386
Mayonnaise, 1 tbsp.	92	18	11	8	5	71
Milk, 1 glass	166	32	20	15	9	128
Milk, skim, 1 glass	81	16	10	7	4	62
Milk shake	421	81	51	38	22	324
Orange, medium	68	13	8	6	4	52
Orange juice, 1 glass	120	23	15	11	6	92
Pancake with syrup	124	24	15	11	6	95
Peach, medium	46	9	6	4	2	35
Peas, green, 1/2 c.	56	11	7	5	3	43
Pie, apple, 1/6	377	73	46	34	19	290
Pie, raisin, 1/6	437	84	53	39	23	336
Pizza, cheese, 1/8	180	35	22	16	9	138
Pork chop, loin	314	60	38	28	16	242
Potato chips, 1 serving	108	21	13	10	6	83
Sandwiches						
Club	590	113	72	53	30	454
Hamburger	350	67	43	31	18	269
Roast beef with gravy	430	83	52	38	22	331
Tuna fish salad	278	53	34	25	14	214
Sherbet, 1/6 qt.	177	34	22	16	9	136
Shrimp, french-fried	180	35	22	16	9	138
Spaghetti, 1 serving	396	76	48	35	20	305
Steak, T-bone	235	45	29	21	12	181
Strawberry shortcake	400	77	49	36	21	308

*From: Konishi, F.: Food and energy equivalents of various activities. J. Am. Diet. Assoc., 46:187, 1965.
[a]Energy cost of walking for 70-kg. individual = 5.2 calories per minute at 3.5 m.p.h.
[b]Energy cost of riding bicycle = 8.2 calories per minute.
[c]Energy cost of swimming = 11.2 calories per minute.
[d]Energy cost of running = 19.4 calories per minute.
[e]Energy cost of reclining = 1.3 calories per minute.

drugs to produce anorexia, most of which have adverse side effects, and administration of bulk agents to satisfy the appetite. Microcrystalline cellulose added to some foods ordinarily limited in most reduction regimens has been acceptable to overweight individuals.[23] Each of these therapies may have some use in individual cases but, in general, such methods used alone do not result in long-term weight loss and weight control.

Regular follow-up contacts are reassuring to the patient and serve as a stimulus to continue the diet treatment. Organizations such as Weight Watchers and Take Off Pounds Sensibly (TOPS) help individuals during the period of adjustment in calorie intake. The person is encouraged with a weekly record showing his progress. A full length mirror will reflect the results too.

Behavior Modification

Behavior modification as a therapy in weight control is only about ten years old but already seems to be more effective than the traditional calorie reduction diet plan method already discussed. Calorie restriction and diet plans focus only on the desired outcome of eating behavior, that is, reduced energy intake. The individual is told what to eat, how much to eat and perhaps when to eat but never *why* to eat. He or she goes home with the diet, tries it for a while and then reverts to old eating habits because the basic eating behavior was not changed. The the person feels guilty because of "failure" with the diet, which generates still another psychological influence on eating that usually leads to regaining of any lost weight. Through behavior modification techniques, the overweight person gains *insight into the factors that influence his or her eating behavior* and learns *methods for controlling the factors or the eating response to them,* so that the end result is new eating habits, weight loss and maintenance of the lower weight.

The following behavior modification techniques have been applied in obesity therapy:[13]

1. *Aversive control:* A real or imagined aversive stimulus such as nausea is associated with a favorite food or eating behavior.

2. *Contingency management:* A positive or negative consequence is attached to a desirable or undesirable eating behavior, depending upon the need of the client. For example, paying a nickel every time one eats a piece of cake is a form of contingency management.

3. *Environmental management:* Changes are made in the environment by the client to aid in or reinforce positive eating behaviors.

4. *Self-monitoring:* Client observes and keeps a constant record of eating behavior or weight change and the antecedents and consequences.

The most important item for beginning modification of eating behavior is a record of that behavior—the *food record* or *food diary.* (See Fig. 27–7.) The food diary, kept by the client to record present eating behavior, includes:[13]

1. Time of eating.
2. Place of eating.
3. Physical position during eating.
4. Presence of others.
5. Activity associated with eating.
6. Mood or emotional state at time of eating.
7. Degree of hunger just before eating.
8. Type and amount of food eaten.

The record kept by the client is then shared with the counselor or therapy group, and the client is made aware of some of the factors that influence his eating behavior. Depending upon which individual behaviors are recognized as problems (that is, those that produce a high-caloric, rapid or frequent intake), some of the following behavioral changes may be decided upon by the client and the counselor:

1. To control the rate of eating:
   Chew every mouthful of food 15 times before swallowing it.
   Set utensils down between each bite of food.
   Wait 15 seconds between each bite of food.
   Prepare a meal and set the table before beginning to eat.
2. To control the frequency of eating:
   Eat in only one place, probably the kitchen or dining room.
   When not eating, make food inconspicuous.
   Eat only when hungry.
   Identify activities other than eating that are enjoyable, and do these instead of eating.
3. To control the amount of food eaten:
   Serve meals on a smaller plate so that it appears as if there is more on it.
   Eat half of everything.
   Write down the amount of everything eaten.

These are only some of the methods that can be used when beginning to control eating behavior. The techniques used should be individualized, depending upon the types of eating

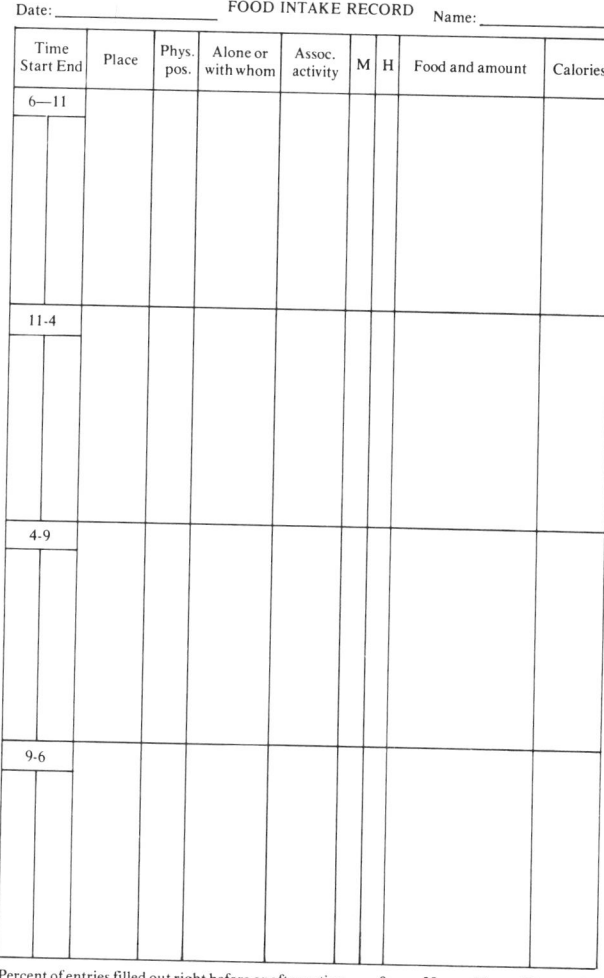

Figure 27-7 Food diary. M = mood. Record mood before beginning to eat and use the first letter of the word that most closely correlates with the mood: Neutral, Content, Tense, Depressed, Angry, Happy, Bored, Fatigued, or Rushed. H = hunger. Record subjective feeling of hunger just before eating on a scale of 0 to 5, with 5 being the most severe. (From: Ferguson, J.: Learning to Eat: Behavior Modification for Weight Control. Palo Alto, California, Bull Publishing Co., 1975.)

behaviors that need to be changed. Behavioral change should be approached in a step-wise fashion. For example, setting utensils down after every fourth bite may be all the person can cope with at first. When this becomes easy, then putting them down after every third bite can be tried, and so on.

Changing any behavior, especially eating behavior, is neither easy nor rapid. While learning new behaviors and changing old ones, people need constant reinforcement and positive feedback. In the beginning, much of this comes from self-observation in the form of daily records that show control over eating behavior. Later, reinforcement will come from comments by others about weight loss or from the development of a more pleasing body image. The counselor or therapy group must give reinforcement and constantly remind the person that perfection is not the goal but rather *improvement* in eating habits. *Weight loss is not the primary goal* but a natural secondary one to the achievement of control over eating behavior.

Exercise

The activity of the patient should also be considered. If the patient is inactive, exercise is prescribed to promote the oxidation of body fat. It aids in restoring muscle tone, good posture and a feeling of well-being. Brisk walking, not strolling, is recommended. This can be done even by the very heavy person who may find other forms of exercise impossible because of his awkward bulk. Daily gymnastic exercises, golf and swimming are advised, too. The type and amount of exercise must be prescribed for the individual patient. The amount of exercise for patients who have complications of cardiovascular diseases and arthritis must be very limited or withheld. Good judgment must be

used when exercises are prescribed, keeping in mind the age and physical condition of the patient. Because the increased activity may stimulate the appetite, the amount of food consumed must be kept under strict control. More likely, however, increased activity will decrease appetite.

Modern living is conducive to more rest and less physical activity. Labor-saving devices and electronic equipment have eliminated much of the daily exercise. A man who lives 2½ miles from work burns up 17 calories driving his car. Cycling would utilize 122 kcal. and walking, 210 kcal. Thus, 193 more kcal. are burned by walking than by riding. The typist working a mechanical typewriter burns up 450 more calories than the person who operates an electric typewriter for a 5-day week; in 8 weeks this can be equivalent to 1 pound of weight, assuming a constant intake.

In general, it should be stressed that the approach to weight reduction is through caloric restriction. The amount of weight that can be lost by daily, regular exercise can be a strong adjunct. A definite distinction must be drawn between weight loss due to temporary dehydration and that following an adequate period of caloric restriction. The patient may find that he has lost several pounds after a brisk session in the gymnasium and so feels free to compensate by overindulgence at the next meal. Perhaps the greatest misunderstanding concerns the distinction between water balance and caloric balance.

Hormonal Therapy

Hormonal therapy for obesity is fraught with mystique, a lack of complete understanding regarding all of its physiological effects, a certain amount of risk and a lack of long-term effectiveness. However, hormones continue to be used and may be valid therapy in some cases.

Thyroid hormone has been used most frequently, based on the erroneous assumption that the obese person has a hypoactive thyroid and therefore a lower BMR. Thyroid hormone given in large enough doses for a long enough period of time will produce weight loss, but the loss is only temporary while therapy lasts. Upon termination of thyroid therapy, weight is quickly regained because of a resulting hypothyroidism, increased appetite developed during therapy or decreased activity that results from muscle weakness and fatigue following treatment.[24] The hazards of thyroid hormone treatment are possible cardiovascular

symptoms, increased urinary excretion of nitrogen and calcium and the loss mainly of lean body mass and not of adipose tissue.

Human chorionic gonadotropin (HCG) is usually given as a daily injection in conjunction with a 500 kcal. diet. The efficacy of this hormone in the treatment of obese persons is doubtful, and its reported usefulness in aiding weight loss and avoiding hunger may be due to a psychological effect—motivation to follow the diet.

Human growth hormone has recently been used in obesity treatment because it depletes body fat and does not produce excess nitrogen excretion. It seems to be effective; however, the supplies of this hormone are small, and it is used only for limited research purposes.

Surgery

Three types of surgery have been used in obesity treatment: surgical removal of adipose tissue, the jejunoileal bypass and, more recently, the gastric bypass. Surgical removal of adipose tissue has been ineffective, since the adipose stores return. The other two surgical procedures are performed fairly frequently.

Jejunoileal Bypass Surgery. This surgery should be restricted to the morbidly obese person who has no other hope for weight reduction, for whom this procedure is a last resort, and whose health is severely jeopardized by the presence of the extreme obesity. An existing condition such as hypertension, diabetes mellitus, degenerative arthritis or pickwickian syndrome can be reason for the surgery; however, the patient should not be emotionally immature, elderly or unrealistic regarding the outcome of the operation.

As the term *jejunoileal bypass* implies, the surgery involves bypassing most of the absorptive capacity of the intestine by connecting the jejunum directly to the terminal ileum. Ten to 20 inches (25 to 50 cm.) of jejunum are measured and then the jejunum is cut. The ileum is measured 4 to 20 inches (10 to 50 cm.) back from the ileocecal valve and may be cut or not cut and then attached to the end of the section of jejunum still attached to the duodenum. (See Fig. 27–8.) The portion of small intestine that has been bypassed (approximately 6 meters or about 20 ft.) is left in the abdominal cavity for physiological reasons, but no food will pass through it. The result of the surgery is a tremendous reduction in the absorptive length of the small intestine, from about 22 ft. (approximately 7 meters) to about 1½ ft. (about ½ me-

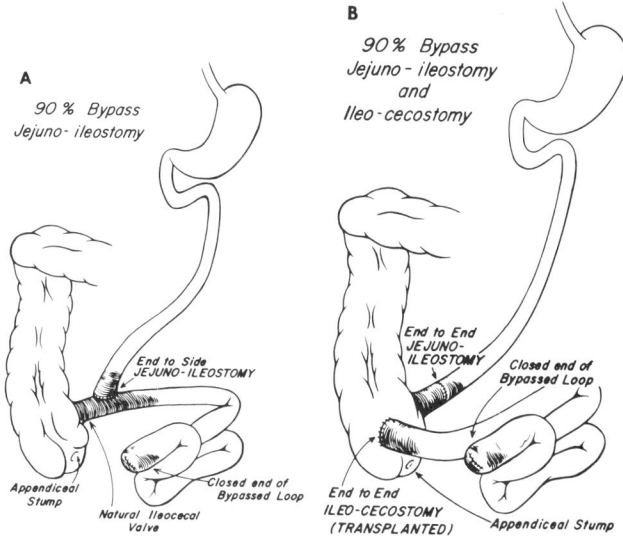

Figure 27–8 *A*, Intestinal bypass: end-to-side jejunoileostomy (Payne procedure). *B*, Intestinal bypass: end-to-end jejunoileostomy (Scott procedure). (From: Soper, R. T., et al.: Gastric bypass for morbid obesity in children and adolescents. J. Pediatr. Surg., *10*:51, 1975. Reproduced by permission.)

ter). Consequently, the patient is put into a chronic state of malabsorption due to reduced absorptive area and reduced transit time (which may be as little as 45 minutes in some patients). Food nutrients, including calories, are "lost" in the feces. The patient is in caloric deficit and loses weight even though he eats the same amount of food he was eating before. However, the person usually decreases his intake somewhat because of the discomfort and diarrhea that accompany overeating.

Weight losses are substantial, ranging from 60 to 100 lb. or more (27 to 45+ kg.) within a year after surgery. The heavier the patient, the faster the rate of weight loss. Most patients continue to lose at the rate of 8 lb. (3.6 kg.) per month, and usually their weight stabilizes about two years after surgery at a point 20 to 25 per cent above their ideal body weights. Where this point will be is determined by the pre-surgical weight of the patient and the length of the intestine left intact after surgery. Weight stabilizes because the remaining intestinal tract hypertrophies and is able to absorb enough nutrients to maintain this weight. For this reason and the fact that eating habits are rarely changed, the person who has his intestine reconnected will almost always regain the lost weight and perhaps gain more.

There are a number of complications of this surgery. Liver failure is the most severe long-term complication, and the patient should be made aware of this and the other major complications that can occur and that are not clearly understood. (See Table 27–4.)

NUTRITIONAL CARE. Nutritional care is as important for these patients as it is for any other person with a malabsorption syndrome. Attention must be given to vitamin and mineral supplements and nutritional counseling to minimize discomfort from diarrhea, cramping, steatorrhea and gas, to prevent complications and to maintain body protein stores.

Food intolerances are very individual although some general advice may be helpful.[8] The patient must be supported and encouraged

Table 27–4 COMPLICATIONS OF INTESTINAL BYPASS SURGERY*

SURGICAL
    Operative death
    Wound infection or dehiscence
    Anastomotic leak
METABOLIC
    Hypocalcemia and tetany
    Hypokalemia and weakness
    Oxalate renal stones
    Risk of osteoporosis
    Dehydration
GASTROINTESTINAL
    Nausea and vomiting
    Diarrhea that may persist
    Abdominal distention
    Cirrhosis
    Malnutrition with risks of hypovitaminosis
MISCELLANEOUS
    Loss of hair
    Arthralgia and arthritis
    Anemia

*From: Bray, G. A.: The overweight patient. Adv. Intern. Med., *21*:267, 1976.

to try adding new foods as the intestine adapts. Jejunoileal bypass patients can receive a great deal of support from each other, and the organization of a group may be very helpful for them.

Potassium supplements (usually in the form of KCl) are necessary because of the very common problem of hypokalemia that results from excessive losses of K^+ because of the profuse diarrhea. As the intestine adapts to its new condition, the number of stools will slowly decrease from 10 to 20 per day right after surgery to 3 to 4 per day by the end of the year after surgery. After the patient is able to eat fruits and vegetables and other potassium-rich foods, the potassium supplements may be able to be decreased and substituted with fruits and vegetables.

Calcium, magnesium and vitamin D may also need supplementation because of poor absorption. Vitamin D may be poorly absorbed as a result of fat malabsorption, and calcium can form calcium soaps with the fatty acids in the gut lumen, which prevents its absorption. The few reported cases of tetany following jejunoileal bypass may have been due to hypocalcemia or hypomagnesemia.

All *vitamins* should be given as supplements, usually in therapeutic doses, in anticipation of poor absorption. A liquid vitamin preparation may be more valuable, considering the reduced transit time in the gut. An encapsulated vitamin preparation may not be digested and absorbed fast enough. Although the terminal ileum remains after most of these surgeries and allows for the absorption of vitamin B_{12}, some authorities still suggest supplementation for two reasons: (1) there may or may not be enough of the terminal ileum left for adequate B_{12} absorption, and (2) there may be bacteria from the "resting gut" in the end-to-side anastomosis that compete with the body for B_{12}.[22]

Protein deficiency is thought to be a factor in the development of fatty liver seen after this surgery. It is somewhat similar to that seen in patients with kwashiorkor.[20] Fatty liver and the low serum albumin and sporadic hair loss observed in some patients are thought to be signs of protein deficiency due to poor absorption and possibly to inadequate protein intake. For this reason, the patient should be counseled to eat a large amount of protein (more than the recommended dietary allowance), possibly 80 to 100 gm. per day. These patients were not amenable to diet changes before, so the counseling must be in the form of suggestion and encouragement.

Because of the steatorrhea that almost always occurs after a high-fat meal, a *low-fat* diet (less than 50 gm. of fat) is suggested for the patient.

Alcohol should be avoided for the first year after surgery and preferably avoided permanently. Alcohol may place a metabolic load on an already overtaxed liver, and these patients will become highly intoxicated after drinking just a small amount of alcohol. For most patients, giving up alcohol is no problem.

Medications are given to help reduce the diarrhea, and creams are recommended to alleviate the anal discomfort associated with diarrhea and frequent bowel movements.

These patients should be checked even after thay have reached a stable weight and assessed periodically for nutritional status through biochemical measurements, dietary history, and clinical examination. (See Chapter 11.)

All investigators have reported that their patients are happy with the surgery and would never go back to their former condition. Solow reports an improvement in patients' self-confidence, self-esteem and body image after substantial weight loss. He found that these patients felt a relief of the constant guilt and helplessness that had accompanied every mouthful they had eaten before. The weight loss appeared to restore a more normal responsiveness to the internal cues of satiety and a sharpening of satiety mechanisms.[28]

Gastric Bypass Surgery. Recently instituted as a treatment for obesity, gastric bypass surgery closes part of the stomach and thus reduces its reservoir capacity. The remaining portion is connected directly to the jejunum via a small opening about 2 cm. in diameter. (See Fig. 27–9.) The main cause of weight loss appears to be the reduced food intake due to the smaller stomach and to the nausea and vomiting that result if the person continues to eat. The operation is not accompanied by the problems of the jejunoileal bypass surgery, but there may be some occurrence of fat malabsorption and dumping syndrome, and an increased incidence of gallstone formation has been reported.[16] As with the jejunoileal bypass, patients usually stabilize at a weight somewhat above their ideal weight. The gastric bypass is probably as effective as the jejunoileal bypass in producing and maintaining weight reduction.

NUTRITIONAL CARE. Nutritional care involves counseling regarding dumping syndrome if it is present (see Chapter 34) and a low-fat diet to avoid steatorrhea and possible gallstone formation. Attention to a food record

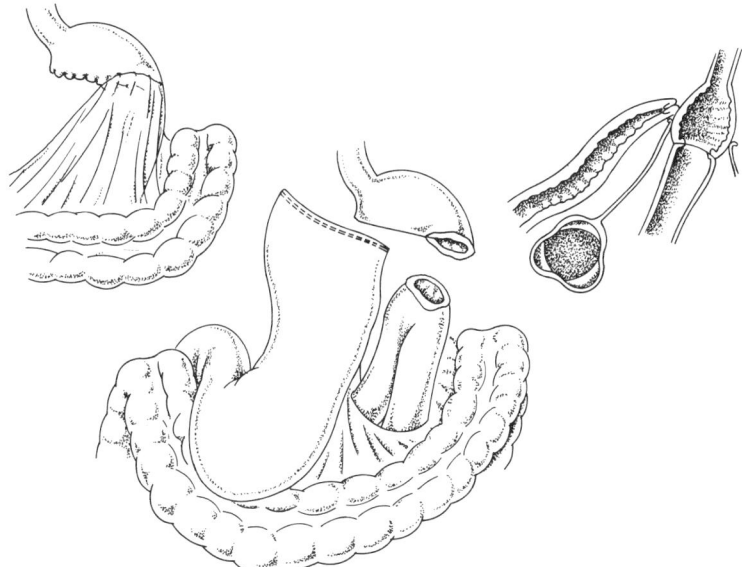

Figure 27–9 Gastric bypass. The upper pouch is small. A 2-cm. opening is made along the greater curvature. The mesocolon is sutured to the stomach above the gastroenterostomy, and the proximal end of the excluded stomach is sutured to the anterior wall of the fundic pouch. (From Mason, E. E.: From giant hernias to gastric bypass. In: Asher, W. L. (ed.): Treating the Obese. New York, Medcom Press, 1974.)

kept after surgery will give the counselor information on how much the patient is consuming, what is being consumed and tolerated and what is being vomited. Recommendations for a more balanced food intake or for mineral or vitamin supplements could be made to maintain nutritional status during this period of weight reduction. Again, this may be impossible or unrealistic, since these patients desired this surgery because they were unable to control their food intake.

Jaw Wiring

Wiring the jaws closed is another method of reducing food intake through physical control rather than through a change in eating or activity habits. The result is that the person can no longer eat solid food but can only take liquids through a straw. Regular dental attention and nutritional care are important while the jaws are wired. *Nutritional care* should include obtaining a dietary history to find out what types of liquids the person is taking. Counseling should include recommendations for liquids so that adequate protein, minerals and vitamins are ingested during the period of weight loss. Rather than only juices, Kool-aid and soda pop, the dieter could be taking nutritious soups, milk, formula diets and vitamin and mineral supplements. The nutrition counselor

can also serve as a valuable source of support and encouragement. The long-term effectiveness or safety of this measure for weight control is unknown.

In the final analysis, many methods may be effective in causing weight loss, but the most important criterion of their success is maintenance of the new lower weight. This is very, very difficult, as reflected by the fact that while more people are dieting now than ever before, the incidence of obesity is not going down. *Proper activity* and *controlled intake* need to be *started early* to insure the most effective form of obesity treatment: *prevention.* See Chapters 14 and 15 for discussion of obesity during growth and development.

UNDERWEIGHT

Almost eclipsed by all the attention focused on obesity in the United States is the effort of some persons to gain weight. The term *underweight* is applicable to persons who are 15 to 20 per cent or more below the normal accepted weight standard or desired weight. Because *underweight is often a symptom or predisposing cause of a disease,* it should receive medical investigation. In underweight individuals the resistance to disease is lowered, the growth during childhood and adolescence is retarded and efficiency is impaired. The person who is

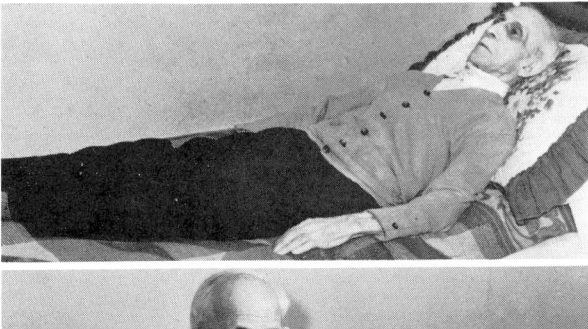

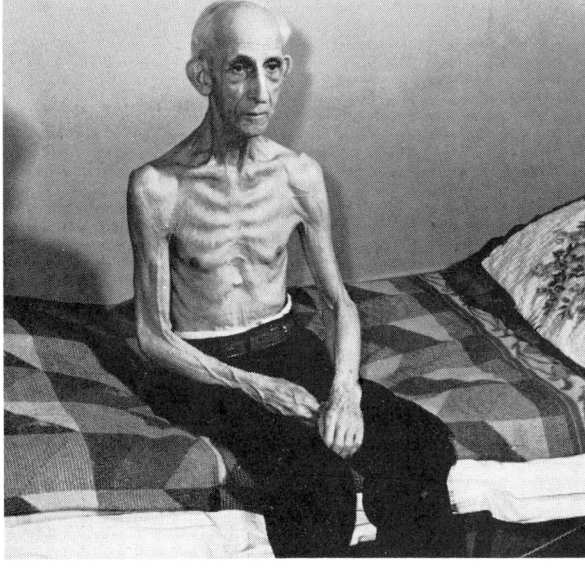

Figure 27–10 Underweight. Resistance to disease is lowered in underweight individuals. (From: S. L. Halpern: Nutrition and chronic disease. Health News, New York State Department of Health.)

seriously underweight often tires easily, is sensitive to cold and complains of feeling weak. (See Fig. 27–10.)

Etiology

Underweight may be caused by (1) an insufficient intake in the quantity and quality of food to meet the needs of the person's activity, (2) poor absorption and utilization of the food consumed, (3) poor choice of food consumed, (4) a wasting disease such as tuberculosis or hyperthyroidism that increases the metabolic rate and (5) psychological or emotional stress or psychological abnormality (anorexia nervosa). (See Chapter 32.) Undernutrition itself may lead to multiple endocrine disturbances. Undernourished individuals may show signs of underfunction of the pituitary, thyroid, gonads and adrenals. Young women with anorexia nervosa, for instance, stop menstruating when they have lost a significant amount of weight.

Treatment

Before starting a program to gain weight, it is necessary to determine the basic cause of the patient's underweight. If a wasting disease is the cause then the disease must be treated, and the diet becomes part of the treatment. Information on the budgeting of foods, marketing, meal planning and preparation may be needed by the patient. If the problem is psychological, the meals are consciously limited by the patient to attract attention and sympathy. Psychological therapy is needed to direct the interests of the patient. In cases of anorexia nervosa, the basic fears and anxieties need to be discovered and removed; at the same time, maximal food intake is encouraged. Faulty absorption of food is a medical problem and must be treated. Probably the most common cause of underweight is an inadequate food intake.

It is frequently more difficult for an underweight individual to gain weight than it is for an obese patient to lose weight. The "set point" theory applies to thin people as well as to overweight individuals. The selection and service of food is important, since the appetite of the underweight person must be teased with eye-appealing and nutritious meals. Well-planned meals at scheduled hours instead of hastily planned, bolted meals are advised. Mealtimes should be periods of leisure and relaxation,

since nervous tension is often part of the problem circle of underweight individuals. If upset, the person should postpone his meal until he has calmed down.

HIGH CALORIE DIETS FOR WEIGHT GAIN

Before a diet is planned with the person, a careful dietary history should be taken. This history of the food intake most likely will reveal the good and poor dietary habits and inadequacies.

The Diet Plan

Calories. In addition to the calories needed to meet the total energy requirement of the body, an allowance of 500 to 1000 additional calories for storage of fat in the adipose tissues should be planned. An acceptable method of determining the patient's daily caloric requirement is simply to calculate his needs on the basis of his present weight. If a person normally needs 2800 kcal. (11,700 kJ.) to maintain present weight, his dietary needs would be 3300 to 3800 kcal. (13,800 to 15,900 kJ.) to gain weight. The intake should be gradually increased to avoid gastric discomfort and periods of discouragement. When a person is offered or expected to ingest more food than he can take at one time, he is apt to be overwhelmed by the amount and be unable to eat very much. The amount of food that could be ingested at one meal should be determined and the rest of the calories supplied in a concentrated supplemental form.

It has been found through experience with patients of both sexes and different ages that men seem to prefer to receive the additional calories through extra portions of the usual foods served at meals, children and adolescents prefer between-meal nourishment, and women seem to favor more concentrated foods, such as the addition of cream to milk when it is served as a beverage. The secret of a successful diet program is to *individualize* the treatment for each patient and to include foods which the patient really enjoys.

Protein. In the average high-calorie diet for the underweight, the daily protein allowance is maintained at the optimum level. A high protein intake of 100 gm. or more may be necessary for replacement and repair of the body tissues. In cases of severe malnutrition caused by the patient's inability to take sufficient food, crystalline amino acids are sometimes given

orally or parenterally. It has been found that, after a certain period of malnutrition, the gastrointestinal tract is incapable of digesting a sufficient amount of protein foods, especially if edema of the gastrointestinal tract is present, and vomiting or diarrhea may result. Sparing the patient's digestion by giving amino acids (protein hydrolysates) will frequently alleviate the difficulty.

Carbohydrates and Fats. The amount of fuel foods, carbohydrates and fats, is increased in the high-calorie diet. The concentrated calorie foods such as butter, fortified margarine, cream, cereals, bread, potatoes and high-calorie desserts are especially advised. A moderate fat allowance is made to increase the palatability of the diet and increase the caloric value without dulling the appetite. Carbohydrates are digested easily and when taken in excess of body needs are readily converted into body fat.

Minerals and Vitamins. The mineral and vitamin allowances should be maintained at an optimum level. Supplements of vitamins, especially the B vitamins, are given as a possible appetite stimulant and to meet the requirement when calories are increased.

For the high-calorie diet this food pattern provides about 3000 kcal., 130 gm. protein and generous amounts of vitamins and minerals. The normal protective diet, outlined in Tables 10–4 and 19–1, is the basis or pattern for the high-calorie diet. Increasing the amounts of the basic foods increases the intake of daily calories, minerals and vitamins. Additional foods such as desserts, candy and special dishes may be enjoyed by the patient if the protective foods are not sacrificed. Eating between meals is encouraged but should not interfere with the patient's appetite for regular meals.

To increase the patient's daily calorie intake, the 500 kcal. step-up is suggested. For example, if the patient is now eating 2500 kcal. (10,450 kJ.) and a diet containing 3000 kcal. (12,550 kJ.) is desired, then a step-up of 500 kcal. (2100 kJ.) is added, or if an increase of 1000 kcal. is desired, then two 500 kcal. step-ups are added (Table 27–5). The high-calorie diet is the adequate normal diet with increased calories. A 500 kcal. increase over the daily caloric requirements should allow for a gain of 1 lb. per week.

Suggestions for Increasing Calories in the Diet

Serve heavy cream instead of light cream.
Include cereal in the breakfast menu with a

Table 27–5 SUGGESTIONS FOR INCREASING CALORIC INTAKES IN STEPS OF 500 KCAL.

ADDITIONAL FOODS	WEIGHT (gm.)	KCAL.	PROTEIN
Plus 500 Kcal.			
(Served between meals and/or before retiring):			
1. 1 cup (8 oz.) half milk and half cream (20%)	242	325	8
1 slice bread	23	60	2
2 pats butter or fortified margarine	14	100	
		Total 485	10
2. 3 cups milk (¾ qt.)	732	Total 480	27
3. 4 slices bread	92	240	8
1 serving List 3 fruit[a]	100	40	
1 egg	50	80	6
1 cup milk (8 oz.)	244	160	9
		Total 520	23
Plus 1000 Kcal:			
(Beverage served between meals and/or before retiring):			
1. 3 cups milk nourishments (¾ qt.), eggnogs and malteds	810	840	39
1 tbsp. jelly	20	55	
2 pats butter or fortified margarine	14	100	
		Total 995	39
2. 3 slices bread	69	180	6
2 servings potato or equivalent	244	160	4
1 egg	50	80	6
3 cups milk (¾ qt.)	732	480	27
2 tbsp. jam	40	110	
		1010	43
Plus 1500 Kcal.:			
(Some served between meals and/or before retiring):			
1. 2 cups (1 pt.) milk nourishment, eggnogs and malteds.	540	560	26
2 cups (1 pt.) half milk and half cream (20%)	484	650	16
1 baked custard	248	285	13
		Total 1495	55
2. 2 cups (1 pt.) milk nourishment (malted milk, etc.)	540	560	26
3 cups milk (¾ qt.)	732	480	27
1 glass fruitade (8 oz.)	240	65	
3 slices bread	69	180	6
1 serving List 3 fruit	100	40	
2 servings potato or equivalent	244	180	6
		Total 1504	65

[a]From Exchange list, Table 25–5.

banana or other fruit, because sugar, cream and cereal offer additional calories.

Butter breakfast toast when it is hot because more butter or margarine can be used. Cinnamon toast, pancakes, waffles and French toast are good alternates for breakfast toast.

Serve jelly and jam along with bread and butter. Add jelly, jam and preserves to cheesecake, puddings and other desserts.

Add cream or undiluted evaporated milk to milk beverages. Malted milk and eggnogs can replace milk.

Add skim milk powder to milk, milk beverages, soups and puddings and on hot cereal.

Add ice cream or whipped cream to desserts and milk beverages.

Serve cream soups instead of clear bouillon.

Eat dried fruits between meals because they are high in calories besides being good sources of minerals and vitamins.

Serve mayonnaise, oil and salad dressings whenever possible with sandwiches, salads and vegetables.

Serve gravy on meat and potatoes.

Add sauce to desserts such as puddings, molded gelatins, custards, rennet puddings, cakes and ice creams.

Consume at least one qt. of milk daily. When possible, substitute cream for one half of the milk, or add non-fat dry milk solids if fat is not well tolerated.

Potatoes, spaghetti, rice, macaroni and noodles may be served twice every day.

Along with a breakfast egg, serve bacon, sausage or ham.

Eat nuts between meals. They are high in fat

content besides being good protein and calorie additions.

Plan a definite eating schedule and then adhere to it. The benefits derived from an improved physical condition will more then repay the effort.

See Appendix Table 3 for additional suggestions.

It may be more difficult for an underweight person to gain 1 lb. a week than for an obese person to lose 1 lb. a week. It is not an easy task for the underweight person to add 500 kcal. to his daily intake of food. He should be involved in planning what and how much additional food he will take at one time and how often he will eat. He usually can suggest what can be added to make the plan appealing.

Behavior modification techniques can be applied to the process of weight gain just as they are used in weight reduction. The basis for thinness is the person's eating behavior, which must be changed to result in a consistently higher caloric intake.

PROBLEMS AND SUGGESTED TOPICS FOR DISCUSSION

1. Define (a) overweight and (b) obesity.
2. Why is obesity becoming a recognized public health problem?
3. Classify obesity and list (a) the direct cause and (b) factors that may influence obesity.
4. What are the principles of a low-calorie diet?
5. Describe various reducing regimens and give the advantages and disadvantages of each.
6. Should all overweight individuals reduce? Explain. (See Young, C. M.: JAMA, 186:903, 1963.)
7. Assist a person who is overweight with the necessary changes in her present dietary pattern to lose 1 lb. per week. Permit her to indicate the changes that she will make.
8. Interview a patient who is obese. How many calories is he consuming to maintain his present weight? How many excess calories is he consuming? How can he improve his diet? Try to follow the patient's progress in the outpatient clinic.
9. Keep a diary of your own eating for two days, making note of the items discussed in this chapter. If you had to lose or gain weight, which behavior would you attempt to change first?
10. How would you help a person who is underweight gain weight? How will he implement the changes?
11. Take a food-consumption history of an underweight patient who is in the hospital or in the outpatient clinic. Calculate the calories. How many calories does he need to reach his ideal or desired weight? How long will it take him to reach the desired weight?
12. List the foods that should be stressed or added to the normal diet to make it a high-calorie diet.

CITED REFERENCES

1. Backman, L., and Hallberg, D.: Small-intestinal length. Acta Chir. Scand., 140:57, 1974.
2. Blackburn, G. L., Bistrian, B. R., and Flatt, J. P.: Role of a Protein Sparing Fast in a Comprehensive Weight Reduction Program. London, Proceedings of the First International Congress of Obesity, October 1974.
3. Bray, G. A.: Effect of caloric restriction on energy expenditure in obese patients. Lancet, 2:397, 1969.
4. Bray, G. A., and Campfield, L. A.: Metabolic factors in the control of energy stores. Metabolism, 24:99, 1975.
5. Brobeck, J. R.: Food intake as a mechanism of temperature regulation. Yale J. Biol. Med., 20:545, 1948.
6. Craig, D. G.: Guiding the change process in people. J. Am. Diet Assoc., 58:22, 1971.
7. Davis, J. D., et al.: Disappearance of a humoral satiety factor during food deprivation. J. Comp. Physiol. Psychol., 75:476, 1971.
8. Dewind, L.: Jejunoileal bypass surgery for obesity. In: Bray, G. A., and Bethune, J. E. (eds.): Treatment and Management of Obesity. New York, Harper and Row, 1974, pp. 142–143.
9. Edholm, O. G., et al.: Food intake and energy expenditure of army recruits. Br. J. Nutr., 24:109, 1970.
10. Flack, R., and Grayer, E. A.: Consciousness-raising group for obese women. Social Work, 20(6):484, 1975.
11. Harper, A. E., Benevenga, N. J., and Wohlhueter, R. M.: Effects of ingestion of disproportionate amounts of amino acids. Physiol. Rev., 50:428, 1970.
12. Hirsch, J., and Knittle, J. L.: Cellularity of obese and nonobese human adipose tissue. Fed. Proc., 29:1516, 1970.
13. Jordan, H. A., and Levitz, L. S.: A behavioural approach to the problem of obesity. In: Silverstone, T. (ed.), Obesity: Its Pathogenesis and Management. Acton, Mass., Publishing Sciences Group, Inc., 1975.
14. Liebowitz, S. F.: Reciprocal hunger-regulating circuits involving alpha- and beta-adrenergic receptors located respectively in the ventromedial and lateral hypothalamus. Proc. Natl. Acad. Sci., 67:1063, 1970.
15. Lytle, L. D., and Messing, R. B.: Appetite in the regulation of food intake for energy (animal and man). Prog. Food Nutr. Sci., 2:49, 1976.
16. Mason, E. E.: From giant hernias to gastric bypass. In: Asher, W. L. (ed.): Treating the Obese. New York, Medcom Press, 1974.
17. Mayer, J.: Why people get hungry. Nutr. Today, 1:2, 1966.
18. Mayer, J., Monello, J. F., and Seltzer, C. C.: Hunger and satiety sensations in men, women, boys and girls. Postgrad. Med., 37(6): A97, 1965.
19. Miller, D. S., Mumford, P., and Stock, M. J.: Gluttony: thermogenesis in overeating man. Am. J. Clin. Nutr., 20:1223, 1967.
20. Moxley, R. T. III, Pozefsky, T., and Lockwood, D. Y.: Protein nutrition and liver disease after jejunoileal bypass for morbid obesity. N. Engl. J. Med., 290:921, 1974.
21. Nisbett, R. E.: Hunger, obesity and the ventromedial hypothalamus. Psychol. Rev., 79:433, 1972.
22. Pi-Sunyer, F. X.: Jejunoileal bypass surgery for obesity. Am. J. Clin. Nutr., 29:409, 1976.
23. Pratt, D. E., et al.: Bulking agents in foods. J. Am. Diet. Assoc. 59:120, 1971.
24. Rivlin, R. S.: Therapy of obesity with hormones. N. Engl. J. Med., 292:26, 1975.
25. Seltzer, C. C., and Mayer, J.: Body build and obesity—Who are the obese? JAMA, 189:677, 1964.
26. Simon, R. I.: Obesity as a depressive equivalent. JAMA, 183:209, 1963.
27. Sims, E. A. H., et al.: Endocrine and metabolic effects of experimental obesity in man. Recent Prog. Horm. Res., 29:457, 1973.
28. Solow, C., Silberford, P. M., and Swift, K.: Psycho-

logical effects of intestinal bypass surgery for severe obesity. N. Engl. J. Med., *290*:300, 1974.

29. Stellar, E.: Hunger in man: Comparative and physiologic studies. Am. Psychol., *22*:105, 1967.

30. Yang, M. U., and Van Itallie, T. B.: Composition of weight lost during short-term weight reduction. J. Clin. Invest., *58*:722, 1976.

31. Young, C. M.: Dietary treatment of obesity: Carbohydrate content and feeding frequency. In Asher, W. L. (ed.): Treating the Obese. New York, Medcom Press, 1974.

32. Young. C. M.: Weight reduction using a moderate fat diet: Clinical response and energy metabolism. J. Am. Diet. Assoc., *28*:410, 1952.

ADDITIONAL REFERENCES

Bortz, W. M.: Predictability of weight loss. JAMA, *204*:99, 1968.

Bray, G. A., and Bethune, J. E. (eds.): Treatment and Management of Obesity, New York, Harper and Row, 1974.

Bruch, H.: Eating Disorders: Obesity, Anorexia Nervosa and the Person Within. New York, Basic Books, 1973.

Bullen, B. A., Reed, R. B., and Mayer, J.: Physical activity of obese and nonobese adolescent girls appraised by motion picture sampling. Am. J. Clin. Nutr., *14*:211, 1964.

A critique of low-carbohydrate ketogenic weight reduction regimens. JAMA, *224*:1415, 1973.

Drenick, E. J.: Prolonged fasting. In: Asher, W. L. (ed.): Treating the Obese. New York, Medcom Press, 1974.

Fabry, P., and Tepperman, J.: Meal frequency—a possible factor in human pathology. Am. J. Clin. Nutr., *23*:1059, 1970.

Ferguson, J.: Learning to Eat: Behavior Modification for Weight Control. Palo Alto, Cal., Bull Publishing Co., 1975. (Leader's manual and student's manual.)

Goldblatt, P. B., et al.: Social factors in obesity. JAMA, *192*:1039, 1965.

Hegsted, D. M.: Energy needs and energy utilization. Nutr. Rev., *32*:33, 1974.

Jordon, H. A.: In defense of body weight. J. Am. Diet. Assoc., *62*:17, 1973.

Leveille, G. A., and Romsos, D. R.: Meal eating and obesity. Nutr. Today, *9*:4, 1974.

Lewis, K. J., and Doyle, M. D.: Nutrient intake and weight response of women on weight-control diets. J. Am. Diet. Assoc., *56*:119, 1970.

Maddox, G. L.: Overweight as a social deviance and disability. J. Health Soc. Behav., *9*:287, 1968.

Mann, G. V.: The influence of obesity on health. N. Engl. J. Med., *291*:178; *291*:226, 1974.

Mayer, J.: Overweight: Causes, Cost, and Control. Englewood Cliffs, NJ, Prentice-Hall, Inc., 1968.

Mayer, J.: Physiology of hunger and satiety: Regulation of food intake. In: Goodhart, R. S., and Shils, M. E. (eds.), Modern Nutrition in Health and Disease. Philadelphia, Lea & Febiger, 1973.

Montague, A.: Obesity and evolution of man. JAMA, *195*:149, 1966.

Moore, M. E., Stunkard, A., and Srole, L.: Obesity, social class, and mental illness. JAMA, *181*:962, 1962.

Pollack, H.: Protein therapy in emaciation. J. Am. Dietet. A., *23*:410, 1947.

Seifrit, E.: The high calorie diet. Am. J. Clin. Nutr., *12*:66, 1963.

Stein, M. R., et al.: Ineffectiveness of human chorionic gonadotropin in weight reduction: A double-blind study. Am. J. Clin. Nutr., *29*:940, 1976.

Stock, A. L., and Yudkin, J.: Nutrient intake of subjects on low carbohydrate diet used in treatment of obesity. Am. J. Clin. Nutr., *23*:948, 1970.

Stunkard, A. J.: The Pain of Obesity. Palo Alto, Cal., Bull Publishing Co., 1976.

Stunkard, A., and Mendelson, M.: Disturbances in body image of some obese persons. J. Am. Diet. Assoc., *38*:328, 1961.

Swendseid, M. E., et al.: Nitrogen and weight losses during starvation and realimentation in obesity. J. Am. Diet. Assoc., *46*:276, 1965.

Symposium on jejunoileostomy for obesity. Am. J. Clin. Nutr., *30*(1), 1977.

Young, C. M.: Planning the low calorie diet. Am. J. Clin. Nutr., *8*:896, 1960.

Young, C. M., et al.: Frequency of feeding, weight reduction and body composition. J. Am. Diet. Assoc., *59*:466, 1971.

UNIT NINE

DISEASES OF THE
CIRCULATORY SYSTEM,
BLOOD AND
BLOOD-FORMING
ORGANS

Chapter 28

NUTRITIONAL CARE FOR PATIENTS WITH CARDIOVASCULAR DISEASES

The United States is reported to have one of the highest death rates from cardiovascular diseases in the world. Coronary disease takes first place, with stroke in second place; combined they account for three fourths of all deaths from cardiovascular diseases. Proper functioning of the cardiovascular apparatus depends upon good nutrition, and diet plays an important role in the management and prevention of heart disease.

CARDIAC DISEASES

Heart Failure

When heart disease results in circulatory failure or heart failure, nutritional care is important in order to maintain homeostasis in the patient. In heart failure the heart cannot maintain an adequate blood supply to the tissues, and this has nutritional ramifications. The symptoms of heart failure vary depending upon the cardiovascular defect. *Acute* heart failure

occurs when the heart suddenly stops pumping, and it usually results in death. *Chronic* heart failure, while not causing immediate death, can adversely affect other organs in the body (such as the liver, kidneys and brain) because of the decreased blood flow. Heart failure that is due to a defect in the heart itself is called *myocardial failure*. Heart failure that is due to circulatory congestion from abnormal salt and water retention is called *congestive heart failure*. (See Fig. 28–1.) There is congestion of the pulmonary or systemic circulations by abnormal amounts of blood. The reduced cardiac output results in decreased blood flow through the kidney and causes increased tubular resorption of sodium and finally an increased retention of water.

Surgery

Many forms of congenital disturbances of the heart and blood vessels are now helped or

579

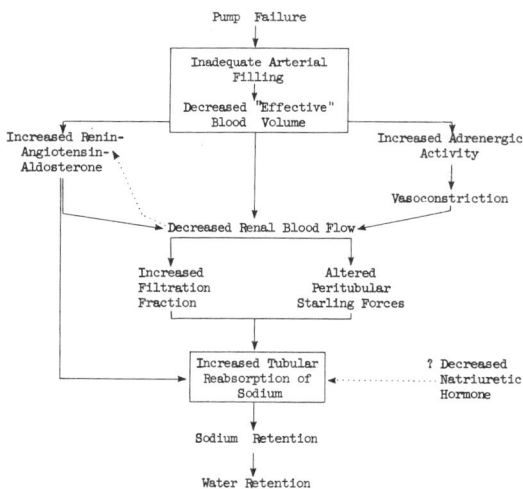

Figure 28–1 Pathogenesis of sodium and water retention in congestive heart failure. (From: del Greco, F.: The kidney in congestive heart failure. Mod. Concepts Cardiovasc. Dis., *44*:47, 1975.)

cured by surgery to the extent that the patient frequently returns to a completely normal life. More recently, the surgical approach to coronary artery disease has produced encouraging results.

However, not all patients with cardiac diseases are candidates for surgery. Ideal candidates must be screened from sufferers who cannot be helped by these operations or for whom the risk is too great. For such less fortunate patients, therapeutic diet and drugs are relied upon to prolong life and give greater comfort.

Principles of Nutritional Care

The purpose of the diet in cardiac disease is to give adequate nourishment with the least possible work effort and muscular strain on the heart and to prevent or eliminate edema.

Energy. Loss of weight results in less work for the heart and improved cardiac efficiency. The patient who is obese usually is given a 1000 to 1200 kcal. diet while bedridden. Those patients of normal weight are permitted calories sufficient to maintain weight slightly below the desired weight level.

Protein. The normal intake of protein (0.8 gm. per kilogram of body weight or about 50 to 60 gm. daily) is adequate for maintenance of body tissues.

Carbohydrate and Fat. The relative proportions of carbohydrate and fat are determined according to the nature and amount of fat and carbohydrate to be included in the diet. (See discussion on atherosclerosis.)

Minerals. All minerals should be provided in normal amounts except when sodium restriction is indicated. The average daily diet provides 2800 to 6000 mg. sodium (2 to 6 gm.), although a liberal intake of salty food or a high content of sodium in drinking water may result in considerably higher sodium levels.

Vitamins. The selection of food to include all vitamins is important. In instances when the intake of deep yellow and dark green vegetables is restricted, the vitamin A intake may be below the recommended allowance. When fat such as butter, whole milk or margarine is omitted, the intake of vitamin A could be low and a vitamin supplement may be indicated.

Stimulants. Since dietary stimulants such as caffeine and theobromine should be avoided in the acute phase of cardiac disease, the patient should not be allowed to have coffee, tea or cola drinks (which contain caffeine) or chocolate or cocoa (which contain theobromine). Very weak tea or herb tea may be allowed but should be served warm rather than hot. Unfortunately, the caffeine content of these beverages varies widely depending on the strength, blend of coffee or tea and method of brewing. Individual coronary care units may have additional "coronary precautions" regarding stimulants.

Food Frequency and Consistency. Frequently the patient can tolerate five or six small meals a day much better than the usual three meals. Large meals can cause increased distention of the stomach and elevation of the diaphragm, thus displacing the heart upward and restricting breathing. Foods commonly considered bulky, gas-forming (p. 485), easily fermented and indigestible can have the same result and cause distress or an acute attack. Other foods may need to be restricted depending upon the individual. It is important to learn from the patient which foods give him gas in order to avoid unnecessary restriction in his diet.[2]

The cardiac patient should not eat when upset, under stress or in a hurry, because at those times there may not be a sufficient supply of blood in the digestive organs to carry on good digestion. Each patient is different, and the dietary management should be planned according to the individual's needs.

Nutritional Care During Acute Cardiac Disease

In acute cardiac disease, which occurs in certain acute infections resulting in endocar-

ditis or carditis, in cardiac failure, after myocardial infarction and after cardiac surgery, the diet is reduced to the minimum nutritional requirements. Dyspnea and chewing are incompatible in the patient with severe congestive heart failure, since they often have to breathe through their mouths. Initially, these individuals should be given soft or liquid food that does not require chewing and should eat or be fed slowly in order to avoid aspiration of food. The frequency of feeding is also important; more frequent and smaller feedings are obviously indicated.

The *Karrell diet,* first used in 1866, consists of 800 ml. of milk (given in four equal feedings) and fulfills many of the aims of the management of acute cardiac failure.[16] This diet provides about 600 kcal. and 500 mg. of sodium. For patients who cannot tolerate milk, variations have been devised, most of them containing 800 ml. of fluids and no free salt. Lonalac is a commercially prepared liquid supplement low in sodium. (See Table 35–5.) Because these diets are nutritionally inadequate, they are prescribed only for a short period of 4 to 7 days. As cardiac compensation increases, salt (sodium) intake and the diet can be liberalized.

Nutritional Care During Chronic Cardiac Disease

In chronic cardiac disease the myocardium and valves of the heart are most likely to be involved. The condition may be (1) *compensated* or (2) *decompensated.* In compensated heart disease the organ is able to maintain almost normal circulation, through its own efforts, by an enlargement of the heart and by an increased pulse rate. In decompensated heart disease the heart is unable to compensate for its disturbance; it is unable to maintain normal circulation to supply nutrients and oxygen to the tissues or to carry away the waste products.

Compensated Heart Disease. The patient's weight should be normal or 10 per cent underweight to help improve the functional state of the vascular system. *Slight underweight* lessens the burden on the heart and thereby improves its efficiency. The well-compensated heart may not require any diet modification other than to avoid obesity. However, mild restriction of sodium is sometimes prescribed to maintain fluid balance.

Decompensated Heart Disease. For patients with decompensated heart disease a rigid diet treatment is usually planned to relieve the present strain and prevent further damage to the organ. These patients, if obese, will experience symptomatic relief following *weight reduction,* which will also serve as an inducement for them to adhere to additional diet restrictions in their supervised regimens, if necessary.

The protein allowance is kept a little high at 60 to 80 gm. Complex carbohydrates should furnish the bulk of the remaining calories, with fat adjusted to type and calorie allowance.

When there is poor circulation to tissues in advanced cardiac disease, the tissues are deprived of nutrients, and the patient can become malnourished and may lose weight. This state of malnutrition can be masked by the concomitant weight gain that results from fluid retention and edema as the heart fails. The patient's face can continue to look puffy and the extremities edematous. For this patient it is important to record the daily weight both before and during therapy, so that as diuresis begins there will be an accurate determination of the person's dry body weight as a starting point for the nutritional care.

In severe heart failure the patient is also less likely to eat and may become malnourished from a decreased intake of nutrients, particularly protein. This problem is made worse by the fact that with greatly reduced renal blood flow proteinuria may exist and can cause a significant loss of body protein.

Vitamins and minerals (except perhaps sodium) are given in normal amounts but may need some supplementation.

SODIUM AND FLUIDS. Edema is the result of impaired cardiac function that causes sodium (and therefore fluids) to accumulate in the tissues (dropsy). Salt (sodium) and sometimes fluids are restricted and adjusted to the patient's individual needs. Theories regarding control of fluid balance emphasize the restriction of sodium, and there is an increasing trend not to limit the fluid intake except in the case of dilutional hyponatremia. When the sodium intake is limited the formation of edema fluid can be prevented, since the mechanisms that usually regulate the sodium concentration in extracellular fluid do not permit the retention of water without sodium. The effect of electrolytes upon the fluid balance is related primarily to the sodium ion rather than to the chloride ion, and dietary recommendations should refer to sodium, rather than to salt.

Sodium Restricted Diets

Nomenclature. The diets commonly called "salt restricted" are really *sodium restricted*

Table 28–1 SODIUM AND SALT IN GRAM AND MILLIEQUIVALENT MEASUREMENTS

MEq. Na$^+$ (Approximate)	Mg. Na$^+$	Gm. NaCl (Approximate)
11	250	0.6
22	500	1.3
43	1000	2.5
65	1500	3.8
87	2000	5.0
130	3000	7.6
174	4000	10.2

diets. Each molecule of salt is approximately 40 per cent (39.3 per cent) sodium. To convert a specified weight of salt or sodium chloride to its sodium equivalent, multiply the weight of salt by 0.40 (0.393). In other words, 10 gm. of sodium chloride contains approximately 4 (3.93) gm. of sodium. Sodium is also measured in milliequivalents (mEq.). See Appendix Table 9 for an explanation of the conversion of mg. of sodium to mEq. of sodium. 1 gm. of sodium is equal to 43.5 mEq. of sodium, and Table 28–1 lists other conversions of sodium in mg. to sodium in mEq. One tsp. of salt contains approximately 2400 mg. or 104 mEq. of sodium.

The Basic Sodium Restricted Diets. Diets representing varying degrees of sodium restriction are prescribed, depending upon the severity of the cardiac or vascular disease and the amount of edema or fluid retention present.

Table 28–2 shows the nutritive value of a basic normal dietary pattern for an adult that provides approximately 500 mg. of sodium daily. The foods included provide nutrients at levels that, except for total iron content for young women, equal or exceed those of the Recommended Dietary Allowances for the normal healthy adult. The iron content can be increased by using sources that contain insignificant amounts of sodium, such as green leafy vegetables (except beet greens, kale, dandelion, mustard greens and spinach), dried fruit, dried beans or dried lentils. Adjustments and substitutions can be made from this basic pattern for the individual's requirements and eating habits.

The calorie content of this basic diet can be increased or decreased to meet the individual requirements by using more or less of the foods low in sodium, such as unsalted cereal foods, bread, potatoes and fat. Sugar and jelly may be used as desired within the calorie allowance. None of these additions will significantly offset the sodium level of the diet. See Appendix Table 9 for sodium content of foods.

DEGREES OF SODIUM RESTRICTION. Diets based on three levels of sodium restriction are classified as follows:

1. *Mild Sodium Restriction.* Containing 2400 to 4500 mg. (100 to 200 mEq.) sodium daily.

2. *Moderate Sodium Restriction.* Containing 1000 mg. (43 mEq.) sodium daily.

3. *Strict Sodium Restriction.* Containing 500 mg. (22 mEq.) sodium daily. (See Table 28–2.)

Diet booklets explaining these three sodium restriction levels have been prepared by the American Heart Association's Nutrition Committee and are available at local heart association offices to distribute to patients as indicated. The sodium-restricted dietary patterns are based on the Exchange Method such as the one used for diabetic dietary patterns (Chapter 25). In each booklet the appropriate calorie level for the patient can be selected from among three levels: 1200 kcal., 1800 kcal. and unrestricted calories. Variety in food selection is possible through food unit lists or exchanges based on the sodium content per serving in the unit. Table 28–3 gives the average sodium values of the food exchanges. Table 28–4 gives the foods included in each exchange list. These lists are especially useful in designing a diet for someone who also needs to control caloric intake or who must also follow a diabetic diet.

Mild Sodium Restriction: 2400 to 4500 Mg. (104 to 196 mEq.) Sodium Daily. For the patient with only moderate heart damage when some control of sodium intake is indicated, a *limited* amount of salt is allowed in cooking; however, no salt is allowed on the tray or at the table. Salty foods such as those listed in Table 28–5 should be omitted.

Moderate Sodium Restriction: 1000 Mg. (43 mEq.) Sodium Daily. For the patient with edema or a tendency to develop edema when following only mild sodium restriction, no salt is added during the preparation of food or at the table, with the exception of allowing either ¼ tsp. salt daily or measured amounts of foods such as regular bakery bread (1 slice contains 150 mg. sodium) and salted butter (2 tsp. contains 100 mg. sodium) to make the diet more palatable. No salty foods such as listed in Table 28–5 are allowed. A diet providing these restrictions will usually increase urine output.

Strict Sodium Restriction: 500 Mg. Sodium (22 mEq.) or Less Daily (Table 28–2). If edema and pulmonary congestion persist despite drugs, medication and moderate sodium

Table 28–2 NUTRITIVE VALUE OF BASIC DIET PATTERN FOR THE SODIUM-RESTRICTED DIET (500 MG. SODIUM)*

FOOD	MEASURE[a]	WEIGHT (gm.)	KCAL.[b]	PROTEIN (gm.)	FAT (gm.)	CARBOHYDRATE (gm.)	MINERALS Na[c] (mg.)	Ca (gm.)	Fe (mg.)	VITAMINS A (I.U.)	THIAMIN (mg.)	RIBOFLAVIN (mg.)	NIACIN (mg.)	ASCORBIC ACID (mg.)
Milk	2 cups (1 pt.)	488	335	17	19	24	244	0.58	0.4	780	0.18	0.84	0.6	6
Meat, fish or poultry	5 oz. (raw) (cooked)	120	365	28	27		104	0.01	3.5	2280[d]	0.30	0.40	6.9	1
Egg	1 medium	54	75	6	6		70	0.03	1.3	550	0.05	0.14	tr.	0
Whole-grain or enriched cereal[e]	1 serving	20	75	2	tr.	16	tr.	0.01	0.6	0	0.11	0.03	0.7	0
Whole-grain or enriched bread (without added sodium)	3 slices	90	250	8	1	47	27	0.07	1.6	0	0.22	0.14	2.0	0
Potato	1 medium	150	125	3	tr.	29	4	0.02	1.0	30	0.14	0.05	1.5	21
Leafy green or yellow vegetable[f]	1 serving	100	30	2	tr.	6	9	0.05	0.9	880	0.08	0.07	0.7	26
Other vegetable[g]	1 serving	100	35	1	tr.	8	4	0.02	0.6	770	0.06	0.06	0.7	17
Citrus fruit	1 serving	100	45	1	tr.	12	1	0.03	0.4	120	0.07	0.03	0.2	47
Other fruit[h]	2 servings	200	125	1	1	32	5	0.02	1.0	120	0.08	0.08	0.8	18
Butter, unsalted	2 tbsp.	30	215		24		3			990				
Totals			1675	69	78	174	471	0.84	11.3	6520	1.29	1.84	14.1	136
Recommended Dietary Allowances:† Woman (51+ years)			1800	46				0.8	10	4000	1.0	1.1	12[j] equiv.	45
Man (51+ years)			2400	56				0.8	10	5000	1.2	1.5	16[j] equiv.	45

*From Sodium-Restricted Diets. A Report of the Food and Nutrition Board. National Research Council. Publication 325, 1954.
†From Recommended Dietary Allowances. Washington, D.C., National Research Council, 1974.
[a] Average values for each food group have been computed according to the percentage distribution of food supplies as described in "Planning Food for Institutions." Agriculture Handbook No. 16, Washington, D.C.: U.S. Dept. of Agriculture, 1951.
Food values used are those published in "Composition of Foods—Raw, Processed, Prepared" by Bernice K. Watt and Annabel L. Merrill. Agriculture Handbook No. 8, Washington, D.C.: U.S. Dept. of Agriculture, 1950.
[b] Calories have been rounded off to the nearest 5. The total calories should be adjusted to the patient's needs by using more or less of cereal foods, bread, potatoes or unsalted fat. Sugar and jelly may be used when there is no calorie restriction.
[c] Values for sodium are those naturally occurring in food before any additions have been made through processing and cookery.
[d] This vitamin A value is reduced to 0 if average of 1 oz. liver per week is omitted.
[e] Includes farina, rolled oats, rolled wheat cereal, wheat meal, puffed wheat, puffed rice, shredded wheat. Quick-cooking cereals and other dry cereals omitted because of high sodium content.
[f] Includes asparagus, green lima beans (not frozen), snap beans, broccoli, brussels sprouts, lettuce and escarole, okra, peas (not frozen), peppers, pumpkin, winter squash, turnip greens and products packed without added sodium. Excludes carrots, kale, beet greens, chard, spinach.
[g] Includes cauliflower, corn, cucumber, eggplant, onion, parsnip, radishes, rutabagas, summer squash, tomatoes and products packed without added sodium. Excludes beets, celery, white turnips.
[h] Includes all fruits other than citrus—fresh, canned or frozen according to consumption data.
[j] Niacin equivalents include sources of the preformed vitamin and the precursor tryptophan. 60 mg. tryptophan equals 1 mg. niacin.

Table 28–3   SODIUM AND NUTRIENT VALUES FOR FOOD EXCHANGE GROUPS

LIST	FOOD GROUP	AMOUNT	Na+ (mg.)	Na+ (mEq.)	PRO (gm.)	CHO (gm.)	FAT (gm.)	KCAL.
1	Milk	see list						
1A	whole milk	1 cup	120	5	8	12	10	170
	skim milk	1 cup	120	5	8	12	–	80
1B	Milk, low sodium	1 cup	7	–	8	12	10	170
	Buttermilk, salted	1 cup	280	13	8	12	3	110
2	Vegetables							
	cooked, raw, fresh, frozen	½ cup	9	–	2	5	–	25
	canned	½ cup	230	10	v a r i a b l e			
3	Fruits	see list	2	–	–	10	–	40
4	Bread or cereal	see list						
	low sodium or made without salt		5	–	2	15	–	70
	salted yeast bread	1 slice	150	7	2	15	–	70
5	Meat, poultry, fresh fish	1 oz. or						
	cooked without salt	see list	25	1	7	–	5	75
	Cheese, cottage (dry)	¼ cup	5	–	7	–	5	75
	cheddar	1 oz.	207	9	7	–	5	75
	Egg	1	70	3	7	–	5	75
6	Fat							
	unsalted	see list	–	–	–	–	5	45
	salted		50	2	–	–	5	45

restriction, sodium should be reduced to 500 mg. (0.5 gm.) or less daily. For strict sodium restriction no salt is added during the preparation of food or at the table, and foods listed in Table 28–5 are avoided.

Severe Sodium Restriction: 250 Mg. (11 mEq.) Sodium Daily. Further reduction in sodium content of the basic diet pattern (Table 28–2) can be accomplished by substituting appropriate amounts of low-sodium whole or non-fat milk (7 mg. sodium per cup) for the regular whole or skim milk (120 mg. sodium per cup). This is necessary to meet the protein and calcium requirements for this diet.

Sodium-deficient milk has been processed to remove most of the naturally occurring sodium. It is usually prepared in powder form, which can be reconstituted; however, a fluid milk preparation is also available. Within the last 10 years the palatability of this milk has been vastly improved. The fluid low-sodium milk is usually available from local dairies. Dietary adequacy is maintained so long as the sodium-deficient milk contains the other nutrients usually present in regular milk. For those who object to the taste of the milk, flavorings such as chocolate, honey, lemon, vanilla, maple and coffee can be added. The milk can also be used in preparing such dishes as soups, custards and puddings.

Low Salt Syndrome. Severe sodium restriction is intended primarily for the hospitalized patient whose sodium tolerance is un-usually low. Caution should be employed to avoid sodium depletion azotemia, which may develop with this regimen. Harmful results may follow drastic and prolonged restriction of sodium intake, and it is important that the patient be watched carefully for evidence of sodium depletion. Grave danger may exist in severely restricting sodium intake in cases of renal insufficiency in which the kidneys cannot excrete dilute urine. Some symptoms of potential salt depletion that must be evaluated are:

1. Complaints of weakness, lassitude, anorexia and vomiting.
2. Mental confusion.
3. Abdominal cramps and aching skeletal muscles.

However, the possibility that the *low sodium syndrome* may occur does not contraindicate the use of a sodium restricted diet when therapeutically indicated.

SOURCES OF SODIUM.   In their natural state, the majority of foods contain varying amounts of sodium, but the main source of sodium in the diet is salt added in food preparation, food preservation and processing and at the table. Other sodium compounds are found in leavening agents (baking powder, baking soda), disodium phosphate (used in some cereals and cheeses), monosodium glutamate (used to enhance food flavor), sodium alginate (used in some ice creams and chocolate milks), sodium benzoate (a preservative), sodium hydroxide (used in food processing), sodium propionate

Text continued on page 590

Table 28–4 SODIUM CONTENT OF FOOD EXCHANGES
(PROCESSED OR PREPARED WITHOUT ADDED SALT)*

MILK (LIST 1)

GROUP A	GROUP B
Regular Milk	*Low-sodium Milk*

Each unit in both groups contains about 170 kcal., 8 gm. protein, 10 gm. fat and 12 gm. carbohydrate. Group A units contain 120 mg. sodium, whereas group B units contain 7 mg. sodium.

1 cup	Evaporated whole milk (reconstituted)		4 tbsp.	Low-sodium dry milk (powder)
[a]2 fat units and 1 cup	Non-fat buttermilk (unsalted–ask dairy)		1 cup	Low-sodium dry milk (reconstituted)
[a]2 fat units and 3 tbsp.[b]	Non-fat dry milk (powder)		[a]2 fat units and 3 tbsp.[b]	Low-sodium non-fat dry milk (powder)
[a]2 fat units and 1 cup	Non-fat dry milk (reconstituted)		[a]2 fat units and 1 cup	Low-sodium non-fat dry milk (reconstituted)
[a]2 fat units and 1 cup	Skim milk		1 cup	Low-sodium whole fresh milk
1 cup	Whole milk			
1 cup	Whole milk buttermilk (unsalted–ask dairy)			

Note: Two units from the meat list may be substituted for not more than one milk unit a day.

[a] If non-fat milk is used, 2 fat units can be added to the diet.

[b] Use the amount specified on package for making one cup of milk–usually 3 or 4 tbsp.

DO NOT USE: Any kind of milk not on list.

Any commercial foods made of milk: ice cream, sherbet, milk shakes, chocolate milk, malted milk, milk mixes, condensed milk.

VEGETABLES (LIST 2)

Use fresh, frozen or dietetic canned vegetables only. Each unit contains about 9 mg. sodium, 25 kcal., 2 gm. protein, 5 gm. carbohydrate and negligible fat.

VEGETABLE UNITS	DO NOT USE:
Each unit is a ½-cup serving.	

VEGETABLE UNITS — *Each unit is a ½-cup serving.*

Asparagus
Broccoli
Brussels sprouts
Cabbage
Cauliflower
Chicory
Cucumber
Eggplant
Endive
Escarole
Green beans
Lettuce
Mushrooms
Okra
Onions
Peas (fresh or low-sodium dietetic canned only)
Peppers, green or red
Pumpkin
Radishes
Rutabaga (yellow turnip)
Squash, summer (yellow, zucchini, etc.)
Squash, winter (acorn, Hubbard, etc.)
Tomato juice (low-sodium dietetic only)
Tomatoes
Turnip greens
Wax beans

DO NOT USE:

Canned vegetables or vegetable juices unless they are low-sodium dietetic.

Frozen vegetables if processed with salt. (Watch out especially for frozen peas and lima beans.) *Read the label.*

Do not use these vegetables in any form:

Artichokes
Beet greens
Beets
Carrots[c]
Celery[c]
Chard, Swiss
Dandelion greens
Hominy
Kale
Mustard greens
Sauerkraut
Spinach
Turnips, white

Do not use salt or MSG in cooking or at the table.

*From: Your 500 Milligram Sodium Diet. New York, American Heart Association, 1970, pp. 38–53, and Appendix Table 12. Refer to Exchange Lists, Chapter 25.

[c] Even though carrots and celery are high in sodium to be used as vegetables, you may use them sparingly to season (for example, one stalk of celery or carrot to a pot of stew) or as garnish.

Table continued on following page

Table 28–4 SODIUM CONTENT OF FOOD EXCHANGES
(PROCESSED OR PREPARED WITHOUT ADDED SALT)* *(Continued)*

FRUIT (LIST 3)

Use fresh, frozen, canned, or dried fruit. Each unit contains about 2 mg. sodium, 40 kcal., negligible protein and fat and 10 gm. carbohydrate.

FRUIT UNITS				DO NOT USE:
1 small	Apple	⅛ medium	Honeydew melon	Crystallized or glazed fruit. Maraschino cherries.
⅓ cup	Apple juice or apple cider	½ small	Mango	
½ cup	Applesauce	1 small	Orange	
4 halves	Apricots (dried)	½ cup	Orange juice	**Do not use salt or MSG in cooking or at the table.**
2 medium	Apricots (fresh)	⅓ medium	Papaya	
¼ cup	Apricot nectar	1 medium	Peach	
½ small	Banana	1 small	Pear	
1 cup	Blackberries	½ cup diced or 2 small		
⅔ cup	Blueberries	slices	Pineapple	
¼ small	Cantaloupe	⅓ cup	Pineapple juice	Note: Read labels on packages of dried and frozen fruit. Sometimes sodium sulfite has been added to dried fruit and salt to frozen fruit.
10 large	Cherries	2 medium	Plums	
1 tbsp.	Cranberries (sweetened)	2 medium	Prunes	
		¼ cup	Prune juice	
⅓ cup	Cranberry juice (sweetened)	2 tbsp.	Raisins	
		1 cup	Raspberries	
2	Dates	2 tbsp.	Rhubarb (sweetened)	
1 medium	Fig			
½ cup	Fruit cup or mixed fruits	1 cup	Strawberries	
½ small	Grapefruit	1 large	Tangerine	
½ cup	Grapefruit juice	½ cup	Tangerine juice	
12	Grapes	1 cup	Watermelon	
¼ cup	Grape juice			

Note: Fresh lemons and limes (and their juice) may be used as desired. They do not count as a unit. Unsweetened cranberries and cranberry juice and unsweetened rhubarb may also be used as desired.

BREAD (LIST 4)
Low-sodium Breads, Cereals and Cereal Products

Each unit contains about 5 mg. sodium, 70 kcal., 2 gm. protein, negligible fat and 15 gm. carbohydrate.

BREAD UNITS		DO NOT USE:
Breads and rolls (yeast) made without salt.		Yeast breads or rolls made with salt, MSG or from commercial mixes.
1 slice	Bread	
4 pieces (3½″ × 1½″ × ⅛″)	Melba toast (unsalted)	
1 medium	Roll	
Breads (quick) made with sodium-free baking powder or potassium bicarbonate and without salt or made from low-sodium dietetic mix.		Quick breads made with baking powder, baking soda, salt, MSG or made from commercial mixes.
1 medium	Biscuit	
1 cube (1½″)	Cornbread	
2 three-inch	Griddle cakes	
1 medium	Muffin	
Cereals (cooked), unsalted Each unit is a ½-cup serving		Quick-cooking and enriched cereals that contain a sodium compound. Read the label.
	Farina	
	Grits	
	Oatmeal	
	Rolled wheat	
	Wheat meal	

Table 28–4 SODIUM CONTENT OF FOOD EXCHANGES
(PROCESSED OR PREPARED WITHOUT ADDED SALT)* (*Continued*)

BREAD (LIST 4) (*Continued*)
Low-sodium Breads, Cereals and Cereal Products
Each unit contains about 5 mg. sodium, 70 kcal., 2 gm. protein, negligible fat and 15 gm. carbohydrate.

BREAD UNITS		DO NOT USE:
	Cereals (dry)	Dry cereals except for those listed as allowed.
¾ cup	Puffed rice	
¾ cup	Puffed wheat	
⅔ biscuit	Shredded wheat	

(You may use other dry cereals—¾-cup serving—*if the label states* that there are no more than 6 mg. of sodium to each 100 gm. of cereal.)

1½ tbsp. uncooked	Barley	Self-rising cornmeal.
2 tbsp.	Cornmeal	Graham crackers or any other crackers except low-sodium
2½ tbsp.	Cornstarch	dietetic.
5 two-inch-square	Crackers (low-sodium dietetic)	Self-rising flour.
2½ tbsp.	Flour	
½ cup cooked	Macaroni	
1 five-inch-square	Matzo (plain, unsalted)	Salted crackers.
		Salted popcorn.
½ cup cooked	Noodles	Potato chips.
1½ cups	Popcorn	Pretzels.
½ cup cooked	Rice, brown or white	
½ cup cooked	Spaghetti	
2 tbsp. uncooked	Tapioca	Waffles containing salt, baking powder, baking soda.
1 three-inch-square section	Waffle, yeast or low-sodium baking powder, and/or your egg for the day	
½ cup cooked	Beans, lima or navy (fresh or dried)	**Do not use salt or MSG in cooking or at the table.**
¼ cup	Beans, baked (no pork)	
⅓ cup or 1 small ear	Corn	
½ cup cooked	Lentils (dried)	
⅔ cup	Parsnips	
½ cup cooked	Peas, split green or yellow, cowpeas, etc. (dried)	
1 small	Potato, white	
½ cup	Potatoes, mashed	
¼ cup or ½ small	Sweet potato	

Note: One unit from the bread list may be substituted for one unit from Group C.

Table continued on the following page

Table 28–4   SODIUM CONTENT OF FOOD EXCHANGES
(PROCESSED OR PREPARED WITHOUT ADDED SALT)* (*Continued*)

MEAT[d] (LIST 5)
Meat, Poultry, Fish, Eggs and Low-sodium Cheese and Peanut Butter
Units allowed per day will average about 25 mg. sodium, 75 kcal., 7 gm. protein, 5 gm. fat and negligible carbohydrate.

MEAT UNITS	DO NOT USE:
Meat or poultry (fresh, frozen or canned low-sodium dietetic)	Brains or kidneys
1 oz., cooked, of any of the following is a unit	Canned, salted, or smoked meat: bacon, bologna, chipped or corned beef, frankfurters, ham, meats koshered by salting, luncheon meats, salt pork, sausage, smoked tongue, etc.

MEAT UNITS:

beef	quail
chicken	rabbit
duck	tongue (fresh,
lamb	cooked without salt)
liver (beef, calf,	turkey
chicken, pork)	veal
pork	

(Beef or calf liver allowed not more than once in two weeks.)

Fish or fish fillets (fresh only)

1 oz., cooked, of any of the following is a unit

bass	eels	salmon
bluefish	flounder	sole
catfish	halibut	trout
cod	rockfish	tuna

1 oz.	Canned low-sodium dietetic fish (tuna or salmon)
¼ cup	Cottage cheese (unsalted)
1	Egg (limit is 1 a day)
1 oz.	Low-sodium dietetic cheese
2 tbsp.	Low-sodium dietetic peanut butter

DO NOT USE:

Frozen fish fillets

Canned, salted, or smoked fish: anchovies, caviar, salted and dried cod, herring, canned salmon,[e] sardines, canned tuna,[e] etc. Shellfish: clams, crabs, lobsters, oysters, scallops, shrimp, etc.

Cheese[e]

Salted cottage cheese

Regular peanut butter

Do not use salt or MSG in cooking or at the table.

[d]See List 5, Table 25–5 to select meats that are also low in fat.
[e]Unless it is low-sodium dietetic.

GUIDE TO BUYING MEAT, POULTRY AND FISH

An average serving of meat, poultry or fish is 3 oz. This is equal to three units.
Because these foods shrink during cooking, you will have to buy more than 3 oz. for a 3 oz. serving.
To have a 3 oz. serving of fish or lean meat without bone—for example, liver or ground beef—you will need to start with 4 oz. raw.
For meat with bone or fat, you will need to buy 5 to 6 oz. of raw meat to give you 3 oz. of lean cooked meat.
Here are some examples to guide you when you shop. One of these will usually give you three meat units:

> 1 pork chop
> 2 rib lamb chops
> leg and thigh of 3-lb. chicken
> half breast of chicken
> 2 meat patties, 2″ diameter, ½″ thick
> 2 thin slices roast meat, each 3″ × 3″ × ¼″

Table 28–4   SODIUM CONTENT OF FOOD EXCHANGES
(PROCESSED OR PREPARED WITHOUT ADDED SALT)* (*Continued*)

FAT (LIST 6)

Each unit contains negligible sodium, about 45 kcal. and 5 gm. fat.

FAT UNITS		DO NOT USE:
⅛ of four-inch	Avocado	Salted butter
1 tsp.	Butter, unsalted	Bacon and bacon fat
(1 small pat)		Olives
1 tbsp.[f]	Cream, heavy (sweet or sour)	Salt pork
		Commercial French or other dressing[g]
2 tbsp.[f]	Cream, light (sweet or sour)	Salted margarine
		Commercial mayonnaise[g]
1 tsp.	Fat or oil for cooking, unsalted	Salted nuts
1 tbsp.	French dressing, unsalted	
1 tsp.	Margarine, unsalted	
1 tsp.	Mayonnaise, unsalted	
6 small	Nuts, unsalted	

[f]Limit is 2 tbsp. a day because cream contains more sodium than the other fats.
[g]Unless it is low-sodium dietetic.

MISCELLANEOUS FOODS (LIST 7)

Each food listed contains small amounts of sodium.

	DO NOT USE:
Sugar, white or brown	
Syrup, honey, jelly, jam, marmalade	Saccharin
	Molasses
	Instant cocoa mixes
Alcoholic beverages	Beverage mixes, including fruit-flavored powder
Cocoa, made with milk from diet	Fountain beverages: Malted milk and their milk preparates
Coffee, regular and instant	Commercial candies
Coffee substitute	Commercially sweetened gelatin desserts
Tea	Regular baking powder
Postum	Regular baking soda
	Barbecue sauce
Candy, homemade without salt	Regular bouillon cubes
Cornstarch	Catsup and sauces
Gelatin	Celery, onion and garlic salts
	Meat sauces, extracts and tenderizers
Cream of tartar	MSG salt
Sodium-free baking powder	Soy or Worcestershire sauce
Potassium bicarbonate	Salt substitutes, unless recommended by physician
Yeast	Mustard, prepared
	Olives, pickles, relishes
Bouillon cube (Low-Na)	Celery leaves, dried or fresh
Spices	Cooking wine
Chives	Horseradish
Flavorings	
Vinegar	
Wine	

Table 28–5 DIETARY SUBSTANCES
GENERALLY TO BE AVOIDED IN SODIUM
RESTRICTION

1. Smoked, processed or cured meats and fish, such as ham, bacon, corned beef, cold cuts, frankfurters, sausage, tongue, salt pork, chipped beef and anchovies.
2. Meat extracts, bouillon cubes and meat sauces.
3. Salted foods, such as potato chips, nuts and popcorn.
4. Prepared condiments, relishes, Worcestershire sauce, catsup, pickles, mustard and olives.
5. Vegetable salts and flakes, such as onion, garlic or celery salt; celery and parsley flakes.
6. Sodium in any form, such as sodium benzoate as a preservative and monosodium glutamate as a flavoring aid.
7. Bread or bakery products unless prepared without salt and other sources of sodium.
8. Frozen fish fillets and shellfish, except oysters.
9. Prepared flours, flour mixes, baking powder and baking soda.
10. Frozen peas and lima beans; sauerkraut in any form.
11. All canned meat and vegetable products unless prepared without salt (dietetic pack).
12. Canned pears, figs and applesauce unless prepared without salt (dietetic pack).
13. Butter, cheese and peanut butter unless prepared without salt.

(used to inhibit growth of mold) and sodium sulfite (used to bleach certain fruits and as a preservative).

The sodium content of water supplies must be known before it is possible to design effective sodium-restricted diets. The amount of sodium in drinking water may vary widely in different localities and is apt to be relatively high where "softening" treatment is employed. Typical water softeners exchange Na^+ ions for calcium and other ions that cause water hardness. Beverages and processed foods also reflect the sodium content of the drinking water where they are manufactured. Various synthetic detergents used as dishwashing aids contain a much higher proportion of sodium than do true soaps, and the residue on dishes should be removed by rinsing. It may be necessary to use distilled or a natural water, low in sodium, when sodium intake is restricted.

The animal protein foods, namely, milk, cheese, eggs, meat, poultry and fish, are relatively high in sodium. Thus, while nutritionally essential, these foods must be used in measured amounts unless they are processed so that most of the naturally occurring sodium is removed. Fruit is low in natural sodium and its use should be encouraged, since frequently the sodium restricted patient also needs to lose weight, and fruits are generally low in calories.

Certain vegetables—beets, beet greens, celery, kale, dandelion greens, carrots, chard, white turnips and spinach—are relatively high in natural sodium (50 to 80 mg. per serving). Prepared foods such as breads, desserts, cakes and cookies vary appreciably in amounts of sodium. In these foods salt must be omitted, an appropriate leavening agent chosen and allowances made for milk and eggs used. Cream of tartar, sodium-free baking powder, potassium bicarbonate and yeast are leavening agents that may be used. Appendix Tables 9 and 13 give the sodium content of certain common basic foods.

Incidental Sources of Sodium. In addition to the sodium in food and water, incidental amounts may be ingested in the form of medicines and dentifrices. Barbiturates, sulfonamides, antibiotics and other drugs, cough medicines, stomach alkalizers, laxatives, tooth pastes and powders and mouthwashes may contain large amounts of sodium. Labels on these items should be read carefully. The San Francisco Heart Association, Inc. has published a complete booklet of the sodium content of medicines.[27]

AVAILABILITY OF SPECIAL LOW-SODIUM FOODS. Many of the more important food items are available as specially prepared low-sodium products. These include:

Low-sodium milk (whole and skimmed)
Unsalted canned meat
Unsalted canned vegetables
Unsalted cheese (cottage, cheddar)
Unsalted butter and margarine
Unsalted bakery products (bread, crackers, cake, cookies)
Low-sodium baking powder

The term "salt free" does not imply necessarily that the product is low in sodium. The food may have a lot of natural sodium. Also, processing, which removes the natural sodium from foods, may remove other nutrients and may require the diet to be appropriately supplemented.

COMMERCIAL SALT SUBSTITUTES. Most salt substitutes are mineral bases consisting of salts other than sodium compounded to simulate sodium chloride in taste. Potassium chloride, calcium chloride and ammonium chloride are used, but it is conceivable that the administration of a substitute containing large amounts of potassium to patients with renal insufficiency or of ammonium to patients with severe liver disease could be harmful. Some salt substitutes advertised as being "low

sodium" contain in fact another salt *and* sodium chloride. They contain *half* as much sodium as regular table salt, and this must be understood by the patient. *These are not salt substitutes.*

Other products classified as vegetized salts are available. They range somewhere between condiments and salt substitutes. Most products have powdered dehydrated vegetables as a base and varied additional ingredients. However, they may contain considerable quantities of sodium and should therefore not be used. Salt substitutes should be used only when recommended by a physician for a particular patient. Generally, it is advisable for the patient to learn to avoid the salt substitutes and to employ other methods, such as the use of herbs and spices, in making the sodium restricted diet more palatable.

IODINE. In areas of the country where iodine intake is largely dependent on the use of iodized salt, the sodium restricted diet should be carefully evaluated for adequate iodine content when prolonged sodium restriction is required. The RDA for adults for iodine is 100 to 130 μg. per day, and one tsp. (5 gm.) of iodized salt contains approximately 380 μg. of iodine. Supplemental iodine in tablet form may have to be provided if the iodine content of the diet and local drinking water is inadequate.

Suggestions for Making the Sodium Restricted Diet Palatable. Every possible means should be used to make the sodium restricted diet palatable. The patient should be encouraged to enjoy the natural flavors of foods. The preparation of food for the sodium restricted diet need not be complicated, but ingenuity should be exercised in developing flavorings that will compensate for the lack of salt. This is particularly important for the patient following a diet of 1000 mg. sodium or less. In addition, these patients are frequently very sick and frightened. A number of recipe manuals and cooking suggestions are available and are listed at the end of this chapter. In general, as in the case of the diabetic diet, the recipes must be related to the daily food allowances from the diet, especially when calories are limited. For example, the milk and egg used in a custard will be deducted from the total day's food allowance.

Many spices, herbs and other seasonings can be used to improve the flavor of low sodium foods. According to Elvehjem and Burns, "Most of the values (of sodium in spices) are below 0.05%, and all are below 0.1% with the exception of allspice, celery seed, dehydrated celery flakes, whole mace and dehydrated parsley flakes. These figures indicate that, with the exception of celery flakes and parsley flakes, the amount of sodium contributed through the usual amount of spices used is insignificant and that most spices can be used safely in low-sodium diets."[8]

Instruction of the Patient. If a sodium restricted or modified fat diet is prescribed, it is not enough to give the patient a list of foods to avoid. The instructions should help the person secure an adequate diet. He must be given assistance in planning menus, in methods of preparing foods at home and in selecting food when eating away from home, since sodium is very prevalent in prepared and packaged foods.

The nurse, dietitian and physician can do much to encourage the patient concerning the necessary modifications in his diet, but real success depends upon the patient's understanding of the importance of the diet and of the need to adhere to it indefinitely.

The patient should be encouraged to experiment with seasoning and flavoring foods. Suggestions and recipe sources, such as those listed at the end of this chapter, will be stimulating and helpful. Cooking classes or demonstrations for a group of patients who need to control their sodium intake can be effective and enjoyable.

VASCULAR DISEASES

Vascular disorders can be classified as hypertensive vascular disease, various forms of arteriosclerosis, diseases of the aorta and vascular disorders of the extremities.

HYPERTENSION

Hypertension or high blood pressure is not a disease but a symptom. It occurs during the course of such maladies as toxic goiter, in certain forms of cardiac disease, in atherosclerosis and kidney disease and during the course of pregnancy. In the majority of cases the cause is not known, and then it is called "essential" or primary hypertension. This is common in the black population.

The effect of hypertension or elevated tension upon the blood vessels is a narrowing of the vessels as their lining becomes thicker in nature's attempt to help the vessel walls withstand the intensified pressure. Unfortunately, the changes in the vessels or tissues alter the flow of blood to the heart and kidneys and ultimately injure these organs. Persons with hypertension also have a greater risk of developing coronary artery disease.

Renin

In the evaluation of the hypertensive patient, plasma renin activity (PRA) frequently is measured to determine whether renin is a factor in the pathogenesis of the hypertension.[25] *Renin* is an enzyme secreted by the juxtaglomerular apparatus of the kidney in response to many cardiovascular factors, such as a fall in blood pressure, sodium depletion or a fall in plasma volume, and it indirectly increases blood pressure. It acts to increase the blood concentration of angiotensin, which is converted to angiotensin II when it circulates through the lungs. Angiotensin II causes an increase in aldosterone secretion, which increases peripheral vascular resistance, and hypertension develops. The PRA level is a useful measure for determining the necessary therapy.

In order to stimulate renin release and prepare the patient for the PRA test, the patient is told to follow a diet very low in sodium for three days prior to the test. The diet contains 10 to 20 mEq. (250 to 500 mg.) of sodium and is shown in Table 28–2. To adapt the diet to a 10 mEq. sodium restriction, omit the milk or substitute low-sodium milk. It is very important that the patient follow this diet closely, and the nurse must help the patient understand the necessity for compliance.

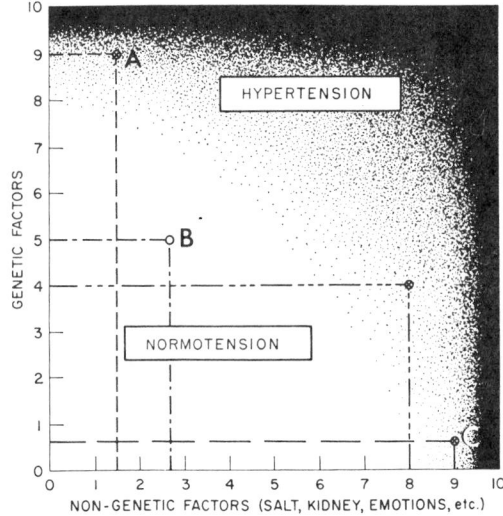

Figure 28–2 Possible relationship between genetic and non-genetic factors in hypertension. *(A)* represents the person with a strong genetic tendency who will develop hypertension when consuming large amounts of salt or who has abnormal kidney function or another medical problem. *(B)* represents the person with less of a genetic predisposition toward hypertension who requires a greater influence from environmental factors (more salt, for instance) before developing hypertension. *(C)* represents the person in whom the genetic tendency to develop hypertension is extremely low. He develops hypertension only after several non-genetic factors are present. (Adapted from: Dahl, L. K.: Salt and hypertension. Am. J. Clin. Nutr., 25:231, 1972.)

Sodium

Dahl[5] has reported that sodium plays a primary role in causing essential hypertension in rats. He also suggests that there is a genetic tendency toward hypertension that is influenced by environmental factors such as kidney function, emotions and salt intake, particularly early in life (see Figure 28–2).

Salt and sodium intake is increasing with the increased use of processed foods and heavily salted snack items. In the early 1970's the sodium content of baby foods, which was shown to be high, was studied very critically, since it seemed possible that an infant could acquire a taste for salt in infancy that would continue into adult life. Baby food manufacturers complied by lowering the salt content of these foods. In 1974 the Committee on Nutrition of the American Academy of Pediatrics recommended "actions that reduce or avoid increasing the present level of salt intake by children in the population at large," even though there is only enough evidence to *suggest* a relationship between salt consumption and hypertension.[3] Dahl suggests that

those with a family history of hypertension restrict sodium intake to 200 to 400 mg. per day and that all others limit intake to a maximum of 2 gm. of sodium per day. The sodium requirement for the healthy human who is not sweating excessively is about 4 to 10 mEq. (92 to 230 mg.) daily, much less than the 200 mEq. or 5 gm. daily that most Americans consume. The body's tolerance for sodium is great—levels as high as 1000 mEq. per day are not toxic.

There is an increased incidence of hypertension in the overweight population that is not understood. Weight reduction causes a lowering of blood pressure that may be due to the decreased salt intake or to other physiological factors.[5]

Prevalence

In the U.S. there is a 20 per cent prevalence of hypertension in adults over 40 years of age, yet many do not know they have it since there are no symptoms. The onset of hypertension in younger individuals is more serious than after middle age. Any attempt to lower the blood

pressure level will help to minimize the stress, strain and degeneration of the tissues. The symptoms start gradually and usually develop into a chronic condition.

Surgery

Surgical treatment is a method of management of essential hypertension. Some excellent results have been reported, especially among comparatively young patients during the early phases of the ailment, from treatment by splanchnicectomy. The long-term results available, however, indicate that side effects following splanchnicectomy may be quite disturbing to the patient, and surgical treatment of hypertension has gradually lost much of its appeal.

Drugs

Antihypertensive drugs have been successfully used in the treatment of hypertension. Various agents are employed—alone and in combination—including those that act centrally, those that produce ganglionic blockade and those that exert peripheral sympatholytic and adrenolytic effects. Unfortunately, side effects are common with the use of every agent currently available, but newer agents are appearing and it is hoped that these side effects can be eliminated.

The thiazide diuretics chlorothiazide (Diuril) and hydrochlorothiazide (Hydro-Diuril) and furosemide (Lasix) potentiate the action of antihypertensive drugs by promoting volume depletion and sodium loss. However, the continued use of chlorothiazide or hydrochlorothiazide may produce hypokalemia, especially in the presence of a high salt intake. Even in those patients taking diuretics, the sodium intake should be restricted to 22 to 87 mEq. (500 to 2000 mg.) for the most effective lowering of blood pressure. Except in the case of a potassium-sparing diuretic, such as spironolactone or triamterene, additional potassium usually is required. Appendix Table 9 gives the potassium values of various foods that contribute potassium to the diet. A KCl supplement can also be used. The Na:K ratio is important, and Langford suggests that the most effective diet for patients using thiazide diuretics contains 50 mEq. each of Na^+ and K^+, although 100 mEq. of each is more realistic. He further has found that patients taking diuretics crave salt because of the increased excretion of sodium in the urine and will eat even more salt unless it is intentionally restricted.[22] Fortunately, many of the foods that are high in potassium (fruits and vegetables, for instance) are also low in sodium.

Other possible effects of the excessive use of diuretics are hyponatremia, hypochloremia, hyperuricemia, and hyperglycemia.

Nutritional Care

Kempner Rice Diet. In 1944 the *Kempner rice diet*[17] was introduced for treatment of both hypertensive vascular disease and kidney disease. The patient consumes daily 10 oz. of dry rice (approximately 1050 kcal.), which is cooked without salt. The remaining 900 to 1000 kcal. are supplied by liberal quantities of sugar and fresh or preserved fruits. Thus, the diet is high in carbohydrate, furnishes about 2000 kcal., 15 to 30 gm. of protein, 4 to 6 gm. of fat and 100 to 150 mg. of sodium daily. Salt is strictly forbidden. Fluids are limited to 700 to 1000 ml. of fruit juices. Tomato juice and vegetable juices are not permitted. Iron and vitamin supplements are given. After reduction of blood pressure and alleviation of the symptoms, the diet is somewhat liberalized. However, it is difficult for a patient to live on this regimen for any length of time, and dietary restriction and manipulation may lead to nutritional deficiencies.

Kempner utilized this method in 213 patients with high blood pressure who exhibited various stages of the disease. After an average period of 62 days on the strict or modified diet, improvement was noted in 64 per cent of the patients. Subsequent investigations carried out by other workers using a more liberal diet that was adequate in protein but equally low in sodium amply demonstrated that sodium restriction was the only important factor.

Sodium Restriction and Weight Control. Today the most common management of hypertension includes the use of diuretics, a moderate dietary sodium restriction (90 to 130 mEq. or 2 to 3 gm. sodium) and weight loss if the patient is overweight. Obesity places an added burden on the heart, and there is general agreement that normal weight is important in relieving the symptoms of hypertension. Protein is not restricted unless there is impairment of renal function. (See Chapter 30.) If cardiac damage has resulted, sodium is restricted even further, to 43 mEq. (1 gm.) or less. A diet with sodium restricted to 500 mg. daily may be necessary to insure maximum therapeutic results. The degree of sodium restriction will depend upon the severity and course of the hypertension. Sodium restricted diets were discussed previously.

ATHEROSCLEROSIS

Atherosclerosis is a form of arteriosclerosis; that is, a thickening of the walls of the arteries. Normally, the blood vessels are smooth-lined tubes. In atherosclerosis small yellow flakes appear on the inner lining of arteries and arterioles that represent early deposits of fatty materials containing *cholesterol, phospholipids* and calcium. (See Chapter 4.) These deposits gradually harden into tough, fibrous bulges called *plaques*. As the plaques in these patches become more numerous, the arteries become roughened and narrowed, the elasticity is lost and the flow of blood through the vessels is curtailed. The arteriosclerotic process does not develop at a uniform rate in all arteries.

Atherosclerosis interferes with the circulation, chiefly to the heart, kidneys and brain. These organs need blood to function efficiently, and when impairment occurs, the effect is noted throughout the system. Atherosclerosis of the coronary arteries—*coronary heart disease* (CHD) or *atherosclerotic heart disease* (ASHD)—underlies most heart attacks. *Stroke,* or *apoplexy,* is often caused by the same condition. The problem of preventing or retarding these attacks or diseases is largely one of preventing or retarding atherosclerosis.

Etiology

The exact origin of atherosclerosis is unknown. Most researchers hold that a variety of factors must be involved and that it is a gradual process that probably begins at birth. Whether it is a disease or a natural process of aging has not been established. Heredity plays a role in that some individuals inherit the tendency to develop atherosclerosis at an earlier age.

Risk Factors

Many risk factors have been identified in trying to unravel the puzzling etiology of CHD, and some are more definitive than others. In summarizing the knowledge concerning risk factors, the Inter-Society Commission for Heart Disease Resources identified three *major* risk factors: hypercholesterolemia, hypertension and cigarette smoking.[26] Some other risk factors are diabetes mellitus, hypertriglyceridemia, obesity, sedentary living, psychosocial tensions and certain dietary factors.

1. *Hypercholesterolemia* in relation to CHD has been studied extensively. It has been shown that people from countries or races that consume large amounts of fat have higher serum cholesterol levels and a greater incidence of coronary and aortic atherosclerosis than those of comparable age who eat less fat.[23] Keys and associates, in studying selected male populations in seven countries, found significant differences in the prevalence of CHD in these populations. These differences were related to serum cholesterol levels, and furthermore, the serum cholesterol variations could be explained by the different proportions of saturated fats in the diets.[18] As the serum cholesterol increases, so does the risk of CHD.

2. *Hypertension* seems to aggravate the atherosclerotic process, especially in the presence of elevated levels of blood lipid. As with the blood lipid level, the correlation between hypertension and risk of CHD is continuous— the higher the blood pressure, the greater the risk of CHD.

3. *Cigarette smoking* is positively correlated with CHD mortality. Carbon monoxide inhaled in cigarette smoke leads to a relative state of hypoxia, which results in an increase in serum lipid levels. Cholesterol-fed rabbits in which hypoxia was induced through inhalation of carbon monoxide showed an increase in lipid accumulation in the arterial walls.[1]

In the final analysis we still do not have definitive evidence that modification of the risk factors will reduce mortality from CHD. However, the Multiple Risk Factor Intervention Trial (MRFIT) was initiated in 1974 to answer this question. In the meantime, there is still enough evidence to warrant a conscientious effort toward modification of the risk factors whenever possible.

Serum Lipids—Cholesterol and Triglyceride

Influence of Non-Dietary Factors. Increasing evidence suggests that blood cholesterol levels are directly related to *exercise*. This evidence thus favors a continued, active life of muscular work. *Sex* and *hormones* have also been mentioned as factors, and atherosclerosis is more common in young males than young females. During the childbearing years women have relatively little cardiovascular disease, and the blood fat levels are relatively low. After menopause there is a greater frequency of such disorders and higher blood cholesterol levels. This suggests that the female sex hormones are a protective factor. *Brief repeated insults* resulting from fever, infection, intense emotional upsets, fatigue, stress and obesity are also

Table 28–6 CONCENTRATIONS OF C, TG OR LDL[a] THAT, IF EXCEEDED, CLEARLY INDICATE HYPERLIPIDEMIA[*, b]

AGE	C (mg. per 100 ml.)	LDL (mg. per 100 ml.)	TG
1–19	230	170	150
20–29	240	170	200
30–39	270	190	200
40–49	310	190	200
50 and up	330	210	200

[a]   C = cholesterol
  LDL = low density lipoproteins
    TG = triglycerides

[b]These values are set high and also allow for lipid increases that occur in Americans as they age. This may not be optimal or normal. Hyperlipidemia deserving attention exists when cholesterol exceeds 200 mg. per 100 ml. plus the person's age in years and triglyceride exceeds 150 mg. per 100 ml.

*From: Fredrickson, D. S., et al.: Dietary Management of Hyperlipoproteinemia. DHEW Publ. No. (NIH) 75-110. Bethesda, Md., National Heart and Lung Institute, 1974.

claimed to be contributing factors. In *certain diseases* such as hypothyroidism, nephrosis, diabetes, obstructive liver disease and pancreatitis there is more lipid in the blood than normally, and atherosclerosis frequently is associated with these conditions. *Pregnancy* and *oral contraceptives containing estrogen* also lead to hyperlipidemia. Serum triglycerides can be elevated by alcohol. Table 28–6 lists the upper limits of normal serum cholesterol and serum triglyceride.

Influence of Dietary Factors

FAT.   The type and amount of fat in the diet influence the serum cholesterol level. Although epidemiological evidence shows that a low fat intake is associated with lower serum cholesterol levels and lower incidence of CHD, it appears that the *type* of fat in a moderate fat diet (30 to 35 per cent of kcal.) is more important than the *amount* of fat.

By substituting highly unsaturated fats (those with multiple double bonds, such as safflower, corn and cottonseed oils) for saturated fats (animal or hydrogenated vegetable fats) in human diets or, in some instances, by adding sufficient amounts of unsaturated fats to a normal fat intake, the total amounts of plasma lipids and serum cholesterol are consistently lowered in a high percentage of cases. However, the removal of saturated fat from the diet is twice as effective as adding an equal amount of polyunsaturated fat in lowering blood

cholesterol. Grande and associates have shown that even when the total fat content of the diet remains the same, subtracting a certain amount of saturated fat has the same effect as adding twice that amount in polyunsaturated fat.[12] Monounsaturated fats were found to be neutral and do not cause a rise or fall of serum cholesterol. Apparently, it is the proportion of saturated to polyunsaturated fatty acids in the total diet consumed that determines the lipid level and, consequently, the vascular deposition of lipids. The Framingham study showed that the polyunsaturated fat to saturated fat ratio (P:S) for the American diet was between 0.3 and 0.4:1.[15] It should be raised to 1:1.

CHOLESTEROL.   Dietary cholesterol does not have as much influence on serum cholesterol level as does the intake of saturated or polyunsaturated fat. A reduction of 100 mg. in dietary cholesterol results in a lowering of only 5 mg. in serum cholesterol when dietary fat is not also altered. However, dietary cholesterol becomes a significant factor when compared with the polyunsaturated fat in the diet, which has a greater lowering effect on serum cholesterol when dietary cholesterol is also reduced. For example, Hegsted and coworkers found that when the only fat in the diet was the highly saturated coconut oil, a 300 mg. cholesterol intake (reduced from the usual American intake of 800 mg.) had little effect, and serum cholesterol increased by 40 mg. per 100 ml. When the dietary fat was monounsaturated olive oil, a 300 mg. cholesterol intake did not affect the serum cholesterol level, and when the dietary fat was polyunsaturated safflower oil with the 300 mg. cholesterol intake, the serum cholesterol level was reduced 35 mg. per 100 ml.[13]

CARBOHYDRATE.   Large quantities of dietary carbohydrate will cause an increase in the amount of serum triglyceride in some people. The liver converts the excess carbohydrate to triglyceride, which may then exceed the clearing capacity of the adipose tissue and result in an increase in serum triglyceride levels. Sucrose and fructose are more effective than starch as inducers of this hypertriglyceridemia. Some people are more sensitive to a carbohydrate load than others, but carbohydrate-induced hypertriglyceridemia seems to be closely related to an impaired glucose tolerance and diabetes mellitus and also to obesity.[28]

DIETARY FIBER.   Pectin, a form of dietary fiber found in fruits, has been found to lower serum cholesterol levels. There is no substantial evidence for the lowering of blood choles-

terol levels by other types of fiber in the diet.[14, 19]

TRACE ELEMENTS. An interesting observation that may possibly link a trace element with coronary heart disease is the reported lower death rate from CHD in areas with a hard water supply.[29] When the water has been softened, the mortality from CHD has increased. A likely difference between hard and soft water that may be important is the increased calcium content of hard water, but this has not been proven.[7]

Recently Klevay has suggested that the zinc:copper ratio in the body becomes abnormal as a result of food choices, hypertension, water hardness and lack of exercise. This zinc-copper imbalance results in an increased serum cholesterol level and thus, increased mortality due to CHD.[20]

OTHER FACTORS. The function of vitamin E in ischemic heart disease is not clear, but at this time there is no evidence to implicate a deficiency of vitamin E. The use of vitamin E supplements is unfounded. Vitamin C may have a function in lipolysis and protection against atherosclerosis, but this is still unclear.

The Prudent Diet for the Prevention of Atherosclerosis

Because many Americans have elevated or moderately elevated blood lipid levels and be-

cause we now possess greater knowledge about the dietary factors that influence blood lipid levels, the Inter-Society Commission on Heart Disease Resources and the American Heart Association have suggested some general guidelines to the public for dietary modification. A diet following these guidelines will lower blood lipid levels and possibly help prevent coronary heart disease. These recommendations have been termed the "Prudent Diet."[4] Table 28–7 summarizes this diet and compares it with the present typical American diet. Recently the Senate Select Committee on Nutrition and Human Needs, in their report, *Dietary Goals for the United States,* endorsed similar guidelines.[30]

To translate these recommendations into eating habits means: (1) eating smaller portions of meat (6 oz. per day) that contains less fat, (2) avoiding all whole-milk dairy products such as ice cream, hard cheeses, cream, butter and whole milk, (3) increasing the intake of fruits and vegetables, which contain virtually no fat, no salt (except in canned vegetables) and no cholesterol and are low in calories, (4) eating breads, cereals and flour products that do not contain large amounts of sugar and fat, (5) restricting eggs and high-cholesterol foods to three times per week, (6) using a polyunsaturated oil for cooking and baking (see Fig. 28–3) and (7) cooking to avoid saturated fats and to include polyunsaturated fats. See Table 28–8 for the translation of these

Table 28–7 COMPARISON OF TYPICAL AMERICAN DIET AND THE AHA PRUDENT DIET*

NUTRIENT	APPROXIMATE COMPOSITION	
	TYPICAL AMERICAN DIET	AHA PRUDENT DIET
Cholesterol	600–700 mg.	300 mg.
Total Calories	Often overconsumption	Reduction to achieve and/ or maintain ideal weight
Total Fat (% of kcal.)	40–42%	35%
Saturated	15%	<10%
Monounsaturated	16–17%	15%
Polyunsaturated	5– 6%	10%
P:S Ratio	0.3–0.4:1	1–1.5:1
Carbohydrate (% of kcal.)	40–45%	50–55%
Starch	20–25%	Increased
Simple sugars	15–20%	Decreased
Protein (% of kcal.)	12–15%	12–15%
Sodium	150–200 mEq.	130 mEq.

*Sources: U.S. Department of Agriculture, Agricultural Research Service, 1974. American Heart Association: Diet and Coronary Heart Disease. New York, AHA, 1973. Connor, S., and Connor, W.: The "Alternative American Diet" for the Prevention of Coronary Heart Disease. Iowa City, Iowa, University of Iowa, Lipid-Atherosclerosis Group. Dahl, L. K.: Salt and hypertension. Am. J. Clin. Nutr., *25*:231, 1972.

Unsaturated   Safflower oil
⬆   Sunflower oil
               Soybean oil
               Corn oil
               Cottonseed oil
               Sesame oil
               Tub margarine, liquid
                 safflower oil
               Mayonnaise
               Tub margarine, liquid
                 corn oil
               Peanut butter
               Stick margarine, liquid
                 corn oil
               Olive oil
               Vegetable shortening,
                 hydrogenated
               Peanut oil
               Tub or stick margarine,
                 hydrogenated or hardened fat
               Lard
⬇   Butterfat
Saturated   Coconut oil

Figure 28–3   Unsaturation of dietary fats and oils.

principles into a diet. This diet is planned using the food exchange lists in Table 25–5.

These proposals are major changes for Americans, and it is difficult to make them in our present environment. The Commission further recommends that the food industry be encouraged to make available leaner meats; processed meats, dairy products, frozen desserts and baked goods reduced in saturated fat, cholesterol and calories; and margarine, shortening, mayonnaise, salad dressing and oil of low saturated fat and cholesterol content. We are beginning to see some of these changes with the development of cholesterol-free egg substitutes, cheeses and breakfast meats, polyunsaturated margarines and statements of fat content on food labels (Fig. 28–4). Appendix Table 4 lists the fatty acid and cholesterol content of some foods.

Even highly motivated individuals will find some of these changes difficult; the process of change will not be sudden and complete. Connor states that it takes two to ten years to make radical changes in one's eating habits and proposes "phases" of diet adjustment that should be individualized.[4] A reasonable change for some people may be the use of a soft or tub margarine instead of regular stick margarine or butter. It is important to know what is reasonable for patients when counseling and helping them to begin the process of dietary modification. (See Chapter 19.)

HYPERLIPOPROTEINEMIA

Hyperlipidemia, or an elevated blood lipid level, is frequently classified into one of various types of *hyperlipoproteinemia*, for which there are specific regimens of nutritional care. All blood lipids (cholesterol, phospholipid and triglyceride) are bound to specific proteins that circulate in the plasma. These proteins transport the lipids into and out of plasma in complexes called *lipoproteins*. An abnormally high level of one or more of these lipoproteins in the blood is called hyperlipoproteinemia.

These lipoproteins may be identified by zonal gel electrophoresis or by ultracentrifugation. Each lipoprotein contains cholesterol, phospholipid, triglyceride and protein in different and characteristic proportions. The plasma lipoproteins are (1) chylomicrons, (2) pre-β-lipoproteins (very low density lipoproteins or VLDL), (3) β-lipoproteins (low density lipo-

Table 28–8   FAT- AND CALORIE-CONTROLLED DIETS*
(Fat = 35 to 40 Per Cent of Total Calories)

FOOD GROUP	1200 KCAL.	1800 KCAL.	2400 KCAL.
Milk Exchanges (non-fat)	2	2	2
Vegetable Exchanges	3 or more	3 or more	3 or more
Fruit Exchanges	3	3	5
Bread and cereal Exchanges	4	7	8
Meat, fish, poultry Exchanges[a]	6	6	7
Eggs[a] (per week)	3	3	3
Fat Exchanges	6	9	15
Sugar, sweets (Kcal.)			200

[a] Meat exchanges may be substituted for egg exchanges (1 exchange = 1 egg). Lean meat exchanges should be used as often as possible.

Ratio of polyunsaturated to saturated fatty acids ranges from 1.1:1 to 1.5:1. Diets planned according to ADA Exchange System and Table 25–4.

*Adapted from: American Heart Association: Planning Fat Controlled Meals for 1200 and 1800 Calories. New York, AHA, 1966; and Planning Fat Controlled Meals for 2000 to 2600 Calories. New York, AHA, 1967.

NUTRITION INFORMATION PER SERVING

Serving size: 1 tbsp.   14 gm.
Servings per container   32 (per lb. container)
Calories   100
Protein   0 gm.
Carbohydrate   0 gm.
Fat   11 gm.
*Percent of calories from
   fat   over 99%
     polyunsaturated   5 gm.
     saturated   2 gm.
*Cholesterol   0 (0 per 100 gm.)

Percentage of U.S. Recommended Daily Allowances (U.S. RDA)
Vitamin A   10%
Vitamin D   15%
  Contains less than 2 per cent of the U.S. RDA of protein, vitamin C, thiamin, riboflavin, niacin, calcium and iron.

Ingredients: Liquid corn oil, partially hydrogenated corn oil, water, salt, non-fat dry milk, vegetable mono- and diglycerides and lecithin, sodium benzoate (0.1%) as a preservative, artificially flavored and colored (carotene), vitamins A and D added.

*Information on fat and cholesterol content is provided for individuals who, on the advice of a physician, are modifying their total dietary intake of fat and cholesterol.

Figure 28–4 Label describing a typical unsaturated margarine.

proteins or LDL) and (4) α-lipoproteins (high density lipoproteins or HDL). Normally most of the plasma cholesterol is found in β-lipoproteins and most of the plasma triglyceride is in the pre-β-lipoproteins. (See Figure 28–5.)

Chylomicrons consist mostly of triglyceride absorbed from the diet. Chylomicrons are synthesized in the intestine and transport dietary triglycerides from the intestine into the plasma. They give a milky appearance to normal plasma after a fatty meal, but their presence in the fasting plasma is indicative of abnormal lipid levels.

The *pre-β-lipoproteins (VLDL)* are composed largely of triglycerides (but also contain some cholesterol) and function to transport triglycerides of endogenous origin, largely from the liver. Virtually all of the triglyceride that is not in chylomicrons is in VLDL.

The function of *β-lipoproteins (LDL)*, which normally carry two thirds of the total plasma cholesterol, is not clear. They apparently represent the plasma residue of VLDL catabolism. By weight, LDL is about 45 per cent cholesterol and 25 per cent protein.

The fourth and smallest group in the lipoprotein family is the *α-lipoproteins (HDL)*. They contain the remainder of plasma cholesterol, and their function is not clear.

When any of the blood lipid levels are abnormally elevated, particularly those of cholesterol or triglyceride, there will also be an elevation in the levels of the particular lipoproteins that transport them.

Classification of Hyperlipoproteinemias

Many different genetic and metabolic factors control lipoprotein concentrations. A hyperlipoproteinemia may be primary and sometimes inherited or may be secondary to some other disease, such as diabetes mellitus, nephrotic syndrome, hypothyroidism, pancreatitis or obstructive liver disease. Six types of hyperlipoproteinemias have been described. Each is classified in terms of the abnormal accumulation of one or more lipoprotein families in the plasma. (See Table 28–9).

Types IIa, IIb and IV are associated with premature atherosclerosis.[21] Because they are fairly common they deserve special attention, particularly now that type II is detectable in neonates by cord blood analysis. Thus, preventive dietary measures can be started early.[11]

The identification and classification of these genetic hyperlipidemias is useful, because what we are witnessing with regard to the incidence of the disease is possibly the influence of environmental factors, particularly

diet, on an inherited or other tendency in some people toward various degrees of abnormal lipid metabolism. This can lead to elevated blood lipid levels and a greater risk of CHD.[24] There may be individual factors that modify or even eliminate the influence of nutrients such as fat among certain people.

Nutritional Care for the Hyperlipoproteinemias

The dietary management of the hyperlipoproteinemias has been carefully formulated and is available upon request from the National Institutes of Health.[10] Appropriate suggestions for using, buying and cooking foods are included. See Table 28–10 for a summary of these diets.

Generally, the purpose of the diets is to reduce the hyperlipidemia and keep the patient asymptomatic. A 15 per cent or greater reduction in serum cholesterol or triglyceride levels means that the diet is successful and should be continued. All persons on these diets should try to achieve or maintain ideal body weight. Weight loss in itself will cause a lowering of serum triglyceride levels in overweight patients. In designing these diets the exchange lists given in Table 25–5 can be used.

Type I Hyperlipoproteinemia. Type I hyper-lipoproteinemia indicates an inability to clear chylomicrons from the blood due to a deficiency of adipose tissue lipoprotein lipase. As a result, the *serum triglyceride* concentration is *extremely high* (more than 1000 mg. per 100 ml.). A very low fat diet, 25 to 35 gm. of fat per day, is effective therapy and results in a clearing of the triglyceride from the serum and prevention of bouts of abdominal pain. Medium-chain triglycerides (MCT) can be used as supplementary fat, since they are absorbed directly into the portal vein and are transported to the liver without requiring chylomicron formation. This source of fat may help to make the diet more palatable.

DIET FOR THE CHILD WITH TYPE I
HYPERLIPOPROTEINEMIA
(4–6 Years of Age, 35–40 lb.) 1400–1600 Kcal.[10]

DAILY FOOD PLAN

---

1 qt. skim milk (fortified with vitamins A and D)
2 oz. cooked poultry, fish or lean trimmed meat[a]
4 servings of vegetable and fruit
4 or more servings of bread or cereal
1 or more servings of potato, rice, etc.
Allowed desserts[b] and sweets

---

[a] Add one additional ounce of meat for the child 6 to 12 years old.
[b] Desserts made with skim milk; also Jello, fruit, fruit ices. MCT oil may be used but adds calories to the diet.

DIET FOR THE ADULT WITH TYPE I
HYPERLIPOPROTEINEMIA
(1700–2000 Kcal.)[10]

DAILY FOOD PLAN

---

1 qt. skim milk (fortified with vitamins A and D)
5 oz. cooked poultry, fish or lean trimmed meat
5 servings of vegetable and fruit including 1 serving citrus fruit, and 1 serving dark green or deep yellow vegetable
6 or more servings whole-wheat or whole-grain bread or cereal
1 or more servings potato, rice, noodles, grits
Desserts[a]
Sugars, sweets
Beverages (non-dairy)

---

[a] Made with skim milk; Jello, fruit, fruit ices. Medium chain triglycerides (MCT) may be used if prescribed by a physician, in which instance adjustment in calories is necessary.

Type II Hyperlipoproteinemia. Type II or hyperbetalipoproteinemia is characterized by an increase in beta lipoprotein (LDL) due either to overproduction or inadequate removal. It is thought to be transmitted as an autosomal dominant trait and is easily diagnosed early in the first or second year of life. It is classified as *type IIa* if the VLDL level is

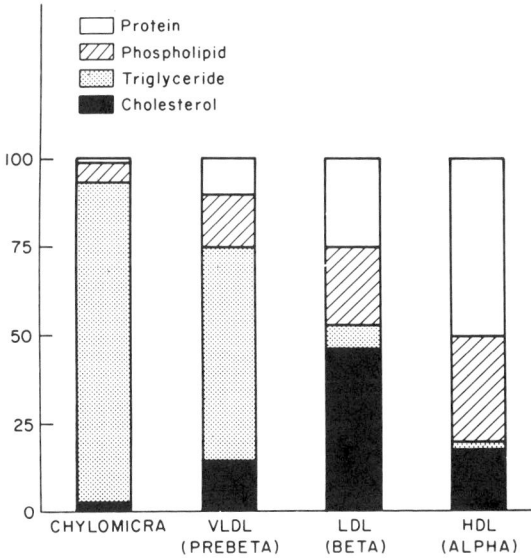

Figure 28–5 Approximate percentage of composition of the four lipoprotein families. VLDL = very low density lipoproteins, LDL = low density lipoproteins, HDL = high density lipoproteins. (From: Levy, R. I., et al.: Dietary and drug treatment of primary hyperlipoproteinemia. Ann. Intern. Med., 77:267, 1972.)

Table 28–9   TYPES OF PRIMARY HYPERLIPOPROTEINEMIA*

TYPE	LIPID ABNORMALITIES	LIPOPROTEIN ABNORMALITIES[a]	USUAL AGE OF EXPRESSION	FAMILIAL FORMS	SOME CLINICAL FEATURES
I	Cholesterol: normal or elevated. Triglyceride: elevated (>1000 mg./100 ml.)	Severe chylomicronemia	Infancy and childhood	Rare and usually familial (recessive)	Bouts of abdominal pain, pancreatitis, eruptive xanthomas, hepatosplenomegaly
IIa	Cholesterol: elevated (300–600 mg./100 ml.). Triglyceride: normal	LDL increased	At birth, if genetic	Most obvious genetic form is expressed in heterozygote, more severe in homozygote; many mild examples are not obviously familial	Premature vascular disease; in familial forms, tendon and tuberous xanthomas
IIb	Cholesterol: elevated (300–600 mg./100 ml.). Triglyceride: elevated (150–400 mg./100 ml.)	LDL increased, plus excess VLDL	At birth, if genetic	Pattern alternates with IIa in families affected with "monogenic" type II; milder defects are sporadic or due to other genetic defects	Severe forms are like IIa; milder IIb patterns tend to be accompanied by glucose intolerance, obesity
III	Cholesterol: elevated (350–800 mg./100 ml.). Triglyceride: usually elevated (150–1000 mg./100 ml.)	VLDL/LDL of abnormal composition	Third decade; often after menopause in women	Frequently familial, genetic mode uncertain	Glucose intolerance, tuberoeruptive or planar xanthomas, premature vascular disease (especially peripheral vascular disease); worsened by alcohol excess
IV	Cholesterol: normal or elevated. Triglyceride: elevated (400–1000 mg./100 ml.)	VLDL increased	Usually third decade or later; can occur in children	Often half of adult close relatives will also have type IV; number of mutants or frequency of familial involvement unknown	Glucose intolerance in about 50%; excess caloric intake common; occasionally eruptive xanthomas; worsened by alcohol excess
V	Cholesterol: elevated. Triglyceride: elevated (>1000 mg./100 ml.)	VLDL increased, chylomicrons present	Adulthood, very rare in children	When familial, more than half of close relatives have either type IV or type V	Bouts of abdominal pain and pancreatitis, eruptive xanthomas, hepatosplenomegaly, excess caloric intake common, hyperuricemia; most patients have glucose intolerance; worsened by alcohol excess

*Adapted from: Levy, R. I., et al.: Dietary and drug treatment of primary hyperlipoproteinemia. Ann. Intern. Med., 77:267, 1972.
[a]LDL = low density lipoproteins; VLDL = very low density lipoproteins.

Table 28–10 SUMMARY OF DIETS AND DRUGS FOR TYPES I–V HYPERLIPOPROTEINEMIA*

	TYPE I	TYPE IIa	TYPE IIb & TYPE III	TYPE IV	TYPE V
Diet Prescription	Low fat (25–35 gm.; 10–15 gm. for a child)	Low cholesterol; polyunsaturated fat increased	Low cholesterol; approximately: 20% cal. Pro. 40% cal. Fat 40% cal. CHO	Controlled CHO (approximately 45% of calories); moderately restricted cholesterol	Restricted fat (30% of calories); controlled CHO (50% of calories); moderately restricted cholesterol
Calories	Not restricted	Not restricted	Achieve and maintain "ideal" weight; reduction diet if necessary	Achieve and maintain "ideal" weight; reduction diet if necessary	Achieve and maintain "ideal" weight; reduction diet if necessary
Protein	Total protein intake not limited	Total protein intake not limited	High protein	Not limited other than control of patient's weight	High protein
Fat	Restricted to 25–35 gm.; kind of fat not important	Saturated fat intake limited; polyunsaturated fat intake increased	Controlled to 40% calories (polyunsaturated fats recommended in preference to saturated fats)	Not limited other than control of patient's weight (polyunsaturated fats recommended in preference to saturated fats)	Restricted to 30% of calories (polyunsaturated fats recommended in preference to saturated fats)
Cholesterol	Not restricted	As low as possible; only source of cholesterol is meat in the diet	Less than 300 mg.; only source of cholesterol is meat in the diet	Moderately restricted to 300–500 mg.	Moderately restricted to 300–500 mg.
Carbohydrate	Not limited	Not limited	Controlled; concentrated sweets restricted	Controlled; concentrated sweets restricted	Controlled; concentrated sweets restricted
Alcohol	Not recommended	May be used with discretion	Limited to 2 servings (substituted for carbohydrate)	Limited to 2 servings (substituted for carbohydrate)	Not recommended
Drug of Choice	None effective at present	Cholestyramine Nicotinic acid[a]	Clofibrate Nicotinic acid[a]	Clofibrate Nicotinic acid[a]	Clofibrate Nicotinic acid[a]

*Adapted from: Fredrickson, D. S., et al.: Dietary Management of Hyperlipoproteinemia. DHEW Publ. No. (NIH) 75-110. Bethesda, Md., National Heart and Lung Institute, 1974.
[a]Nicotinic acid has the unpleasant side effects of cutaneous flushing and pruritus, which limit its usefulness.

$$\frac{\text{gm. of linoleic acid}}{\text{gm. of saturated fat}} = \text{P:S ratio}$$

Example:

$$\text{P:S ratio for vegetable fat} = \frac{0.4 \text{ gm. linoleic acid}}{1 \text{ gm. saturated fat}} = 0.4$$

$$\text{P:S ratio for corn oil} = \frac{2.7 \text{ gm. linoleic acid}}{0.5 \text{ gm. saturated fat}} = 5.4$$

Figure 28–6 Calculation of polyunsaturated:saturated fat ratio (P:S).

normal and as *type IIb* if the VLDL level is elevated along with that of LDL. Type IIa is characterized by elevated cholesterol levels, and type IIb shows elevated levels of both triglyceride and cholesterol. Mild forms of IIa can be due to dietary indiscretion, and more severe forms are genetic in origin. The treatment involves lowering the intake of cholesterol to less than 300 mg. per day (100 to 150 mg. per day for children) and modifying the fat intake to produce a high polyunsaturated to saturated fatty acid ratio (P:S of about 2). (See Fig. 28–6 for calculation of P:S ratio.)

To follow this diet the patient must eat lean meat, including fish and poultry (without skin), limited to not more than 9 oz. per day, and beef, lamb, ham and pork, limited to a 3 oz. portion three times a week. Whole-milk dairy products and eggs are omitted. An intake of at least 1 tsp. of oil high in polyunsaturated fat is recommended for every ounce of meat. See Figure 28–3 for the most unsaturated oils. When beef, lamb or pork is selected, 2 tsp. of oil is recommended for each ounce of meat. Recipes are available from local heart associations for low-fat cooking and cooking with oil.

DIET FOR THE CHILD WITH TYPE IIa HYPERLIPOPROTEINEMIA
(4–6 Years of Age, 35–40 lb.)[10]
1400–1600 Kcal.

DAILY FOOD PLAN

1 qt. skim milk (fortified with vitamins A and D)
Cooked poultry, fish or lean trimmed meat
4 servings of vegetables and fruit; including 1 serving citrus fruit,[a] 1 serving dark green or deep yellow vegetable[b]
4 or more servings of whole-grain or enriched bread or cereal[c]
1 or more servings of potato, rice, etc.
Allowed fat
Allowed desserts
Sugars and sweets

[a]One serving of citrus fruit is recommended daily to provide adequate vitamin C.
[b]One dark-green or deep-yellow vegetable is recommended daily to provide adequate vitamin A.
[c]Enriched cereal or bread should be included in the diet to provide adequate vitamin B complex and iron.

DIET FOR THE ADULT WITH TYPE IIb HYPERLIPOPROTEINEMIA
1700–2000 Kcal.[10]

DAILY FOOD PLAN

1 pt. or more skim milk (fortified with vitamins A and D)
Cooked poultry, fish or lean trimmed meat[a]
5 servings of vegetable and fruit[b] including 1 serving dark green or deep yellow vegetable[c]
7 or more servings of bread or cereal[d]
1 or more servings of potato, rice, etc.
Fat[a]
Desserts and sweets made with skim milk, egg whites, oil and sugar substitute.[e]

[a]To restrict the saturated fat, the meat, which is the principal source of saturated fats, must be limited to not more than 9 oz. (well trimmed, cooked) per day. Limit beef, lamb and pork to 3 oz. portions 3 times per week. Fish and poultry without skin are naturally lower in fat and should be used in place of meat as often as possible. For each 3 oz. of cooked meat consume 3 tsp. of polyunsaturated fat.
[b]One serving of citrus fruit is recommended daily to provide adequate ascorbic acid.
[c]One dark green or deep yellow vegetable is recommended daily to provide adequate vitamin A.
[d]Enriched cereal or bread should be included in the diet to provide adequate vitamin B complex and iron. Use Exchange lists, Table 25–5, for calculation.
[e]To maintain calories at this level, it will be necessary to omit additional desserts and sweets.

People with Type IIb have elevated serum triglyceride levels and hypercholesterolemia. Because the elevation of VLDL level is affected by carbohydrate intake, the diet for this type also includes weight reduction and carbohydrate limitation. The diet for Type III will probably benefit most Type IIb patients.

Type III Hyperlipoproteinemia. Type III is a pattern associated with the presence in the plasma of an abnormal form of beta-lipoprotein, "broad" beta-lipoprotein, due to a block in the metabolism of VLDL to LDL. Consequently, serum triglyceride and cholesterol levels are elevated. This type of hyperlipoproteinemia is usually familial and apparently transmitted as a recessive trait. The initial diet therapy is a reduction in weight to the desired level. The cholesterol intake is maintained at

DIET FOR THE ADULT WITH TYPE III
HYPERLIPOPROTEINEMIA
2000 Kcal.[10]

DAILY FOOD PLAN[a]	LIST
2 3-oz. servings of poultry, fish or lean trimmed meat	5
3 servings skim milk	1
8 servings bread, cereal	4
15 servings allowed fat[b]	6
3 servings fruit, unsweetened	3
Vegetables (as desired)	2

[a] Use Exchange List for calculation, Table 25–5.
[b] Avoid saturated fats.

less than 300 mg. per day. The amount of fat is limited to not more than 40 per cent of the total calories. Polyunsaturated fat, vegetable oil and special margarine are recommended. The amount of carbohydrate is restricted to not more than 40 per cent of the total calories. Sugars and starches as used in desserts and sweets are eliminated. Because of the fat and carbohydrate restriction, protein is high at about 20 per cent of calories. Alcohol is restricted, since it is a source of endogenous triglyceride production. The dietary plan is similar in form and food groups to the diabetic pattern.

Type IV Hyperlipoproteinemia. Type IV is a common lipoprotein pattern and is often asso-

DIET FOR THE ADULT WITH TYPE IV
HYPERLIPOPROTEINEMIA
2000 Kcal.[10]

DAILY FOOD PLAN[a]	LIST
2 3-oz. servings poultry, fish or lean trimmed meat	5
Egg, cheese, liver[b]	
3 servings skim milk	1
8 servings bread, cereal, etc.	4
15 servings allowed fat (polyunsaturated)[c]	6
3 servings fruit	3
Vegetables (as desired)	2

[a] Use Exchange List for calculation, Table 25–5.
[b] Egg allowance: 3 egg yolks per week. Include egg yolk in cooking or baking; *or* 2 oz. of shrimp in place of 1 egg yolk; *or* 2 oz. of liver, heart or sweetbreads for 1 egg yolk. Two oz. of cheddar-type cheese may be used once per week.
[c] All vegetable oil (except coconut), special margarine, salad dressings without sour cream or cheese, mayonnaise.

ciated with diabetes mellitus and possibly premature atherosclerosis. It is characterized by an increase in endogenous triglyceride and pre-beta-lipoprotein (VLDL). Cholesterol level may be normal or only slightly elevated. About 50 per cent of patients have abnormal glucose tolerance tests. Diet therapy stresses reduction in weight to the desired level, since at the desired weight the individual nearly always has lower (or normal) triglyceride concentrations than when he was heavier. Carbohydrate and alcohol restrictions are recommended. The cholesterol content of the diet is moderately restricted to 300 to 500 mg. per day. The fat is only modified to emphasize polyunsaturated fat and is only restricted in accordance with calorie reduction. Concentrated sweets and empty calories are eliminated from the diet.

Type V Hyperlipoproteinemia. The type V pattern is a familial trait and is usually secondary to acute metabolic disorders such as diabetic acidosis, pancreatitis, alcoholism and nephrosis. It is characterized by a mixed hyperlipidemia. Both exogenous (chylomicrons) and endogenous glyceride (pre-beta-lipoproteins) accumulate in the fasting plasma. Plasma triglyceride levels are markedly elevated, and abnormal glucose tolerance is frequently associated with this type. Diet therapy stresses caloric restriction and maintenance of desired body weight. The amount of fat is restricted to 25 to 30 per cent of the calories, with unsaturated fats predominating; protein is high at 20 to 25 per cent of the calories and carbohydrate is modified to 40 to 50 per cent. Concentrated sweets and empty calories are eliminated, and alcohol is not recommended. Cholesterol is restricted to 300 to 500 mg. per day. Lack of adherence to the diet and eating a high-fat meal will result in chylomicronemia and abdominal pain.

For individuals diagnosed as having a hyperlipoproteinemia for which a therapeutic diet is required, it is important to keep all nutrient requirements in mind, not just those nutrients that must be restricted. If certain nutrients are lacking, appropriate supplements are indicated. For example, the diet for type I (a low-fat diet) can be low in the fat-soluble vitamins and iron. Dark green and deep yellow vegetables 3 to 4 times per week are recommended, as well as liver occasionally. In fact, water-soluble forms of the fat-soluble vitamins may have to be given to remedy the lack of absorption in the absence of fat.

DIET FOR THE ADULT WITH TYPE V
HYPERLIPOPROTEINEMIA
2000 Kcal.[10]

DAILY FOOD PLAN[a]	LIST
2 3-oz. servings of poultry, fish or lean trimmed meat; egg, cheese, shellfish[b]	5
4 servings skim milk	1
11 servings bread, cereal, etc.	4
9 servings allowed fat[c]	6
3 servings fruit	3
Vegetables (as desired)	2

[a] Use Exchange List for calculation, Table 25–5.
[b] Egg allowance: 3 egg yolks per week. Includes egg yolks in cooking or baking; or 2 oz. of shrimp for 1 egg yolk; or 2 oz. of liver, meat or sweetbreads for 1 egg yolk. Two oz. cheddar-type cheese once per week may be used.
[c] All vegetable oil (except coconut), special margarine, salad dressing without sour cream or cheese, mayonnaise.

Summary of Diets for Hyperlipoproteinemia

In summarizing practical nutritional care for patients with hyperlipidemias, Fredrickson states that the treatment for any person with moderately elevated levels of serum triglyceride and cholesterol is a weight-controlling diet that is low in saturated fat and cholesterol and liberal in polyunsaturated fat and that avoids simple sugars and alcohol. If after a month on this diet the serum triglyceride level is still higher than 300 mg. per 100 ml., clofibrate (a triglyceride-lowering drug) may be used. If the triglyceride level has fallen but the serum cholesterol concentration remains high, then the diet should be even further restricted in cholesterol and saturated fat, and cholestyramine, a bile sequestrant, may be required.[9] See Chapter 21 for the nutritional implications of using these drugs.

PROBLEMS AND SUGGESTED TOPICS FOR DISCUSSION

1. Interview cardiac patients to learn the foods that cause distention. What is your conclusion?
2. Name some substitutes for salt that can be used safely in flavoring salt-poor food.
3. When is salt restricted for a cardiac patient? Study the diet prescribed for cardiac patients in your institution.
4. Secure the dietary pattern of a person with compensated heart disease and determine the approximate intake of sodium. How may it be modified to the level of 1000 mg.?
5. Obtain a diet history from a patient with congestive heart failure. Determine how much a 500 mg. sodium diet would deviate from his usual pattern.

6. Check the food intake of a patient on the ward who is recovering from an acute heart attack. Is it adequate? Should it be adequate in calories, carbohydrates, proteins, minerals and vitamins? Give reasons for your answer.
7. Obtain a diet history from a patient who is suffering with hypertension. Calculate the average daily intake of food. Is the amount normal or excessive? What is his usual sodium intake? Modify the diet to make it correct in all factors.
8. Assist a person with any one of the diets given for hyperlipoproteinemia. What changes did he need to make in his customary habits?

RECIPES AND MEAL PLANNING FOR SODIUM RESTRICTED DIETS

American Heart Association, local office or 44 East 23rd St., New York, New York, 10010. Booklets: Your Sodium-Restricted Diet 500 mg.; 1000 mg.; Mild Restriction.
Field, F.: Gourmet Cooking for Cardiac Diets. New York, Collier Books, 1962.
Payne, A. S., and Callahan, D.: Low Sodium–Fat Controlled Cookbook. Revised. Boston, Little, Brown and Company, 1960.
Planning Low Sodium Meals: The Nutrition Foundation, Inc., 99 Park Avenue, New York, New York, 10016.

RECIPES AND MEAL PLANNING FOR FAT CONTROLLED DIETS

American Heart Association booklets: Planning Fat-Controlled Meals for Unrestricted Calories and Planning Fat-Controlled Meals for 1200 and 1800 kcalories.
American Heart Association Cookbook, 2nd ed. New York, David McKay Co., Inc., 1976.
Cavanna, E., and Welton, J.: Gourmet Cookery for a Low Fat Diet. Revised, Englewood Cliffs, New Jersey, Prentice-Hall, Inc., 1961.
Connor, W. E., et al.: The Alternative Diet Book. Iowa City, Iowa, Univ. of Iowa Publications Order Dept., 17 W. College Street, Iowa City, 52240, 1976.
Keys, A., and Keys, M.: Eat Well and Stay Well. Garden City, New York, Doubleday & Co., Inc., 1959.
Rosenthal, S.: Live High on a Low Fat Diet. Philadelphia, J. B. Lippincott Company, 1962.
Stead, E. S., and Warren, G. K.: Low Fat Cookery. 2nd ed. New York, McGraw-Hill Book Co., Inc., 1959.

CITED REFERENCES

1. Astrup, P., and Kjeldsen, K.: Carbon monoxide, smoking, and atherosclerosis. Med. Clin. North Am., 58:323, 1974.
2. Barnes Hospital: Handbook of Nutrition Care, 5th ed. St. Louis, Barnes Hospital, 1975, p. 166.
3. Committee on Nutrition, American Academy of Pediatrics: Salt intake and eating patterns of infants and children in relation to blood pressure. Pediatrics, 53:115, 1974.
4. Connor, S.: The "Alternative American Diet" for the Prevention of Coronary Heart Disease. (Abstract). 57th Meeting, American Dietetic Association, Philadelphia, 1974.

5. Dahl, L. K.: Salt and hypertension. Am. J. Clin. Nutr., *25*:231, 1972.
6. del Greco, F.: The kidney in congestive heart failure. Mod. Concepts Cardiovasc. Dis., *44*:47, 1975.
7. Diet and Coronary Heart Disease. Report of the Advisory Panel of the British Committee on Medical Aspects of Food Policy (Nutrition) on Diet in Relation to Cardiovascular and Cerebrovascular Disease. London, Her Majesty's Stationer's Office, 1974. In: Nutrition Today, *10*(1):16, 1975.
8. Elvehjem, C. A., and Burns, C. H.: Sodium content of commercial spices. JAMA, *148*:1033, 1952.
9. Fredrickson, D. S.: It's time to be practical. Circulation, *51*:209, 1975.
10. Fredrickson, D. S., et al.: Dietary Management of Hyperlipoproteinemia: A Handbook for Physicians and Dietitians. DHEW Publ. No. (NIH) 75–110. Bethesda, Md., National Heart and Lung Institute, 1974.
11. Glueck, C. J., et al.: Neonatal familial type II hyperlipoproteinemia: Cord blood cholesterol in 1800 births. Metabolism, *20*:597, 1971.
12. Grande, F., Anderson, J. T., Keys, A.: Diets of different fatty acid composition producing identical serum cholesterol levels in man. Am. J. Clin. Nutr., *25*:53, 1972.
13. Hegsted, D. M., et al.: Quantitative effects of dietary fat on serum cholesterol in man. Am. J. Clin. Nutr., *17*:281, 1965.
14. Jenkins, D. J., et al.: Effect of pectin, guar gum and wheat fiber on serum cholesterol. Lancet, *1*:1116, 1975.
15. Kannel, W. B., and Gordon, T., (eds.): The Framingham Study: Diet and the Regulation of Serum Cholesterol. Section 24, U.S. Dept. of HEW, Public Health Service, 1970.
16. Kark, R. M., and Oyama, J. H.: Nutrition and cardiovascular-renal diseases. In: Goodhart, R. S., and Shils, M. E., (eds.): Modern Nutrition in Health and Disease. Philadelphia, Lea & Febiger, 1973, p. 889.
17. Kempner, W.: Compensation of renal metabolic dysfunction: Treatment of kidney disease and hypertensive vascular disease with rice diet. N. Carolina Med. J., *6*:61, 1945 and *6*:117, 1945.
18. Keys, A., (ed.): Coronary heart disease in seven countries. Circulation, *41*:suppl. 1, 1970.
19. Keys, A., Grande, F., and Anderson, J. T.: Fiber and pectin in the diet and serum cholesterol concentration in man. Proc. Soc. Exp. Biol. Med., *106*:555, 1961.
20. Klevay, L. M.: Coronary heart disease: The zinc/copper hypothesis. Am. J. Clin. Nutr., *28*:764, 1975.
21. Kuo, P. T.: Hyperlipidemia and coronary artery disease. Med. Clin. North Am., *53*:351, 1974.
22. Langford, H. G.: Rationale for Diets Modified in Sodium and Potassium. Paper presented at the 57th Meeting of the American Dietetic Association, Philadelphia, 1974.
23. McGill, H. C., Jr., (ed.): Geographic Pathology of Atherosclerosis. Baltimore, Williams & Wilkins, 1968.
24. Motulsky, A.: The genetic hyperlipidemias. N. Engl. J. Med., *294*:823, 1976.
25. Peart, S. W.: Renin-angiotensin system. N. Engl. J. Med., *292*:302, 1975.
26. Report of the Inter-Society Commission for Heart Disease Resources. Circulation, *42*, Dec. 1970; Revised April 1972.
27. San Francisco Heart Association: Sodium in Medicinals. SFHA, 421 Powell, San Francisco, 1973.
28. Scheig, R.: Diseases of lipid metabolism. In: Bondy, P. K., and Rosenberg, L. E., (eds.): Duncan's Diseases of Metabolism, 7th ed. Philadelphia, W. B. Saunders Co., 1974, p. 382.
29. Schroeder, H. A.: Municipal drinking water and cardiovascular death rates. JAMA, *195*:81, 1966.
30. Select Committee on Nutrition and Human Needs of the U.S. Senate: Dietary Goals for the United States. Washington, U.S. Government Printing Office, 1977.

ADDITIONAL REFERENCES

American Spice Trade Association: The art of seasoning low sodium diets. Hospital Management, *89*:80, 1960.
Brown, H. B.: Food patterns that lower blood lipids in man. J. Am. Diet. Assoc., *58*:303, 1971.
Christakis, G., et al.: Effect of the anti-coronary club program on coronary heart disease. Risk-factor status. JAMA, *198*:129, 1966.
Lees, R. S., and Wilson, D. E.: The treatment of hyperlipoproteinemia. N. Engl. J. Med., *284*:186, 1971.
Levy, R. I., et al.: Dietary and drug treatment of hyperlipoproteinemia. Ann. Intern. Med., *77*:267, 1972.
Mueller, J. F.: A dietary approach to coronary artery disease. J. Am. Diet. Assoc., *62*:613, 1973.
Ponsati, L. P., et al.: Comprehensive evaluation of fatty acids in foods. J. Am. Diet. Assoc., I. Dairy products, *66*:482, 1975; II. Beef products, *67*:35, 1975; III. Eggs and egg products, *67*:111, 1975; IV. Nuts, peanuts and soups, *67*:351, 1975; V. Unhydrogenated fats and oils, *68*:224, 1976. VI. Cereal products, *68*:335, 1976; VII. Pork products, *69*:44, 1976; VIII. Finfish, *69*:243, 1976; IX. Fowl, *69*:517, 1976; X. Lamb and veal, *70*:53, 1977.
Prior, I. A. M.: The price of civilization. Nutrition Today, *6*:2, 1971.
Yudkin, J., and Morland, J.: Sugar intake and myocardial infarction. Am. J. Clin. Nutr., *20*:503, 1967.

Chapter 29

NUTRITIONAL CARE FOR PATIENTS WITH DISEASES OF THE BLOOD AND BLOOD-FORMING ORGANS

PHYSIOLOGY AND FUNCTION OF THE BLOOD

Blood transports nutrients, oxygen, hormones, electrolytes, cellular excreta and other substances to and from all parts of the body. It is life itself, and any disease or disorder of the blood or blood-forming organs affects the body as a whole. The red and white blood cells and the blood platelets are the constituents usually concerned in diseases of the blood-forming organs.

In the normal, healthy individual the blood amounts to approximately 5 to 6 per cent of the body weight. The concentration of red blood cells (erythrocytes) is approximately 4,500,000 per cu. mm. in women and 5,000,000 per cu. mm. in men. The white blood cells (leukocytes) are fewer in number than the erythrocytes; the ratio is approximately 1 to 500.

THE ANEMIAS

Anemia is a condition in which there is a deficiency in the size or number of erythrocytes or in the amount of hemoglobin they contain. Nutritional factors of greatest importance in anemias are deficiencies of iron, vitamin B_{12}, and folic acid.

Classification. Formerly, the anemias were classified into primary and secondary types; however, it is known now that anemia is never primary. It is always secondary to some pathological state in the patient. Anemia may be classified according to cell size and hemoglobin content.[17] (See Table 29–1.)

ANEMIAS RESULTING FROM ACUTE HEMORRHAGE

Following an acute hemorrhage in a formerly healthy individual, the body replaces plasma within a few days. However, the speed with which the hemoglobin is restored depends largely upon the type of diet ingested. An adequate normal diet rich in foods containing iron, ascorbic acid and protein is essential. Liquids are mandatory to replace the fluid lost through hemorrhage and consequently lost from the tissues. In cases of very serious hemorrhage, restoration of blood volume by transfusion may be necessary.

NUTRITIONAL ANEMIAS

The anemias that result from an inadequate intake of iron, protein, certain vitamins (B_{12}, folic acid, pyridoxine, ascorbic acid), copper and other heavy metals are frequently termed nutritional anemias. The deficiency may be caused by inadequate ingestion, defective absorption, imperfect utilization, injury to the bone marrow or increased requirement, as in pregnancy or adolescence. Stores of these nutrients may be reduced, and in periods of increased need there may be biochemical or clinical effects. A further reduction in nutrient stores may result in anemia, the final stage of deficiency. The most common types of nutritional anemias in this country are due to iron deficiency or folic acid deficiency. However, not infrequently a combined type of anemia is present. There appears to be an interde-

Table 29–1   MORPHOLOGICAL CLASSIFICATION OF ANEMIA*

MORPHOLOGICAL TYPE OF ANEMIA[a]	UNDERLYING ABNORMALITY	CLINICAL SYNDROMES	TREATMENT
I. Macrocytic (MCV>94, MCHC>31)			
Megaloblastic	Vitamin B_{12} deficiency	Pernicious anemia, etc.	Vitamin B_{12}
	Folic acid deficiency	Nutritional megaloblastic anemias, sprue and other malabsorption syndromes.	Folic acid
	Inherited disorders of DNA synthesis	Orotic aciduria, etc.	According to nature of disorder
	Drug-induced disorders of DNA synthesis	Chemotherapeutic agents	Stop offending drug
		Anticonvulsants, oral contraceptives	Folic acid
Non-megaloblastic	Accelerated erythropoiesis	Hemolytic anemia	Treatment of underlying disease
	Increased membrane surface area	Hepatic disease, obstructive jaundice, post-splenectomy	
	Obscure	Myxedema	
		Hypo- and aplastic anemia, etc.	
II. Hypochromic-microcytic (MCV<80, MCHC<31)			
	Iron deficiency	Chronic loss of blood, inadequate diet, impaired absorption, increased demands, etc.	Ferrous sulfate and correction of underlying cause
	Disorders of globin synthesis	Thalassemia, along or with a hemoglobinopathy	Non-specific
	Disorders of porphyrin and heme synthesis	Pyridoxine-responsive anemia, etc.	Pyridoxine
	Other disorders of iron metabolism		
III. Normochromic-normocytic (MCV 82–92, MCHC>30)			
	Recent blood loss	Various	Transfusion, iron Correct underlying condition
	Overexpansion of plasma volume	Pregnancy Overhydration	Restore homeostasis
	Hemolytic diseases		According to nature of disorder
	Hypoplastic bone marrow	Aplastic anemia Pure red cell aplasia	Transfusions Androgens
	Infiltrated bone marrow	Leukemia, multiple myeloma, myelofibrosis, etc.	Chemotherapy, etc.
	Endocrine abnormality	Hypothyroidism, adrenal insufficiency, etc.	Treatment of underlying disease
	Chronic disorders		Treatment of underlying disease
	Renal disease	Renal disease	Treatment of underlying disease
	Liver disease	Cirrhosis	Treatment of underlying disease

*From: Wintrobe, M. M., et al.: Clinical Hematology, 7th ed. Philadelphia, Lea & Febiger, 1974, p. 547.

[a]MCV (mean corpuscular volume) = volume of one red cell expressed in femtoliters (fl.).

MCHC (mean corpuscular hemoglobin concentration) = concentration of hemoglobin expressed in gm. per deciliter (dl.).

pendence between iron deficiency and folic acid deficiency. Iron deficiency precipitates folic acid deficiency, possibly by increasing the folic acid requirement. The increased hemolysis of red blood cells that occurs in iron deficiency would increase the amount of folate needed to regenerate them.[10] For a long period, diet has been recognized as a remedial agent in overcoming nutritional anemia.

Iron Deficiency Anemias

Etiology. This form of anemia is characterized by a reduced concentration of hemoglobin in the blood and a depletion of total body iron content. The three causes of iron deficiency anemia are (1) chronic blood loss, such as from a chronically bleeding peptic ulcer or bleeding hemorrhoids or from parasites or malignancy, (2) faulty iron intake or absorption and (3) increased requirement for growth of blood volume, which occurs in infancy, puberty, pregnancy and lactation.

During infancy, a close relationship exists between diet and iron deficiency. At puberty, as well as in infancy, there is an acceleration of growth and an increase in the amount of circulating hemoglobin. This type of anemia is often present in growing children or in women losing blood during menstruation when their iron intake is inadequate. In the adult male, however, iron deficiency anemia is, with few exceptions, ascribed to blood loss. While loss of blood is a natural process in females, adequate stores of iron should be made available to meet such demands.

During pregnancy, there is an increased need for iron to supply the growing fetus. During lactation, there is a loss of iron in milk secretion, which probably is similar in quantity to the loss in the menstrual flow. Unless iron is provided to replace the amount lost or to build new hemoglobin, iron deficiency anemia will develop. Sometimes gastrointestinal disturbances such as diarrhea, achlorhydria or intestinal disease, which interfere with the absorption, will prevent iron from entering the blood stream in the required amount, even though the dietary intake of iron is adequate. When such a condition exists, the individual may maintain a low hemoglobin level for years.

Clinical Findings. Iron deficiency has been categorized by the stages of deficiency: (1) iron stores depletion, (2) iron deficiency without anemia and (3) iron deficiency with anemia.[4]

In the early stage, ferritin and hemosiderin (storage forms of iron) are depleted, and iron absorption increases. The *total iron binding capacity (TIBC)* of transferrin rises as iron stores in the bone marrow and liver decrease. When iron stores are depleted, the level of plasma iron falls. There may also be depletion of iron-containing enzymes in the tissues. Finally, in stage three the hemoglobin falls, and the erythrocytes become smaller *(microcytic)* and contain less hemoglobin *(hypochromic)*. (See Figure 29–1.) The mean corpuscular volumn (MCV), mean corpuscular hemoglobin (MCH) and mean corpuscular hemoglobin concentration (MCHC) are all below normal (Table 29–1).

A symptom that is possibly a sign of early iron deficiency is a reduction in immunocompetence and therefore an increased propensity to infection. However, the association of immunological changes with iron deficiency is still controversial. The dispute centers around the fact that iron is required for microbial growth. Serum with a high iron content enhances microbial growth; therefore, it seems likely that iron deficiency would protect against it. On the other side are the observations made by several investigators that cell-mediated immunity and the phagocytic activity of neutrophils are impaired in iron-deficient subjects.[3, 9] However, others have found no change in phagocytic activity in such cases.[8] Chandra suggests that the outcome of the exposure of an iron-deficient person to an infective challenge probably depends upon the host defense mechanisms as well as upon the effect of the person's iron status on the growth of the infecting organism.[2]

Patients with iron deficiency usually adapt to their slowly progressing disease, and frequently they see a physician only when another symptom or problem arises. Most patients develop symptoms from anemia when their hemoglobin level approaches 7 to 8 gm. per 100 ml. Fatigue, although popularly thought to be an early symptom of iron deficiency anemia, has not been correlated with decreased hemoglobin levels.[5] Several behavioral symptoms of iron deficiency, such as fatigue, weakness, anorexia and pica (which seem to respond to iron therapy much before the anemia is cured), may be due to tissue depletion of iron-containing enzymes and not to the decreased level of blood hemoglobin.[12]

As iron deficiency anemia becomes more severe, defects develop in the structure and function of the epithelial tissues, especially of the tongue, nails, mouth and stomach. Fingernails become thin and flat, and eventually

HOW IRON DEFICIENCY EVOLVES:

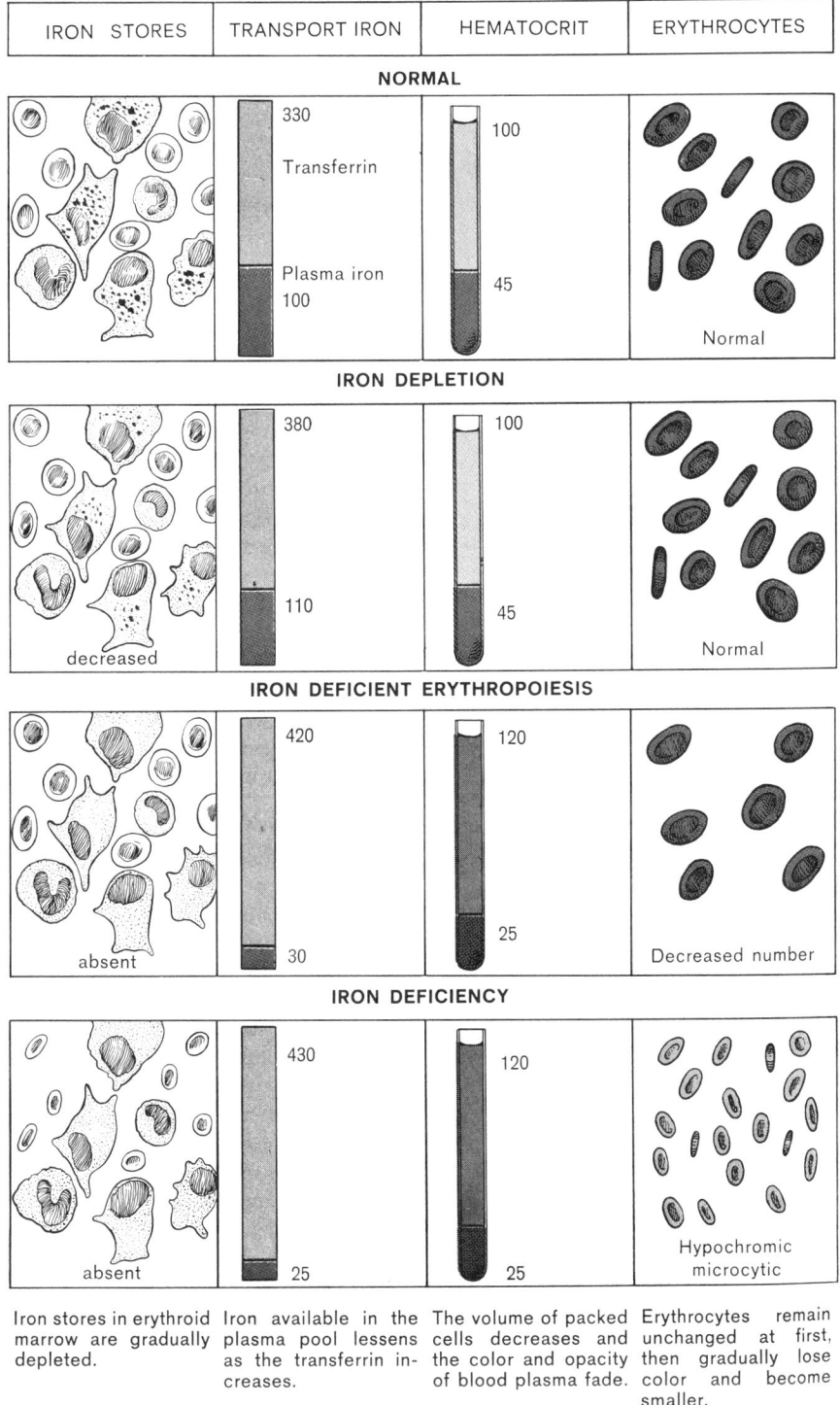

IRON STORES	TRANSPORT IRON	HEMATOCRIT	ERYTHROCYTES

NORMAL

330
Transferrin
Plasma iron
100

100
45

Normal

IRON DEPLETION

380
110

decreased

100
45

Normal

IRON DEFICIENT ERYTHROPOIESIS

420
30

absent

120
25

Decreased number

IRON DEFICIENCY

430
25

absent

120
25

Hypochromic
microcytic

Iron stores in erythroid marrow are gradually depleted.

Iron available in the plasma pool lessens as the transferrin increases.

The volume of packed cells decreases and the color and opacity of blood plasma fade.

Erythrocytes remain unchanged at first, then gradually lose color and become smaller.

Figure 29–1   How iron deficiency evolves. (From: Finch, C. L.: Iron metabolism. Nutrition Today, 4:2, Summer 1969.)

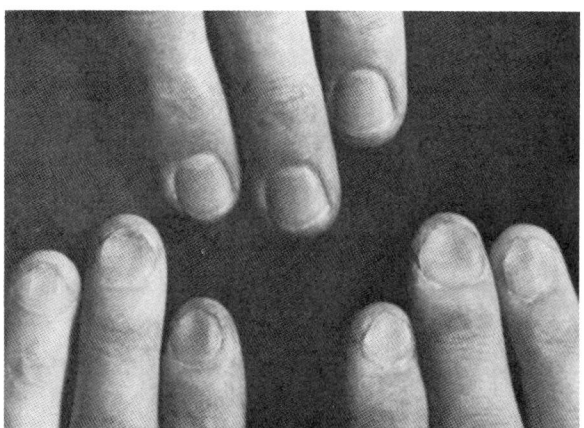

Figure 29–2 Fingernails of an iron-deficient adult (below) compared with those of a normal subject. (From: Rosenbaum, E., and Leonard, J. W.: Nutritional iron deficiency anemia in an adult male. Ann. Intern. Med., *60*:683, 1964, p. 684.)

koilonychia (spoon-shaped nails) develops. (See Figure 29–2.) Mouth changes include atrophy of the lingual papillae, burning and redness and, in severe cases, a completely smooth, waxy and glistening appearance to the tongue. Angular stomatitis may also develop, as well as a form of dysphagia (difficulty in swallowing). Gastritis occurs frequently and may result in achlorohydria. Progressive, untreated anemia results in cardiovascular and respiratory changes that can eventually end in cardiac failure.

Treatment. Treatment should focus primarily on the underlying disease leading to the anemia. This may be very difficult to determine. Repletion of iron stores, which is treatment of the symptom, is rather simple in comparison.

MEDICATION. Today, the chief treatment for iron deficiency anemia consists of oral administration of inorganic iron, preferably ferrous iron, in adequate dosage over a proper time interval. The most widely used preparation is *ferrous sulfate*, and the dose is calculated in terms of the amount of elemental iron provided. Iron is best absorbed when the stomach is empty; however, it also causes the greatest gastric irritation at this time. Even though food decreases the absorption of iron by 40 to 50 per cent, it is still better to take iron after a meal. Gastrointestinal side effects can also be minimized by increasing the dosage slowly over a few days until the required amount is reached and by giving the iron in at least 3 doses per day. Adults should take 100 to 200 mg. of elemental iron daily, and children should receive 1.5 to 2.0 mg. elemental iron per kg. of body weight, depending upon the severity of the anemia and their tolerance of the iron. Enteric-coated iron preparations reduce gas-

trointestinal side effects by preventing rapid dissolution of iron, but at the same time they may allow the iron to bypass the jejunum, which is the most active site of iron absorption. Ascorbic acid greatly increases iron absorption through its capacity to maintain iron in the reduced state.

The response to iron treatment usually occurs in one to three weeks, with an increased number of reticulocytes being the first sign. Blood hemoglobin level increases, and then epithelial changes are corrected. Iron therapy should be continued for six months, even after hemoglobin levels have been restored, to allow for repletion of body iron reserves.

Parenteral administration of iron may be necessary for patients who are unable to take it orally because of gastrointestinal symptoms or an inability to absorb iron or who lose iron (blood) too rapidly to be replaced by oral intake.

NUTRITIONAL CARE. In addition to medication, foods that contain a high percentage of iron should be provided, especially when the anemia is caused by faulty ingestion of iron. Liver, kidney, beef, tripe, egg yolk, dried fruits (apricots, peaches, prunes, raisins), dried peas and beans, nuts, green leafy vegetables (beet greens), molasses, whole-grain breads and cereals and fortified cereals rank highest among the iron-rich foods. (See Appendix Table 8 for a more complete list; also see Tables 10–12 and 20–6.) Beef, fish, liver, lamb and poultry should be included, since it is known that heme iron (which these foods contain) is better absorbed than non-heme iron. If the patient's digestion is impaired, the foods should be simple and easily digested, including those foods that have been suggested and outlined for the soft diet. Anorexia, if present, must be considered when

selecting food or planning the diet. Attractive food service and individual preferences should be considered to stimulate a desire for food.

IRON TOXICITY. An overdose of iron medication, seen occasionally in children who eat iron tablets thinking they are candy, can be fatal in doses of 3 to 10 gm.[6] Death can occur in 12 to 48 hours from the irritative action of iron—mucosal ulceration and bleeding, hypoxia, metabolic acidosis, alveolar and hepatic damage and renal failure. Treatment consists of oral or intravenous administration of deferoxamine, which chelates with iron and allows its excretion by the kidneys. Calcium disodium EDTA (ethylenediamine-tetraacetate) can also be used.

Protein Deficiency Anemia

Protein is essential for the proper production of hemoglobin and red blood cells. It appears that in protein deficiency, the body decreases erythropoiesis and diverts the available amino acids to the synthesis of other, more urgently needed proteins, and anemia results. In less severe protein-deficient states, hemoglobin formation may take precedence over other body protein needs. The anemias of kwashiorkor may be complicated by deficiencies of iron and other nutrients and by associated infections, parasitic infestation and malabsorption. Patients usually suffer from multiple deficiencies, such as of iron, folic acid and, less frequently, vitamin B_{12}, when their diet is lacking in protein. In such cases, administration of folic acid, iron, vitamin B_{12}, or a combination, along with a normal, well-balanced diet, will usually bring good response.

An individual on a normal adequate diet usually ingests an adequate amount of protein. However, in nephrotic conditions in which there is an extensive urinary loss of protein, the amount of food protein must be increased above the normal requirements. Anemia can result in this situation also.

Copper Deficiency Anemia

While copper and other heavy metals are essential for the proper formation of hemoglobin, the amounts needed are so minute that they are amply supplied by the normal adequate diet.

Copper plays a role in iron metabolism. The copper-containing protein *ceruloplasmin* is essential for normal mobilization of iron from its storage sites to the plasma. In the copper-deficient state iron cannot be released, and this leads to low serum iron and hemoglobin levels even in the presence of normal iron stores. Other consequences of copper deficiency suggest that copper proteins are also needed for utilization of iron by the developing erythrocyte and for optimal functioning of the erythrocyte membrane.

Copper deficiency is only likely in infants who are fed cow's milk instead of human milk or a prepared infant formula or in an adult or child with a malabsorption syndrome.

Pyridoxine-Responsive Anemia

A sideroblastic anemia that responds to vitamin B_6 therapy has been reported. This is a severe microcytic, hypochromic anemia in the presence of high serum iron and tissue iron levels. Transferrin saturation is increased. Frequently, this condition is not due to a pyridoxine deficiency but is an inherited sex-linked anemia. The synthesis of heme appears to be impaired because of an inherited defect in the formation of ALA (D-aminolevulinic acid), a substance involved in heme synthesis. Pyridoxal-5-phosphate is necessary in this reaction; hence, upon administration of pyridoxine the anemia responds. The iron that cannot be used for heme synthesis is stored in the mitochondria of immature red blood cells, which are then called *sideroblasts*. These iron-laden mitochondria do not function normally, and the development and production of red blood cells becomes ineffective. The symptoms are those of anemia and iron overload. The neurological and cutaneous manifestations of vitamin B_6 deficiency are not observed.

Treatment. Treatment consists of a therapeutic trial dose of pyridoxine of 50 to 200 mg. per day, which is 25 to 100 times the RDA. If the anemia responds, pyridoxine therapy is continued for life. However, the anemia is only partially corrected; normal red blood cell morphology is never achieved. Patients respond to this treatment in varying degrees, and some may achieve normal hemoglobin levels.

Pyridoxine is widely distributed in foods. Meat, liver, vegetables and whole-grain cereals and breads are good sources.

Vitamin Deficiency Megaloblastic Anemias

There is an interrelationship between the metabolism of folic acid to folinic acid, and

vitamin B_{12} and folic acid; a deficiency of any one will interfere with the normal development of erythrocytes and lead to anemia. Vitamin B_{12} and folic acid are essential for the synthesis of nucleoproteins required in the development of erythrocytes. Ascorbic acid is believed to function as a protector of reduced folates from oxidative destruction in the body. Ascorbic acid also influences the rate of iron absorption and the release of iron from transferrin to the tissues.

Folic Acid Deficiency Anemia

ETIOLOGY. This anemia is present in tropical sprue (Chapter 23), in some pregnant women (Chapter 13) and in infants born to mothers who have the deficiency (Chapter 14), and it may respond dramatically to folic acid therapy. Poor eating habits of long duration or faulty absorption and utilization of folic acid are believed to be the most frequent cause of the disorder. Additional causes are shown in Table 29–2. Normal body stores of folate are depleted rapidly (within two to four months) on a folate-deficient diet, and anemia is soon evident.

CLINICAL FINDINGS. Because of their interrelated roles in protein synthesis, a deficiency of either vitamin B_{12} or folic acid will result in the same clinical sign—a megaloblastic bone marrow and anemia. In the deficient state red blood cell protein cannot be synthesized properly, and a large (macrocytic) immature (megaloblastic) blood cell is the result. This state is characterized by a decreased number of erythrocytes, leukocytes and platelets.

Folate deficiency anemia is manifested by very low serum folate and red blood cell (RBC) folate levels, less than 3 mg. per liter and less than 100 mg. per liter, respectively. Serum levels of vitamin B_{12} are lowered moderately. To differentiate B_{12} deficiency anemia from folate deficiency anemia, both serum folate and B_{12} levels should be measured. There are several other tests that can be used, among which is the FIGLU (formiminoglutamic acid) urinary excretion test. Excretion of FIGLU is increased in folic acid deficiency and to a lesser extent in B_{12} deficiency. (See Chapter 11.) Other symptoms of folate deficiency and B_{12}

Table 29–2 PATHOGENETIC CLASSIFICATION OF THE CAUSES OF MEGALOBLASTIC ANEMIA*

I. Vitamin B_{12} deficiency
  A. Dietary deficiency (rare)
  B. Lack of Castle's intrinsic factor
    1. Pernicious anemia
      a. Congenital form
      b. Adult form
    2. Gastrectomy
      a. Total
      b. Partial
    3. Ingestion of caustic materials
  C. Functionally abnormal intrinsic factor
  D. Biologic competition
    1. Small-bowel bacterial overgrowth
      a. Small-bowel diverticulosis
      b. Anastomoses and fistulae
      c. Blind loops and pouches
      d. Strictures
      e. Scleroderma
      f. Achlorhydria
    2. Fish tapeworm disease
  E. Familial selective vitamin B_{12} malabsorption (Imerslund's syndrome)
  F. Drug-induced vitamin B_{12} malabsorption
  G. Chronic disease of the pancreas
  H. Zollinger-Ellison syndrome
  I. Diseases especially affecting the ileum
    1. Ileal resection and bypass
    2. Regional enteritis
II. Folate deficiency
  A. Dietary deficiency
  B. Increased requirements

    1. Cirrhosis
    2. Pregnancy
    3. Infancy
    4. Diseases associated with rapid cellular proliferation
  C. Congenital folate malabsorption
  D. Drug-induced folate malabsorption
    1. Anticonvulsants
    2. Oral contraceptives
  E. Extensive intestinal resection, jejunal resection
III. Combined folate and vitamin B_{12} deficiency
  A. Tropical sprue
  B. Gluten-sensitive enteropathy
IV. Inherited disorders of DNA synthesis
  A. Orotic aciduria
  B. Lesch-Nyhan syndrome
  C. Thiamin-responsive megaloblastic anemia
  D. Deficiency of enzymes required for folate metabolism
    1. N^5-methyl tetrahydrofolate transferase
    2. Formiminotransferase
    3. Dihydrofolate reductase
  E. Congenital megaloblastic anemia responsive to large doses of folate and vitamin B_{12}
V. Drug-induced disorders of DNA synthesis
  A. Folate antagonists (e.g., methotrexate)
  B. Purine antagonists (e.g., 6-mercaptopurine)
  C. Pyrimidine antagonists (e.g., cytosine arabinoside)
VI. Erythroleukemia

*From: Wintrobe, M. M., et al.: Clinical Hematology, 7th ed. Philadelphia, Lea & Febiger, 1974, p. 574.

Table 29–3   CLINICAL PICTURE OF THE MEGALOBLASTIC ANEMIAS*

SYMPTOMS
Weakness, tiredness
Dyspnea
Sore tongue
Paresthesia (B_{12} deficiency only)
Diarrhea (especially folate deficiency)
Constipation (especially B_{12} deficiency)
Irritability and forgetfulness (especially folate deficiency)
Anorexia
Syncope
Headache
Palpitation

SIGNS
Anemia, leukopenia, thrombocytopenia, with macroovalocytes (normal MVC = 87 ± 5 cu. μ) and "hypersegmented
   polys" (normal "Arneth count"; 2 lobes = 20–40%; 3 lobes = 40–50%; 4 lobes = 15–25%; 5 lobes = 0–5%; 6 lobes = 0–
   0.1%; more than 6 lobes = 0) (normal "lobe average" = 3.17 ± 0.25) (Rule of Fives: When 100 neutrophils are counted,
   the presence of five or more with five or more lobes means hypersegmentation.)
Morphologic "red herrings": congenital hypersegmentation (approx. 1% of population); hypersegmentation with renal
   disease; twinning deformities; macrocytes of pyruvate kinase deficiency, aplastic anemia, reticulocytosis
Fever
Icterus
Glossitis
   Acute
   Chronic atrophic
Neurologic damage (only B_{12} deficiency damages myelin)
   Vibration sense diminished
   Position sense diminished; ataxia
   Impaired mentation, paranoid ideation
Malabsorption
Achylia gastrica (primary with B_{12} deficiency; secondary with folate deficiency)
Splenomegaly (in approximately $^1/_3$ of cases, if looked for radiologically)
Weight loss (especially folate deficiency)
Pigmentation
Postural hypotension (especially B_{12} deficiency)
Low serum vitamin B_{12} or folate level
Elevated serum lactic dehydrogenase (LDH)
Elevated urine formiminoglutamate (FIGLU)
Methylmalonic aciduria (B_{12} deficiency only)
High serum iron, increased saturation of iron-binding capacity of serum, increased bone marrow iron stores

*From: Goodhart, R. S., and Shils, M. E.: Modern Nutrition in Health and Disease. Philadelphia, Lea & Febiger, 1973, p. 239.

deficiency can be used to differentiate between them. (See Table 29–3.)

TREATMENT. Before initiating treatment it is important that the megaloblastic anemia be properly diagnosed. Administration of folate in the presence of a B_{12} deficiency could correct the megaloblastic anemia, but it will not correct the B_{12} deficiency, which will continue and cause progressive nerve disease.

To replenish folate stores, 1 mg. of folate given orally every day for two to three weeks is recommended. To maintain repleted stores, the person should have an intake of at least 50 to 100 μg. of pure folic acid every day, either in his food or in a supplement. One half to 1 cup of orange juice supplies between 50 and 100 μg. of folic acid.[15] See Appendix Table 5 for the folate content of some other foods.

Symptomatic improvement, such as increased alertness, cooperativeness and appetite, may be apparent before the hematological values are back to normal. After the anemia is corrected, the patient should be instructed about ways to include folate in the diet. Liver, asparagus, dried beans, brewer's yeast, spinach, wheat bran, dark green vegetables and whole-wheat bread are all good sources of folate. Since folate is destroyed by heat, fruits and vegetables should be eaten fresh, if possible, or with very little cooking. See Chapter 12 for further discussion of folic acid deficiency.

Scurvy. The macrocytic anemia of scurvy may be the result of the ascorbic acid deficiency, which interferes with the conversion of folic acid to folinic acid. In such cases, ascorbic acid and folic acid therapy plus an

adequate diet high in protein and ascorbic acid are indicated. Not all anemia in scurvy is true macrocytic anemia requiring folic acid therapy. Some scorbutic anemia will respond to ascorbic acid therapy alone, while some may be the result of iron deficiency. The normal adequate diet with increased amounts of protein of high biological value will carry the necessary vitamins, unless there is also evidence of vitamin deficiency.

Pernicious and Other Macrocytic Anemias

ETIOLOGY. Macrocytic megaloblastic anemia due to vitamin B_{12} deficiency is only rarely caused by inadequate B_{12} intake. One example is the strict vegetarian who has no intake of vitamin B_{12} because B_{12} is found only in foods of animal origin. Other causes are shown in Table 29–2.

A more common cause of B_{12} deficiency is pernicious anemia. Pernicious anemia is attributed to a deficiency of vitamin B_{12} due to the lack of the *intrinsic factor* (IF), a glycoprotein in the gastric juice, which is necessary for absorption of this vitamin from food. Since B_{12} is involved in DNA synthesis, its lack results in defective synthesis and defective maturation of red blood cells. Although the disease was formerly considered fatal, it can now be treated successfully and controlled.

The most popular method for testing B_{12} absorption is the Schilling urinary excretion test. After an oral dose of radioactive B_{12} is given, excretion of B_{12} will be low in patients with pernicious anemia, because the B_{12} was not absorbed. When the same test is repeated with IF also given orally, the urinary excretion becomes almost normal, because the B_{12} is absorbed. A deficiency of vitamin B_{12} due to factors other than pernicious anemia, such as non-tropical sprue, will be reflected in decreased urinary excretion of B_{12} in the Schilling test that will remain unchanged upon administration of IF.

CLINICAL FINDINGS. Pernicious anemia affects not only the blood but the gastrointestinal tract and the peripheral and central nervous systems as well. The symptoms are paresthesia, especially numbness and tingling in the hands and feet, diminution of senses of vibration and position, poor muscular coordination, poor memory and hallucinations. This B_{12} neuropathy is due to inadequate myelinization of the nerves. If it continues long enough it may be irreversible, even with treatment.

Vitamin B_{12} deficiency has been reported to impair the microbicidal activity of leukocytes, the cells involved in phagocytosis. The function of leukocytes in folic acid–deficient individuals was not impaired. Therefore, B_{12} appears to play a specific role separate from that of folic acid in the production of the intermediates necessary for normal cell metabolism and function.[7]

METHYLFOLATE TRAP. Deficiency of vitamin B_{12} can result in a deficiency of folic acid by causing the entrapment of folate as 5-methyltetrahydrofolate. (See Fig. 29–3.) The lack of B_{12} means that methyltetrahydrofolate is unable to release its methyl group and become tetrahydrofolate (THFA), the optimal substrate for folate polyglutamate synthesis in the cell. The cells are thus deprived of tetrahydrofolate, and other folate coenzymes cannot be synthesized. Hence, a folic acid deficiency results.

TREATMENT. In 1926 Minot and Murphy[11] reported the effectiveness of liver therapy in pernicious anemia. Soon after, active concentrates of liver suitable for clinical use were developed, and by 1936 relatively purified extracts of liver were available for intramuscular injection, in addition to those preparations that had been developed earlier for oral administration. They were also effective in other macrocytic anemias such as the anemia of sprue and the macrocytic anemia of pregnancy. The intrinsic factor in liver extracts unites with the extrinsic factor, vitamin B_{12}, to form an antianemic factor that is stored in the liver until it is needed by the bone marrow for the maturation of red blood cells. Before liver extract was introduced, large quantities of raw and cooked liver were fed daily to the patients. This was most distasteful and difficult to take, because the patient afflicted with pernicious anemia has a very poor appetite. Today, treatment usually consists of intramuscular or subcutaneous injections of vitamin B_{12} daily for one week. After response, the frequency of injection is reduced until remission can be maintained on injections given 6 to 8 times per year. Oral doses of B_{12} without intrinsic factor may also be effective in very large doses, because about 1 per cent of B_{12} is absorbed by diffusion without the presence of IF.

Response is evidenced by improved appetite, alertness and cooperativeness followed by improved hematological results, as seen by marked reticulocytosis. Neurological improvement may take six months or more. The shorter the duration of the B_{12} deficiency, the greater the neurological response. Neurological mani-

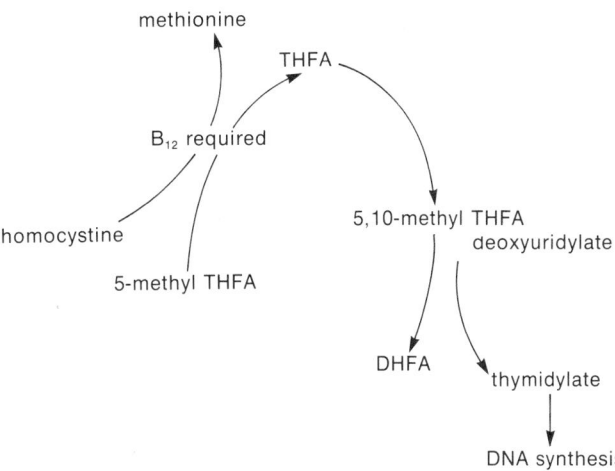

Figure 29–3 Methylfolate trap. Deficiency of vitamin B_{12} can result in a deficiency of folic acid because folate is trapped in the form of 5-methyltetrahydrofolate (5-methyl THFA), which cannot be converted to tetrahydrofolate (THFA) by the vitamin B_{12}–dependent pathway.

festations of B_{12} deficiency that have been present less than three months before treatment are usually reversible.

NUTRITIONAL CARE. The normal or general house diet, with increased amounts of protein, iron and vitamins, is advised for pernicious anemia in addition to vitamin B_{12} and other medication indicated. The high-protein diet (1.5 gm. of protein per kg. of body weight) is desirable both for liver function and blood regeneration. Since the green leafy vegetables contain both iron and folic acid, the diet will contain increased amounts of these necessary components. Liver should be included frequently because it carries a good supply of iron, vitamin B_{12}, folic acid and other important nutrients. Meats (especially beef and pork), eggs, milk and milk products are particularly rich in viitamin B_{12}. It should be remembered that the total patient must be treated, not just his blood. For example, diarrhea may also be present and will have to be treated.

Consult Table 20–6 for a listing of foods rich in iron and protein. Also refer to Appendix Table 8 and review the material on folic acid and vitamin B_{12} in Chapter 8.

SICKLE CELL ANEMIA

Sickle cell anemia (SCA) is an inherited hemolytic anemia in which the hemoglobin is defective and the erythrocytes are sickle-shaped. It occurs most frequently in populations (such as the black population) that can trace their origins to areas of endemic malaria, and it manifests itself clinically in persons homozygous for the gene. It is usually diag-

nosed toward the end of the first year of life and has degrees of severity that depend upon the amount of abnormal hemoglobin and the number of erythrocytes with the characteristic odd shape.

Clinical Findings. In addition to the usual symptoms of anemia, sickle cell anemia is characterized by "crises." These are painful occlusions of the small blood vessels due to the abnormal shape of the erythrocytes. The occlusions frequently occur in the abdomen, causing acute, severe abdominal pain. The hemolytic anemia and vaso-occlusive disease result in impairment of liver function, hepatitis, jaundice, gallstones and deteriorating renal function. Growth slows to below normal. Because of the constant hemolysis of erythrocytes and release of iron, iron stores in the liver are increased.

Treatment. There is no specific treatment for SCA other than relief of pain, and maintenance of homeostasis during a crisis and possibly administration of an exchange transfusion. It is important that SCA not be mistaken for iron deficiency anemia and treated with iron supplements. Iron stores are already in excess in the SCA patient so the diet should be low in iron, with iron-rich foods such as liver, iron-fortified formula and iron-fortified cereals excluded.

The diet should be *low in fat* (less than 30 per cent of kcal.) because of the liver disease and possible gallbladder complications. It should also be *high in folate* (400 to 600 μg.) because the increased production of erythrocytes needed to replace the cells being continuously destroyed also increases the body's folic acid requirements. Administration of folate supplements (250 μg. per day) is also recommended.[16]

The symptoms of sickle cell disease, such as delayed onset of puberty and hypogonadism in males, low body weight, rough skin and poor appetite, are similar to those seen in people with zinc deficiency. Prasad and colleagues examined 36 men and women with SCA and found significantly decreased levels of zinc in erythrocytes, plasma and hair as compared with normal subjects. They also found an increased urinary excretion of zinc. They postulate that the decreased zinc nutriture could be due to the hemolysis of erythrocytes, which contain zinc, and to the resulting hyperzincuria. When a dose of 660 mg. of zinc sulfate (more than 20 times the RDA for zinc) was given daily to these patients, the young men grew and developed sexually, all but one patient gained weight and the healing of ulcers was improved.[14] It has also been shown that zinc can increase the oxygen affinity of both normal and sickle-shaped erythrocytes.[1] Thus, a deficiency of zinc in SCA patients may intensify the anemia of sickle cell disease.

Zinc supplementation appears to be beneficial in the management of sickle cell disease, but the long term effects of such high doses are unknown. For example, since zinc competes with copper for binding sites on proteins, the use of high doses of zinc may precipitate a copper deficiency, and this possibility should be kept in mind.[13]

DISEASES OF THE WHITE BLOOD CELLS

Therapy for diseases of the white blood cells can be successful only if the agent depressing the formation of bone marrow is removed or the causative factor is corrected. Blood transfusions are the chief palliative treatment. Diet therapy has not been found to have direct influence.

LEUKEMIA

Leukemia is the best known example of white blood cell disease, with crowding of the erythrogenic tissue and subsequent anemia. The disease is a type of cancer of the blood-forming organs. (See Chapter 36.) There is an abnormally large production of leukocytes or white blood cells. The normal white count is between 7500 and 10,000; in leukemia it increases to 300,000 or more. Many of these cells are abnormal, a sign that the blood-forming organs are overworking. The white cells are manufactured in bone marrow, spleen, lymph glands and the liver.

Etiology and Classification. The etiology of leukemia is unknown. Leukemia may be classified as (1) acute, (2) chronic myeloid, and (3) chronic lymphatic. The acute variety is most common in children and runs a shorter course than the milder or chronic type, which attacks adults and is more prevalent. The prognosis is almost invariably poor. However, newer forms of therapy have made life substantially more comfortable for these patients, and a high percentage of those who respond to therapy have a remission following treatment.

Treatment. Life expectancy has been increased somewhat for patients with the acute form through the use of drug therapy, combined with supportive therapy, for complications such as hemorrhage, infection and anemia. ACTH, cortisone or the antimetabolite products amethopterin (methotrexate) and 6-mercaptopurine, as well as prednisone and prednisolone, are the most frequently used of the steroid compounds. Remedies are also available for chronic leukemia, including the nitrogen mustard compound chlorambucil, which works on lymphocytic tissue, as well as ACTH, cortisone, radioactive phosphorus, total body radiation (x-ray) and specific alkylating agents such as triethylenemelamine (TEM) and busulfan, which acts on granulocytic tissue. The best results have been obtained with acute leukemia in children.

In addition, transfusions, antibiotics, iron, folic acid and vitamin B_{12} are given as supportive therapy.

Nutritional Care. Nutritional care for patients with cancer is discussed in Chapter 36.

PROBLEMS AND SUGGESTED TOPICS FOR DISCUSSION

1. Discuss the functions of hemoglobin.
2. Study the effect of nutritional anemia and pernicious anemia on the metabolic processes of the body. What are the causes of iron deficiency anemia?
3. Describe the absorption, transport and storage of iron.
4. How much dietary iron, ascorbic acid and protein do you ingest daily? How adequate is your intake of these nutrients?
5. Interview a patient with iron deficiency anemia. How can he improve his diet?
6. Obtain a dietary history of a person with pernicious anemia or of a postgastrectomy patient.
7. What role does vitamin B_{12} play in the treatment of pernicious anemia? How does the treatment of pernicious anemia differ from that of folic acid deficiency anemia?
8. Why is it often advisable to give folic acid when antimetabolic drugs are used in the treatment of leukemia?

CITED REFERENCES

1. Brewer, G., and Oelshlegal, F. J., Jr.: Antisickling effects of zinc. Biochem. Biophys. Res. Commun., *58*:854, 1974.
2. Chandra, R. K.: Iron and immunocompetence. Nutr. Rev., *34*:129, 1976.
3. Chandra, R. K., and Saraya, A. K.: Impaired immunocompetence associated with iron deficiency. J. Pediatr., *86*:899, 1975.
4. Committee on Iron Deficiency, Council on Foods and Nutrition, American Medical Assn.: Iron deficiency in the United States. JAMA, *203*:61, 1968.
5. Elwood, P. C.: Evaluation of the clinical importance of anemia. Am. J. Clin. Nutr., *26*:958, 1973.
6. Greenblatt, D. J., Allen, M. D., and Koch-Weser, J.: Accidental iron poisoning in children. Clin. Pediatr., *15*:835, 1976.
7. Kaplan, S. K., and Basford, R. E.: Effect of vitamin B_{12} and folic acid deficiencies on neutrophil function. Blood, *47*:801, 1976.
8. Kulapongs, P., et al.: Cell mediated immunity and phagocytosis and killing function in children with severe iron-deficiency anemia. Lancet, *2*:689, 1974.
9. Macdougall, L. G., et al.: The immune response in iron-deficient children: Impaired cellular defense mechanisms with altered humoral components. J. Pediatr., *86*:833, 1975.
10. McKibbin, J. M., and Stare, F. J.: Nutrition in blood regeneration. J. Am. Diet. Assoc., *19*:331, 1943.
11. Minot, G. R., and Murphy, W. P.: Treatment of pernicious anemia by special diet. JAMA, *87*:470, 1926.
12. Pollitt, E., and Leibel, R. L.: Iron deficiency and behavior. J. Pediatr., *88*:372, 1976.
13. Prasad, A. S.: Trace elements in sickle cell disease. JAMA, *235*:2396, 1976.
14. Prasad, A. S., et al.: Zinc deficiency in sickle cell disease. Clin. Chem., *21*:582, 1975.
15. Streiff, R. R.: Folate levels in citrus and other juices. Am. J. Clin. Nutr., *24*:1390, 1971.
16. Trubowitz, S.: The management of sickle cell anemia. Med. Clin. North Am., *60*:933, 1976.
17. Wintrobe, M. M., et al.: Clinical Hematology, 7th ed. Philadelphia, Lea & Febiger, 1974, p. 546.

ADDITIONAL REFERENCES

Alperin, J. B.: Effect of vitamin B_{12} therapy in a patient with folic acid deficiency. Am. J. Clin. Nutr., *15*:177, 1964. Control of Nutritional Anemia with Special Reference to Iron Deficiency. WHO Technical Report Series No. 580. Geneva, WHO, 1975.

Cook, J. D., and Monsen, E. R.: Food iron absorption in human subjects. III. Comparison of the effect of animal proteins on non-heme iron absorption. Am. J. Clin. Nutr., *29*:859, 1976.

Ellison, A. B. C.: Pernicious anemia masked by multivitamins containing folic acid. JAMA, *173*:240, 1960.

Finch, C. A.: Iron metabolism. Nutrition Today, *4*:2, 1969.

Goldsmith, G. A.: Nutritional anemias with special reference to vitamin B_{12}. Am. J. Med., *25*:680, 1958.

Herbert, V.: Folic acid and vitamin B_{12}. *In*: Goodhart, R. S., and Shils, M. E. (eds.): Modern Nutrition in Health and Disease, 5th ed. Philadelphia, Lea & Febiger, 1973.

Lukens, J. N.: Iron deficiency and infection. Am. J. Dis. Child., *129*:160, 1975.

Moore, C. V.: Iron and hypochromic anemia. Prog. Food Nutr., *1*:245, 1975.

Nutritional Anemias. WHO Technical Report Series No. 503. Geneva, WHO, 1972.

Review. Zinc deficiency in sickle cell disease. Nutr. Rev., *33*:266, 1975.

Serjeant, G. R., Galloway, R. E., and Gueri, M. C.: Oral zinc sulfate in sickle cell ulcers. Lancet, *2*:891, 1970.

Streiff, R. R., and Little, A. B.: Folic acid deficiency in pregnancy. New Eng. J. Med., *276*:776, 1967.

Tandon, B. N., et al.: Protein deficiency and anemias. Am. J. Clin. Nutr., *21*:813, 1968.

Wilson, T. H.: Intrinsic factor and B_{12} absorption. Nutr. Rev., *23*:33, 1965.

UNIT TEN

RENAL DISEASE

Chapter 30

NUTRITIONAL CARE FOR PATIENTS WITH DISEASES OF THE KIDNEY

PHYSIOLOGY AND FUNCTION OF NORMAL KIDNEYS

The kidneys maintain the chemical homeostasis of all body fluids. Their chief functions are to regulate and conserve nutrients and water and to excrete waste products. Blood entering the kidneys reaches the arterioles and enters the nephrons. Approximately 1.2 liters of whole blood pass through the kidneys each minute, about one fourth of the total cardiac output.

Each nephron is composed of a glomerulus surrounded by a membrane (Bowman's capsule) and the tubules (which include the convoluted tubules, Henle's loop and the distal tubules). Blood is supplied through the capillaries. Approximately one fifth of the water from plasma is filtered through the nephron, forming a glomerular filtrate of fluid, electrolytes and low-molecular-weight proteins and carbohydrates. At various points along the tubules, certain elements are selectively reabsorbed or secreted. A number of factors influence the selection of elements to be reabsorbed. The final fluid leaving the nephron is water that contains a high concentration of waste metabolites. The reabsorbed essential elements are returned to the blood.

Ultimately, the waste products proceed into large channels and finally arrive in the funnel-shaped, central edge of the area known as the renal pelvis. Now the waste products are ready to be sent to the bladder for accumulation and then elimination as urine. (See Fig. 30-1.)

Water makes up the greatest percentage of the waste product. The quantity is related to the amount taken into the body and the amount excreted through the skin and lungs in the process of temperature regulation, but normally it averages 1 to 2 liters daily. Urine usually consists of approximately 95 per cent water and 5 per cent solutes.

Water reabsorption from the distal tubules and collecting duct is controlled by the small peptide hormone *vasopressin,* or *antidiuretic hormone (ADH),* which is made by the cells of the hypothalamus and stored in the pituitary. When there is a fall in the total blood volume, the hypothalamus stimulates the secretion of ADH, which increases the reabsorption of water. The hormone is not released when the blood volume is high and thus allows diuresis to take place.

A minimum urinary volume of approximately 600 ml. (obligatory fluid) is required for the excretion of the average load of solids. A greater volume is required for the excretion of increased loads.

About 60 per cent of the solute load is nitrogenous waste, and inorganic salts make up the other 40 per cent. Of the *nitrogenous wastes,* urea predominates; uric acid, creatinine and ammonia are present in small amounts. The amount of urea present depends upon the diet. A high protein intake or a high intake of protein of low biological value (LBV) (i.e., high in non-essential amino acids) increases the urea output. A lower consumption of protein de-

618

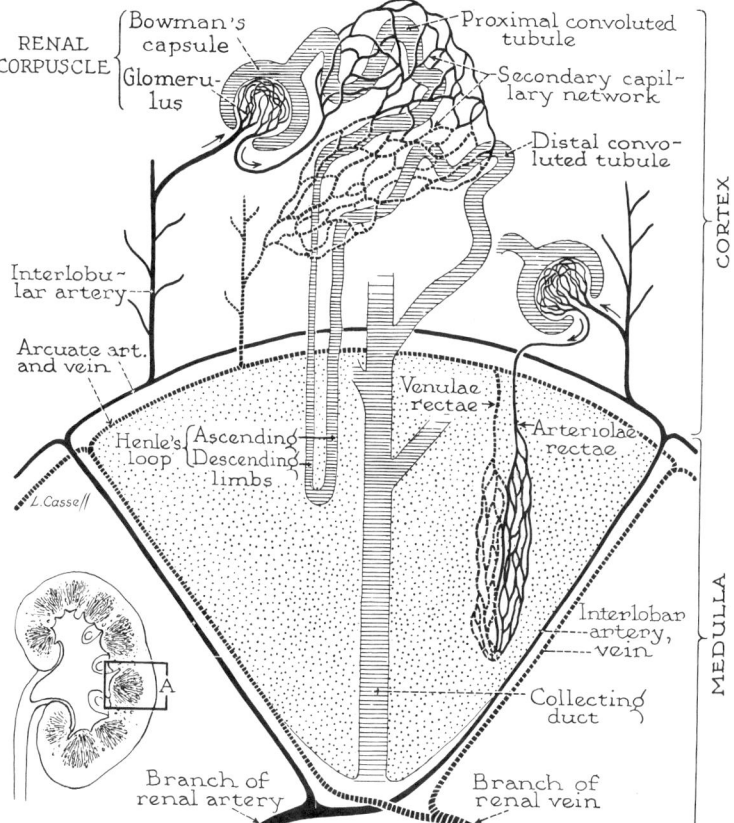

RENAL CORPUSCLE {Bowman's capsule / Glomerulus

Proximal convoluted tubule

Secondary capillary network

Distal convoluted tubule

CORTEX

Interlobular artery

Arcuate art. and vein

Henle's loop {Ascending Descending limbs

L.Cassell

Venulae rectae

Arteriolae rectae

Interloban artery, vein

Collecting duct

MEDULLA

A

Branch of renal artery

Branch of renal vein

Figure 30–1 Diagram of renal tubule or nephron. Inset A shows the location of the renal tubule in the kidney. (King and Showers.)

creases the urea content. If these normal waste products are not eliminated appropriately, they collect in abnormal quantities in the blood.

Of the *inorganic salts,* sodium chloride predominates; phosphate and sulfate salts of calcium, sodium, potassium and magnesium are present in small amounts. In the balance of minerals, some sodium is reabsorbed from the distal tubules and is exchanged for potassium or H^+.

Throughout this process of waste elimination, the kidney maintains a chemical homeostasis in the body, balances the amounts of body fluids and maintains the normal pH of body fluids, thus keeping an acid-base balance. In addition, the kidney performs some non-excretory functions:

1. The kidney controls blood pressure through the *renin-angiotensin* mechanism. Cells in the Bowman's capsules (known as the juxtaglomerular apparatus) react to decreased blood volume and secrete renin, a proteolytic enzyme. Renin acts in the plasma to form angiotensin I, which is converted to angiotensin II, a powerful vasoconstrictor and a potent stimulus of aldosterone secretion by the ad-

renal gland. Thus aldosterone is secreted, sodium is reabsorbed, and blood pressure is returned to normal.

2. The kidney is further involved in the production of *erythropoietin,* which is a critical determinant of erythroid activity in the bone marrow. A deficiency of erythropoietin results in the severe anemia present in chronic renal disease.

3. The kidney maintains *calcium-phosphorus-bone homeostasis* and equilibrium by making the active form of Vitamin D_3, which is needed for regulation and maintenance of the system. For this reason, osteodystrophy is a common, complex and usually inevitable outcome of renal disease. This will be discussed later in the chapter.

Diseases of the kidney, whether acute or chronic, have many causes. The origin of the disease and the portion of the nephron it affects will determine the symptoms and subsequently the treatment. Depending on the type, kidney diseases may produce (1) nephrotic syndrome, with significant protein loss, (2) decreased overall renal function, in which the remaining nephrons cannot handle the metabolic load, or

(3) a combination of the two. Objectives of nutritional care will depend on the abnormality to be treated.

NEPHRITIS

Nephritis, or Bright's disease (named after the English physician who was the first to describe it), is now used as a general term to indicate any altered kidney function caused by either a diffuse inflammation or a degenerative change.

Classification

Although there are many ways to classify nephritis, the following grouping by the primary area of the kidney affected seems to be the most functional. This method of looking at nephritis divides it as follows:

1. *Glomerulopathies*—acute, subacute and chronic—affect the glomeruli and have many underlying causes.
2. *Tubular disorders*—acute, chronic or obstructive.
3. *Vascular diseases,* such as arteriosclerosis of the large arteries, intermediate and small artery diseases and renal vein thrombosis.
4. *Interstitial nephritis*—acute or chronic—may be caused by pyelonephritis, drugs, analgesic abuse, heavy metals or papillary necrosis.

In this chapter, a few of these conditions will be discussed.

GLOMERULONEPHRITIS (ACUTE)

Etiology and Characteristics

Acute glomerulonephritis is characterized by inflammation of the capillary loops in the glomeruli of the kidney, with varying degrees of hematuria, edema, hypertension and nitrogen retention (*azotemia*). A decreased amount of urine is excreted (*oliguria*), and it is highly concentrated. Because of the red blood cells that appear in the urine, the disease has been termed *hemorrhagic nephritis.* Anorexia and lethargy are present; nausea and vomiting are usual. Edema of the soft tissues may be either minimal or massive.

The disorder occurs most frequently in children and young adults and is often a sequel to an inflammatory reaction or infection in the body, especially of the upper respiratory tract.

The causative organisms are numerous, but *Streptococcus* is the most common.

Objectives and Principles of Nutritional Care

The treatment of acute glomerulonephritis attempts to maintain good nutritional status while allowing time for the disease to cure itself spontaneously. There is no reason to restrict protein or potassium intake unless uremia or hyperkalemia develops. Sodium is restricted to 10 to 15 mEq. daily during the oliguric phase, and this is continued until there is no evidence of congestion or edema. When diuresis occurs, it is important to replace all fluid lost. The sodium-retaining phase has passed; thus, sodium restriction is no longer necessary.

GLOMERULONEPHRITIS (CHRONIC)

The acute stage of nephritis may develop into a chronic form. However, the majority of patients with chronic glomerulonephritis give no history of having had the acute condition.

The patient usually experiences headaches and frequent urination during the night. Variable amounts of albumin and casts are present in the urine. There may be a latent period lasting for several years, during which the patient feels well. In this period optimum nutrition should be maintained. The latent stage may be followed by a nephrotic stage, but as the disease progresses hypertension, proteinuria, a lowered serum protein level and edema develop. Since the kidneys are unable to excrete all of the urea and the other metabolic wastes that are being formed, these products are retained in the blood. Eventually, uremic symptoms such as lethargy and anorexia result from the increasingly toxic levels of waste products.

Objectives and Principles of Nutritional Care

The primary objectives of nutritional care are (1) to minimize the production of urea and metabolic waste products, (2) to restore good nutritional status, replace protein lost in urine and return serum protein to normal levels by providing adequate protein and calories, (3) to prevent edema and control hypertension and (4) to maintain potassium balance. Depending on the stage of the disease, nutritional care is the same as that for nephrotic syndrome or chronic renal failure.

NEPHROTIC SYNDROME (NEPHROSIS)

Nephrotic syndrome is a term used to designate a variety of pathological conditions characterized by edema, proteinuria, hypoalbuminemia, altered glomerular filtration rate (GFR) and hypercholesterolemia. Hypertension and hematuria may also occur, depending on the diseased state of the kidney. There is an *increased capillary permeability* in the glomeruli and probably throughout the body. Several forms of renal disease may be associated with the nephrotic syndrome, all having in common an effect on the glomeruli to such a degree that protein is filtered through the usual barriers. Clinically, the kidneys are usually able to function adequately in the excretion of urea and other metabolic waste products, but the severe loss of protein from the plasma continues. Sometimes the protein deficit is so great that tissue wastage and malnutrition result (Fig. 30–2), and plasma albumin concentrations of less than 1 gm. per 100 ml. are common. The reduced serum albumin level causes a transudation of fluid from the circulating blood into the surrounding tissue, resulting in edema and decreased blood volume. The decreased volume, in turn, causes an increased reabsorption of sodium.

A familial form of nephrosis occurs in young children; 80 per cent of these cases occur in the age group under 15 years, with the peak incidence at the age of three and one half years. This is discussed in Chapter 38.

Objectives and Principles of Nutritional Care

The primary objective of the diet treatment in nephrotic syndrome is to replace the albumin and other protein that is lost from the plasma into the urine. Patients with a severe protein deficiency already established who have a continued protein loss may require months of carefully supervised nutritional care.

The diet should provide sufficient protein and calories to maintain a positive nitrogen balance, with an increase in the plasma albumin concentration and the disappearance of edema. Thus the diet should be designed to provide 1.5 gm. protein per kg. body weight per day and to replace the protein lost in the urine in a 24-hour

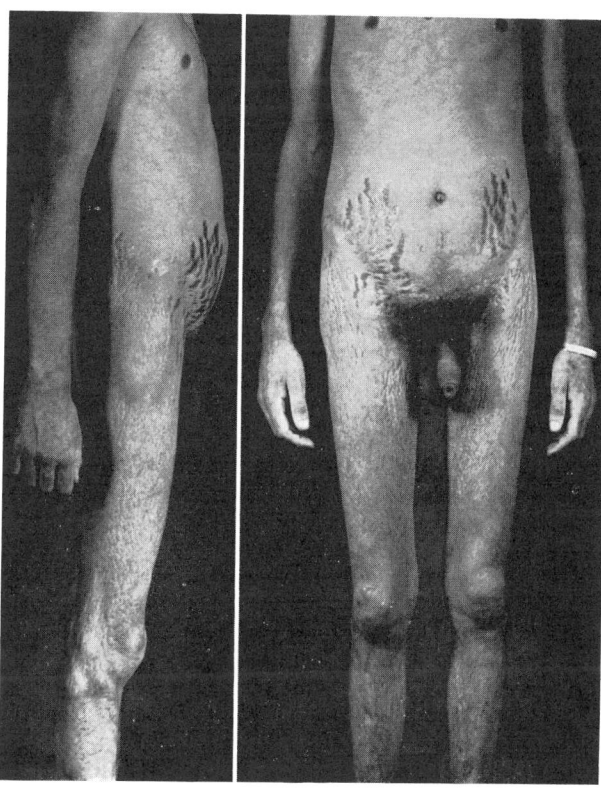

Figure 30–2 Nephrotic syndrome, malnutrition, and "lipoid nephrosis" in 18-year-old male. Photographs show severe tissue wasting and abdominal striae following diuresis and weight loss from 223 to 125 pounds in 6 foot, previously husky youth who had ascites, severe pedal edema, and massive proteinuria. (From Kark, R. M., and Oyama, J. H.: Nutrition and cardiovascular-renal disease. In: Goodhart, R. S., and Shils, M. E. [eds.]: Modern Nutrition in Health and Disease, 5th ed., Philadelphia, Lea and Febiger, 1973, p. 874.)

period. (Several 24-hour urine collections are needed to determine the maximum protein output). There are times when the amount of protein in the urine is greater than the maximum daily plasma albumin regeneration, and in such cases it becomes virtually impossible to make up the protein deficit.

Eighty per cent of the protein should be from sources of high biological value to allow for optimal use of the protein. Fuel sources should be provided to prevent utilization of protein for energy. Therefore, calorie intake should be from 35 to 50 kcal. per kg. body weight per day.

Because of the tubular reabsorption mentioned previously, it is essential to restrict sodium in the diet. The level of intake can be established by measuring the patient's 24-hour output and merely replacing the daily loss. The amount may vary from 40 to 90 mEq. per day.

There is little evidence to suggest that dietary control of cholesterol and fat alters the patient's hyperlipidemia. The extent of the hypercholesterolemia and hyperlipidemia in the individual patient will determine whether fat and cholesterol modification is necessary.

High-Protein, Sodium-Restricted Diets. The protein foods in the daily diet may be increased to 1 qt. milk, 3 eggs and 1/2 lb. meat, fish or poultry. A diet that must be high in protein yet also low in sodium may require the use of special low-sodium protein sources such as low-sodium milk. By replacing the quart of regular whole fluid milk in the diet with modified low-sodium milk, the sodium content of the diet can be lowered by 480 mg. In recent years low-sodium milks have been greatly improved and are very palatable, both as a beverage and when used in cooking. A special low-sodium protein supplement, Lonalac (Mead Johnson), may be used to increase the protein content of the diet still further. Table 30–1 gives a diet containing 120 gm. protein and 74 mEq. sodium. The sodium can be reduced to about 50 mEq. if low-sodium milk is used. If salt-free bread is also used, the diet will contain only about 23 mEq. of sodium. Unsalted nuts, legumes, low-sodium canned meat products and other specially processed low-sodium products are valuable adjuncts to the diet.

Parenteral Protein. In some circumstances, particularly in the presence of pronounced anorexia, nausea or vomiting, oral administration of protein in sufficient amounts to correct the protein deficit may not be possible. In these cases protein hydrolysates or amino acids may be given parenterally.

Table 30–1 HIGH PROTEIN, LOW SODIUM DIET[a]

(Approximately 120 gm. protein, 74 mEq. [1700 mg.] sodium, 2800 kcal.)

SAMPLE MENU

Breakfast

Stewed prunes
Cooked Wheatena
Poached eggs, 2
Toasted whole-wheat bread, 1 slice
Sweet butter
Milk, 8 oz.
Coffee

Lunch

Cream of pea soup
Cold sliced roast lamb, 4 oz.
Cooked spinach
Sliced tomato salad
Whole-wheat bread, 1 slice
Sweet butter
Vanilla ice cream
Milk, 8 oz.

Dinner

Swiss steak, 4 oz.
Mashed potatoes
Baked squash
Whole-wheat bread, 1 slice
Sweet butter
Fresh fruit cup
Milk, 8-oz.

Bedtime

Eggnog

[a]This diet is prepared and served without added salt.

NEPHROSCLEROSIS

Nephrosclerosis refers to disorders involving the renal blood vessels, including arteriosclerosis and essential or malignant hypertension.

Nutritional Care

The diet prescribed for nephrosclerosis should be as much like the adequate normal diet (Chapter 10) as possible. The obese patient should lose weight gradually until normal weight is reached. The loss in weight is essential to lessen the work of the circulatory system.

As renal function decreases, protein in the diet should be adjusted proportionately. In cases of severe kidney damage, the nutritional

care is the same as that for chronic renal failure. (See page 626.)

Fluids are forced unless there is retention by the kidneys, in which case fluid intake is correlated with output.

A low-sodium diet and diuretics are used to control the hypertension. The basic sodium-restricted diets outlined in Chapter 28 can be adjusted to meet the individual needs of the patient.

UREMIA IN RENAL FAILURE

Uremia is a toxic condition caused by the retention of urinary constituents in the blood: urea, creatinine, uric acid, potassium, organic acids and other end products of protein metabolism. The name indicates that urea is the waste product retained in the greatest amount. The term *azotemia* refers only to excess urea and other nitrogenous bodies in the blood. Uremia is a result of the severe progressive loss of renal function that is seen in acute and chronic renal failure, and it is characterized by weakness, anorexia, nausea, vomiting, pruritus, twitching, neuropathy, mental disturbances and, in advanced cases, stupor and coma. Nitrogen retention, measured by the concentration of urea nitrogen, is an indication of the severity of the loss of kidney function. The symptoms and degree of severity are not dependent on a specific level of blood urea nitrogen (BUN) but rather on how rapidly the BUN level rises and on the individual's tolerance of the chemical changes. Some patients may have severe uremic symptoms at BUN levels of 50 mg. per dl., while others show few symptoms at levels greater than 100 mg. per dl. If advanced as far as the coma stage, the condition is grave and usually fatal.

History and General Principles of Protein Nutrition in Renal Failure and Uremia

The primary problem in managing the uremia of kidney failure is to reduce the amount of nitrogenous waste that must be excreted by the kidney and yet maintain a positive nitrogen balance. Nitrogenous wastes are reduced by restricting the intake of protein enough so that there is no "extra" protein to be metabolized and no excess nitrogen to be removed. Ideally, all the protein or nitrogen will be used by the body for enzyme and hormone synthesis, muscle and tissue repair and general body mainte-

nance. The second and more difficult phase is to provide enough protein to maintain nitrogen balance. This problem was first investigated by three Italian researchers, Giordano, Giovannetti and Maggiore, who showed that it was possible to produce positive nitrogen balance and yet reduce blood urea nitrogen levels in uremic patients. These doctors fed their patients a high-calorie diet containing 24 gm. of protein, of which at least 70 per cent was complete protein of high biological value (HBV) containing all of the essential amino acids. Protein of low biological value (LBV), which contains mostly non-essential amino acids, was kept to a minimum. See Table 30–2 for a description of the Giovannetti diet.

The efficacy of this diet is based on the following principles: (1) when the essential amino acid requirements are supplied, a positive nitrogen balance can be maintained, (2) when the amount of protein containing non-essential amino acids is minimal, the urea from the amino acid pool is utilized to make the non-essential amino acids as they are needed and (3) when adequate calories are supplied, protein is not used for energy, but rather is spared and used only for tissue synthesis, repair and maintenance. If sufficient calories are not provided then protein is metabolized for energy, which means that nitrogen must be removed as the carbon skeleton is shunted into the Krebs cycle for oxidation and energy (ATP) production. The nitrogen thus removed must be metabolized to urea in the liver, and the body is left with a supply of urea that must be excreted. In renal failure urea excretion is deficient or non-existent, and uremia develops.

These principles of dietary management, developed over 15 years ago, still form the basis of today's nutritional care in the presence of uremia. Present research is seeking better methods of providing the essential amino acids. One such attempt involves supplementing the diet with the carbon skeletons of essential amino acids (the alpha-hydroxy and alpha-keto

Table 30–2 MODIFIED GIOVANNETTI DIET

(20 gm. protein, 1500 mg. potassium)

1 egg
¾ cup (6 oz.) milk *or* 1 additional egg *or* 1 oz. meat
½ lb. low-protein bread
Vegetables and fruits to provide:
    4–6 gm. protein
    1300–1900 mg. potassium (see Table 30–7)
Fats and sweets as desired (see Table 30–7) to supply adequate calories

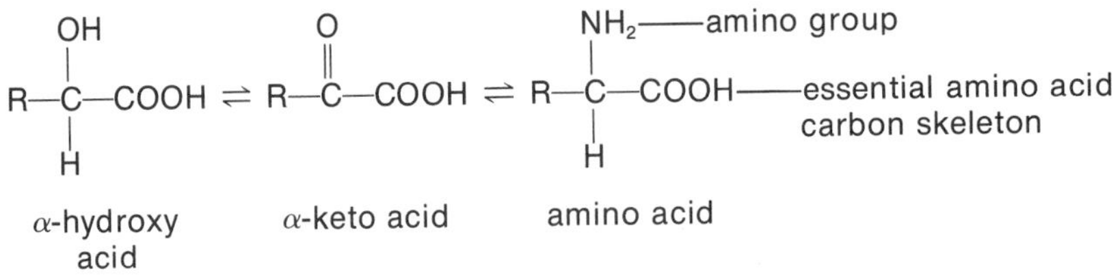

$$\underset{\substack{\text{α-hydroxy} \\ \text{acid}}}{R-\overset{\displaystyle OH}{\underset{\displaystyle H}{C}}-COOH} \;\rightleftharpoons\; \underset{\text{α-keto acid}}{R-\overset{\displaystyle O}{C}-COOH} \;\rightleftharpoons\; \underset{\text{amino acid}}{R-\overset{\displaystyle NH_2}{\underset{\displaystyle H}{C}}-COOH}$$

NH₂——amino group

essential amino acid carbon skeleton

Figure 30–3 Formation of an amino acid.

acids). The hydroxy acid corresponding to methionine has been used for years as a feed supplement to promote growth in animals. It is known that only the skeleton structure of essential amino acids is needed and that the uremic person can use the excess nitrogen in urea to form not only the non-essential amino acids but the essential ones as well. (See Fig. 30–3.) The deterrents to using this method at present are the cost, availability and palatability of the alpha-hydroxy and alpha-keto acids.

It is now accepted that *histidine* is an essential amino acid for the uremic adult; therefore, any essential amino acid supplements would need to include histidine for optimal nitrogen balance. *Arginine* has also been found to produce a more positive nitrogen balance in uremic patients, but it is not yet available in essential amino acid supplements. Methods of providing essential amino acids separate from the diet have been sought, so that dietary protein does not have to be restricted to those containing all of the essential amino acids (eggs, meat, milk). If the essential amino acids could be provided in liquid (Amin-Aid, McGaw Labs) or tablet form,[13] then the diet could contain more incomplete proteins (vegetables, cereals, bread) and be more acceptable to the patient. Again, the problem is one of cost and palatability, but the future should bring improvement. Use of these products in addition to a low-protein diet might enable uremic patients to be managed without dialysis or with less frequent dialysis.

Adequate calories are essential in the dietary treatment of uremia to prevent oxidation of protein for energy and keep the protein for tissue maintenance. Providing calories at the level of 35 to 55 kcal. per kg. IBW is difficult because of the protein, sodium and potassium restrictions. In addition, the anorexia and nausea that occur with uremia deter the patient from consuming the sufficient calories. The caloric intake requires special attention by nurses, dietitian-nutritionists and physicians caring for patients with renal diseases.

ACUTE RENAL FAILURE

Acute renal failure (ARF) is characterized by a sudden reduction in glomerular filtration rate (GFR) and an alteration in the ability of the kidney to excrete waste products and preserve the internal milieu. It is usually associated with oliguria (defined as excretion of less than 400 ml. of urine in 24 hours). Its duration varies from a few days to several weeks, and it may develop in previously healthy kidneys from a number of causes. These causes are usually divided into three categories: (1) inadequate renal perfusion (pre-renal), (2) diseases within the renal parenchyma (intrinsic) and (3) obstruction (post-renal). See Table 30–3 for specific causes.

Acute renal failure has two distinct phases. The first is the *oliguric phase,* during which extensive catabolism and tissue destruction take place. Hemodialysis is used to reduce the acidosis, correct the uremia and lower the rapidly increasing hyperkalemia.

This oliguric phase is followed by a recovery period, referred to as the *diuretic phase,* during which the urinary volume may double each day. For several days renal function remains poor, and uremia continues to be a problem, with rising BUN levels. Dialysis may still be necessary for treatment. The major concern during this period is the excessive loss of fluid, sodium and potassium. It is of utmost importance to measure the daily loss of each to provide for appropriate replacements.

Nutritional Care

Nutritional care in acute renal failure is particularly important, because the patient is suffering not only from uremia, metabolic acidosis and fluid and electrolyte imbalance but usually also from physiological stress (e.g., infection, tissue destruction or poisoning), which increases protein needs. The problem of balancing protein and caloric needs with treatment of acidosis and excessive nitrogenous waste is a complicated and delicate one.

Table 30–3   SOME CAUSES OF ACUTE RENAL FAILURE

I. Pre-renal
  Severe dehydration
  Circulatory collapse
II. Intrinsic
  Acute glomerulonephritis of any cause
    Post-streptococcal infection
    Systemic lupus erythematosus
  Vascular disorders
    Malignant nephrosclerosis
    Bilateral renal infarction
  Severe infection
  Nephrotoxicity
    Antibiotics, analgesics
  Acute tubular insufficiency
III. Post-renal
  Obstruction
    Benign prostatic hypertrophy
    Carcinoma of bladder or prostate
    Uretero-vesical stricture

Fluid and Sodium Balance. The diet should be planned to help regulate the water balance and the adjustment of the various mineral salts, especially sodium and potassium. In both the oliguric and diuretic phases, fluid intake is extremely important and is regulated according to the volume of urine excreted. Intake therefore should replace the output in urine, vomitus or diarrhea, with an additional amount to account for the usual daily insensible losses due to skin and respiratory evaporation. See Table 30–4 for this calculation. While the steps in calculating the fluid intake are relatively simple, fluid balance continues to be a difficult daily management problem due to the variation in the patient's status. His insensible fluid loss, for instance, may be very high because of infection and high fever. On the other hand, the patient may easily become overloaded with fluid as a result of a catabolic decrease in lean body weight and the consequently greater endogenous production of water.

During the diuretic phase it is often very difficult to keep up with the patient's water and sodium excretion. The amounts lost in 24 hours must be carefully monitored, and replacements should be given to avoid hypovolemic shock. Often intravenous administration of normal saline is required.

Sodium is restricted depending on the level of urinary excretion. In the oliguric phase when the output is very low, the intake is kept as low as possible, about 20 to 40 mEq. per day.

Potassium Balance. In ARF potassium is not excreted, and its level in serum may also rise because of tissue destruction and the movement of K^+ out of the cells. For this reason, potassium intake must be restricted as much as possible, to 30 to 50 mEq. per day. Exchange resins such as Kayexalate in sorbitol are used to treat the high K^+ concentration. However, it is important to remember that this drug exchanges sodium for potassium. For every gram of Kayexalate used, 1 mEq. of K^+ is removed and 1 mEq. of Na^+ is added. This could aggravate edema that is already present. Sorbitol is used because it is an unabsorbed sugar that induces diarrhea and so aids the removal of the resin and K^+ from the body. Peritoneal dialysis or hemodialysis is used when the need to reduce the serum potassium level is urgent.

During the diuretic phase of ARF, it is possible for the patient to lose large amounts of potassium and become hypokalemic. KCl may then be added to the dietary intake.

Protein. At the onset of acute renal failure, when few patients can tolerate oral feedings because of vomiting and diarrhea, I.V. preparations have been used to reduce protein catabolism. Giving carbohydrate alone (for example, 100 gm. over a 24-hour period) will only reduce protein breakdown by 50 per cent. The preferred treatment is parenteral administration of essential amino acids such as Freamine-E (McGaw) in glucose. This will reduce protein catabolism and urea production to a minimum until the patient can tolerate oral feeding. Since aggressive treatment using dialysis can rapidly reduce uremic symptoms, this parenteral nutritional support may only be necessary for a short period of time, if at all. After dialysis is discontinued, protein catabolism and high BUN levels are controlled by protein and caloric intake.

At this point, regulation of the protein con-

Table 30–4   SAMPLE CALCULATION OF FLUID REQUIREMENTS FOR A TYPICAL PATIENT IN ACUTE RENAL FAILURE

Measured urine output of previous 24 hr.	−200 ml.
Insensible water loss in 24 hr.	−1000 ml.
(Varies with room temperature, room humidity and body temperature)	
Water loss in vomitus	−100 ml.
Total water loss in 24 hr.	−1300 ml.
Water produced by metabolism in 24 hr.	+500 ml.
(Provided catabolism and weight loss are not occurring)	
Water requirements for 24 hr.	800 ml.
Water in usual diet in 24 hr.	500 ml.
Additional fluid intake needed in 24 hr.	300 ml.

Table 30–5   NUTRITIONAL CARE DURING
ACUTE RENAL FAILURE

NUTRIENT	AMOUNT
Protein	0.5 gm./kg. IBW, increasing as GFR returns to normal. 80% should be HBV protein.
Calories	40–55 kcal./kg. body weight.
Potassium	20–50 mEq./day in oliguric phase (depending on urinary output, dialysis and serum K^+ level); replace losses in diuretic phase.
Sodium	20–40 mEq./day in oliguric phase (depending on urinary output, edema, dialysis and serum Na^+ level); replace losses in diuretic phase.
Fluid	Replace output from the previous day plus 500 ml. (approximately equal to fluid in food).

tent of the diet is important, but authorities differ regarding the amount of protein to include. Some recommend 0.2 to 0.3 gm. protein per kg. per day,[2] but others feel that this is too low. A good method is to limit protein to the minimum of 0.5 gm. per kg. IBW per day in the beginning to reduce uremia by decreasing nitrogen metabolism and retention. Gradually the amount is increased as the kidneys show signs of improvement and the GFR returns to normal. The protein intake eventually reaches the RDA of 0.8 gm. per kg. IBW per day or even higher if there has been much tissue wasting.

Reducing protein intake to 0.5 gm. per kg. per day means that a 70-kg. man will eat only 35 gm. of protein per day. Eighty per cent, or 28 gm., should be HBV protein, which means that the diet should include 4 oz. of meat, fish or poultry *or* 1 egg, 2 oz. of meat, fish or poultry and 1 cup of milk. Consequently, this allows only 7 gm. of protein to be obtained from other protein-containing foods in a diet—breads, cereals, vegetables and fruits. Exchange lists (p. 630) may be used to aid in the planning of the diet.

Calories.   Calorie needs are high (approximately 50 kcal. per kg. IBW per day) in order to provide positive nitrogen balance under stress situations. Alternative fuel sources that will prevent the use of protein for energy production must come from a high intake of carbohydrate and fat. In addition to the usual dietary sources of refined sweets and fats, special high-calorie, low-protein and low-electrolyte formulas have been developed to add to the diet. Borst was the first to develop such a product when he concocted the butterball (butter and sugar).[7] Some of the modern products are Controlyte (Doyle), Polycose (Ross), Cal-

Power (General Mills) and Hycal (Beecham). The liquid products contain 70 to 85 kcal. per oz., and the powders contain approximately 140 kcal. per oz. Special recipes have been developed that are low in protein and electrolytes and extremely high in calories. (See the list of cookbooks at the end of this chapter.) Table 30–5 summarizes nutritional care during acute renal failure.

CHRONIC RENAL FAILURE

Renal disease can progress relentlessly until chronic renal failure develops and finally uremia appears. As illustrated in Figure 30–4, a person may lose almost 85 per cent of renal function before experiencing symptoms of uremia and renal failure. Frequently, by the time the person sees a physician or the diagnosis has been made, disease has been raging in the kidneys for years. With chronic renal failure comes a myriad of problems related to the kidney's inability to excrete waste products, reabsorb nutrients, maintain fluid and electrolyte balance, produce hormones and perform other metabolic functions. As the failure grows more severe and as more nephrons die, the kidney can no longer compensate for their loss, and symptoms become apparent.

Nutritional Care

Nutritional care aims to make up for the work no longer being done by the nonfunctioning nephrons. The goals of nutritional care in chronic renal failure are:

1. To prevent deficiency and maintain good

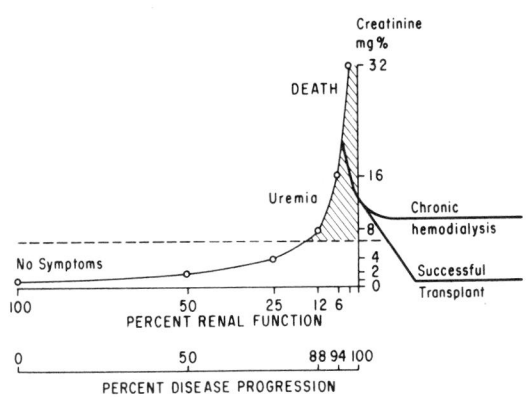

Figure 30–4   Natural course of renal failure. (From: de St. Jeor, S. T., et al.: Low Protein Diets for the Treatment of Chronic Renal Failure. Salt Lake City, Utah, University of Utah Press, 1970, p. 4.)

nutritional status (and growth, in the case of children) through adequate protein, calorie, vitamin and mineral intake.

2. To minimize uremia by controlling the protein intake while still maintaining a positive nitrogen balance.

3. To control edema and electrolyte imbalance by controlling sodium, potassium and fluid intake.

4. To prevent or retard the development of renal osteodystrophy by controlling calcium, phosphorus, magnesium and vitamin D intake.

5. To enable the patient to eat a palatable, attractive diet that fits into his lifestyle as much as possible.

Even with the development of dialysis methods and transplantation techniques, nutritional care remains an important therapy for patients with chronic renal failure. Such care is essential to enhance dialysis, maintain optimal nutritional status and prevent complications. Through good nutritional care, the patient will be able to minimize the symptoms of uremia prior to beginning a dialysis treatment program, making dialysis less traumatic. In each of the following sections, the need to modify nutritional care for the dialysis patient will be discussed.

Fluid and Sodium. The kidney's ability to handle sodium and water in the patient with chronic renal failure changes and must be assessed frequently through measurement of urinary sodium excretion, urine output, blood pressure, presence of edema, serum sodium level and dietary intake. The diet and fluid intake are then modified accordingly. In the early stages of renal failure, nephrons may not be able to concentrate urine, and large quantities of fluid and sodium may be lost daily and will have to be replaced. As the failure worsens, the kidney may only be able to produce 400 to 500 ml. of dilute urine per day (oliguria). At this point, fluid restriction is necessary.

Many patients with chronic renal failure may be *losing* sodium. Examples of diseases with a salt-losing tendency are polycystic disease of the kidney, chronic obstructive uropathy, chronic pyelonephritis and analgesic nephropathy. Other renal diseases, such as chronic glomerulonephritis, can have a *salt-losing phase*. To prevent hypotension, hypovolemia, cramps and further deterioration of renal function, extra sodium may be required. Measurement of the urinary sodium concentration of patients receiving a known amount of sodium should be made several times to assess the sodium excretion of patients who are still excreting urine.

The diet should be matched to the sodium and fluid excretion. Usually this is 87 to 130 mEq. (2 to 3 gm.) or higher of sodium per day, which may be found in a normal diet without added salt. In some cases sodium intake will need to be increased above normal. Sodium can be increased by adding salt or salty foods such as bouillon (one cube contains 20 mEq. of sodium).

Patients with hypertension and edema may need a restricted sodium and restricted fluid intake. Again, intake should be matched to the urinary sodium excretion. Since fluid in the diet is approximately 500 to 800 ml., the diet will replace the 500-ml. insensible water loss (insensible water loss of 1000 ml. offset by water of metabolism of 500 ml.). Additional fluid is given to replace urinary loss.

In the *anuric* patient (without urine) who is maintained with dialysis, sodium intake and fluid intake are regulated to allow for weight gain from edema of 1 lb. (0.5 kg.) per day between dialyses. This means a sodium intake of 87 to 90 mEq. (2 gm.) per day and a fluid intake of 500 ml. per day plus the additional 500 ml. from the diet. An 87 to 90-mEq. sodium diet with protein limitations allows for light salting of foods during cooking but no additional salt at the table and no salted, smoked or cured meat or fish, salted snack foods, bouillon and canned soups or foods canned in brine. See Chapter 28 for the diet plan for an 87 to 90 mEq. (2 gm.) sodium diet. An interdialysis weight gain of one half pound (0.25 kg.) per day would necessitate the intake of only 250 ml. of fluid daily plus the amount received from food. Sodium intake should be adjusted to equal the amount lost in 24 hours plus 35 mEq. In educating patients about fluid balance, the dietitian must deal with their constant complaints of thirst. Suggestions such as to suck on a few ice chips to stretch a fluid requirement or to use a spray mouth wash to take away the dryness may help.

Patients must be taught to measure their fluid intake and urine output, to examine their eyelids and ankles for edema, to weigh themselves regularly each morning and to record their weight. Occasionally (in about 10 per cent of patients), hypertension is not alleviated even after meticulous attention is paid to fluid and water balance. Usually in these cases hypertension is being perpetuated by the presence of a high level of renin secreted by the kidney and requires medication for control.

Fluid and sodium requirements can increase in the presence of perspiration, vomiting or fever. Hypotension and the possibility of clotting at the shunt site must be avoided by

scrupulous attention to fluid and sodium intake.

Potassium. Potassium usually requires restriction, depending upon the individual's body size, the 24-hour urinary potassium excretion, the serum K^+ level and the frequency of dialysis. The patient receiving less frequent dialysis cannot tolerate a high potassium intake. Potassium intake is usually 40 to 65 mEq. (1.5 to 2.5 gm.) per day. For the patient with no urine excretion who is maintained with dialysis, the diet usually includes 51 mEq. (2 gm.) of potassium. This is a moderate restriction from the usual intake of 75 to 100 mEq. (3 to 4 gm.) of potassium for most Americans. See Appendix Table 9 for the potassium content of foods. The exchange lists on page 630 show the potassium content for groups of food.

Rarely, a chronic renal failure patient may require additional potassium because of hypokalemic nephropathy (K^+-losing tendency). Those who are taking diuretics may be losing potassium in the urine. The amount lost in a 24-hour period should be measured and replaced. The potassium may be added to the diet, added to the dialysate or given as potassium supplements.

Protein. In chronic renal failure, as the GFR decreases and fewer nitrogenous waste products are excreted, it becomes necessary to control the level of protein intake while continuing to maintain a positive nitrogen balance. A mild protein restriction is usually initiated when the kidney function has decreased to about 25 per cent of normal, and protein is decreased further as renal function continues to decline, as measured by creatinine clearance. Therefore, the renal failure patient may restrict his protein intake in stages as failure progresses. Authorities do not agree on the exact amount of protein recommended at each stage of deterioration, but the plan shown in Table 30–6 is representative.

When protein restriction is started, at least 75 per cent of the protein intake should be of high biological value (HBV), or complete proteins to assure that the essential amino acid requirements are met. The body then uses its extra nitrogen to synthesize the non-essential amino acids and thus reduces the amount of urea that must be removed.

Dialysis is a drain on protein in the body, and the daily protein intake should be increased to compensate for this. Losses of 10 to 30 gm. of protein can occur during a 24-hour peritoneal dialysis, with an average of 1 gm. per hour. Hemodialysis results in a similar loss of approximately 1 gm. of protein for every hour of dialysis. Patients receiving once-weekly peritoneal dialysis or twice-weekly hemodialysis should have an intake of at least *0.75 gm. protein per kg. body weight* per day, while those receiving hemodialysis three times per week should ingest *1 gm. protein per kg. body weight* per day. However, the patient's serum BUN and serum creatinine levels, uremic symptoms and weight should be monitored and the diet adjusted accordingly.

An example of a dietary protein calculation is as follows:

Example: A 60-kg. anuric female receiving hemodialysis 3 times per week should be eating 60 gm. of protein per day. If 75 per cent of this protein is to be of high biological value, then 46 gm. of protein should be in the form of eggs, meat, fish, poultry, milk or cheese. A likely combination of these foods to *contribute 46 grams of HBV protein* would be the following:

Table 30–6 PROTEIN INTAKE ACCORDING TO DEGREE OF RENAL FAILURE*

CREATININE CLEARANCE (ml./min./1.73m.²)	PROTEIN INTAKE (gm./kg. IBW/day)
30–20	0.75–0.8
10–19	0.5 –0.75
<10	0.5
Hemodialysis	0.75–1.0

*From: Section of Nephrology, Department of Internal Medicine, Rush-Presbyterian-St. Luke's Medical Center, Chicago, Illinois.

FOOD	GM. PROTEIN
1 egg	7
2 oz. chicken	14
3 oz. beef	21
½ cup milk	4

The remaining 14 gm. is obtained from the LBV protein in our diets that we enjoy so much: breads and cereals, vegetables, fruit, potatoes, pasta and desserts. An example of a combination of foods that would provide this *14 gm. LBV protein allowance* is the following:

FOOD	GM. PROTEIN
3 slices bread	6
¾ cup cereal	3
½ cup mashed potatoes	2
½ cup carrots	1
½ cup peas	1
1 small glass orange juice	0.5
1 large apple	0.5

The tedium of the diet comes from the patient's awareness that he must not only control his intake of HBV protein but must also restrict other foods containing LBV protein, and he does not have the freedom of substitution. He cannot, for example, use 3 slices of toast (6 gm. of incomplete protein) to replace a morning glass of milk (6 gm. of complete protein) without increasing his BUN concentration. One way to add variety and calories to the diet is to include protein-free or low-protein products such as those discussed on page 626. In addition, low-protein flour and flour products such as pasta, bread, muffins, cereal and baking mix are available from General Mills and other companies. Wheat flour is treated to remove the proteins gliadin and gluten so that only the starch remains. Recipes using this wheat starch have to be modified, and the foods made with it are different from those made with regular flour. While these products are expensive and require extra effort in preparation, patients should be informed about them and given the opportunity to try them. Flavor and texture can often be improved by adding margarine, jelly, honey, spices, and lemon or peppermint flavoring. Many recipe books and tasty recipes are now available. (See the list at the end of this chapter.)

Table 30–7 contains the exchange lists quantified for protein, sodium, potassium and calories that are used in designing a diet for patients who must have controlled intakes. Table 30–8 shows how these exchanges might be combined to construct diets to meet various requirements. Tables 30–9 and 30–10 present sample menus.

Calories. Caloric intake must be adequate in order to spare protein for tissue protein synthesis and prevent its metabolism for energy. Calories provided by foods other than protein are very important for patients with chronic renal failure, just as they are in cases of acute renal failure. Depending on the patient's present nutritional status and degree of stress, between *35 and 50 kcal. per kg. body weight* should be provided.

Patients with chronic renal failure who require tube feeding may be given a product such as Amin-Aid (McGaw), which contains only the essential amino acids plus histidine in the amount required and which when mixed with water provides amino acids, carbohydrate and a few electrolytes. Another possible source of protein may be electrodialyzed whey (milk protein [lactalbumin] treated to remove the electrolytes), which when combined with glucose and water provides HBV protein with adequate calories and few electrolytes. The palatability of these products is low, and as soon as possible the patient should be encouraged to eat the low-protein, high-calorie diet with controlled sodium and potassium intake. A third possible means of nutritional support not yet extensively used is parenteral administration of the essential amino acids. These techniques can also be used in patients with acute renal failure.

Calcium, Phosphorus and Vitamin D. A major complication of chronic renal failure is metabolic bone disease or renal osteodystrophy. The disease is essentially of three types: *osteomalacia,* or bone demineralization, *osteitis fibrosa cystica,* caused by hyperparathyroidism, and *metastatic calcification* of joints and soft tissues.

As the GFR decreases, phosphorus is retained in the plasma, resulting in a decrease in serum calcium. Normally, a low calcium level with a high phosphorus level would trigger: (1) the release of parathyroid hormone (PTH) from the parathyroid glands and (2) the release of 1,25-dihydroxycholecalciferol, also known as 1,25-$(OH)_2$ Vitamin D_3, the chief active metabolite of vitamin D from the kidney. The PTH would act with 1,25-$(OH)_2 D_3$ (a calcium mobilizer) to reabsorb calcium from the bone, raising the serum level to normal. Simultaneously, the 1,25-$(OH)_2 D_3$ would be absorbing Ca^{++} in the gut to replace the calcium ions lost from the bone and to keep serum Ca^{++} within normal range. (Chapter 8 discusses the activities of 1,25-$(OH)_2 D_3$ more fully.)

Cholecalciferol is first converted in the liver to 25-hydroxycholecalciferol, and 1-hydroxylation occurs in the kidney to make it an active vitamin (1,25-$[OH]_2 D_3$). Renal failure prevents this process from being completed. In fact, it has been shown in patients with renal failure that there is reduced absorption of calcium from the intestine, supposedly because of inadequate amounts of 1,25-$(OH)_2 D_3$.[6] There-

Text continued on page 637

Table 30–7   EXCHANGE LISTS FOR DIETS WITH CONTROLLED PROTEIN, SODIUM AND POTASSIUM*

FOOD	APPROXIMATE AMOUNT	PRO-TEIN (gm.)	CAL-ORIES	SODIUM (mEq.) Unsalted	SODIUM (mEq.) Salted	POTAS-SIUM (mEq.)	FLUID (ml.)	PHOS-PHORUS (mg.)	CAL-CIUM (mg.)
Egg	1	7	75	3.0	5.0	2.0	35	110	27
Meat	1 oz.	7	75	1.0	3.0[a]	2.5	20	Varies (50–100)	25
Fat	Varies	–	35	–	2.0	–	1	–	1
Milk Product	Varies	4	Varies	2.5	2.5	4.0	70	110	125
Bread	1 slice	2	70	0.5	6.0	1.5	10	20	20
Potato	½ cup	2	70	0.5	10.0[b]	7.0	80	50	20
Cereal	½ cup	2	70	0.5	10.0[b]	1.5	Varies	Varies (5–80)	5
Vegetable									
Group 1	Varies	1	20	0.3	10.0[b]	3.0	60	30	26
Group 2	Varies	1	20	0.8	11.0[b]	5.0	80	20	23
(Average value)				(0.5)		(4.0)	(70)		
Fruit									
Group 1	Varies	0.5	60	–	–	2.5	80	15	12
Group 2	Varies	0.5	60	–	–	5.0	75	15	12
(Average value)						(3.0)	(80)		
Low-Protein Bread	1 slice (40 gm.)	0.2	115	0.5	–	0.3	10	20	–
CHO Supplement	Varies	–	120	–	–	1.0	Varies	–	–
Beverage (coffee, tea)	1 cup	–	–	–	–	2.0	240	–	–
Salt	1 tsp.	–	–	–	86	–	–	–	–

[a] Moderately salted during preparation, approximately ½ tsp. salt per lb. of meat.
[b] Moderately salted during preparation or processing, approximately ⅛ tsp. salt per ½ cup.

Meat Group (Unsalted)

Protein	7.0 gm.
Sodium	1.0 mEq.
Potassium	2.5 mEq.
Calories	75
Water	20 ml.
Calcium	25 mg.
Phosphorus	Varies

FOOD	AMOUNT	WEIGHT (gm.)
Meat (unsalted)		
Beef, lamb, liver, pork, veal	1 oz.	30
Fowl (unsalted)		
Chicken, duck, turkey	1 oz.	30
Fish (unsalted, fresh or frozen)		
Fish	1 oz.	30
Clams	2 oz.	50
Oysters	2½ oz.	50
Shrimp	1 oz.	30
Egg (unsalted, 3 mEq. sodium)	1 medium	50
Cheese (unsalted)		
Cheese	1 oz.	30
Cottage cheese	¼ cup	50
Peanut butter (unsalted)	2 tbsp.	30

Omitted: Salted meat, fish, fowl, cheese, peanut butter; other organ meats; other shellfish.

Table 30–7 EXCHANGE LISTS FOR DIETS WITH CONTROLLED PROTEIN, SODIUM AND POTASSIUM (*Continued*)

Fat Group (Unsalted)

Protein	–
Sodium	–
Potassium	–
Calories	35
Water	1 ml.
Calcium	1 mg.
Phosphorus	–

FOOD	AMOUNT	WEIGHT (gm.)
Margarine	1 tsp.	5
Mayonnaise	1 tsp.	5
Cooking fats or oils	1 tsp.	5

Omitted: Salted butter or margarine; commercial salad dressings.

Milk Group

Protein	4.0 gm.
Sodium	2.5 mEq.
Potassium	4.0 mEq.
Calories	Varies
Water	70 ml.
Calcium	125 mg.
Phosphorus	110 mg.

FOOD	AMOUNT	WEIGHT (gm.)
Milk	½ cup	120
Evaporated or condensed milk	¼ cup	60
Yogurt	½ cup	120
Powdered whole milk	2 tbsp.	14
Half and half (coffee cream)	½ cup	120
Light whipping cream	⅔ cup	160
Heavy whipping cream	¾ cup	180
Sour cream	½ cup	120
Ice cream	½ cup	100
Ice milk	⅓ cup	80
Sherbet	1 cup	240
Custard	¼ cup	60

Omitted: Commercial buttermilk, powdered skim milk, instant dairy mixes, non-dairy cream substitutes

Bread Group (Unsalted)

Protein	2.0 gm.
Sodium	0.5 mEq.
Potassium	1.5 mEq.
Calories	70
Water	Varies
Calcium	20 mg.
Phosphorus	Varies

FOOD	AMOUNT	WEIGHT (gm.)
Bread (unsalted)	1 slice	25
Cereal (unsalted; calcium = 5 mg.)		
Cooked	½ cup	100
Dry, flake	⅔ cup	20
Dry, puffed wheat or rice	1½ cups	20
Dry, biscuit	1	25

Table continued on the following page

Table 30–7 EXCHANGE LISTS FOR DIETS WITH CONTROLLED PROTEIN, SODIUM AND POTASSIUM (*Continued*)

FOOD	AMOUNT	WEIGHT (*gm.*)
Crackers (unsalted)		
Crackers	6	20
Melba toast	4	15
Flour Products (unsalted)		
Flour	2 tbsp.	20
Cornmeal	2 tbsp.	25
Macaroni, noodles, spaghetti		
Dry	½ oz.	15
Cooked	¼ cup	50
Rice		
Dry	1 oz.	30
Cooked	½ cup	100
Vegetable (unsalted)		
Brussels sprouts	¼ cup	50
Corn[c]	⅓ cup	80
Corn grits	½ cup	100
Lima beans	¼ cup	50
Parsnips[c]	½ cup	100
Peas	¼ cup	50
Potato[c]	½ cup	100
Sweet potato, fresh or canned[c]	½ cup	100
Miscellaneous		
Milk or sweet chocolate	1 oz.	30
Pie crust (unsalted)	⅛ pie (9″)	135
Popcorn	1 cup	14

Omitted: Breads, rolls or crackers made with salt, baking powder or baking soda; self-rising flour; instant, quick-cooking or ready-to-eat cereals processed with salt or sodium compound; commercially prepared mixes; dried beans or peas, commercially frozen peas.

[c]Potassium = 3–9 mEq.

Vegetable Groups (unsalted)

Group 1		
	Protein	1.0 gm.
	Sodium	0.3 mEq.
	Potassium	3.0 mEq.[d]
	Calories	20
	Water	60 ml.
	Calcium	25 mg.
	Phosphorus	30 mg.

VEGETABLE	AMOUNT	WEIGHT (*gm.*)
Asparagus, fresh, frozen, canned	¼ cup	50
Bean sprouts	½ cup	50
Beans (green or wax), canned	½ cup	100
Broccoli, fresh or frozen	¼ cup	50
Carrots, canned	½ cup	100
Cauliflower, fresh or frozen[e]	¼ cup	50
Collards, cooked	¼ cup	50
Dandelion greens, cooked	¼ cup	50
Endive[e]	½ cup	50
Escarole[e]	4 leaves	50
Lettuce[e]	¼ small head	100
Mustard greens, cooked	¼ cup	50
Okra	¼ cup	50
Onions[e]	½ cup	50
Pepper, green, cooked	¼ cup	50
Radishes	10	100
Rutabaga, fresh or frozen	⅓ cup	80
Spinach, cooked	¼ cup	50
Squash	⅓ cup	80

[d]Potassium restrictions: cooked vegetables, drained.
[e]May be eaten raw in amounts specified.

Table 30–7 EXCHANGE LISTS FOR DIETS WITH CONTROLLED PROTEIN, SODIUM AND POTASSIUM (*Continued*)

Vegetable groups (unsalted)

Group 2		
	Protein	1.0 gm.
	Sodium	0.8 mEq.
	Potassium	5.0 mEq.[d]
	Calories	20
	Water	80 ml.
	Calcium	25 mg.
	Phosphorus	20 mg.

VEGETABLE	AMOUNT	WEIGHT (gm.)
Beans (green or wax), fresh or frozen	½ cup	100
Beets, fresh, frozen, or canned	½ cup	100
Cabbage, fresh[e]	½ cup	100
Carrots, fresh or frozen	¼ cup	50
Cucumber[e]	½ cup	100
Eggplant[e]	½ cup	100
Mushrooms, fresh[e]	2 large or 5 small	50
Pepper, green, fresh[e]	⅓ cup	80
Pumpkin	⅓ cup	80
Tomato, fresh or canned[e]	½ cup or 1 small	100
Tomato juice, canned	½ cup	120
Turnip greens, cooked	⅓ cup	80
Watercress[e]	10 sprigs	50

Omitted: Vegetables processed or prepared with salt, sodium, or sodium compound; any vegetable not listed.

[d] Potassium restrictions: cooked vegetables, drained.
[e] May be eaten raw in amounts specified.

Fruit Groups

Group 1		
	Protein	0.5 gm.
	Sodium	–
	Potassium	2.5 mEq.
	Calories	60
	Water	80 ml.
	Calcium	12 mg.
	Phosphorus	15 mg.

FRUIT	AMOUNT	WEIGHT (gm.)
Apple	1 (2″ diameter)	80
Apple juice	½ cup	120
Applesauce	½ cup	100
Blackberries	¼ cup	50
Blueberries	½ cup	100
Cantaloupe	¼ small	50
Cherries, canned or frozen	⅓ cup	80
Coconut, fresh or dried	½ oz.	15
Cranberries, fresh	½ cup	100
Cranberry juice	2 cups	480
Dates	2	15
Grapefruit, fresh	½ small	100
Grapefruit sections, canned	½ cup	100
Grapes, canned	⅓ cup	80
Grapes, fresh	⅓ cup or 10	50
Grape juice	¼ cup	60
Grape juice drink	1 cup	240
Honeydew melon	¼ small	50
Lemon juice	½ cup or 1 lemon	100
Loganberries	⅓ cup	80

Table continued on the following page

TABLE 30–7 EXCHANGE LISTS FOR DIETS WITH CONTROLLED PROTEIN, SODIUM AND POTASSIUM (*Continued*)

	Fruit Groups	
Group 1	Protein	0.5 gm.
	Sodium	–
	Potassium	2.5 mEq.
	Calories	60
	Water	80 ml.
	Calcium	12 mg.
	Phosphorus	15 mg.

FRUIT	AMOUNT	WEIGHT (gm.)
Mango, fresh	1 medium	70
Orange-apricot drink	½ cup	120
Peach, frozen	½ cup	100
Peach nectar	⅔ cup	160
Pear, fresh	1 small	80
Pear, canned	¾ cup	150
Pear nectar	¾ cup	180
Pineapple, canned	½ cup	100
Pineapple, fresh or frozen	⅓ cup	80
Pineapple-grapefruit drink	⅔ cup	160
Pineapple-orange drink	⅔ cup	160
Plums, canned	3	80
Raisins	2 tbsp.	15
Raspberries, frozen	⅓ cup	80
Strawberries, frozen	½ cup	100
Tangerine	2 small	80
Watermelon	½ cup	100

Group 2	Protein	0.5 gm.
	Sodium	–
	Potassium	5.0 mEq.
	Calories	55
	Water	75 ml.
	Calcium	12 mg.
	Phosphorus	15 mg.

FRUIT	AMOUNT	WEIGHT (gm.)
Apricots	1 medium	80
Apricot nectar	½ cup	120
Banana, fresh	½ small	60
Blackberries, fresh	⅓ cup	80
Figs, canned	½ cup	100
Figs, fresh	1 large	50
Fruit cocktail, canned	½ cup	100
Grapefruit juice	½ cup	120
Melon balls, frozen	⅓ cup	80
Nectarines, fresh	1 small	80
Orange, fresh	1 small	80
Orange juice, fresh, frozen or canned	½ cup	120
Papaya, fresh	⅓ cup	80
Peaches, fresh or canned	2 halves	100
Persimmon, fresh	½ small	60
Pineapple juice	½ cup	120
Plums, fresh	2 small	80
Prune juice	½ cup	120
Prunes	2 small	15
Raspberries	⅓ cup	80
Rhubarb	⅓ cup	80
Strawberries, fresh	½ cup	100

Omitted: Any fruit not listed.

Table 30–7   EXCHANGE LISTS FOR DIETS WITH CONTROLLED PROTEIN, SODIUM AND POTASSIUM (*Continued*)

Low-Protein Bread Group (Unsalted)[f]

Protein	0.2 gm.
Sodium	0.5 mEq.
Potassium	–
Calories	115
Water	10 ml.
Calcium	–
Phosphorus	20 mg.

FOOD	AMOUNT	WEIGHT (gm.)
Low Protein Products		
Bread	1 slice	40
Pasta, cooked	1½ cups	135
Rusk	2 slices	20
Low Protein Bread		
(made with low protein bread mix)	1 slice	40

[f] Recipes for other low protein products should be calculated individually. Wheat starch, cornstarch, arrowroot and tapioca may be used in preparation of breads and desserts.

Carbohydrate Supplement Group (CHO Supplement)

Protein	–
Sodium	–
Potassium	1 mEq.
Calories	120
Water	Varies
Calcium	–
Phosphorus	–

FOOD	AMOUNT	WEIGHT (gm.)
Sugar and syrups		
Sugar	2½ tbsp.	30
Honey	2 tbsp.	40
Jelly or jam	2 tbsp.	40
Syrup (table blends)	2 tbsp.	40
Candy		
Fondant or sugar mints	3	30
Gumdrops	3 large	30
Hard candy, unfilled	6 pieces	30
Jelly beans	20	60
Lollipops, unfilled	1 medium	30
Fruit desserts		
Cranberry (sauce or relish)	2 tbsp.	80
Fruit ice	⅔ cup	140
Popsicle	1 twin bar	130
Flavored beverages		
(carbonated, fruit flavored; Kool Aid; lemonade)	1 cup (8 oz.)	240
Flour products		
Cornstarch or tapioca	¼ cup	30

Beverage (Values Should Be Calculated Individually)

BEVERAGE	AMOUNT	WEIGHT (gm.)	POTASSIUM (mEq.)
Coffee, tea	1 cup	240	2

Table continued on the following page

Miscellaneous	
ALLOWED	OMITTED
Pepper; spices and herbs except "Omitted"; fresh celery (no more than 2 tbsp.); fresh garlic, onion powder or juice; horseradish root, powdered mustard; vinegar; unsalted white sauce made with milk allowance; flavoring extracts.	Salt[g], seasoned salts, mixed spices; baking powder, baking soda; parsley, dried celery products; bottled meat sauces, catsup, prepared mustard or horseradish, meat extracts, meat tenderizers, monosodium glutamate; pickles; gravy; commercial soups; commercially prepared dessert mixes; cocoa; nuts; olives; salt substitutes unless approved by physician.

[g]Allowed when specifically calculated.

*Adapted from: Mayo Clinic Diet Manual, 4th ed. Philadelphia, W. B. Saunders Co., 1971, pp. 80–86.

Table 30–8 FOOD EXCHANGE COMBINATIONS FOR CONTROLLED PROTEIN, SODIUM AND POTASSIUM DIETS*

DIET	MEAT	FAT	MILK OR MILK PRODUCTS[a]	BREAD	LOW PROTEIN BREAD	VEGETABLE	FRUIT	CARBOHYDRATE SUPPLEMENT	BEVERAGE	SALT (Shaker)[b]
30 Gm. protein, 45 mEq. potassium, 1500 ml. fluid										
20 mEq. Na	3	11	1	1	6	2[c]	4	6	3	–
40 mEq. Na	3	11	1	1	6	2[c]	4	6	3	¼ tsp.
90 mEq. Na	3[c]	11[c]	1	1[c]	6	2[c]	4	6	3	¼ tsp.
50 Gm. Protein: 65 mEq. potassium, 1800 ml. fluid										
20 mEq. Na	5(4[c])	8	1	2	5	3	6	5	3	–
40 mEq. Na	5(4[c])	8	1	2	5	3	6	5	3	¼ tsp.
90 mEq. Na	5[c]	8[c]	1	2[c]	5	3(1[c])	6	5	3	¼ tsp.
70 Gm. Protein: 85 mEq. potassium, 2200 ml. fluid										
20 mEq. Na	5	6	4	6	–	4	6	6	3	–
40 mEq. Na	5(4[c])	6[c]	4	6	–	4	6	6	3	–
90 mEq. Na	5[c]	6[c]	4	6[c]	–	4	6	6	3	–
100 Gm. Protein: 95 mEq. potassium, 2200 ml. fluid										
30 mEq. Na	9	6	4	6	–	4	5	4	3	–
40 mEq. Na	9	6[c]	4	6	–	4	5	4	3	–
90 mEq. Na	9	6[c]	4	6[c]	–	4	5	4	3	⅛ tsp.
120 Gm Protein: 95 mEq. potassium, 2300 ml. fluid										
90 mEq. Na	11[c]	6[c]	6	7	–	3	4	2	3	¼ tsp.

*From: Mayo Clinic Diet Manual, 4th ed. Philadelphia, W. B. Saunders Co., 1971, p. 79.

[a]A half cup of half-and-half is included in all diets (4 gm. protein, 14 gm. fat, 6 gm. carbohydrate, 165 kcal.). When other milk products are included, the nutritive composition of the diet should be reevaluated.

[b]In place of salt allowance, the equivalent in salted foods may be given.

[c]Foods salted in preparation or processing.

Table 30–9 SAMPLE MENU 1 FOR PROTEIN-, SODIUM- AND POTASSIUM-CONTROLLED DIET

(40 mg. protein, 800 mg. (35 mEq.) sodium, 1500 mg. (38 mEq.) potassium, 1500 cc. fluid, 2500 + kcal.)*

MEAL	PROTEIN (gm.)	KCAL.	Na (mg.)	K (mg.)	FLUID (cc.)	P (mg.)
Breakfast						
½ cup orange juice	0.5	60	–	250	110	15
½ cup unsalted oatmeal	2.0	70	7	25	85	20
½ cup light coffee cream	3.5	250	52	150	95	95
1 unsalted poached egg	7.0	88	66	70	35	110
1 slice regular toast	2.0	70	130	25	10	20
4 tsp. unsalted butter or margarine	–	180	–	–	–	–
1 tbsp. jelly	–	48	–	–	–	–
6 oz. coffee	–	–	–	–	180	–
3 tsp. sugar	–	48	–	–	–	–
10:00 A.M. Snack						
4 oz. high-calorie supplement[a]	–	273	–	–	60	–
Lunch						
1 oz. unsalted beef patty	7.0	73	25	135	20	50
1 hamburger bun	2.0	70	130	25	10	20
1 tbsp. low-sodium mayonnaise	–	106	–	28	–	–
Sliced tomato and lettuce	2.0	35	5	200	100	50
1 tbsp. low-sodium French dressing	–	88	–	10	–	–
1 sugar cookie	1.0	35	65	12	5	10
4 oz. lemonade	–	40	–	–	120	–
3:00 P.M. Snack						
4 oz. high-calorie supplement	–	273	–	–	60	–
Dinner						
1 oz. unsalted broiled chicken	7.0	73	25	135	20	50
⅓ cup unsalted mashed potatoes with 4 tsp. unsalted	2.0	35	5	200	100	50
butter or margarine	–	180	–	–	–	–
2 slices bread, regular	4.0	140	260	50	20	40
4 tsp. unsalted butter or margarine	–	180	–	–	–	–
1 tbsp. jelly	–	48	–	–	–	–
½ cup fruit cocktail	0.5	60	–	175	110	15
8 oz. lemonade	–	80	–	–	240	–
Bedtime Snack						
4 oz. high-calorie supplement	–	273	–	–	60	–
Totals	40.5	2876	770	1490	1440	563

*From: Manual of Clinical Dietetics. Downers Grove, Ill., Johnson Printers, 1975, Sec. V p. 15.

[a]Cal-Power is used as a high-calorie supplement. If the patient desires water instead of a high-calorie supplement, the calorie level of the diet will be decreased.

fore, the active role that vitamin D_3 plays in maintaining serum Ca^{++} levels is reduced, and PTH is constantly being secreted. Furthermore, PTH usually works with vitamin D_3 to mobilize the bone Ca^{++}. In the absence of the vitamin, more PTH is required to do the same amount of work, and the end result is hyperparathyroidism and osteomalacia, or bone demineralization. The excessive action of PTH results in osteitis fibrosa cystica, with its characteristic dull, aching bone pain. See Figure 30–5 for an illustration proposed by Bricker and associates[5] to explain the development of hypocalcemia, hyperphos-

phatemia and resulting bone disease in chronic renal failure.

Even though in response to PTH the serum calcium level is elevated, the serum phosphate concentration will remain high as the GFR falls lower. If the product of serum calcium level (mg. per 100 ml.) multiplied by serum phosphate level (mg. per 100 ml.) is greater than 70, *metastatic calcification* is imminent. Clinical management aims to keep the product below 70 by preventing transient elevations in serum phosphate concentration.

In essence, calcium and phosphorus intake must be controlled to as great a degree as pos-

Table 30-10   SAMPLE MENU 2 FOR PROTEIN-, SODIUM- AND POTASSIUM-CONTROLLED DIET*

(60 gm. protein, 2000 mg. (87 mEq.) sodium, 2000 mg. (51 mEq.) potassium, 1500 cc. fluid, 2500 + kcal.)

MEAL	PROTEIN (gm.)	KCAL.	Na (mg.)	K (mg.)	FLUID (cc.)	P (mg.)
Breakfast						
½ cup orange juice	0.5	60	–	250	110	15
½ cup oatmeal	2.0	70	197	25	85	20
½ cup light coffee cream	3.5	250	52	150	95	95
1 poached egg	7.0	88	130	70	35	110
2 slices regular toast	4.0	140	260	50	20	40
6 tsp. unsalted butter or margarine	–	270	–	–	–	–
1 tbsp. jelly	–	48	–	–	–	–
6 oz. coffee	–	–	–	–	180	–
3 tsp. sugar	–	48	–	–	–	–
10:00 A.M. Snack						
4 oz. high-calorie supplement[a]	–	273	–	–	60	–
Lunch						
2 oz. unsalted beef patty	14.0	146	50	270	40	100
1 hamburger bun	2.0	70	130	25	10	20
1 tbsp. mayonnaise	–	106	84	28	–	–
Sliced tomato and lettuce	2.0	35	5	200	100	50
1 tbsp. French dressing	–	88	210	10	–	–
1 sugar cookie	1.0	35	65	12	5	10
5 oz. lemonade	–	50	–	–	150	–
3:00 P.M. Snack						
4 oz. high-calorie supplement	–	273	–	–	60	–
Dinner						
2 oz. unsalted broiled chicken	14.0	146	50	270	40	100
⅓ cup mashed potatoes	2.0	35+	300	200	100	50
2 slices bread	4.0	140	260	50	20	40
4 tsp. unsalted butter or margarine	–	180	–	–	–	–
1 tbsp. jelly	–	48	–	–	–	–
½ cup fruit cocktail	0.5	60	–	175	110	15
6 oz. lemonade	–	60	–	–	180	–
Bedtime Snack						
¾ cup orange sherbet	2.0	70+	7	25	100	20
1 slice poundcake	2.0	70	130	25	10	20
Totals	60.5	2859	1930	1835	1510	705

*From: Manual of Clinical Dietetics, Downers Grove, Ill., Johnson Printers, 1975, Sec. V p. 16.

[a] Cal-Power is used as a high-calorie supplement. If the patient desires water instead of a high-calorie supplement, the calorie level of the diet will be decreased.

sible to avoid aggravation of the delicate situation posed by hyperparathyroidism, phosphate retention and hypocalcemia in renal failure. In practical terms, *calcium intake* is kept *high* and *phosphorus intake* is kept *low*. This is a problem as far as food is concerned, since most of the high-calcium foods—milk and milk products—are also high in phosphorus. Consequently, methods other than dietary ones must be relied upon.

Calcium is increased by giving calcium supplements in the form of calcium carbonate, lactate or gluconate along with the 300 to 500 mg. of calcium provided in the diet. For dialysis patients, 6 to 8 mg. of calcium is added to the dialysate bath so that a smaller amount of serum calcium is drawn off during dialysis. As much as 100 mg. Ca^{++} can be infused in a six-hour dialysis. The earlier calcium supplementation is started, the better for the patient in order to prevent hyperparathyroidism.

Phosphate intake is lowered by restricting it in the diet to 1000 mg. or less and by using phosphate-binding resins such as Basaljel or Amphojel. These aluminum hydroxide products (also used as antacids) bind with phosphate and prevent its absorption from the gut. Frequently, patients have to take large amounts (40 tablets per day) of the resins to keep their serum phosphate levels in control. Taken by themselves the resins may be distasteful, so recipes for cookies and other products that

incorporate the aluminum hydroxide have been developed. Because of potential *hypermagnesemia,* which can exacerbate the already existent bone disease, magnesium-containing antacids such as Maalox, Gelusil or Mylanta should not be used.

As with calcium supplementation, the initiation of these phosphate reduction therapies as soon as possible is advantageous in order to delay hyperparathyroidism and bone disease. Unfortunately, most patients do not have any symptoms during the early phase of hyperparathyroidism and are not attentive about following a modified diet, taking the calcium supplements or taking the phosphate binders; however, they should be encouraged to do so.

Vitamin D is given only when the hypocalcemia of renal failure is severe or causing osteomalacia. However, because so little vitamin D_3 is changed into its active form (1,25-$[OH]_2 D_3$) in the renal failure patient, large amounts (10,000 to 30,000 units daily) must be given. The dangers inherent in the use of these large doses of vitamin D_3 are hypercalcemia and hypermagnesemia from overdosage and metastatic calcification from combined hyper-

calcemia and hyperphosphatemia. Vitamin D should be used carefully, with attention to the development of hypercalcemia. Such hypercalcemia could be difficult to treat because of the accumulation of vitamin D in the body, which would perpetuate the condition and the vitamin D toxicity even after discontinuing its administration.

Far more effective would be the administration of 1,25-$(OH)_2 D_3$ directly. However, at this time this hormone is available only for experimental purposes. Analogs such as 1-α-$OH D_3$ and 1-α,25-$(OH)_2 D_3$, which have similar configurations, have been produced and are much more readily available and much less expensive.

Hemodialysis or peritoneal dialysis does not alleviate osteodystrophy. However, it can reduce the progression of the disease because the infused calcium results in decreased PTH secretion. Patients must still be responsible for following a low-phosphorus diet and for taking the aluminum hydroxide binders, however.

Fluoride. High levels of fluoride in the serum of the uremic patient seem to aggravate the existing bone disease by enhancing bone

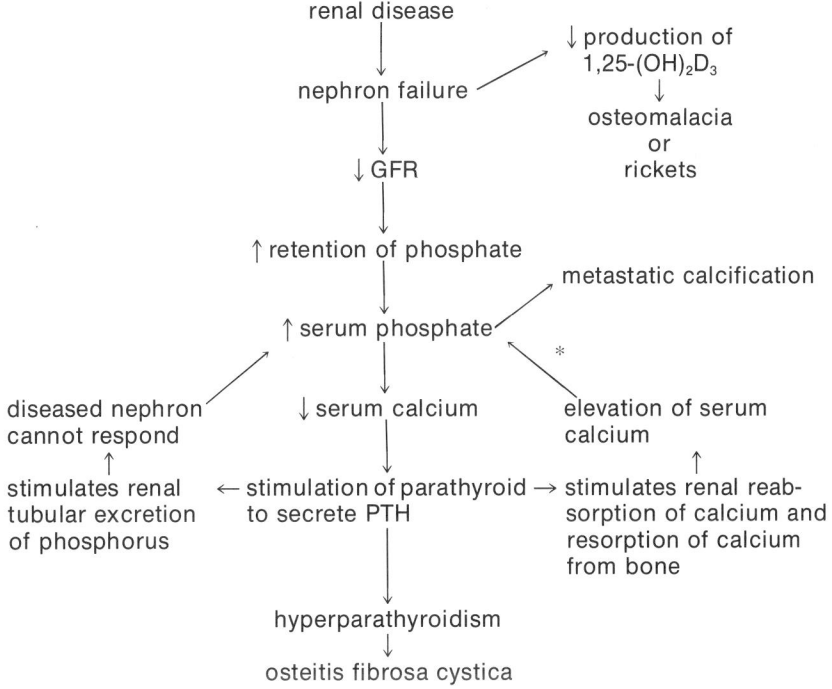

*As the disease worsens, the elevation in serum calcium level no longer causes a drop in serum phosphate level.

Figure 30–5 Development of renal osteodystrophy in chronic renal failure. (Adapted from: Bricker, N. S.: The pathogenesis of the uremic state. An exposition of the "trade off" hypothesis. N. Engl. J. Med., *286*:1093, 1972.)

demineralization. Increased serum fluoride levels in dialyzed uremic patients have been reported and may possibly be attributed to the fluoride content of the dialysate bath. It is recommended that water from fluoridated supplies be deionized before using it in dialysis.[15]

Aluminum. There is evidence that aluminum can be absorbed from the gut, and in fact it is found in increased concentrations in the tissues of uremic patients taking aluminum hydroxide phosphate-binding resins.[4, 9] It has been postulated that the increased levels of aluminum found in the brain tissue of these patients *may* be a cause of the encephalopathy occasionally seen in renal patients.[1] However, until more proof is available, aluminum-containing phosphate resins continue to be used for lack of a better therapy. Another way to reduce aluminum ingestion would be to lower the aluminum in the dialysis bath through deionization of the water.

Iron. The anemia of chronic renal failure usually stabilizes and is relatively asymptomatic, manifesting itself only in complaints of fatigue. It is treated with oral iron supplementation and androgens, anabolic steroids that stimulate erythropoiesis. In addition, sources of iron in the diet such as liver, meat (particularly beef), eggs and some dark green vegetables may be used. Blood transfusion is not recommended because of (1) its depression of erythropoiesis by organs other than the kidney that are still functioning in the renal patient, (2) the possibility of overexpansion of the blood volume, (3) the risk of hepatitis and (4) the introduction of tissue antigens that may complicate a possible kidney transplant.

Vitamins. Although many studies of uremic patients have been conducted to determine their vitamin requirements, the existing data leaves much to be desired. Many vitamin deficiencies have symptoms that coincide with the symptoms of uremia and may in fact be the cause of some of them.

One of the several causes for vitamin deficiency in uremia is the decreased intake due to the restriction of protein and potassium in the diet. Water-soluble vitamins are usually abundant in both high-potassium foods such as citrus fruits and vegetables and high-protein foods such as meat and milk. When compared with normal diets, restricted protein and potassium diets tend to be low in folacin, niacin, riboflavin and vitamin B_6; ascorbic acid is marginal. With frequent episodes of anorexia or illness, the vitamin intake is decreased even further.

Altered metabolism and excretory function as well as drug administration may alter the vitamin levels. Little is known about gastrointestinal absorption in uremia, but it may be significantly decreased. It is possible that uremic toxins interfere with the activity of some vitamins. For example, the phosphorylation of pyridoxine (vitamin B_6) and its analogs may be inhibited.

Water-soluble vitamins are also lost during dialysis. In general, most of the B-complex vitamins, i.e., folic acid, thiamin, riboflavin, nicotinic acid, pantothenic acid and biotin, as well as ascorbic acid, are dialyzable. Since vitamin B_{12} is protein-bound, losses during dialysis are minimal.

At present, no vitamin supplement is available that fits the needs of the uremic patient or of the patient receiving dialysis. A supplement of vitamin B complex with vitamin C is often used. Additional supplements of folic acid and pyridoxine are given.

Carbohydrate. Glucose intolerance with both hyperglycemia and hypoglycemia is frequently observed in patients with chronic renal failure. It seems to reflect a delayed and erratic action of insulin due to a resistance by the tissues to the action of insulin or to an insulin antagonism by the products of uremia. In any case, this glucose intolerance rarely requires administration of insulin and never requires control of the carbohydrate in the diet.

Lipid. There are lipid changes in renal failure patients. Concentrations of serum triglycerides are elevated, usually without elevation of serum cholesterol levels. Causes for the hyperlipidemia are unknown but may be related to insulin resistance, impaired lipoprotein lipase activity, metastatic calcification and hypertension. At this time there is no indication to modify the diet in an attempt to reduce the lipemia, even though cardiovascular disease is by far the most frequent cause of death in patients maintained on long-term hemodialysis.

GROWTH IN CHILDREN WITH CHRONIC RENAL FAILURE

Growth in children with chronic renal failure is retarded owing to chronic acidosis, hypernatremic dehydration, hypertension, undernutrition and osteodystrophy. However, growth can be renewed or maintained if the child consumes enough calories (100 kcal. per kg. per day) and enough protein. (See Fig. 30–6.) The recommendation for dietary protein is at least 1 to 2 gm. per kg. per day, although this may not

C. W. (^{51}Cr EDTA GFR = 10ml/min/1.73m^2)

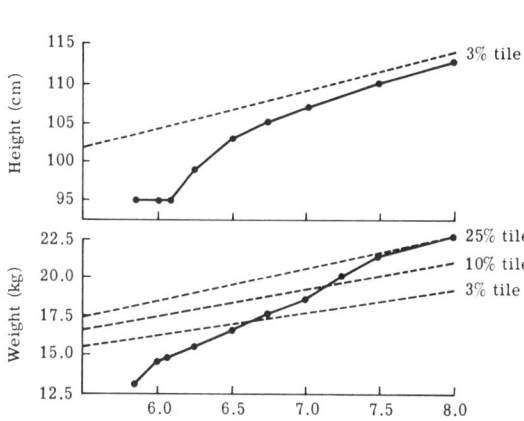

Age (years)

Figure 30–6 Height and weight of a 6-year-old girl with renal failure due to obstructive uropathy. After a one-month period on peritoneal dialysis, she was given a diet containing 2.5 gm./kg. body weight protein (74% of which was first class) and consumed at least 100 kcal./kg. body weight. She began to grow one month after starting this diet; during the period shown, the blood urea remained above 100 mg./100 ml. (From Chantler, C., and Holliday, M. A.: Growth in children with renal disease with particular reference to the effects of calorie malnutrition: a review. Clin. Nephrol., 1:230, 1973.)

be possible in cases of severe uremia. It has been suggested that children's diets be routinely supplemented with the essential amino acids because their needs for them for growth are greater on a per kilogram basis than are those of adults.[3, 10] Special encouragement, creativity and attention are required to help the child with chronic renal failure to consume the necessary calories. The atmosphere in the home must be as free from anxiety and tension as possible to avoid causing a poor food intake.

PSYCHOLOGICAL SUPPORT

Patients with renal failure must deal not only with conflicting feelings about prolonging their lives with a machine but also with the fact that their lives are no longer the same. They become "marginal" people who are partially ill and partially well. They must take certain medications, can no longer eat what they please and must devote several hours per week to being dialyzed. Even then, they do not feel "perfect" or completely well and have to live with progressive bone disease, clots or infection at the shunt site and anorexia or nausea. By being especially sympathetic to their feelings of thirst, their anorexia when faced with eating, the taste changes due to uremia, and the tedium

of the diet, the nurse, dietitian-nutritionist, physician and social worker can help dialysis patients cope with their new way of life.

Those who work with renal dialysis patients must be aware of both the often-present depression and the frequent denial of illness and overindependence of these patients, who are trying to live with chronic illness and the threat of death.

TRANSPLANTATION

A successful kidney transplant can result in normal health if no permanent damage has been done to other organs due to the previous kidney failure. Nutritional care consists of controlling carbohydrate intake to counteract the effect of taking corticosteroids and controlling sodium intake to counteract the fluid retention tendencies of steroid therapy.

During periods of rejection and compromised function, uremia may develop, requiring dietary management. In transplant patients hyperparathyroidism may continue to be a problem, and severe bone disease may develop.

NEPHROLITHIASIS OR RENAL CALCULI

Nephrolithiasis is a condition characterized by the presence of renal calculi. Renal calculi, or kidney stones, may form in either the kidney or the bladder. They look like pebbles, although their appearance varies depending upon the constituents. Some have a smooth surface and others are jagged. They vary in size from fine gravel to those that fill the renal pelvis. (See Fig. 30–7.)

Etiology

How renal calculi materialize continues to be a mystery, although many theories have been suggested. Certain diseases seem to favor the precipitation of gravel. These include disorders that bring about increased parathyroid secretion, with a loss of calcium phosphate in the urine. If this loss is excessive the particles of the substance may gather in amounts sufficient to produce a calculus. Vitamin A, systemic infections, metabolic disturbances, hormone imbalances, inadequate fluid intake and lesions that obstruct the flow and produce stasis of urine are considered causative factors. Immobilization favors the formation of calcium

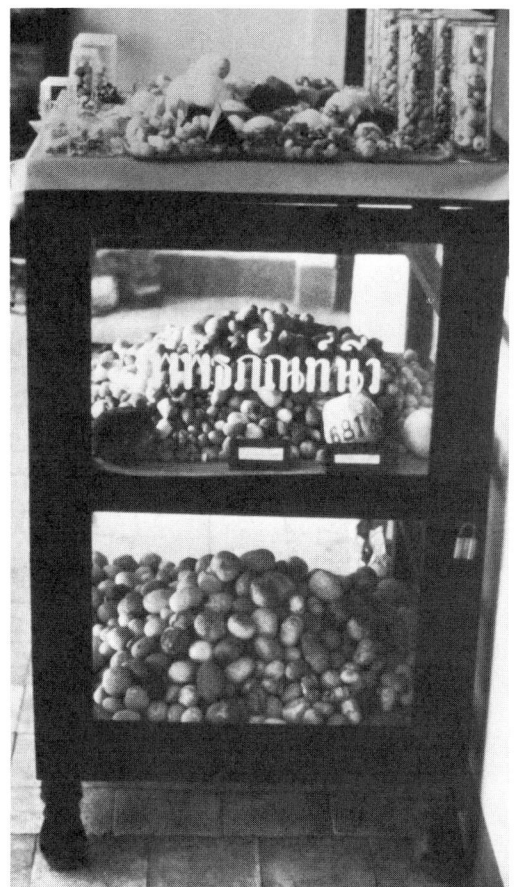

stones, because of large increases in the excretion of calcium.

Types of Stones

Vermooten[17] divides renal calculi into three basic types: (1) *organic calculi*, such as uric acid, cystine and xanthine stones, which result from some metabolic disturbance, (2) *alkaline earth stones*, such as calcium or magnesium ammonium phosphates or carbonates, which are generally secondary to urinary tract infection and (3) *calcium oxalate stones*, which usually are not associated with infection.

The types of stone that may develop depend largely upon the concentration of the constituent in the urine and the acidity or alkalinity of the urine. Normally, urine is slightly acid. The pH of urine depends upon the character of the diet. If the diet consists largely of acid-

forming foods, a very acid urine is produced. Diets consisting mainly of base-forming foods yield an alkaline urine. Stones composed chiefly of uric acid and cystine appear most frequently in an abnormally acid urine. Stones appearing in an alkaline urine are composed of phosphates, carbonates and oxalates.

Nutritional Care

Although medicine has largely replaced the use of therapeutic diets for the treatment of renal calculi, specific diets are still recognized and advocated by a number of authorities as a preventive measure against the recurrence of stones, especially following surgical removal. Urinary calculi recur in a significant number of patients; therefore, prophylactic programs are desirable.

The type of diet prescribed is determined by the acidity or alkalinity of the urine and by the variety of stone. Fluids are encouraged (3000 to 4000 ml. or more daily) to prevent concentration of the urine, which is believed to favor precipitation of the stone-forming minerals.

Regardless of the diet prescribed, it must be an adequate one. Renal calculi are a chronic condition, and the diet treatment must be carried on indefinitely.

Calcium-containing Calculi. Of all renal calculi, 90 to 95 per cent contain calcium salts as the predominant crystalline component. A urine that is high in calcium (*hypercalciuria*, or a urine calcium level greater than 4 mg. per kg. body weight in 24 hours) predisposes to the formation of calcium oxalate, calcium phosphate and calcium carbonate stones. Conditions that favor calcium stone formation are (1) overindulgence in foods high in calcium, such as large quantities of milk (for example, milk or milk and cream therapy for patients with peptic ulcer), (2) excessive intake of proprietary antacids that contain calcium salts, (3) excessive vitamin D intake, which will mobilize calcium and so increase urinary excretion, (4) general body immobilization following fractures or extended bed rest, (5) hyperparathyroidism and (6) osteoporosis.

Idiopathic hypercalciuria is found in approximately 40 per cent of patients with calcium stones, possibly due to faulty renal tubular reabsorption or conservation of calcium. Thiazide diuretics have been used to treat idiopathic hypercalciuria. They reduce the renal excretion of calcium and thus the possibility of a calcium renal stone.[12] Cellulose phos-

phate or aluminum hydroxide gel can be used to reduce gastrointestinal absorption of calcium.[14] Milk, cheese and other milk products are limited (1 to 2 cups of milk daily), and the diet usually contains 400 mg. or less of calcium. There is some danger of calcium deficiency if this diet regimen is continued indefinitely. Fortified vitamin D milk is excluded, as well as other D-fortified dairy products.

The protein content of the diet should be high normal in an attempt to promote deposition of calcium in the bones. Acid ash foods favoring production of an acid urine might help to keep the calcium salts in solution.

Calcium Oxalate Stones. When oxalates predominate, the condition is known as hyperoxaluria. Hyperoxaluria commonly results from ilial disease or intestinal resection due to increased absorption of oxalates.[8, 16] There is no generally accepted dietary regimen for patients with recurrent calcium oxalate stones. The diet therapy is to avoid large quantities of foods high in calcium (Appendix Table 7) and high in oxalates. Oxalate stones are extremely resistant to treatment, and clinical experience has demonstrated that oxalate calculi may recur even after strict elimination of dietary oxalate intake. This may be due to endogenous production, independent of an exogenous food supply. Fluids are forced in order to reduce the concentration of calcium and oxalate ions in the urine. Foods high in oxalate include:

FOODS OMITTED
(High Oxalic Acid Content—0.002 to 0.9%)

Asparagus	Rhubarb
Beet greens	Raspberries
Spinach	Black tea
Sorrel	Chocolate
Dandelion greens	Cocoa
Cranberries	Coffee
Figs	Gelatin
Gooseberries	Pepper
Plums	

FOODS RESTRICTED
(Moderate Oxalic Acid Content)

Milk: 1 pint daily.
Not more than one serving daily of the following foods:

Oranges	Brussels sprouts
Pineapple	Potatoes
Strawberries	Tomatoes
Beans	Beets

According to studies by Gershoff,[11] vitamin B_6 (pyridoxine) deficiency causes increased production of oxalates. The administration of this vitamin to individuals on diets that presumably were adequate in vitamin B_6 sharply decreased oxalate production. Experimentally, calcium oxalate stones have been produced in animals fed a low pyridoxine and magnesium diet and prevented by increasing the dietary levels of these two nutrients. Magnesium, it is believed, aids in keeping the oxalate in solution and prevents precipitation of oxalates and stone formation. Vitamin B_6 increases citric acid secretion, and this may keep oxalates in solution.

Calcium Phosphate Stones. The principles of dietary treatment for calcium oxalate stones are virtually the same ones used for stones consisting largely of calcium combined with phosphate. The diet is the normal adequate diet with moderately low calcium and low phosphorus contents. Foods generally considered high in phosphate that should be limited are: milk and milk products, eggs, organ meats (brain, heart, liver, sweetbreads, kidney), sardines, fish roe, whole-grain bread and cereal, bran, oatmeal, brown and wild rice, wheat germ, nuts, soybeans and meat in general. (See Table 7–2 for the phosphorus content of foods.)

Zinsser,[18] however, warns that in using low-phosphorus diets there is a possibility that citrate stones can be formed as a result of a rise in citrate excretion in the presence of inadequate phosphorus intake. Thus, the reduction in phosphorus intake as a treatment for the condition is fraught with hazard.

Uric Acid Stones. When kidney stones containing uric acid—an end product of purine metabolism—have been found to occur in an acid medium, the *high alkaline ash diet* is sometimes prescribed. While acidifying or alkalinizing agents are more effective and have largely replaced the high-alkaline and high-acid diets, the diet should support the medication used.

An attempt is made to keep the pH of the urine above 7, or alkaline. If urinary alkalinization alone does not prove adequate, the purine intake restriction may be tried, along with anabolic drugs. (See the low-purine diet in Chapter 26.) Proteins may be restricted to 0.8 gm. per kg. ideal body weight. *Allopurinol,* a drug that prevents the synthesis of uric acid, has been used with success.

Cystine Stones. If the sulfur-containing amino acid cystine is not broken down in the body and appears in the urine (cystinuria), it

may form stones. Cystine stones, formed because of an inborn error of metabolism, are very rare.

A low-protein diet is sometimes used but has not been shown to be very effective. All protein contains cystine (and methionine, from which cystine may be formed) in varying amounts, and it is especially high in milk and milk products. Alkalinizing agents or the high alkaline ash diet, or both, are recommended to keep the urine at pH of 7.2 or above.

Acid and Alkaline Ash Diets

Acid-Base Balance in Foods. The potential acidity or alkalinity of foods means the reaction the food will yield ultimately after being burned in the body. The acids of most fruits and vegetables are utilized in the body and yield an alkaline or basic ash, owing to their high potassium, calcium and magnesium contents. Thus, a diet rich in vegetables and fruits will form bicarbonate and hence decrease urine acidity. Hence, fruits and vegetables, except prunes, plums, cranberries and corn, are restricted in an acid ash diet. On the other hand, a diet containing large amounts of proteins, which in their course of metabolism yield acids such as sulfuric and phosphoric, will increase the urine acidity. Foods that are not acid in taste, such as cereals, meat, fish, egg and bread, become strongly acid when their end products reach the blood and urine owing to their high phosphorus, iron and sulfur contents. However, the normal, healthy individual always maintains a slightly alkaline reaction in the blood and other tissues regardless of the diet. (See Appendix Table 11 for a listing of alkali-producing, acid-producing and neutral foods.)

Salt (sodium) is sometimes restricted in the acid ash diet because sodium is alkaline, and some authorities believe it has a buffering action. Baking powder and soda products may also be prohibited. Salt substitutes contain an alkaline radical and cannot be used. Foods high in acid ash include eggs, meat, fish, poultry, bread, cereal and cereal products. There is a moderate restriction on milk (1 pint daily) and milk products. Cranberry juice is an excellent urine acidifying agent.

An alkaline ash diet is sometimes used to treat uric acid and cystine stones. The principle of the diet is to restrict enlargement of already present calculi that form in an acid medium or to prevent other stones from forming. Foods high in alkaline ash include fruits and vegetables, which should predominate—except prunes, plums, cranberries and corn. Milk, while usually considered alkaline, is limited to 1 pint daily because a considerable amount of the calcium in milk is excreted in the feces with the remainder excreted in the urine, and its effect on the acidity or alkalinity of urine is controversial. Meat, fish, poultry, eggs, bread, cereal and cereal products are somewhat restricted.

The patient may find it difficult to change his dietary pattern. A person who has been in the habit of eating large portions of meat and the acid ash–forming foods must learn to like and ingest more vegetables and fruits and much less meat.

PROBLEMS AND SUGGESTED TOPICS FOR DISCUSSION

1. What is the function of the kidneys? Describe the "functioning units." What does the urine from a normal, healthy individual contain?
2. What are the objectives and principles of dietary treatment in acute glomerulonephritis? What is the purpose of the low-protein diet?
3. When is fluid restriction indicated? When is salt (sodium) restriction indicated? When is potassium restriction indicated?
4. Which salt substitutes are not allowed in renal diseases? Why? Using Appendix Table 9, list foods high in potassium and foods high in sodium.
5. What foods are allowed patients with uremia? What are some of their nutritional problems?
6. Obtain a diet history from a patient with chronic glomerulonephritis and outline a meal plan. Assist him in making the necessary adjustments in his dietary pattern.
7. Outline a diet for the following amounts of protein, in each case keeping the calories to at least 2500 daily: (a) 20 gm., (b) 40 gm., (c) 60 gm., (d) 100 gm. and (e) 150 gm.
8. Obtain a diet history from a patient with nephrotic syndrome. Analyze the food history, noting the amount of fat, protein and calories. What are the objectives and principles of diet therapy?
9. Plan a menu pattern with a patient who has kidney stones. A high acid ash diet is prescribed. Observe the daily urine analysis made by the laboratory and note the pH of the urine. Compare with the average normal pH of urine. What are the principles of the dietary treatment?
10. Outline a typical diet for a man with calcium oxalate kidney stones. What is the purpose of the diet?
11. Plan a diet with a person who is receiving hemodialysis. The diet ordered is 60 gm. protein, 800 mg. sodium and 1800 mg. potassium. Fluids are restricted to 1000 ml. What would you do about the patient's calcium and phosphorus intakes?
12. Plan a diet for a patient who has recurrent calcium stones. The diet is low in calcium (600 mg.) and not excessive in vitamin D (no vitamin D–fortified foods).
13. List foods restricted and foods allowed in a high acid ash diet; do the same for a high alkaline ash diet. When might each diet be used?

COOKBOOKS AND MANUALS FOR PATIENTS WITH RENAL FAILURE

de St. Jeor, S. T., et al.: Low Protein Diets for the Treatment of Chronic Renal Failure. Salt Lake City, University of Utah Press, 1970.

Cost, J. S.: Dietary Management of Renal Disease. Thorofare, N. J., Charles B. Slack, Inc., 1975.

Jones, O.: Diet Guide for Patients on Chronic Dialysis. DHEW Pub. No. (NIH) 76–685. Bethesda, Md., Artificial Kidney-Chronic Uremia Program, National Institute of Arthritis, Metabolism and Digestive Diseases, National Institutes of Health, 1976.

Margie, J. D., et al.: The Mayo Clinic Renal Diet Cookbook. New York, Golden Press/Western Publishing Co., Inc., 1974.

Spitzer, M. E., et al.: A Renal Failure Diet Manual Utilizing the Food Exchange System. Springfield, Ill., Charles C Thomas, 1976.

U.S. Public Health Service: Living with End-Stage Renal Failure. A Book for Patients. Washington, D.C., U.S. Government Printing Office, 1976.

Kidney Foundation of Illinois: Fun with Food for Dialysis Patients. Illinois Council on Renal Nutrition, 127 N. Dearborn, Chicago, Ill., 60602, 1977.

CITED REFERENCES

1. Alfrey, A. C., LeGendre, G. R., and Kaehny, W. D.: The dialysis encephalopathy syndrome: Possible aluminum intoxication. N. Engl. J. Med., 294:184, 1976.

2. Anderson, C. F., et al.: Nutritional therapy for adults with renal disease. JAMA, 223:68, 1973.

3. Aronson, S. A., et al.: Essential amino acids in the treatment of advanced uremia: 22 months experience in a 5 year old girl. Pediatrics, 56:538, 1976.

4. Berlyne, G. M., et al.: Hyperaluminaemia from aluminum resins in renal failure. Lancet, 2:494, 1970.

5. Bricker, N. S.: The pathogenesis of the uremic state. An exposition of the "trade off" hypothesis. N. Engl. J. Med., 286:1093, 1972.

6. Brickman, A. S., et al.: Impaired calcium absorption in uremic man: Evidence for defective absorption in the proximal small intestine. J. Lab. Clin. Med., 84:791, 1974.

7. Borst, J. G. G.: Protein katabolism in uraemia: effects of protein-free diets, infections, and blood transfusions. Lancet, 1:824, 1948.

8. Chadwick, V. S., Modha, K., and Dowling, R. H.: Mechanism for hyperoxaluria in patients with ileal dysfunction. N. Engl. J. Med., 289:172, 1973.

9. Clarkson, E. M., et al.: The effect of aluminum hydroxide on calcium, phosphorus and aluminum balances, the serum parathyroid hormone concentration and the aluminum content of bone in patients with chronic renal failure. Clin. Sci., 43:519, 1972.

10. Diaz, M., Kleinknecht, C., and Broyer, M.: Growth in experimental renal failure. Kidney Int., 8:349, 1975.

11. Gershoff, S. N., and Prien, E. L.: The effect of daily MgO and vitamin B_6 administration to patients with recurring calcium oxalate kidney stones. Am. J. Clin. Nutr., 20:393, 1967.

12. Kaplan, R. A., and Pak, C. Y. C.: Diagnosis and management of renal calculi. Tex. Med., 70:88, 1974.

13. Lee, H. A., et al.: Amino acid tablet substituted diets in the management of chronic renal failure. Nutr. Metab., 17:154, 1974.

14. Pak, C. Y. C., Delea, C. S., and Bartter, F. C.: Successful treatment of recurrent nephrolithiasis (calcium stones) with cellulose phosphate. N. Engl. J. Med., 290:175, 1974.

15. Rao, T. K. S., and Friedman, E. A.: Fluoride and bone disease in uremia. Kidney Int., 7:125, 1975.

16. Stauffer, J. Q., Humphreys, M. H., and Weir, G. J.: Acquired hyperoxaluria with regional enteritis after ileal resection. Ann. Intern. Med., 79:383, 1973.

17. Vermooten, V.: Some aspects of the medical management of renal calculi. JAMA, 157:783, 1955.

18. Zinsser, H. H.: Urinary calculi. JAMA, 174:2062, 1960.

ADDITIONAL REFERENCES

Abram, H. S.: Psychiatric reflections on adaptation to repetitive dialysis. Kidney Int., 6:67, 1974.

Aluminum intoxication (letters to the editor). N. Engl. J. Med., 294:1129, 1976.

Bailey, G. L., and Sullivan, N.: Selected-protein diet in terminal uremia. J. Am. Diet. Assoc., 52:125, 1968.

Bergstrom, J., et al.: Improvement of nitrogen balance in uremic patient by addition of histidine to essential amino acid solutions given intravenously. Life. Sci., 9:787, 1970.

Berlyne, G. M. (ed.): Nutrition in Renal Disease. Baltimore, Williams & Wilkins Co., 1968.

Berlyne, G. M., et al.: The dietary management of acute renal failure. Q. J. Med., 36:59, 1967.

Berlyne, G. M., Shaw, A. B., and Nilwarangkur, S.: Dietary treatment of chronic renal failure. Experiences with modified Giovanetti diet. Nephron, 2:129, 1965.

Burton, B. T.: Current concepts of nutrition and diet in diseases of the kidney. J. Am. Diet. Assoc., 65:623, 1974.

Close, J. H.: The use of amino acid precursors in nitrogen accumulation diseases. N. Engl. J. Med., 290:663, 1974.

Coe, F. L., and Kavalach, A. G.: Hypercalciuria and hyperuricosuria in patients with calcium nephrolithiasis. N. Engl. J. Med., 291:1344, 1974.

Curtis, J. R., and Williams, G. B.: Clinical Management of Chronic Renal Failure. Oxford, England, Blackwell Scientific Publications, 1975.

Dudrick, S. J., Steiger, E., and Long, J. M.: Renal failure in surgical patients. Treatment with intravenous essential amino acids and hypertonic glucose. Surgery, 68:180, 1970.

Giovannetti, S., and Maggiore, Q.: A low-nitrogen diet with proteins of high biological value for severe uraemia. Lancet, 1:1000, 1964.

Hansen, G. L. (ed.): Caring for Patients with Chronic Renal Disease. Philadelphia, J. B. Lippincott Co., 1972.

Harlan, W. R., Jr., et al.: Proteinuria and nephrotic syndrome associated with chronic rejection of kidney transplants. N. Engl. J. Med., 277:769, 1967.

Hughes, J., et al.: Oxalate urinary tract stones. JAMA, 172:774, 1960.

Kark, R. M., and Oyama, J. H.: Nutrition and cardiovascular-renal diseases. In: Goodhart, R. S., and Shils, M. E. (eds.): Modern Nutrition in Health and Disease, 5th ed. Philadelphia, Lea & Febiger, 1973.

Keto analogs of essential amino acids in treatment of human diseases. Nutr. Rev., 34:41, 1973.

Kopple, J. D., and Swendseid, M. E.: Nitrogen balance

and plasma amino acid levels in uremic patients fed an essential amino acid diet. Am. J. Clin. Nutr., *27*:806, 1974.

Kopple, J. D., and Swendseid, M. E.: Histidine deficiency anemia in renal failure. Clinical Research, *21*:266, 1973.

Lindner, A., et al.: Accelerated atherosclerosis in prolonged maintenance hemodialysis and renal transplant patients. Am. J. Dis. Child., *130*:957, 1976.

Merrill, A. J.: Nutrition in chronic renal failure. Am. J. Clin. Nutr., *4*:497, 1956.

Niwa, T., et al.: Plasma level and transfer capacity of thiamin in patients undergoing long-term hemodialysis. Am. J. Clin. Nutr., *28*:1105, 1975.

Overly, V. A., and Greenwood, M. L.: Developing wafers and biscuits of varying protein content. J. Am. Diet. Assoc., *45*:342, 1964.

Pennisi, A. J., et al.: Hyperlipidemia in pediatric hemodialysis and renal transplant patients. Am. J. Dis. Child., *130*:957, 1976.

Possible aluminum intoxication. Nutr. Rev., *34*:166, 1976.

Prien, E. L.: Studies in urolithiasis. III. Physiochemical principles in stone formation and prevention. J. Urol., *73*:627, 1955.

Richards, P., et al.: Utilisation of ammonia nitrogen for protein synthesis in man, and the effect of protein restriction and uraemia. Lancet, *2*:845, 1967.

Schoolwerth, A. C., and Engle, J. E.: Calcium and phosphorus in diet therapy of uremia. J. Am. Diet. Assoc., *66*:460, 1975.

Silverberg, D. S., et al.: Effects of 1,25-dihydroxycholecalciferol in renal osteodystrophy. Can. Med. Assoc. J., *112*:190, 1975.

Tsaltas, T. T.: Dietetic management of uremic patients. Extraction of potassium from foods for uremic patients. Am. J. Clin. Nutr., *22*:490, 1969.

Chapter 31

NUTRITIONAL CARE FOR PATIENTS WITH FOOD ALLERGY

ALLERGY

Definition

Allergy may be defined as an adverse immunological reaction to a substance that is harmless in similar amounts to the majority of people. Allergies are many and varied. In this text the discussion will be limited to food allergy. *Food allergy,* or a reaction to food, can affect the gastrointestinal tract, in which case it is called a *gastrointestinal allergy,* or it can affect any other body system. Food allergy is an immune reaction and must be differentiated from *food intolerance,* which may be due to an enzyme deficiency, digestive problem or psychological reaction. It is estimated that allergies affect about 5 per cent of the population.

MECHANISMS OF ALLERGY AND FOOD INTOLERANCE

The immunological principles of an allergic response will be reviewed briefly.

The offending substance, called the *allergen* or *antigen,* may gain access to the body by *ingestion, inhalation, direct contact* or *injection* (drugs, serum). The allergen, usually a protein, passes through the gastrointestinal mucosa (in the case of a food allergy) and is perceived by the host's immune system in the body's circulation. The first time the antigen appears in the circulation there is no clinical allergic response to it, but it stimulates the production of *antibodies* (Ab) of one or more classes of *immunoglobulins* (Ig): IgA, IgE, IgG or IgM. The antibodies remain attached to cells or circulate in the body. The next time the antigen (Ag) appears in the circulation, it will form a complex with its specific antibody, and these complexes may then act on serum and cells to give the biological effects of an allergic reaction. Allergic responses include the production of anaphylatoxins, kinins or histamine, which can cause inflammatory reactions and shock. Individual organs respond in different ways to the antigen-antibody complexes. The various types of antibodies, when combined with their specific antigens, usually cause certain types of reactions. (See Table 31–1.) However, *even though antibodies can cause an allergic reaction, their presence does not necessarily mean that clinical symptoms of an allergic response will follow.* It is for this reason that measuring a person's serum immunoglobulin levels is unlikely to help to diagnose a food allergy or predict the occurrence of one later in life.

IgA, which coats the intestinal tract, seems to be somewhat protective against the development of food allergy. Practically speaking, if highly allergenic foods are not introduced until after an infant has developed intestinal IgA (age 7 months), food allergies are less likely to develop. Before this age the infant's gastrointestinal tract is more permeable to dietary proteins, which may enter circulation and stimulate the production of antibodies.

In addition to this antibody component of the

Table 31–1 RELATION OF IMMUNOLOGICAL FACTORS TO SYMPTOMS OR SIGNS*

ANTIBODIES	SYMPTOMS OR SIGNS	TIMING
IgE	Rhinitis, asthma, urticaria, abdominal pain, "rash"	Immediate (minutes)
IgG, IgM	Urticaria, inflammation, edema, eczema, asthma	Early (hours)
IgA	Malabsorption, enteropathy	Intermediate (days)
IgG, IgM	Nephritis, arthritis, fever, "rash"	Late (weeks)
Cellular	Unknown effects	

*From: May, C. D.: Food allergy. In: Fomon, S. J.: Infant Nutrition, 2nd ed. Philadelphia, W. B. Saunders Co., 1974, p. 440.

immune reaction, the body also contains a *cellular* component that does not depend on antibodies. This type of reaction is sometimes referred to as *delayed hypersensitivity*.

The role of cellular immunity in food allergy reactions is still unclear, but it may account for a chronic allergic response and stress state—the allergic tension-fatigue syndrome.[1] The person, usually a child, has the typical allergic look: dull facies, infraorbital circles and an allergic gape.

Symptoms that occur immediately after ingestion of a certain food obviously are easier to diagnose as being due to a food allergy than are delayed symptoms such as diarrhea. Uncooked foods are more likely to induce immediate allergic reactions. A delayed reaction may be caused by one of the digestive products of the food, which would explain why the patient may not have a positive response to a skin test using the whole food.

Etiology

Various factors are involved in the development of allergy, including age, type of allergen, nature of ingested protein, intestinal permeability and other individual characteristics. It is possible that the tendency to allergy is inherited, although the inheritance is seldom specific.

Manifestations

Several manifestations of allergy may appear in the same individual, varying from a minor reaction such as slight eye or nose itching or rash to severe gastrointestinal symptoms such as diarrhea, vomiting and cramping. Stunted growth and malnutrition are sometimes traced to an allergy. Bronchial asthma, hay fever, dermatitis, urticaria, eczema, acne, migraine headaches, canker sores and cardiovascular disorders are some of the observed manifes-

tations of an allergy that may be caused by foods. Anorexia and food aversion may be due to an allergy to one or more common foods. Clinical symptoms of food allergy are listed in Table 31–2.

ALLERGENS OTHER THAN FOOD

Most people who are allergic to one or more foods are usually sensitive to one or more of the common inhalants as well. House dust, feath-

Table 31–2 CLINICAL MANIFESTATIONS OF FOOD ALLERGY*

RESPIRATORY

Allergic rhinitis	Bronchitis
Allergic cough	Serous otitis media
Asthma	

GASTROINTESTINAL

Canker sores	Diarrhea
Cheilitis	Dyspepsia (belching,
Colic	flatulence, etc.)
Colitis (ulcerative	Stomatitis
and functional)	Vomiting

CUTANEOUS

Angioedema	Pruritus
Atopic dermatitis	Purpura
Contact dermatitis	Urticaria

NEUROLOGICAL OR PSYCHOSOMATIC

Deafness	Personality changes
Epilepsy	Vertigo (Meniere's
Migraine	syndrome)
Neuralgias	Visual (amblyopia)

MISCELLANEOUS

Arthralgia	Idiopathic fever
Arthritis	Intermittent hydroarthrosis
Enuresis	Menstrual irregularity

*From: Tuft, L.: Allergy Management in Clinical Practice. St. Louis, C. V. Mosby Co., 1973, p. 143.

ers, animal hair, horse dander, pollens, molds, grain dust, silk, wool, bacteria, plant oils or resins, drugs, cosmetics and tobacco smoke are potent allergens. Many of them are met in everyday living and are difficult to avoid.

COMMON FOOD ALLERGIES

A person may become allergic to a food or other allergen at any age, but usually begins to have symptoms in childhood. A very early allergic reaction (in the first five days of life) means that the neonate was probably sensitized *in utero* because of the mother's overindulgence in allergenic foods such as eggs or milk. The sensitivity may wear off, or the person may become desensitized and entirely free from the disturbance that affected him in childhood. Foods that belong to the same botanical group may produce a similar allergic reaction, for example, cabbage and cauliflower or orange and grapefruit. Furthermore, an allergic individual who experiences a reaction to a given food may on another day eat the same food without reaction. This may be due to his general physical condition and the complexity of immune reactions. An allergic response may occur only when the individual is fatigued or emotionally upset. These are some of the numerous observations that baffle allergists.

Protein

Any food can produce allergic manifestations. However, it is believed that protein is the important factor in food allergy, although the offending food may contain only a minute amount of it. Among the *most common offenders are wheat, milk, eggs, fish, shellfish, strawberries, tomatoes* and *chocolate.* Others to be considered are pork, oranges, spices, condiments, nuts, corn, asparagus, spinach, cabbage, celery, onion, garlic and rhubarb. The ingestion of the smallest quantity of an offending food may produce symptoms or reaction; therefore, it is necessary for the allergic individual to analyze prepared foods and food combinations before eating them. For example, sausage may contain wheat, and the small amount of wheat could cause an allergic disturbance.

Milk Intolerance. It has been found that 30 per cent of the people who suffered from an idiosyncrasy to some foods were uncomfortable after taking milk and cream. This is important for the nurse to know since she helps to feed and care for the sick. When a patient says

he cannot drink milk, he should not be told he is "imagining things" or that "milk is a health food" or that he "must drink at least a pint a day." Although milk is an excellent, nutritious food, a patient may be allergic to it. If milk is the offender, then cheese, ice cream and any product made with milk must also be omitted. However, thoroughly boiled milk or evaporated milk, having had the offending proteins denatured, may sometimes be consumed without evoking symptoms.

Although there are five proteins in milk, the one that most frequently causes allergic reactions is beta-lactoglobulin. This protein is not present in breast milk, which makes breast feeding particularly suitable for infants with a family tendency to allergy.

Breast milk may induce an allergic response in an infant if the mother eats strawberries, oranges, crab, eggs or milk. The antigens formed in response to these foods may pass into the breast milk, and the second time the infant feeds he will have an allergic response.

An infant allergic to cow's milk should be given soya formula. If this is not tolerated either, Nutramigen or Pregestimil should be tried. See Chapter 23 for discussion of lactose or milk sugar intolerance.

In other instances, intolerance to milk may be due to the action of the milk protein of fresh cow's milk on the gastrointestinal mucosa. The protein damages the mucosa and results in a breakdown of mucosal cells, a loss of blood and iron deficiency anemia. This occurs fairly frequently in children under 18 months of age who are drinking fresh cow's milk rather than heat-treated evaporated milk. It is still not known whether this intolerance is caused by an antigen-antibody reaction.

Other Allergens in Food

A food contaminant such as trace amounts of penicillin in cow's milk may also be an allergen. An allergen may be one of the many substances added to processed foods. These substances, such as artificial colors, artificial flavors, spices and other food additives, should always be tested for in cases of unexplained allergy.

Food History

A carefully detailed food history (see Chapter 11) should be taken for every individual suspected of having an allergy. The food history often discloses specific food allergies through the listing of disliked foods or foods

that disagree with the patient. In addition, patients should be asked about their cigarette smoking and use of aspirin, antacids, chewing gum, lozenges and laxatives, which may contain substances that cause an allergic reaction.

Food Diary

If a patient keeps a food diary and records the foods eaten preceding the appearance of allergic symptoms, the data will be useful for diagnosis.

TESTS FOR ALLERGY

In addition to the food history and food diary, other aids employed to establish a diagnosis of food allergy are (1) skin tests and (2) elimination diets.

Skin Tests

The most popular and best known of the skin tests is the *scratch test*. A series of scratches are made on the patient's arm or back, and a solution containing the suspected offending allergen is dropped into each scratch. If the person is allergic to any of the solutions used, welts or wheals surrounded by a red inflamed area may develop within a few minutes, or there may be a delayed reaction that will not manifest itself for a day or so. The greater the area of the reaction, the more potent the allergen is to the patient. Some foods do not react well in the skin tests and may produce negative results in some allergic individuals, or a food may exhibit a positive result without causing allergic symptoms, so the scratch test cannot be relied upon for complete accuracy. However, when properly interpreted it may throw some light on the diagnostic problem.

Another skin test, the *patch test,* is administered by applying the suspected antigen on a filter paper and placing the paper on a certain patch of skin and then covering with cellophane. Readings are made in two to four days.

In the *intradermal test* a solution of food extracts is injected into the superficial layers of the skin. The interpretation and the accuracy of the reactions are similar to those described for the scratch and patch tests.

The *Rinkle provocative food test* requires that the patient avoid all suspected allergenic foods for four days. On the fifth day one of the foods is eaten in moderate amounts, or an intracutaneous injection of the food extract is given. A positive result is the induction of symptoms within 10 to 20 minutes using the extract or within 24 hours using the food itself.

Elimination Test Diets

An elimination diet may be defined as an allowance of foods that have rarely produced sensitivity in human patients. Because of the fallibility of skin tests, the use of trial diets for suspected food allergy is considered the most reliable test. The objective of using an elimina-

Table 31–3 FOODS ALLOWED IN CEREAL-FREE ELIMINATION DIET (ROWE)*[a]

Tapioca	Apricots
White potatoes	Grapefruit[d]
Sweet potatoes or yams	Lemon
Soybean potato bread[b]	Peaches
Lima bean potato bread[b]	Pineapples
	Prunes
Soy milk (Mull-Soy)[c]	Pears
	Cane or beet sugar
Lamb	Salt
Chicken, fryers,	Sesame oil (not Chinese)
roosters and capon	Soybean oil
(no hens)	Willow Run oleo-
Bacon	margarine[e]
Liver (lamb)	Gelatin (Knox's) with
	flavoring of allowed
	fruits and juices
Peas	White vinegar
Spinach	Vanilla extract
Squash	Lemon extract
String beans	Corn starch-free baking
Tomatoes	powder[e]
	Baking soda
	Cream of tartar
Artichokes	
Asparagus	Maple syrup or syrup
Carrots	made with cane
Lettuce	sugar flavored with
Lima beans	maple

*From: Rowe, A. H., and Rowe, A., Jr.: Food Allergy: Its Manifestations and Control and the Elimination Diets. Springfield, Ill., Charles C Thomas, 1972, p. 46.

[a]This diet was revised in 1970.

[b]If a baker trusted and supervised by the physician is not available, it is best to make these bakery products at home by our recipes. Bray's, 3764 Piedmont Avenue, Oakland, California, has cooperated with us for over 35 years.

[c]Mull-Soy (free of corn glucose) may be used. It may cause indigestion. Other soy milks contain corn sugar. Neo-Mull-Soy (Borden's) contains sucrose and is more palatable than Mull-Soy.

[d]The canned fruits should be preserved with cane sugar and not corn sugar. Water-packed fruits may be used and sweetened with cane sugar syrup.

[e]A baking powder containing tapioca or potato starch instead of corn starch and no tartaric acid and also Willow Run oleomargarine can be obtained from Bray's, 3764 Piedmont Avenue, Oakland, California.

Table 31–4 FOODS ALLOWED IN FRUIT-FREE, CEREAL-FREE ELIMINATION DIET (ROWE)*

Tapioca (pearl)[a]	Lamb
White potatoes	Bacon
Potato starch	Chicken (no hens)
Sweet potatoes or yams	
Soybean-potato bread	Cane or beet sugar
Lima bean-potato bread	Willow Run oleomargarine[b]
Neo-Mull-Soy (Borden's)	Soybean oil
	Gelatin (Knox)
Cooked carrots	Salt
Squash	Syrup made with cane
Artichokes	sugar (no maple syrup)
Peas	Corn-free, tartaric acid[c]-
Lima beans	free baking powder[d]
String beans	

*From: Rowe, A. H., and Rowe, A., Jr.: Food Allergy: Its Manifestations and Control and the Elimination Diets. Springfield, Ill., Charles C Thomas, 1972, p. 49.

[a]Minute tapioca contains citric acid (not allowed in this diet).

[b]Kosher margarine is allowed if it contains no cow's milk or its products or if allergy to its vegetable oil is not present.

[c]Tartaric acid is made from grapes (not in this diet).

[d]For corn-free baking powder, see Table 31–3.

tion diet is to eliminate the symptoms and arrive at a baseline from which to start trying to determine the food causing the reaction.

The elimination test diets most frequently used are those devised by Rowe,[3] outlined in Tables 31–3 to 31–5. He has devised a series of three different test diets that are based on a few carefully selected foods chosen from those that have been found least likely to cause allergic symptoms.

The patient is placed on the diet that, on the basis of the diet history, food diary and skin tests, is least likely to produce allergy symptoms. The diet is followed for at least three weeks, unless severe adverse reactions occur in the meantime. If there is no change in symptoms and no positive reaction, another diet is tried for a similar period until all the diets have been used. (See Fig. 31–1.) If at the end of the trial diets no change in symptoms occurs and no new reaction appears, all foods on the combined diets may be used, and the allergy is probably caused by an allergen other than food. However, should relief of symptoms appear while the patient is on any one of the trial diets, he is kept on the diet for another week or so. Gradually other foods are added to the basic diet, one at a time every 10 days, with close observation of the development of symptoms. Wheat, eggs and milk are the foods added at the conclusion of the test because these three foods have been found to cause allergy symptoms most frequently. If the patient shows allergic

symptoms following the addition of a specific food to the basic diet, that food (or foods) is suspected of causing the allergy.

The elimination diets are useful only if followed faithfully. This means that the patient and his family must have a clear understanding of the diet and be instructed about reading food labels. Thorough, careful discussions with a dietitian-nutritionist are necessary to achieve this. The elimination diet may not be adequate for the patient, but during a short period of testing this can be overlooked. However, if the diet continues for several weeks adequate supplementation with vitamins and minerals may be needed.

Testing for food allergies is not easy, since children and adults allergic to one food are frequently allergic to many foods. In addition, what appears at first to be an allergy to one component of a food, such as the protein in an infant formula, may really be to another component, such as the corn oil used in the formula.

Table 31–5 FOODS ALLOWED IN MINIMAL ELIMINATION DIETS*

I. To eliminate beef, all cereals and fruits, soybeans and lima beans and most of the vegetables in one or both of the diets in Tables 31–3 and 31–4.

Lamb	Salt
White potatoes	Sugar
Pearl tapioca	Water
Carrots	Neo-Mull-Soy[b]
Peas	
Cottonseed or sesame oil[a]	

II. To eliminate all cereals, legumes, meat, vegetables and fruits.

Chicken	Salt
Turkey	Sugar
Rice	Water
Pearl tapioca	Neo-Mull-Soy[b]
Cottonseed or sesame oil[a]	

III. To eliminate all meat and fowl, all cereals, legumes, vegetables and fruits.

Fin fish	Cake and cookies
Crab	Willow Run oleo-
Eggs	margarine
Pearl tapioca	Sugar
	Salt
	Water
	Neo-Mull-Soy[b]

*From: Rowe, A. H., and Rowe, A., Jr.: Food Allergy: Its Manifestations and Control and the Elimination Diets. Springfield, Ill., Charles C Thomas, 1972, p. 53.

[a]Chinese sesame oil is made from roasted sesame seeds and is not acceptable.

[b]Neo-Mull-Soy (Borden's) or other soy products, if tolerated, can be used in any of these minimal diets. Neo-Mull-Soy can be diluted with water and cane sugar and salt can be added to taste and taken three times a day to increase calories if allergy to soy is absent.

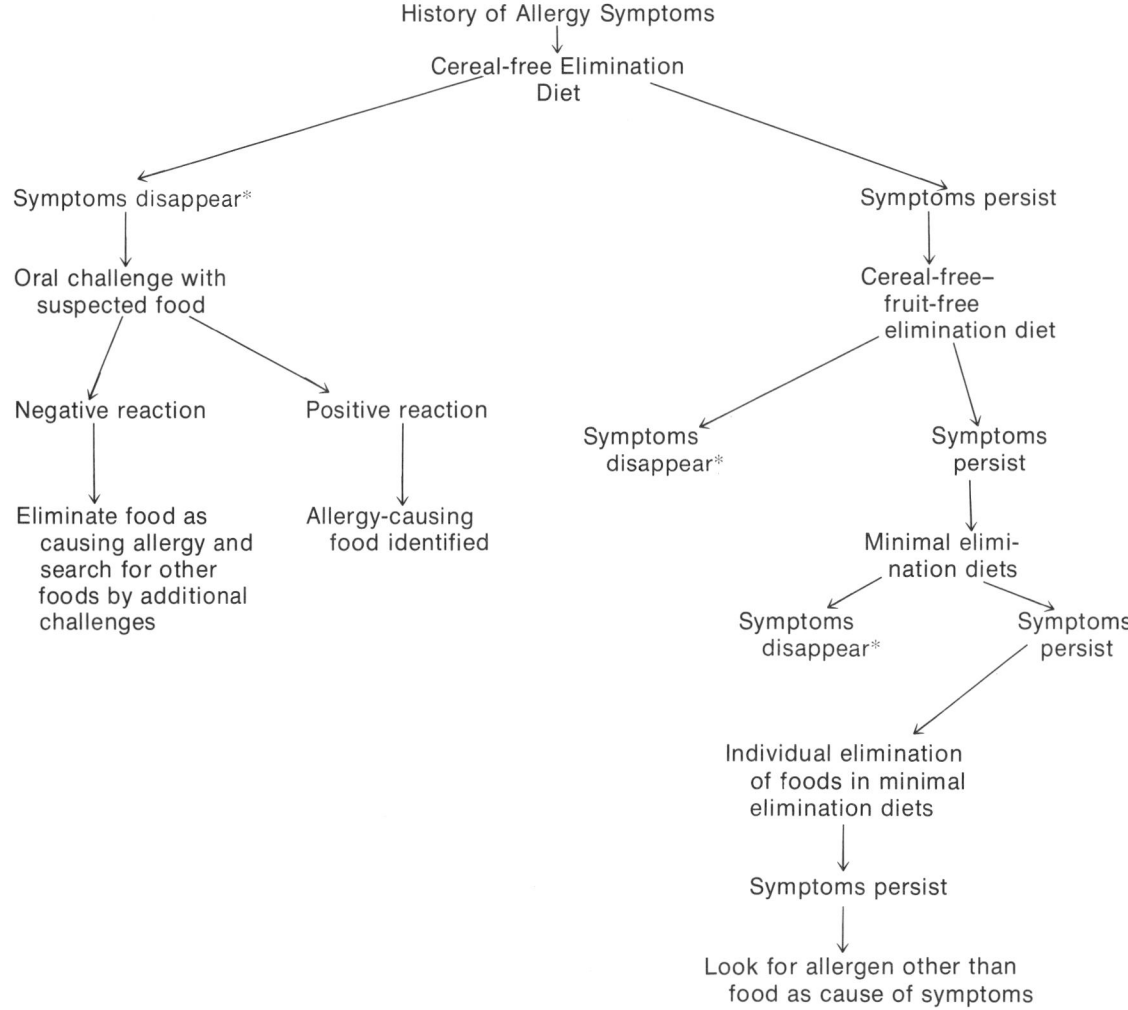

Figure 31–1   Dietary elimination—oral challenge scheme. *Each time symptoms disappear, the sequence illustrated on the far left is followed.

TREATMENT OF ALLERGY

Removal of the offending food or foods from the diet and desensitization are two possible methods of treatment for allergy. In patients with severe allergic manifestations, the hormones corticotropin and cortisone have been found to be highly efficient drugs for the symptomatic *control* of all types of allergies. They are not used to replace treatment directed against the cause of the allergy but to relieve severe acute symptoms. The symptoms return promptly upon cessation of the drug.

Desensitization

To develop tolerance for the offending food, the food allergen is excluded from the diet for an indefinite period. The length of time to build up the tolerance varies with the individual; it may be weeks, months or years, or it may never occur. Following the period of complete abstinence from the offending food, tiny amounts are given by mouth and the size of the servings gradually increased until average food portions are tolerated by the patient.

A patient will more likely develop a tolerance for a mild allergen than for a food that has produced severe symptoms. If the offending allergen is a protective food such as milk, meat or eggs, desensitization is important. Seasonal foods such as strawberries may not be worth the bother of desensitization.

Elimination Diet Treatment

The importance of elimination diets in the diagnosis of an allergy has been discussed. Elimination diets are also prescribed in the treatment of an allergy. Some patients may find

it necessary to avoid continuously certain foods to which they are hypersensitive. Following are outlined the more common food allergy diets,[4] listing the foods to avoid for each.

MILK-FREE DIET

Avoid

Milk, buttermilk and cream, alone and in prepared foods, as ice cream, sodas, milk sherbet, Bavarian cream mousses, custards, gravies, cream sauces, soups, chowders.

Prepared flour mixes for home cooking.

Malted milk, hot chocolate or cocoa prepared with milk.

Cheese.

Evaporated, powdered and condensed milks (bakery products such as pies, breads and cakes containing small amounts of cooked milk can often be tolerated).

Butter and oleomargarine can usually be permitted in modest amounts. (Traces of milk are present.)

Study the label on packaged foods for evidence of milk or milk products content.

EGG-FREE DIET

Avoid

Eggs: fresh, frozen and powdered, cooked in any form.

Egg-containing foods, such as:

Soups and broths made with egg.

Prepared flour mixes for home cooking.

Waffles, doughnuts, pretzels.

Pancakes, griddle cakes, pastries, French toast.

Macaroons, meringues, frostings.

Cakes and cookies, unless known to be egg-free.

Breads with glazed crust.

Foods breaded with egg mixture.

Sausages, croquettes and meat cakes containing egg as binder.

Poultry, especially chicken, if fricasseed or in broth.

Salad dressings, unless known to be egg-free; Hollandaise, mayonnaise and egg sauces.

Ice cream and sherbets, unless known to be egg-free.

Custards, cream candies, fondants, Bavarian cream.

Marshmallows.

Baking powder containing egg white.

Prepared drinks containing egg or egg powder for insomnia or underweight.

Study the labels on packaged foods for evidence of egg in any form.

Avoid virus vaccine made in egg, such as vaccines for influenza, spotted fever, yellow fever.

SEAFOOD-FREE DIET

Avoid

Fish and shellfish, fresh, canned, smoked, pickled; fish liver oils and concentrates in vitamin preparations.

Fish and shellfish stews, bisques, broths, soups, salad, hors d'oeuvres, caviar.

Licking labels, which may contain a fish glue adhesive.

Injections of fish origin in the treatment of varicose veins.

WHEAT-FREE DIET

Avoid

White, whole-wheat and cracked wheat flour in breads, waffles, griddle cakes, doughnuts, muffins, pastries, pies, cakes, crackers, spaghetti, macaroni, dumplings, pretzels, zwieback, noodles.

Corn bread, unless known to be wheat-free.

Soy bread, unless known to be wheat-free.

Rye bread, unless known to be wheat-free.

Gluten bread.

Breakfast cereals, dry or cooked, containing wheat, whole wheat; cream soups, Farina or bran.

Custards, gravies and sauces containing wheat.

Coffee substitutes containing wheat; beer; ale.

Prepared meats, such as sausages, frankfurters, meat loaf, croquettes made with wheat.

Prepared mixes for biscuits, muffins, pastries, pie crusts, cookies.

Study the label on prepared foods for evidences of wheat or wheat product content.

NUT-FREE DIET

Avoid

Nuts of all types, also peanuts (although a member of the bean family), cottonseed meal in health and laxative breads, soybean bread.

Nut crumbs on cookies, cake icings, ice cream.

Candies containing nuts.

Salad oils, lard substitutes, margarines made of coconut, soybean, cottonseed or peanut oils. (Olive oil permitted.)

Individuals highly sensitive to nuts are often allergic to seeds, such as cottonseed, flaxseed, mustard (by external application in poultices as well as when ingested as food), beans and peas. Legumes such as peas, beans and lentils are often allergenic factors in the patient sensitive to nuts, but some patients tolerate legumes such as peanuts despite high degrees of nut sensitivity.

Instructing the Patient

Patients who follow an elimination diet program for a long period require careful supervision. It is not sufficient to instruct the patient to omit specific offending foods. The essential, nutritious foods should be included in the diet if possible. If foods such as milk, meat or eggs are eliminated, adequate substitutions or supplements must be made. Malnutrition must be guarded against when the diet is severely restricted.

A number of procedures have been advocated for the treatment of foods to render them less antigenic. One of these procedures is the denaturation of food. This is done by chemical treatment or by heat and is both simple and useful. For example, denatured milk (boiled, evaporated and powdered) is valuable prophylactically.

INFANT WITH ALLERGY

If it is determined that an infant has a food allergy, it is best to keep him on breast milk, if possible, while looking to the mother's diet for possible allergens that may have passed into her milk. If the infant is on cow's milk formula, the allergy is likely to be to cow's milk protein, and a soy formula should be used. However, 20 per cent of infants found to be allergic to cow's milk are also allergic to soy milk.[2] If soy formula is not tolerated, a hypoallergenic formula such as Nutramigen or Pregestimil, in which the protein is in the form of protein hydrolysate, may be tried. If the infant cannot tolerate either of these formulas, a meat base formula such as Gerber's MBF may be used. If this too is unsuccessful, a formula may have to be devised using a specific meat, such as pureed lamb, and glucose.

PROGNOSIS

The prognosis for allergy varies with the individual. Some patients are cured, others improved, while still others receive very little aid through treatment. The patient must be impressed with the fact that continuous adherence to the program is necessary to obtain beneficial results. The duration of the treatment depends upon the individual; it may be weeks, months or years.

The patient should have careful, frequent checkups to avoid the unnecessary exclusion of foods and to ingest an adequate diet to correct mistakes. Psychosomatic medicine enters into the treatment of allergy, since some patients prefer clinging to symptoms rather than getting well; others develop the emotional tension typical in any recurrent disease.

PREVENTION OF FOOD ALLERGY

Although it is not a foolproof way to prevent food allergy, delaying the introduction of highly allergenic foods into the diets of infants with a family history of allergy is a wise precaution. The early feeding of solid foods to an infant with an immature gastrointestinal tract invites absorption of an allergen and possible sensitivity. Giving foods such as wheat, eggs, oranges, chocolate, fish and nuts should be postponed. Meats should not be started before 6 to 9 months of age, and lamb and veal, the least allergenic, should be tried first. Breast feeding until this age is also recommended.

PROBLEMS AND SUGGESTED TOPICS FOR DISCUSSION

1. What are the most common allergenic foods? List suitable substitutions that can be made for each of these foods to keep the diet nutritionally adequate.
2. What are the common methods used to diagnose a food allergy? What is the procedure for using the Rowe Elimination Test Diets?
3. Plan menus for one week for a patient instructed to follow the fruit-free, cereal-free elimination diet (Table 31–4). Check for adequacy.
4. If a patient is allergic to milk, what foods in what amounts will supply 800 mg. calcium?
5. Obtain a dietary history of a patient suspected of having a food allergy who is in the hospital or in the outpatient clinic.
   (a) List the foods to which he may be hypersensitive.
   (b) Have the patient plan three days' menus.
   (c) Analyze the nutritional adequacy of the menus, considering calories, proteins, calcium, iron and the vitamins.
   (d) How could the patient desensitize himself to the allergen?

PATIENT EDUCATION MATERIALS

Allergy Recipes, 5th ed. Chicago, The American Dietetic Assn., 430 N. Michigan Avenue, 60611, 1969.

Baking for People with Food Allergies. Home and Garden Bulletin No. 147, U.S.D.A. Washington, D.C., U.S. Government Printing Office, 1975.

Frazier, C. A.: Coping with Food Allergy. New York, Quadrangle/The New York Times Co., 1974.

Joseph, L., and Mills, A. S.: A Doctor Discusses Allergy Fact and Fallacies. Chicago, Budlong Press Co., 1973.

Sainsbury, I. S.: The Milk-Free and Milk-Free, Egg-Free Cookbook. Springfield, Ill., Charles C Thomas, 1974.

Wheat, Milk and Egg Free Recipes. Consumer Services Department, The Quaker Oats Company, Chicago, Illinois, 60654.

CITED REFERENCES

1. Crook, W. G.: The allergic tension-fatigue syndrome. Pediatr. Ann., *3*:69, 1974.
2. Gerrard, J. W., et al.: Cow's milk allergy: Prevalence and manifestations in an unselected series of newborns. Acta Paediatr. Scand. [Suppl.] *234*:1, 1973.
3. Rowe, A. H., and Rowe, A., Jr.: Food Allergy: Its Manifestations and Control and the Elimination Diets. Springfield, Ill. Charles C Thomas, 1972.
4. Wohl, M. G., and Goodhart, R. S.: Modern Nutrition in Health and Disease, 3rd ed. Philadelphia, Lea & Febiger, 1964.

ADDITIONAL REFERENCES

Bronsky, E. A., et al.: Evaluation of the provocative food test technique. J. Allergy, *47*:104, 1971.

Felleson, J. A.: The clinical ecology unit. RN, *40*:49, 1977.
Frazier, C. A. (ed.): Current Therapy of Allergy. New York, Medical Examination Publishing Co., Inc., 1974, pp. 204–223.
Lymphocyte hypersensitivity in cow's milk protein intolerance. Nutr. Rev., *35*:39, 1977.
May, C. D.: Food allergy. In: Fomon, S. J.: Infant Nutrition, 2nd ed. Philadelphia, W. B. Saunders Co., 1974, pp. 435–458.
Rinkle, H. J., et al.: The diagnosis of food allergy. Arch. Otolaryngol., *79*:78, 1964.
Rowe, A. H.: Elimination Diets and the Patient's Allergies. Philadelphia, Lea & Febiger, 1944.
Tuft, L.: Allergy Management in Clinical Practice. St. Louis, C. V. Mosby Co., 1973, pp. 132–153.
Woodruff, C. W.: Milk intolerances. Nutr. Rev., *34*:33, 1976.
Zanjanian, M. H.: The intestine in allergic diseases. Ann. Allergy, *37*:208, 1976.

UNIT TWELVE

DISEASES OF THE NERVOUS SYSTEM AND MENTAL ILLNESS

Chapter 32

NUTRITIONAL CARE FOR PATIENTS WITH DISEASES OF THE NERVOUS SYSTEM AND MENTAL ILLNESS

The state of the nervous system is largely dependent upon the state of nutrition of the individual. Minor disturbances, such as forgetfulness, irritability, uneasiness and disorderly thinking, as well as gross mental changes, may develop from poor nutrition. Following prolonged nutritional inadequacy, lesions appear in both the central and peripheral nervous systems. For the most part these changes are reversible when the nutritional deficiency is corrected. However, there is very little evidence that increasing the intake of nutrients to hundreds of times the RDA will enhance mental functioning. Several mental disorders benefit from proper nutritional care in conjunction with other forms of therapy. Epilepsy, multiple sclerosis, anorexia nervosa, and other disorders will be discussed in this chapter.

NEURITIS AND POLYNEURITIS

Etiology

Polyneuritis is a term applied to any condition in which there is a symmetrical involvement of the peripheral nerves, and it is usually

believed to be the result of some nutritional, toxic or metabolic disturbance. It is inflammatory in nature. Frequently, the cause is unknown, and most of the treatment must be of the symptoms only. Polyneuropathy may result from a deficient intake of any one of the B vitamins: thiamin, niacin, pyridoxine (vitamin B_6), vitamin B_{12} or pantothenic acid. There is some evidence that folate deficiency may also cause neuropathy rather than only causing hematological changes as previously thought.[20, 26] Polyneuropathy is exhibited occasionally by alcoholics, and it may be associated with stomach and liver symptoms. These individuals neglect to eat and thereby set the foundation for the vitamin deficiency. Apparently alcohol requires thiamin to be metabolized, and when large quantities of alcohol are taken there is a greater demand for this vitamin. By eating an adequate diet the needs are met, but when meals are replaced by alcohol, the thiamin reserve is exhausted quickly. (See Chapter 24.)

When there is *interference with absorption* of these vitamins for long periods of time, the nerves frequently suffer. Replenishing the miss-

ing vitamins does not necessarily cure the patient, because in many instances either the tissue structures have degenerated beyond repair or the period of treatment is too short.

Nutritional Care

Treatment is dependent on the basic disorder. Biochemical assessment of the status of suspected nutrients (Chapter 11) will determine which nutrient deficiency is causing the neuritis. In most cases the cause will be multiple deficiencies that have existed for a long time. If the diet is inadequate in one nutrient, it is usually deficient in many. In addition, if malabsorption is causing the neuritis, it will usually affect many nutrients.

The diet must be adequate and contain liberal amounts of vitamins. Supplementary vitamins, particularly of the B complex, are supplied as indicated. Parenteral vitamin B_{12} is of value in some cases; for example, for the neurological involvement in pernicious anemia. In a thiamin deficiency the administration of thiamin hydrochloride (100 mg. a day) should be beneficial. The mental symptoms of pellagra respond specifically to administration of niacin.

Establishment of an improved dietary regimen—with high intake of the protective foods—to be carried out throughout life is the important aim in therapy of any of the neurological manifestations of nutritional deficiencies. Many of the patients are elderly, with early personality deterioration; some are from poverty-stricken areas and have the further complication of marginal mental ability. Understanding, patience and skill are required to cope with the patient's psychological, financial and other problems in order to change his eating habits.

EPILEPSY

Epilepsy is one of the oldest known and most dreaded diseases. The name comes from the Greek word for "seizure," and in ancient times the seizing was believed to be the work of spirits. It is defined as a chronic functional disease of nervous origin, characterized by seizures or attacks in which there is sometimes loss of consciousness with a succession of tonic or clonic convulsions. The attacks vary in frequency, occurring several times daily in some instances. With other patients, a year or two may elapse between episodes. If severe convulsions appear, the disorder is labeled *grand mal,* which is French for "great sickness" or "major attack." When seizures are mild, the condition is called *petit mal,* meaning "little sickness" or "minor attack." The attack may last from a few seconds to 20 minutes. Epilepsy may be the result of a variety of lesions of the central nervous system, which are still not understood. It is estimated that approximately 1 per cent of the total population of the United States have epilepsy. Electroencephalography has aided physicians to a better understanding of the disease.

Nutritional Care

Anticonvulsant medications have largely superseded diet therapy in the treatment of epilepsy. An adequate, well-balanced diet with avoidance of excess food or fluid intake, in addition to use of drugs, is the treatment of choice. However, for a few individuals who do not tolerate drugs well or who do not respond to anticonvulsant medication, the ketogenic diet may be helpful in controlling *petit mal* seizures. It is more effective in young children, possibly because the brain of a younger individual has a greater capacity to oxidize ketone bodies than does the brain of an adult.

Ketogenic Diet. This is a diet constructed to produce a state of ketosis in the patient. It is now thought that the anticonvulsant effect of the diet is due to the high plasma levels of ketone bodies.[18] The diet is extremely low in carbohydrates and high in fats, so that a ketogenic-antiketogenic ratio of 3:1 is maintained. In older children the ratio may be 4:1 to keep them in ketosis. The ratio is of the fat to non-fat calories in the diet.

The ketogenic diet can be calculated using either regular dietary fat or medium-chain triglycerides (MCT). (See Chapter 4 for a definition of MCT.) Using dietary fat to construct a diet with a ketogenic-antiketogenic ratio of 3:1 or 4:1 means that the fat content of the diet must be extremely high—80 to 90 per cent of the calories. (The usual diet contains 40 per cent of the calories as fat.) Protein and carbohydrate each contribute about 7 per cent of the calories. These extremely high-fat diets are unpalatable and difficult for a child to follow.

The second method, using medium chain triglycerides, became possible with the development of MCT oil about 15 years ago. Unlike dietary fat, MCT oil is more rapidly absorbed and is transported directly to the liver. This accounts for its more rapid induction of ketosis

in the child. As a result, a smaller amount of fat is needed, and dietary fat need not be so high. The diet using MCT is more flexible and palatable because more protein and carbohydrate are allowed, and yet the diet is still as effective.[18] Another advantage is that serum cholesterol levels are not elevated, as happens frequently with the traditional ketogenic diet.

The method for calculating the ketogenic diet is given in Table 32–1. Calories are determined first; most children require 75 to 90 kcal. per kg. per day, depending on their activity. After the calorie requirement has been determined, the amount of MCT oil needed is calculated, then the dietary fat, protein and carbohydrate allowances are computed. Protein should be at least 1 gm. per kg. per day, which is the minimum needed for proper growth. The RDA for protein is 1.5 gm. per kg. per day.

To simplify the choosing of food to contribute the necessary nutrients, the diabetic exchange lists (Table 25–5) are used. Table 32–2 gives an example of the food exchanges included in a ketogenic diet using MCT oil for a four year old child. The oil can be used in skim milk, fruit juice, casseroles, salad dressings and sandwich spreads.

The child may feel hungry during the first few days while growing used to the diet, but weight should be the criterion used to judge whether the diet is adequate. He or she may also experience nausea and vomiting if ketosis becomes excessive. This condition can be relieved by giving orange juice. Symptomatic hypoglycemia is rare, but all children should be tested for a tendency to ketotic hypoglycemia before starting the diet.

If rapid ketosis is desired, the treatment starts with a period of fasting. During the 2 to 3 days of fasting, the patient is permitted a very restricted daily diet of water, broth, tea and 6 to 8 oz. of orange juice. After the fasting period the prescribed ketogenic diet is given to the patient.

If no further attacks are noticed after the diet has been followed for a period of three months, then the carbohydrate intake may be increased gradually in steps of 5 gm., until 50 to 60 gm. of carbohydrates are tolerated daily. Of course, the fats in the diet are reduced proportionately

---

Table 32–1   CALCULATION OF KETOGENIC DIET USING MCT FOR AN
EPILEPTIC 4 YEAR OLD CHILD*

Child: age = 4 yr., weight = 20 kg.
1. Establish caloric requirement:
     20 kg. × 80 kcal./kg./day = 1600 kcal./day
2. Determine amount of MCT oil to be given—50 to 70% of total calories, depending on the amount needed
     to induce ketosis in the individual child:
     60% of 1600 = 960 kcal. from MCT
     1 gm. MCT = 8.3 kcal.
     960 ÷ 8.3 = approximately 116 gm. MCT (115.6)
     116 × 8.3 = 963 kcal.
     15 ml. (1 tbsp.) MCT = 14 gm.
     116 ÷ 14 = 8.3 tbsp. (8 tbsp. + 1 tsp.) MCT
3. Determine calories to be provided by foods exclusive of MCT:
     1600 − 960 = 640 kcal.
4. Establish protein intake according to recommended allowance and patient's desires:
     RDA = 1.5 gm./kg./day
     20 kg. × 1.5 gm./kg./day = 30 gm. protein
   For this child, protein intake is set at 41 gm./day.
     41 gm. protein × 4 kcal./gm. = 164 kcal. from protein
5. Estimate maximum calories to be given in form of carbohydrate:
     19% of 1600 = no more than 304 kcal.
     304 kcal. ÷ 4 = no more than 76 gm. carbohydrate
     74 gm. carbohydrate × 4 kcal./gm. = 296 kcal.
6. Estimate maximum calories to be given in form of protein and carbohydrate combined:
     29% of kcal. × 1600 kcal. = no more than 464 kcal. from protein and carbohydrate
     164 + 296 kcal. = 460 kcal. from protein + carbohydrate
7. Estimate minimum calories to be given as fat exclusive of MCT oil:
     10% × 1600 kcal. = 160 kcal. from other fats
     20 gm. of fat × 9 kcal./gm. = 180 kcal. from fat exclusive of MCT
8. After determining above dietary requirements, the dietary pattern can be calculated using the Exchange
     Lists, as shown in Table 25–5. See Table 32–2.

---

*Adapted from: Signore, J. M.: Ketogenic diet containing medium-chain triglycerides. J. Am. Diet. Assoc., *62*:285, 1973.

Table 32–2   KETOGENIC DIET USING MCT OIL FOR A 4 YEAR OLD CHILD[a]

FOOD	EXCHANGES	PROTEIN (gm.)	FAT (gm.)	CHO (gm.)
Skim milk	2	16	–	24
Lean meat	2½	17	8	–
Fruit	1	–	–	10
Vegetable	2	4	–	10
Bread	2	4	–	30
Fat	2½	–	12.5	–
MCT oil[b] 116 gm = 8 T. + 1 tsp.				
Total MCT = 116 gm.		41	20.5	74

[a]Calories from foods exclusive of MCT = 960. Total calories including MCT = 1600.
[b]1 gm. MCT oil = 8.3 kcal.

to maintain the desired number of calories. A state of ketosis must always be maintained, as shown by diacetic acid and acetone in the urine. Urinalysis will indicate the effectiveness of the diet. Both types of ketogenic diets, and even anticonvulsive medication, lose some of their anticonvulsant effect over time.

Stimulants.   Stimulants such as tea and coffee may be restricted; generally, beer and alcohol are forbidden as they tend to precipitate seizures.

Minerals and Vitamins.   Great care must be exercised to prevent any nutritional deficiencies, especially in calcium, iron and the water-soluble vitamins (B vitamins and vitamin C) and vitamin D. A supplement of 10,000 I.U. of vitamin D should be given per week, as well as a daily dose of a preparation containing calcium, the vitamin B complex and vitamin C.

Drugs

When the ketogenic diet has been used exclusively in cases of epilepsy, it has been reported to be only partially successful. Several years ago more progress was noted if the sedative phenobarbital was prescribed. Some patients showed more improvement with a combination of the ketogenic diet plus medication.

More recent research has introduced additional drugs that have proved effective and safe when used under medical supervision. Patients who are helped lose the defeatist attitude usually associated with this disease. Dilantin was the first of the new drugs, and since then several others have been introduced. The anticonvulsants are somewhat selective in the way they work, and different ones are used to control different kinds of seizures. Dilantin, for example, is more effective in controlling convulsions, whereas Tridione is used to prevent blackouts in petit mal epilepsy. Each new drug

has been used to control seizures in some individuals who were helped only a little or not at all by previous medications. As a result of research, the treatment of epilepsy has advanced further during the past 25 years than during the preceding 25 centuries. The currently available medications can enable 80 to 85 per cent of epileptics to lead an essentially normal life. Evaluation of the effectiveness of the chemicals continues.

Nutritional Implications of Anticonvulsant Drug Therapy.   The anticonvulsants, when taken for periods of time ranging from several months to several years, affect the nutritional status of the child. An osteomalacia, *anticonvulsant rickets,* is frequently seen in children taking phenobarbital, Primidone, or phenytoin. It is thought that these drugs, through hepatic enzyme induction, decrease the activation of 25-hydroxy vitamin D_3 so that it cannot be further converted to 1,25-dihydroxy vitamin D_3 in the kidney. Since 1,25-$(OH)_2$ D_3 acts on the gut to facilitate calcium absorption, calcium absorption is reduced. (Vitamin D is discussed in Chapter 8.) The inadequate calcium absorption leads to osteomalacia. It is thought that phenytoin also affects calcium absorption directly, and the drug does lower serum folate levels. Low serum folate and vitamin B_{12} levels and megaloblastic anemia may be present.[21]

The person taking anticonvulsants should probably receive at least 1000 I.U. of vitamin D per day or whatever amount is required to maintain normal serum levels of 25-OH D_3. Regular exposure to sunlight will also help to prevent rickets. If folic acid is given to correct low serum folate levels, there may be a deterioration of seizure control. Although the reason is not clear, anticonvulsive agents in the presence of folate supplements are less effective in some people. The relationship between folate

metabolism, anticonvulsive drugs and epileptic seizures needs further study.[6, 27] (See Chapter 21.)

MULTIPLE SCLEROSIS

Multiple sclerosis is a central nervous system disease of unknown etiology affecting the myelinated nerve fibers and the muscles they innervate. It develops as an acute disease without warning and runs an intermittent course characterized by exacerbations at intervals of weeks, months or years. There is destruction of the fatty myelin sheaths that surround the nerves in different parts of the brain and spinal cord. This insulating material is replaced by scar tissue, and there are many such areas (multiple) of nerve degeneration (sclerosis). The condition may appear at any age but usually does so between the ages of 20 to 40. It is more common in temperate climates, especially in the northern European countries such as the British Isles, Iceland, the Low Countries, northern and central France, Germany, Poland and Czechoslovakia.

Etiology

Many theories have been advanced about the cause of multiple sclerosis. The most promising one seems to be that it is a slow virus disease or, more likely, a virus-induced immune disease.[30] However, it also seems that many other factors are involved, such as vascular condition, heredity, metabolic alterations and disturbed immune mechanisms.

A metabolic alteration involving fatty acid metabolism has attracted attention for over 20 years. Abnormal fatty acid metabolism may help set the stage for a pathogenic agent to attack the central nervous system (CNS). Thompson reported that the level of linoleic acid (a polyunsaturated fatty acid) in the serum of multiple sclerosis patients was lower than in control subjects. It seems that the more severe the recent clinical deterioration, the lower the level of linoleic acid.[31] In a well-controlled study, investigators found that the clinical course of the disease was improved if the diet was supplemented with linoleic acid rather than oleic acid (a saturated fatty acid).[23]

Nutritional Care

The patient should have a well-balanced and adequate diet to meet all the requirements of normal nutrition for his age, activity and desired weight. When activity is limited owing to nerve degeneration, the patient should carefully control his weight. Because of the crippling nature of the disease, every opportunity for rehabilitation should be taken to make life more livable and worthwhile. Present capabilities and potentialities of each patient should be developed to the maximum. The patient should be given feeding aids and taught to use them, rather than be made to feel helpless by being fed.

Fat. There is no proven nutritional care that will improve the course of multiple sclerosis; however, Swank reported convincing evidence from a 20 year study that a low-fat diet maintained over a long period of time tends to retard the disease process and to reduce the incidence of new attacks.[29] He recommends a fat intake of 10 gm. of saturated (animal) fat and 40 to 50 gm. of a polyunsaturated oil (8 to 10 tsp.) daily. At least 1 tsp. should be cod liver oil. A 10 gm. saturated fat diet is given in Table 32–3. Protein is kept at normal levels (60 to 70 gm.), and carbohydrate is supplied to meet calorie needs. At this time there is not enough evidence to say definitely that a low-saturated-fat diet will improve the course of multiple sclerosis. However, it would not hurt a patient to follow such a diet after receiving some dietary counseling to assure that the diet is adequate. A diet very low in animal fat restricts meat, usually to less than 2 oz. per day, and therefore deficient intakes of protein, iron, B vitamins and trace minerals such as zinc may result from it.

Excessive physical and emotional stress should be avoided. Currently no medication has been proved to be consistently beneficial, although steroid treatment during periods of exacerbation or relapse may be helpful.

HYPERKINETIC BEHAVIOR SYNDROME

Hyperkinetic behavior in children is an ill-defined disorder. When is an active child hyperactive? Although there is disagreement on the precise definition of hyperkinetic behavior, most authorities agree that the following are major features of such behavior: excessive gross motor activity, impulsiveness, low tolerance to frustration, short attention span and easy distraction. Any or all of these can be present in the hyperkinetic or hyperactive child.

Table 32–3 TEN GRAM ANIMAL FAT DIET

(Polyunsaturated vegetable oils are allowed; animal fats are restricted.)

FOOD CLASS	FOODS INCLUDED	FOODS OMITTED
Beverages	Coffee, coffee substitutes, tea, skim milk, buttermilk made from skim milk. At least 4–5 glasses of milk per day.	Whole milk, 2% milk, low-fat milk, chocolate milk, cream, half and half.
Breads	Enriched white, rye, whole-wheat breads; Italian or French breads; hard rolls, saltines, graham crackers, melba toast.	Commercial pancakes, waffles, hot breads, snack crackers.
Cereals	Hot and ready-to-eat.	None
Condiments	All	None
Desserts	Angel food cakes, white cake, fruit whips, gelatin and rennet desserts, puddings made with skim milk; sherbets, fruit ices and other desserts made with allowed foods.	Ice cream, pastries and other desserts made with butter, cream, half and half, whole milk, 2% milk or egg yolks.
Fats	Corn oil, safflower oil, soybean oil, cottonseed oil only; soft or liquid margarines; non-dairy creamers.	Butter, stick margarine, lard, shortenings, hydrogenated vegetable oils; coconut oil and all others not allowed.
Fruits and fruit juices	Canned, cooked, fresh or frozen.	Avocado.
Meats and substitutes	2 oz. daily of lean meats, fish, poultry without skin, and eggs only; one egg is equal to 1 oz. of meat. Use as desired: egg whites, cottage cheese made from skim milk, dry cottage cheese, fat-free cheeses or those made with skim milk or allowed oils; vegetable protein substitutes; egg substitutes; dried beans, lentils and peas.	Fatty meats, fish and poultry, such as duck, goose, luncheon meats; canned fish packed in oils; bacon, sausages, frankfurters and organ meats; all cheeses except those allowed.
Potatoes and substitutes	White and sweet potatoes; macaroni, rice, noodles and spaghetti.	Potato chips; pastas made with eggs, such as egg noodles.
Soups	Fat-free broths, consommés and bouillons; cream soups made with skim milk; other soups made with allowed foods.	All others.
Sweets	Hard candies, gum drops, marshmallows, jams, jellies, sugars and syrups.	Candies made with chocolate, coconut, cream, fats and nuts.
Vegetables and vegetable juices	Canned, cooked, fresh or frozen.	Any vegetables prepared with a butter, cream or cheese sauce.
Miscellaneous	Vinegar, fat-free gravies, salad dressings made with allowed oils, pickles, olives; nuts: hazel, hickory, pecans, walnuts; cocoa.	Coconut; rich gravies and sauces; nuts, except those allowed.

A child may be hyperkinetic for a variety of physiological or psychological reasons and should always be thoroughly examined and evaluated before any kind of treatment is started. Therapies encompass stimulant medication, behavior modification, psychotherapy, special classroom situations, megavitamin therapy and the Feingold diet. All of these have been tried with various degrees of success, but claims for the Feingold diet have probably attracted the most attention.

The Feingold Diet

In 1973 Dr. Feingold proposed that some children are hyperactive because they are sensitive to salicylates and artificial flavors and colors in their food. His hypothesis seems to have originated from his observations that in some people salicylates cause allergic reactions such as urticaria and asthma. When he treated the allergy by removing the salicylates from the diet, he noted a behavior change in

addition to the disappearance of the allergic symptoms. Since many patients who are allergic to salicylates also react to artificial colors, specifically yellow FD and C number 5, he postulated that the food colors may also have a behavior effect similar to that of the salicylates in those people sensitive to them. He applied this hypothesis to children with hyperkinetic behavior. Based upon his anecdotal clinical observations, he published a popular book in which he presented both the hypothesis and the salicylate-free, artificial color-free and artificial flavor-free diet, which he claims has been successful in improving behavior in 30 to 50 per cent of the hyperactive children he has treated.[12]

No convincing experimental work is available to confirm Feingold's claims of success with his diet. Harley and his colleagues have conducted a controlled study to test the Feingold hypothesis.[14] They found that the Feingold diet did not cause a consistent or significant reduction in hyperactive behavior in the children, as assessed from the observations of parents, teachers and trained classroom observers or the results of neuropsychological tests. Nine of the 46 children who showed the best, although not significant, response to the diet were then challenged with special candy bars and cookies containing all of the certified artificial food colors and others without artificial coloring, in an attempt to "turn on" and "turn off" their hyperactive behavior. Again, the results were negative.[13] In addition, many of the foods that Feingold eliminates from the diet because they contain salicylates are in fact salicylate-free.[1] Connors, who also tested the hypothesis but under less rigorous conditions, concluded that the diet may be effective in a small subgroup of hyperactive children, but he also reported that the diet produced poorer nutritional intake than the child's regular diet, particularly for vitamin C, since the diet omits many fruits.[7]

Feingold's hypothesis has not been experimentally confirmed, and the claims for its success by Feingold and the press may be primarily attributable to a placebo effect rather than to the characteristics of the diet. If the diet is to be used, attention should be paid to its possible nutritional inadequacies, and there should be some nutritional counseling and vitamin supplementation, if necessary.

ANOREXIA NERVOSA

Anorexia nervosa (AN) is a disorder usually seen among teenage girls that seems to be becoming more common, irrespective of the increased medical awareness of it.[4, 9] However, it has also been seen in men and older women. The typical anorexia nervosa occurs among girls from upper middle class families. Most of these families appear to be stable and happy, and frequently only after long periods of psychotherapy do subtle problems become apparent. An "atypical" or secondary form of anorexia nervosa may be associated with a hypothalamic tumor.

Definition

Although this disorder has been recognized since the 19th century (Gull described it in 1874), there is still uncertainty as to whether it is primarily a psychological disorder, primarily a physical disorder of hypothalamic or pituitary function, or a combination of both. The hypothalamic-pituitary dysfunction may result from psychogenic stress or may be secondary to the malnutrition and starvation that result from the condition.

Physically, these patients exhibit a refusal to eat, loss of 25 per cent or more of body weight with emaciation (many lose up to 35 per cent of their body weight), amenorrhea (cessation of menstruation), overactivity (often vigorous exercise), downy hair over normally hairless parts of the body, cold extremities, hypotension, insulin insensitivity and lowered basal metabolic rate (BMR).

Psychologically, according to Bruch, there is a distortion of body image, so that these girls frequently overestimate their size by 60 per cent, saying "I'm fat" when obviously they are underweight. They also are obsessed with dieting to lose weight and deny that they are already painfully emaciated. Second, there is a distorted perception of stimuli arising in the body, so that hunger, appetite and satiation are not perceived correctly, and they do not feel fatigue or other changes. Third, these patients have a sense of personal ineffectiveness. Secondary to these three major psychological problems is a distorted attitude toward food that may include an aversion to carbohydrates in particular. This attitude can alternate with food binges, guilt at having eaten, self-induced vomiting or use of cathartics, secrecy or denial regarding food habits and overactivity or rigorous exercise.

Etiology

Proposed causes for this psychological and behavioral pattern are that (1) the individual

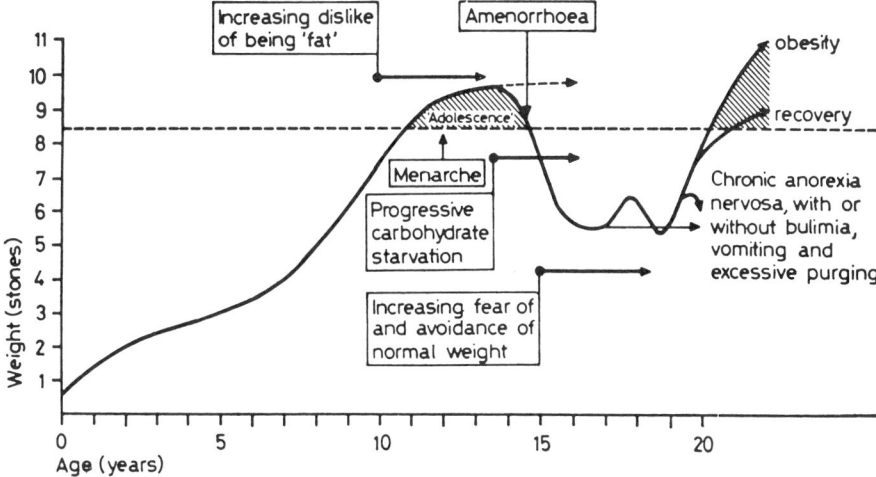

Figure 32–1   Some typical developments found in a series of 82 patients with primary anorexia nervosa or weight phobia. One stone equals 14 lb. (From: Crisp, A. H.: Anorexia nervosa. In: Silverstone, T., and Barraclough, B. (eds.): Contemporary Psychiatry. Br. J. Psychiatry, Special Publication No. 9, 1975.)

wants to exert control over some aspect of her life, (2) she equates increasing body weight during adolescence with maturity and is afraid of the onset of womanhood and (3) she has an obsessive desire for slimness due to societal pressure. Usually there is a precipitating event, such as the first actual or threatened separation from parents or a first attempt at a sexual relationship. Figure 32–1 shows the usual progression of this disease.

Because body functions other than food intake, such as thermoregulation, menstruation, basal metabolic rate and activity, are also affected in this disorder, many postulate that the cause is an organic lesion in the hypothalamus.[19, 22, 32] On the other hand, the hypothalamic dysfunction and other endocrine abnormalities may be secondary to the starvation, malnutrition or psychiatric illness. For instance, amenorrhea commonly occurs when a woman falls below a critical body weight. To illustrate, although the average age at menarche has decreased from 16.5 to 12.5 years over the last 125 years, the mean weight of girls at menarche has remained unchanged, showing that weight seems to be a critical factor for endocrine function. The area of endocrine and neurophysiological factors is being looked at with renewed interest and may give more answers about the pathogenesis of anorexia nervosa.

Treatment

Although usually she will not admit it initially, the patient with severe anorexia nervosa is seriously ill and requires prompt attention. Treatment should include *both* nutritional rehabilitation and psychotherapy.

Psychotherapy.   If the underlying problems of the individual and her family are not corrected, release from the hospital or treatment center after nutritional rehabilitation will only result in a relapse into abnormal behavior and weight loss. However, most authorities agree that some weight gain should be initiated before effective psychotherapy can be started. Individual psychotherapy begins with determining the underlying psychological reasons for the behavior. The patient's family should also be involved in therapy.

Nutritional Rehabilitation and Weight Gain.   Hospitalization is usually required in order to separate the patient from family stresses and to control her eating environment. Some have used this situation for forced feeding and medication, usually with little success.[8, 10] Others use the hospital setting as a way to establish an atmosphere in which the anorexia nervosa patient can eat. Bruch and others feel that this can be done by providing a protective, non-punitive environment. The patient is relieved of decision-making by not having to choose clothing (wearing only pajamas) or food (having her meals chosen and provided for her). Having the AN patient select a menu of food for the next day, as is usual in hospitals, is frequently too great a task. Many AN patients will refuse to eat solid foods but may drink liquids. A nourishing, high-caloric, high-protein liquid (see Table 35–7) should be tried, with a comment to the patient that this

will save making a decision and that it is required for all hospitalized patients in order to maintain fluid intake and is not a punishment. A patient who flatly refuses to eat will have to be fed with a tube or by intravenous hyperalimentation.

BEHAVIOR MODIFICATION. Some groups have employed behavior modification techniques by which the patient is denied all privileges unless he or she gains a certain amount of weight each day. One technique is to deny the AN patient any kind of activity until a certain weight gain is achieved. This usually is a good motivation because activity is so important to these patients. As the weight gain continues, more and more activity and privileges are allowed. The behavior modification technique seems effective for inducing weight gain, and gains of as much as 6 lb. per week have been reported.[3] However, Bruch has warned against the serious repercussions of this technique with *some* severely anorexic patients. "Its very efficiency increases the inner turmoil of patients who feel tricked into relinquishing control over their bodies and lives." This compounds the patient's feeling of all pervasive ineffectiveness, which is one of the root problems in the development of anorexia nervosa.[5]

Prognosis

Follow-up studies of treated patients showed that two thirds recovered after several years of treatment.[8, 10] Criteria of recovery agreed upon by most clinicians are: reasonable and stable weight in the individual, reasonable diet and eating habits, no vomiting, regular menstruation and healthy adolescent behavior, including peer heterosexual relationships. Fifteen to 20 per cent of patients who have this disorder eventually die from it.

NUTRITION AND MENTAL FUNCTION

Because so little is known regarding the functioning of the brain, especially in relation to nutrients and nutrient intake, this has been an area ripe for exploitation and full of misleading statements. Great claims have been made for various vitamins as being able to improve memory, enhance intelligence or change moods. None of them have been proven unequivocally, except in cases where the person was vitamin-deficient to begin with.

Neurotransmitters

Considerable research has shown that the concentration of some of the neurotransmitters in the brain are influenced by diet. *Neurotransmitters* are the substances present in the neurons of mammals that, when released, will transmit signals across synapses to other neurons in the brain or to muscle cells or secretory cells outside the brain. Four primary amines are serotonin, dopamine, norepinephrine and acetylcholine, which are synthesized from amino acids.* Dopamine and norepinephrine are synthesized from tyrosine and phenylalanine (phenylalanine is metabolized to tyrosine), serotonin is synthesized from tryptophan, and acetylcholine is synthesized from choline.

Food consumption influences the levels of tyrosine, choline and tryptophan in the brain, and the brain's synthesis of the neurotransmitters depends on the level of these precursors. However, the relationships are not direct, since insulin is involved in the control of serum levels of amino acids.

A high-protein meal increases brain tyrosine level and brain dopamine accumulation. It does not elevate the concentrations of brain tryptophan and serotonin. A high-carbohydrate or protein-free meal will increase the brain tryptophan level and thus the serotonin level. A protein that contains high levels of choline, such as eggs or meat, will increase the concentration of brain acetylcholine. An increase in the level of brain neurotransmitters will be physiologically significant only if it is also correlated with a change in the amount of neurotransmitters secreted into synaptic clefts. Whether or not this occurs is still not known. However, concentrations of brain neurotransmitters are already being manipulated with clinical effect. For example, most authorities agree that drugs that block dopamine receptors are useful in treating psychoses, and drugs that stimulate these receptors are being used to treat Parkinson's disease. Drugs that increase brain norepinephrine levels in synapses have antidepressant effects. Tryptophan and choline themselves, as isolated proteins, and not as part of the diet, are also being used. This "precursor therapy" has been tried in treatment of insomnia, depression, Huntington's chorea[2] and tardive dyskinesia.[11] Tryptophan at bedtime appears to be an effective hypnotic

---

*Other possible neurotransmitters are epinephrine, gamma-amino butyric acid (GABA) and glycine.

agent.[34] Perhaps drinking the traditional glass of hot milk (carbohydrate) increases the tryptophan level in the brain and is really a rather scientific practice.

ORTHOMOLECULAR PSYCHIATRY

Orthomolecular psychiatry is a form of treatment used for schizophrenia. Although anecdotal clinical reports of success have been given by its proponents,[16, 24] in clinically controlled trials other investigators have been unable to reproduce their results.[33]

The term *orthomolecular psychiatry,* coined by Linus Pauling in 1968, means "the achievement and preservation of good mental health by the provision of the optimum molecular environment for the mind, especially the optimum concentrations of substances normally present in the human body, such as the vitamins."[25] He claims that certain people require larger quantities of some vitamins than others do for optimal mental function. Orthomolecular psychiatry relies on several therapeutic components: nicotinic acid, vitamin C, vitamin B_6, other water-soluble vitamins such as vitamin B_{12}, trace minerals, an antihypoglycemia diet, electroconvulsive therapy (ECT) and conventional psychotropic drugs such as the phenothiazines. Large doses of vitamins (10 to 500 times the RDA) are used. Some say that these are not physiological doses and that, when used in these amounts, vitamins should be considered drugs.

In 1973 an American Psychiatric Association (APA) Task Force report rejected orthomolecular psychiatry on the grounds that it is unsubstantiated by scientific evidence and uses questionable clinical methods and that its results are non-reproducible in controlled studies. The value of orthomolecular psychiatry is not a settled issue, and it remains extremely controversial. As we learn more about the brain and how it functions, perhaps this high-level nutrient intake will prove to be valuable therapy.

MENTAL ILLNESS

One out of every two hospital beds in the United States is reported to be occupied by a patient suffering from mental illness. These patients are often in a poor nutritional state and require sympathy and understanding on the part of the entire hospital team—nurse, dietitian and physician—to encourage the ingestion of a balanced diet. Food served in an attractive and pleasant environment will often stimulate the patient to eat. Many psychiatric disorders follow prolonged periods of tension, worry and anxiety, during which intelligent and adequate food intake was neglected. The patient may be overweight as a result of compulsive eating during anxiety periods or thin and emaciated from lack of interest in eating. Both types of patients require discerning guidance to meet their emotional needs and metabolic requirements.

As previously pointed out, mental symptoms such as forgetfulness, confusion, depression and anxiety may result from dietary inadequacies. For example, deficiencies of folate and vitamin B_{12} are associated with sleeplessness, forgetfulness and irritability, and these symptoms disappear within 24 hours of starting therapy.[15]

Methods of therapy, such as the tranquilizers or shock treatment or both, along with psychotherapy, are restoring many patients to a normal life who were once considered hopeless. Special attention should also be given to the nutrition of these patients because some of them can be helped by restoration of nutritional status. Vitamin supplements and a good, nutritious diet have relieved many patients of symptoms arising from the nervous system. Many of the drugs used to control mental disorders interact with nutrients to cause nutritional deficiencies or metabolic problems. For example, monoamine oxidase inhibitors used to treat depression can interact with tyrosine in food and cause a hypertensive reaction. (See Chapter 21.)

Food has many meanings for people. These vary with individuals in health and illness. Ross[28] states that food is the "root of psychopathologies." From early childhood food forms the basis of many motives and behaviors. Emotions are expressed in how one responds to food. Feelings of defiance, helpless submission or self-contempt, demands for love and affection and many other underlying emotions may be expressed or acted out through overeating or rejection of food. Fears and anxieties associated with eating certain foods that will "hurt" or "poison" him and feelings of guilt and unworthiness about eating *with* the family are related to the underlying cause of the illness. These feelings may be relieved by permitting the patient to discuss the problem, to participate in the preparation of food or to select his food along with others in whom he has confidence.

Feeding patients "means a good deal more than simply supplying a balanced diet rich in protein and vitamins and balanced in minerals, fats and carbohydrates. It offers a way of reaching them on the level of satisfying a simple human need and thereby also offering them in an unthreatening way the opportunity of rebuilding relationships with their fellowman."[17]

PROBLEMS AND SUGGESTED TOPICS FOR DISCUSSION

1. Obtain a food intake history from a patient suffering with neuritis. Calculate the vitamin content of the food history. Compare the calculation with the Recommended Dietary Allowances. What changes are needed to correct low intakes of nutrients? Are the caloric and protein intakes appropriate?
2. What is the objective of the ketogenic diet for epilepsy? Plan a food prescription for an epileptic patient who is going on a ketogenic diet. The patient is a 14 year old schoolgirl who weighs 135 pounds, and her height is 5 feet 2 inches. Using the food prescription as a basis, make out a meal plan.
3. Talk with a patient who has anorexia nervosa. Describe what she looks like and how she acts. What is her weight? How much is she underweight for her height?
4. Plan a menu for one day for a 35 year old woman with multiple sclerosis who has difficulty in chewing and in feeding herself.
5. List typical dietary problems encountered in the mentally ill patient.

CITED REFERENCES

1. Ashoor, S., and Chu, F. S.: Analysis of Salicylic Acid and Methyl Salicylate in Fruits and Almonds (unpublished manuscript). Madison, Wisconsin, Food Research Institute, University of Wisconsin, 1977.
2. Bird, E. D., and Iverson, L. L.: Huntington's chorea. Post-mortem measurement of glutamic acid decarboxylase, choline acetyltransferase and dopamine in basal ganglia. Brain, 97:457, 1974.
3. Blinder, B. J., Freeman, D. M. A., and Stunkard, A. J.: Behavior therapy of anorexia nervosa: Effectiveness of activity as a reinforcer of weight gain. Am. J. Psychiatry, 126:8, 1970.
4. Bruch, H.: Anorexia nervosa. Dietetic Currents, 4 (2), 1977.
5. Bruch, H.: Perils of behavior modification in treatment of anorexia nervosa. JAMA, 230:1419, 1974.
6. Cerebrospinal folate levels in epileptics and their response to folate therapy. Nutr. Rev., 32:70, 1974.
7. Connors, C. K., et al.: Food additives and hyperkinesis: A controlled double-blind experiment. Pediatrics, 58:154, 1976.
8. Crisp, A. H.: A treatment regime for anorexia nervosa. Br. J. Psychiatry, 112:505, 1965.
9. Crisp, A. H., Palmer, R. L., and Kalucy, R. S.: How common is anorexia nervosa? A prevalence study. Brit. J. Psychiatry, 128:549, 1976.
10. Dally, P., and Sargant, W.: Treatment and outcome of anorexia nervosa. Br. Med. J., 2:793, 1966.
11. Davis, K. L., Berger, P. A., and Hollister, L. E.: Choline for tardive dyskinesia (letter). N. Engl. J. Med., 293:152, 1975.
12. Feingold, B. F.: Why Your Child is Hyperactive. New York, Random House, 1974.
13. Harley, J. P.: Personal communication. April 1977.
14. Harley, J. P., et al.: Hyperkinesis and food additives: Testing the Feingold hypothesis. American Psychiatric Assn. Meeting, September 1976.
15. Herbert, V., and Tisman, G.: Effects of deficiencies of folic acid and vitamin B_{12} on central nervous system function and development. In Gaull, G. E. (ed.): Biology of Brain Dysfunction, Vol. 1. New York, Plenum Press, 1973, pp. 380 and 387.
16. Hoffer, A.: Niacin Therapy in Schizophrenia. Springfield, Ill., Charles C Thomas, 1962.
17. Hunscher, M. A.: Nutritional needs of mentally ill geriatric patients. J. Psychiatr. Nurs., 1:220, 1963.
18. Huttenlocher, P. R.: Ketonemia and seizures: Metabolic and anticonvulsant effects of two ketogenic diets in childhood epilepsy. Pediatr. Res., 10:536, 1976.
19. Katz, J. L., et al.: Toward an elucidation of the psychoendocrinology of anorexia nervosa. In: Sachar, E. J. (ed.): Hormones, Behavior, and Psychopathology. New York, Raven Press, 1976, pp. 263–283.
20. Manzoor, M., and Runcie, J.: Folate responsive neuropathy: Report of 10 cases. Br. Med. J., 1:1176, 1976.
21. March, D. C.: Handbook: Interactions of Selected Drugs with Nutritional Status in Man. Chicago, The American Dietetic Assn., 1976, pp. 49–53.
22. Mecklenburg, R. S., et al.: Hypothalamic dysfunction in patients with anorexia nervosa. Medicine, 53:147, 1974.
23. Millar, J. H. D., et al.: Double-blind trial of linoleate supplementation of the diet in multiple sclerosis. Br. Med. J., 1:765, 1973.
24. Osmond, H., and Hoffer, A.: Massive niacin treatment in schizophrenia: Review of nine year study. Lancet, 1:316, 1962.
25. Pauling, L.: Orthomolecular psychiatry. Science, 160:265, 1968.
26. Pincus, J. H., Reynolds, E. H., and Glaser, G. H.: Subacute combined system degeneration with folate deficiency. JAMA, 221:496, 1972.
27. Reynolds, E. H.: Folate and epilepsy. In: Bradford, H. F., and Marsden, C. D. (eds.): Biochemistry and Neurology. New York, Academic Press, 1976, pp. 247–252.
28. Ross, M.: Food in the mental hospital. J. Am. Diet. Assoc., 40:318, 1962.
29. Swank, R. L.: Multiple sclerosis: Twenty years on a low fat diet. Arch. Neurol., 23:460, 1970.
30. Symposium on multiple sclerosis. Br. Med. Bull., 33:2, 1977.
31. Thompson, R. H. S.: A biochemical approach to the problem of multiple sclerosis. Proc. R. Soc. Med., 59:269, 1966.
32. Warren, M. P., and Vande Wiele, R. L.: Clinical and metabolic features of anorexia nervosa. Am. J. Obstet. Gynecol., 117:435, 1973.
33. Wittenborn, J. R., Weber, E. S. P., and Brown, M.: Niacin in the long-term treatment of schizophrenia. Arch. Gen. Psychiatry, 28:308, 1973.
34. Wyatt, R. J., et al.: Effects of L-tryptophan (a natural sedative) on human sleep. Lancet, 2:842, 1970.

ADDITIONAL REFERENCES

Neuritis

Cohn, H., et al.: Neurological manifestations in nutritional impairment. Am. J. Dig. Dis., 21:281, 1954.

Editorial: Nerve conduction in vitamin B_{12} deficiency. JAMA, *194*:189, 1965.

Epilepsy
Dodson, W. E., et al.: Management of seizure disorders: Selected aspects. Part II. J. Pediatr., *89*:695, 1976.
Freund, G., and Weinsier, R. L.: Standardized ketosis following medium chain triglyceride ingestion. *Metabolism, 15*:980, 1966.
Lasser, J. L., and Brush, M. K.: An improved ketogenic diet for treatment of epilepsy. J. Am. Diet. Assoc., *62*:281, 1973.
Schaefer, K., von Herrath, D., and Kraft, D.: Disordered calcium metabolism during anticonvulsant treatment. Ger. Med., *3*:140, 1973.
Signore, J. M.: Ketogenic diet containing medium-chain triglycerides. J. Am. Diet. Assoc., *62*:285, 1973.

Multiple Sclerosis
Alter, A., Yamoor, M., and Harshe, M.: Multiple sclerosis and nutrition. Arch. Neurol., *31*:267, 1974.
Editorial: Low-fat diet in multiple sclerosis. JAMA, *177*:702, 1961.
Maugh, T. H. III.: Multiple sclerosis: Genetic link, viruses suspected (research news). Science, *195*:667, 1977.
Mertin, J., and Meade, C. J.: Relevance of fatty acids in multiple sclerosis. Br. Med. Bull., *33*:67, 1977.
Olson, W. H.: Diet and multiple sclerosis. Postgrad. Med., *59*:219, 1976.

Hyperkinetic Behavior Syndrome
Feingold, B. F.: Hyperkinesis and learning disabilities linked to artificial food flavors and colors. Am. J. Nurs., *75*:797, 1975.
Lucas, B., and Sells, C. J.: Nutrient intake and stimulant drugs in hyperactive children. J. Am. Diet. Assoc., *70*:373, 1977.
National Advisory Committee on Hyperkinesis and Food Additives: Report to the Nutrition Foundation. New York; The Nutrition Foundation, 1975.
Ross, D. M., and Ross, S. A.: Hyperactivity: Research, Theory, and Action. New York, John Wiley & Sons, 1976.
Spring, C., and Sandoval, J.: Food additives and hyperkinesis: A critical evaluation of the evidence. J. Learning Disabilities, *9*:28, 1976.

Anorexia Nervosa
Agras, W. S., et al.: Behavior modification of anorexia nervosa. Arch. Gen. Psychiatry, *30*:279, 1974.
Bruch, H.: Eating Disorders: Obesity, Anorexia Nervosa and the Person Within. New York, Basic Books, 1973.
Crisp, A. H.: Anorexia Nervosa. Br. J. Psychiatry, Special Publ. No. 9, p. 150, 1975.
Crisp, A. H., and Stonehill, E.: Relation between aspects of nutritional disturbances and menstrual activity in primary anorexia nervosa. Br. Med. J., *3*:149, 1971.

Frisch, R. E., and Revelle, R.: Height and weight at menarche and a hypothesis of critical body weights and adolescent events. Science, *169*:397, 1970.
Gull, W. W.: Anorexia nervosa. Trans. Clin. Soc. London, *7*:22, 1874.
Halmi, K. A., Powers, P., and Cunningham, S.: Treatment of anorexia nervosa with behavior modification. Arch. Gen. Psychiatry., *32*:93, 1975.
Kellett, J., Trimble, M., and Thorley, A.: Anorexia nervosa after the menopause. Br. J. Psychiatry, *128*:555, 1976.
Lucas, A. R., Duncan, J. W., and Piens, V.: The treatment of anorexia nervosa. Am. J. Psychiatry, *133*:1034, 1976.
Lupton, M.: Biological aspects of anorexia nervosa. Life Sci., *18*:1341, 1976.
Schmidt, M. P. W., and Duncan, B. A. B.: Modifying eating behavior in anorexia nervosa. Am. J. Nurs., *74*:1646, 1974.

Nutrition and Mental Function
Fernstrom, J. D., and Wurtman, R. J.: Nutrition and the brain. Sci. Am., *230*:84, 1974.
Fernstrom, J. D.: Effects of the diet on brain neurotransmitters. Metabolism, *26*:207, 1977.
Fernstrom, J. D., and Lytle, L.: Corn malnutrition, brain serotonin and behavior. Nutr. Rev., *34*:257, 1976.
Growdon, J. H., Cohen, E. L., and Wurtman, R. J.: Treatment of brain disease with dietary precursors of neurotransmitters. Ann. Intern. Med., *86*:337, 1977.
Kolata, G. B.: Brain biochemistry: Effects of diet (research news). Science, *192*:41, 1976.
Wurtman, R. J., and Fernstrom, J. D.: Control of brain neurotransmitter synthesis by precursor availability and nutritional state. Biochem. Pharmacol., *25*:1691, 1976.

Orthomolecular Psychiatry
Committee on Nutrition, American Academy of Pediatrics: Megavitamin therapy for childhood psychoses and learning disabilities. Pediatrics, *58*:910, 1976.
Hawkins, D., and Pauling, L. (eds.): Orthomolecular Psychiatry: Treatment of Schizophrenia. San Francisco, W. H. Freeman & Co., 1973.
Leff, D. N.: Megavitamins and mental disease. Med. World News, *16*:71, 1975.
Megavitamin and orthomolecular therapy in psychiatry: Excerpts from a report of the American Psychiatric Association Task Force on Vitamin Therapy in Psychiatry. Nutr. Rev., Suppl. *32*:44, 1975.
Pauling, L. et al.: On the orthomolecular environment of the mind: Orthomolecular theory. Am. J. Psychiatry, *131*:1251, 1974.
Winter, S. L., and Boyer, J. L.: Hepatic toxicity from large doses of vitamin B_3 (nicotinamide). N. Engl. J. Med., *289*:1180, 1973.
Wittenborn, J. R.: Premorbid adjustment and response to nicotinic acid. In: Serban, G. (ed.): Nutrition and Mental Functions. New York, Plenum Press, 1975, pp. 213–224.

UNIT THIRTEEN

DISEASES OF THE MUSCULOSKELETAL SYSTEM

Chapter 33

NUTRITIONAL CARE FOR PATIENTS WITH DISEASES OF THE MUSCULOSKELETAL SYSTEM

Diseases of the musculoskeletal system usually affect the nutritional status of the individual by altering dietary intake. Arthritis can make the processes of food preparation and eating very difficult and painful. Dental caries and periodontal disease can make the inflicted individual omit foods that require mastication and thus jeopardize the adequacy of his dietary intake. Immobilization, also discussed in this chapter, can affect food intake but also affects body metabolism and nutritional requirements.

ARTHRITIS

Arthritis may be defined as inflammation of the joints. It has been estimated that at least 20 million people in the United States are afflicted with arthritis of one kind or another. About 5 million suffer from rheumatoid arthritis and another 12 million have some type of osteoarthritis.[2]

Arthritis may be acute or chronic. Any acute attack is of short duration but may recur and develop into a chronic condition. When acute arthritis involves multiple joints, rheumatic fever is a likely cause, particularly in a young person. Arthritis may also be secondary to another disease, such as systemic lupus erythematosus, ulcerative colitis or gout. Rheumatoid and degenerative arthritis are the most common forms of chronic arthritis, and of these two rheumatoid is the more severe.

RHEUMATOID ARTHRITIS

The etiology of rheumatoid or atrophic arthritis is unknown. It is a chronic, debilitating and frequently crippling disease that has tremendous personal, social and economic effects.

Any joint may be affected, but multiple involvement of the small joints of the extremities, most frequently the proximal interphalangeal joints, hands and feet, is the rule. Pain, stiffness and swelling are the common complaints (Fig. 33–1). The swelling or puffiness is caused by the accumulation of fluid in the lining membranes of the joints and inflammation of the surrounding tissues. Several cellular and chemical mediators, including prostaglandins, are probably involved in the inflammatory process.

The incidence of rheumatoid arthritis is re-

668

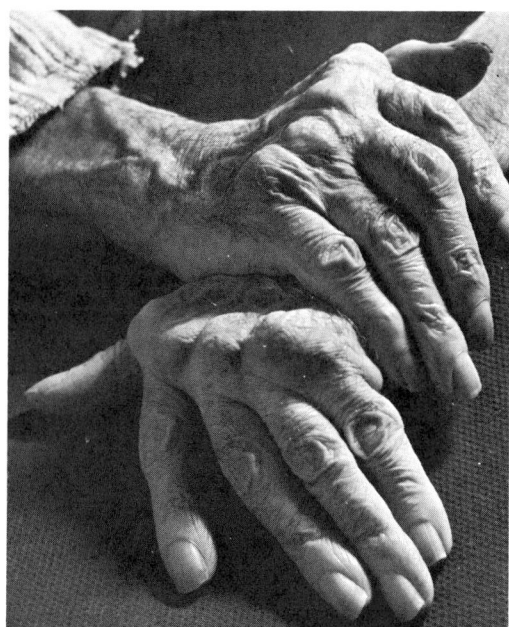

Figure 33–1 A patient with advanced rheumatoid arthritis. Note the twisted hands and the puffiness of the metacarpal joints, typical of the disease. (Courtesy of George E. Pickow, Three Lions, Inc.)

ported to increase twofold in the later decades of life and may reach 15 per cent in females over 60 in some population studies. The average age of onset is 35 years, followed generally by numerous remissions and exacerbations. It occurs much more frequently in females than in males, the proportion averaging three to one. While patients with rheumatoid arthritis are frequently underweight, those with osteoarthritis are often overweight. Because of the chronic disability and pain that accompany arthritis, these individuals are often given unwise or even harmful dietary advice. They become easy prey to the solicitous neighbor, food faddist or charlatan who offers quick and easy cures. The nurse, nutritionist and physician must be alert to this and use every opportunity available to stress good health habits, including a well-balanced diet.

Nutritional Care

Numerous diets have been devised for the treatment of rheumatoid arthritis. At one time or another a low-carbohydrate diet, a high-protein diet, the B-complex vitamins, vitamin C, vitamin A and sulfur have been advocated.

The use of massive therapeutic doses of vitamin D is not recommended because this form of treatment resulted in severe and some-times fatal calcification of the kidneys. Potent vitamin D preparations are capable of causing damage because of the effect of vitamin D on calcium and phosphorus metabolism.

At present, the trend is to treat rheumatoid arthritis with a normal well-balanced diet, with calories adjusted to maintain the patient's weight at normal standards. Since the condition is a chronic disease that frequently hinders the preparation and eating of adequate meals, measures should be used to improve the general health of the patient. It is important to survey the person's dietary pattern and eating habits. The teaching is focused on how the person's intake may be improved in order to have a well-balanced diet and to maintain weight at the desired level.

Low serum pyridoxal (vitamin B_6) levels have been reported in these patients.[14, 16] The low levels may be due to the drug therapy, or the gastric mucosal lesions commonly seen in rheumatoid arthritis patients may increase the need for pyridoxal-5-phosphate.[14] However, when serum pyridoxal levels were raised after B_6 supplementation, clinical symptoms of arthritis did not change.[16]

Low levels of ascorbic acid in white blood cells are also frequently seen in rheumatoid arthritis patients. Possibly this is due to their ingestion of large quantities of aspirin, although how this occurs is unclear.[13] A vitamin C deficiency state may exist in some individuals with cutaneous bruising that improves when they begin to take a vitamin C supplement.[8]

Hypochromic anemia is found frequently associated with arthritis, but it does not always respond well to the administration of iron. However, there is a dramatic response to the transfusion of whole blood.

It is reported that up to 50 per cent of people with rheumatoid arthritis overcome the disease process spontaneously. This is encouraged through a well-directed daily pattern of living, including a well-balanced diet.

Hormones and Drugs

The symptoms of rheumatoid arthritis are usually controlled by large daily doses of aspirin, which is the mainstay of treatment. The side effects of chronic aspirin ingestion are gastrointestinal problems, audiological problems and increased bleeding time (slowing of the clotting mechanism). The gastrointestinal problems can frequently be alleviated by taking the aspirin with food, milk or an antacid.

In 1949 rheumatoid arthritis was found to

respond dramatically to two hormones, corticotropin (ACTH) and cortisone. Corticotropin is released by the pituitary gland and acts by stimulating the adrenal cortex to release cortisone, which relieves pain and stiffness in patients with rheumatoid arthritis. Since then, several synthetic variations of cortisone or of the adrenocorticosteroids, such as prednisone, methylprednisone, hydrocortisone, dexamethasone and betamethasone, have been produced. They are very effective in reducing inflammation and can be given as local injections or taken orally. However, side effects such as cushingoid symptoms, sodium retention, and potassium excretion, gastrointestinal complications, diabetes mellitus, osteoporosis and others are common. Oral corticosteroids are only used after aspirin and other nonsteroidal anti-inflammatory drugs such as indomethacin have not proved to be effective. Nutritional care, in the form of sodium restriction, potassium supplementation or a diabetic diet, may be needed for patients taking steroids. See Chapters 21 and 26 for discussion of the nutritional implications of steroid therapy.

Antimalarial drugs are sometimes of benefit in inducing a remission if other drugs are ineffective. The therapy must be continued for at least six months, and the side effects are serious.

Gold salt therapy can also cause a remission of rheumatoid arthritis. Again, at least six months of therapy are necessary, and toxicity must be continually monitored by measurement of serum gold levels. There are significant dermatological, hematological and renal side effects of this treatment.

OSTEOARTHRITIS (DEGENERATIVE OR HYPERTROPHIC ARTHRITIS)

Osteoarthritis, also known as hypertrophic and degenerative arthritis, is the most common form of arthritis and is almost universal among older people. It probably does not have a single cause but seems to develop from the stresses and strains experienced during the course of one's life. It may follow injuries and other diseases of the joints and be influenced by congenital and mechanical derangements of the joints. Numerous studies have established that the primary lesion is degeneration of the articular cartilage.

The joints most likely to be attacked are the distal interphalangeal joints, the thumb joint and especially the joints that bear the bulk

of the weight: the knees, hips, ankles and spine. In the beginning there is stiffness, usually on arising from a chair or after standing. Later definite soreness may be experienced, which is worse when motion is first attempted but, after warming up, is less noticeable. One or more joints may be affected, and usually symptoms are confined to the afflicted parts. In this respect, the condition differs from rheumatoid arthritis, in which the general health may suffer.

Nutritional Care

Diet is important, especially if weight reduction is necessary. Excess weight means an added burden for the weight-bearing joints. Symptoms have been known to disappear completely after the loss of unnecessary pounds. Thus, the main dietary treatment is to try to acquire and maintain normal weight. (See Chapter 27.) Weight reduction is especially difficult for these patients because the disease limits their exercise potential and caloric expenditure.

Drugs

Except for the oral corticosteroids, the same medications used in rheumatoid arthritis are used to treat osteoarthritis. Corticosteroids may be given as local injections.

Rest, Heat and Physical Therapy

For both osteoarthritis and rheumatoid arthritis the patient should be encouraged to lie down at least once during the day. This takes weight off the joints and allows them to rest. There should also be a regular exercise period, and massage and heat can also relieve pain.

GOUT

Gout is included in the classification of arthritis because of the frequent occurrence of crippling of the joints. In this textbook it is discussed in Chapter 26; it is caused by an inborn error of metabolism.

PROLONGED IMMOBILIZATION

Nutritional Implications

Protein. Prolonged bed rest can result in the development of negative nitrogen balance.

Immobilization of a healthy person leads to an appreciable increase in nitrogen loss. Nitrogen losses in healthy, immobilized subjects average 55 gm. over a 6-week period or as much as 2 to 3 gm. of nitrogen per day when the diet would normally be adequate in protein and calories. To replace 2 to 3 gm. of nitrogen lost, an additional 15 to 20 gm. of protein is needed (N lost × 6.25). On the other hand, debilitated, chronically ill patients will excrete less nitrogen because their bodies adapt to the stress, but they will still be in negative nitrogen balance and nutritionally depleted.

During immobilization the prevention of skin breakdown, decubitus ulcers, infection and negative nitrogen balance requires optimum protein in quantity and quality, sufficient calories and ascorbic acid. A minimum of 70 to 100 gm. of protein (1.2 gm. per kg.) per day is recommended for the average patient, and some patients may require more.

Helping the immobilized patient to avoid skin breakdown is a challenge to nursing care. Adequate dietary management, turning and positioning of the patient and provision of passive exercise for him will help to prevent the adverse metabolic effects of immobility. For more discussion of metabolic response to stress, see Chapter 35.

Calories. The calorie requirement of the individual is of prime importance and is adjusted from time to time according to energy needs. The energy requirement in the acute phase following bone fractures or other types of accidents is usually high. There is a loss of weight due largely to anorexia and the failure of food intake and to the catabolic response on the part of the body to the noxious, toxic or mechanical agents that produced the condition. In the chronic phase and when weight has reached the ideal level, the caloric intake is adjusted to meet requirements for activity. For instance, during physical therapy, which is often required for the rehabilitative process, hard work is involved, and calories should be sufficient to furnish the energy for metabolic demands.

On the other hand, the patient with hemiplegia, quadriplegia or another type of paralysis has a tendency to gain weight. Besides having a decreased caloric expenditure, his intake may be increased because of a need for alternative means of gratification, which may be found in food. Both factors lead to obesity. Once the patient becomes obese, it is difficult to get him to be mobile again. Weight loss is necessary to relieve the load on the muscles during physical rehabilitation and mobilization of the patient.

Vitamins and Minerals. Optimum dietary intake of vitamins and minerals is essential. It has been observed that patients with chronic illness or under stress lose potassium, a mineral important to muscle contraction and strength. (See Chapter 7.)

CALCIUM. Calcium is lost from the bones (osteopenia) following a fracture and during periods of complete bed rest of a few weeks or more. Normally, bone integrity and homeostatic balance are maintained by the weight-bearing and muscle tension produced by normal motion and activity. With immobilization a deossification of bone occurs (Fig. 33–2), and in some patients there is hypercalcemia, hypercalciuria and metastatic calcification of soft tissues such as the kidney. In addition, kidney and bladder calculi can result. Hypercalcemia, although an unusual complication, seems to be more frequent in the immobilized adolescent. This is not surprising considering the bone growth activity of this age group. The clinical symptoms of hypercalcemia are more apparent in a patient who also has a low level of serum albumin, which normally binds calcium. When not bound, more calcium is available in its biologically active form.

The symptoms of immobilization hypercalcemia can occur immediately or insidiously and include anorexia, nausea and vomiting, abdominal cramps, constipation, headache, malaise, lethargy and sometimes polydipsia and polyuria. If these symptoms are not treated, renal insufficiency, hypertension, seizures and hearing loss can result. Hyman and colleagues hypothesize that immobilization hypercalcemia may be more common than is now realized and that vague complaints of anorexia, nausea and abdominal cramps from immobilized patients may be due to hypercalcemia.[7]

The treatment of choice for serum hypercalcemia is mobilization as soon as possible. A diet low in calcium does not seem to be effective in decreasing serum calcium concentration.[7] The calcium intake should remain at a normal level of 600 to 800 mg. per day.

Phosphate supplements have been shown to decrease the level of serum calcium in immobilized patients in the first weeks following immobilization but not after that.[6] Phosphate therapy also does not decrease the bone resorption. It still is not clear whether this therapy is of any value for treating hypercalcemia.

Other therapy includes the use of diuretics

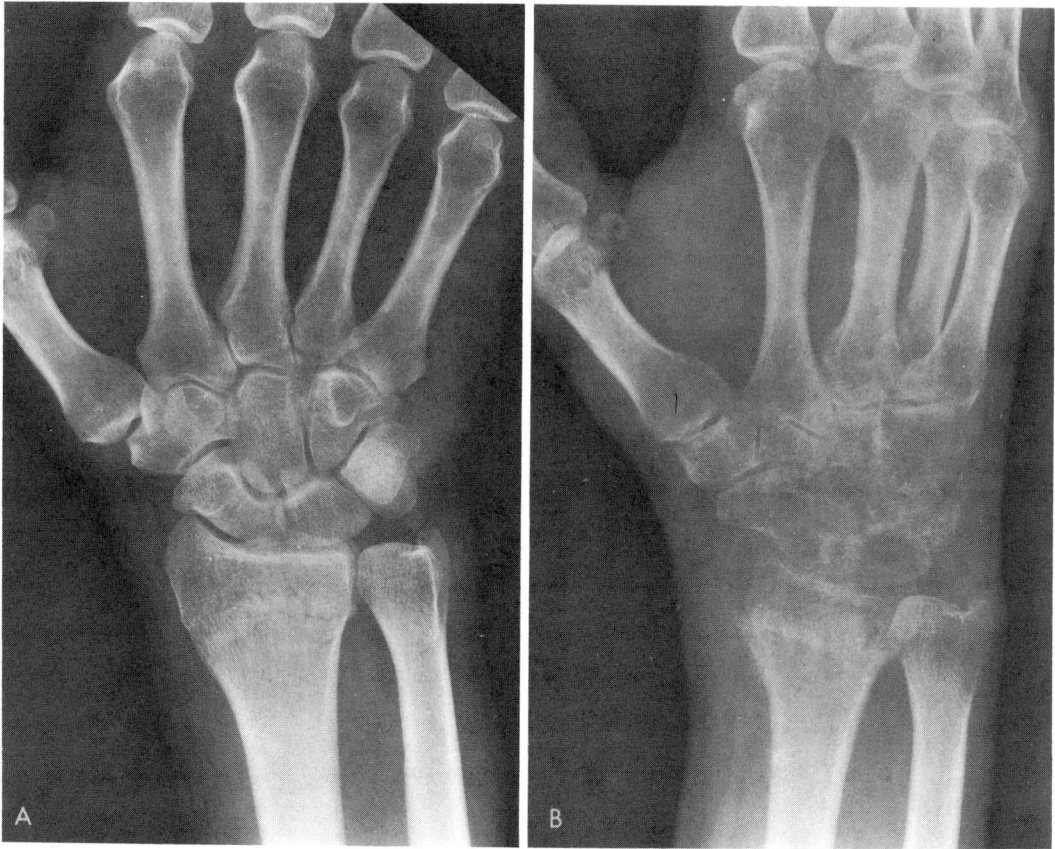

Figure 33–2 *A,* Roentgenogram of the carpal area shortly after fracture of the distal radius. The part was immobilized by a plaster cast. *B,* Roentgenogram of the same area several weeks after immobilization. Note the disuse atrophy of the carpal bones. (From Aegerter, E. E., and Kirkpatrick, J. A.: Orthopedic Diseases: Physiology, Pathology, Radiology, 4th ed. Philadelphia, W. B. Saunders Co., 1975, p. 32.)

and of up to 3 or 4 liters per day of saline fluids to dilute the calcium concentration. Hypomagnesemia and hypokalemia must be watched for when using this therapy.

Bowel and Bladder Training

As mentioned, calciuria may precipitate the formation of urinary calculi (Chapter 30). Poor bladder function may cause urinary infection and may influence the formation of urinary calculi by alkalinizing the urine. An acid ash diet can be used to keep the urine acid. (The acid ash diet is described in Chapter 30.) A high fluid intake is necessary in the prevention and treatment of infection and urinary calculi. Diminished thirst sensation has been observed in these patients. Therefore close attention must be paid to be sure that the person has sufficient fluid intake.

During bladder training for the immobilized patient, fluid is given at regularly spaced inter-

vals throughout the day, and recording the time, type and amount given must be a routine procedure.

During bowel training, a high-fiber diet served at regular intervals is desirable, but too much fiber may cause fecal impaction. Foods causing watery stools should be avoided. A regular time should be set for defecation. For constipated individuals, prune juice given in large amounts may be helpful. (See Chapter 23.)

Feeding the Disabled Patient

All the suggestions of ways to encourage the appetite and provide the essential nutrients apply here. The psychology of feeding is especially important, since most chronically ill and disabled individuals are limited in activity and hence have a greater amount of leisure time to focus attention on meals. Planning the diet with the patient around his customary eating pattern usually attracts his interest and motivation. A

review of his food intake periodically discloses how well the person is following the principles of therapy recommended.

One of the aims in the rehabilitation of the person is to help him become as self-sufficient and productive as possible. The training process usually begins in the hospital or rehabilitation center, depending upon the nature of the illness or injury. His follow-up nursing care in the home may be supervised by the community health nurse. The importance of nutrition is stressed from the beginning. Persons who have difficulty in feeding themselves and in swallowing are often depressed because of this handicap. Food placed on the unaffected side of the mouth beyond the tip of the tongue in paralyzed patients can usually be tasted and swallowed. If the patient is unable to swallow or ingest enough food, tube feedings are available to supply adequate nutrition. Mechanical devices are available for those individuals who have difficulty in using ordinary eating utensils. The Lowman and Klinger[9] reference discusses these. (See Fig. 33–3.) Kitchens have been renovated to heights that are convenient for people in wheelchairs. Guides for streamlining kitchen tasks are available.

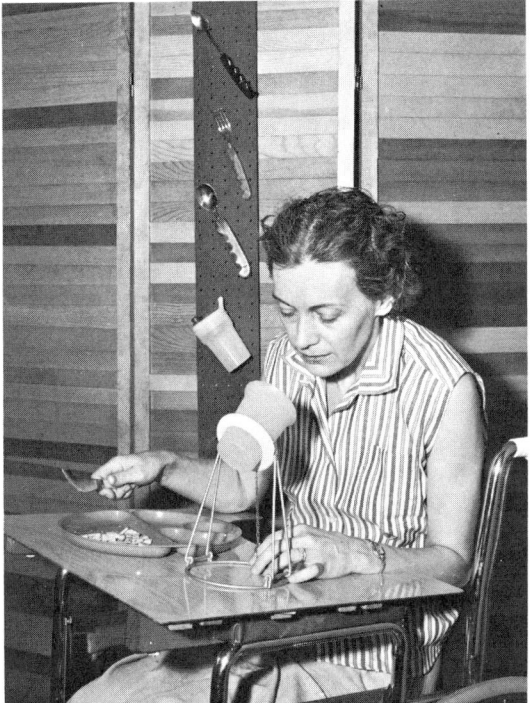

Figure 33–3 Multiple sclerosis patient learning the use of feeding aids at the Treatment Center of the National Multiple Sclerosis Society, Nassau County Chapter, 834 Willis Avenue, Albertson, New York. (Photo by Miyata.)

DENTAL CARIES

Tooth decay is the most prevalent chronic disease in the United States and occurs among all populations throughout the world. Some primitive people such as older Eskimos, some Pacific islanders, Greenlanders and South Africans, who live in remote areas of the world under native or natural conditions, are freer from dental caries than are more civilized people. When these persons come into contact with civilization, they frequently experience an increased incidence of tooth decay. This is believed to be due, in major degree, to a change in their diets, specifically to an increase in their consumption of simple sugar.[15]

Etiology

Dental caries are characterized by demineralization of the inorganic portion and dissolution of the organic substance of teeth. Dental caries are recognized as an infection caused by the cariogenic *Streptococcus mutans*. The carious process begins with the production of acid by bacterial enzymatic action on carbohydrates in the dental plaque, and these organic acids cause decalcification of the enamel. Proteolytic degradation and demineralization

of the dentin follow. (See Fig. 33–4.) It has been shown that three factors must be present simultaneously for dental caries to develop: (1) food, particularly carbohydrate, in the oral environment; (2) a caries-prone tooth and (3) bacteria on the surface of the tooth in the *plaque,* an adherent microbial matrix on the tooth surface.

No one knows why some individuals are more afflicted with dental caries than others. Hereditary influences have been demonstrated in experimental animals. We know that among humans some families have good teeth, whereas others do not. As yet ill-understood

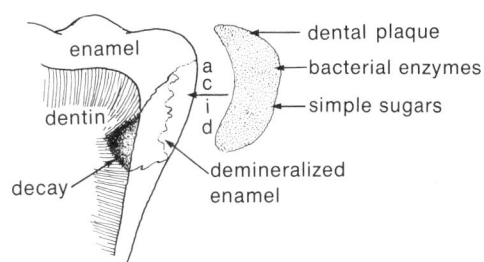

Figure 33–4 Formation of dental caries.

hormonal, immunological and nutritional factors in both the pre-eruptive and post-eruptive phases of tooth development affect later caries development.

Carbohydrates. The current, dominant theory is that decay is caused by a chemical-bacterial action, acting from outside directly upon the enamel and dentin of the teeth. The cariogenic bacteria apparently prefer sucrose, but they can also act upon other sugars to produce an extracellular polysaccharide, dextran, and acids. The acids dissolve the calcium in the tooth to form a cavity. Starches produce very little or no decay in experimental animals and man.[10]

An extensive experiment on the relationship between tooth decay and the form in which carbohydrate is taken was carried out in Vipeholm, Sweden.[5] Under institutional circumstances, patients were given a variety of carbohydrate supplements to the basic, highly nutritious diet. When sucrose in solution was added to the diet over prolonged periods of time, there was practically no increase in the incidence of dental caries. However, when the sugar was fed in the form of sticky candies that adhered to the teeth, the incidence of dental caries increased far above that during the preliminary control period. As soon as these candy supplements were stopped, tooth decay quickly dropped to the control level. In other groups of patients, the sugar was fed in breads, or in less sticky candies. More severe effects were observed than with sugar in solution, but the effects were less severe than with the sticky candies. It is logical to conclude from these observations that the longer the carbohydrate is retained in the oral cavity and available to bacteria for fermentation, the greater the possibility of tooth decay. Thus, the physical characteristics of the carbohydrates determine to a large extent their influence on dental caries.

Frequency of eating is an important factor in caries causation, and between-meal eating is to be discouraged unless noncariogenic foods are consumed. A marked increase in caries development occurs when sweets are consumed between meals.

The rate at which carbohydrate and other bacterial substrate is cleared from the teeth is also important in determining the extent of caries formation. Adequate salivary secretion is an important factor. Vigorous mastication promotes salivary production. For example, patients with damaged salivary function, such as those receiving radiotherapy for cancer,

usually develop an increased number of dental caries.

Protein. Protein is important in dental health because of its role in the development of teeth, salivary glands, oral epithelium, lips, palate and maxillary and mandibular bone. Because tooth development involves the formation of a protein matrix that becomes mineralized, adequate protein must be available during the critical periods of tooth formation. We do not know exactly when these periods of increased protein need occur, but it is probably throughout gestation and during periods of childhood and adolescence. Protein and minerals must be adequate during these times to permit proper development, tooth mineralization and maximum resistive capabilities to later microbial challenge. (See Fig. 33–5.)

Menaker and Navia have shown that the offspring of rats who received a protein-deficient diet during pregnancy had increased susceptibility to caries due to dental and salivary gland abnormalities that could be attributed to protein deficiency during gestation.[11] Part of the salivary gland abnormality was a decrease in the ability to synthesize and secrete salivary proteins, some of which may be antimicrobial agents such as secretory IgA or lysozyme, which are defense mechanisms against microbial invasion.

Fat. Fats form a protective film on the surface of the tooth, have an antimicrobial action

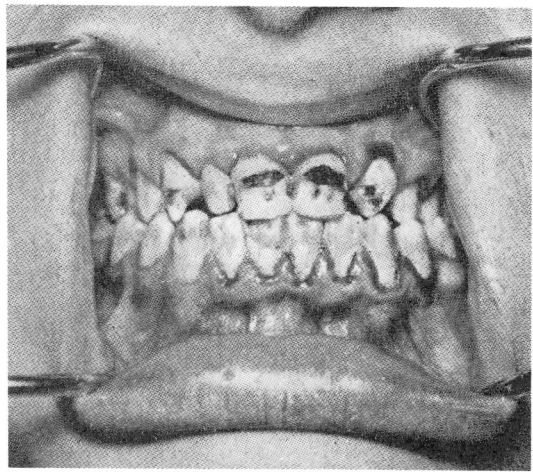

Figure 33–5 Excessive enamel hypoplasia of the anterior teeth of a 16-year-old girl caused by severe malnutrition at the age of 6 months. The marked gingivitis on lower anterior gingiva cleared up quickly as a result of vitamin C therapy. (From: Cahn, L. R.: Pathology of the Oral Cavity. Baltimore, The Williams & Wilkins Co.)

and thereby decrease the caries-producing potential of carbohydrates.

Calcium and Phosphorus. The importance of minerals in the diet, more specifically calcium and phosphorus, has been discussed elsewhere (Chapter 7). Since these minerals make up a large percentage of the enamel and dentin of teeth, an ample amount must be supplied in the diet if the teeth are to be sound. Since major calcification of bones and teeth takes place during the last two months of gestation, it is important that the mother's calcium and phosphorus intake be adequate during this period. It appears that the calcium : phosphorus ratio is important, and phosphorus seems to have a protective effect.

Fluoride. The incidence of dental caries and its relation to the fluoride content of the drinking water has been studied. It would appear from the extensive studies made by the U.S. Public Health Service that minute amounts of fluoride taken during the first 8 to 12 years of life (the period when the dentin and enamel of the permanent dentition are being formed) will reduce the incidence of dental caries by as much as 65 per cent. This increased resistance is believed to be carried over into later life to an appreciable degree. Before the eruption of teeth, fluoride is incorporated into bone in the mineralization process. After eruption it can be applied to the tooth surface, where it is absorbed and so increases the fluoride content of the superficial layers of enamel. It has a protective effect against bacterial action by retarding demineralization and enhancing remineralization. It converts the crystal hydroxyapatite normally present in teeth to fluoroapatite, which is much more resistant to acid demineralization. During gestation the infant does not benefit from the fluoride intake of the mother because fluoride does not cross the placenta in sufficient amounts.[4] The optimal effect of fluoride ingestion is achieved when it is taken in from birth to 18 years of age.

Following favorable results from years of water fluoridation in well-controlled studies[3] in Evanston, Illinois, Newburgh, New York, and elsewhere, fluoride is now being added to the drinking water in a number of cities and communities as a prophylactic agent to reduce the incidence of dental caries. Virtually every authoritative public health and medical organization recommends fluoridation, including the American Medical Association, the American Dental Association and the American Academy of Pediatrics. The level considered to be most protective is 0.7 to 1.2 parts fluoride per million parts of drinking water. When fluoride exceeds 1.5 ppm., as occurs naturally in some areas, mottling of the enamel is apt to occur. (See Fig. 7–8 and the discussion of fluoride in Chapter 7.)

Vitamins. There is no definite evidence that vitamin A is concerned directly with dental caries, but it is a vital factor in the formation of dental enamel and dentin.

There is also no conclusive evidence that lack of any of the B-complex vitamins brings increased susceptibility to decay; however, painful teeth may be due to a neuritis that is secondary to vitamin B deficiency.

Vitamin C is known to be important in building teeth and in maintaining health of gums and other structures, and changes in gum tissue are characteristic of scurvy. However, there has not been satisfactory evidence that susceptibility to decay is reduced by giving vitamin C to individuals on a diet that is partially deficient in vitamin C. Nor has it been found that scurvy makes a person more subject to tooth decay.

Vitamin D may help in caries prevention because it is involved in the calcification of teeth. It promotes greater deposition of calcium and phosphorus, the minerals in teeth.

Prophylactic Nutritional Care

There seems to be agreement that diet and the incidence of dental caries are closely related. The adequate normal diet (Chapter 10) should be followed, with restriction of foods containing readily adherent, fermentable carbohydrates such as sticky candy or other concentrated sweets. Jams, jellies, candies, sugar, heavily sugared beverages or soft drinks and all excessive sweets should be discouraged. (See Table 33–1.) The intake of nonadherent, rough, coarse foods such as raw carrots, lettuce, celery, apples and most fruits and vegetables, which clean the teeth by friction, is suggested to aid control of dental caries. The longer food is in contact with the teeth, the greater the reaction. Thus, it is claimed that the thicker and more gelatinous foods are more likely to cause dental caries than those of thinner consistency.

Since an acid bath is formed on the teeth after every food ingestion, the decalcification can be inhibited for the most part if proper oral hygiene is followed and if the "acid bath" exposures are not too frequent. Brushing the teeth or rinsing the mouth, or both, immediately after each meal or snack will remove the food particles and reduce the reactions. Dentists have discovered that most of the

Table 33–1   APPROXIMATE SUGAR CONTENT OF POPULAR FOODS *

FOOD		AMOUNT	SUGAR CONTENT[a] (tsp.)
Candy[b]	Chocolate bar	1 average size	7
	Chocolate cream	1 average size	2
	Chocolate fudge	1½″ sq. (15 to 1 lb.)	4
	Chocolate mints	1 med. (20 to 1 lb.)	3
	Marshmallow	1 average (60 to 1 lb.)	1½
	Chewing gum	1 stick	½
Cakes and	Chocolate cake	1/12 cake (2 layer, iced)	15
Cookies	Angel food cake	1/12 of lg. cake	6
	Sponge cake	1/10 of avg. cake	6
	Cream puff (iced)	1 avg. custard-filled	5
	Doughnut, plain	3″ diameter	4
	Macaroons	1 lg. or 2 sm.	3
	Gingersnaps	1 med.	1
	Molasses cookies	3½″ diameter	2
	Brownies	2″ × 2″ × ¾″	3
Ice Cream	Ice cream	⅛ qt. (½ cup)	5–6
	Sherbet	⅛ qt. (½ cup)	6–8
Pie	Apple	1/6 med. pie	12
	Cherry	1/6 med. pie	14
	Raisin	1/6 med. pie	13
	Pumpkin	1/6 med. pie	10
Soft Drinks	Sweet carbonated beverage	1 bottle, 6 oz.	4⅓
	Ginger ale	6 oz. glass	3⅓
Milk Drinks	Chocolate	1 cup, 5 oz. milk	6
	Cocoa	1 cup, 5 oz. milk	4
	Eggnog	1 glass, 8 oz. milk	4½
Spreads and	Jam	1 level tbsp.	3
Sauces	Jelly	1 level tbsp.	2½
	Marmalade	1 level tbsp.	3
	Syrup, maple	1 level tbsp.	2½
	Honey	1 level tbsp.	3
	Chocolate sauce (thick)	1 level tbsp.	4½
Cooked Fruits	Peaches, canned in syrup	2 halves, 1 tbsp. syrup	3½
	Rhubarb, stewed, sweetened	½ cup	8
	Apple sauce (unsweetened)	½ cup, scant	2
	Prunes, stewed, sweetened	4 to 5 med., 2 tbsp. juice	8
Dried Fruits	Apricots, dried	4 to 6 halves	4
	Prunes, dried	3 to 4 med.	4
	Dates, dried	3 to 4 pitted	4½
	Figs, dried	1½ to 2 sml.	4
	Raisins	¼ cup	4
Fruits and	Fruit cocktail	½ cup, scant	5
Fruit Juices	Orange juice	½ cup, scant	2
	Pineapple juice, unsweetened	½ cup, scant	2³/₅
	Grapefruit juice, unsweetened	½ cup, scant	2¹/₅
	Grapefruit, sweetened	½ cup, scant	3⅔

* From: American Dental Association, 211 E. Chicago Avenue, Chicago, 60611.

[a] 100 gm. sugar = 20 tsp. = ½ cup = 3½ oz. = 400 calories.

[b] Candy is from 75 to 85 per cent sugar. Popular candy bars are likely to weigh from 1 to 5 oz. and may contain 5 to 20 tsp. of sugar. Adapted from current publications on food values. Courtesy of Dr. Herman Becks, University of California.

chemical reaction takes place within 15 minutes after the meal is started.

Nursing Bottle Caries

This syndrome is commonly seen in children who are given a bottle of milk or sugared liquid to nurse when they go to bed. There is rampant decay of the upper front teeth that begins shortly after the teeth erupt, and if uncontrolled, decay may spread throughout the upper jaw. The lower front teeth usually are spared due to the protective position of the tongue and lip during sucking.

As the child falls asleep with the nipple of the bottle resting against the palate, the liquid spreads over the upper and the lower back teeth. As it covers the teeth it forms a medium that encourages the growth of bacteria. In addition, when the child is asleep the salivary secretion and swallowing decrease, thus adding to the cariogenic environment.

Parents should be told very early about the possibility of caries development caused by a bedtime bottle and should be counseled against this practice. A bottle of water or a pacifier can be given if the child insists. It is important not to start the nursing bottle habit; Rosenstein found that many children who have nursing bottle syndrome as infants develop the later habit of eating carbohydrate snack foods continually throughout the day.[12]

Dietary Factors

There is an important relationship between nutrition and dental caries during the development of the teeth. The greatest hope in preventive dentistry lies in developing teeth that have a high resistance to tooth decay—highly mineralized teeth with a low solubility of enamel. Close adherence to an adequate diet throughout the period of tooth development is of major importance in attaining this goal. This applies both to children and to women during pregnancy and lactation. The minerals from the mother's reserves are drawn upon to meet the demands of the growing, calcifying teeth and bones of the child.

It has been demonstrated that the early development of the teeth is influenced by the amount of calcium, phosphorus, fluoride and vitamins in the diet. Consequently, these substances should be supplied in adequate amounts in the diet during pregnancy and for the infant, the growing child and the adult. An ample supply of vitamin D should be provided daily throughout the period of growth and development. A highly desirable factor in the overall diet planning for the attainment of maximum caries resistance is the availability of a fluoridated water supply.

The status of teeth is often reflected in the general health of an individual. Poorly formed, missing or painful teeth may result in the consumption of an inadequate diet and the bolting of food, followed by impaired digestion and poor health. Many physicians and dentists believe the poisonous products from decayed teeth to be among the causes of chronic diseases that involve the heart, the kidneys and the joints.

Denture patients are apt to avoid foods that are difficult to chew and will resort to soft foods. They tend to avoid meat, raw vegetables, fruit and salads. In counseling these patients the person's dietary pattern is obtained, an evaluation of the adequacy of the dietary practice is determined and a plan within his limitations is developed that will enable him to consume a more adequate diet.

PERIODONTAL DISEASE

Etiology

Much of the confusion about the role of nutrition in the etiology of periodontal disease is due to the fact that a great deal of the research in this area has not been well-conducted because of the many-faceted nature of the disease and its slow progression. It appears that the primary etiological factor in the development of periodontal disease is plaque, which progresses to tartar and dental calculus. This acts as a local irritant to the periodonteum, which becomes inflamed.[1] Also important are several host factors such as age; immunological, nutritional and endocrinological status; local oral irritants; faulty tooth restorations; poor tooth alignment and traumatic occlusion of the teeth. It has been suggested that a low calcium intake and high phosphorus intake may cause a secondary hyperparathyroidism that results in mobilization of calcium from the dental alveoli and periodontal disease. It is unlikely that this is a primary etiological factor, but it might contribute to the progression of the disease.[1]

Unlike dental caries disease, which is closely associated with Western civilization and dietary sucrose, periodontal disease is seen more frequently in malnourished, underprivileged populations. Although periodontal disease is not a nutritional deficiency disease, all would

agree that malnutrition may predispose the host to periodontal disease or modify its severity and progression. The defense mechanisms of the gingival fluid, epithelial barrier and saliva can be affected by nutritional intake and status.

It is impossible to say that there is no role for nutrition in periodontal disease, yet it is equally wrong to say that the nutritional status of the host is always a factor. Nutrition seems to affect tissue resistance, the interaction between tissues and oral microbial agents and the chemical environment of the oral tissues. Each patient should be evaluated individually, and nutritional status should be one of the host factors assessed. (See Chapter 11.)

Nutritional care is particularly important in preparation for and after periodontal surgery, when adequate nutrients are needed to regenerate tissue and maintain an immune response to prevent infection. Chapter 34 discusses the nutritional requirements for wound healing. If the procedure or the wound prevents normal dietary intake for longer than three days, a complete, nutritional liquid diet should be designed and recommended for the patient.

PROBLEMS AND SUGGESTED TOPICS FOR DISCUSSION

1. Make a survey in your hospital of patients who are suffering with arthritis. Classify the types of arthritis. Obtain a diet history from a patient with rheumatoid arthritis. Analyze the diet history for carbohydrate, protein, fat, calories, minerals (calcium, phosphorus and iron) and vitamins. Calculate a meal plan based on the diet treatment outlined in this text for rheumatoid arthritis.
2. Plan a high-calorie diet with an underweight patient who has rheumatoid arthritis with extensive crippling of the hands. Use easy-to-handle and easy-to-eat foods.
3. Plan a reduction diet with an obese patient in your hospital who is suffering with osteoarthritis. Follow his or her progress.
4. Discuss the effects of prolonged immobilization on nutritional status and requirements.
5. Visit the dental clinic in your hospital and obtain a diet history from a patient with severe dental caries. Analyze the diet. Assist the patient to plan the correct nutritious diet and include suggestions for tooth decay prevention.
6. Find out the fluorine content of the water in your community and give a report. Is it low, adequate or excessive?

CITED REFERENCES

1. Alfano, M. C.: Controversies, perspectives, and clinical implications of nutrition in periodontal diseases. Dent. Clin. North Am., 20:519, 1976.
2. Arthritis—The Basic Facts. New York, The Arthritis Foundation, 1976.
3. Ast, D. B., and Fitzgerald, B.: Effectiveness of water fluoridation. J. Am. Dent. Assoc., 65:581, 1962.
4. De Paola, D. P., and Kuftinec, M. M.: Nutrition in growth and development of oral tissues. Dent. Clin. North Am., 20:441, 1976.
5. Gustafsson, B. E., et al.: The Vipeholm dental caries study. The effect of different levels of carbohydrate intake on caries activity in 436 individuals observed for five years. Acta Odontol. Scand., 11:232, 1954.
6. Hulley, S. B., et al.: The effect of supplemental oral phosphate on the bone mineral changes during prolonged bed rest. J. Clin. Invest., 50:2506, 1971.
7. Hyman, L. R., et al.: Immobilization hypercalcemia. Am. J. Dis. Child., 124:723, 1972.
8. Katz, W. A.: Rheumatic Diseases, Diagnosis and Management. Philadelphia, J. B. Lippincott Co., 1977, p. 429.
9. Lowman, E. W., and Klinger, J. L.: Aids to Independent Living: Self-Help for the Handicapped. New York, McGraw-Hill Book Co., 1969, chapters 1 and 2.
10. Massler, M.: Nutrition and dental decay. Food and Nutrition News, 39(5), 1968. (Published by National Live Stock and Meat Board, Chicago, Illinois.)
11. Menaker, L., and Navia, J. M.: Effect of undernutrition during the perinatal period on caries development in the rat. Parts II, III and IV. J. Dent. Res., 52:680–692, 1973.
12. Rosenstein, S. H.: Systemic and environmental factors in rampant caries. N.Y. State Dent. J., 32:400, 1966.
13. Sahud, M. A., and Cohen, R. J.: Effect of aspirin ingestion on ascorbic acid levels in rheumatoid arthritis. Lancet, 1:937, 1971.
14. Sanderson, C. R., Davis, R. E., and Bayliss, C. E.: Serum pyridoxal in patients with rheumatoid arthritis. Ann. Rheum. Dis., 35:177, 1976.
15. Schaeffer, O.: When the Eskimo comes to town. Nutr. Today, 6(6):8, 1971.
16. Schumacher, H. R., Bernhart, F. W., and György, P.: Vitamin B6 levels in rheumatoid arthritis: Effect of treatment. Am. J. Clin. Nutr., 28:1200, 1975.

ADDITIONAL REFERENCES

Arthritis
Aegerter, E. E., and Kirkpatrick, J. A.: Orthopedic Diseases, 4th ed. Philadelphia, W. B. Saunders Co., 1975.
Bienenstock, H., and Fernando, K. R.: Arthritis in the elderly. An overview. Med. Clin. North Am., 60:1173, 1976.
Brassell, M. P.: Arthritis nursing. In: Katz, W. A.: Rheumatic Diseases: Diagnosis and Management. Philadelphia, J. B. Lippincott Co., 1977, pp. 1000–1010.
DePaola, D. P., and Alfano, M. C.: Diet and oral health. Nutrition Today, 12(3):6, 1977.
Howard, M. S.: Energy-saving kitchen. J. Am. Diet. Assoc., 39:201, 1961.
Kaye, R. L., and Pemberton, R. E.: Treatment of rheumatoid arthritis. Arch. Intern. Med., 136:1023, 1976.
Katz, W. A.: Rheumatic Disease: Diagnosis and Management. Philadelphia, J. B. Lippincott Co., 1977.
Ragan, C., and Farrington, E.: The clinical features of rheumatoid arthritis. JAMA, 181:663, 1962.
Symposium on arthritis in older persons. J. Am. Geriatr. Soc., 25:49, 1977.
The diet of patients with arthritis. Nutr. Rev., 21:203, 1963.

Immobilization

Wolf, A. W., et al.: Immobilization hypercalcemia. A case report and review of the literature. Clin. Orthop., *118*:124, 1976.

Dental Health

Brown, W. E., and König, K. G. (eds.): Cariostatic mechanisms of fluorides. Caries Res., *11*(Suppl. 1), 1977.

Bunting, R. W., Jay, P., and Hard, D. G.: A report of the successful control of dental caries in three public institutions. J. Am. Dent. Assoc., *18*:672, 1931.

Drain, C. L., and Boyd, J. D.: Dietary control of dental caries. J. Am. Dent. Assoc., *17*:738, 1930.

Enwonwu, C. O.: Nutrition and dental health. Nutrition News, *39*(1), 1976. (Published by National Dairy Council, Chicago, Illinois.)

Fass, E. N.: Is bottle feeding of milk a factor in dental caries? J. Dent. Child., *29*:245, 1962.

Freeland, J. H., Cousins, R. J., and Schwartz, R.: Relationship of mineral status and intake to periodontal disease. Am. J. Clin. Nutr., *29*:745, 1976.

Mellanby, M.: The chief dietetic and environmental factors responsible for the high incidence of dental caries: Correlation between animal and human investigations. Br. Dent. J., *49*:769, 1928.

Navia, J. M.: Prevention of dental caries: Agents which increase tooth resistance to dental caries. Int. Dent. J., *22*:427, 1972.

Newbrun, E.: The safety of water fluoridation. J. Am. Dent. Assoc., *94*:301, 1977.

Nizel, A. E.: Nutrition in Preventive Dentistry: Science and Practice. Philadelphia, W. B. Saunders Co., 1972.

Protein deficiency and tooth and salivary gland development. Nutr. Rev. *32*:24, 1974.

Shaw, J. H.: Nutrition and dental caries. JAMA, *166*:633, 1958.

Slavkin, H. C.: Current concepts in nutrition, molecular biology and the prevention of periodontal disease. In: Hazen, S. P. (ed.): Diet, Nutrition and Periodontal Disease. Report on the proceedings of a Workshop. Chicago, American Society for Preventive Dentistry, 435 N. Michigan Ave., 60611, 1975.

Symposium on nutrition. Dent. Clin. North Am., *20*(3), 1976.

Symposium. Nutrition in tooth formation and dental caries. JAMA, *177*:304, 1961.

Walsh, D. C.: Fluoridation: Slow diffusion of a proved preventive measure. N. Engl. J. Med., *296*:1118, 1977.

Weiss, R., and Trithard, A.: Between-meal eating habits and dental caries experience in preschool children. Am. J. Public Health, *50*:1097, 1960.

UNIT FOURTEEN
PHYSIOLOGICAL STRESS

Chapter 34

NUTRITIONAL CARE FOR PATIENTS HAVING SURGERY, TRAUMA OR BURNS

The nutritional care before and after surgery plays an important role in the success of the operation as well as in the welfare and comfort of the patient. The duration of disability following surgery, trauma or burns can be significantly shortened, wound healing improved, the number of infections and complications lessened and mortality reduced by providing adequate nutritional support to the patient.

PREOPERATIVE NUTRITIONAL CARE

The actual preoperative nutritional care given a patient will depend largely upon the situation in which the operation is to be performed. If it is an emergency operation, there is little or no time for preliminary dietary treatment. In elective cases, particularly for patients having recent previous surgery, malabsorption, prolonged immobilization, chronic alcoholism, or bizarre eating habits, a nutritional assessment should be made. The patient should be brought to the best possible nutritional state for the operation. Illness and disease prior to surgical intervention may cause patients to restrict their food intake for days or weeks, predisposing them to nutritional depletion and weight loss. In some instances vomiting, diarrhea and bleeding may have contributed further

to the patient's depletion, with marked losses of sodium, chloride, potassium and iron. In other cases there may have been a long period of malabsorption due to disease, and the patient may be depleted in protein, vitamins and minerals.

Preoperative diagnostic procedures and blood tests frequently require that the patient fast or receive clear liquids only, a situation that acts against optimal nutritional intake. On the other hand, patients who are extremely overweight are poor operative risks, and they should lose weight prior to surgery.

Carbohydrate and Protein. In elective surgery it is advisable to administer a diet adequate in calories, high in carbohydrate (300 gm.) content and with ample protein (150 gm.) for a period of 7 to 14 days prior to the operation. The length of the time of preparation is in direct proportion to nutritional depletion or weight loss in the patient. In extreme malnutrition, preoperative preparation may require up to a month. Even using the most intensive means of nutritional rehabilitation, intravenous hyperalimentation, the maximum weight gain possible is 1 to 1½ lbs. per day.

Extra amounts of carbohydrate spare the protein and enable the liver to store glucose and glycogen, an action that exerts a protective function on the liver and helps to prevent postoperative ketosis and vomiting. The added pro-

tein improves the postoperative physiological status.

Vitamins and Minerals. Selection of foods to provide the minerals (especially calcium, zinc and iron) and the vitamins (fat-soluble and water-soluble) is important. See Chapter 7 for further discussion of these requirements.

Food. It is important that the stomach be empty of food at the time of the operation. If food remains in the stomach there is danger of aspiration of vomitus during the induction of anesthesia or upon awakening. In elective cases no food is allowed by mouth for at least six hours prior to surgery. This is usually managed routinely by allowing a light meal the night before the operation and nothing after midnight. In emergency cases it is advisable to perform gastric lavage to remove the stomach contents before starting the anesthesia.

For intestinal surgery the colon should be free of residue to prevent postoperative distention. Low-fiber foods or a liquid diet are given for two to three days preceding the operation, and the patient is given an enema a few hours before going to the operating room. A chemically defined or elemental liquid diet is appropriate for preoperative therapy because it is nutritious yet leaves minimal residue.

Fluids. It is of utmost importance to the safety of the patient that no operation be attempted when the patient is dehydrated. In an emergency fluids can be given parenterally, if there is insufficient time to administer them orally.

In general, intravenous infusions (preoperative, during the operation and postoperative) are administered to maintain fluid and electrolyte balance. Having a needle in the vein during an operation also permits the immediate administration of blood in the event of serious hemorrhage. In cases in which deficiency of specific nutrients may be present, it is important to supplement the infusion appropriately. This is especially true with vitamins C and K. Glucose may be required if the liver glycogen stores are inadequate, as in alcoholic patients. Glucose is also used to avoid insulin shock in diabetic patients.

POSTOPERATIVE NUTRITIONAL CARE

Since it should be individualized and related to the type of surgery performed, the nutritional care for patients following surgery will vary. For example, a patient who had a major stomach operation receives different care from

that given to a patient who underwent a limb amputation.

Whereas the importance of adequate postoperative nutrition is well recognized, oral feeding in the first 24 to 48 hours following surgery can precipitate vomiting and subsequent ileus. Blood, fluids and electrolytes are lost from the body during surgery and further loss could occur through vomiting and drainage. To prevent dehydration and shock during the immediate postoperative period, fluid and electrolytic balances are maintained by intravenous, subcutaneous or rectal infusion.

Although some surgeons may be very specific about the postoperative diet orders for their patients, there are some general principles applicable to all patients who have undergone surgery.

Calories and Protein. For the elective surgical patient the energy requirement postoperatively will increase by only 10 per cent providing that there are no complications. However, if the surgery was preceded by multiple fractures or trauma, the energy requirement will increase 10 to 25 per cent. See Table 35–4 for the increased energy requirements of stressful clinical situations, such as infection, surrounding surgery.

Moderate or severe tissue damage caused either by injury or surgery also leads to an increased excretion of nitrogen and often to considerable loss of body protein. Sepsis, fever, infection, poor circulation and trauma accelerate nitrogen loss further.

If there are not enough carbohydrates and fats to supply calories in the diet, protein must be broken down to carbohydrate and fat to provide energy needs. If there are exudates or discharges, such as occur in peritonitis or open wounds, much nitrogen may be lost daily (6.25 gm. of protein is required to replace 1 gm. of nitrogen lost). There may be some loss of nitrogen through hemorrhage or through excretion from the kidneys. In general, the caloric requirement for most postoperative patients is 35 to 45 kcal. per kg. ideal body weight per day, and the protein intake should be 1 to 1.5 gm. per kg. ideal body weight per day.

Depletion of body protein is very serious. It causes edema, inhibits wound healing, makes the body more vulnerable to infection, renders the liver more liable to toxic damage, impedes regeneration of hemoglobin, prevents resumption of normal gastrointestinal activity and delays the return of muscular strength. It is largely responsible for postoperative weakness and slow recovery.

Vitamins. Ascorbic acid deficiency is associated with the delay or prevention of wound healing and with chronic, non-healing cutaneous ulcers. Vitamin C is required for the formation of collagen precursors and collagen, and 1000 mg. or more daily may be required in extreme conditions. Vitamin A deficiency may also interfere with wound healing because vitamin A is necessary for normal epithelialization. It also helps to prevent gastric stress ulceration. Vitamin K deficiency is characterized by a decrease in prothrombin content of the blood, with a resultant defect in clotting. It is therefore of particular interest in surgery. The B vitamins (thiamin, riboflavin and niacin) provide essential coenzyme factors to metabolize carbohydrate and protein and can be rapidly depleted after major trauma. The requirement for thiamin is doubled in hypermetabolic states such as fever, trauma or hyperthyroidism. Other members of the B-complex vitamins play important metabolic roles in stress conditions.

A healthy person having minor surgery usually does not require vitamin supplements. Patients fasting longer than four days before or after surgery and those having major surgery, especially if poorly prepared for it, usually require therapeutic doses of vitamins.

Minerals. There is evidence that the administration of zinc helps the process of wound healing in patients who have low serum zinc levels. Although its specific role in wound healing is unclear, zinc seems to be necessary for amino acid metabolism and synthesis of collagen precursors. In some patients after adrenalectomy and in those receiving long-term corticoid therapy, there will be decreased serum zinc levels and poor wound healing. Zinc will increase the rate of wound healing in these patients.

Fluids. Immediately following an operation the patient should be supplied with sufficient fluids to maintain normal water and electrolyte balance. At this time, the patient may experience more or less difficulty with the intake of large quantities of water by mouth, and fluids are usually administered intravenously. In many instances, fluids can be given by mouth as soon as the patient has recovered from the anesthesia.

Food. The introduction of food following surgery will depend upon the condition of the patient's gastrointestinal tract. As soon as bowel sounds return after the operation, the patient should be given a clear liquid diet for a few meals. Then a full liquid diet can be given for a day or so, followed by a regular diet or the diet the patient was receiving prior to surgery. To meet the all-important calorie, protein and carbohydrate needs, generous amounts of high-quality protein foods, such as milk, meat and eggs, and simple carbohydrate foods are needed. When the patient cannot tolerate adequate amounts of such foods, protein in the form of supplemental liquids should be given. See Chapter 35.

NUTRITIONAL CARE FOLLOWING GASTROINTESTINAL SURGERY

GASTRIC SURGERY

After gastric surgery, such as partial or total gastrectomy, vagotomy, pyloroplasty, or the Billroth I or II procedure (see Fig. 34–1), all fluids and foods by mouth are withheld for 24 to 48 hours. A parenteral feeding formula made up of glucose, vitamins and minerals and perhaps amino acids may be administered for the first few days and gradually reduced as oral feeding is resumed. The first types of fluids allowed by mouth are ice, which is held in the mouth, or infrequent sips of water. Some patients tolerate warm water better than iced or cold water. When vomiting ceases, larger amounts of fluids may be served. Bland foods can be chosen from those outlined in Table 22–5. More important is offering the patient those foods he likes and can tolerate. By the tenth postoperative day, most patients can tolerate solid foods.

Nutritional impairment frequently occurs after gastrectomy, and many patients have difficulty regaining normal preoperative weight due to one or all of the following: (1) inadequate food intake related in most instances to the dumping syndrome, (2) malabsorption of ingested food, specifically fat and protein or (3) increased metabolic requirements, especially for protein. Patients who have had a total or nearly total gastrectomy often have difficulty in taking large amounts of food and may need to make a permanent habit of eating several small meals a day.

The Dumping Syndrome

The dumping syndrome is a complex physiological response to the presence of undigested food in the jejunum. Following gastric surgery, some patients who have had two thirds or more

COMMON GASTRIC SURGERIES

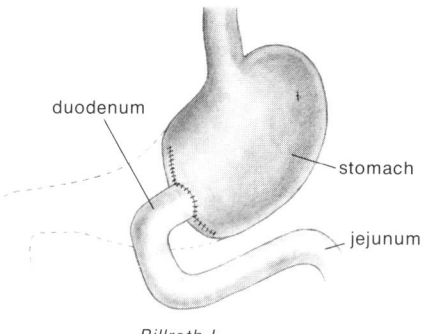

duodenum

stomach

jejunum

Billroth I

gastroduodenostomy
Less dumping than
with Billroth II.

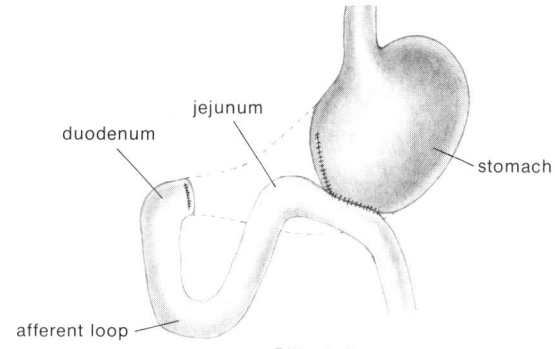

jejunum

duodenum

stomach

afferent loop

Billroth II
gastrojejunostomy

Sequelae such as steatorrhea, weight
loss, dumping, vomiting and bacterial
overgrowth occur more often with the
Billroth II procedure.

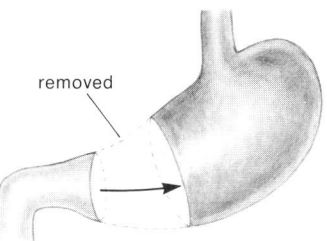

removed

Partial Gastric Resection

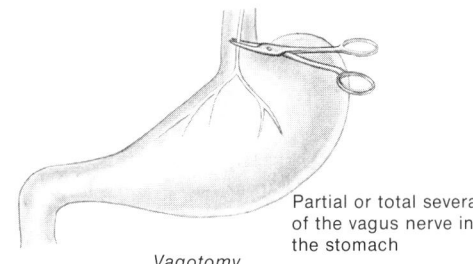

Partial or total severance
of the vagus nerve innervating
the stomach

Vagotomy

Depending on the extent of the
vagotomy, HCl secretion is reduced
and gastric emptying is slowed.
Dumping syndrome does not follow
this surgery.

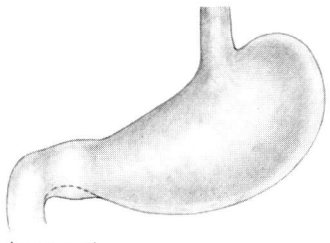

nlargement
f pyloric sphincter

Pyloroplasty

Duodenal reflux frequently
follows this surgery.

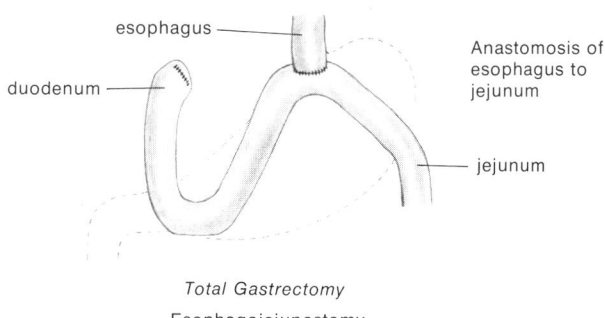

esophagus

duodenum

Anastomosis of
esophagus to
jejunum

jejunum

Total Gastrectomy
Esophagojejunostomy

Figure 34–1 Gastric surgical procedures. (Adapted from: Luckman, J., and Sorensen, K. C.: Medical-Surgical Nursing: A Psychophysiologic Approach. Philadelphia, W. B. Saunders Co., 1974, p. 1091.)

of the stomach removed and have advanced to the full diet regimen may experience the dumping syndrome. After food is swallowed, it is "dumped" into the jejunum about 10 to 15 minutes after ingestion instead of being gradually released in small amounts, and it does not have the benefit of the stomach's participation in the digestive process. Most patients who

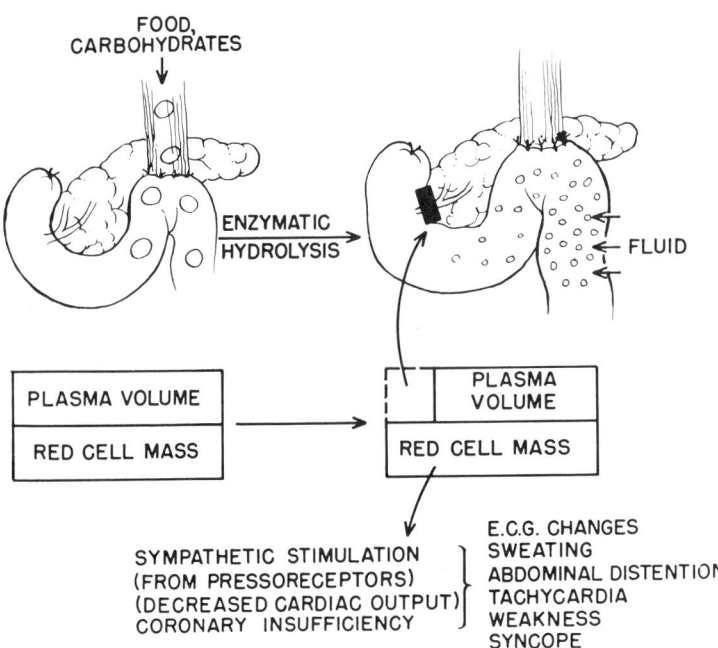

FOOD, CARBOHYDRATES

ENZYMATIC HYDROLYSIS

FLUID

PLASMA VOLUME

RED CELL MASS

PLASMA VOLUME

RED CELL MASS

SYMPATHETIC STIMULATION
(FROM PRESSORECEPTORS)
(DECREASED CARDIAC OUTPUT)
CORONARY INSUFFICIENCY

E.C.G. CHANGES
SWEATING
ABDOMINAL DISTENTION
TACHYCARDIA
WEAKNESS
SYNCOPE

Figure 34-2 Changes occurring in dumping syndrome. (From: Vanamee, P.: Nutrition after gastric resection. JAMA, *172*:2045, 1960. Courtesy of Dr. Parker Vanamee and JAMA.)

undergo this type of surgery develop a new pouch through nature's stretching of the remaining stomach tissue. The ingested foods and liquids are prepared for absorption in the gastric pouch exactly as in the original stomach. However, many patients still develop symptoms of the dumping syndrome.

Symptoms. Some individuals complain of abdominal fullness, nausea and, at times, crampy abdominal pain followed by diarrhea within 15 minutes after eating. Others feel warm, dizzy, weak and faint; their pulse races and they break into a cold sweat. Lying down immediately after eating lessens these symptoms because food remains longer in the stomach pouch. Physiologically, the changes are explained by Figure 34-2.

Rapid entry of ingested nutrients into the jejunum and their subsequent hydrolysis lead to a hypertonic intestinal content. This hypertonic material is rapidly diluted by fluid drawn from the plasma and extra-cellular fluid and leads to a sharp drop in circulating blood volume. Drop in blood volume, decrease in cardiac output and perhaps dilatation of the jejunum lead to a sympathetic vasomotor response producing sweating, tachycardia, electrocardiographic changes and weakness. Serotonin, a vasoconstrictor, and vasoactive kinins, histamine and prostaglandins are thought to be released because of the hyperosmolarity of the jejunal chyme. These substances cause the cramping, hypermotility and diarrhea of the dumping syndrome.

Alimentary Hypoglycemia

Symptoms of hypoglycemia, such as weakness, perspiration, hunger, nausea, anxiety and tremors, can occur from one to two hours after the meal is ingested, in patients who have had gastrectomies. This hypoglycemia is due to the rapid digestion and absorption of the food (especially of carbohydrate) that has been dumped into the duodenum. The glucose rapidly enters the blood stream and causes a postprandial elevation in blood glucose and an overproduction of insulin, which results later in hypoglycemia.

Malabsorption

Following the Billroth II procedure in particular, there is steatorrhea in addition to dumping and hypoglycemia. This is due to pancreatic insufficiency and defective digestion. Because food bypasses the duodenum, the secretion of secretin and pancreozymin by the duodenal mucosa is reduced. Since these two hormones stimulate the pancreas to secrete its enzymes and bicarbonate, there is little pancreatic exocrine secretion when they are not present. Furthermore, pancreatic atrophy and some fibrosis occur.[11]

Anemia

Anemia may develop after gastric surgery, possibly due to iron deficiency caused by bleed-

ing from recurrent ulcers or by impaired iron absorption. Because of rapid stomach emptying, which prevents thorough mixing of food with gastric HCl, iron is not changed to the absorbable ferrous form. Also, because of the surgery, the iron bypasses the duodenum, where 50 per cent of iron absorption takes place.

Iron absorption is improved if the patient lies down after eating or taking an iron preparation. This slows gastric emptying so that the duodenal environment will be more acidic for a longer time and this will enhance iron absorption. For convenience, iron medication and a snack could be taken before bed.

Vitamin B_{12} deficiency may cause the anemia. Because there is a reduced amount of gastric mucosa, intrinsic factor is not produced in quantities adequate to allow complete B_{12} absorption, and pernicious anemia develops. Bacterial overgrowth in the proximal small bowel or in the afferent loop (see Fig. 34–1) binds B_{12} and competes with the body for absorption. The result is a macrocytic anemia that should be treated with B_{12} injections.

Anemia can also result from folate deficiency as part of the general malabsorption syndrome.

Nutritional Care

Because of the problems that accompany eating, post-gastrectomy patients frequently do not eat enough, have diarrhea from the increased intestinal activity and become underweight, malnourished and frustrated. The prime objective of nutritional care is to restore nutritional status and pleasant living for the patient.

Protein and fats are better tolerated than carbohydrates because they are more slowly hydrolyzed into osmotically active substances. Simple carbohydrates—lactose, sucrose and dextrose—are rapidly hydrolyzed and should be limited, but complex carbohydrates such as starches can be included. Liquids enter the jejunum rapidly, and for that reason should only be taken between meals, without food.

Basically, the diet is moderate in fat (30 to 40 per cent of calories), low in simple carbohydrates and high in protein (20 per cent of calories), with the purpose of achieving or maintaining the optimal weight and nutritional status of the patient. Diabetic exchange lists (Tables 25–4 and 25–5) can be used to calculate the carbohydrate intake and to teach the patient about carbohydrate control.

Milk in small amounts is apt to be tolerated better than in large amounts, although some patients may not tolerate it at all. Dried skim milk or various casein hydrolysates may be used and be well tolerated.

Each diet must be adjusted to the patient, based on a careful dietary and social history. Table 34–1 gives the general nutritional care required for patients after gastric surgery.

Alexander[1] recommends the use of a high-protein drink in addition to the normal intake. This allows for a large intake of calories without adverse symptoms. After several years of trial, he found a combination of casein and soy protein to be the most suitable: 2.5 oz. soy protein-casein mixed in 24 oz. water.

GALLBLADDER AND COMBINED ABDOMINOPERINEAL RESECTIONS

Following surgery such as removal of the gallbladder or combined abdominoperineal resections, oral feedings are usually resumed with the return of bowel sounds, and the patient gradually progresses from a liquid to a solid diet. If enteral feeding, either by tube or by mouth, is not possible by the seventh postoperative day, some form of intravenous nutritional support should be started. Some patients who have had the gallbladder removed may be more comfortable on the low-fat diet for several weeks. The usual full liquid diet, moderate in fat (70 to 100 gm. per day), may have to be modified.

Table 34–1 NUTRITIONAL CARE FOR PATIENTS SUFFERING FROM DUMPING SYNDROME AND ALIMENTARY HYPERGLYCEMIA

DUMPING SYNDROME
High-protein, moderate-fat, high-calorie diet.
  1.5–2 gm. protein per kg. ideal body weight (IBW).
  35–45 kcal. per kg. IBW.
Use medium-chain triglycerides if steatorrhea is present.
Lie down for an hour or so after eating.
Drink liquids only between meals.
Avoid those foods known to cause individual problems.
Eat small meals of 4–5 oz. in size.

ALIMENTARY HYPOGLYCEMIA
Avoid concentrated sweets such as candy, sugar, cola drinks, cookies, cakes and ice cream unless made with sugar substitute.
Have concentrated forms of sugar available in the event of hypoglycemia 1–2 hr. after meals.
Eat small meals six times per day.

After pancreatic surgery, the patient usually requires a diet restricted in concentrated sugar to prevent hyperglycemia; pancreatic enzymes with meals; vitamin and mineral supplementation and, possibly, bile salt replacement.

SMALL BOWEL RESECTION

Patients undergo small or large bowel resection for treatment of cancer, diverticulitis, ileitis, local abscess, perforation, mesenteric vascular accidents or obstruction. When more than two thirds of the small bowel is removed, severe metabolic problems and malnutrition are very likely to occur. Weight loss, muscle wasting, diarrhea, rapid gastrointestinal transit time and malabsorption of calcium, zinc, magnesium, fats and iron are common. The syndrome is commonly referred to as *"short bowel syndrome."* The nutritional care for this condition is complex and must be aggressive and anticipatory. Figure 6–9, which shows the sites of absorption of various nutrients, will be helpful in formulating proper nutritional care for these patients.

Malabsorption

Protein nutrition is usually not a problem because protein absorption is efficient even in short lengths of otherwise normal intestine. Absorption may be decreased initially but improves with time. Glucose is also easily absorbed if adequate amounts of intestinal enzymes are present.

Fats are poorly absorbed, and malabsorption may exist for some time, in contrast with the adaptation exhibited by carbohydrate and protein absorption. Besides causing steatorrhea, the unabsorbed fatty acids may saponify calcium and magnesium in the intestine, form "soaps" and prevent the absorption of these two minerals. Fat-soluble vitamins are also poorly absorbed.

Certain other nutrients, such as vitamin B_{12}, which are absorbed mainly in the ileum, will have to be given parenterally if too much of the ileum has been removed. See page 502 for further discussion of the malabsorption syndrome.

Other Effects

Three disorders are secondary to small bowel resection. First, there is *hypersecretion of gastric acid* because there is no inhibitory effect on gastric acid secretion by small intestinal secretions. The gastric acid hypersecretion injures the remaining proximal mucosa and reduces absorption. It also inactivates pancreatic lipase and trypsin, so that fat and protein maldigestion and malabsorption result, and causes an acidic diarrheal stool. Second, *gastrointestinal motility and peristalsis are increased.* Third, in some patients there is *bacterial overgrowth* of unknown etiology.[2] These three complications should be considered in planning nutritional care.

Adaptation of the Remaining Small Bowel

Provided that adequate nutrition is provided both parenterally and enterally for a period of several months, the remaining small bowel will increase its absorptive surface area through dilatation and cellular hypertrophy and hyperplasia.[9] It appears that the nutritional support cannot be entirely parenteral and that nutrients in the gastrointestinal tract stimulate the beginning of the hyperplasia. Gastrin may also be involved in this process.[10] For this reason, oral intake should be started as soon as it can be tolerated, even though most of the nutritional intake comes from parenteral support.

If 15 to 18 in. (38 to 46 cm.) or more of the small bowel is remaining, most likely the person will eventually be able to support himself nutritionally by oral intake alone. If he has less than this remaining, he will probably require permanent parenteral nutrition to supplement his oral intake. See Chapter 35, which discusses permanent parenteral nutrition for patients living at home.

Nutritional Care

In the *first stage* after surgery, nutritional support is totally by parenteral means and may be the only nutritional intake for several weeks or months. Oral feedings at this stage promote hypermotility, diarrhea and fluid and electrolyte loss. The diarrheal stool in this stage is acidic and frequent, and good perianal hygiene is necessary to prevent excoriation.

The *second stage* after surgery begins with a cautious trial of isotonic fluid about four weeks post-operatively, if 20 to 30 per cent (48 to 84 in.) of the small bowel remains. If less than this of the bowel remains, oral intake may have to be postponed another month or so. In this stage small bowel adaptation will take place as the bowel is presented with nutrients by the oral route. Liquids are taken first and then, with a

great deal of support from the dietitian and nurse, the patient begins the slow return to a normal diet. At this point, dilute feedings of an elemental diet are appropriate if the patient can tolerate them. More liquids are added, then some solid foods and later a greater variety of foods. The patient should be told that there will be temporary setbacks and that he or she may not tolerate some foods one week that were tolerated the week before. The patient should not get discouraged, and the diet should just be simplified for a while. If a food is not tolerated at one time, it should be tried again several weeks later. As the oral intake increases, parenteral nutritional support is decreased, but only to the level where the patient can still maintain weight or gain weight if necessary. Antidiarrheal agents and potassium supplements are necessary.

Within three to six months after the bowel resection, it is usually possible to provide the entire intake by mouth, and the patient enters *stage three*. More foods are introduced into the diet. It is helpful if the patient keeps a food diary that can be shared with the nurse and dietitian, who can help to correlate the patient's digestive problems with possible dietary intake. During this stage it is advisable to avoid alcohol and caffeine for at least a year following surgery, because they stimulate gastrointestinal activity. Six to eight small meals daily are usually better tolerated than three larger meals.

Many of these patients receive narcotics for several months postoperatively to decrease gastrointestinal motility. They can become addicted to these drugs, and this should be monitored; narcotic requirements should decrease progressively after surgery. Excessive use of narcotics manifests itself as abdominal distention, cramping, vomiting, poor dietary intake and progressive weight loss. The situation must be differentiated from dietary intolerance and treated accordingly.

ILEOSTOMY OR COLOSTOMY

An ileostomy is frequently performed to treat severe ulcerative colitis, Crohn's disease or colonic cancer. The entire colon, rectum and anus can be removed *(ileostomy)* or just the rectum and anus *(colostomy)*, so that the intact intestine must be brought through the abdominal wall to allow for defecation. The opening, or *stoma*, eventually becomes about the size of a nickel. The output from the stoma will depend on its location in the colon. The consistency of the stool from an ileostomy will be liquid, while that from a colostomy can range from mushy to fairly well-formed. (See Fig. 34–3.)

Patients who have an ileostomy or colostomy learn to observe their stools to determine which foods to eliminate in order to have good control of bowel movements. Each person must learn which foods to avoid, and this differs with individuals. Usually corn and dried beans are not tolerated. The nurse and dietitian can be of great assistance in helping to establish good eating habits and an adequate dietary intake.

One of the biggest concerns of the patient with an ileostomy is odor. The usual ileostomy stool has a weakly acidic odor that is not unpleasant. A malodorous stool is usually caused by steatorrhea or by bacteria acting on particular foodstuffs to produce odorous gas. Items that seem to be particular odor-causers are onions, cabbage, highly spiced foods, fish, antibiotics and some vitamin-mineral supplements. Persistent odor may be due to poor stoma hygiene or to an ileostomy complication that allows bacterial overgrowth in the ileum. Deodorants are available, but placing an aspirin in the ostomy pouch is almost as effective.[5]

Gas production is another gastrointestinal function that is more noticeable in the ostomy patient. The pouch can become tense and distended, and accidental dislodgment is likely. The nutritional recommendations in Chapter 23 for reducing flatulence may be helpful.

Ileostomy adaptation does occur, and fecal losses will lessen and stools will become firmer.

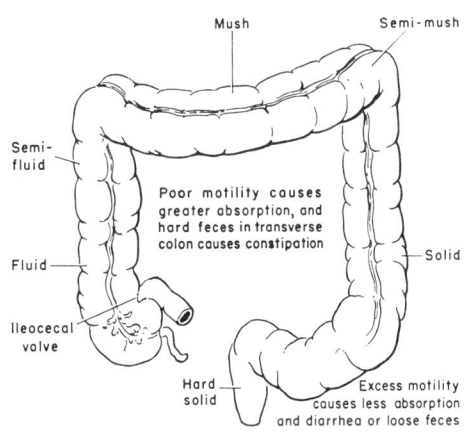

Figure 34–3 As the feces move from the ileocecal valve to the anus, water is absorbed and the feces become more solid. The characteristics of the output from a colostomy will depend on its location in the colon. (From: Guyton, A. C.: Textbook of Medical Physiology, 5th ed. Philadelphia, W. B. Saunders Co., 1976, p. 864.)

This usually happens in 7 to 10 days. It does not happen to the same extent in patients who have an ileal resection in addition to the ileostomy. Their ileal output will be about 2 to 5 times greater than that of the patient who has only an ileostomy.[6]

The patient with a normal, well-functioning ileostomy will not become nutritionally depleted. However, in instances of high ileal output and chronic ileostomy diarrhea, fluid and electrolyte losses can occur and will need replacement. Patients who also have an ileal resection will need vitamin B_{12} supplementation. A B_{12} depletion may result in patients with only an ileostomy if there is an imbalance in small bowel flora and vitamin B_{12} absorption.

Since it is possible for a food bolus to get caught in the ileum at the point where it narrows as it enters the abdominal wall, it is important to caution the patient to avoid very fibrous vegetables and to chew all food well. Other than this, ileostomy and colostomy patients should be encouraged to follow their normal diet, omitting only those particular foods known to cause them problems.

Patients with a colostomy or an ileostomy require considerable sympathetic understanding from the nurse and the entire medical, surgical and dietary team. It is difficult for the person to accept his condition and the problems involved in maintaining bowel regularity. Plans to have these patients meet other people who have undergone similar surgery will help them to adjust to the new problems by comparing and discussing the difficulties involved. Eventually most patients are aided by the realization that in the future they will not have frequent gastrointestinal illness, multiple hospitalizations or chronic disabilities.

RECTAL SURGERY

Following rectal surgery such as hemorrhoidectomy, nutritional care should be directed toward maintaining an intake that will allow for wound repair, prevent frequent stools so that the wound can heal and prevent infection of the wound by feces. A minimal-residue diet and the use of constipating drugs are indicated. Elemental diets or chemically defined diets are effective because they are lowest in residue, but nutritious oral diets are available. Using these diets, stool volume and frequency can be reduced to as little as 50 gm. every six days. Such diets can make the surgical construction of a temporary diverting colostomy unnecessary.[4] Chapter 35 discusses chemically

defined diets. The minimal-fiber diet in Table 23–4 can be started by about the tenth day postoperatively, depending on the severity of the surgery. A normal diet is resumed when it can be tolerated, and the patient is instructed about eating a high-fiber diet to avoid constipation. Table 23–2 gives a high-fiber diet.

FISTULA OF THE INTESTINAL TRACT

A *fistula* is an abnormal passage between two internal organs or leading from an internal organ to the surface of the body. Fistulas occur as a result of prenatal developmental error or are caused by trauma or inflammatory or malignant disease processes. Fistulas of the intestinal tract can be serious threats to the nutritional status of the patient because large amounts of fluid and electrolytes are lost, and malabsorption and infection can occur. Fluid and electrolyte balance must be restored, infection brought under control and aggressive nutritional support provided to allow for closure of the fistula and wound. It is absolutely necessary to start total parenteral nutrition or a minimal-residue, chemically defined diet within a few days after the fistula appears. (See Chapter 35.) These feeding methods will allow time for the physician to search for any undrained abscesses. Only after all other sites of infection have been treated will the fistula close and the patient make progress in weight gain and protein synthesis.

TONSILLECTOMY

Following a tonsillectomy, very cold and very mild-flavored foods bring the most comfort to the patient and offer the most protection against bleeding of the surgical area. Because the convalescent period is comparatively short, the nutritional adequacy of the diet is not so important.

For the first 24-hour postoperative period, these foods are recommended:

Cold milk
Milk beverages, such as malted milk and eggnogs
Chocolate and vanilla ice cream
Fruit ice
Pear, peach or prune juice

The following foods are usually added to the diet by the second day. Warm fluids and food may be started and cautiously replaced by hot foods as healing progresses.

Strained soups
Jellied consommé
Enriched refined cooked cereals
Soft-cooked or poached egg
Milk toast (no crust)
Soft puddings, custard, milk-rennet puddings
  and gelatin desserts
Mashed potatoes and strained vegetables
Finely ground chicken or meat in broth or gravy;
  creamed fish
Fruit purée (whips)

The patient will gradually return to the normal diet within a week to ten days.

SURGERY OF THE MOUTH OR ESOPHAGUS

After extensive surgery of the mouth or esophagus, parenteral feedings are usually administered at first, followed by feedings given by nasogastric tube or by direct tube feeding into the jejunum or stomach, depending on the operative area. Since the patient may have to stay on such a schedule for a long period or even permanently, it is of utmost importance that the formula be adequate in all nutrients. In either tube feedings or liquid diets, variety can be obtained by liquefying normally solid foods, such as potatoes, chopped meat, vegetables and fruit purées, in a food blender or by forcing them through a sieve and adding liquids. An additional advantage of tube feeding whole foods to the long-term patient is that several trace minerals, for which at present there are no recommended allowances, are included naturally. (See Table 35–8.) Commercial preparations of strained baby foods are widely available for use when labor or the special devices needed for preparation are lacking.

The success of giving adequate nourishment to these patients is largely dependent upon the attention and encouragement the patients receive. Attractive dishes and service are important to stimulate appetites.

NUTRITIONAL CARE FOLLOWING FRACTURES AND OTHER MECHANICAL TRAUMA

Following fractures of the long bones there is an increase in protein breakdown in well-nourished individuals, which is aggravated still further by prolonged immobilization in bed. The loss of protein (loss of nitrogen) is accompanied by losses of potassium, phosphorus and sulfur. Development of osteoporosis will coincide with loss in calcium due to immobilization. Severe functional imbalance and loss of fluids and electrolytes may take place.

In addition, there is a 10 to 20 per cent increase in energy requirements, which may go as high as 50 per cent if the patient also has an infection. Figure 34–4 summarizes the metabolic changes that take place after an injury or burn.

Nutritional Care

Replacement of losses is the aim of diet therapy. During the first four to five days after the injury it is necessary to maintain blood volume and electrolyte balance, and aggressive nutritional support is not important in this period. About 400 to 600 kcal. are supplied as intravenous glucose, and a 3 per cent amino acid solution may also be used. After this time, attention should be focused on nutritional support to help the patient resist infection, heal the wound, regain muscular strength and prevent weight loss. Protein, calories and all other nutrients should be supplied in liberal amounts. About 150 gm. of protein and 3000 kcal. are recommended. The calorie intake would not have to be this high in overweight patients, since their caloric reserve in the form of fat is greater. Nitrogen balance could probably be achieved in these patients with 2000 kcal.

If the patient cannot eat an adequate amount at meals, high-protein, high-calorie beverages can be served between meals. A tube feeding is necessary for comatose patients or for patients unable to take food by the normal route. In cases of gastrointestinal injury, the tube will have to be placed at a point below the injury so that food can still be absorbed. If the tube is located in the jejunum or lower, a chemically defined formula diet that requires minimal digestion is used. Sometimes pancreatic enzymes or bile salt solutions will be given with the meals. These will assure digestion and absorption of nutrients if the pancreas or biliary tract has been injured.

Parenteral nutrition is indicated if adequate nutrition by the gastrointestinal route is impossible. It may be given as either peripheral vein supplementation or central vein total nutrition. (See Chapter 35.) If the injury results in renal failure, the essential amino acids should be given intravenously to prevent uremia and additional catabolism of protein. (See Chapter 30.)

Fractures heal poorly when the tissues are depleted. A liberal amount of protein in the diet

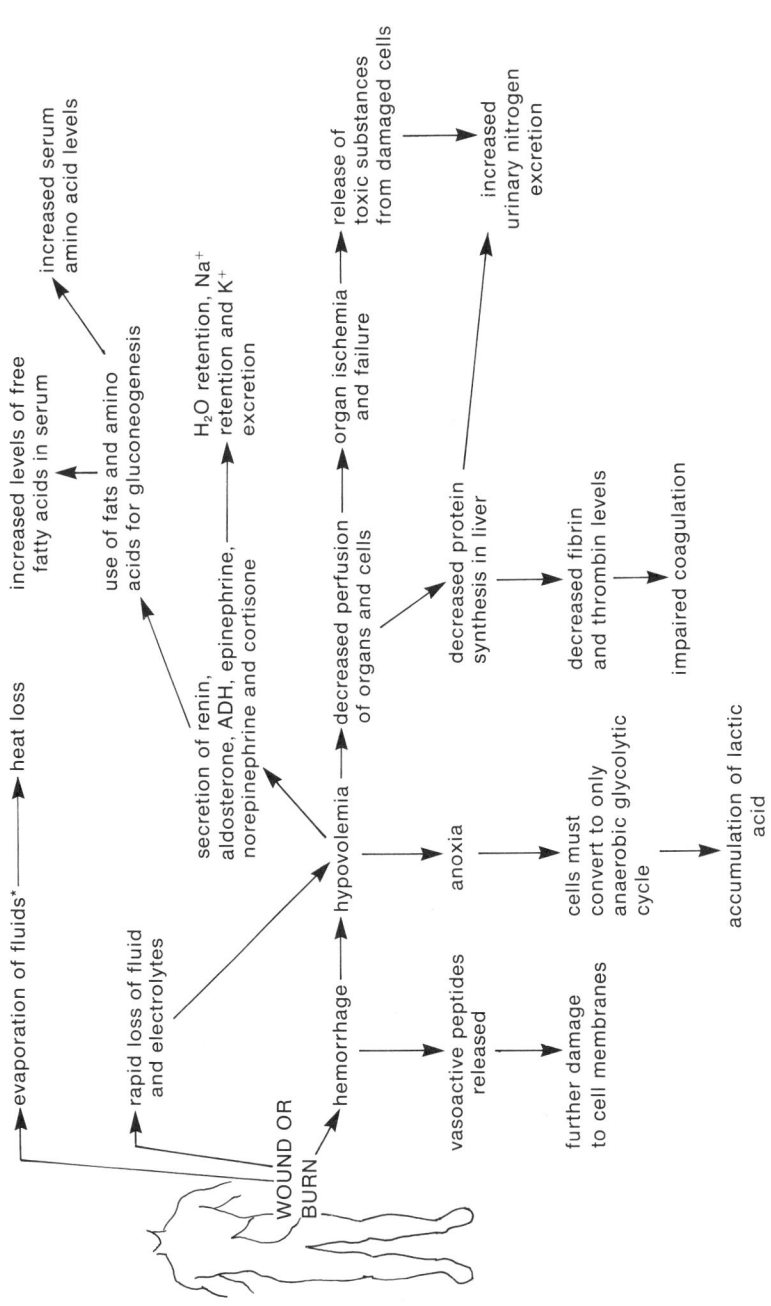

Figure 34–4 Physiological and metabolic changes after an injury or burn. The extent of these changes depends on the severity of the trauma.

*Mainly occurs in the patient with extensive burns

favors deposition of calcium in the bones and the formation of good callus.

NUTRITIONAL CARE FOLLOWING EXTENSIVE BURNS

Severe burns present a difficult problem in nutritional therapy because of the quantity of nutrients required, neurohormonal catabolic changes, gastrointestinal dysfunction, increased insensible water loss, increased heat loss and anorexia. (See Fig. 34–4.) Nitrogen excretion following major burns is considerably greater than that following multiple fractures or elective surgical operations, and vast quantities of protein can be lost, depending upon the extent and depth of the burn. If infection develops, the nitrogen losses are even greater.

In addition to losses of protein, fluid and electrolytes (especially potassium and sodium chloride) are lost through exudation. Anemia may be an additional problem.

Fluid and Electrolyte Replacement

In the average adult with burns over 50 per cent of the body surface area (BSA), the hourly fluid loss may be more than 10 times greater than normal. The "rule of nines" or the Lund and Browder chart[7] can be used to determine the percentage of BSA burned. The initial consideration in treatment is fluid and electrolyte replacement. Seven to 10 liters per day may be needed.

The provision of adequate fluid and electrolytes is paramount for maintaining circulatory volume and preventing acute renal failure. If the burns are treated by soaking with silver nitrate, electrolytes will be leached out through the burn wound, which necessitates continuous replacement of fluids and electrolytes.

The anemia that results from severe burns necessitates giving therapeutic doses of iron. Prevention of tissue depletion is essential for successful skin grafting. Studies also suggest that burn wound healing is enhanced by the administration of zinc in the form of zinc sulfate.

Nutritional Care

In the first five to seven days after being burned, the patient is hypercatabolic and will not retain much of the protein given to him, so nutrition is not the focus of attention in this first week. However, after a week nutritional support should be started. For six to eight weeks

following a burn, the patient has a high rate of metabolism. The resting metabolic rate may be increased as much as 50 to 125 per cent. The increase in metabolism is caused by the increased release of catecholamines and is directly related to the extent of the burn.

Calories and Protein. Calorie requirements depend on the weight of the individual before being burned and the extent of the injury. The minimum caloric requirements are determined by the following formula:[3]

25 kcal./kg. IBW/day + 40 kcal. × % total BSA burned

This example illustrates the application of the formula:

83-kg. man burned in an automobile accident
50% of BSA has been burned
Caloric requirements = 25 kcal. × 83 kg. + 40 kcal. × 50
= 2075 kcal. + 2000 kcal.
= 4075 kcal. per day

A formula to determine protein requirements is as follows:

1 gm. protein/kg. IBW + 3 gm. protein × % total BSA burned

Using the same example, this man's protein requirements are:

Protein requirements = 1 gm. protein × 83 kg. + 3 gm. protein × 50
= 83 gm. protein + 150 gm. protein
= 233 gm. protein

Every effort should be made to prevent the loss of more than 10 per cent of the patient's pre-burn weight. If profound weight loss ensues, death is inevitable. The high-protein, high-calorie, high-vitamin diet should be started as soon as cardiac output has been restored, diuresis occurs and gastrointestinal motility returns. Efficient protein utilization requires simultaneous administration of potassium, especially in the burned patient who has had large potassium losses. Phosphorus requirements may also be increased.

Supplementary between-meal beverages that are high in protein and calories are necessary, because the patient is usually unable to take an adequate amount of the regular foods.

Table 34–2 NUTRITIONAL CARE FOR BURNED PATIENTS

1. Hospitalization in a warm environment with 20 to 30 per cent humidity.
2. Covering of wounds to prevent fluid loss.
3. Calorie allowance of 50 to 90 kcal./kg. pre-burn weight/day, depending on the extent of the burn or the presence of infection.
4. Protein allowance of 2 to 3 gm./kg. pre-burn weight/day, or more, depending on the extent of the burn or presence of infection.
   Adult: 1 gm. protein/kg. IBW + 3 gm. protein × % total BSA burned
   Child: 3 gm. protein/kg. IBW + 1 gm. protein × % total BSA burned
5. Vitamin and mineral supplementation.
6. Physical therapy to promote muscle nitrogen retention.
7. Antacids and frequent feedings to prevent development of Curling's ulcers.
8. Use of supplements, tube feedings, parenteral nutrition or a combination of these as necessary to meet the patient's requirements.
9. Service of attractive, appetizing food in a pleasing, supportive environment.

See Table 35–5. The patient's weight and his calorie and protein intakes must be recorded. Intake should be 50 to 90 kcal. per kg. pre-burn weight per day and 2 to 3 gm. or more protein per kg. per day. If a week after the burn the patient cannot eat enough food to meet these requirements, a method of artificial feeding should be started. Most patients with burns over 40 per cent or more of their BSA cannot meet their needs by oral intake alone.

Tube feedings are given if the patient is unable to eat or drink the large quantity of food required. However, tube feedings may also have to be supplemented by intravenous nutrition, since only 3000 or so calories can be given in a tube feeding. Milk-based tube feedings may cause diarrhea because of post-traumatic lactose intolerance. Total parenteral nutrition may be necessary in some cases. (See Chapter 35.)

Vitamins should be supplied in amounts that are 5 to 10 times the RDA. At least 1 gm. of vitamin C is needed daily.

Ancillary Measures

Administration of *human growth hormone* can increase the effectiveness of intravenous feeding regimens because it increases the level of insulin, an anabolic hormone.

Physical therapy facilitates the incorporation of nitrogen into muscle, and provision of a *warm environment* minimizes heat loss and the expenditure of kcalories to maintain body temperature. The room should be 30°C., about 5 degrees higher than the usual hospital room temperature of about 25°C.

Antacids should be given to patients with burns covering more than 35 per cent of BSA to prevent formation of Curling's ulcer in the gastric or duodenal mucosa. Although the reason for the development of this ulcer is unknown, it appears that through ischemia there is a break in the gastric mucosa, which when aggravated by excessive gastric acid secretion develops into an ulcer. The administration of antacids has been shown to be effective in preventing these ulcers.[8] Table 34–2 summarizes nutritional care for burned patients.

PROBLEMS AND SUGGESTED TOPICS FOR DISCUSSION

1. List the principles of preoperative and postoperative nutritional care and give the reasons for this care.
2. Interview a patient who has had a partial or total gastrectomy. Does he or she have symptoms of the dumping syndrome? Alimentary hypoglycemia? Malabsorption? Describe the patient's symptoms. What changes would you recommend in the present diet?
3. Keep a record of the food ingested in one day by a patient who has had a colostomy. Is the intake meeting the patient's nutritional requirements? What changes will need to be made? Are there any nutrients that this patient may not be absorbing properly because of the surgery?
4. Prepare a nutritional care plan for a patient with burns over 25 per cent of her body. Define the nutritional requirements and how they will be met. What teaching will be necessary?

CITED REFERENCES

1. Alexander, H. C.: A protein dietary supplement for the severe dumping syndrome. Surg. Gynecol. Obstet., *141*:863, 1975.
2. Curreri, P. W., and Richmond, D.: Nutritional management following massive small bowel resection. Dietetic Currents, *1*(4), 1974.
3. Curreri, P. W., et al.: Dietary requirements of patients with major burns. J. Am. Diet Assoc., *65*:415, 1974.
4. Gordon, P. H.: The chemically defined diet and anorectal procedures. Can. J. Surg., *19*:511, 1976.
5. Hill, G. L.: Ileostomy: Surgery, Physiology, and Management. New York, Grune & Stratton, 1976, p. 59.
6. Hill, G. L.: Impairment of "ileostomy adaptation" in patients after ileal resection. Gut, *15*:982, 1974.

7. Lund, C. L., and Browder, N. C.: The estimation of areas of burns. Surg. Gynecol. Obstet., *79*:352, 1944.
8. McAlhany, J. C., Czaja, A. J., and Pruitt, B. A.: Antacid control of complications from acute gastroduodenal disease after burns. J. Trauma, *16*:645, 1976.
9. Scheflan, M., et al.: Intestinal adaptation after extensive resection of the small intestine and prolonged administration of parenteral nutrition. Surg. Gynecol. Obstet., *143*:757, 1976.
10. Stimulus for hyperplasia of the small bowel. Nutr. Rev., *34*:345, 1976.
11. Tympner, F., et al.: The function of the exocrine pancreas after exogenous and endogenous stimulation in Billroth II patients. Acta Hepatogastroenterol., *23*:444, 1976.

ADDITIONAL REFERENCES

Surgical Conditions
American College of Surgeons, Committee on Pre and Postoperative Care: Manual of Surgical Nutrition. Philadelphia, W. B. Saunders Co., 1975.
Bury, K.: Carbohydrate digestion and absorption after massive resection of the small intestine. Surgery, *135*:177, 1972.
Himal, H. S., et al.: The importance of adequate nutrition in closure of small intestinal fistulas. Br. J. Surg., *61*:724, 1974.
Gurry, J. F., and Ellis-Pegler, R. B.: An elemental diet as preoperative preparation of the colon. Br. J. Surg., *63*:969, 1976.
Lee, P. W. R., et al.: Zinc and wound healing. Surg. Gynecol. Obstet., *143*:549, 1976.
Mason, E. E.: Fluid, Electrolyte and Nutrient Therapy in Surgery. Philadelphia, Lea & Febiger, 1974.
McClelland, R. N.: Surgical treatment of peptic ulcer and postgastrectomy complications. In: Dietschy, J. M., and Sanford, J. P. (eds.): Disorders of the Gastrointestinal Tract, Disorders of the Liver, Nutritional Disorders. New York, Grune & Stratton, Inc., 1976, pp. 102–111.
Scott, H. W., et al.: The dumping syndrome. Gastroenterology, *37*:194, 1959.
Tilston, W. J.: The effects of environmental conditions on the metabolic requirements after injury. In: Lee, H. A. (ed.): Parenteral Nutrition in Acute Metabolic Illness. New York, Academic Press, 1974, pp. 167–177.
Trunkey, D., Grzyb, S., and Sheldon, G. F.: Nutrition and Trauma. Intake: Perspectives in Nutrition. Norwich, New York, Eaton Laboratories, 1973.
Vanamee, P.: Nutrition after gastric resection. JAMA, *172*:2045, 1960.
Webster, M. W., and Corey, L. C.: Fistulae of the intestinal tract. Curr. Probl. Surg., *13*(6), 1976.
Wright, H. K., and Tilson, M. D.: Postoperative Disorders of the Gastrointestinal Tract. New York, Grune & Stratton, 1973.

Burns
Artz, C. P.: Guide to assessment and management of burns. Hospital Medicine, *13*:105, 1977.
Davies, J. W. L., and Liljedahl, S. O.: The effect of environmental temperature on the metabolism and nutrition of burned patients. Proc Nutr. Soc., *30*:165, 1971.
Feller, I., et al.: The team approach to total rehabilitation of the severely burned patient. Heart Lung, *2*:701, 1973.
Larkin, J. M., and Moylon, J. A.: Complete enteral support of thermally injured patients. Am. J. Surg., *131*:722, 1976.
Liljedahl, S. O., and Birke, G.: The nutrition of patients with extensive burns. Nutr. Metab., *14*(Suppl.):110, 1972.
Moncrief, J. A.: Burns. N. Engl. J. Med., *288*:444, 1973.
Newsome, T. W., Mason, A. D., and Pruitt, B. A.: Weight loss following thermal injury. Ann. Surg., *178*:215, 1973.
Wilmore, D. W., et al.: Catecholamines: Mediator of the hypermetabolic response to thermal injury. Ann. Surg., *180*:653, 1974.

Chapter 35

THE METABOLIC STRESS RESPONSE AND METHODS FOR PROVIDING NUTRITIONAL CARE TO STRESSED PATIENTS

In the previous chapter the physiological stress associated with surgery, trauma and burns and the nutritional care necessary for these conditions were discussed. In this chapter we will explore the metabolic response to physiological stress and the effect of infection or starvation added to this stress. Parenteral and enteral feeding techniques to meet the high nutritional requirements of these conditions will also be discussed. These techniques can be used to meet the nutritional needs of patients who are either unable or unwilling to take regular food or who cannot meet their nutritional requirements with the usual oral intake.

STARVATION

Adaptive Response to Starvation

It is important to understand the normal response to starvation before discussing the response when physiological stress is also present. In the normal adult the available stored energy amounts to about 200 gm. of glycogen, 6000 gm. of protein and 15,000 gm. of fat. Obviously, the fat component varies the most among individuals. When a person starves, the glycogen stores are used first as glycogenolysis takes place for the synthesis of blood glucose. These stores, which supply about 800 kcal., are usually exhausted within 15 to 20 hours. After that, protein from skeletal muscles is mobilized, converted to glucose in the liver and released into the blood stream to maintain the blood glucose level. Initially, the body may use as much as 75 gm. of protein per day in maintaining the blood glucose concentration. This protein must have the nitrogen (N) removed before it can be converted into glucose, and this nitrogen is excreted in the urine. Consequently, urinary nitrogen excretion is increased, which reflects a negative nitrogen balance of about -12 mg. N per day (1 gm. N = 6.25 gm. of protein). (Chapter 5 discusses nitrogen balance and its calculation.) Shown below is a method for estimating nitrogen balance:

ROUGH ESTIMATION OF NITROGEN (N) BALANCE

Nitrogen balance = nitrogen intake − nitrogen output

$$\text{Nitrogen intake} = \frac{\text{protein in gm. consumed by patient in 24 hr.}}{6.25 \text{ gm. protein/1 gm. nitrogen}}$$

Nitrogen output = gm. urinary urea N in 24 hr. + 1.5 gm. N (2.0 gm. N for men)

Nitrogen intake > nitrogen output = *positive* nitrogen balance = patient in state of anabolism with synthesis of body tissue protein exceeding breakdown of tissue protein

Nitrogen intake = nitrogen output = nitrogen *balance* = build-up of tissue protein is equal to breakdown of tissue protein.

Nitrogen intake < nitrogen output = *negative* nitrogen balance = patient in state of catabolism with breakdown of tissue protein exceeding synthesis of tissue protein

In the fasting body, muscle protein is metabolized first, then the protein in digestive enzymes and last, liver protein.

This use of body protein for energy is very costly, so the body adapts by using a more dispensable body energy store—fat. This process of adaptation takes 3 to 4 days, but soon the body is mobilizing fatty acids for energy and using only about 25 gm. of protein per day for energy. A look at the patient's nitrogen balance at this point shows that it has decreased to only −4 gm. N.

Besides using fatty acids directly for energy and converting some to glucose, the liver also converts some fatty acids to ketone bodies. In the next stage of adaptation, all tissues of the body, including the brain, can metabolize ketones for energy. Seventy per cent of the brain's energy needs can be supplied by the oxidation of ketones rather than of glucose. In this stage, the urinary nitrogen loss will become even less, and the negative nitrogen balance will decrease further, to −2 to −4 gm. N per day. In the final phase of starvation, fat stores are used up, and the entire energy requirement must be met by visceral organ and plasma proteins. Depletion of these proteins is signaled by edema and finally results in death.

Healthy humans of normal weight will not tolerate the loss of more than 35 to 40 per cent of their body weight. Losses of this size (about 300 gm. of nitrogen in the male and 200 gm. of nitrogen in the female) represent a loss of 1200 to 1800 gm. of body protein, about one third of the total body protein. This is fatal. In a person who is depleted or underweight prior to starvation, a lesser body weight loss will be fatal.

The process of conversion to the economical utilization of stored fat for energy depends on a progressive decrease in circulating insulin, which falls from a basal level of 16 to 20 μU. per ml. to less than 12 μU. per ml. When this happens, fatty acid mobilization and ketone body production are promoted. Severe ketonemia will stimulate insulin secretion, however, and since insulin strongly inhibits ketogenesis, a feedback control exists that prevents ketosis from reaching pathological levels. This is not the situation with diabetics, who have no insulin to control the ketogenesis when it becomes excessive. Table 35–1 summarizes the phases of starvation and the changes that take place in a person who is fasting completely but is otherwise healthy.

Starvation Added to Physiological Stress

While the totally fasting healthy person adapts to an economical utilization of body fat with a conservation of body protein to the greatest possible extent, the person who has had trauma, burns, surgery, infection or shock does not adapt as well to starvation. In this situation, the body exhibits a *stress response* that is protective and necessary for the body yet is very catabolic. Eventually the body adapts to both the stress and the starvation so that the nitrogen loss decreases, but it never decreases as much as it will in a starving person who has no other stress.

NUTRITION AND INFECTION

Laboratory, clinical and field observations have demonstrated that the severity and outcome of infection are frequently worsened by malnutrition. When patients are given diets inadequate in protein, it is very likely that they will develop a lowered resistance to infection. This will interfere with the production of antibodies and lymphocytes, which play an im-

Table 35–1 STAGES OF STARVATION

STAGE I (Days 2–4)		STAGE II (Days 20–40)		STAGE III (Ketoadaptation)
Increase in urinary N loss from use of tissue protein for gluconeogenesis	A D A	Decrease in urinary N loss as protein conservation takes place	A D A	Decrease in urinary N loss as glucose-burning tissues adapt to ketone metabolism
Negative nitrogen balance: −12–15 gm. N/day	P T A T I O N	Negative nitrogen balance: −4 gm. N/day	P T A T I O N	Negative nitrogen balance: −2 to −4 gm. N/day
		Reduction in BMR		In absence of dietary intake, total urinary N is a measure of gluconeogenesis
		Body fat utilization at maximum		
		Serum fatty acids ↑		
		Serum ketones ↑		
		Serum insulin (basal) ↓		

portant role in both natural and acquired immunity. Serum antibodies or immunoglobulins in malnourished people may be normal, but the production of specific antibodies may be impaired. If this is the case, immunization programs for malnourished children may be ineffective because these children do not have the proper amino acids for antibody synthesis in response to the vaccination. T-lymphocyte or cell-mediated immunity may also be impaired. This can be demonstrated in children with protein-energy malnutrition who do not show a tuberculin-positive reaction following vaccination.

In animal experiments and clinical studies, deficiencies of protein and vitamins have been found to reduce the phagocytic activity of white blood cells and to lower resistance. It appears that the intracellular killing of the infective organism by the phagocyte is impaired by these deficiencies.

A number of vitamin deficiencies can alter the immunocompetence of the host. Deficiencies of vitamins A and C and of niacin impair tissue integrity, wound healing, fibroblastic response to trauma, walling off of abscesses, collagen formation and thus, the body's resistance to the invasion of infective organisms. Lysozymes, which help to destroy pathogenic microorganisms, are present in tears, sweat and saliva, and their levels in the body are reduced in malnutrition, particularly when vitamin A is deficient.

Infection reduces blood levels of vitamin A. Considerable research has been carried out on the relationship between vitamin A and the common cold, pulmonary tuberculosis and other infectious diseases. Apparently, vitamin A deficiency may play a role in reducing natural resistance, but the administration of the vitamin during the course of an infection has little, if any, beneficial effect unless a deficiency is present.

Vitamin C may have a role in the white blood cell response to infection, but this is only a speculation. It seems to depend on the timing and type of infection. See Chapter 8 for a discussion of this theory.

Vitamin B_6 and pantothenic acid deficiencies cause depressed antibody formation in humans.

No doubt future research will support current evidence that people who have inadequate diets also have a decreased resistance to infection and will elucidate the mechanisms whereby nutritional deficiencies influence the body's resistance to infectious diseases.

Effect of Infection on Nutritional Requirements

Increased Metabolic Rate. Fever is usually present with infection. According to DuBois,[7] there is an elevation of approximately 13 per cent in the metabolic rate for each rise of 1°C. in body temperature, or 7.2 per cent for each degree Fahrenheit. Sometimes the increase is as much as 40 per cent when a patient has a temperature of 40°C., or 104°F. If the patient is restless, delirious or coughing, the total energy need is increased further because of increased activity.

An easy method to determine the metabolism of a patient with fever, suggested by DuBois, is:

1. Determine the normal basal metabolic rate (1400 to 1800 kcal. per day) and then add 7 per cent of the BMR for each degree Fahrenheit (13 per cent for each degree Celsius) of elevation of temperature above normal.

2. If there is sepsis, add another 10 per cent of the BMR.

3. If the patient is restless, add another 10 to 30 per cent of the BMR.

This method will give a sufficiently accurate caloric allowance or energy requirement for a patient with fever.

Catabolism. During the early part of the century it was established that severe bacterial infections, such as typhoid fever, pneumonia, malaria and tuberculosis, cause severe and prolonged loss of nitrogen, chiefly as a result of the toxic destruction of intracellular protein. Studies[19] have shown that mild and asymptomatic viral invasion, such as that produced by yellow fever vaccine or mild chickenpox in children, will produce adverse nitrogen balance effects, even when the patient is receiving an apparently adequate protein intake.

The catabolic response to infection begins after the onset of fever. (See Fig. 35–1.) This catabolism is reflected in negative nitrogen, potassium, magnesium, phosphate, sulfate and zinc balances that persist into convalescence. If the infection is severe and prolonged there will be muscle wasting and weight loss as muscle protein is catabolized for energy. Eventually, however, a stable negative nitrogen balance is reached. As mentioned in the discussion of the catabolic stress response, there is a hyperglycemia due to decreased secretion of insulin and tissue resistance to insulin. This explains why diabetics who normally have their conditions in good control become hyperglycemic during an infection and require more insulin.

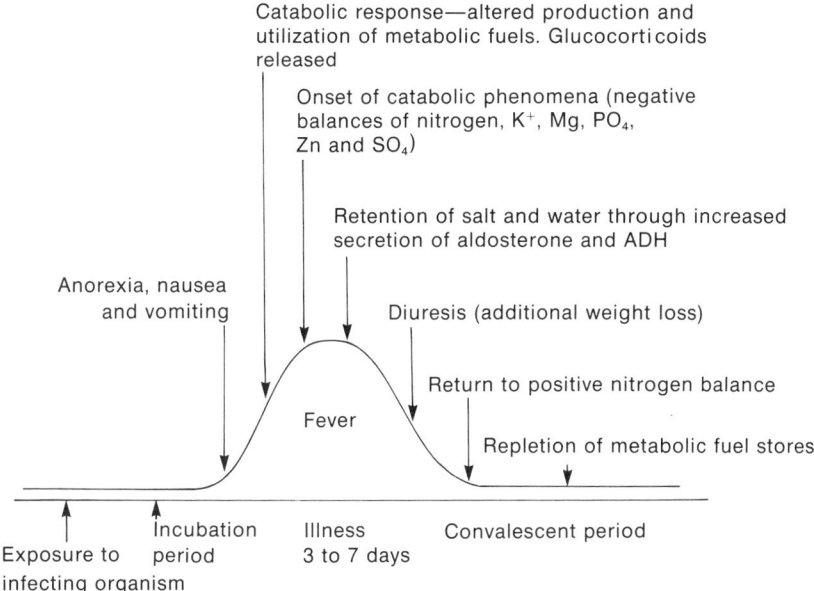

Catabolic response—altered production and
utilization of metabolic fuels. Glucocorticoids
released

Onset of catabolic phenomena (negative
balances of nitrogen, K^+, Mg, PO_4,
Zn and SO_4)

Retention of salt and water through increased
secretion of aldosterone and ADH

Anorexia, nausea
and vomiting

Diuresis (additional weight loss)

Return to positive nitrogen balance

Fever

Repletion of metabolic fuel stores

Exposure to
infecting organism

Incubation
period

Illness
3 to 7 days

Convalescent period

Figure 35–1   Timing of catabolic response to infection. (Adapted from: Beisel, W. R.: The influence of infection or injury on nutritional requirements during adolescence. In: McKigney, J. I., and Munro, H. N. (eds.): Nutrient Requirements in Adolescence, Cambridge, Mass., MIT Press, 1976, p. 259.)

In addition to the wastage of nutrients caused by this catabolic response, there are additional gastrointestinal losses from vomiting and diarrhea. Nutrient intake is diminished because of anorexia and the common practice of withholding food from an ill person and possibly because of malabsorption, as in the case of gastrointestinal infection. Demands on the host's defense system to synthesize phagocytes, leukocytes, immunoglobulins and nonspecific proteins further increase protein requirements.

Nutritional Care

Calories and Protein.   During the acute phase of infection it is difficult to maintain positive nitrogen balance because of the patient's anorexia and the catabolic stress response, which promotes tissue protein breakdown. However, after the body adapts in 3 to 4 days it may be possible to achieve positive nitrogen balance, depending upon the severity of the infection.[2] Protein must be supplied at levels of 0.8 to 1.0 gm. per kg. ideal body weight per day. (See the section later in this chapter on administration of amino acids into a peripheral vein when the patient is unable to eat.) Orally, protein can be supplied in the form of meat, fish, poultry or soups and broths made from proteins such as casein, soy isolate and hydrolyzed protein.

After the catabolic phase subsides, an anabolic phase follows, during which calories and protein should be provided at higher than normal levels. Protein should be increased to 1.5 to 2.0 gm. per kg. and calories to 35 to 45 kcal. per kg. to restore nitrogen losses. The nutritional goal is to put the patient into positive nitrogen balance.

Fluids.   Fluids are of major importance in the treatment of infections. Any fluids that appeal to the patient are satisfactory. As a rule, very sweet liquids are not appealing and frequently cause gastric disturbance as well as distention in the abdominal region. Carbonated beverages (such as ginger ale) and lemonade that is not too sweet seem to be favorites. Protein-containing fluids would be preferable because they help to spare other body protein. If the patient is nauseated and vomiting and too ill to take fluids by mouth, liquid may be given parenterally. Often 3 to 4 liters of fluids are required daily to facilitate the elimination of toxins and to replace water lost through excessive perspiration.

Vitamins.   Fevers increase vitamin requirements, especially of the B-complex vitamins, ascorbic acid and vitamin A. As the calorie need increases, thiamin, riboflavin and niacin requirements also increase. Antibiotics and drugs may interfere with the intestinal synthesis of the B-complex vitamins. Vitamin supplements are usually advised during the illness and convalescence.

Minerals. Loss of sodium and potassium because of fever may be considerable during the acute phase of illness. Unless contraindicated, salty broth, soups and additional sodium and potassium in foods usually replenish the loss. A full liquid or regular diet usually supplies enough potassium. An inadequate intake of food may be supplemented by fruit juices and milk, which are good sources of potassium.

Sometimes patients with infections develop anemia, but this is due to a redistribution of iron in the body's defense against infection rather than to a deficient iron intake.

Meal Plan. Frequent small liquid feedings are usually best tolerated in the beginning. Occasionally, tube feedings (p. 703) may be necessary if the patient has no appetite. The full liquid diet (Table 20–9) is served to the patient as soon as it is tolerated. Such a diet contains food that is easily and quickly digested. Protein supplements may be added in varying amounts to fruit juice, milk or soup. Many patients do better when they eat a regular diet with protein and calorie adjustments to meet the individual requirements. They experience less anorexia, nausea and vomiting. See Table 35–2 for increased protein content of the daily meal plan.

Since most patients with fevers have poor appetites, it is important that special attention be given to the selection of food. An attempt should be made to appeal to the appetite through the careful choice of color, temperature and texture of different foods. Often the person can suggest a food or foods that are appealing. The foods should be easily digested, good sources of protein, and of concentrated food value, such as cereal, whole-grain or enriched bread, potatoes, ice cream, custards, cheese, milk, cream, eggs and fruit juices. Meat and leafy green and yellow vegetables should be included as soon as tolerated. In-between feedings, such as high-calorie beverages that furnish calories and protein and additional fluids, are recommended. Examples are hot chocolate and malted milk with whipped cream, eggnogs and fruit juices with added sugar or lactose. The average high-calorie diet contains approximately 3000 kcal. However, it may be necessary to provide as many as 5000 kcal. if the patient is very restless and if there is great toxic destruction along with high temperature. The aphorism to "starve a fever and feed a cold" is false.

To increase the daily protein and calorie intake in 500 kcal. steps, the plan in Table 27–5 is suggested. The additional milk, eggs and bread will increase the protein intake as well as the calories. Additional menu may be served when practical and advisable. For example, the normal general hospital diet for an individual is calculated to be approximately 2000 kcal. If a diet of 2500 kcal. is desired, a step-up of 500 kcal. is added; or if 3000 kcal. are desired, then two such supplements are added. The choice of food for the addition of calories will be governed by the preference and tolerance of the patient. When the appetite is very poor, small meals and a concentrated supplement are tolerated best. Patients are often overwhelmed by the quantity of food served on the high-calorie, high-nutrient diets.

The dietary and fluid intakes are important concerns of those caring for patients with infection and fever. Observations by the nurse will help to determine the type of diet that best meets the individual needs of the patient.

THE CATABOLIC RESPONSE TO STRESS

A person subjected to stress is one upon whom external forces (often severe) are acting. Examples of such forces are war wounds, industrial injuries, starvation, surgical operations, burns, infections, extreme heat and extreme cold. There are many variables involved that relate to nutrition, such as the severity of the injury, the previous state of nutrition of the individual and the nutrients consumed following stress.

The catabolic stress response is characterized by a *sympathetic nervous reaction*. The sympathetic activity causes release of glucagon by the pancreas and of glucocorticoid and epinephrine by the adrenals. (See Fig. 34–4.) These substances inhibit the release of insulin and antagonize its actions. The net effect of this response is a reduced concentration of serum insulin, hyperglycemia and a resistance to insulin by the peripheral tissues, causing a pseudodiabetic state. The lack of insulin in response to glucose and the tissue resistance to insulin action prevent muscle tissue from utilizing glucose, and a local fuel deficit develops. To satisfy its requirements for energy, skeletal muscle oxidizes the branched-chain amino acids (leucine, isoleucine and valine) from its own tissues. As this protein is mobilized for

Table 35–2 INCREASED PROTEIN CONTENT OF THE DAILY MEAL PLAN*†

DAILY MEAL PLAN *To increase the protein content of the day's meals from 100 gm. to 125 or 150, use the allowances of dried milk solids indicated in columns 2 and 3.*	PROTEIN CONTENT IN GRAMS		
	100 gm. (approx.)[a]	*125 gm. (approx.)*[b]	*150 gm. (approx.)*[c]
BREAKFAST			
Fruit juice, citrus, ½ cup	0.5	0.5	0.5
Cereal, enriched, ½ cup, cooked or prepared, with	2.5	2.5	2.5
½ cup whole milk	4.2	4.2	4.2
Plus 2 tbsp. dried non-fat milk solids	–	6.0	6.0
Egg, 1	6.5	6.5	6.5
Bread (white, enriched or whole-wheat), 1 slice	2.5	2.5	2.5
Butter or enriched margarine (as desired)			
Whole milk, 1 cup	8.5	8.5	8.5
LUNCH			
Meat, poultry, fish, 2 oz. cooked; or cheese	15.2	15.2	15.2
Salad, ½ cup (with dressing)	0.5	0.5	0.5
Cooked vegetable, green or yellow, ½ cup	2.0	2.0	2.0
Bread (white, enriched or whole-wheat), 1 slice	2.5	2.5	2.5
Butter or enriched margarine (as desired)			
Simple dessert,[d] fruit	0.5	0.5	0.5
Whole milk, 1 cup	8.5	8.5	8.5
Plus 2 tbsp. dried non-fat milk solids	–	6.0	6.0
MIDAFTERNOON SNACK			
Whole milk, 1 cup	–	8.5	8.5
Plus 2 tbsp. dried non-fat milk solids	–	–	6.0
Graham crackers, 2	–	–	2.5
DINNER			
Meat, poultry, fish (liver once a week); or cheese:			
4 oz. raw weight; 3 oz. cooked	22.8	22.8	22.8
Cooked vegetable, ½ cup	2.0	2.0	2.0
Potato	2.0	2.0	2.0
Plus 2 tbsp. dried non-fat milk solids	–	6.0	6.0
Bread (white, enriched or whole-wheat), 1 slice	2.5	2.5	2.5
Butter or enriched margarine (as desired)			
Simple dessert,[d] pudding	4.5	4.5	4.5
Plus 2 tbsp. dried non-fat milk solids	–	–	6.0
Whole milk, 1 cup	8.5	8.5	8.5
EVENING SNACK			
Whole milk, 1 cup	8.5	8.5	8.5
Plus 2 tbsp. dried non-fat milk solids	–	–	6.0
Total Gm. Protein	104.7	131.2	151.7

*Source of calculations: Turner, D. F.: Handbook of Diet Therapy, 5th ed. Chicago, University of Chicago Press, 1970. If additional calories are needed to maintain body weight, concentrated foods such as sugar, jelly, sauces and salad dressings may be added.

†To make these meal plans low in sodium, omit all salt in cooking and at the table, omit the cheese, substitute unsalted butter or fortified margarine and replace all or part of the whole milk and dried non-fat milk solids with low sodium milk, available in fresh fluid and canned forms and in powdered whole milk (Lonalac, Mead Johnson) and powdered skim milk (Cellu, Chicago Dietetic Supply House).

[a]2400 kcal.

[b]2700 kcal.

[c]3000 kcal.

[d]Desserts: custards, puddings, plain ice cream, fruit.

Table 35–3   CATABOLIC RESPONSE TO STRESS

IMMEDIATE RESPONSE	ADAPTIVE RESPONSE
Ventromedial hypothalamic activity ↑	VMH activity ↓
Sympathetic activity ↑	Sympathetic activity more specific
Epinephrine release ↑	Serum glucagon ↑
Serum glucagon ↑	Glucocorticoids normal
Glucocorticoid release ↑	Serum insulin in response to glucose challenge ↓
Serum insulin in response to glucose challenge ↓	Growth hormone normal
Peripheral tissue resistance to insulin	
Growth hormone ↑	
	These changes, after a few days of constant stress, result in:
These nervous and hormonal changes result in:	Serum glucose ↓
Hyperglycemia	Plasma fatty acids ↑
Inability of skeletal muscle to utilize glucose even though hyperglycemia is present	Ketonemia
	Ketonuria
Breakdown of skeletal muscle protein	Less breakdown of skeletal muscle protein
Ileus	Return of appetite
Anorexia	Urinary nitrogen excretion ↓
Urinary nitrogen excretion ↑	Mineralocorticoids normal; diuresis ensues
Mineralocorticoid release ↑, causing fluid and sodium retention and potassium excretion	

energy, the excess NH_3 that results from the oxidation is attached to pyruvate and carried back to the liver as the amino acid alanine. Alanine stimulates the pancreas to secrete glucagon, which induces gluconeogenesis and ureagenesis in the liver and clears the blood of alanine, glycerol and lactate. The basal level of insulin initially has an antilipolytic effect, so that the body does not adapt by oxidizing fatty acids and ketones for energy.

Sympathetic nervous activity also stimulates the release of mineralocorticoids from the adrenal gland. These cause fluid and sodium retention and potassium excretion.

Protein catabolism during this phase does not take place solely to meet energy requirements. The amino acids mobilized from the skeletal muscles are also used by the liver to synthesize the proteins needed during stress: immunoglobulins, leukocytes and lymphocytes to fight infection, hemoglobin or albumin to replace blood loss, collagen to begin tissue healing and the enzymes necessary to make all of these proteins. The catabolic response differs from the starvation response because the initial mobilization of protein comes from the skeletal muscles, whereas in simple starvation the visceral protein is used first, and mobilization of peripheral skeletal protein does not begin until after 3 to 4 days.

The net effect of the catabolic stress response is a hormonal environment that protects and defends the body at the expense of skeletal muscle (see Table 35–3). It is a beneficial response to stress that includes negative nitrogen balance as a necessary side effect. During this catabolic response, which lasts 5 to 8 days, there is loss of nitrogen, sulfur, phosphorus, potassium, magnesium, zinc and creatine.

If stress continues, the body's sympathetic activity should also continue. If the sympathetic response stops when the body is still under stress, it indicates that the stress is overpowering the body, and this is a bad prognostic sign.

Assuming that the stress continues and that the body can maintain its sympathetic response and overcome the stress, the body will adapt somewhat to prolonged stress and enter an *adaptive catabolic phase.* (See Table 35–3.) The prominent feature of this stage is that the body uses a smaller amount of skeletal protein for its energy needs and adapts to using fatty acids and ketone bodies for energy, so that the nitrogen balance is not quite as negative. The blood glucose level is lower, and this is the clinical sign that the body has entered the adaptive phase. Serum fatty acid concentrations are higher. At this point, nutritional support should definitely be started either orally or parenterally if it has not already begun. Administration of amino acids via peripheral vein (1.5 gm. per kg. IBW) or orally in the form of complete protein is necessary if the patient cannot tolerate a completely oral intake or total parenteral nutrition.

Nutritional intake in this adapted phase is more efficiently utilized because the levels of epinephrine and glucocorticoids do not an-

tagonize the action of insulin. Calories and protein given at this time can be used more efficiently.

Sudden development of hyperglycemia means that the stress has increased and that the patient has again entered a catabolic stress response phase, with increased sympathetic activity and insulin resistance.

As the stress is relieved through treatment or by its own natural course, the sympathetic response decreases and the parasympathetic activity increases. The patient begins to feel hungry, a sign that he is feeling better. Nutritional care should be aimed at putting the patient into anabolism and restoring the tissue protein lost during stress.

Nutritional Care

Since the body does not adapt to its starvation fat economy unless the stress, trauma or infection is alleviated, the primary emphasis of nutritional care should be removal of the stress (draining the abscess, covering the burns, treating the infection, and so on). However, if the stress cannot be removed, nutritional support should be started. If support is not provided and the patient continues to use lean body mass for necessary protein synthesis, the consequences are severe. Eventually protein synthesis declines, and weakness, loss of immunocompetence, hypoalbuminemia, failure of wound healing, further infection, decubitus ulcers from skin breakdown, respiratory insufficiency from respiratory muscle weakness,

and eventually multiple organ failure and death result.

The turn to anabolism should be promoted by offering food and nutrients as soon as the patient's blood glucose level begins to fall and gastrointestinal function returns. The patient should not be without nutritional support longer than 5 days following physiological trauma.[8]

The nutrients should be provided in the correct form and by the most efficient route—enteral or parenteral. During convalescence, the amounts of nutrients should be high in order to promote anabolism. The calorie intake should be balanced with the protein intake for the most efficient utilization of protein.

If the goal of nutritional therapy is reached, the patient will achieve positive nitrogen balance (p. 694). Another way to evaluate the nutritional care is to use the nutritional index as presented in Chapter 20. A daily comparison of the patient's *actual intake* with his *determined requirements* for protein and calories will give an index, either positive or negative, as to whether the nutritional care is meeting his requirements.

Calories. The caloric requirement should be determined first and depends on the increase in metabolic expenditure caused by the patient's clinical situation. Rutten and coworkers have defined degrees of increased metabolic expenditure by measuring the daily urinary urea nitrogen loss.[18] (See Table 35–4.) Appearance of 5 to 10 gm. of urea nitrogen in the urine in 24 hours means the energy requirement is 0 to 10

Table 35–4 CLASSIFICATION OF CATABOLISM*†

CLINICAL SITUATION	DEGREE OF CATABOLISM	UREA = N (gm./day)	INCREASE OF RESTING METABOLIC RATE OVER BMR (%)	TOTAL CALORIC REQUIREMENT[a] (kcal.)
Person in bed	1° (Normal)	<5	None	1800
Uncomplicated surgery	2° (Mild)	5–10	0–20	1800–2200
Multiple fractures or trauma	3° (Moderate)	10–15	20–50	2200–2700
Acute major infections or major burns	4° (Severe)	>15	50–125	2700–4000 or more

*Adapted from: Rutten, P., et al.: Determination of optimal hyperalimentation infusion rate. J. Surg. Res., *18*:477, 1975.

†Classification of patients according to the following: (1) obligate nitrogen loss (N obg.) expressed in gm. urea-N per 24 hr.; (2) energy expenditure expressed as per cent increase of the resting metabolic expenditure over calculated basal energy expenditure.

[a]This total caloric resting metabolic requirement includes the amount needed for activity, about 20 per cent since these patients usually are not active, and 10 per cent for specific dynamic action (SDA). This is a rough estimate for a 70-kg. man and depends on the patient's size.

per cent above the basal requirement, while 10 to 15 gm. of urinary urea nitrogen in 24 hours indicates a 20 to 50 per cent increase. Patients with urinary urea nitrogen losses of more than 15 gm. in 24 hours have energy requirements 50 to 125 per cent above the basal need. The increase in energy and protein requirements is directly related to the output of urinary urea nitrogen (N) and the N output of other sites such as draining wounds or burns. In those patients without burns or large surface wounds, the N loss can be estimated by adding 1.5 gm. of N for women and 2.0 gm. of N for men to the urinary urea N per 24 hours.

Using several patients with mild to moderate degrees of catabolism, it was determined that calories provided at a level of 54 per cent above basal need, or 1.54 × BEE (basal energy expenditure), would provide enough calories to prevent breakdown of body tissues and to promote anabolism and the repair of the body tissues in most patients. Burned or other severely traumatized patients will require more than this. For most patients, provision of calories to equal 1.54 × BEE gives about 40 to 45 kcal. per kg. ideal body weight (IBW), and this amount will put patients into anabolism and rehabilitate them. A level of 1.22 × BEE, or about 30 to 35 kcal. per kg. IBW, will maintain most patients and prevent negative nitrogen balance if they are already rehabilitated.[3] Most surgical patients have a resting energy expenditure of about 20 per cent above their basal expenditure.

Protein. The optimal protein intake for depleted, stressed adults is 16 per cent of total calories. This level, in the presence of 40 to 45 kcal. per kg., promotes positive nitrogen balance and the restoration of lean body mass or of protein reserves.[4] A few calculations show that if 16 per cent of the total caloric intake comes from protein, then the nitrogen to kcalorie ratio is 1 gm.:150 kcal. Therefore, the nitrogen requirement in grams can be determined from the calorie requirement by dividing the kcal. required by 150. The protein requirement can be determined by dividing the kcal. by 24.

Example: Ms. L's basal energy requirements = 1400 kcal. She has had a long bout with ulcerative colitis, followed by surgery with a resulting ileostomy.
Urinary urea N/24 hr. = 15 gm.
Her energy requirements = 54% over basal = 1400 + 756 = 2156 kcal.
Her protein requirements = 16% of kcal. = 2156 × 0.16 = 345 kcal.

Protein requirements in gm. = 345 kcal. ÷ 4 kcal./gm. protein = 86 gm. protein
Her requirements calculated using the nitrogen: calorie ratio of 1:150 or the N:Protein ratio of 24:
2156 kcal. ÷ 150 kcal./gm. N = 14.37 gm. N
2156 kcal. ÷ 24 kcal./gm. pro = 90 gm. protein
This is very close to the 86 gm. determined by the first method.
14.37 gm. N × 6.25 gm. pro/gm. N = 90 gm. protein, also very close to the 86 gm. determined by the first method.

Initial weight gain when the stressed patient switches from negative to positive nitrogen balance is really a reflection of body water retention. Following the initial gain, weight gain is minimal in spite of the continued positive nitrogen balance, because spontaneous diuresis keeps body water level down. Restoration of lean tissue and fat usually occurs at the rate of 250 gm. or ½ lb. per day with optimal nutritional support. Rates greater than this reflect an undesirable water retention.

Vitamins and Minerals. Vitamins should be given at high levels, and a supplement is probably justified. Mineral intake will depend on the patient's prior nutritional status and mineral losses during stress.

LIQUID NUTRITION FOR ENTERAL FEEDING

The preferable and most palatable method for providing nutrition to meet the increased demands of the catabolic patient and of the patient who has come through a catabolic period is through abundant, nutritious and frequent meals and supplements. With the multitude of additional methods now available for feeding, the appearance of wasted, cachectic patients in our hospitals is no longer tolerable. Table 35–2 gives the amounts of foods needed to provide protein intakes of 100, 130 and 150 gm. and calorie intakes of 2400, 2700 and 3000 kcal.

NUTRITIONAL SUPPLEMENTS

When a sufficient quantity of food is not eaten at meals, calorie and protein concentrates can be administered as between-meal drinks. Nutritional supplements are usually not adequate in all nutrients and are not meant to provide complete nutrition. Powdered dried skim milk contains approximately 35 per cent protein of high biological value and provides 3 gm. of protein and 27 kcal. per tablespoon. Eight oz. of whole milk provides 160 kcal. and 8 gm. of protein. Although milk is an inexpensive

and convenient protein supplement, many patients may not tolerate it because of a lactose intolerance either primary (many non-Caucasians) or secondary to gastrointestinal disease. Milk is used frequently for liquid feedings because it is one of the few liquid forms of a complete protein. Casein and lactalbumin can be added to dried skim milk powder to increase its protein content at low cost. However, there are now several formulas on the market that are not milk-based and are suitable as nutritional supplements or for complete nutritional support.

Other forms of concentrated protein that can be used are powdered whole eggs and powdered dried egg albumin. The choice of a nutritional supplement will depend on the cost, availability, use and palatability of the product and on the patient's disease, extent of hypermetabolism and nutritional requirements. The composition and indications for use of available nutritional supplements are given in Table 35–5.

COMPLETE NUTRITIONAL FORMULAS

Liquid feedings that provide all nutritional requirements are used in the nutritional care of patients unable to take solid food because of dysphagia, gastrointestinal obstruction or oral surgery. These patients need to have their food dispersed in water. Table 35–6 outlines the situations requiring artificial feeding techniques and the recommended type of formula for each.

Tube Feedings

Because of gastrointestinal surgery, unconsciousness or esophageal obstruction that prevents oral intake, some patients require liquid feeding through a tube. Other patients cannot meet their nutritional requirements through oral intake alone and require additional nourishment through a tube.

The compositions of some commercial formulas that are suitable for tube feedings are given in Table 35–7. Commercial products save time in preparation, are less likely to be contaminated and are of a known composition, but they are not quite as flexible in meeting patient needs as tube feedings prepared especially for the individual. However, more and more products of special composition and function are becoming available.

Feedings may be made from a mixture of the foods served in the adequate normal diet, finely homogenized in a mechanical blender and strained to ensure passage through the tube, or food combinations planned to meet specific therapeutic needs may be used. Formulas made from whole foods have the advantage of including trace minerals and vitamins that are naturally present in whole foods but may not be added to a chemically defined formula diet. Table 35–8 gives a typical formula made from whole foods.

Composition

When evaluating a feeding formula it is useful to look at its osmolality, caloric concentration and protein, carbohydrate, fat, vitamin and mineral composition.

Osmolality. *Osmolality* is a measure of the osmotically active particles per kg. of the solvent in which the particles are dispersed, which in this case is water. Osmolality is expressed as milliosmoles of solute per kg. of solvent or mOsm./kg. The osmolality of normal body fluids is about 275 to 298 mOsm. per kg. Solutions taken into the body that have an osmolality greater than this are hyperosmolar and cause water to be drawn into those areas where the hyperosmolar solutions are. Most tube feedings are hyperosmolar, and they will cause water to be drawn into the gastrointestinal tract if given too rapidly. See Table 35–7 for the osmolality of feeding formulas.

Calories. Feedings usually provide 1 kcal. per ml. when mixed full strength according to directions. In other words, the volume needed to give 1000 kcal. is 1000 ml. Some formulas such as Ensure Plus (Ross Labs) contain more than 1 kcal. per ml., and thus only 676 ml. are required to give 1000 kcal. Other formulas such as Nutramigen have a lower concentration of calories and require 1500 ml. to give 1000 kcal. The calorically dense formulas are meant for severely debilitated patients requiring very high calorie and protein intakes.

Protein. The protein content of formulas varies from 9 to 24 per cent of the calories. It is usually provided by a complete protein and may be partially hydrolyzed into peptide fragments or into the individual amino acids for easier digestion. The protein source can be casein (milk protein), puréed beef, egg albumin, skim milk powder, soy protein, hydrolyzed casein or amino acids. Formulas that contain the whole protein are much more palatable than those containing hydrolyzed protein or amino acids, and they are also cheaper. Many formulas are milk-based and have casein as the primary protein source because it is complete and easily digested and will make a solution

Table 35–5　COMPOSITION AND USE OF LIQUID NUTRITIONAL SUPPLEMENTS[*][a]

NUTRIENT, AMOUNT AND USE	AMIN-AID (McGaw)	CAL-POWER (General Mills)	CASEC (Mead Johnson)	CHO-FREE (Syntex)	CITRO-TEIN (Doyle)	CONTRO-LYTE (Doyle)	DP HIGH P.E.R. PROTEIN (General Mills)	EMF (Control Drugs)	GEVRAL (Lederle)	HY-CAL (Beecham)	LIPOMUL-ORAL (Upjohn)
Protein (gm.)	9.4	0.6	237.6	46.9	60.5	Trace	206.0	250.0	170.9	0.1	0.1
Fat (gm.)	31.7	0	5.4	91.3	2.6	48.0	10.0	0	5.7	0.1	111.1
Carbohydrate (gm.)	168.6	272.0	0	0.5	184.2	143.0	21.0	0	66.8	244.1	1.1
Sodium (mEq.)	2.88	2.39	6.00	41.34	45.80	1.30	22.40	53.00	18.57	2.41	2.90
Potassium (mEq.)	2.88	0.70	2.10	59.21	26.80	0.20	9.90	5.10	3.65	0.07	0.09
Amount Needed to Give 1000 Kcal.	213 gm. dry weight or 489 ml. standard dilution	550 gm. liquid	270 gm. dry weight	1304 ml. undiluted	263.4 gm. dry weight	198 gm. dry weight	258 gm. dry weight	500 ml. liquid	284.8 gm. dry weight	407 ml. liquid	166.7 ml. liquid
Use	Formula for renal failure therapy	Carbohydrate source	Protein source	Low carbohydrate formula	Calorie supplement	Low-protein, low-electrolyte calorie source	Protein supplement, low electrolytes	Protein source	Protein-calorie supplement	Carbohydrate source	Fat source

[*]From: Shils, M. E., Bloch, A. S., and Chernoff, R.: Liquid formulas for oral and tube feeding. Clinical Bulletin, 6:151, 1976.
[a]Amounts of nutrients provided per 1000 kcal.

Table 35–5 COMPOSITION AND USE OF LIQUID NUTRITIONAL SUPPLEMENTS (*Continued*)

NUTRIENT, AMOUNT AND USE	LIPROTEIN (*Upjohn*)	LOFENA-LAC (*Mead Johnson*)	LONALAC (*Mead Johnson*)	LYTREN (*Mead Johnson*)	MCT OIL (*Mead Johnson*)	PEDIALYTE (*Ross*)	POLYCOSE (*Ross*)	PROBANA (*Mead Johnson*)	SUMACAL (*Hosp. Diet Prod.*)
Protein (gm.)	82.7	32.5	53.0	0	0	0	0	60.0	0
Fat (gm.)	64.3	39.0	54.7	0	120.5	0	0	32.0	0
Carbohydrate (gm.)	22.1	130.0	74.2	253.0	0	250.0	235.0	118.0	250.0
Sodium (mEq.)	8.00	21.00	1.70	100.00	0	150.00	12.00	40.50	10.40
Potassium (mEq.)	42.46	25.50	48.08	83.30	0	100.00	0.30	46.50	1.15
Amount Needed to Give 1000 Kcal.	183.7 gm. dry weight	1500 ml. standard dilution	1500 ml. standard dilution or 196 gm. dry weight	268 gm. dry weight or 3333 ml. standard dilution	120.5 gm. liquid	5000 ml. liquid	250 gm. dry weight	1500 ml. standard dilution	360 ml. liquid
Use	Calorie source	Low-phenylalanine formula	Low-sodium, high-protein source	Calorie & electrolyte source	Medium-chain triglycerides	Calorie & electrolyte source	Oligosaccharides	High-protein banana powder formula for celiac condition & diarrhea	Concentrated carbohydrate source, low electrolytes

Table 35–6   SITUATIONS REQUIRING ARTIFICIAL FEEDING TECHNIQUES

PHYSIOLOGICAL PROBLEM	RECOMMENDED FEEDING	CLINICAL SITUATION OR DISORDER

Inability to ingest food	Liquid feedings: whole food or milk-based formula
	Route of administration:
	  Tube
	    nasogastric
	    gastrostomy
	    jejunostomy
	  Oral
		Carcinoma of esophagus or stomach
		Dental or oral surgery
		Inflammatory disease of esophagus
		Coma

Inability to digest food	Predigested or chemically defined diet
	  Amino acids and peptides
	  Glucose and dextrins
	  Minerals and vitamins
	Route of administration:
	  Oral
	  Tube
		Pancreatitis
		Enzyme deficiency
		Biliary tract disease

Decreased ability to absorb food	Chemically defined diet
	  Route of administration:
	    Oral
	    Tube
		Radiation therapy
		Sprue
		Inflammatory bowel disease
		Short bowel syndrome

Inability to absorb food	Peripheral vein nutritional support Total parenteral nutrition	

Inability to handle colonic residue	Chemically defined diet
	  Route of administration:
	    Oral
	    Tube
	Peripheral vein nutritional support
	Total parenteral nutrition
		Inflammatory bowel disease
		Presurgical preparation
		Ileostomy, colostomy
		Draining fistula

Inability to meet nutritional requirements fully with normal foods	Liquid feeding
	  Oral supplement
	  Tube feeding
	Peripheral vein nutritional supplementation
	Central vein nutritional supplementation
		Major surgery
		Burns
		Trauma
		Extended fever
		Anorexia of chronic illness
		Anorexia nervosa

of low viscosity. The hydrolyzed form of casein is a good source of peptides for a patient with protein maldigestion or malabsorption who needs a somewhat digested form of protein.

Fat. The fat in most commercial formulas is corn, soy or safflower oil, and the amount may range from 1 to 47 per cent of the calories. A few products contain medium-chain triglycerides (MCT) and thus are easier to digest, and these should be used in cases of fat malabsorption. Alternatively, a fat-free formula can be used, with small amounts of fat (10 gm. per liter) added each day in order to increase the fat intake gradually. Fat added to a feeding is important because it increases the calories yet does not increase the osmolality of the formula. It also gives the patient a feeling of satiety.

Carbohydrate. The many possible sources of carbohydrate in a liquid feeding range from puréed fruits and vegetables to corn syrup solids, fructose, sucrose and lactose. The carbohydrate source greatly affects the palatability of the formula, and the amount of carbohydrate affects its osmolality. See Table 35–7 for the carbohydrate sources of common formulas.

Vitamins and Minerals. Most commercially available liquid diets are fortified with vitamins and minerals to meet the Recommended Dietary Allowances when a certain volume is taken. (See Table 35–7.) However, the allowances are designed for healthy people and are only guidelines to the vitamin and mineral needs of the ill person. Home-prepared or institutionally prepared formulas should have vitamins and minerals added, since some of these formulas may not be adequate depending on the choice of foods used in the feeding. The use of a multivitamin and mineral supplement is advised. Additional vitamins would have to be added in cases of vitamin deficiency or excessively high requirements. For some patients, electrolytes may also need to be added to replace losses.

Defined Formula Diets or "Elemental Diets"

These formulas are designed for easy digestion and absorption, and they leave minimal residue in the bowel. Stool passage is markedly reduced or stopped with the use of these formulas. These diets do contain known quantities of purified substances, but the substances are not truly elements, and the name "elemental diet," although widely used, is erroneous. It is true, however, that the protein and carbohydrate used in these diets are in simpler forms than those found in normal diets and in tube feedings formulated from whole foods. The carbohydrate is present in the form of glucose or dextrins (disaccharides and oligosaccharides) and the protein in the form of amino acids or peptides. There is very little fat, or else it is present in the form of MCT or is partially digested into mono- or diglycerides. (See Table 35-7C.) Because nutrients are present in simple forms, little digestion is required, and these formulas are especially suited for cases of steatorrhea and malabsorption caused by disease, short bowel syndrome, radiation therapy or antibiotic damage to the intestinal tract. Patients with as little as 100 cm. of remaining jejunum can be maintained with defined formulas because the nutrients are so easily absorbed.

It was once thought that the protein in these products had to be supplied in the form of amino acids, but it has been shown that the dipeptides and tripeptides are better absorbed in patients with malabsorption syndrome.[16] The dextrins, glucose and the oligosaccharides do not need pancreatic amylase for digestion. Very little fat is present, usually only enough to prevent essential fatty acid deficiency. (The exception is Flexical, by Mead Johnson.) All of the products are supplemented with vitamins and minerals to meet the RDA.

These products can be taken orally, although they are better tolerated when given through a tube. They are somewhat unpalatable when taken by mouth because of the peptides and amino acids. However, if they are to be taken orally, they should be offered to the patient with a positive attitude and not with a look of disgust on the face of the nurse or clinical dietitian. Their palatability may be greatly improved by using various flavors and by serving them chilled, "on the rocks" or in fruit juice.

High-nitrogen defined formula diets that contain more protein are available for severely traumatized, burned or very depleted patients who require a higher percentage of calories from protein. See Table 35–9 for factors to consider when choosing a feeding formula.

Administration

The method and route of administration of a tube feeding will determine the type of formula to be used and how it will be tolerated by the patient. The route may be by nasogastric, esophagostomy, gastrostomy or jejunostomy

Text continued on page 714

Table 35–7   COMPLETE NUTRITIONAL FORMULAS*

A. Contain Milk and Intact Protein[a]

NUTRIENT AND AMOUNT[b]	COMPLEAT B (Doyle)		FORMULA 2 (Cutter)	MEATBASE FORMULA 142 (Hosp. Diet Prod.)[c]	C.I.B.[d, e] (Carnation)
Protein (gm.)	40.0		37.5	33.0	55.2
Protein source	Beef Non-fat milk		Non-fat milk Beef	Beef Soy protein isolate Non-fat milk	Non-fat milk Soy protein Na caseinate
Fat (gm.)	40.0		40.0	48.2	27.6
Fat source	Corn oil		Corn oil Egg yolks	Corn oil	Milk fat
Carbohydrate (gm.)	120.0		122.5	107.6	124.1
Carbohydrate source	Sucrose Maltodextrin Vegetables Fruits Orange juice	23.0 ⎫ ⎬ 73.4 ⎭	Sucrose Vegetables Orange juice Farina Dextrose	Dextrose Fruit Vegetables	Sucrose Corn syrup solids Lactose
Lactose	24.4		37.5		84.0
Volume to Give 1000 kcal. (ml.)	1000		1000	667	880
Minerals					
Calcium (mg.)	625.0		720.0	646.8	1206.9
Phosphorus (mg.)	1687.5		560.0	710.2	972.4
Magnesium (mg.)	250.0		100.0	264.0	403.5
Iron (mg.)	11.3		12.6	11.9	15.9
Iodine (μg.)	93.8		75.0	100.0	129.3
Copper (mg.)	1.3		1.0	1.7	2.0
Manganese (mg.)	2.5		0.2		
Zinc (mg.)	9.4		7.5	9.9	13.7
Sodium (mEq.)	67.9		26.1	31.5	37.0
Potassium (mEq.)	33.7		45.1	27.1	63.3
Chloride (mEq.)	22.9		53.5		
mOsm./kg.	490		435–510	725	
Volume Needed to Meet 100% RDA Including Vitamins (ml.)	1600		2000	1000	1373

*From: Shils, M. E., Bloch, A. S., and Chernoff, R.: Liquid formulas for oral and tube feeding. Clinical Bulletin, 6:151, 1976.

[a] "Compleat B," "Formula 2" and "Meatbase Formula 142" are *moderate residue;* all others are *low residue.*

[b] Amounts of nutrients provided per 1000 kcal.

[c] This is only one of a variety of formulas offered by Hospital Diet Products Corp.

[d] Vanilla flavor used.

[e] Whole milk added.

Table 35–7 COMPLETE NUTRITIONAL FORMULAS (*Continued*)

A. Contain Milk and Intact Protein [a] (Continued)

MERITENE LIQUID[d] (*Doyle*)	MERITENE + MILK[d, e] (*Doyle*)	NUTRI-1000[d] (*Syntex*)	SUSTACAL LIQUID[d] (*Mead Johnson*)	SUSTACAL + MILK[d, e] (*Mead Johnson*)	SUSTAGEN + WATER[d] (*Mead Johnson*)
60.0 Conc. skim milk Na caseinate	65.1 Non-fat milk Whole milk	38.0 Skim milk	60.3 Conc. skim milk Na + Ca caseinate Soy protein	60.3 Non-fat milk Whole milk	60.0 Non-fat milk Whole milk Ca caseinate
33.3 Vegetable oil Mono & diglycerides	32.5 Milk fat	52.0 Corn oil	23.0 Soy oil	24.4 Milk fat	8.6 Milk fat
115.0 Corn syrup solids Sucrose	112.0 Corn syrup solids 14.4	95.6 Sucrose 30.7 Corn syrup solids 14.8	137.8 Sucrose 97.2 Corn syrup solids 25.4	134.4 Sucrose 36.2 Corn syrup solids 11.8	171.4 Corn syrup solids 104.7 Glucose 9.3
56.7	97.5	50.1	16.7	85.8	57.3
1000	995	960	1000		600
1250.0	2168.6	1150.0	1000.0	1611.2	1828.6
1250.0	1807.2	900.0	916.7	1333.4	1371.4
333.3	361.4	200.0	375.0	375.0	228.6
15.0	16.3	9.0	16.7	16.7	10.3
125.0	136.1	75.0	138.9	138.9	85.7
1.7	1.8	1.0	1.9	1.9	1.1
3.3	3.6	1.3	2.8	2.8	2.9
12.5	13.5	7.5	13.9	13.9	11.4
39.8	39.3	21.7	40.2	40.2	29.8
42.7	71.1	35.9	52.7	64.8	51.3
47.0	64.6	31.0	43.8	37.6	
700–750	690	500	625	756	1334
1200	1095	1920	1080		1050

Table continued on the following page

Table 35–7 COMPLETE NUTRITIONAL FORMULAS (*Continued*)

B. Intact Protein, Protein Isolates—Low Lactose, Low Residue

NUTRIENT AND AMOUNT[b]	ENSURE[d] (*Ross*)	ENSURE PLUS[d] (*Ross*)	ISOCAL (*Mead Johnson*)	ISOMIL[f] (*Ross*)	LOLACTENE (*Doyle*)	MULL-SOY[f] (*Syntex*)
Protein (gm.)	35.0	36.6	32.5	30.0	66.2	48.0
Protein source	Na + Ca caseinate 30.6 Soy protein 4.4	Na + Ca caseinate Soy protein	Na caseinate Soy protein	Soy protein isolate L-methionine	Non-fat dry milk Na caseinate	Soy flour
Fat (gm.)	35.0	35.5	42.0	54.0	23.5	55.5
Fat source	Corn oil	Corn oil	Soy oil 33.6 MCT 8.4	Soy oil Coconut oil Corn oil	Vegetable oil Mono & diglycerides	Soy oil
Carbohydrate (gm.)	136.7	133.2	125.0	102.0	132.4	79.5
Carbohydrate source	Corn syrup solids 98.3 Sucrose 38.4	Corn syrup solids Sucrose	Corn syrup solids	Corn syrup Sucrose	Corn syrup solids 27.3 Sucrose 10.4 Glucose 46.7 Galactose 46.7	Sucrose Invert sucrose
Lactose	0	0	0	0	<4.0	0
Volume to Give 1000 kcal. (ml.)	943	676	960	1500	1250	1500
Minerals						
Calcium (mg.)	500.0	422.5	600.0	1050.0	2353.0	1875.0
Phosphorus (mg.)	500.0	422.5	500.0	750.0	2058.8	1250.0
Magnesium (mg.)	200.0	211.3	200.0	75.0	441.2	117.2
Iron (mg.)	9.0	9.5	9.0	18.0	19.9	15.6
Iodine (μg.)	75.0	70.4	75.0	225.0	166.2	234.4
Copper (mg.)	1.0	1.1	1.0	0.8	2.2	1.6
Manganese (mg.)	2.0	1.4	2.5		4.4	2.2
Zinc (mg.)	15.0	15.9	10.0	7.5	16.5	12.5
Sodium (mEq.)	30.4	30.6	21.7	19.6	47.9	28.1
Potassium (mEq.)	30.8	32.5	32.1	27.3	79.0	66.1
Chloride (mEq.)	28.2	30.2	28.2	22.4	57.2	
mOsm./kg.	450	600	350		670	252
Volume Needed to Meet 100% RDA Including Vitamins (ml.)	1920	1920	1920		1150	

[f] Infant formula.

Table 35–7   COMPLETE NUTRITIONAL FORMULAS (*Continued*)

B. *Intact Protein, Protein Isolates—Low Lactose, Low Residue* (Continued)

NEO MULL-SOY[f] (*Syntex*)	PRECISION HN (*Doyle*)	PRECISION ISOTONIC (*Doyle*)	PRECISION LR (*Doyle*)	PRECISION MOD N (*Doyle*)	PORTAGEN (*Mead Johnson*)	PROSOBEE[f] (*Mead Johnson*)
27.0 Soy protein isolate L-methionine	41.7 Egg white solids	30.0 Egg white solids	23.7 Egg white solids	32.5 Egg white solids	35.0 Na caseinate	37.5 Soy protein isolate L-methionine
52.5 Soy oil	0.5 Vegetable oil Mono & di-glycerides	31.3 Vegetable oil Mono & di-glycerides	0.7 Vegetable oil Mono & di-glycerides	31.0 Vegetable oil Mono & di-glycerides	47.7 MCT 41.0 Corn oil 5.5 Lecithin 1.3	50.0 Soy oil
96.0 Sucrose	206.7 Maltodex-trin 193.9 Sugar 12.8	150.0 Maltodextrin Sugar	224.7 Maltodex-trin 209.4 Sugar 15.3	150.0 Maltodex-trin 114.2 Sugar 35.8	115.0 Maltodex-trin 83.5 Sucrose 28.8 Other 2.5	100.0 Sucrose 62.0 Corn syrup solids 38.0
0	0	0	0	0	<0.3	0
1500	950	1042	900	825	1000	1500
1250.0	333.3	667.0	526.3	500.0	937.8	1185.0
950.0	333.3	667.0	526.3	500.0	604.4	795.0
120.0	133.3	266.0	210.5	200.0	208.4	111.0
15.6	6.0	12.0	9.5	9.0	18.8	18.8
234.4	50.0	100.0	78.9	75.0	72.9	72.0
0.6	0.7	1.3	1.1	1.0	1.6	0.9
4.0	1.3	2.7	2.1	2.0	3.1	1.7
4.8	5.0	10.0	7.9	7.5	9.4	8.0
26.2	40.6	34.8	27.5	37.0	20.4	27.0
41.2	22.2	25.6	20.2	19.2	32.1	28.5
14.1	32.0	30.1	28.2	25.4	24.2	18.0
275	557	300	500–545	395	357	258
	2950	1560	1710	1650	960	

Table continued on the following page

Table 35–7   COMPLETE NUTRITIONAL FORMULAS (*Continued*)

C. Hydrolyzed Protein, Amino Acids—Low Lactose, Low Residue

NUTRIENT AND AMOUNT[b]	FLEXICAL (*Mead Johnson*)	NUTRAMIGEN[f] (*Mead Johnson*)	PREGESTIMIL[f] (*Mead Johnson*)	VIVONEX (*Eaton*)	VIVONEX HN (*Eaton*)
Protein (gm.)	22.4	32.5	32.5	20.4	45.6
Protein source	Hydrolyzed casein Amino acids	Hydrolyzed casein	Hydrolyzed casein	Crystalline amino acids	Crystalline amino acids
Fat (gm.)	34.0	39.0	41.0	1.4	0.9
Fat source	Soy oil 27.4 MCT 6.6	Corn oil	MCT 36.6 Corn oil 5.2	Safflower oil	Safflower oil
Carbohydrate (gm.)	154.0	130.0	130.0	226.3	202.4
Carbohydrate source	Sugar 100.9 Dextrin 48.4 Citrate 4.7	Sucrose 93.6 Tapioca starch 36.4	Glucose 91.0 Tapioca starch 39.0	Glucose oligo-saccharides	Glucose oligo-saccharides
Lactose	0	0	0	0	0
Volume to Give 1000 kcal. (ml.)	1000	1500	1500	1000	1000
Minerals					
Calcium (mg.)	600.0	945.0	945.0	443.3	266.6
Phosphorus (mg.)	500.0	705.0	705.0	443.3	266.6
Magnesium (mg.)	200.0	111.0	111.0	194.3	116.7
Iron (mg.)	9.0	18.8	18.8	5.6	3.3
Iodine (μg.)	75.0	72.0	72.0	80.0	48.0
Copper (mg.)	1.0	0.9	0.9	1.1	0.6
Manganese (mg.)	2.5	1.7	1.7	1.6	0.9
Zinc (mg.)	10.0	6.3	6.3	6.9	3.7
Sodium (mEq.)	15.2	21.0	21.0	37.4	33.5
Potassium (mEq.)	32.0	25.5	25.5	30.0	18.0
Chloride (mEq.)	35.2	19.5	19.5	50.8	52.4
mOsm./kg.	723	443	590	500[g]	850
Volume Needed to Meet 100% RDA Including Vitamins (ml.)	2000			1800	3000

[g]Unflavored.

Table 35–8   STANDARD BLENDED TUBE FEEDING USING WHOLE FOODS*

(1 Liter)

FOOD	AMOUNT
Strained meat	1 jar (100 gm.) Select a variety.
Egg[a]	1 (50 gm. frozen egg or 30 gm. powdered egg)
Applesauce	⅔ cup (200 gm.)
Strained mixed vegetable	1 jar (200 gm.)
Instant mashed potato	2 tbsp. (50 gm.)
Powdered skim milk	1 cup (60 gm.)
Vegetable oil	1 tbsp. (15 gm.)
Orange juice (or vitamin C supplement)	½ cup (100 gm.)
Water	1½ cups (400 cc.)

INGREDIENT	AMOUNT (gm.)	KCAL.	PRO. (gm.)	FAT (gm.)	CHO (gm.)	VIT. A (I.U.)	VIT. C (mg.)	NIACIN (mg.)	RIBOFLAVIN (µg)	THIAMIN (mg.)	CA (mg.)	P (mg.)	FE (mg.)	NA[b] (mg.)	K[b] (mg.)
Strained meat	100	97	14.5	4.3	–	–	4	3.7	151	0.01	8	81	1.6	192	234
Egg	50	78	6.0	5.5	–	570	–	–	140	0.05	26	50	1.1	59	62
Applesauce	200	182	0.4	0.2	48	80	2	–	20	0.04	8	10	1.5	4	130
Strained vegetable	200	82	2.8	0.2	17	7134	3	1.0	54	0.08	30	56	1.6	504	244
Instant mashed potato	50	182	3.6	0.3	42	–	32	5.4	30	0.11	17	86	0.8	40	800
Powdered skim milk	60	215	21.4	0.4	31	18	4	0.5	1060	0.2	777	603	0.4	315	1034
Vegetable oil	15	126	–	14.0	–	–	–	–	–	–	–	–	–	–	–
Orange juice	100	45	0.7	0.1	11	200	45	0.3	10	0.9	9	16	0.1	1	186
Total		1007	49.4	25.0	149	8002	90	10.9	1465	1.39	875	902	7.1	1115	2690

*From: Chicago Dietetic Association, Inc.: Manual of Clinical Dietetics. C.D.A., Downers Grove, Ill., 1976, Sec. 3, p. 14.
[a]The use of fresh raw eggs should be discouraged because of salmonella hazard. Use cooked egg custard (½ cup), salmonella-free frozen or powdered eggs or canned baby egg yolks.
[b]Various degrees of sodium restriction are achieved by using low-sodium vegetables, meat and milk. Potassium restriction is achieved by reducing or omitting the orange juice and mashed potato.

Table 35–9 FACTORS TO CONSIDER WHEN
SELECTING A FEEDING FORMULA

Form of protein, fat and carbohydrate in the formula as
related to patient's absorptive capacity (e.g., peptides
vs. whole protein).
Type of carbohydrate (e.g., lactose) used.
Sodium and potassium content, particularly when contemplating use for patients with compromised hepatic, renal
or cardiac function.
Recommended uses of the formula.
Caloric and protein density (i.e., kcal./ml. and gm. protein/
ml.) when contemplating use for a debilitated patient.

---

tube. (See Fig. 35–2.) A smaller tube is more
comfortable for a nasopharyngeal feeding but
may also require the use of a defined formula
diet, which has a lower viscosity. Commercially available tube feedings will flow through
a number 12 French tube; defined formula diets
will flow through a number 8 tube; and the tube
feeding made in a blender, because of its thick
consistency, requires use of a number 16
French tube for administration. (See Fig.
35–3.)

Continuous drip administration of the feeding at about 80 to 150 cc. per hour is ideal.
However, this does restrict the patient's activity. If feeding is given in batches, 200 to 350 cc.
should be given in not less than 10 to 15 minutes, and this should be mixed with or followed
by one half that amount of water. The additional water after feeding is important to prevent hypertonic dehydration from solute overload. The water is also used for careful rinsing
of the tube, since the protein in the feeding tends
to coagulate when it comes in contact with
gastric HCl.

In the first few days, the feeding should be
diluted to at least half strength, and not more
than 50 to 100 cc. should be given at a time, or
40 to 60 cc. per hour in the case of continuous
drip administration. This enables the patient to
develop tolerance gradually to the osmolality
of the formula, which is usually hyperosmolar
(greater than 350 mOsm. per kg.). This gradual
administration is especially important with defined formula diets, which have osmolalities of
800 to 1200 mOsm. per kg. when the formula is
taken at full strength. In these cases, it is wise
to dilute the formula even further and start with
one-quarter strength and then gradually increase to full strength and the required amount
within four to five days. The gastrointestinal
tract can adapt to accommodate a hyperosmolar formula when the formula is given in a way
that increases the osmolality slowly. Initially,
cramping and diarrhea may occur as the
hyperosmolar formula draws water into the intestinal tract. Debilitated patients, those with
gastrointestinal disorders, those being fed by
gastrostomy and jejunostomy tubes and those
whose gastrointestinal tracts have been without food for a long period of time are more
likely to be intolerant of the hyperosmolar formula and to require special attention. *Remember: when a patient is not taking a formula
full strength or is not taking the recommended*

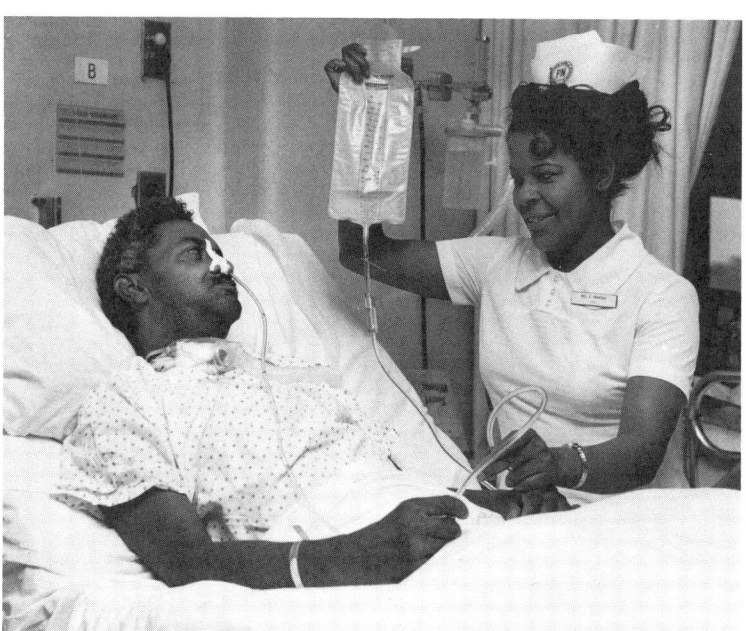

Figure 35–2 Tube feeding
administered through a nasogas-
tric tube. (Courtesy of Graduate
Hospital of the University of
Pennsylvaina. Photo by Paul
Axler.)

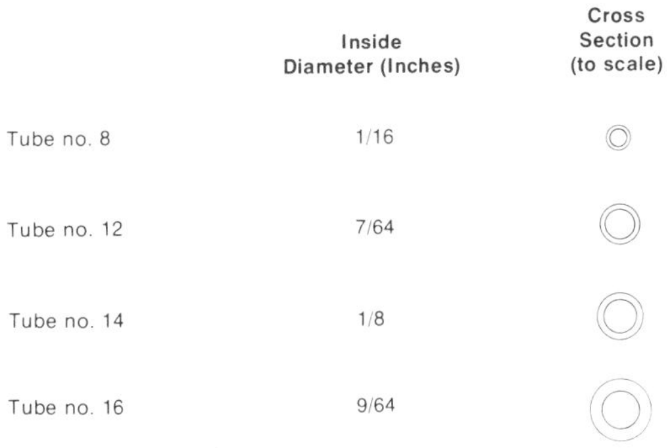

	Inside Diameter (Inches)	Cross Section (to scale)
Tube no. 8	1/16	◎
Tube no. 12	7/64	◎
Tube no. 14	1/8	◎
Tube no. 16	9/64	◎

Figure 35–3 A view of the inside diameters of commonly used nasogastric tubes suggests certain precautions; the number 8 tube is the most comfortable for the adult patient. Non-viscous formulas, such as soluble elemental diets, will flow freely through the lumen of this tube. Other prepackaged tube feedings may or may not flow readily through a number 8 tube, depending in part upon the method of administration and the physicochemical properties of the feeding. As a result, the feeding may have to be overdiluted if an inappropriately small tube is used, causing substantial reduction in daily nutrient intake by the patient. As an alternative, a tube of larger diameter may be used so that the formula can be given undiluted, but this will probably be less comfortable for the patient. (From: Gormican, A.: Tube feeding: an overview. Dietetic Currents, 2(2), 1975. Published by Ross Labs, Columbus, Ohio.)

amount, neither his energy needs nor his needs for vitamins and minerals are being met, and a supplement will be necessary. Eventually, six feedings per day of 300 to 400 cc. each spaced at intervals of three hours will permit administration of 1800 to 2400 kcal. per day, with an additional 1000 cc. of water as a minimum.

The nurse should record the *actual* formula intake of the patient, any incidents of vomiting or diarrhea and any signs of hypertonic dehydration or inadequate feeding. Assessment of hydration is particularly important in comatose, weak, very ill or frightened patients who are unable to communicate their feelings of thirst. Patients with tracheostomies who are unable to express their thirst are typical of those who may become dehydrated from a tube feeding. Renal or cardiovascular disease that causes malfunction of a patient's water elimination and retention mechanism is also likely to cause dehydration. The amount of water given to a tube-fed patient should be increased if insensible water loss is great owing to fever, perspiration or fistula drainage or if the formula is high in protein or electrolytes. Hypernatremia, dehydration and azotemia have been reported in tube-fed patients. See Table 35–10 for a list of factors that should be monitored routinely for the tube-fed patient.

The feeding should not be administered to a patient who is prone unless the head and thorax are elevated at least 30 degrees from the horizontal for at least 1 hour after feeding. This prevents possible aspiration of the formula into the lungs. The tube should be properly positioned in the stomach and not in the duodenum or jejunum, unless it is supposed to be there. The patient's stomach contents should be suctioned out before a new feeding is administered to make sure that there is only minimal residue from the previous feeding. Excessive residue may indicate an obstruction or digestive problem that should be resolved before the feeding is continued.

Diarrhea and cramping may be reduced by giving the tube feeding after it has reached room temperature or by warming it in hot water. Unused formula should be kept refrigerated and should not be used after 24 hours. If diarrhea continues even after dilution of the formula, it may be due to a lactose intolerance, either transitory or permanent, and a lactose-free formula such as Isocal (Mead Johnson) or Ensure (Ross Labs) should be tried. The addition of applesauce, pectin or Kanana-Banana flakes or the use of Probana, all good sources of pectin, may help to bring the diarrhea under control. Methylcellulose (a bulking agent) or paregoric, Kaopectate or Lomotil (antidiarrheal agents) can be added to the feeding just before administration. After the patient has become stabilized on the tube feeding, constipation may develop because of the low fiber content of the formula and the large amounts of milk used. Stool softeners or cathartics may then be necessary.

The goal of tube feeding is to put the patient into positive nitrogen balance or at least into nitrogen balance. Refer to the beginning of this chapter for a method to calculate roughly the N balance of a patient. The usual problem is not whether the patient is receiving nutritional support but whether he or she is getting *enough* support. Daily use of the nutritional

Table 35–10 FACTORS TO MONITOR IN ROUTINE MANAGEMENT OF TUBE-FED PATIENTS

Weight (at least three times per week)
Signs of edema
Signs of dehydration
Fluid intake and output records
Records of calorie, protein, fat, carbohydrate, mineral and vitamin intakes
Blood urea nitrogen (BUN) level
Urine glucose concentration
Serum glucose concentration
Serum electrolyte concentrations

index (Chapter 20), particularly for protein and calories, is also a valuable guide.

Patients who are being tube-fed need a great deal of encouragement to help them adjust to the situation. When administering the nourishment, the nurse can be of great assistance in establishing pleasant associations with the feedings. Prior to meal time, the feeding should be placed in an attractive pitcher on a neat, clean tray. When able, the patient should be given every encouragement to learn the procedure and to feed himself with the nurse's supervision.

PARENTERAL FEEDING

Maintenance of fluid balance and prophylaxis against nutritional depletion should be started during the first 24 hours after major surgery, trauma, burns or infection. As a general rule, each patient should receive a minimum of from 2500 to 3500 ml. of fluid daily, provided there is normal kidney function and no excessive or abnormal loss of fluid or electrolytes. Sodium and water have a tendency to be retained following surgery or trauma, and excessive sodium chloride should be avoided during the first 48 hours. There is also an increase in potassium and nitrogen excretion in the urine in the first 24 to 48 hours, and if the patient is unable to take fluid orally in 24 hours, potassium should be added to the basic intravenous fluid.

Intravenous Glucose and Intravenous Amino Acids

The usual regimen of fluid therapy is administration of a 5 per cent glucose solution intravenously, which gives the patient 50 gm. of glucose per liter, or about 100 to 150 gm. of glucose per day, or 400 to 600 kcal. This clinical practice is based on Gamble's observation while on a life raft that he could reduce ketosis and conserve water and salt in starving men by providing 100 gm. of carbohydrate daily.[10] This is true; however, it was also assumed that ketosis, known to be harmful to the diabetic patient, is also detrimental to the normal human being, which is not necessarily so. It is now known that, besides preventing ketosis and some protein breakdown, the administration of glucose during fasting prevents the body from adapting to conserve its body protein. As was mentioned in the discussion of starvation, the adaptation of the body that allows fat

mobilization and decreased use of body protein for energy is dependent upon a drop in the level of serum insulin. A constant infusion of glucose as D_5W (5 per cent dextrose in water) stimulates the pancreas to release insulin, and the body is never allowed to adapt to starvation with a protective ketosis.

The long-term effects of ketosis are unknown, but it appears that ketosis is not harmful for the normal human, as it is for the diabetic. The normal body has a feedback mechanism that stimulates the release of insulin and prevents ketonemia from becoming excessive, while diabetics do not have this mechanism.

Several researchers have shown that nitrogen balance improves even more when 3 per cent amino acids are given (either alone or in combination with glucose or fat) than when 5 per cent glucose is given by itself.[6, 12, 13] Second, it seems that the protein loss during stress is even less if the patient is given amino acids alone, without glucose or fat. Blackburn and others have been able to maintain nitrogen balance in patients by providing 30 to 60 gm. of amino acids daily via a peripheral vein.[5, 11, 13]

Three per cent amino acids instead of glucose can be given intravenously in a peripheral vein when it is known that the patient will be unable to eat for a few days during the catabolic phase. In these first few days, when the patient is hypercatabolic, the amino acids will be converted to glucose and used for energy, and they seem to help spare body protein. The amino acids, usually given at about 1 to 1.5 gm. per kg. ideal body weight (IBW), maintain visceral protein mass (organ and serum proteins). The precise mechanism by which this occurs is still unclear. It may be that a hypoinsulinemia develops that allows endogenous fat mobilization. The insulin level would be high enough to allow the utilization of protein but not high enough to inhibit lipolysis. Dispensable fat stores, rather than expensive protein and lean body mass, are used for energy. This therapy is controversial. Critics state that, for the patient who cannot eat for 2 to 3 days, the amount of protein saved by administration of 3 per cent amino acids (about 1 lb. or 0.5 kg.), is not worth the expense of giving the amino acids.

Each liter of 3 per cent amino acids contains 30 to 35 gm. of protein. When administered, the amount given is increased slowly from 1 liter the first day to 2 liters the second day and 3 liters the third day if necessary.

This form of parenteral nutrition is not a long-term therapy for the debilitated patient

who has no fat stores. Patients who are unable to eat for more than five days require more aggressive alimentation in the form of total parenteral nutrition.

The 3 per cent amino acid therapy has also been used in starvation treatment for obesity. (See Chapter 27.) The patient fasts, remains in ketosis and thus does not feel hungry. He receives 1.5 gm. protein per kg. IBW either intravenously or orally and thus maintains body protein while using excessive fat tissue for energy. In some cases, positive nitrogen balance can be maintained in the presence of negative calorie balance. Electrolytes, vitamins and minerals are also included in this therapy.

Besides intravenous administration of the necessary amino acids as a 3 per cent solution, protein can and should be given orally if possible. Meat, fish or fowl protein can be used, or tryptophan-enriched collagen or soy protein isolate can be added to water and given as a high-protein broth.

For the routine postoperative "clean" surgical patient, who will only be unable to eat for two to three days, 5 per cent glucose given intravenously is still the preferred therapy. However, for the patient who must be without oral intake longer than this and who has adequate fat stores, intravenous administration of isotonic amino acids might be considered. This procedure avoids the risk associated with insertion of the total parenteral nutrition (TPN) catheter into the superior vena cava. However, even when combined with glucose, this peripheral alimentation as used at present cannot meet the patient's complete calorie needs. If the patient is still not eating after 10 to 14 days of peripheral intravenous therapy, total parenteral nutrition using the superior vena cava should be considered.

TOTAL PARENTERAL NUTRITION (TPN)

This method of feeding has also been called *intravenous hyperalimentation* because so many more calories above normal requirements can be provided by it. For many patients, however, it is not hyperalimentation but merely normal alimentation—the maintenance of nutritional status or achievement of ideal body weight after being underweight.

By providing all nutrients intravenously, positive nitrogen balance can be attained and sustained for a prolonged period of time.

Indications for Use

This method of feeding is used for individuals who are debilitated and malnourished, with a weight loss of 10 per cent of body weight or more, and who are unable to obtain adequate nutrition orally or by peripheral intravenous feedings. A functioning gastrointestinal tract is always used in preference to intravenous nutrition if the patient can obtain an adequate intake by this route.

Patients with short bowel syndrome, bowel obstruction, inflammatory bowel disease or hypermetabolic states in which the gastrointestinal tract is completely or partially unusable benefit from this form of nutritional support. It is useful for patients with cancer who are malnourished but who still have a chance of responding to oncological treatment if they can be nutritionally rehabilitated. It is also useful in the treatment of neonatal abnormalities (see Chapter 37), extreme cachexia, anorexia, pulmonary diseases in which aspiration of food is a danger and in acute hepatic and renal failure, when the composition of the amino acid intake must be manipulated (for instance, the TPN for a hepatic patient with encephalopathy can be low in phenylalanine and high in tyrosine). Unlike the usual parenteral feeding of glucose, which at most provides 600 kcal. per day, total parenteral nutrition can supply enough calories for anabolism—up to 5000 kcal. or more per day if necessary. This is possible because the concentrated solution is administered through a polyvinyl or siliconized rubber catheter inserted into a large vein, the superior vena cava, where the hypertonic solution can be rapidly diluted by the large volume of blood. If such a concentrated solution were given in a peripheral vein, phlebitis would develop in 4 to 8 hours.

Nutrient Requirements and Composition of Formula

The body is less effective in using calories and nutrients provided by vein, so a greater amount must be given to keep the patient in positive nitrogen balance.

The composition of a typical TPN solution is shown in Table 35–11. It is a concentrated liquid that, at the usual strength, provides 1 kcal. per cc. or 1000 kcal. per liter of solution and about 42 gm. of protein per liter. The calorie:protein ratio of this solution is about 24 kcal. for every gram of protein—perfect for protein synthesis and anabolism.

Table 35–11 ADULT HYPERALIMENTATION
SOLUTION PREPARATION*

UNIT PREPARATION OF BASE SOLUTION	AMOUNT
Bulk Method (pharmacy)	
165 gm. anhydrous dextrose U.S.P. + 860 ml. 5% dextrose in 5% protein hydrolysate	
Sterilization through 0.22μ membrane filter under laminar-flow filtered-air hood	
Volume	1000 ml.
Calories	1000 kcal.
Glucose	208 gm.
Hydrolysates[a]	43 gm.
Nitrogen	6.0 gm.
Sodium	8 mEq.
Potassium	14 mEq.
Single Unit Method (ward or pharmacy)	
350 ml. 50% dextrose + 750 ml. 5% dextrose in 5% protein hydrolysate	
Aseptic mixing technique under laminar-flow filtered-air hood	
Volume	1100 ml.
Calories	1000 kcal.
Glucose	212 gm.
Hydrolysates[a]	37 gm.
Nitrogen	5.25 gm.
Sodium	7 mEq.
Potassium	13 mEq.
Additions to Each Unit of Base Solution (average adult)	
Sodium (⅔ chloride, ⅓ acetate)	40–50 mEq.
Potassium (chloride)	30–40 mEq.
Magnesium (sulfate)	8–12 mEq.
Optional	
Calcium (gluconate)	4–9 mEq.
Phosphate (potassium acid salt)	15–20 mEq.
Routine Additions to Only One Unit Daily (average adult)	
Multiple vitamin infusion	5 ml.
Optional Additions to One Unit (as indicated by serum studies)[b]	
Phytonadione (vitamin K_1)	5–10 mg.
Cyanocobalamin (vitamin B_{12})	10–30 μg.
Folic acid	0.5–1.5 mg.
Iron (dextriferron)	1.0–3.0 mg.

*From: Dudrick, S. J.: Total intravenous feeding: when nutrition seems impossible. Drug Therapy, February 1976, pp. 11–20.

[a] Micronutrients such as zinc, copper, manganese, cobalt and iodine are present as contaminants in hydrolysate solutions but may be given in plasma transfusions once or twice weekly if desired.

[b] Alternatively, may be given intramuscularly in weekly dosages.

Protein. Protein is provided by crystalline amino acids or protein hydrolysates, although the crystalline amino acids are preferable because more of their protein is available for use and they cannot cause an allergic reaction. Since the usual TPN solution contains 42 gm. of protein per liter, most patients require at least 2 to 3 liters per day in order to meet their protein requirements of 1 to 1.5 gm. protein per kg. IBW per day. Infants require at least 2.5 gm. protein per kg. IBW. (See Table 35–12.)

Calories. The caloric source in a TPN formula is usually a 50 per cent solution of glucose, which has a much higher osmolality than the usual 5 per cent glucose solution administered in peripheral intravenous therapy. The amount of glucose is usually 500 ml., or one half of a liter of TPN solution. This provides 250 gm. of glucose or 1000 kcal. per liter of TPN solution (250 gm. glucose × 4 kcal. per gm. glucose = 1000 kcal.). To this is added the calories provided by the protein in the mixture (42.5 gm. protein × 4 kcal. per gm. protein = 170 kcal.), so that the final solution contains 1170 kcal. per liter or about 1200 kcal. per 1000 cc., which is usually remembered as 1 kcal. per cc. Most patients require at least 2 to 3 liters per day to meet their caloric requirements of 35 to 50 kcal. per kg. per day. Four liters per day is about the maximum amount of fluid that can be given. Some patients in catabolic states (e.g., those with burns or severe trauma) who have exaggerated nutritional requirements of 5000 to 8000 kcal. per day will require a more concentrated solution. This can be achieved by using additional glucose or Intralipid.

Fat. Fat in a form suitable for intravenous use is now available in this country. Such products had been banned for about 10 years because of some bad experiences. The fat source Intralipid is much more suitable than previous ones and has been shown to be safe. The addition of fat can increase the caloric concentration of the TPN fluid considerably, and the addition of small amounts also prevents essential fatty acid (EFA) deficiency, which has been reported in babies and severely depleted adults receiving TPN.[9] The signs of EFA deficiency are: light, flaky and perhaps reddened skin lesions that appear on the scalp, arms and legs; thrombocytopenia; increased hemolysis; impaired wound healing; and growth retardation in the case of infants. (See Chapter 12 for further discussion.) To cure or prevent the deficiency state, Intralipid can be given in the TPN fluid 2 to 3 times per week. If Intralipid cannot be added to the TPN solution and cannot be taken orally, some success in relieving essential fatty acid deficiency may be achieved by rubbing sunflower seed oil or another highly polyunsatured oil into the skin.[17]

Table 35–12   RECOMMENDED DAILY REQUIREMENTS OF PARENTERALLY FED PATIENTS[a]

NUTRIENT	CHILD (per kg.)	ADULT—NORMAL (per kg.)	ADULT—HIGH (per kg.)	INFANT (per kg.)
Energy	50–60 kcal.	25–30 kcal.	50–60 kcal.	90–125 kcal.
Water	100 ml.	25–30 ml.	50–60 ml.	90–125 ml.
Amino Acids	2 gm.	1 gm.	2 gm.	2.5 gm.
Glucose	5 gm.	2 gm.	5 gm.	25–30 gm.
Fat[b]	3 gm.	2 gm.	3 gm.	4 gm.

[a]Based on ideal body weight
[b]Where fat is not used, add 4 gm. per kg. per day of carbohydrate.

Electrolytes.   Electrolytes are added to the solution as they are required by the patient. They must be added to promote efficient tissue weight gain. Table 35–11 gives the electrolyte content of a typical solution. Potassium is especially important because as the patient enters anabolism, glucose and potassium move into the cells, and the potassium requirement may be increased.

Phosphate is also important because, in the presence of high-calorie feedings, dangerous hypophosphatemia can develop. Calcium is necessary to balance the phosphate infusion.

Vitamins and Other Minerals.   Vitamins are added to the intravenous feedings as a multiple vitamin infusion (MVI). Five cc. daily is the usual dosage, although some people prescribe 10 cc. The vitamin infusion is not ideal, however, because it is not formulated for TPN use. The amounts of fat-soluble vitamins in this preparation should be decreased and given at levels of two-thirds the RDA, because those allowances were developed for oral intake. The amounts of water-soluble vitamins in the formula should be increased and given at 1.5 to 2 times the RDA, because when given intravenously they are excreted more rapidly. Since folic acid and vitamin B_{12} are not present in this vitamin preparation, they must be added separately. Folic acid is added to 1 liter of fluid each day, and vitamin B_{12} is added to 1 liter once every three weeks. A committee of the Department of Foods and Nutrition of the American Medical Association has proposed a formulation for an intravenous vitamin supplement.[1] Vitamin K, iron, zinc, copper and other trace minerals are added when necessary, although Solomons and associates recommend routine supplementation with trace minerals.[20] Incidences of zinc deficiency in patients receiving long-term TPN have been reported, as well as a chromium deficiency in a woman who received TPN for three and one half years. It resolved itself when chromium was added to the TPN solution.[14]

Administration

Insertion of the TPN catheter into the superior vena cava is a surgical technique performed under sterile conditions with a draped field. The patient is given local anesthesia. Once placement of the tube in the inferior vena cava has been confirmed, administration of TPN can begin. Because the TPN solution is hyperosmolar and a very concentrated source of glucose, it must be administered slowly at first. Usually, 1 liter is given in 24 hours using a constant drip infusion maintained by gravity or a pump. Blood glucose, urine glucose and electrolyte levels are watched closely. The second liter is given in 12 hours, followed by the third liter bottle in another 12 hours. This regimen of two liters per 24 hours is continued for the next several days until it becomes apparent from monitoring of the blood glucose and urine glucose concentrations, urinary output, blood urea nitrogen (BUN) level and electrolyte levels that the patient is stable and the insulin response is sufficient. Table 35–13 lists the clinical factors that should be monitored in the patient receiving TPN. The amount of solution can then be increased by giving 1 liter every 8 hours (3 bottles in 24 hours) and then 1 liter every 6 hours (4 bottles in 24 hours). Four liters per day is the maximum that most patients can tolerate. Patients requiring more than 4000 kcal. per day will probably require the addition of some fat to the solution to increase its caloric concentration. The solution should be administered at a steady rate. If the administration falls behind, the administration rate should be corrected. Do not attempt to "catch up," because an excessive glucose load will result. When hyperalimentation is no longer needed, it is important to decrease the amount infused

Table 35–13 VARIABLES TO BE MONITORED DURING INTRAVENOUS HYPERALIMENTATION*

| VARIABLES TO BE MONITORED | SUGGESTED FREQUENCY[a] | |
	INITIAL PERIOD	LATER PERIOD
Growth Variables		
Weight	Daily	Daily
Length (infants only)	Weekly	Weekly
Head circumference (infants only)	Weekly	Weekly
Metabolic Variables		
Blood		
Plasma electrolytes (Na^+, K^+, Cl^-)	Daily	3/week
Blood urea nitrogen	3/week	2/week
Plasma total calcium and inorganic phosphorus	3/week	2/week
Blood glucose	Daily	3/week
Plasma transaminases	3/week	2/week
Plasma total protein and fractions	2/week	Weekly
Blood acid-base status	Daily	3/week
Hemoglobin	Weekly	Weekly
Ammonia	2/week	Weekly
Magnesium	2/week	Weekly
Urine		
Glucose	4–6/day	2/day
Specific gravity or osmolarity	2–4/day	Daily
General Measurements		
Volume of infusate	Daily	Daily
Oral intake (if any)	Daily	Daily
Urinary output	Daily	Daily
Prevention and Detection of Infection		
Clinical observations (activity, temperature, etc.)	Daily	Daily
WBC[b] count and differential	As indicated	As indicated
Cultures	As indicated	As indicated

*From: Winters, R. W., and Wilmore, D. W.: Evaluation of the patient. In: White, P. L., Nagy, M. E., and Fletcher, D. C. (eds.): Total Parenteral Nutrition. Acton, Mass., Publishing Sciences Group, Inc., 1974, p. 48.

[a]*Initial period* refers to that period in which a full glucose intake is being achieved; *later period* implies that the patient has achieved a steady metabolic state. In the presence of metabolic instability, the more intensive monitoring outlined under *initial period* should be followed.

[b]WBC = white blood cell.

gradually to prevent hypoglycemic shock. Oral intake should also be well established and should increase as the TPN decreases.

Some patients receiving TPN still feel hungry and, if possible, they can take some food orally. If complete bowel rest is required, however, the patient should not be given anything, not even water, by mouth but can only suck on ice chips.

TPN should be given in amounts to allow a daily weight gain of one quarter to one half lb. (0.1 to 0.2 kg.). This seems to be the limit for the amount of body tissue that can be synthesized in 24 hours. A weight gain greater than this indicates fluid retention, and the intake of TPN solution should be reduced. Once ideal weight is achieved, the TPN intake should be adjusted to maintain it.

Care of the TPN Catheter Site

Care of the catheter site requires special attention by the nurse because it is an easy entrance for microorganisms into a major vein. The dressings around the site and the tubing from the catheter to the TPN bottle should be changed 2 to 3 times per week. The area around the catheter insertion site should be cleansed with an antiseptic during each dressing change, and antibiotic ointment should be applied to the catheter site. The area is then covered with sterile dressings. The TPN catheter should not be used for any procedures other than TPN administration. The catheter is not removed until it is no longer needed or until there is indication of an infection at the catheter tip where it enters the vein (usually evidenced by a fever).

Exercise

Skeletal muscle protein synthesis is enhanced if the muscles are exercised. For example, in states of protein depletion the heart muscle is spared until the end, apparently because it receives constant exercise. Exercise and physical therapy are very useful for the patient who is being nutritionally rehabilitated. They are an important part of the total therapy and allow efficient use to be made of the nutritional support being provided to the patient.

Cyclic Hyperalimentation

Cyclic hyperalimentation is a method of parenteral nutrition whereby the patient is fed amino acids and glucose parenterally for 10 to 14 hours and amino acids only, either orally or parenterally, for the remainder of the 24-hour period.[15] This technique is valuable when (1) oral intake is not adequate to meet the patient's nutritional needs but total parenteral support is not necessary, (2) the patient is ambulatory or at home and does not want the encumbering I.V. bottle during the day or (3) essential fatty acid deficiency must be prevented.

It is postulated that cyclic hyperalimentation follows the body's normal intake of nutrients more closely, so that for a period of every day, usually at night during sleep, there is no nutritional intake. Second, cyclic hyperalimentation prevents essential fatty acid deficiency because, during the period without hyperalimentation, the person uses some fatty acids from fat stored for energy and thus receives linoleic acid. Third, liver function returns to normal, and fourth, a lower caloric intake is required to maintain nitrogen balance because some of the patient's fat stores are used.

Total Parenteral Nutrition at Home

The patient who will never recover gastrointestinal tract function but who is free of disease can be maintained indefinitely with TPN. Patients have been kept alive and have returned to normal lives and work using this method. Such a person usually receives infusions for 5 to 7 nights per week while sleeping, depending upon the requirements needed to maintain weight. The infusion is gradually decreased in the last few hours in order to prevent hypoglycemia in the non-alimentary period.

Table 35-14   POTENTIAL COMPLICATIONS OF HYPERALIMENTATION

SUBCLAVIAN CATHETERIZATION
- Pneumothorax
- Hemothorax
- Hydrothorax
- Tension pneumothorax
- Subcutaneous emphysema
- Brachial plexus injury
- Subclavian artery injury
- Subclavian hematoma
- Central vein thrombophlebitis
- Arteriovenous fistula
- Thoracic duct injury
- Hydromediastinum
- Air embolism
- Catheter embolism
- Catheter misplacement
- Cardiac perforation; tamponade
- Endocarditis

INFECTION AND SEPSIS
- Catheter entrance site
  - Contamination during insertion
  - Long-term catheter placement
- Catheter seeding from blood-borne or distant infection
- Solution contamination

METABOLIC COMPLICATIONS
- Dehydration from osmotic diuresis
- Hyperosmolar, nonketotic, hyperglycemic coma
- Rebound hypoglycemia on sudden cessation of treatment
- Hypomagnesemia
- Hypocalcemia
- Hyperphosphatemia and hypophosphatemia
- Hyperchloremic metabolic acidosis
- Azotemia
- Hyperammonemia
- Electrolyte imbalance

Complications

Although TPN appears to be the answer to many clinical nutritional problems, it is not without risk. Some of the complications are listed in Table 35-14. The risk to the patient should always be balanced against the benefit of TPN, and patients receiving it should always be monitored closely.

PROBLEMS AND SUGGESTED TOPICS FOR DISCUSSION

1. Describe what is happening metabolically in a healthy person who is fasting. Talk with a healthy person who has fasted and try to find out how he felt during the first 2 days of the fast and after about 1 week of fasting.
2. Give reasons for emphasis on (a) adequate protein therapy, (b) adequate fluid therapy, (c) adequate electrolyte therapy and (d) adequate calorie therapy in a patient with an infection.
3. Describe the catabolic stress response. How does it protect the body during stress?
4. Become familiar with the various types of tube feedings

used for patients. What do they contain? Determine whether what the patient actually receives meets his nutritional needs.

5. Talk with a patient who is receiving a defined formula diet. What is his or her reaction to it? How much is he or she taking? Does the patient need this form of therapy?

6. Under what conditions would intravenous hyperalimentation be indicated?

CITED REFERENCES

1. American Medical Association, Nutrition Advisory Group: Statement on Guidelines for Multivitamin Preparations for Parenteral Use. Chicago, A.M.A., 1975.

2. Bistrian, B. R., Blackburn, G. L., and Scrimshaw, N. S.: Effect of mild infectious illness on nitrogen metabolism in patients on a modified fast. Am. J. Clin. Nutr., 28:1044, 1975.

3. Blackburn, G. L., and Bistrian, B. R.: Nutritional care of the injured or septic patient. Surg. Clin. North Am., 56:1195, 1976.

4. Blackburn, G. L., and Bistrian, B. R.: Protein-calorie curative therapy. In: Sneider, H.: Nutritional Support in Medical Practice. New York, Harper & Row, 1976.

5. Blackburn, G. L., et al.: Peripheral intravenous feeding with isotonic amino acid solutions. Am. J. Surg., 125:447, 1973.

6. Blackburn, G. L., et al.: Protein-sparing therapy during periods of starvation with sepsis or trauma. Ann. Surg., 177:588, 1973.

7. DuBois, E. F., and Chambers, W. H.: Calories in medical practice. Handbook of Nutrition. Chicago, American Medical Association, 1943, pp. 55–70.

8. Dudrick, S. J., et al.: Total Parenteral Nutrition (videotape). Network for Continuing Medical Education, Houston, Texas, 1976.

9. Fleming, C. R., Smith, L. M., and Hodges, R. E.: Essential fatty acid deficiency in adults receiving total parenteral nutrition. Am. J. Clin. Nutr., 29:976, 1976.

10. Gamble, J. L.: Physiological information gained from studies on the life raft ration. Harvey Lect., 42:247, 1947.

11. Gazzaniga, A. B., et al.: Endogenous caloric sources and nitrogen balance. Arch. Surg., 111:1357, 1976.

12. Greenberg, G. R., et al.: Protein-sparing therapy in postoperative patients. N. Engl. J. Med., 294:1411, 1975.

13. Hoover, H. C., et al.: Nitrogen-sparing intravenous fluids in postoperative patients. N. Engl. J. Med., 293:172, 1975.

14. Jeejeebhoy, K. N., et al.: Chromium deficiency, glucose intolerance, and neuropathy reversed by chromium supplementation in a patient receiving long-term parenteral nutrition. Am. J. Clin. Nutr., 30:531, 1977.

15. Maini, B., et al.: Cyclic hyperalimentation: an optimal technique for preservation of visceral protein. J. Surg. Res., 20:515, 1976.

16. Matthews, D. M., and Adibi, S. A.: Peptide absorption. Gastroenterology, 71:151, 1976.

17. Press, M., Hartop, P. J., and Prottey, C.: Correction of essential fatty acid deficiency in man by cutaneous application of sunflower seed oil. Lancet, 1:597, 1974.

18. Rutten, P., et al.: Determination of optimal hyperalimentation infusion rate. J. Surg. Res., 18:477, 1975.

19. Scrimshaw, N. S.: Malnutrition and infection. Borden's Review, 26(2), 1965.

20. Solomons, N. W., et al.: Plasma trace metals during total parenteral alimentation. Gastroenterology, 70:1022, 1976.

ADDITIONAL REFERENCES

American College of Surgeons: Manual of Surgical Nutrition. Philadelphia, W. B. Saunders Co., 1975.

Barker, H. G.: Supplementation of protein and caloric needs in the surgical patient. Am. J. Clin. Nutr., 3:466, 1955.

Barron, J.: Tube feeding with liquified natural foods. Henry Ford Hospital Med. J., Vol. 1, June 1953.

Blackburn, G. L., et al.: Restoration of the visceral component of protein malnutrition during hypocaloric feedings. Clin. Res., 23:315A, 1975.

Border, J. R., et al.: Multiple systems organ failure: muscle fuel deficit with visceral protein malnutrition. Surg. Clin. North Am., 56:1147, 1976.

Broviac, J. W., and Scribner, B. H.: Prolonged parenteral nutrition in the home. Surg. Gynecol. Obstet., 139:24, 1974.

Cahill, G. F.: Starvation in man. N. Engl. J. Med., 282:668, 1970.

Clowes, G. H. A. (ed.): Response to infection and injury. II. Metabolism. Surg. Clin. North Am., 56(5), 1976.

Colley, R., and Phillips, K.: Helping the patient with hyperalimentation. Nursing '73, 3:6, 1973.

Copeland, E. M., et al.: Intravenous hyperalimentation in cancer patients. J. Surg. Res., 16:241, 1974.

Dudrick, S. J., Copeland, E. M., and MacFayden, B. V.: Long-term parenteral nutrition: its current status. Hospital Practice, 10:47, May 1975.

Dudrick, S. J., and Rhoads, J. E.: New horizons for intravenous feeding. JAMA, 215:939, 1971.

Dudrick, S. J., et al.: Can intravenous feeding as the sole means of nutrition support growth in the child and restore weight loss in the adult? Ann. Surg., 169:974, 1969.

Dudrick, S. J., et al.: Long-term total parenteral nutrition and growth, development, and positive nitrogen balance. Surgery, 64:134, 1968.

Engle, F. L., and Jaeger, C.: Dehydration with hypernatremia, hyperchloremia and azotemia complicating nasogastric tube feeding. Am. J. Med., 17:196, 1954.

Fason, M. F.: Controlling bacterial growth in tube feedings. Am. J. Nurs., 67:1246, 1967.

Felig, P.: Intravenous nutrition: fact and fancy. N. Engl. J. Med., 294:1455, 1976.

Fischer, J. E. (ed.): Total Parenteral Nutrition. Boston, Little, Brown & Co., 1976.

Flatt, J. P., and Blackburn, G. L.: The metabolic fuel regulatory system: implications for protein-sparing therapies during caloric deprivation and disease. Am. J. Clin. Nutr., 27:175, 1974.

Gault, A. M., et al.: Hypernatremia, azotemia and dehydration due to high protein tube feeding. Ann. Intern. Med., 68:778, 1968.

Good, R. A., et al.: Nutritional deficiency, immunologic function and disease. Am. J. Pathol., 84:599, 1976.

Gordon, J. E.: Synergism of malnutrition and infectious disease. In: Beaton, G. H., and Bengoa, J. M. (eds.): Nutrition in Preventive Medicine. Geneva, Switzerland, WHO, 1976, pp. 193–209.

Gormican, A.: Tube feeding. An overview. Dietetic Currents, 2(2), 1975.

Gormican, A., and Liddy, E.: Nasogastric tube feedings. Postgrad. Med., 53:71, 1973.

Jeejeebhoy, K. N., et al.: Total parenteral nutrition at

home: studies in patients surviving 4 months to 5 years. Gastroenterology, *71*:943, 1976.

Kaminski, M. V.: Enteral hyperalimentation. Surg. Gynecol. Obstet., *143*:12, 1976.

Kaminski, M. V.: Parenteral Hyperalimentation: Prevention and Treatment of Complications. A Policy and Procedure Manual. Washington, D.C. Walter Reed General Hospital, Hyperalimentation Registry, 1974.

Krehl, W. A.: Tube feeding. JAMA, *169*:1153, 1959.

Kubo, W., et al.: Fluid and electrolyte problems of tube-fed patients. Am. J. Nurs., *76*:912, 1976.

McFarlane, H.: Nutrition and Immunity. In: Present Knowledge in Nutrition, 4th ed. New York, The Nutrition Foundation, Inc., 1976.

Mecray, P., Jr.: Nutrition and wound healing. Am. J. Clin. Nutr., *3*:461, 1955.

Mitty, W. F., Nealon, T. F., and Grossi, C.: Use of elemental diets in surgical cases. Am. J. Gastroenterol., *65*:297, 1976.

Porte, D., and Robertson, R. P.: Control of insulin secretion by catecholamines, stress, and the sympathetic nervous system. Fed. Proc., *32*:1792, 1973.

Riella, M. C., et al.: Essential fatty acid deficiency in human adults during total parenteral nutrition. Ann. Intern. Med., *83*:786, 1975.

Schwartz, P. L.: Ascorbic acid in wound healing: a review. J. Am. Diet. Assoc., *56*:497, 1970.

Scribner, B. H., et al.: Long-term parenteral nutrition. JAMA, *212*:457, 1970.

Shils, M. E.: A program for total parenteral nutrition at home. Am. J. Clin. Nutr., *28*:1429, 1975.

Shils, M. E., Bloch, A. S., and Chernoff, R.: Liquid formulas for oral and tube feeding. Clin. Bull., *6*:151, 1976.

Skillman, J. J., et al.: Improved albumin synthesis in postoperative patients by amino acid infusion. N. Engl. J. Med., *295*:1037, 1976.

Smith, A. V.: Nasogastric tube feedings. Am. J. Nurs., *57*:1451, 1957.

Vanamee, P.: Parenteral nutrition. In: Present Knowledge in Nutrition, 4th ed. New York, The Nutrition Foundation, Inc., 1976.

Walike, B. C., and Walike, J. W.: Lactose content of tube feeding diets as a cause of diarrhea. Laryngoscope, *83*:1109, 1973.

White, P. L., and Nagy, M. E. (eds.): Total Parenteral Nutrition. Acton, Mass., Publishing Sciences Group, Inc., 1974.

Wolstenholme, G. E. W., and O'Connor, M.: Nutrition and Infection. Boston, Little, Brown & Co., 1968.

UNIT FIFTEEN

NEOPLASTIC DISEASE

Chapter 36

NUTRITION, DIET AND CANCER

Dorice M. Czajka-Narins, Ph. D.*

Definition

Today *cancer, tumor* and *neoplasia* are terms used interchangeably. The term *tumor* was applied to all masses before the natures of various types of lesions were understood. The suffix *-oma* was used to denote the lesion. Eventually, swellings due to known causes, especially those due to infection, were excluded, and use of the term was limited to those masses of unknown cause that apparently arose by unrestrained growth of the individual's own cells. Excessive growth can be invasive rather than manifested as a mass. *Neoplasia* means an uncontrolled, progressive multiplication of cells.

Tumors can be classified on the basis of the cell of origin and their behavior as benign, intermediate and malignant. A *benign* tumor is circumscribed, usually well encapsulated, and affects the host either by pressure atrophy or by obstruction. A *malignant* tumor, or cancer, invades surrounding tissue and releases cells that are carried to other parts of the body to set up secondary growth, or metastases. Malignant tumors produce a number of effects on the host, including mechanical pressure and obstruction, destruction of tissue, hemorrhage, infection, anemia, cachexia, hormonal abnormalities and other changes, such as muscle weakness, which cannot be explained. Tumors with patterns of behavior that do not fall into either category are classified as *intermediate* tumors. Intermediate tumors are locally invasive but do not metastasize.

*Associate Professor, Clinical Nutrition, Rush University, Chicago, Illinois.

Mode of Action

According to one theory, tumorigenesis or carcinogenesis is a two-stage process involving initiation and promotion. In the *initiation* stage, normal cells are transformed into tumor cells by interaction with a virus, chemical or as yet unknown agent. This interaction involves alteration of DNA. Most errors in DNA replication are corrected by the body's repair mechanisms. It is not known definitely whether the repair mechanisms can reverse the effects of an inductive agent in some people but not in others. During the *promotion* stage, initiated cells multiply to form a discrete tumor. The effect of diet and nutrition on both the initiation and promotion stages of tumor development is currently the subject of intense scrutiny.

Our knowledge of nutrition related to cancer, although limited, is in two general areas: (1) nutrition in the etiology of cancer and (2) the role of nutrition in patients who have cancer. The second area can be subdivided into (a) the nutritional effects of cancer, (b) the nutrition disorders resulting from cancer treatment and (c) the nutritional therapy for cancer patients.

NUTRITION IN THE ETIOLOGY OF CANCER

If the estimate that 80 to 90 per cent of cancer is related to environmental factors is correct, then the majority of human cancer may be potentially preventable. An example of the influence of environmental factors is the observation that migrants from one culture to

another show a shift in cancer pattern from that of the old habitat to that of the new one. Migrants to the United States develop bowel and breast cancer more often even though they come from areas where these cancers are uncommon. Cancer is the second leading cause of death in the United States, and according to preliminary data 360,000 people died of various forms of cancer in 1975, and there were 665,000 new cancer patients. Therefore, if environmental factors can be specifically defined and this knowledge applied, the potential ramifications for treatment and prevention of cancer are tremendous.

One environmental factor possibly involved in carcinogenesis is the diet. Food additives or contaminants have been suspected to be causes of cancer for a number of years, but that foods themselves may facilitate cancer development is a more recent concept. Subsequent studies have shown positive correlations between dietary components and cancer; however, *correlation is not cause.*

The diet may also contain precursor compounds that are converted into carcinogens. *Nitrates* and *nitrites* can be converted to *nitrosamines,* which are powerful carcinogens. Conclusive data on the absorption, distribution, metabolism and excretion of nitrites and nitrates in humans, however, are not available. Nitrites are present naturally in spinach, beets and drinking water and are added during the processing of some meats such as bacon. In Chile, nitrate in the water supply has been linked to stomach cancer. American data have not supported this relationship.[3]

Different nutrients affect cancer differently, and one nutrient can have different effects on different types of cancer. Unfortunately, this area is largely unexplored, and the available data frequently appear to conflict, so that practical suggestions for preventive nutrition cannot be formulated.

Calories

In general, studies of experimentally induced tumors in animals show that chronic calorie restriction inhibits the growth of most tumors. However, hepatic tumors are stimulated by such restriction, while adrenal adenomas are unaffected. How does caloric restriction inhibit tumor growth? According to one theory, mitotic activity is inhibited by the limited amount of carbohydrate and carbohydrate intermediates available for energy production. Other theories postulate that changes in hormones produced by caloric restriction inhibit tumorigenesis by a complex but unknown mechanism.

For both humans and animals, body weight appears to be related to tumor risk. A retrospective study of 8293 college men classified according to their athletic participation revealed that more major athletes (lettermen) died from neoplasms than did non-athletes.[23] When all the men dying from cancer were compared, major athletes were found to die at younger ages than minor athletes or non-athletes did. The findings suggest that the heavier the athlete in college (i.e., the major athletes and lettermen), the younger the age of death from the neoplasm. Studies using rats also demonstrate that the incidence of various types of tumors is consistently greater in heavier animals.

Lipid

In 1941, studies of experimental carcinogenesis in rats showed that increasing the dietary lipid from low (2 to 5 per cent) to moderate levels (20 to 27 per cent) produced more tumors, and the tumors appeared earlier.[5] However, increasing the lipid from moderate levels to high levels (61 per cent) did not produce a similar increase in tumors. More recently, Carroll and Khor[8, 9] examined the effect of fat in the diet by feeding rats diets containing either 0.5 per cent or 20 per cent corn oil both before and after administration of the carcinogen 7,12-dimethylbenzanthracene (DMBA). There was a greater incidence of tumors in the animals fed 20 per cent corn oil after DMBA administration. The amount of fat fed before DMBA administration was not found to be related to the induction of cancer. These findings suggest that a high-fat diet may be important in the promotion stage of tumor development. However, high-fat diets do not produce an increase in the incidence of all experimental tumors, thus confounding most conclusions about the role of fat in carcinogenesis.

Extensive epidemiological data show a positive correlation between the amount of fat in the diet and the incidence of some neoplasms. High-fat Western diets are associated with intestinal cancer in both males and females and with cancer of the breast (Fig. 36–1) in females.[7]

Concomitant with changes in the amount of fat in the diet is usually a change in the amount

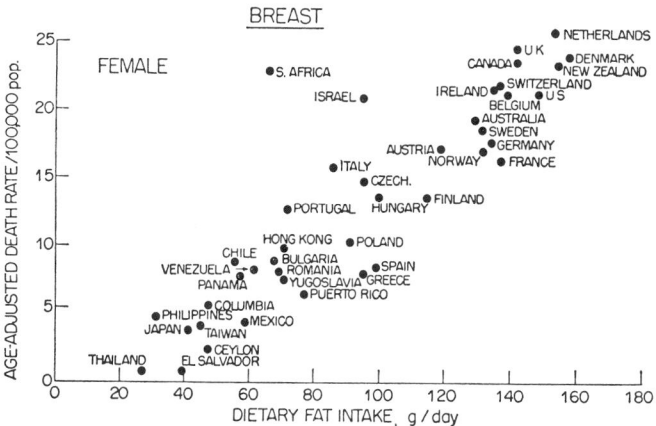

Figure 36–1 Positive correlation between per capita consumption of dietary fat and age-related mortality from cancer of the breast. (From: Carroll, K. K., and Khor, H. T.: Dietary fat in relation to tumorigenesis. Prog. Biochem. Pharmacol., *10*:308, 1975.)

of fiber. Alterations in the fiber intake can lead to changes in the composition of the feces and in the type of bacteria in the intestinal tract and alterations in the bile salt metabolism. Therefore, some of the effects of a high-fat diet may be due to alterations in these other variables. The relatively low lipid content and high fiber content of the typical Seventh Day Adventist (vegetarian) diet have been suggested to account for the relatively low incidence of certain types of cancer in this group. On the other hand, populations such as Indians and Eskimos, who consume large amounts of fat with or without fiber intake, are not usually prone to colonic cancer.

Tumor growth appears to be affected by the type of lipid as well as by the amount of lipid ingested. In animals, tumors are more readily induced when the diet contains lipid high in polyunsaturated fatty acids. One retrospective study in humans showed a higher incidence of fatal cancers in individuals whose diets were four times higher in polyunsaturated fatty acids and 50 per cent lower in cholesterol than in those on the control diet. However, subsequent studies of diets high in polyunsaturated fatty acids do not confirm these findings. Obviously, more controlled studies are needed on the effect of a diet high in polyunsaturated fatty acids on tumorigenesis.

The mechanism by which a high fat intake may facilitate tumor development may be hormonal. Certain hormone-dependent mammary tumors in rats require estrogen and prolactin for continued growth. In addition, a high fat intake raises the concentration of serum prolactin and thus might promote tumor growth. However, studies of plasma concentration of prolactin in women of various ethnic backgrounds suggest that elevation *per se* does not increase the risk of breast cancer in humans.[17]

Protein

Mortality from lymphoma and the consumption of animal protein, particularly beef protein, are positively correlated.[13] Understanding of the role of protein in tumor development is complicated by the fact that most diets high in protein are also high in meat, which raises the fat content and lowers the fiber content of the diet. Epidemiological data indicate that those countries in which the intake of animal protein is increasing are also experiencing a concurrent rise in mortality from colonic cancer. However, the interaction between beef intake, fat intake and the incidence of colonic cancer is not at all clear.

The effect of protein on experimental carcinogenesis depends on the tissue of origin and the type and malignancy of the tumor, as well as on the type of protein and the caloric adequacy of the diet. Certain amino acid deficiencies inhibit some but not all tumors. Plasma amino acid concentrations and urinary amino acid excretion are altered in some patients with cancer, but the significance of these changes is not known.

Although the role of immunity in tumorigenesis is still questionable, the mechanism by which calories and protein affect the growth of tumors may involve cell-mediated immunity. Cell-mediated immunity is depressed when protein and caloric intake are inadequate. Since cell-mediated immunity may be a defense against cancer, factors that alter cellular immunity could affect tumorigenesis. The effects of endocrine function (enhance-

ment of tumorigenesis) seem to be in opposition to those of cell-mediated immunity (depression of tumorigenesis).

Vitamins

Deficiencies of some vitamins enhance tumor growth; deficiencies of other vitamins suppress it. Conversely, excesses of some vitamins enhance tumor growth, while excesses of others are inhibitory. The relationships are complex, knowledge of them is sparse, and many more studies are needed.

Vitamin A. Some data suggest that vitamin A may be protective against cancer. Theories state that vitamin A may stimulate the immune system, inhibit the binding of the carcinogen to DNA or control premalignant epithelial cell differentiation. High dietary levels of retinoids (forms of vitamin A) have some protective effect in preventing chemical carcinogenesis in epithelial tissues. On the other hand, vitamin A deficiency in animals enhances their susceptibility to the chemical induction of some tumors. Since natural retinoids in the large doses required to produce this protective effect are also toxic and are largely deposited in the liver where they would have limited usefulness, the clinical application seems remote. Synthetic analogs of the vitamin have been suggested as therapeutic agents, based on the successful prevention of some cancers in animals. The future practical use of these analogs will depend on the availability of synthetic retinols and on the results of more extensive studies.

Epidemiological data suggest that relatively low dietary intakes of vitamin A are correlated with high incidence of cancer of the stomach, nasopharynx and lung when a correction is made for smoking habits. Plasma vitamin A and beta-carotene levels, indicators of the nutritional status of the vitamin in an individual, are low in patients with tumors of the alimentary tract.[4]

Vitamin C. Ascorbic acid may also influence tumorigenesis. In one study of the vitamin C status of patients with malignant disease it was found that 92 per cent had leukocyte ascorbic acid levels less than the lower limit of normal range, and 60 per cent had very low levels.[20] Physical signs compatible with subclinical scurvy were seen in some patients with the lowest levels. Another study of cancer patients confirmed the low leukocyte ascorbic acid levels, and further, found that patients with bone metastases had lower vitamin C values than patients without bone metastases,[2] even though both groups were receiving vitamin supplements. These and other data suggest that large doses of vitamin C may retard collagen breakdown and, possibly, metastases.

So far, only one clinical trial of the effects of high doses of ascorbic acid on patients with advanced cancer has been conducted.[6] One hundred terminal cancer patients received a vitamin C supplement (usually 10 gm. per day by intravenous infusion for about 10 days and orally thereafter) as their only definitive form of treatment. Their progress was compared to matched control patients. Supplementation with vitamin C led to an increase in patient's life expectancy and improvement in the quality of their lives. Further controlled trials are necessary before this treatment can be recommended, however.

Vitamin C may protect the gastrointestinal tract by preventing the conversion of sodium nitrite to nitrosamine. This idea also needs further study to obtain confirmatory data.

Other Vitamins. Very little information is available on any relationship between the other vitamins and the etiology of cancer. Alterations in vitamin metabolism occur in patients with advanced malignancy or as a result of chemotherapy. These alterations will be discussed later.

Minerals

Most minerals that have been implicated as causative agents in tumor development are contaminants not required by the body and usually are not consumed in large amounts. Whether esential minerals such as sodium, potassium, calcium, magnesium, zinc and selenium in large amounts are carcinogenic is still controversial. Deficiencies of iodine and magnesium are associated with thyroid cancer and thymoma, respectively. Significantly lower death rates from cancer were found in states that had high selenium levels in both males and females; however, the difference was greater for males than females. Clinically, the significance is unclear but may be related to the males being heavier smokers and more frequently exposed to industrial pollution.

Fiber

In recent years much attention has been focused on the possible protective role of fiber in the prevention of cancer of the large bowel (colon and rectum). This interest has stemmed

from the observation that the incidence of colonic cancer is lower among Ugandans who
consume a diet high in unabsorbable fiber, than
among Western populations who consume a
diet low in fiber. As was mentioned earlier, no
single component of the diet can change independently of other components. Consequently, dietary fiber intake affects meat, fat
and refined carbohydrate intakes, so that it is
difficult to study one variable alone. In addition, dietary fiber affects intestinal microflora
and bile salt metabolism, which also seem to be
involved in bowel carcinogenesis. Therefore, it
is unreasonable at this point to say that dietary
fiber intake is the only variable influencing the
incidence of colonic cancer.

Intestinal Microflora

Changes in diet appear to alter the pattern of
intestinal microflora. Higher numbers of certain anaerobes and lower counts of *Streptococcus* and other aerobic microorganisms were
found in fecal specimens of individuals consuming a high-fat, high-meat diet or a high-beef
diet. Other investigators found no significant
differences, however. In addition to the variation in the number and types of microorganisms
found in some individuals, there are differences
in the metabolism of the microorganism of
people following various dietary regimens.
There also are variations in persons who have
cancer compared with those without cancer.

NUTRITIONAL EFFECTS OF CANCER

The most striking effect of cancer in many
patients is malignant *cachexia*. Cancer cachexia
is clinically manifested by anorexia, marked
asthenia, significant loss of body fat and protein, anemia, water and electrolyte abnormalities and increased basal metabolism rate.
The clinical spectrum of cachexia ranges from
the patient with an undiagnosed neoplasm who
consults the physician because of a small
weight loss to the patient with end-stage disease
who has marked weakness and muscle wasting.

Anorexia

Anorexia, or hypophagia, can occur as an
early manifestation or may appear as the
malignant neoplasm grows and spreads. There
seems to be a relationship between anorexia
and the hypothalamic centers involved in regulating hunger and satiety.

Tumor growth affects the ability of the host
to meet his or her increased nutrient needs by
causing malabsorption, hypoglycemia, imbalance of amino acids and altered activity of the
hypothalamus. Any one or a combination of
these may cause anorexia. Since the mechanism of hunger and satiety is largely hypotheti-
cal, it compounds the problem of understanding anorexia in the patient with cancer.

Certain substances have been isolated from
the serum of starving animals that will produce
anorexia in other animals. Further, peptides of
low molecular weight in the hypothalamus also
have roles in brain function, so it seems reasonable to postulate that peptides, nucleotides
and other low-weight metabolites may be responsible for the development of anorexia in
the patient with cancer.[27] These metabolites
may also produce their anorexic effect by react-
ing with central nervous system sensor and
responder cells.

In animals, anorexia begins at a very early
stage of tumor growth. These animals show an
impairment of appetite response to food dilution and a change in diurnal activity and feeding
pattern before overt cachexia appears. Dietary
intake begins to decline when the tumor makes
up only 3 to 5 per cent of the total body mass.[22]
Overt cachexia can appear in a human with a
tumor of less than 0.01 per cent of his total
body weight. At the time of the recurrence or
spread of cancer, about 15 per cent of patients
have significant anorexia, and another 25 per
cent complain of early satiety despite their
feelings of hunger at the beginning of a meal.[29]

Anorexia leads to weight loss, which debili-
tates the patient and causes secondary complications that include weakness, decubiti, ulcers,
fluid and electrolyte abnormalities, decreased
resistance to infection, apathy and further dis-
interest in food. Anorexia should receive special attention from the nurse and dietitian-nutritionist, and every effort should be made to
help the patient overcome it. Insulin, once used
as an appetite stimulant, can cause acute hypoglycemia and is therefore not recommended.
Alcohol may be a better appetite stimulant.

Changes in Taste Perception

Many patients with cancer complain of decreased or altered taste sensation. A preference for higher concentrations of sucrose solutions is seen in both animals and humans.[14] In
one study, sweet recognition thresholds were
elevated during 5-fluorouracil therapy and became normal after termination of the treat-

ment.[10] Patients with cancer also show a lower threshold to bitter taste, which may be the basis for their common aversion to meat. The bitter taste of meat may result from the presence of small amounts of amino acids in it that are not detected by persons without cancer.

Zinc deficiency, known to cause changes in taste, has been suggested as one possible cause of hypogeusia in patients with cancer. Abnormalities of taste in patients with other diseases can be corrected with oral zinc therapy,[15] but unfortunately it was not determined if these patients had a pre-existing zinc deficiency. (See page 137 for discussion of zinc deficiency as it affects taste acuity). Zinc therapy is probably warranted for those patients with hypogeusia who also have evidence of zinc deficiency.

The relationship between weight loss and food intake and the patient's perception of loss of appetite is unclear. In a study of patients who lost weight, those with abnormalities of taste had an increased incidence of weight loss compared with patients who had normal taste acuity. Weight loss in patients with normal taste acuity was due to an anatomical interference with G.I. function or the adverse effects of chemotherapy, or to pain or hypermetabolism.[19]

Metabolic Changes

Asthenia, or loss of energy, has been noted in patients with cancer. It is more difficult to measure changes in the spontaneous activity of humans with cancer than it is to measure the decline in motor activity and food intake that occurs in animals with the disease. In these host animals there is no conclusive evidence of an increase in total metabolic rate, but there does appear to be a change in the metabolic pattern. The basal or resting rates of these animals are increased, while energy attributable to spontaneous motor activity is reduced compared with that of normal animals of the same size that have the same food intake. Some human subjects with malignant disease have an increased basal metabolic rate (BMR). This increase in energy needs is similar to that of a patient undergoing elective surgery, about 10 per cent. Other reports indicate a significantly lower BMR in the presence of active disease. Rather than being contradictory, these differences may have occurred because the patients were studied at different stages of the disease process.

Waterhouse studied energy metabolism in a very limited number of patients but obtained some interesting results.[30] She found that many of the adaptive mechanisms normally seen in semistarved patients (Chapter 35) were impaired in patients with uncontrolled cancer. The loss of enzyme adaptation for energy conservation was implied by the body's failure to reduce caloric expenditure, its continued utilization of amino acids for gluconeogenesis and its inability to oxidize exogenous glucose normally.

Protein metabolism is also altered by the presence of a tumor in the host. Initially, tumor tissue and visceral tissue both appear to be spared at the expense of peripheral tissue, which is broken down and metabolized. Eventually hypoalbuminemia, a non-specific abnormality, develops as one indicator of visceral depletion. The mean serum albumin concentration in a series of 222 cancer patients was 2.9 gm. per dl., compared with 4.0 gm. per dl. in normal adults.[21] Patients with widespread disease had lower values than patients with localized carcinomas. Similar results have been reported by other investigators. The major pathophysiological mechanism is decreased albumin synthesis, although in some patients the loss of protein into the gastrointestinal tract may also be important. Although the levels of synthesis of some proteins are reduced, the production of others is well maintained or even increased.

With effective cancer therapy, nitrogen retention occurs in normal tissue, and during tumor regression nitrogen may even be drawn from the tumor and incorporated into body tissue.

NUTRITIONAL DISORDERS RESULTING FROM CANCER TREATMENT

Therapeutic techniques such as radiation treatment, surgery or drug therapy may in turn induce nutritional problems. Table 36–1 summarizes some of the problems that may be consequences of treatment. It must always be remembered that there may be psychological as well as physiological effects of the treatment that can exacerbate the problem.

Radiation Treatment

The epithelium of the small intestine is second only to the bone marrow in its sensitivity to radiation. Irradiation of the abdomen can cause extensive damage to the intestine, which re-

Table 36–1 POTENTIAL SIDE EFFECTS OF CANCER TREATMENT THAT MAY CAUSE NUTRITIONAL PROBLEMS

RADIATION TREATMENT
    Nausea, vomiting and general loss of appetite
    Loss of taste and dysphagia
    Dental problems
    Obstruction
    Diarrhea; malabsorption resulting from bowel damage
SURGICAL TREATMENT
    Dependence on tube feeding as a result of resection of oropharyngeal area
    Malabsorption resulting from resection of segments of gastrointestinal tract
    Dumping syndrome resulting from gastrectomy
    Hypoglycemia resulting from gastrectomy
    Altered water and electrolyte balance resulting from ileostomy and colostomy
    Diabetes mellitus resulting from pancreatectomy
CHEMOTHERAPY TREATMENT
    Fluid and electrolyte imbalance resulting from hormonal treatment
    Gastrointestinal damage resulting from antimetabolites and other agents
    Nausea, anorexia and vomiting resulting from antimetabolites and other agents
    Anemias resulting from drugs

sults in diarrhea, steatorrhea, malabsorption and obstruction. (Chapter 23 discusses nutritional care for patients with malabsorption.) Nausea and vomiting can also result from radiation therapy.

Radiotherapy to the oropharyngeal region can destroy the sense of taste, leading to a condition that has been described as "mouth blindness." Decreased salivation can create discomfort during mastication. Other undesirable side effects are mucositis, dental caries, progressive periodontal disease and osteoradionecrosis. A treatment regimen has been developed that significantly reduces morbidity from therapeutic irradiation of the jaws.[24] During the pre-irradiation period, the patient's oropharyngeal area is evaluated by radiographic and oral examination, and then non-salvageable teeth are extracted and an oral hygiene regimen is begun. During the irradiation period, the patient has weekly prophylaxis with fluoridated polishing paste and is given pain relievers. After radiation therapy, the regimen includes examination of the mouth and neck for detection of recurrent or new neoplastic disease, fluoridation prophylaxis, restoration procedures as needed and reinforcement of oral hygiene procedures.

Liver tissue in adults is supposedly quite radioresistant. However, in small children the liver is very susceptible to radiation damage, and patients receiving long-term therapy should be monitored regarding nutritional deficiencies that may result from reduced or altered liver function (see Chapter 24.)

Surgery

Radical surgery in the head and neck region often interferes with chewing and swallowing and may necessitate prolonged tube feeding. Excision or resection of various segments of the gastrointestinal tract cause dumping syndrome and malabsorption of varying degrees. Without proper attention and nutritional care, this syndrome can result in a malnourished, cachectic, uncomfortable and frustrated patient. (See Chapter 34.)

Massive bowel resection with a residual length of three feet or less presents very serious and long-term problems in maintaining adequate nutritional status and water and electrolyte balance (see Chapter 34). Clinical studies of normal subjects and of those who have undergone ablation of varying lengths of the small intestine indicate that, except for vitamin B_{12}, all nutrients can be absorbed in the proximal small bowel if at least 100 cm. (40 in.) remains after surgery. Fortunately, the remaining bowel hypertrophies to accommodate its new role. Removal of the ileocecal valve, which moderates the passage of the intestinal contents, causes diarrhea and interferes with electrolyte and water absorption.

Pancreatectomy results in maldigestion and malabsorption due to loss of pancreatic digestive enzymes and in diabetes mellitus due to decreased production of insulin and other hormones. The malabsorption can be improved by oral intake of pancreatic enzymes, and the diabetes is treated with insulin and adjustment of the diet (see Chapter 25).

Chemotherapy

Chemotherapeutic drugs can cause nausea, anorexia and vomiting, as well as malabsorption, diarrhea and stomatitis. (See Table 36–2.) Folic acid antagonists affect all areas of rapid cellular proliferation, such as bone marrow and the intestinal mucosa. The intestinal alterations are much like those seen in sprue (Chapter 23) and result in a decrease in absorption of carbohydrate, fat, protein and other nutrients.

Fluorinated pyrimidines such as 5-fluorouracil affect the intestinal mucosa, producing stomatitis and diarrhea. The return of high sweet recognition thresholds to normal after termination of treatment with

Table 36–2 CANCER CHEMOTHERAPEUTIC AGENTS THAT CAN ADVERSELY AFFECT DESIRE FOR FOOD*

DRUG	Stomatitis	Nausea	Vomiting	Diarrhea	Oral Ulcerations	Constipation	Ulceration of Buccal Mucosa	Gingivitis	Metallic Taste	Prolonged Anorexia	Abdominal Pain	Glossitis
Actinomycin D	X	X	X	X	X							
Bleomycin	X	X	X									
Cyclophosphamide		X	X									
Cytarabine		X	X	X	X							
Doxorubicin	X	X	X	X								
5-Fluorouracil	X	X	X	X	X							
Hydroxyurea	X	X	X	X		X	X					
Melphalan		X	X									
6-Mercaptopurine	X	X	X									
Methotrexate	X	X	X	X	X			X				
Nitrogen mustard		X	X	X					X			
Nitrosoureas		X	X							X		
Vinblastine	X	X	X	X		X					X	X
Vincristine		X	X			X					X	

*From: Visconti, J. A.: Drug-Food Interaction: Nutrition in Disease. Columbus, Ohio, Ross Laboratories, 1977, p. 18.

5-fluorouracil suggests that the drug itself may produce some changes in taste acuity.[10] Secondary effects of drugs include anemia and loss of protein, calcium and potassium in the urine. Some forms of chemotherapy may lead to a deficiency state that shows characteristics of a mixed B-complex vitamin deficiency and neurological disturbances that presumably are a consequence of these deficiencies. Between periods of chemotherapy the patient should be rehabilitated nutritionally if the gastrointestinal tract is functioning properly. (Drug-nutrient interactions are discussed more fully in Chapter 21.)

The increased amount of breakdown products from the drug's destruction of cancer cells places an additional burden on the kidneys. Frequently the drugs themselves are highly toxic both to nephrons and bladder. Diarrhea and fever, which sometimes accompany the treatment, also increase the need for extra fluids. Patients taking alkylating agents should increase their intake of fluids to prevent kidney damage. For example, patients taking Cytoxan should receive 2 to 3 liters of fluids daily to prevent hemorrhagic cystitis.

NUTRITIONAL CARE FOR PATIENTS WITH CANCER

Will improved intake of protein and calories improve the condition of the patient with cancer? Pessimism in this area stemmed from animal studies which demonstrated that spontaneous tumor growth occurs more readily in well-nourished animals and that protein undernutrition slowed the rate of tumor growth. However, very few reports suggest that improvement of nutritional status stimulates tumor growth in humans. Although there is still no evidence that aggressive nutritional management prolongs survival, it does appear to improve the quality of life and allow the patient to better tolerate the demands made on his body

both by the disease and the therapies given for the disease.

Early in the management of metastatic cancer a complete nutritional history should be obtained by the dietitian. With this information, changes in weight, food consumption, meal composition and other factors can be evaluated. Efforts to encourage patients to eat must be aggressive, persevering and compassionate.

Every effort should be made to maintain an adequate oral intake by the patient. Food is more than calories and nutrients: it means normalcy and having some control over one's environment. Eating what and as much as he or she wants has psychological values for the patient. It must be recognized constantly by all members of the treatment team that there are differences among patients and that one approach will not work with all individuals.

The patient should be the guide for what foods will be eaten and how well they are seasoned. Cold food, such as sandwiches, cottage cheese and salad plates, is frequently better accepted.[10, 16, 28] Aromas from hot foods sometimes aggravate nausea. Lemons and dill pickles are requested frequently by children and appear to curb nausea.[16] Popsicles are sometimes accepted when patients can not tolerate other food.

Patients with stomatitis prefer their food at room temperature. Highly seasoned and spicy foods should be avoided, but this does not necessarily mean that the food should be bland. Rinsing the mouth with a local anesthetic such as lidocaine before meals may help patients who have pain while swallowing. Soft and moist foods may make the meal easier to eat, as do soup, milk or other liquids with the meal. Patients should be prepared for a possible weight loss. If oral intake is not adequate to maintain weight, additional measures may be necessary.

Forced Feeding

The earliest attempt to counteract the weight loss associated with tumor growth in humans was forced feeding.[26] Significant weight gains were achieved during the period of forced feeding; however, weight loss was just as rapid when feeding was discontinued. In about half the patients, forced feeding had a detrimental effect.

Tube Feeding

Another method is tube feeding using a nasogastric, esophagostomy, gastrostomy or jejunostomy tube. Fine-bore tubes are well tolerated by most patients but require a finely dispersed formula. In some hospitals, a tube feeding is prepared by blending puréed and liquid foods, in which case a larger tube is required. (See Chapter 35.) Since flavors and odors are important to the patient, real foods are used. At the M. D. Anderson Hospital (Houston, Texas) the patient receives a tray with three glasses of formula, juice, coffee, cream, sugar, milk and salt.[16] The patient is encouraged to season the formula and add cream and sugar to the coffee before tube-feeding himself. Some patients were seen to take small amounts of the puréed foods or liquids by mouth in addition to taking the rest as a tube feeding.

Defined formula or elemental diets, although almost as low in viscosity as water, are expensive and hyperosmolar, and their use is indicated only when the patient has intestinal malabsorption, short bowel syndrome or intolerance to a larger feeding tube. To prevent diarrhea, cramping and gas, the strength of the formula should be increased gradually to develop tolerance. Usually half strength is recommended for the first two days, three-fourths strength for the next two days and finally full strength on the fifth day. These diets are frequently best served cold, and the patient is instructed to sip them slowly to prevent a bolus of hyperosmotic solution from reaching the small intestine. Because of their unpleasant taste, these formulas are best used as tube feedings. The administration of tube feedings is discussed more fully in Chapter 35.

Intravenous Hyperalimentation

If oral or tube feeding is ineffective or impossible, total parenteral nutrition (TPN) is the alternative (see Chapter 35). Parenteral nutrition alone can achieve weight gain, increased strength and activity and positive nitrogen balance together with bowel rest.[25] Bowel rest significantly reduces the physical, mechanical and chemical trauma produced by the passage of food, digestive juices and feces through the alimentary tract. The essential nutrients are applied directly to the cells, thus improving their rate of regeneration. By using TPN to maintain the patient in good nutritional status it is possible to increase the total deliverable dose of anticancer agents and to reduce their toxic gastrointestinal side effects. Hyperalimentation has also been used to rehabilitate patients nutritionally so that the risk involved with sur-

gical treatment or radiation therapy becomes acceptable.

Hyperalimentation allows a planned course of radiation therapy to be delivered to previously malnourished and poor-risk patients. The patients who responded best to radiation therapy had gained an average of 13 lb.; the patients who responded least well had only gained an average of 4.9 lb.[11]

Although multiple factors affect immunocompetence, nutritional rehabilitation using TPN restored delayed hypersensitivity in 13 of 17 patients with cancer.[12] These patients were subsequently treated by chemotherapy, surgery or radiotherapy. Response to chemotherapy occurred only in those patients whose skin tests were positive. The surgical patients whose skin tests were positive initially or whose skin tests converted to normal had uncomplicated recoveries. However, although their nutritional rehabilitation was considered adequate, none of the patients who were treated with radiotherapy developed or retained a positive skin test. This study of a limited number of patients suggests that generalized malnutrition is the cause of the absence of delayed hypersensitivity in the cancer patient.

Patient Rehabilitation

Concern for the patient with cancer should not stop when he or she is no longer acutely ill. It must continue until the patient has returned to a useful life. If at all possible, patients should be encouraged to serve themselves between meals from a snack pantry, and ideally, they should go through a cafeteria line and select their own food. These alternatives are available in some hospitals. A dietitian-nutritionist could be on hand to guide selections, and patients could get together to encourage each other. Since most hospitals are not structured for this arrangement, perhaps the first step would be to allow the patients to select their own diets from a menu as soon as possible. The American Cancer Society has published a booklet of suggestions and high-protein recipes that can be given to patients to help them maintain their dietary intake at home.[11] These recipes are selected for their protein and calorie content as well as for economy of cost and preparation time. Table 36–3 summarizes recommendations for feeding the patient with cancer.

Misconceptions in Nutritional Care

As can be anticipated from the obvious lack of knowledge about nutrition related to cancer, the area of nutritional care for cancer patients is fraught with mystique, misunderstanding and unsubstantiated claims. The most recent and most popularized example of this harmful situation is *Laetrile*.

The use of Laetrile for cancer has been reviewed by Jukes.[18] Laetrile, or more properly, amygdalin, is a cyanogenetic glycoside found in the seeds of apricots, peaches and plums. Upon hydrolysis, glucose and a mandelonitrile are produced. The mandelonitrile decomposes

Table 36–3 SUMMARY OF NUTRITIONAL PROBLEMS AND CARE FOR PATIENTS WITH CANCER

MECHANICAL PROBLEMS
    A. Due directly to cancer:
        Anorexia, weight loss, changes in taste acuity, obstruction, malabsorption.
    B. Due to treatment of cancer:
        Nausea, vomiting, diarrhea, dryness in swallowing, fear of aspiration of food, lack of necessary secretions, excision of functional organs.
PSYCHOLOGICAL PROBLEMS
    Fear of pain and treatment; panic about anorexia, nausea and weight loss.
    Disfiguration due to surgical procedures.
    Unnaturalness of nasogastric tube or TPN apparatus.
    General depression and low morale.
SUGGESTIONS FOR NUTRITIONAL CARE
    Get good nutritional history early and monitor changes in nutritional status.
    Record likes, dislikes, tolerances, pattern of intake and other food patterns as well as anthropometric data.
    Discuss alternative methods of patient management with the health team.
    Discuss diet, procedures and other concerns with patient.
    Involve the patient. Have patient record his own weight and intake and make calorie estimation. Let patient choose favorite supplement. If tube feeding or TPN is used, explain it carefully to patient. If using puréed foods in tube feeding, allow patient to season them. Be sensitive to his or her needs and comments. If possible, place patients who are receiving the same diet together. Visit patient regularly.
    Make terminally ill patient comfortable. Give whatever food he or she desires, in whatever form is desired.

---

into benzaldehyde and cyanide, either spontaneously or by the action of an enzyme. Laetrile is not a vitamin but has been identified mistakenly as vitamin B_{17} by some people in order to avoid the federal requirements concerning food additives. Legislation has been passed in some states to make Laetrile legal to use. In controlled studies, Laetrile has been shown to have no effect on tumor growth. In the popular literature, cases of improvement of patients who take the drug daily—frequently after having other forms of treatment—have been reported. Unfortunately, the popular literature never describes the patients who died or who did not improve as a result of taking this drug. The controversy over Laetrile illustrates that victims of incurable diseases are often susceptible to manipulation and exploitation by quacks.

SUMMARY

The role of nutrition and diet in the etiology of cancer is unclear at the present time. Much additional research is needed before definite suggestions to alter the diet of large segments of the population can be made. Our knowledge of the role of nutrition in the treatment of patients with cancer is somewhat better. Well-nourished patients can cope with the disease better than malnourished patients can. Aggressive, understanding support of the patient can aid substantially in improving his or her nutritional status before, during and after therapy. The suggestions included here are just a starting point, because each patient must be treated individually.

PROBLEMS AND SUGGESTED TOPICS FOR DISCUSSION

1. Discuss the role of calorie intake in the etiology of cancer.
2. Explain the etiological role of fat in the development of cancer.
3. Assess the nutritional status of a patient receiving cancer treatment. Does he or she exhibit any biochemical or clinical signs of malnutrition? Evaluate the dietary intake. Is it adequate? Will there need to be changes as the cancer treatment continues?
4. Interview a patient receiving chemotherapy or radiotherapy. Ask about any changes in taste perception he or she is experiencing. Have these changes affected dietary intake?

CITED REFERENCES

1. American Cancer Society: Nutrition for Patients Receiving Chemotherapy and Radiation Treatment. New York, American Cancer Society, Inc., 1974.
2. Basu, T. K.: Significance of vitamins in cancer. Oncology, *33*:183, 1976.
3. Berg, J. W.: Nutrition and cancer. Semin. Oncol., *3*:17, 1976.
4. Bjelke, E.: Dietary vitamin A and human lung cancer. Int. J. Cancer, *15*:561, 1975.
5. Boutwell, R. K., Brush, M. K., and Rusch, H. P.: The stimulating effect of dietary fat on carcinogenesis. Cancer Res., *9*:741, 1949.
6. Cameron, E., and Pauling, L.: Supplemental ascorbate in the supportive treatment of cancer. Prolongation of survival times in terminal cancer. Proc. Natl. Acad. Sci. USA, *73*:3685, 1976.
7. Carroll, K. K., and Khor, H. T.: Dietary fat in relation to tumorigenesis. Prog. Biochem. Pharmacol., *10*:308, 1975.
8. Carroll, K. K., and Khor, H. T.: Effect of level and type of dietary fat on incidence of mammary tumors induced in female S-D rats by 7,12-dimethylbenz[α]anthracene. Lipids, *6*:416, 1971.
9. Carroll, K. K., and Khor, H. T.: Experts of dietary fat and dose level of 7,12-dimethylbenz[α]anthracene on mammary tumor incidence in rats. Cancer Res., *30*:2260, 1970.
10. Carson, J. A. S., and Gormican, A.: Taste acuity and food attitudes of selected patients with cancer. J. Am. Diet. Assoc., *70*:361, 1977.
11. Copeland, E. M., et al.: Intravenous hyperalimentation as an adjunct to radiation therapy. Cancer, *39*:609, 1977.
12. Copeland, E. M., MacFadyen, B. Jr., and Dudrick, S. J.: Effect of intravenous hyperalimentation on established delayed hypersensitivity in the cancer patient. Ann. Surg., *184*:60, 1976.
13. Cunningham, A. S.: Lymphomas and animal protein consumption. Lancet, *2*:1184, 1976.
14. DeWys, W. D., and Walters, K.: Abnormalities of taste sensation in cancer patients. Cancer, *36*:1888, 1975.
15. Henkin, R. I.: Newer aspects of copper and zinc metabolism. In: Mertz, W., and Cornatzer, W. E. (eds.): Newer Trace Elements in Nutrition. New York, Marcel Dekker, 1971, pp. 297–308.
16. Hepedus, S., and Pelman, M.: Dietetics in a cancer hospital. J. Am. Diet. Assoc., *67*:235, 1975.
17. Hill, P., et al.: Prolactin levels in populations at risk for breast cancer. Cancer Res., *36*:4102, 1976.
18. Jukes, J. H.: Laetrile for cancer. JAMA, *236*:1284, 1976.
19. Klipstein, F. A., and Smarth, G.: Intestinal structure and function in neoplastic disease. J. Am. Dig. Dis., *14*:887, 1969.
20. Krasner, N., and Dymock, I. W.: Ascorbic acid deficiency in malignant diseases: a clinical and biochemical study. Br. J. Cancer, *30*:142, 1974.
21. Mider, G. B., Alling, E. L., and Morton, J. J.: The effect of neoplastic and allied diseases on concentrations of plasma protein. Cancer, *3*:56, 1950.
22. Morrison, S. D.: Control of food intake in cancer cachexia: a challenge and a tool. Physiol. Behav., *17*:705, 1976.
23. Polednak, A. P.: College athletics, body size and cancer mortality. Cancer, *38*:382, 1976.
24. Regezi, J. A., Courtnem, R. M., and Kerr, D. A.: Dental management of patients irradiated for oral cancer. Cancer, *38*:994, 1976.
25. Souchon, E. A., et al.: Intravenous hyperalimentation as an adjunct to cancer chemotherapy with 5-fluorouracil. J. Surg. Res., *18*:451, 1975.
26. Terepka, A. R., and Waterhouse, C.: Metabolic ob-

servations during the forced feeding of patients with cancer. Am. J. Med., *20*:225, 1956.

27. Theologides, A.: Anorexia-producing intermediary metabolites. Am. J. Clin. Nutr., *29*:553, 1976.
28. Theologides, A.: Nutritional management of the patient with advanced cancer. Postgrad. Med., *61*:97, 1977.
29. Theologides, A., Ehlert, J., and Kennedy, B. J.: Food intake of patients with advanced cancer. Minn. Med., *59*:526, 1976.
30. Waterhouse, C.: How tumors affect host metabolism animals. Ann. N.Y. Acad. Sci., *230*:86, 1974.

ADDITIONAL REFERENCES

Alcantara, E. N., and Speckmann, E. W.: Diet, nutrition and cancer. Am. J. Clin. Nutr., *29*:1035, 1976.

Bull, D. M.: Nutrition and tumor immunity: divergent effect of antitumor antibody. Cancer Res., *35*:3317, 1975.

Burkitt, D. P.: Epidemiology of cancer of the colon and rectum. Cancer, *28*:3, 1971.

Burkitt, D. P.: Relationships between diseases and their etiological significance. Am. J. Clin. Nutr., *30*:262, 1977.

Copeland, E. M., et al.: Intravenous hyperalimentation in patients with head and neck cancer. Cancer, *35*:606, 1975.

DeWys, W. D.: Abnormalities of taste as a remote effect of a neoplasm. Ann. N.Y. Acad. Sci., *230*:427, 1974.

Dreizen, S., et al.: Oral complications of cancer radiotherapy. Postgrad. Med., *61*:85, 1977.

Ederer, F., et al.: Cancer among men on cholesterol-lowering diets. Lancet, *2*:203, 1971.

Fassett, D. W.: Nitrates and nitrites. In: Toxicants Occurring Naturally in Foods. Washington, D.C., National Academy of Sciences, 1973, pp. 7–25.

Feldman, J. M., Plonk, J. W., Admiral, J., and Sidbury, J. B.: Plasma amino acids in patients with carcinoid syndrome. Cancer, *38*:2127, 1976.

Goldrick, R. B., et al.: Do polyunsaturated fats predispose to malignant melanoma? Med. J. Aust., *1*:987, 1976.

Hill, M. J.: Metabolic epidemiology of dietary factors in large bowel cancer. Cancer Res., *35*:3398, 1975.

Hopkins, G. J., and West, C. E.: Possible roles of dietary fats in carcinogenesis. Life Sci., *19*:1103, 1976.

Kamm, J. J., et al.: Effect of ascorbic acid in amine-nitrate toxicity. Ann. N.Y. Acad. Sci., *258*:169, 1974.

Maugh, T. H.: Vitamin A: potential protection from carcinogenesis. Science, *186*:1198, 1975.

Morrison, S. D.: Generation and compensation of the cancer cachetic process by spontaneous modification of feeding behavior. Cancer Res., *36*:228, 1976.

Ota, D. M., et al.: The effect of protein nutrition on host and tumor metabolism. J. Surg., Res., *22*:181, 1977.

Phillips, L. L.: Role of life-style and dietary habits in risk of cancer among Seventh Day Adventists. Cancer Res., *35*:3513, 1975.

Reddy, B. S., Mastromarino, A., and Wynder, E. L.: Further leads on metabolic epidemiology of large bowel cancer. Cancer Res., *35*:3403, 1975.

Reichenback, D. D.: Autopsy incidence of diseases among Southwestern American Indians. Arch. Pathol. *84*:81, 1967.

Schaefer, O.: Medical observation and problems in the Canadian arctic. Can. Med. Assoc. J., *81*:386, 1959.

Schreier, A. M., and Lavenia, J.: The nurse's role in nutritional management of radiotherapy patients. Nurs. Clin. North Am., *12*:173, 1977.

Schwartz, M. K.: Role of trace elements in cancer. Cancer Res., *35*:3481, 1975.

Shils, M. E.: Nutrition and neoplasia. In: Goodhart, R., and Shils, M. (eds.): Modern Nutrition in Health and Disease, 5th ed. Philadelphia, Lea & Febiger, 1973.

Sporn, M. B.: Retinoids and carcinogenesis. Nutr. Rev., *35*:65, 1977.

Theologides, A.: The anorexia-cachexia syndrome: a new hypothesis. Ann. N.Y. Acad. Sci., *230*:14, 1974.

Waldmann, T. A., Broder, S. D., and Strober, W.: Protein-losing enteropathies in malignancy. Ann. N.Y. Acad. Sci., *230*:306, 1974.

Walker, A. R. P., and Burkitt, D. P.: Colonic cancer—hypotheses of causation, dietary prophylaxis and future research. Am. J. Dig. Dis., *21*:910, 1976.

Walter, J. B.: Introduction to the Principles of Disease. Philadelphia, W. B. Saunders Co., 1977.

Wiseman, C., McGregor, R. F., and McCredie, K. B.: Urinary amino acid excretion in acute leukemia. Cancer, *38*:219, 1976.

Wynder, E. L.: Status of research on nutrition and cancer: concluding remarks. Cancer Res., *35*:3548, 1975.

UNIT SIXTEEN
DISEASES OF INFANCY AND CHILDHOOD

Chapter 37

NUTRITIONAL CARE FOR THE LOW-BIRTH-WEIGHT AND HIGH-RISK NEONATE

Newborn infants considered to be high-risk are those who are of low birth weight, those born to diabetic mothers, premature infants with problems related to prematurity, infants who are ill or those afflicted with a congenital abnormality. Unable to adapt to their environment after birth, these infants require intensive care to support their respiratory and cardiovascular function, metabolic homeostasis and body temperature until they can function independently. As can be imagined, the care of these fragile babies is complex and delicate.

Previously, most of these infants died, but because of our more complete understanding of the neonate's physiological requirements and the development of sophisticated perinatal centers, more of these infants are surviving. Improved methods of ventilatory assistance enable the infant to meet this primary need. Then fluid balance and nutritional needs become important. This chapter will discuss the nutritional care for babies who are separated prematurely from the materno-placental supply line or who are not able to feed successfully on their own because of various problems. Knowledge in the field of neonatology and about the care for high-risk infants is growing rapidly as the search for the optimal techniques in all areas, including nutrition, continues.

BORN TOO SMALL VS. BORN TOO SOON

An infant who weighs less than 2500 gm. (5 ½ lb.) at birth is classified as being of *low birth*

weight (LBW), while an infant weighing less than 1500 gm. (3½ lb.) at birth is frequently referred to as being of *very low birth weight (VLBW).* An infant may be of low birth weight due to a shortened *period* of gestation, which means that he or she is premature, or because of a retarded *rate* of growth, which makes him or her *small for gestational age (SGA).*

Whether the LBW infant is premature or SGA, or both, is determined from: (1) calculation of the length of gestation using the date of the mother's last menstrual period, (2) a detailed neurological examination, since the central nervous system development is related to the gestational age, (3) the size of the fetus as determined by palpation, ultrasound cephalometry or measurement of fetal abdominal circumference and (4) the birth weight of the infant.

The infant who is *small for gestational age* is defined as one who weighs less than the 10th percentile of the standard weight for that gestational age. This is usually a valid test, although sometimes an infant can only be recognized as SGA when compared with normal siblings who supposedly have the same genetic potential. See Figure 37–1 for a standard for intrauterine growth. A *premature* infant is one born before 38 weeks' gestation. If the length and weight of a premature infant are between the 10th and the 90th percentiles on the intrauterine growth grid, the infant is considered to be *appropriate size for gestational age (AGA).* Below the 10th percentile, he or she is also considered to be small for gestational age.

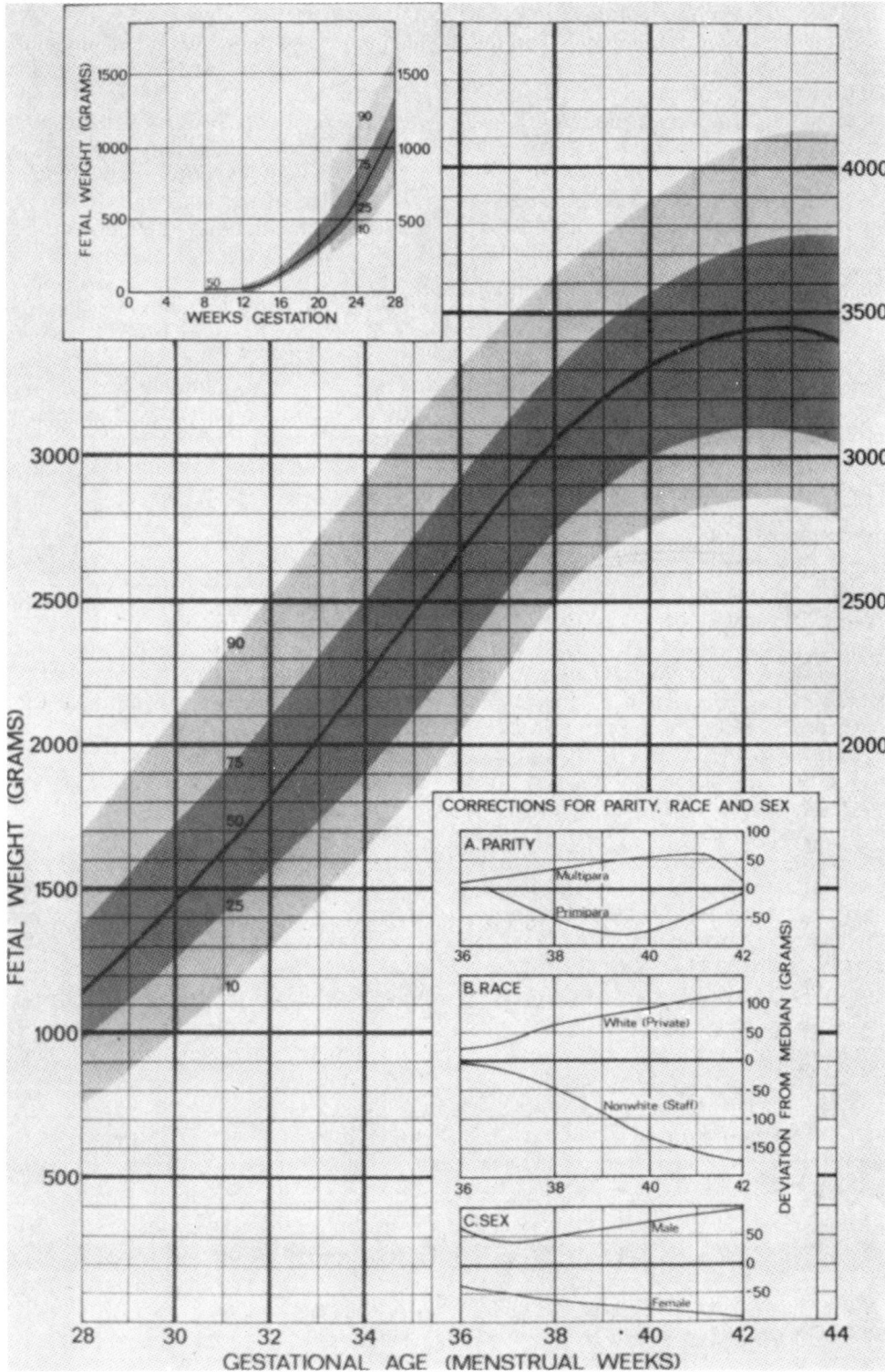

Figure 37–1   Intrauterine growth chart. The 50th (median), 10th, 25th, 75th and 90th percentiles of fetal weight in grams throughout pregnancy and correction factors for parity, race (socioeconomic) and sex derived from 31,202 prostaglandin-induced abortions and "spontaneous" deliveries are graphed. (From: Brenner, W. E., Edelman, D. A., and Hendricks, C. H.: A standard of fetal growth for the United States of America. Am. J. Obstet. Gynecol., *126*:555, 1976.)

The infant who is both premature and SGA has the greatest risk of complications and the least chance for survival. This infant tolerates labor poorly and is more likely to suffer neonatal asphyxia, aspiration of amniotic fluid, polycythemia, hypothermia and massive pulmonary hemorrhage. If the infant does survive, he or she is more likely to have developmental problems or be below normal in physical or mental functioning when older. The prognosis for these infants is discussed more fully later in the chapter.

FETAL GROWTH RETARDATION

The SGA infant, or light-for-date baby (as he or she is sometimes called), is suffering from fetal growth retardation. This can be due to *intrinsic factors,* that is, abnormalities in the fetus that limit its potential for growth, or to *extrinsic factors* that, by malnourishing the fetus, limit the substances needed for growth. Two major extrinsic factors are: uteroplacental insufficiency, which limits both nutrients and oxygen, and inadequate maternal dietary intake, which limits the nutrient supply to the fetus. Extrinsic factors appear to have more influence on the growth of the fetus than the intrinsic factors do, particularly when the extrinsic factors are severe, as in the case of very deficient maternal nutrition.[23] Intrinsic factors such as genetic abnormalities or infectious agents tend to cause early growth retardation, which is reflected in a reduced number of cells, or *hypoplastic* growth. Extrinsic factors usually restrict fetal growth later in the gestation period and influence both cell number and cell size to produce *hypotrophic* growth. These phases of growth are discussed in Chapter 13.

The SGA infant who is malnourished because of placental insufficiency receives inadequate amounts of all nutrients, including oxygen, and this infant illustrates hypotrophic growth. Growth is asymmetrical, which means that the size of the liver and other organs is reduced more than that of the brain. The brain and heart size and body length are preserved to the greatest possible extent and suffer only minimal reduction. Growth retardation resulting from protein restriction is symmetrical, with a reduction in all organs consistent with a decrease in total body mass. This type of growth retardation is more hypoplastic and seems to be more severe and more detrimental to later growth and development. (See Table 37–1.)

PHYSIOLOGICAL CHARACTERISTICS OF PREMATURE AND SGA INFANTS

The premature or SGA infant has not had the chance to develop fully *in utero* and therefore is physiologically different from the term infant weighing 2500 gm. or more. These physiological differences give this infant a greater risk of developing problems than the term AGA infant has.

There also are differences between a baby who is of low birth weight because of prematurity and one who is of low birth weight because of fetal growth retardation. In most cases the management of both types is the same, but certain complications are more likely in one group than in the other. Table 37–2 lists some

Table 37–1   CLINICAL DIFFERENTIATION BETWEEN HYPOPLASTIC AND HYPOTROPHIC SGA INFANTS*

HYPOPLASTIC	HYPOTROPHIC
Global reduction in all measurements.	Weight reduction > length reduction.
	Head circumference usually least affected and may be within normal percentiles.
Do not always appear wasted.	Redundant skin folds usual.
Liver palpable, sometimes enlarged.	Liver usually small.
Congenital anomalies common.	Congenital anomalies usually absent.
Possible evidence of intrauterine infection, e.g., chorioretinitis, jaundice, hepatosplenomegaly.	Spleen not usually enlarged.
	Fundi normal.
Hematocrit value commonly normal.	Hematocrit value usually raised.
Placenta small, rarely enlarged (e.g., in cytomegalovirus infection).	Placenta may be normal or occasionally show extensive recent infarcts.
Hypoglycemia and hypoproteinemia in proportion to immaturity.	Hypoglycemia and hypoproteinemia are common features.

*From: Goodwin, J. W., Godden, J. O., and Chance, G. W.: Perinatal Medicine: The Basic Science Underlying Clinical Practice. Baltimore, The Williams & Wilkins Co., 1976, p. 278.

Table 37–2 CHARACTERISTICS OF PRETERM AND SGA INFANTS*

	PRETERM	SGA
Cause	Short gestation	Intrauterine malnutrition (placental insufficiency)
Dangers	Respiratory distress syndrome Hypothermia Infection Intraventricular or subarachnoid hemorrhage	Hypoglycemia Hypocalcemia Hypothermia
Length	Crown-heel less than 45 cm.	May be more than 45 cm.
Head circumference	Less than 33 cm.	Often more than 33 cm.
Skin	Thin, red	Dry, folds of lax skin
Muscle tone	Poor, frog-like posture	Variable

*From Brown, R. J. K., and Valman, H. B.: Practical Neonatal Pediatrics, 3rd ed. Oxford, England, Blackwell Scientific Publications, 1975, p. 33.

characteristics of each group. In general, the SGA infant is slightly more mature in terms of enzyme development (respiratory enzymes, for instance) than the premature infant. The SGA baby will usually be thin, with a head large for body size but appropriate for gestational age because nature tries to preserve the growth of this important organ.

Major physiological differences between term infants and all low-birth-weight infants account for the more aggressive nutritional care required for LBW babies. First, the low-birth-weight infant enters the world with fewer metabolic reserves than does the term AGA infant. Because most of the infant's glycogen is stored in the fetal liver in the last four weeks of gestation, the premature infant has not had time to build up these stores, and the SGA infant has not had any extra glucose or amino acids to store. Fat deposits are also reduced because most fat deposition in the fetus takes place in the last six weeks of pregnancy. In a small, premature infant weighing 1000 gm., fat may make up only 1 per cent of body weight, in contrast to the full-term infant, whose fat makes up about 16 per cent of body weight. The infant's caloric reserves in the forms of glycogen and fat are minimal, making the period during which this neonate can exist without an exogenous caloric intake short indeed. For example, the caloric reserves available from fat are 90 kcal. per kg. for a 1000-gm. neonate, 670 kcal. per kg. for a 2500-gm. neonate and 1440 kcal. per kg. for a 3500-gm. neonate. Since even the full-term neonate can use up his glycogen stores in the first two to three hours of life, the fat reserves become an important

source of calories for energy, especially if, for some reason, formula or milk intake cannot begin within the first few hours after birth. Based on resting metabolic requirements of 40 to 55 kcal. per kg. per day, Heird and associates[24] estimate that without being fed, the 1000-gm. neonate could live for 4 days, the 2000-gm. neonate for 12 days and the full-term neonate for 33 days. However, these are unrealistically long periods of time, because the caloric requirements upon which these figures are based do not allow for growth, biochemical maturation, activity or response to stress such as hypothermia or respiratory distress syndrome but only for minimal survival. All healthy neonates, and especially low-birth-weight neonates, should be given some kind of nutritional support as soon as possible and at least within the first eight hours following birth.

Second, the low-birth-weight neonate, and particularly the premature neonate, has immature respiratory, cardiovascular, gastrointestinal, hepatic and renal systems that make maintenance of homeostasis and metabolic balance difficult. The immaturity of respiratory and cardiovascular systems can lead to hypoxia, respiratory acidosis, labored breathing and increased caloric requirements. Immaturity of the gastrointestinal system decreases the efficiency of digestion and absorption of nutrients, especially in the premature infant. Gastric emptying time is delayed, and the stomach capacity is small. In 13 infants weighing 1200 to 2000 gm., the average anatomical capacity of the stomach was 22 ml.[38] Such infants have an inability to absorb fat due to decreased secretion of pancreatic lipase and bile acid. Lactase

may also be deficient, since it does not reach full activity in the fetus until just before term.[43] Trypsin and amylase activity may also be low. Protein digestion does not seem to be affected significantly; fat, calcium and perhaps the fat-soluble vitamins and trace minerals are the nutrients most likely to be poorly absorbed. Because the renal system is immature, the renal solute load, or the amount of electrolytes and protein breakdown products excreted by the kidney, must be lower than normal. The urine osmolality of LBW infants should be between 75 and 300 mOsm. per kg. body weight per day. (See Chapter 9 for an explanation of osmolality.)

Third, the neonate with few fat reserves also has a smaller number of brown fat reserves. By uncoupling oxidative phosphorylation so that heat instead of chemical energy (ATP) is produced, the metabolism of brown fat normally enables the neonate to maintain body temperature. Consequently, the neonate who has minimal fat reserves is prone to hypothermia, which can be a tremendous drain on the infant's caloric reserves because it greatly increases calorie requirements. However, infants of less than 36 weeks' gestation have a limited sweat response to heat, and the 30 week old fetus has none, so that these infants are also prone to overheating by the environment.

Fourth, neonates of less than 32 to 34 weeks' gestation have immature sucking and swallowing reflexes, so that feeding by the oral route is a challenge, if not an impossible task. Regurgitation is a frequent problem, and aspiration is a danger because of the infant's immature cough reflex and weak respiratory muscles. Respiratory and cardiovascular difficulties frequently add to the problems of providing nutrition by the oral route.

Fifth, these babies have a high frequency of intrapartum asphyxia, aspiration of meconium, congenital anomalies and other problems resulting from immaturity or retarded growth that increase the difficulty of feeding and of maintaining homeostasis.

FETAL METABOLISM VS. NEONATAL METABOLISM

To further understand the nutritional and metabolic problems of the high-risk infant, it is helpful to compare fetal metabolism with neonatal metabolism and discuss the differences that allow the neonate to live independently when all systems are functioning well. The SGA or premature fetus must struggle to survive in the world with body systems that have not yet made the adjustments necessary to live outside the uterus.

The greatest amount of substrate supplied to the fetus *in utero* is glucose, and the evidence suggests that glucose is its principal source of energy. In the fetus the enzymes that regulate glycogenolysis and gluconeogenesis (mechanisms that maintain blood glucose) are not necessary. The fetal blood glucose level is maintained by the mother, assuming that she is eating adequately. It appears that only small amounts of fat (triglycerides, fatty acids, phospholipids and cholesterol) cross the placenta and that the fetus synthesizes its own lipids from precursors. Essential fatty acids must be transferred to the fetus, but how this happens is not clear. It appears that only in conditions of intrauterine malnutrition or fetal hypoglycemia does the fetus mobilize its lipid deposits for energy, and as would be expected, babies suffering from intrauterine malnutrition have reduced deposits of subcutaneous fat. In the normal gestation the dominant process is anabolism and fat deposition.

Amino acids probably are transported actively across the placenta, since plasma amino acid levels in the fetus are higher than those in the mother. However, the fetal plasma amino acid levels are dependent upon maternal levels of plasma amino acids, which reflect the mother's protein intake. In order to build protein tissue the fetus needs protein, and failure to receive sufficient quantities results in fetal growth retardation, as already discussed. Fetal growth is particularly sensitive to restriction of the maternal protein intake.

Besides protein that comes from across the placenta, the near-term fetus probably receives about 10 to 15 per cent of its protein requirements from the amniotic fluid, which it swallows and digests while *in utero*. This protein may be an important supplement, as suggested by the fact that fetuses in whom esophageal or intestinal atresia impedes swallowing or digestion commonly suffer intrauterine growth retardation.[22]

Insulin in fetal metabolism is more important as an anabolic hormone promoting growth than as a regulator of blood glucose, since the maternal insulin controls the blood glucose level both for herself and the fetus. The fetal pancreatic islet cells begin to function at the end of the first trimester, and the insulin secretion that results may be a major factor causing the increased fetal growth rate in the second and third trimesters.

At birth the fetus's environment changes forever. Out of the womb and disengaged from the placenta, the neonate must now rely on its own organs for breathing, regulation of internal temperature and maintenance of fluid and electrolyte balance and of glucose levels and nutritional homeostasis.

To prepare for separation from the maternal supply of glucose at birth, the fetus deposits glycogen in its liver, so that at term the liver and cardiac glycogen concentrations are high. Besides the glycogen stores, the hepatic enzymes for glycogenolysis and gluconeogenesis, which are necessary for metabolizing glycogen to glucose to maintain blood glucose levels, appear shortly before birth in the term infant. The premature or SGA infant, who has not had enough time or nutrients to develop adequate glycogen stores, obviously will have a difficult time regulating blood glucose levels and so is prone to hypoglycemia. As mentioned earlier, glycogen stores in the full-term neonate can be depleted within the first two to three hours of life because of the neonate's high metabolic rate; those in the small infant are depleted even sooner.

Glycogenolysis (breakdown of glycogen) proceeds under both aerobic and anaerobic conditions, but when hypoxia is present, only the anaerobic mechanism can be used for making energy or ATP. This is less efficient than aerobic metabolism and explains why hypoxia in these infants results in a more rapid use of glycogen reserves for energy and a greater potential for hypoglycemia.

The SGA infant in particular has a large brain-to-liver ratio, which results in demands for glucose by the brain too great to be met by the small number of liver stores. If the neonate is not fed and its glycogen stores are depleted, it then begins to metabolize fatty acids from its fat stores for glucose and energy. Ketones may also be metabolized; it is known that they can be utilized by the neonatal brain. Levels of both plasma fatty acids and plasma ketone bodies rise shortly after birth. The very small LBW infant, who has no fat deposits, must draw on tissue protein for energy after the glycogen reserves are depleted.

NUTRITIONAL REQUIREMENTS

Timing of the First Feeding

It is now accepted that for any neonate, and particularly for the LBW or high-risk infant, some form of feeding should be attempted within the first few hours of life in order to provide for the infant's high fluid and caloric needs and to avoid hypoglycemia. However, neonatologists disagree on the methods to be employed in initiating early feeding. The infant who weighs 1500 gm. or more, has matured beyond 33 weeks' gestation and does not have respiratory distress syndrome (RDS) or some other complication can usually be fed like the term neonate, except that initial feedings will have to be smaller and more frequent and increased gradually. Feedings are usually started by three hours of age. For smaller infants who are unable to feed orally or who have RDS or some other problem, the timing and method of introduction of feeding varies widely, depending on the philosophy of the neonatologist and the policy of the nursery. Some advocate total parenteral nutrition (concentrated glucose and protein, discussed later in this chapter) immediately if oral feeding cannot be started within the first 12 to 24 hours. Others recommend a more conservative approach, withholding TPN or oral feeding until the complication is resolved or at least until the infant's condition is stable. The neonate in this case is usually given intravenously 10 per cent solution of glucose in water, which is not enough to meet caloric requirements, and no protein is included. TPN or oral feeding is usually started on the third day of life.

Fluid

The LBW infant requires more water on a per-kg. basis than the term infant does, and in the first few days of life he or she may require as much as 200 ml. per kg. per day. The amounts of fluid presented in Table 37–3 are only guidelines for fluid administration; it is still important to monitor the infant's hydration by testing the osmolality of the urine, noting any clinical signs of dehydration and recording the fluid intake and urine output. Fluid requirements are increased by phototherapy, radiant heat treatment, high environmental temperature and increased gastrointestinal losses. Adequate fluid intake is crucial because water makes up a large percentage of the LBW infant's body weight, and such infants have limited ability to concentrate urine. If the infant cannot tolerate the oral intake of water or milk, 10 per cent glucose should be given intravenously to meet both the fluid and some of the caloric requirements.

Table 37–3 SUGGESTED RATES OF FLUID ADMINISTRATION FOR LOW-BIRTH-WEIGHT INFANTS (ml./kg./24 hr.)*a

AGE (Days)	BIRTH WEIGHT		
	<1000 Gm.	1000 to 1500 Gm.	1500 to 2500 Gm.
1	100–120	80–100	60– 80
2	140–160	110–130	90–110
3+	180–200+	140–180	120–160

*From: Roy, R. N., and Sinclair, J. C.: Hydration of the low-birth-weight infant. Clin. Perinatol., 3:407, 1976.

aThese are suggested as starting points only. Appropriate downward or upward adjustment may be necessary. Route of administration is not stipulated and will vary for each individual. Volumes quoted are total parenteral plus gastrointestinal intake.

Calories

The LBW infant's metabolic rate is high. The resting metabolic requirement is 50 to 60 kcal. per kg. per day, to which must be added 50 to 60 kcal. per kg. per day for response to cold stress, activity, growth and specific dynamic action (see Chapter 2). The total caloric expenditure then is 100 to 120 kcal. per kg. per day, three times that of an adult and higher than the term infant's expenditure. However, the caloric requirements of LBW infants will vary, and some infants who are SGA are likely to require more than 130 kcal. per kg. per day.

Protein

Protein is extremely important for the LBW infant because of the tremendous protein accretion that would have taken place at this time if the infant had remained in utero and that should continue during the early weeks of life. To illustrate the magnitude of the deposition of protein as tissue in the later stages of pregnancy, the 20 to 22 week old fetus has accrued only 23 gm. of protein, while the term infant has stored 500 gm. of protein. Protein is the nutrient that most influences neonatal growth.

There is controversy about the exact requirements for protein, but an acceptable figure for LBW infants is 3 to 4 gm. per kg. per day, and the VLBW infant or the infant with any kind of stress needs the upper limit of this range.[13] The protein tolerance of a premature infant can be exceeded when the intake is above 4.5 gm. per kg. per day. Excessive protein intake manifests itself in high plasma amino acid concentrations and a high blood urea nitrogen (BUN) level. The capacity for amino acid degradation, amino acid clearance by the kidneys and amino acid incorporation into protein is exceeded and growth is not enhanced when protein is given at this level.[34]

Cystine[42] and tyrosine[40] may be essential for the LBW infant but not for the term neonate. This is probably because of immature enzyme systems in the liver of the LBW infant. In the older infant with mature systems, these amino acids can be synthesized.

Concentration of Formula

The most critical problem in feeding the LBW infant is to meet the tremendous calorie and protein needs within the confines of the limited fluid volume that these infants can tolerate. Unfortunately, it is frequently impossible to meet these needs for several days or even weeks after birth. While the term infant may require 150 ml. of milk (100 kcal.) per kg. of body weight, the LBW infant may require 200 ml. (140 kcal.) per kg. body weight.

The natural tendency is to concentrate the formula for the LBW infant so that it gives more protein and calories in a smaller volume. However, this can present too large an osmotic load to the immature gastrointestinal tract and a large renal solute load to the immature renal system. Unfortunately, there is no ideal formula to meet these requirements as there is for the term infant. Breast milk and most formulas contain 67 kcal. per 100 ml. (20 kcal. per oz.), and this may not be adequate for some premature infants if they cannot take a large enough amount. If weight gain is unsatisfactory, a formula containing 81 to 90 kcal. per 100 ml. (24 to 27 kcal. per oz.) can be used. These formulas are more concentrated in protein and electrolytes and may exceed the infant's renal concentrating capacity of 400 mOsm. per liter. Infants receiving these formulas must be monitored more closely for hypernatremia, elevated BUN levels and dehydration. Formulas can be further concentrated up to 100 kcal. per 100 ml. (30 kcal. per oz.) but only if the infant is also receiving parenteral fluids.

Formulas with enteric osmotic loads of 400 mOsm. per liter or less are better tolerated. Similac, Enfamil and Isomil, at concentrations of 80 kcal. per 100 ml., or 24 kcal. per oz., have enteric solute loads of less than this, but formulas concentrated to 27 to 30 kcal. per oz. usually present higher loads.

The renal solute load from a formula should be 300 to 400 mOsm. per liter. Faster-growing

infants, such as very small neonates, will retain more of the potential renal solute load, and use it for growth and synthesis of new tissue. Thus the renal solute load of a particular formula for these infants will be lower.

Minerals

Providing an adequate calcium intake is another difficult problem of feeding the LBW infant, and hypocalcemia is common. Calcium requirements are high because of rapid skeletal growth, poor gastrointestinal absorption and endogenous fecal excretion of calcium.[3] Calcium absorption depends on the gestational age of the neonate and increases with postnatal age. None of the formulas now available provide calcium in amounts adequate to meet the needs of the LBW infant. Fomon suggests that the calcium content of formulas should be 250 to 300 mg. per 100 kcal., which is about three times that found in most formulas.[19] Whether it is possible to make such a formula is questionable.

Nutritional rickets is seen in very small premature infants and may be due to the inadequate calcium intake. Calcium supplements given early in life can improve bone mineralization, especially when the infant is not receiving an adequate amount of formula.[15]

Because the LBW infant is born with low iron stores, iron should be added to the diet as soon as the infant begins to gain weight. A dose of 5 to 10 mg. of iron from ferrous sulfate should be given daily when the infant is gaining 20 gm. per day, and 15 mg. of iron should be given when the infant is gaining more than 20 gm. per day.

Shaw postulates that the body's deficit of these minerals may be only one aspect of a much wider problem of mineral malabsorption that includes magnesium, copper, and zinc.[39]

Vitamins

Vitamin requirements are not known but are assumed to be similar to those of a term infant. However, commercially prepared formulas that supply an adequate intake of vitamins for the term infant may, because of the small quantity of formula taken, supply inadequate amounts for the LBW infant. Therefore, multiple vitamin supplementation is necessary. It is particularly important to meet requirements for fat-soluble vitamins because of low fetal stores, a high rate of utilization and poor absorption due to gastrointestinal immaturity. Vitamins D, E (see section on hemolytic anemia in this chapter) and K immediately after birth (see page 304) and folic acid are especially important.

Ideal Formula for the Low-Birth-Weight Infant

As mentioned before, there is no ideal formula for the LBW infant, mainly because there are no generally accepted criteria for the growth of these babies. Therefore, the exact nutritional requirements cannot be defined. It is known that the protein-to-calorie ratio should be high and that large amounts of minerals must be supplied without causing an unnecessarily high renal solute load. Available formulas do not have optimal amounts of protein, calories and calcium and do not provide the benefits to the fetus of intrauterine nutriture. The smaller the infant and the more rapid its rate of growth, the more inadequate present formulas are.

For the LBW infant weighing more than 1.5 kg., there is evidence to show the superiority of breast milk because of its protein quality, fat quality, immune factors and osmolarity. (See Chapter 14.) There also seems to be a lower incidence of necrotizing enterocolitis among breast-fed LBW neonates. IgA in breast milk given for even as little as 24 hours seems to protect the neonate from necrotizing enterocolitis. The milk must be fresh, less than 8 hours old, unheated and unrefrigerated.

Some argue that the protein content of human milk is not high enough to promote growth equivalent to intrauterine growth, which at present is the goal in the management of these infants. The advantages of breast milk may, however, outweigh this possible deficiency in its use for LBW infants.

A mother should be encouraged to breast-feed an infant who weighs 2000 gm. or more and can suck effectively. If this is not possible, the mother can express her milk so that it may be given to the infant by bottle, gavage or tube. The fact that the infant is receiving her milk can be very important to the mother, who, because her infant was of low birth weight and had to be separated from her, may feel helpless and inadequate. Producing milk for her infant may be the only way she can show love for it at this time and may give her great satisfaction. To increase the intake of protein and minerals and meet the requirements for LBW infants, Fomon recommends supplementing breast milk with an additional 1 to 2 bottles daily of a more concentrated formula.[19]

If the mother does not want to breast-feed her infant, then a formula that has been "humanized" to make its composition close to that of breast milk should be used. These formulas, such as SMA (Wyeth) and Similac PM 60/40 (Ross), have been modified so that the ratio of casein to lactalbumin protein is 60 to 40, similar to that in human milk. Some formulas such as Portagen and Pregestimil (Mead Johnson), which use medium chain triglycerides (MCT), are more completely absorbed by the LBW infant and would appear to provide more calories. However, the higher fat intake does not seem to promote greater weight gain. The caloric concentration of a formula should be 80 to 100 kcal. per 100 ml., and the protein content should be 2.8 gm. per 100 kcal.

Elemental or Chemically Defined Formulas

Some neonatal intensive care centers have used elemental or defined formulas composed of glucose, amino acids and very little fat or MCT in an attempt to provide a more readily absorbable formula for the LBW infant. The hypertonicity of these formulas has been proposed as the cause of the increased incidence of necrotizing enterocolitis seen in infants who receive these formulas, while others state that they help to avoid the occurrence of the disease. These formulas can provoke osmotic diarrhea, hypertonic dehydration and amino acid imbalance in rare cases.

METHODS OF FEEDING

Parenteral Supplementation by Peripheral Vein

Because of limited gastrointestinal function and a small stomach capacity, most LBW infants and all infants weighing less than 1500 gm. need to be given some fluid and calories by the parenteral route. Usually 10 per cent glucose is given, with added electrolytes and vitamins and sometimes amino acids. Early administration of calories and fluid is especially important in infants who have cyanosis due to respiratory, cardiac or central nervous system distress that may delay oral feeding. Because of the limit on fluid volume, complete caloric requirements usually cannot be met by peripheral vein intake, and this method should only be used as short term supplementation. About 0.6

kcal. per ml. of infusate can be supplied using a peripheral vein; if a central vein, which can tolerate a more osmotic infusate, is used, 1 kcal. per ml. of infusate can be supplied. Central vein nutrition or total parenteral nutrition is discussed later in this chapter and also in Chapter 35.

Oral Feeding

Before giving any type of oral fluid to any LBW neonate, pharyngeal coordination and the patency of the gastrointestinal tract should be tested. This can be done about four to six hours after birth. The first fluid given should always be sterile water, which is less damaging to bronchoalveolar epithelia should the neonate aspirate the fluid. Depending upon the size of the infant, the first feeding can range from 4 to 20 ml.

The infant who is able to suck and swallow should be fed like the normal term neonate but may need to be fed more frequently (every 1 to 2 hours) because of the small stomach capacity. Initially the infant may be unable to suck at the breast but able to suck from a bottle. If given a bottle feeding, the head of the bed should be raised and the infant placed on its right side to allow easier emptying of stomach contents into the duodenum and drainage of any regurgitated formula from the side of the mouth. If the mother desires to breast-feed, the infant should be graduated to the breast as soon as possible.

Tube Feeding

The infant who is unable to suck or swallow, who is dyspneic, septic or lethargic, or whose caloric requirements cannot be met by the usual oral feeding, is given *catheter* or *gavage* feedings hourly at first and then every two to three hours. With gavage feeding a short tube is inserted through the mouth or nose and into the infant's stomach. The mouth is the preferred entrance for the tube, and the infant does not have to be able to swallow. The first feeding is 4 to 6 ml., which is increased by 1 to 2 ml. every other feeding. If vomiting or distention occurs, the volume of the feeding is reduced, and the infant may have to be fed more frequently. Crosse has given a good description of gavage or catheter feeding.[11] If after four days the total caloric intake, including parenteral supplementation, has not reached 80 kcal. per kg. per day, other options for feeding the infant should be considered. Table 37–4 presents a feeding regimen for AGA premature

Table 37–4   FEEDING REGIMEN FOR PREMATURE AGA INFANTS*

DAY OF LIFE	UNCOMPLICATED		COMPLICATED[a]
	Less than 1.5 kg. *33 Weeks' Gestation*	*1.5–2.5 kg.* *33–38 Weeks' Gestation*	
1	65–150 ml./kg./day of $D_{10}W$[b] with vitamins (MVI)[c] and folic acid intravenously.	65–150 ml./kg./day of $D_{10}W$ with MVI and folic acid intravenously. Gavage or nipple feeding with 20 kcal./oz. formula, if tolerated.	65–150 ml./kg./day, plus amount to replace fluid losses, of $D_{10}W$ with MVI and folic acid intravenously.
2	80–150 ml./kg./day of $D_{10}W$ less volume of gavage feeding of 20 kcal./oz. formula. Oral vitamins and folic acid.	80–150 ml./kg./day of $D_{10}W$ less volume of gavage or nipple feedings of 24 kcal./oz. formula. Oral vitamins and folic acid.	80–150 ml./kg./day, plus amount to replace fluid losses, of $D_{10}W$ with MVI and folic acid intravenously.
3	100–200 ml./kg. of $D_{10}W$ less volume of gavage feeding of 24 kcal./oz. formula.	Same as column 2.	Same as uncomplicated 1.5-kg. premature infant on day 2.
4	If total intake is less than 80 kcal./kg./day, consider options.[d]	Same as column 2.	Same as column 2.
7	If total intake is less than 100 kcal./kg./day, consider options.[d]	Same as column 2.	Same as column 2.
10	If no weight gain, a more aggressive effort must be made to increase intake of calories and protein	Same as column 2.	Same as column 2.

*Adapted from: Rickard, K., and Gresham, E.: Nutritional considerations for the newborn requiring intensive care. J. Am. Diet. Assoc., 66:592, 1975.

[a]The complicated group consists of infants presenting medical and surgical management problems that require a delay in alimentation.

[b]$D_{10}W$ = 10 per cent dextrose in water.

[c]MVI = M.V.I. Multi-Vitamin Infusion (USV Pharmaceutical).

[d]Options to be used with infants taking less than 80 to 100 kcal./kg./day:
   1. Continuous intragastric tube feeding.
   2. Continuous intrajejunal tube feeding.
   3. Manipulation of formula concentration.
   4. Peripheral vein nutritional supplementation if feeding limitation of 7 days or less is anticipated.
   5. Total parenteral nutrition if feeding limitation of more than 7 days is anticipated. Certain surgical problems such as short bowel syndrome will require earlier institution of TPN.

infants; SGA infants who are not premature would probably progress at a faster rate.

Another form of tube feeding uses an indwelling nasogastric (NG) or nasojejunal (NJ) tube to feed formula, breast milk or other mixture. The infant's gastrointestinal tract must be functioning if these procedures are to be used. The nasogastric tube, usually a size 5 or 8 French polyethylene tube, is passed through the nose and into the stomach. A bolus feeding can be given every two hours or a constant drip can be maintained, which would allow for a larger intake. One problem with using this technique is that the limited capacity of the stomach may cause regurgitation and possible aspiration of the feeding. A nasojejunal feeding tube can be used to prevent this, particularly with infants who have respiratory distress syndrome. The tip of this tube is placed in the jejunum and the formula is dripped into it. A Silastic rather than a polyethylene tube is preferable, since in the environment of the duodenum a polyethylene tube stiffens and may cause duodenual perforation.[6] Other problems associated with this method are abdominal distention, vomiting, diarrhea, changes in the intestinal flora and decreased absorption, particularly of fat, as compared to fat absorption using nasogastric feeding.[36] However, equal assimilation of nutrients may be achieved by increasing the volume of the feeding into the jejunum.

The continuous drip tube feeding has the advantages of reduced nursing time, decreased amount of handling of the infant and provision of a constant source of glucose. Reduced handling of the infant may not be an advantage, however, since stimulation by physical contact seems necessary for the infant's optimal growth. The volume of the initial feeding is 60 ml. per kg. per 24 hr., and it is gradually increased in steps of 30 ml. per kg. per 24 hr., as tolerated, to a maximum of 300 ml. per kg. per 24 hr.

The head of the incubator bed should be elevated to help prevent regurgitation, and mittens should be placed over the baby's hands to prevent him or her from removing the tube. Particular attention should be paid to the infant's nose and to the position of the tube so that it does not cause stretching of the nares.

The infant's tolerance to regular oral feedings should be tested before tube feeding is discontinued. Sterile water is always used first. The frequency and amount of oral feedings are increased gradually until the infant is taking 100 to 120 kcal. per kg., and then the tube is removed.

Total Parenteral Nutrition

Total parenteral nutrition (TPN) using a central vein such as the superior vena cava (see Fig. 37–2) or the umbilical vein to the inferior vena cava is another option that can be used to meet the infant's nutritional needs. Generally, TPN is reserved for infants who are unable to take any nourishment orally or in whom oral intake and peripheral vein supplementation after several days still do not meet their nutritional requirements. Other candidates for TPN are babies born with anomalies of the gastrointestinal tract, premature infants in whom the gastrointestinal tract is not yet functioning, babies who have complications that limit oral intake or increase nutritional requirements and infants with chronic intractable diarrhea.

TPN can be invaluable in treating diarrhea and breaking the diarrhea-malnutrition cycle. Diarrhea results in loss of nutrients, which leads to malnutrition, which in turn causes changes in intestinal epithelia and leads to diarrhea, poor absorption and malnutrition. Providing nutrition via the parenteral route helps to resolve the disorder and save the life of the child. Keating reported that, of 16 patients ranging from 2½ to 12 weeks of age who had intractable diarrhea, in whom all diagnostic tests were negative and who were managed with total parenteral nutrition, only one died of sepsis. One year later all 15 survivors had normal gastrointestinal function, except for six black infants who were lactose-intolerant.[26] Total parenteral nutrition allows the gastrointestinal villi to regain their normal morphology and absorptive function and maintain nutritional intake.

TPN for the low-birth-weight infant is still under investigation and is not part of the routine management of these infants. TPN can produce satisfactory growth and nitrogen balance, but whether or not the short- and long-term outcome of LBW infants is favorably affected has not been determined. One of the problems that arises when attempting to answer this question is that a large number of very-low-birth-weight babies would be needed to demonstrate the effectiveness or ineffectiveness of the method, and this would require the cooperation of several neonatal centers.[25]

When TPN is used in the LBW infant the

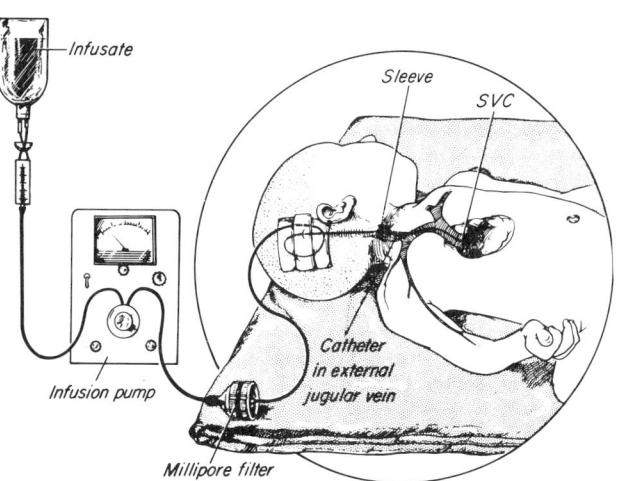

Figure 37–2 System for long-term TPN in a neonate. Infusion pump ensures uniform hourly flow rate of the amino acid-glucose infusion. The Millipore circuit will remove any microorganisms that may have contaminated the system. The silicone or polyvinyl catheter is inserted by cutdown into the external jugular vein and directed into the superior vena cava (SVC). It is secured in place by a silicone rubber sleeve or with sutures, and the other end of the catheter is directed subcutaneously using a needle so that it emerges through a small incision in the parietal scalp behind the ear. The end of the catheter is taped to the skin. (From: Ghadimi, H. (ed.): Total Parenteral Nutrition: Premises and Promises. New York, John Wiley & Sons, 1975, p. 453.)

optimal caloric intake appears to be 110 to 120 kcal. per kg. per day, although 80 kcal. per kg. per day may be adequate for some infants. Calories are provided by glucose or Intralipid (a fat emulsion), or both. When administering large amounts of glucose by vein (especially to VLBW infants) it is important to check for hyperglycemia, which can occur because of limited insulin secretory capacity, sluggish pancreatic response, tissue insensitivity to insulin or inadequate functioning of other glucose-controlling hormones such as glucagon, glucocorticoids, catecholamines and growth hormone.

Intralipid, which contains twice the number of calories found in an equal volume of glucose, allows for administration of more calories in a smaller volume than can be achieved with glucose. However, in attempting to meet the caloric needs, too much fat can be given, and the maximal clearance rate of fat from the blood stream can be exceeded. Plasma Intralipid levels rise and hyperlipidemia ensues. The tolerance to an Intralipid load is lower in SGA infants, premature infants of less than 32 weeks' gestation and acutely ill infants. The use of heparin in these infants will help to promote Intralipid clearance. All the effects of hyperlipidemia in these infants are not known, but in jaundiced infants it may increase the amount of bilirubin unbound from albumin and promote kernicterus.[1] Two to 4 gm. of Intralipid per kg. per day are recommended for parenteral nutrition.

Protein requirements for intravenous nutrition appear to be about 1.2 to 2.5 gm. per kg. per day. Because certain amino acids may be essential only to the premature infant, because the optimal proportion of non-essential to essential amino acids is unknown, and because the LBW infant's hepatic enzyme systems that metabolize amino acids are immature, the ideal amino acid composition for protein in the intravenous formula is not known. The needs when I.V. protein is given are probably different than when protein is taken orally. Ghadimi recommends a formula composed from individual amino acids that is tailored to meet the needs of the LBW infant.[21]

Trace minerals and essential fatty acids are also important, although we do not know the specific requirements. If fat emulsions are used, the essential fatty acid needs will be met; otherwise, periodic blood or plasma transfusions or the cutaneous application of sunflower seed oil will prevent a fatty acid deficiency.[20] Transfusions can also meet the

Table 37–5 USUAL COMPOSITION OF INFUSATE*

CONSTITUENT	AMOUNT (Per Day)
Nitrogen source	2.5 gm./kg.
Glucose	25–30 gm./kg.
NaCl	3–4 mM./kg.[a]
KH_2PO_4	2–3 mM./kg.[b]
Ca gluconate	0.25 mM./kg. (0.5 mEq./kg.)
$MgSo_4$	0.125 mM./kg. (0.25 mEq./kg.)
MVI	1 ml.
Vitamin B_{12}	50 μg.
Folic acid	50–75 μg.
Vitamin K_1	250–500 μg.
Total volume of infusate	130 ml./kg.

*From: Heird, W. C., and Winters, R. W.: Total parenteral nutrition: the state of the art. J. Pediatr., 86:2, 1975.

[a] mM = millimole.

[b] KH_2PO_4 should be limited to 2 mM./kg./day; additional potassium should be provided as KCl.

needs for trace minerals, or trace minerals can be added to the intravenous fluid. See Table 37–5 for the composition of a typical infusate used for infants.

Commercially available vitamin preparations for intravenous use are not well adapted to infant requirements. One ml. of multiple vitamin infusion (MVI) per day is used, but this must be supplemented with vitamins K and B_{12} and folic acid and sometimes with vitamin D.

Metabolic complications of total parenteral nutrition include hypophosphatemia, hyperchloremia, metabolic acidosis, azotemia, hyperammonemia, hypovitaminosis, hypervitaminosis, essential fatty acid deficiency and trace mineral deficiencies. See Table 35–13 for those measurements that should be monitored to avoid these complications in the neonate.

When administering TPN, attempts to encourage oral intake should be continued, if possible. As the infant increases oral intake, TPN is decreased, and when the infant takes 110 kcal. per kg. per day orally TPN should be discontinued. Peripheral vein nutrition as a supplement may still be necessary.

POTENTIAL FOR GROWTH AND ANTICIPATED GROWTH RATE

During the first few weeks or months of life, the goal in the management of LBW infants has always been to mimic the intrauterine growth by promoting a weight gain of 30 gm. per day.

According to Brenner, the mean fetal weight gain between the 28th and 36th week of gestation is 187.5 gm. per week. or 27 gm. per day.[8] For the 37th through 40th weeks, the rate of weight gain is about 23 gm. per day. To maintain the intrauterine growth rate, the LBW infant should gain about 25 to 30 gm. per day after making an adjustment to the extrauterine environment during the first few days of life. The VLBW infant should be expected to grow at a faster rate if adequate nutrition can be provided, which usually is impossible at first. Considering the limitations of present feeding methods and formulas, a 20-gm. daily weight gain is probably a more realistic goal for these infants during the first weeks.[35]

Whether it is optimal for them or not, all neonates lose some weight after birth. Lowest weight should be reached between two and eight days after birth and should be no more than a 5 to 10 per cent reduction from birth weight. The SGA infant should lose no more than 5 per cent. Birth weight should be regained within one to two weeks.

Most neonatal intensive care nurseries use the growth grid of Dancis and associates[12] (Fig. 37–3) to plot the early weight gain of LBW infants. This grid was established over thirty years ago, when perinatal care was not as advanced as it is today. For this reason, the curve depicting weight loss after birth, particularly for infants weighing less than 1000 gm. at birth,

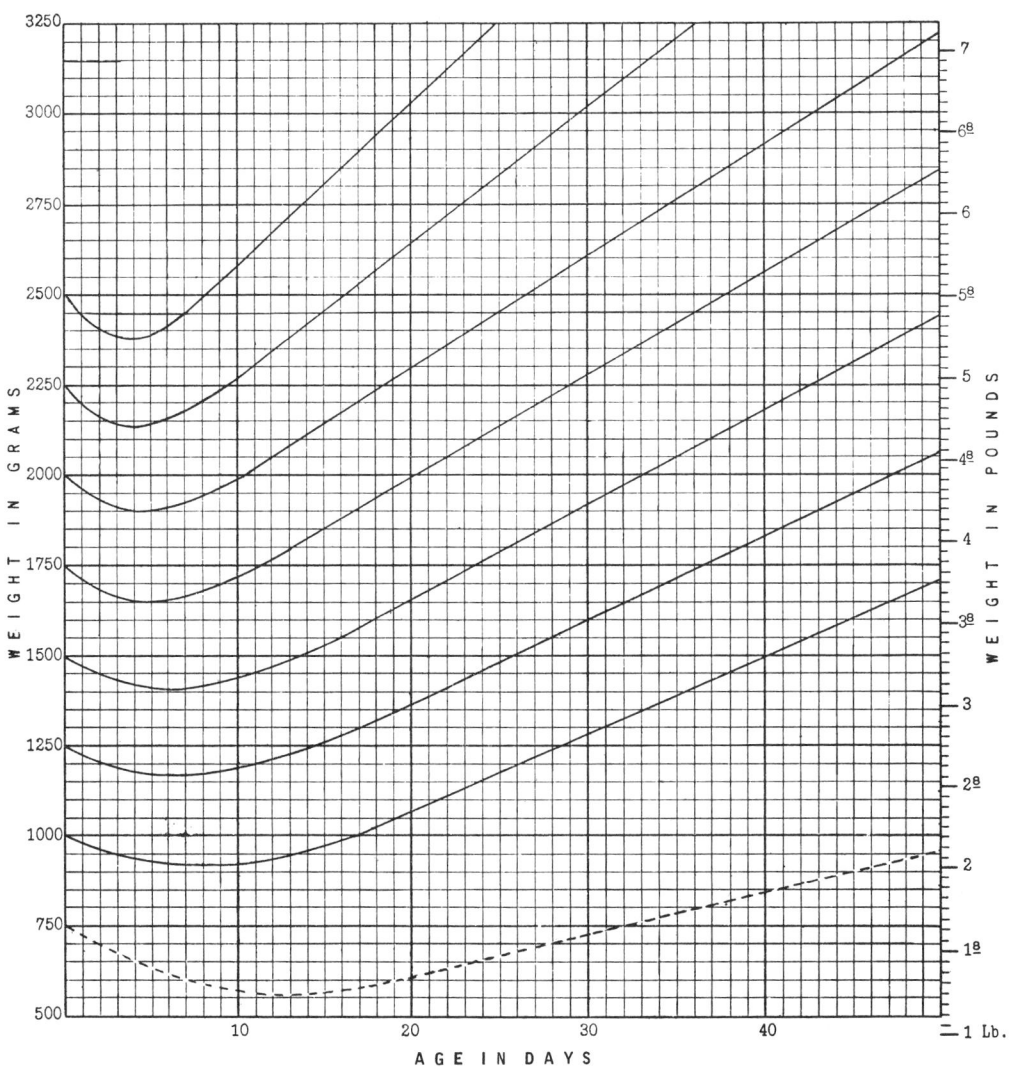

Figure 37–3 Weight chart for premature infants. (From: Dancis, J., O'Connell, J., and Holt, L.: A grid for recording the weight of premature infants. J. Pediatr., *33*:570, 1948.)

is probably a little too low, and the weight of these infants most likely should not be allowed to fall to this level.

Weight gain has always been the standard by which to measure growth and thus, the extent to which the infant's nutritional requirements are being met. This is partially due to the convenience of measuring weight gain. However, weight gain is not the sole criterion for assessing the fulfillment of nutritional requirements and may not be the best one. A great part of weight gain can result from fluid retention rather than from tissue growth.

There is also some doubt about whether faster weight gain and faster growth are desirable. Rats who grow faster die younger (see discussion of longevity in Chapter 16), and rapid early weight gains may predispose a person to later obesity (see discussion of adipose cellularity in Chapter 27).

During the first year of life, the healthy premature infant who is the appropriate size for gestational age (AGA) will grow at the same rate as the full-term infant of the same *post-conceptional* age if the AGA infant's nutritional requirements in the neonatal period are met. The standard for evaluating growth can be the same as that used for term infants as long as age is calculated from the expected date of delivery and not from the actual premature delivery date. For example, an infant born after 36 weeks' gestation instead of after 40 weeks' would be plotted on the *intrauterine* growth chart (Fig. 37–1) for its first four weeks of growth and on the *neonatal* or infant growth chart (Appendixes 24 to 27) beginning in the fourth week of life. At the age of 10 weeks the child would be evaluated for growth as if he or she were a six week old infant. This correction should continue throughout the first year of life. The infant's growth could also be plotted on the growth grid for premature infants (Fig. 37–3). During the first year of life the child will grow the same as normal children with regard to length, but weight will probably remain lower, at about the 50th percentile. By preschool age the child who was a premature infant is of normal height and has a normal head circumference but probably is slender.

The SGA infant must have a period of accelerated or "catch-up" growth in order to reach the size of other children the same age. This growth begins soon after birth if adequate nutrition is provided. Head growth is faster than growth in length or weight, especially if the infant is also premature. When postnatal nutrition is adequate, the SGA infant takes advantage of it and grows at a faster rate than the term infant, sometimes doubling his or her birth weight in five weeks instead of in five months as the term infant does. This period of "catch-up" growth seems to be most rapid at six to nine months post-term but continues throughout the first year of life. If the accelerated growth is sufficient, then the SGA infant will be the same size as other children the same age; if it is insufficient the child will remain small. The growth rate during this period of "catch-up" growth is related to the degree of retardation of the preceding intrauterine growth. The greater the growth retardation, the faster the "catch-up" growth, providing that adequate amounts of nutrients are available. Early nutrition for the SGA infant or the ill premature infant is of paramount importance during the critical growth period to allow for maximum growth of the skeletal system and the central nervous system.

The pattern of intrauterine growth retardation and the effect of adequate or inadequate postnatal nutrition on the extent of "catch-up" growth are still not completely understood. However, it appears that the hypotrophic neonate (who has an adequate number of cells), although physically small, has a good prognosis for physical and intellectual development provided that he or she survives the neonatal period without complications and that adequate nutritional intake is maintained. The prognosis is not good for the infant with hypoplastic growth, which produces an inadequate number of cells. However, at this point we cannot differentiate clinically between the two types of growth retardation, and even if we could, all their ramifications for an infant's development are not completely understood.

COMMON PROBLEMS OF THE PREMATURE OR SGA INFANT

Hypoglycemia

Estimates of the incidence of neonatal hypoglycemia range from 29 per cent in a group of SGA infants to 67 per cent in small premature infants.[28] Other infants prone to hypoglycemia are those born of toxemic or diabetic mothers and those in neonatal distress.

Hypoglycemia in the neonate is usually defined as a blood glucose level less than 20 mg. per 100 ml. in low birth weight and preterm infants and less than 30 mg. per 100 ml. in term infants. Others feel that a value below 40 mg.

per 100 ml. in any neonate indicates hypoglycemia that should be treated.

In all neonates, the concentration of blood glucose falls during the first 4 to 6 hours following birth. It remains low for 7 to 10 days and then reaches adult levels. Factors that increase the neonate's use of blood glucose and thus produce hypoglycemia are increased muscular activity, as occurs in respiratory distress syndrome (RDS), or hypothermia, both of which increase energy requirements.

The clinical manifestations of hypoglycemia in the neonate are tremors in the extremities followed by listlessness, hyperirritability, failure to suck well, unstable thermoregulation and, in severe cases, apnea, convulsions and coma. The first sign, tremors, can appear within an hour after birth. Prolonged intractable symptomatic hypoglycemia results in brain damage and mental retardation, and other evidence shows that even brief periods of hypoglycemia in the neonate may be detrimental to later intellectual growth.

The blood glucose concentration of the LBW neonate should be measured frequently using a microtechnique. With early feeding, blood glucose can be maintained at a normal level, especially if feedings are supplemented with 10 per cent glucose given intravenously.

Hyperbilirubinemia

Hyperbilirubinemia develops in a neonate because his liver is presented with large amounts of red blood cell breakdown products that cannot be metabolized rapidly enough. The breakdown of red blood cells that occurs naturally after birth results in the formation of bilirubin. This must be bound to albumin for transport to the liver, where it is conjugated by liver enzymes and excreted as bile. When all the bilirubin cannot be bound to albumin, and when its conjugation is decreased because of overloaded liver enzyme systems, hyperbilirubinemia results. The excess bilirubin can then diffuse into the extravascular compartments, including the cerebrospinal fluid and the brain, because the blood-brain barrier is permeable to unconjugated bilirubin during the first few days of life. Hyperbilirubinemia is a serious condition and requires treatment because brain damage (kernicterus) and death can result from it.

The younger and smaller the fetus, the greater the level of serum bilirubin. This is because preterm infants and some SGA infants have increased rates of hemolysis following birth, immature liver enzyme systems, poor binding capacities for bilirubin (low serum albumin levels) and more permeable blood-brain barriers.

Phototherapy, or exposure of the infant to ultraviolet light, is frequently used to treat hyperbilirubinemia. The light causes a decomposition of bilirubin so that it becomes water-soluble and can then be excreted, but the photodecomposition products can be toxic to the gut. They may shorten gastrointestinal transit time[37] so that gastrointestinal loss of water is increased.[32] Further dehydration may occur, since phototherapy causes a 40 per cent increase in insensible water loss. Some of the photodecomposition products may inhibit intestinal lactase. Bakken has found that lactase function in these infants is lowered and that the resultant diarrhea from feeding lactose-containing formulas is resolved when lactose-free mixtures are used.[2] This is necessary only while the babies are receiving phototherapy, and after it is discontinued, feedings of breast milk or cow's milk formula can be resumed. Phototherapy seems to be enhanced by the administration of riboflavin, perhaps because the infant's requirement for this nutrient is increased when receiving this treatment.[33] Early oral feeding for those infants who can tolerate it causes increased intestinal mobility and can reduce the enterohepatic reabsorption of bilirubin. In the fasting neonate, conjugated bilirubin that is excreted in biliary fluids will stagnate in the intestinal lumen, where bacteria and enzymes have a longer time to unconjugate it. The unconjugated bilirubin is then reabsorbed into the blood stream and overloads the liver.[7]

Hemolytic Anemia and Vitamin E

Low-birth-weight infants have a high risk of developing vitamin E (alpha-tocopherol) deficiency because they are born with minimal stores of the vitamin. Vitamin E does not easily cross the placenta, and most placental transfer of the vitamin occurs in the last weeks of pregnancy. Second, because of the decreased secretion of bile salts and pancreatic lipase by the immature gastrointestinal tract, the absorption of significant amounts of this fat-soluble vitamin is more difficult and less likely than that seen in the term infant.

Hematopoietic tissue is turning over rapidly, and since red cell membrane stability requires vitamin E, a hemolytic anemia is one of the first signs of vitamin E deficiency. Usually a serum

tocopherol level of less than 0.9 mg. per 100 ml. is associated with hemolysis. The hemolytic anemia usually develops at 6 to 10 weeks of age, depending upon (1) the content of polyunsatured fat in the infant's formula, which increases the need for the antioxidant vitamin E (see Chapter 8), (2) whether the infant is breast-fed or given evaporated milk formula, because human milk contains more vitamin E than cow's milk (commercial formulas are now fortified with vitamin E) and (3) whether the infant is also given iron in the formula or as a supplement. Iron appears to catalyze the oxidative breakdown of red blood cell lipids and also interferes with the absorption of vitamin E from the gut. Premature babies given iron but not vitamin E supplements are more anemic than other premature babies. The rate of hemoglobin decline in LBW babies of gestational ages between 28 weeks and 40 weeks was greatest in those receiving iron, followed by those receiving no supplements, followed by those receiving iron and vitamin E, and it was least in those receiving only vitamin E.[29]

To prevent vitamin E deficiency and hemolytic anemia, oral doses of vitamin E should be given in the water-soluble form for maximum absorption. A daily supplement of 0.5 mg. per kg. of α-tocopherol daily is recommended for premature infants. There is no agreement on the optimal time for starting iron supplementation, but most often it is begun very soon after birth.

PROGNOSIS FOR PHYSICAL AND INTELLECTUAL DEVELOPMENT

The prognosis for optimal physical and intellectual development for a particular premature or SGA infant is difficult to evaluate, and studies report conflicting results. Most of the health problems of these infants appear during the first year of life, and if an infant survives the first year he or she will probably live to adulthood, although the quality of physical and mental development cannot be predicted easily.

In evaluating reported attempts to determine the outcome for a group of premature or SGA infants, one should consider: (1) the composition of the population sample (for example, the neonatal mortality rate is *lower* for black LBW infants than for white ones[4, 31]), (2) the way in which the mortality rate is expressed, (3) the treatment methods used in perinatal life, (4) the duration of follow-up studies, (5) whether the infants were grouped into very-low-birth-weight and low-birth-weight categories and (6) whether those infants who died were also included in the statistics.[18]

The duration of the follow-up studies is important because certain developmental abnormalities do not become apparent until seven to eight years of age. Abnormal physical growth patterns and severe neurological and intellectual defects can usually be determined by age two; however, minor neurological defects and aberrations of vision and hearing are usually not detectable until ages four to six, when the child begins school. Behavior disorders, intelligence level and specific learning disorders are detected at about the age of seven or eight.

Since the introduction of neonatal intensive care in the early sixties and improved techniques of nutrition, ventilatory assistance and heart rate and body temperature monitoring, the percentage of infants who survive the neonatal period (the first 28 days of life) has increased. One report by Stewart from a neonatal center in England reported a mean neonatal survival rate of 23 per cent for infants weighing 1000 gm. or less at birth who were born between 1966 and 1970 and a rate of 39 per cent for similar infants born between 1971 and 1975.[41] Although the survival rate is improving it is still discouragingly low, and every effort should be made to provide good prenatal care that will help to prevent prematurity and low birth weight in newborns.

The same investigators also looked at the long-term sequelae of infants born between 1966 and 1974 and found a 7 per cent incidence of major handicaps and a 15 per cent incidence of minor handicaps. These figures provide even more reason to prevent low birth weight and, for those infants in whom it cannot be prevented, to provide perinatal care in neonatal intensive care centers to improve their prognosis.

It appears that the most vulnerable period for neurological development in the human infant is the last trimester of pregnancy and the first few months of postnatal life.[17] Malnutrition in early postnatal life can produce later deficits in learning ability and in adult stature.[5, 27] It is possible that both myelinization and the integrative aspects of brain development may be vulnerable to malnutrition up to 2½ years of age.[14, 16]

In a retrospective study of a group of premature infants and SGA infants of both LBW and VLBW who were born in the period between 1960 and 1962 it was found that their results on several intellectual performance tests given at ages five, six and seven years were significantly

poorer than those of a random sample of other children the same age. Very low birth weight infants performed less well than LBW infants. Neligan concludes that it is better for a baby's later development to be born prematurely than to be born small for gestational age.[30]

After studying a group of 42 high-risk neonates born in 1971 and 1972 and placed in a neonatal intensive care nursery, Calame found 71 per cent of them to be normal at age three, although the incidence of neurological sequelae and developmental abnormalities (29 per cent) was four times greater than that of a normal infant population. His findings confirmed that, in SGA infants, neurological handicaps are more likely to occur if severe RDS or cerebral distress is also present. All mentally deficient children in this study experienced cerebral distress in the neonatal period. Neonatal cerebral distress remains the most serious adverse prognostic situation for high-risk infants with regard to their later neural development.[10]

Even though the prognosis for LBW infants is improving, later developmental problems still occur in many of these children. Now that the lives of the smallest and most at-risk babies are being saved, health professionals must be concerned with the quality of these lives. Stewart recommends optimal care for all infants born after 24 weeks' gestation or longer. However, if it becomes evident that the infant has an abnormality, such as a large intraventricular hemorrhage, that is certain to lead to a major handicap, then the means of sustaining life should be withdrawn.[41] Since the likelihood that later developmental problems will occur is higher in LBW infants and neonates with complications than in a group of term infants, health professionals must be prepared to conduct developmental problem–detection programs and intervention programs to deal with possible difficulties. Environmental factors also affect the development of these children and, as for any child, should be made as positive as possible.

An important way to improve the prognosis for these children is to ensure that the maternal-infant bond is formed to the greatest possible extent. This can be done by encouraging the mother to come into the nursery to feed her infant and help with its care. If she would like to breast-feed her infant and the infant can suck, she should be encouraged to do so. If the infant is being fed by gavage or tube she can be encouraged to express her milk and bring it to the nursery to be used for the child. It is postulated that failure to form the maternal-infant attachment due to prolonged separation of the mother and her baby in this critical early period is the reason for the higher incidence of abused babies among preterm infants.[9]

The cost of maintaining low-birth-weight or high-risk neonates until they can survive independently is astronomical compared with the cost of good prenatal care, including good nutrition, which can help to reduce the likelihood of having a low-birth-weight or high-risk infant. The existence of neonatal intensive care units should not become an excuse for less-than-optimal prenatal care. Even the highest quality neonatal intensive care unit cannot equal the best environment for the fetus—the uterus of a healthy, well-nourished woman with a well-functioning placenta.

PROBLEMS AND SUGGESTED TOPICS FOR DISCUSSION

1. Learn about an infant in the neonatal intensive care unit of your hospital. (a) What was his or her birth weight? Present weight? (b) Was he or she premature? Small for gestational age? (c) How is he or she being fed? (d) Describe his or her nutritional requirements. Are they being met? If not, what are your recommendations?
2. Read the chart of a neonate who has a clinical problem related to low birth weight. How is this problem affecting the infant's nutritional requirements? What do you recommend as proper nutritional care?
3. Talk with a mother who is breast-feeding her LBW infant. Is she having any problems? If so, what recommendations might you give her? How would you estimate whether the nutritional needs of her infant are being met?
4. What is the policy of the intensive care nursery regarding vitamin and mineral supplementation for low-birth-weight infants? Give the dosage and frequency for each vitamin and mineral.

CITED REFERENCES

1. Andrew, G., Chan, G., and Schiff, D.: Lipid metabolism in the neonate. II. The effect of Intralipid on bilirubin binding *in vitro* and *in vivo*. J. Pediatr., 88:279, 1976.
2. Bakken, A. F.: Temporary intestinal lactase deficiency in light-treated jaundiced infants. Acta Paediatr. Scand., 66:91, 1977.
3. Barltrop, D., Mole, R. H,. and Sutton, A.: Absorption and endogenous faecal excretion of calcium by low birthweight infants on feeds with varying contents of calcium and phosphate. Arch. Dis. Child., 52:41, 1977.
4. Behrman, R. E.: The fetus and newborn infant. In: Vaughn, V. C., and McKay, R. J. (eds.): Nelson Textbook of Pediatrics, 10th ed. Philadelphia, W. B. Saunders Co., 1975, p. 322.
5. Berglund, G., and Rabo, E.: A long-term follow-up investigation of patients with hypertrophic pyloric stenosis with special reference to the physical and mental development. Acta Paediatr. Scand., 62:125, 1973.

6. Boros, S. J.: Duodenal perforation: a complication of neonatal nasojejunal feeding. J. Pediatr., *85*:107, 1974.

7. Brans. Y. W.: Neonatal nutrition. An overview. Postgrad. Med., *60*:113, 1976.

8. Brenner. W. E.. Edelman, D. A., and Hendricks, C. H.: A standard of fetal growth for the United States of America. Am. J. Obstet. Gynecol., *126*:555, 1976.

9. Brown, R. J. K., and Valman, H. B.: Practical Neonatal Paediatrics, 3rd ed. Oxford, England, Blackwell Scientific Publications, 1975, p. 43.

10. Calame, A., et al.: Psychological and neurodevelopmental outcome of high risk newborn infants. Helv. Paediatr. Acta, *31*:287, 1976.

11. Crosse, V. M., and Hill, E. E.: The Preterm Baby and Other Babies with Low Birth Weight, 8th ed. Edinburgh, Churchill Livingstone, 1975, pp. 88–118.

12. Dancis, J., O'Connell, J., and Holt, L.: A grid for recording the weight of premature infants. J. Pediatr., *33*:570, 1948.

13. Davidson, M., et al.: Feeding studies in low-birth-weight infants. I. Relationship of dietary protein, fat, and electrolytes to rates of weight gain, clinical courses, and serum chemical concentrations. J. Pediatr., *70*:695, 1967.

14. Davison, A. N., and Dobbing, J.: Myelination as a vulnerable period in brain development. Br. Med. Bull., *22*:40, 1966.

15. Day, C. M., et al.: Growth and mineral metabolism in very-low-birth-weight infants. II. Effects of calcium supplementation on growth and divalent cations. Pediatr. Res., *9*:568, 1975.

16. Dobbing, J.: The later growth of the brain and its vulnerability. Pediatrics, *53*:1, 1974.

17. Dobbing, J., and Sands, J.: Quantitative growth and development of the human brain. Arch. Dis. Child., *48*:757, 1973.

18. Fitzhardinge, P. M.: Follow-up studies on the low birth weight infant. Clin. Perinatol., *3*:503, 1976.

19. Fomon, S. J., Ziegler, E. E., and O'Donnell, A. M.: Infant feeding in health and disease. In: Fomon, S. J.: Infant Nutrition, 2nd ed. Philadelphia, W. B. Saunders Co., 1974, p. 506.

20. Friedman, Z., et al.: Correction of essential fatty acid deficiency in newborn infants by cutaneous application of sunflower-seed oil. Pediatrics, *58*:650, 1976.

21. Ghadimi, H.: Newly devised amino acid solutions for intravenous administration. In: Ghadimi, H. (ed.): Total Parenteral Nutrition: Premises and Promises. New York, John Wiley & Sons, 1975, p. 407.

22. Gitlin, D., et al.: The turnover of amniotic fluid protein in the human conceptus. Am. J. Obstet. Gynecol., *113*:632, 1972.

23. Harding, P. G. R.: Fetal growth and nutrition. In: Goodwin, J. W., Godden, J. O., and Chance, G. W. (eds.): Perinatal Medicine: The Basic Science Underlying Clinical Practice. Baltimore, Williams & Wilkins Co., 1976, p. 258.

24. Heird, W. C., et al.: Intravenous alimentation in pediatric patients. J. Pediatr., *80*:351, 1972.

25. Heird, W. C., MacMillan, R. W., and Winters, R. W.: Total parenteral nutrition in the pediatric patient. In: Fischer, J. E. (ed.): Total Parenteral Nutrition. Boston, Little, Brown & Co., 1976, p. 268.

26. Keating, J. P.: Parenteral nutrition in infants with malabsorption. In: Winters, R. W., and Hasselmeyer, E. G. (eds.): Intravenous Nutrition in High Risk Infants. New York, John Wiley & Sons, 1975.

27. Klein, P. S., Forbes, G. B., and Nader, P. R.: Effects of starvation in infancy (pyloric stenosis) on subsequent learning abilities. J. Pediatr., *87*:5, 1975.

28. Lubchenco, L. O., and Bard, H.: Incidence of hypoglycemia in newborn infants classified by birth weight and gestational age. Pediatrics, *47*:831, 1971.

29. Melhorn, D. K., Gross, S., and Childers, G.: Vitamin E–dependent anemia in the premature infant. I. Effects of large doses of medicinal iron. J. Pediatr., *79*:569, 1971.

30. Neligan, G. A., et al.: Born Too Soon or Born Too Small: A Follow-Up Study to Seven Years of Age. (Clinics in Developmental Medicine, No. 61.) Philadelphia, J. B. Lippincott Co., 1976, pp. 81–85.

31. North, A. F., and Mac Donald, H. M.: Why are neonatal mortality rates lower in small black infants than in white infants of similar birth weight? J. Pediatr., *90*:809, 1977.

32. Oh, W., and Karecki, H.: Phototherapy and insensible water loss in the newborn infant. Am. J. Dis. Child., *124*:230, 1972.

33. Pascale, J. A., et al.: Riboflavin and bilirubin response during phototherapy. Pediatr. Res., *10*:854, 1976.

34. Rassin, D. K., et al.: Milk protein quantity and quality in low-birth-weight infants. II. Effects of selected aliphatic amino acids in plasma and urine. Pediatrics, *59*:407, 1977.

35. Rickard, K., and Gresham, E.: Nutritional considerations for the newborn requiring intensive care. J. Am. Diet. Assoc., *66*:592, 1975.

36. Roy, R. N., et al.: Impaired assimilation of nasojejunal feeds in healthy low-birth-weight newborn infants. J. Pediatr., *90*:431, 1977.

37. Rubaltelli, F. F., and Largajolli, G.: Effect of light exposure on gut transit time in jaundiced newborns. Acta. Paediatr. Scand., *62*:146, 1973.

38. Scammon, R. E., and Doyle, L. O.: Observations on the capacity of the stomach in the first ten days of postnatal life. Am. J. Dis. Child., *20*:516, 1920.

39. Shaw, J. C. L.: Evidence for defective skeletal mineralization in low-birthweight infants: the absorption of calcium and fat. Pediatrics, *57*:16, 1976.

40. Snyderman, S. E.: The protein and amino acid requirements of the premature infant. In: Jonxis, J. H. P., Visser, H. K. A., and Troelstra, J. A. (eds.): Nutricia Symposium: Metabolic Process in the Fetus and Newborn Infant. Leiden, Stenfert Kroese, 1971, p. 128.

41. Stewart, A. L., et al.: Prognosis for infants weighing 1000 gm. or less at birth. Arch. Dis. Child., *52*:97, 1977.

42. Sturman, A. J., Gaull, G., and Raiha, N. C. P.: Absence of cystationase in human fetal liver. Is cystine essential? Science, *169*:74, 1970.

43. Younaszai, M. K.: Gastrointestinal function during infancy. In: Fomon, S. J.: Infant Nutrition, 2nd ed. Philadelphia, W. B. Saunders Co., 1974.

ADDITIONAL REFERENCES

Abitbol, C. L., et al.: Plasma amino patterns during supplemental intravenous nutrition of low-birth-weight infants. J. Pediatr., *86*:766, 1975.

Barness, L. A., and Pitkin, R. M. (eds.): Symposium on nutrition. Clin. Perinatol., *2*(2), 1975.

Book, L. S., Herbst, J. J., and Jung, A. L.: Necrotizing enterocolitis in infants fed an elemental formula. Pediatr. Res., *8*:379, 1974.

Bryan, H. B., et al.: Intralipid: its rational use in the parenteral nutrition of the newborn. Pediatrics, *58*:787, 1976.

Chen, J. W., and Wong, P. W. K.: Intestinal complications of nasojejunal feeding in low-birth-weight infants. J. Pediatr., 85:109, 1974.

Cockburn, F.: Intravenous feeding of the newborn. Clin. Endocrinol. Metabol., 5:191, 1976.

Colle, E., et al.: Insulin responses during catch-up growth of infants who were small for gestational age. Pediatrics, 57:363, 1976.

Davies, P. A., and Tizard, J. P. M.: Very low birthweight and subsequent neurological defect. Dev. Med. Child. Neurol., 17:3, 1975.

Editorial: PVC, plasticisers, and the paediatrician. Lancet, 1:1172, 1975.

Felig, P.: Maternal and fetal fuel homeostasis in human pregnancy. Am. J. Clin. Nutr., 26:998, 1973.

Filler, R. M., Eraklis, A. J., and Das, J. B.: Total parenteral nutrition in pediatrics: rationale and clinical experience. In: Ghadimi, H. (ed.): Total Parenteral Nutrition: Premises and Promises. New York, John Wiley & Sons, 1975, pp. 445–482.

Fitzhardinge, P. M., and Steven, E. M.: The small-for-date infant. II. Neurological and intellectual sequelae. Pediatrics, 50:50, 1972.

Gabbe, S. G., and Quilligan, E. J.: Fetal carbohydrate metabolism: its clinical importance. Am. J. Obstet. Gynecol., 127:92, 1977.

Gross, S.: Hemolytic anemia in premature infants: relationship to vitamin E, selenium, glutathione peroxidase, and erythrocyte lipids. Semin. Hematol., 13:187, 1976.

Heird, W. C.: Nasojejunal feeding: a commentary. J. Pediatr., 85:111, 1974.

Human milk in premature infant feeding: summary of a workshop. Pediatrics, 57:741, 1976.

Jones, M. D., and Battaglia, F. C.: Intrauterine Growth Retardation. Am. J. Obstet. Gynecol., 127:540, 1977.

Kennell, J., Trause, M. A., and Klaus, M.: Evidence for a Sensitive Period in the Human Mother in Parent-Infant Interaction. Ciba Foundation Symposium No. 33. Amsterdam, Associated Scientific Publishers, 1975.

Klaus, M. H., and Fanaroff, A. A.: Care of the High-Risk Neonate. Philadelphia, W. B. Saunders Co., 1973.

MacKeith, R., and Wood, C.: Infant Feeding and Feeding Difficulties, 5th ed. Edinburgh, Churchill Livingstone, 1977, pp. 197–208.

Melhorn, D. K., and Gross, S.: Vitamin E–Dependent anemia in the premature infant. II. Relationships between gestational age and absorption of vitamin E. J. Pediatr., 79:581, 1971.

Miller, S. A.: Nutrition in neonatal development of protein metabolism. Fed. Proc., 29:1497, 1970.

Oski, F. A., and Barness, L. A.: Vitamin E deficiency: a previously unrecognized cause of hemolytic anemia in the premature infant. J. Pediatr., 70:211, 1967.

Pagliara, A. S., et al.: Hypoglycemia in infancy and childhood, I and II. J. Pediatr., 82:365, 558, 1973.

Roy, N. R., and Sinclair, J. C.: Hydration of the low-birth-weight infant. Clin. Perinatol., 2:393, 1975.

Stewart, A. L., and Reynolds, E. O. R.: Improved prognosis for infants of very low birthweight. Pediatrics, 54:724, 1974.

Tantibhedhyangkul, P., and Hashim, S. A.: Medium-chain triglyceride feeding in premature infants: effect on fat and nitrogen absorption. Pediatrics, 55:359, 1975.

Vitamin E therapy in premature babies. Nutr. Rev., 33:206, 1975.

Widdowson, E. M.: Trace elements in human development. In: Barltrop, D., and Burland, W. L. (eds.): Mineral Metabolism in Pediatrics. Philadelphia, F. A. Davis Co., 1969.

Winters, R. W., and Hasselmeyer, E. G. (eds.): Intravenous Nutrition in the High Risk Infant. New York, John Wiley & Sons, 1975.

Young, D. S., and Hicks, J. M.: The Neonate: Clinical Biochemistry, Physiology and Pathology. New York, John Wiley & Sons, 1976.

Chapter 38

NUTRITIONAL CARE IN DISEASES OF INFANCY AND CHILDHOOD

The nutritional needs of a child who is ill are the same as or greater than those of a well child of the same age and development. Special consideration should be given to children who are receiving therapeutic regimens, to help them meet their normal nutritional needs for growth and development as well as their particular therapeutic requirements. Maintaining optimal nutritional status of the sick child plays an important part in the control of the disease and the rate of recovery.

A child's response to illness and hospitaliza-

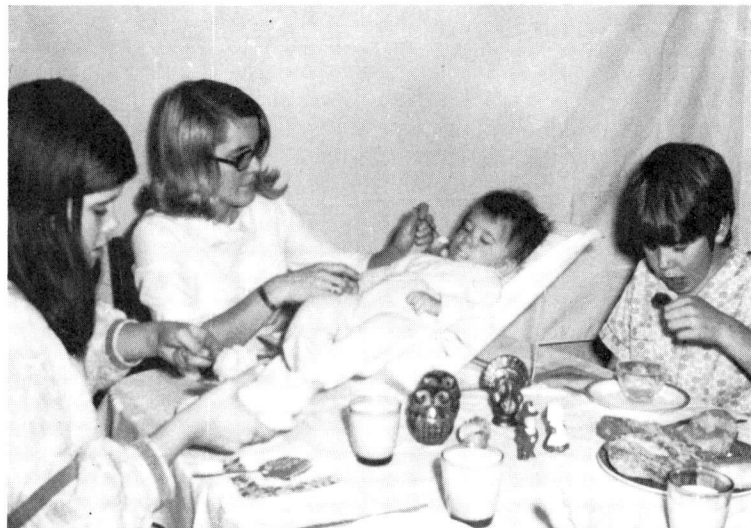

Figure 38–1 These children are obviously enjoying their breakfast under the supervision of an understanding nurse.

tion may lead to undesirable changes in eating behavior. Usually this is not a serious problem, and when feeling better the child will return to regular eating habits. Food must be served attractively and taste good to the sick child. At this time a child's desire for particular foods should be catered to as much as possible. If the appetite is poor, small meals served more frequently may be helpful, and ingenuity in meal planning and meal preparation may stimulate the appetite. Participation by the nurse in mealtime activities encourages the child to eat (Fig. 38–1). Frequently a hospitalized child, such as a newly diagnosed diabetic child, must learn to eat in a new way. Education of the child can begin in the hospital at mealtime if he or she feels up to it. Children are usually interested in learning and desire to participate in activities such as learning to identify foods and even to prepare them to fit their new diets (Fig. 38–2). Children usually can identify the foods that they believe to be good and those that they usually ingest. The nurse or dietitian accepts the child's suggestions and reinforces those that are appropriate. Using this approach the nurse or dietitian learns about the child's normal habits and the changes that may be necessary later.

Because emotional factors are involved with the child being separated from parents and the trauma of medical or surgical treatments, it is often difficult to alter food habits or introduce new foods. Any required education about dietary changes should always be followed up by counseling visits with the child and his parents after the child has returned home.

ACUTE INFECTIONS

Children suffering from acute infections of short duration, such as the common cold, measles, pneumonia or chickenpox, usually have impaired appetites. While it is not essential to insist that the nutritional requirements be met for the few days of the infection and fever, ketosis must be guarded against. (Consult Chapter 35 for discussions of the effect of infection on protein status and the requirements for

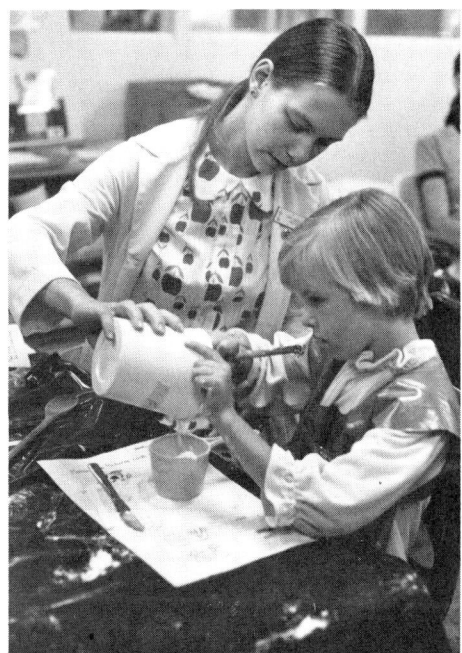

Figure 38–2 Dietitian helping a hospitalized child learn to prepare meals for her new diet. Courtesy of Lutheran General Hospital, Des Plaines, Illinois.

calories and protein during this time.) During the first day or two of the illness, it is advisable to serve either small amounts of food or none at all, but fluids are supplied in quantities to meet the child's need. The infant's formula may be diluted with water, and when the fever subsides, the regular feeding formula is resumed in order to supply the required calories as soon as possible. The liquid diet prescribed for children includes fruit juices, soups, broth and milk as tolerated. As the fever subsides, the appetite usually improves, and the food intake can be increased accordingly. During convalescence, foods rich in protein, vitamins and minerals are advisable, and gradually the child can begin to consume his normal diet.

CHRONIC INFECTIONS

It is essential that adequate nutrition be maintained in children who have infections of long duration, such as rheumatic fever and tuberculosis. Chronic infections can be very debilitating if the child remains in negative nitrogen balance with tissue protein breakdown day after day. (See Chapter 35.)

REGURGITATION AND VOMITING

Regurgitation, or spitting up, is common in infants who take too much milk or swallow air. Burping should be practiced to give the baby a chance during each nursing to get rid of swallowed air.

Vomiting is a symptom of many disturbances that may or may not be serious. In a baby, vomiting of a whole feeding or a large portion of it is often an early sign of infectious disease. However, it may also be caused by indigestion, fatigue or overexcitement. A child who has eaten a meal while overtired, overexcited,

Table 38–1 COMPOSITION OF A TYPICAL FLUID[a] FOR ORAL ADMINISTRATION OF GLUCOSE AND ELECTROLYTES

INGREDIENTS: Water, dextrose, sodium lactate, potassium chloride, magnesium chloride, calcium chloride and sodium chloride.

PROVIDES:

Sodium	30 mEq./l.	Lactate	28 mEq./l.
Potassium	20 mEq./l.	Dextrose	50 gm./l.
Calcium	4 mEq./l.	Calories	6/fl. oz.
Magnesium	4 mEq./l.	Calories	20.3/100 ml.
Chloride	30 mEq./l.		

[a] Pedialyte. (Ross Laboratories, Columbus, Ohio.)

angry or frightened may be unable to digest food well, and vomiting is nature's way of removing the undigested material. Such vomiting is not serious. Sometimes the condition results from an imbalance of food constituents in the formula, particularly from too much fat, which delays normal emptying of the stomach.

Persistent vomiting, especially when accompanied by diarrhea, will cause an imbalance of electrolytes and create a serious condition that demands immediate attention. The cause should be determined and feedings and fluids adjusted accordingly.

DIARRHEA

Occasional diarrhea is common in infancy and childhood. The most frequent causes are contamination or spoilage of food, too much carbohydrate (sugar) or fat in the formula, irritants such as cathartics and allergic reactions to specific foods. However, the modern safeguards against contamination of foods (especially milk)—refrigeration, improved socioeconomic conditions, public education and the effects of antibiotic drugs—reduce the incidence of diarrhea from these causes in developed countries.

In the developing countries acute diarrheal diseases are commonly associated with the weaning period. Some are identified with a specific organism but the majority are not. The condition is listed among the first five causes of high infant mortality and, in many countries, ranks first in children under the age of two. Supplementary foods of low nutritive value, prepared under unsanitary conditions, are usually started during the latter part of the first year, and diarrhea follows.

The result of diarrhea is loss of water, electrolytes and nutrients. Usually no food is given until the diarrhea subsides. However, water, glucose and electrolytes (sodium and potassium) are given, either by mouth or parenterally, to prevent dehydration and ketosis. A bottled preparation such as Lytren (Mead Johnson) or Pedialyte (Ross) (Table 38–1) or a specially prepared glucose-salt solution (Table 38–2) can be given orally.

When feedings are resumed, the diet is built up gradually, starting with skim milk, cooked cereals, toasted white bread and fruit and vegetable juices; then a soft diet and finally the normal or regular diet for the age and development of the child is resumed. An infant formula such as Pregestimil, Nutramigen or Portagen, in which the nutrients are present in an easily

Table 38–2 GLUCOSE-SALT SOLUTION FOR REHYDRATION FOLLOWING ACUTE DIARRHEA*

To 1 liter of water add:
3.5 gm. sodium chloride
2.5 gm. sodium bicarbonate
1.5 gm. potassium chloride
20.0 gm. glucose
The solution should be made up fresh every 24 hours.

*From: The rehydration treatment of acute diarrhea with inexpensive oral fluids. Clin. Pediatr., *15*:1095, 1976.

absorbable form, is recommended for infants with diarrhea. (See Table 35–7.) Skim milk can also be used if tolerated. As the condition improves, regular formula or whole milk can be used.

Pectin, apple or banana flakes may be given in amounts suitable for the age of the child. These substances have antidiarrheal properties. For further discussion of the nutritional care for patients with diarrhea, see Chapter 23.

CONSTIPATION AND COLIC

Constipation is a fairly common disturbance of infancy and childhood. As a rule the bottle-fed baby has fewer stools than the breast-fed baby. Human milk is higher in carbohydrate (lactose) than cow's milk and tends to be more laxative. Feces that are hard and expelled with difficulty should be reported to the physician. Sometimes constipation alternates with the uncontrolled passage of loose stools. This can become a distressing situation for older children and their families. It is also a more serious condition and may be indicative of Hirschsprung's disease or other intestinal disorder.

Treatment varies with the cause. Constipation is most often caused by restricted or inadequate food intake or poor eating habits. In the case of the formula-fed infant, the amount of sugar can be increased or the type of sugar used in the formula can be changed. The breast-fed infant may have a supplementary bottle of fruit juice added to the feeding schedule. In infants receiving supplementary foods or for young children, the diet may include fruit juice (prune, orange), vegetable juice (tomato), fruit purées or fruits (prunes, apricots, applesauce, figs), vegetable purées or vegetables and whole-grain cereals, which may be added to or increased in the diet, depending upon the age level. For older children the suggestions outlined in Chapter 23 may be followed.

Intestinal Colic

In infancy colic is a fairly frequent result of chronic constipation. Other causes are irritation or inflammation of the digestive tract, the swallowing of air (resulting in distention), the use of cathartics, and cold. The taking of warm food may give temporary relief, but correction of the diet is necessary to relieve the constipation and distention.

PYLORIC STENOSIS

Pyloric stenosis of infancy is not uncommon. The condition is serious, and unless recognized and treated in the early stages, it has a high rate of mortality. It usually occurs during the first two months of life.

Mild cases are often treated successfully with continuous gastric suction or frequent lavage. Between aspirations, the infant is given small amounts of formula or is breast-fed. Some infants so affected may require parenteral hyperalimentation to correct dehydration, acid-base imbalance and malnutrition. However, if no definite improvement results, surgery is generally advised.

Babies are usually fed at intervals of four hours. If vomiting occurs and a large part of the feeding is lost, the infant should be re-fed because re-feedings are often retained. The nutritional status of the infant is usually poor because of nausea and limited food intake. Experience has demonstrated that artificially fed infants frequently show improvement when given thick cereal feedings every four hours. Some formula-fed babies show improvement when fed human milk.

PEPTIC ULCERS

Peptic ulcers occur more frequently in infants and children than was believed formerly. The majority of cases reported are diagnosed only when complications appear, and most cases occur with no obvious cause. The stress-inducing factors of modern urban society could be one cause of the increase in the occurrence of peptic ulcers at an early age, according to a survey of hospital and medical case records of children under 16 years of age.[23] Peptic ulceration in infants and children was also found to be associated with steroid therapy or a serious underlying illness.[28] Some babies are bothered by colic after eating and others vomit after being fed, and their abdomens become tender and distended. Children's symptoms are closely al-

lied to those of adult patients; i.e., they have pain in the upper abdomen, more marked when the stomach is empty, that is relieved by food or antacid medication. Chapter 22 discusses the nutritional care for peptic ulcers.

ULCERATIVE COLITIS

Ulcerative colitis frequently appears in the pediatric age group. Although chronic ulcerative colitis is basically the same at all ages, the disease is usually more severe and treatment is less satisfactory in children than in adults. Because of its chronic, regressive nature, its occurrence at a time of active growth and its severe associated complications, the disease requires careful evaluation and active medical treatment, with early surgical intervention when indicated.

The psychological and social problems that can develop when this disease occurs in children also require empathy and attention from the medical staff. These patients are usually underweight and under emotional stress. Parents of these children may be overprotective or overaggressive in forcing them to compete beyond their desire or ability. Ulcerative colitis may occur after failure to meet a challenge or after an outburst of emotion or a severe stress.

Care should be aimed at helping the child obtain sufficient calories and an adequate intake of essential nutrients to provide for growth and to maintain good nutritional status. (See Chapter 23.)

MALABSORPTION

As noted earlier, in malabsorption the products of digestion available to the body are blocked because the absorbing surface of the small intestine is greatly reduced or malfunctioning. The microvilli are fewer and misshapen. The structural polarity of the epithelial cells is lost, and the intracellular enzymes that are responsible for the metabolism of epithelial cells are destroyed. With too few villi and microvilli, fat and fatty substances such as cholesterol and the lipid-soluble vitamins (A, D, K and E) are poorly absorbed. A study of several children with malabsorption due to celiac disease, lymphangiectasia, abetalipoproteinemia, cystic fibrosis and obstructive jaundice showed that they all had deficient levels of serum vitamin E.[22] In addition, unabsorbed fats can combine with minerals, particularly with calcium and trace minerals, to form "soaps," which further prevent their absorption.

The fat-soluble vitamins may be given parenterally or orally. If taken by mouth, very large doses are required. Smaller doses may be used if the vitamins are given in a water-soluble form.

Medium-chain triglycerides (MCT), which are hydrolyzed more rapidly than long-chain triglycerides, are used to supply the needed calories. The fatty acids enter the epithelial cells and are moved into the portal circulation without a change in character. Portagen and Pregestimil are two formulas that contain MCT. MCT oil is also available and can be blended with skim milk, fruit juices and mayonnaise or used in place of table oil in recipes for foods such as cookies, pancakes and French toast. Besides MCT, foods that can be used in a low-fat diet for fat malabsorption are listed on p. 514.

In diseases such as celiac sprue, protein and carbohydrates are also poorly absorbed, resulting in excessive fecal nitrogen loss as well as steatorrhea. The chyme containing amino acids, dipeptides, and glucose, maltose, sucrose and lactose molecules cannot be transferred from lumen to blood because of inadequate villi, misshapen carriers and insufficient pumps. Sodium, water and potassium are apt to stay in the lumen and be lost with the diarrhea.

Screening tests for malabsorption are available. The xylose tolerance test is used in screening for carbohydrate malabsorption. Measurement of the serum carotene level is used in screening for typical celiac sprue. The vitamin B_{12} absorption test of Schilling is used for screening patients with ileal disease or with extensive bacterial colonization of the small intestine.[17] See Chapter 23 for a more complete discussion of malabsorption.

CELIAC DISEASE

Idiopathic celiac disease has been defined as "a state of malnutrition induced by a poorly understood chronic functional disorder of intestinal assimilation."[16] It is believed to be a genetically transmitted deficiency. The age of onset varies between 4 months and 16 years, with the majority of cases occurring between the first and third years. In the adult, celiac disease is referred to as *non-tropical sprue* or *gluten-sensitive enteropathy* (Chapter 23).

The intestinal epithelium cannot tolerate a glutamine-rich polypeptide derived from gluten; an immune reaction may be involved. In celiac disease, pathological changes occur in

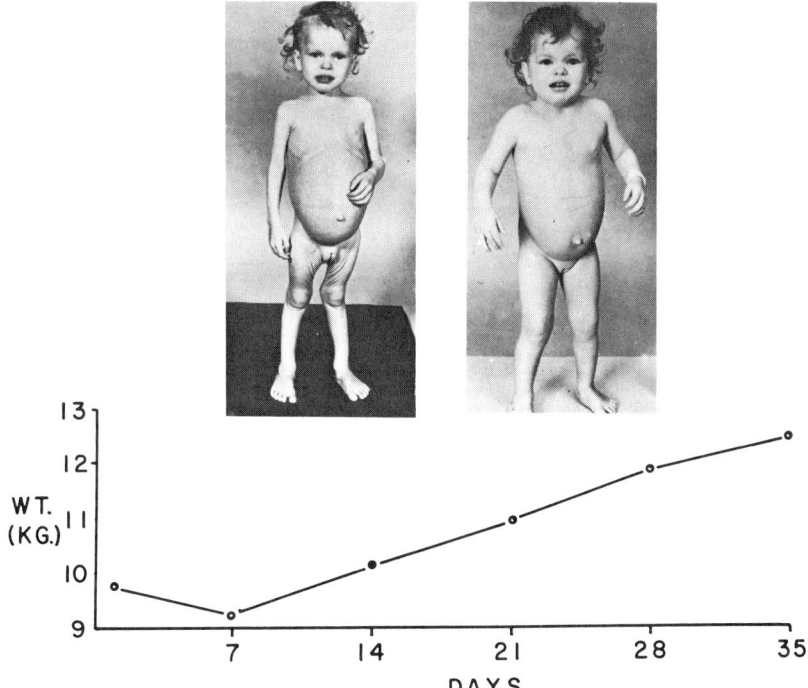

Figure 38–3 A 2½ year old child, with gluten-sensitive enteropathy (celiac syndrome) upon admission to the hospital (left) and after 35 days on gluten-free diet (right). The diagram shows the child's weight gain. (Courtesy of P. A. di Sant'Agnese, M.D., and JAMA, *180*:308, 1962.)

the epithelium and lamina propria, affecting the absorption of the nutrients.[17] The absorbing and secretory surfaces of the small intestine are greatly reduced.

Symptoms. The chief symptom is bulky, foamy, pale and foul-smelling stools resulting from an excess of unabsorbed fat and from carbohydrate fermentation. The patient shows weakness, underweight, malnutrition, retarded growth, a bulging, distended abdomen and excessive irritability. (See Fig. 38–3.)

Associated with the increased bowel activity is the failure to utilize vitamins and minerals. Rickets complicates the condition, and iron deficiency anemia may be one of the striking symptoms. When the storage of vitamin K is interfered with, bleeding tendencies arise. There is also a vitamin B deficiency that leads to symptoms of a red tongue and mouth. Scurvy and hypoproteinemia may also occur.

Gluten. A sensitivity to the gluten or protein fraction, *gliadin,* in wheat, oats, barley and rye flours or cereals is responsible for the symptoms of diarrhea and steatorrhea of celiac disease. The protein-bound glutamine in any given protein is also responsible for the symptoms. The gliadin fraction of the protein appears to cause a latent malabsorption syn-

drome as well. Both glutamine and gliadin are present in the protein of wheat, rye, barley and oats but are low in that of rice, corn and buckwheat.

Nutritional Care

Usually the child requires additional calories, protein, fat in the form of MCT, and supplemental administration of vitamins A and D (in water-soluble form) and iron. Calcium may be needed to treat tetany and vitamin B_{12} and folate to treat macrocytic anemia. The omission of gluten-containing cereals (wheat, oats, barley and rye) from the diet requires careful planning so as to avoid them in the preparation of foods. Gluten constitutes approximately 10 per cent of the weight of wheat flour. Wheat flour is often an ingredient in frankfurters, gravies, soups and meat loaf, so reading product labels is important.

The response to gluten restriction is not immediate. The child with very severe celiac disease requires two to six weeks of treatment before improvement becomes evident. Usually appetite returns first, vomiting and diarrhea disappear, and stools become normal in color and consistency. Gradually, deficiency states

clear, and there is a steady gain in weight (Fig. 38–3). The anemia responds more slowly.

For the child in a state of crisis, treatment may begin with intravenous replacement of fluid and electrolytes. A formula made with skim milk or an easily digested formula such as Pregestimil, Nutramigen or Portagen (Mead Johnson) is given until the diagnosis of gluten-induced enteropathy is established. Then a gluten-free, high-protein, low-fat diet is given as tolerated. Within a few weeks a normal, high-calorie diet that excludes gluten is indicated.

Table 23–8 lists foods suitable for a gluten-free diet. Corn and rice cereal products and flour are used. Lists of cookbooks with recipes for foods without wheat or wheat flour are included at the end of Chapters 23 and 31.

There is no rule of thumb for timing the reintroduction of gluten into the diet of the patient with celiac disease. The severity of the disease usually has a high correlation to the degree of sensitivity to gluten. The gluten-free regimen probably should be continued far beyond the point of symptomatic relief in order to reduce the likelihood of malabsorption difficulties developing later in life. Liberalizing the diet too rapidly may lead to serious and often sudden setbacks that are more difficult to correct than the initial episode. The child's height-weight curve provides a reliable guide to his or her ability to tolerate gluten and to continue to absorb enough to maintain growth. Most authorities seem to believe that true cure is rare, and prefer to speak of remission in a patient who may develop a tolerance to gluten. Celiac disease can reappear in adult life.

CYSTIC FIBROSIS OF THE PANCREAS (MUCOVISCIDOSIS)

Cystic fibrosis of the pancreas is a congenital disease of unknown etiology that is associated with pancreatic exocrine dysfunction. The pancreatic acini are replaced by fibrotic tissue, cysts, mucous and, eventually, fat. Sometimes hepatic biliary channels become plugged, and this can lead to cirrhosis and portal hypertension. It generally is a disease of children, although it may present itself in adulthood.

Deficiency or total lack of pancreatic enzymes—trypsin, lipase and amylase—leads to poor digestion and absorption of foodstuffs. Steatorrhea and malabsorption result. The stools are bulky, greasy and foul-smelling, and, since a large portion of the ingested food is lost in the feces, the appetites of these patients are characteristically ravenous. Despite an apparently adequate nutritional intake, malnutrition is often marked (see Fig. 38–4). Due to the steatorrhea, deficiencies of vitamins A, K and E (as detected by biochemical tests) result from fecal loss of lipid-soluble vitamins. Usually the presence of high sodium chloride concentrations in the sweat ($\geq$ 60 mEq. per liter) aids in the diagnosis of the disease.

Nutritional Care

A diet of simple, easily digested and absorbed foods is prescribed. Carbohydrate is in the form of simple sugars (mono- and disaccharides), since starches are poorly tolerated. The protein should be high: 3 to 4 gm. per kg. per day. Fat is restricted or eliminated, (see p. 514) and supplements of the fat-soluble vita-

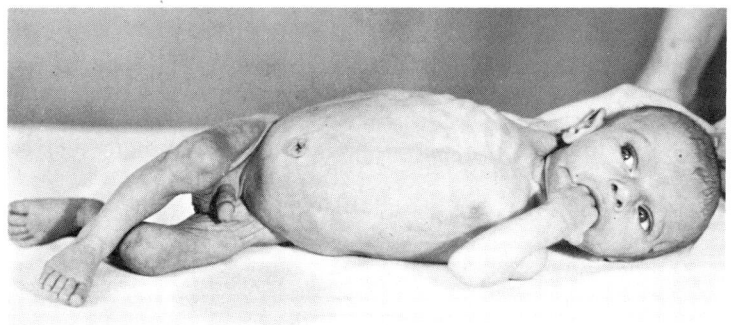

Figure 38–4 Three month old child with cystic fibrosis of the pancreas. He had loose stools, failed to gain weight and was fretful and irritable but had a good appetite. Although the muscles were well developed, there was a complete absence of subcutaneous fat. The abdomen was prominent. No enzymes were found in the duodenal juice. He was first given skim milk, banana powder, dried milk protein and large doses of vitamin A. Later he was given 1 gm. of powdered pancreatin before each feeding of evaporated milk formula. He improved rapidly and at three years, after being maintained on a high-calorie, low-fat diet and pancreatin, appeared to be relatively normal. (Andersen, D. H.: J. Pediatr., 15:10, 1939.)

mins (in water-soluble form) are given daily to treat the deficiencies and to compensate for amounts lost in the stools. The following doses are recommended: 5000 to 10,000 I.U. of an oily preparation or 2000 I.U. of a water-miscible preparation of vitamin A, 1000 I.U. of vitamin D, 1 mg. per kg. per day of vitamin E (α-tocopherol) and 1 mg. per day of a water-soluble analog of vitamin K_3 (menadione).[12] Calories should be high (150 kcal. per kg. body weight per day), as should protein, to promote normal growth. Pancreatic enzymes (Viokase or Cotazym) are given with each feeding to promote digestion. Constipation is frequently a problem and can be resolved by reducing the dosage of pancreatic enzymes or by giving a mild laxative such as Colace. Mineral oil should not be used.

Extra salt is given to offset the characteristic excessive loss of sodium chloride in perspiration, especially in the summer.

A formula with a mixture of vegetable oils is better tolerated than a formula with butterfat, which is less easily digested. However, if the steotorrhea continues, Portagen (a formula containing medium-chain triglycerides as the fat source), can be used. Allan and colleagues have reported increased rates of growth in children with cystic fibrosis after introduction of this easily digested form of fat into their diets.[1] With good care of the respiratory complications that accompany the disease, the cystic fibrosis patient can be expected to grow at about the 50th percentile rate even if there has been a period of malnutrition in infancy. These children demonstrate marked "catch-up" growth.[10]

MALNUTRITION

Malnutrition is usually thought of in reference to children. Malnourished children do not get adequate food materials needed by their bodies, either because they do not ingest sufficient food to supply their needs or because they have faulty digestion, absorption or assimilation. Protein-calorie malnutrition in preschool children is probably the most common and important current nutritional problem in the world.

Over half the world's population is the victim of hunger or inadequate nutrition in one form or another, and the principal victims are infants and children. Millions die in their early years because they do not get adequate food, especially protein. When a baby is weaned at about one year old to a diet of starchy foods—gruel of

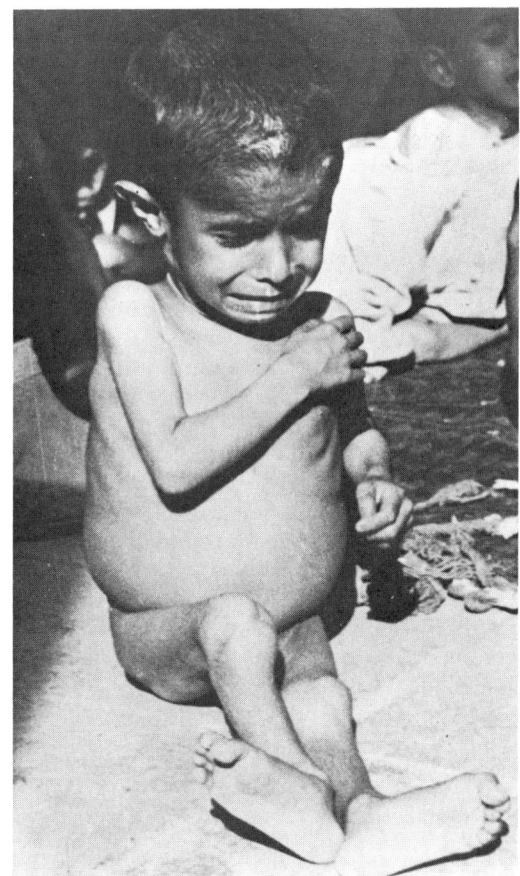

Figure 38–5 An Iranian girl admitted in an advanced stage of malnutrition to a foundling home in Teheran. After 12 months of treatment she became a normal, lively child. (Courtesy FAO.)

rice, sweet potato, maize or manioc—he or she invariably is a sick child by two years of age. Weaning may come even earlier if the mother becomes pregnant again or if she is influenced to use a prepared formula rather than to continue to nurse her infant. (See Fig. 38–5.)

World health organizations such as WHO, FAO, UNICEF and related organizations are constantly working to combat malnutrition in children in developing countries, but this multifaceted problem is not easily remedied. Figure 12–27 provides a good summary of the multitude of factors that contribute to malnutrition.

The National Nutrition Survey (1968–70), the Health and Nutrition Examination Survey (1971–72), the Preschool Nutrition Survey (1968–70) and the White House Conference on Food, Nutrition and Health (1969) have identified undernourished and malnourished groups in the United States. (See p. 372.) The passage

of the National Child Nutrition Act of 1970 showed recognition of the need for nutrition education in addition to feeding programs. The WIC (Women, Infants and Children) feeding program, started in 1974, is aimed at preventing malnutrition in young children as well as in pregnant women and their unborn fetuses.

MARASMUS

Marasmus, or severe malnutrition, is an infantile atrophy resulting from semistarvation. It is characterized by gross underweight resulting from a lack of calories rather than from a lack of any specific food (Fig. 38–6). It is, however, associated with insufficient protein intake, as is kwashiorkor. Often it occurs in patients who have infectious diseases. Children with kwashiorkor develop rounded cheeks because of edema, while those with marasmus have shrunken and wizened faces. Anorexia, diarrhea, vomiting or a combination frequently accompanies marasmus. Kwashiorkor and marasmus are discussed in more detail on pages 265 to 271, and the different clinical symptoms are presented in Table 12–8.

Nutritional Care

Mild cases of protein-energy malnutrition (PEM) can be treated on an outpatient basis with an adequate diet, education in the home for the mothers and others who care for the child, and treatment of the usually coexistent infections. Treatment of severe PEM requires hospitalization.

Initially, fluid and electrolyte imbalances are corrected and treatment of the infections is started. Later the objective of treatment is to raise the level of the child's nutritional status as rapidly as possible. Skim milk is usually the basis of diet treatment, or Pregestimil (Mead Johnson) can be used at first and followed by skim milk, regular formula or whole milk. Patients may have to be tube-fed in the beginning, but as they become rehydrated and gain strength, their appetites will return and they can take nourishment by themselves. This usually takes 2 to 3 days.

Depending upon their clinical condition and tolerance, patients should receive 125–150 kcal. per kg. per day and 3 to 4 gm. of protein per kg. per day. Many recommend caloric intakes as high as 200 kcal. per kg. per day, especially in cases of marasmus or chronic starvation. Because of the small volume of liquid that these children can take initially, most formulas should be modified and given at a strength of 1 kcal. per ml. To reach this concentration, the standard commercially prepared liquid formula concentrate (133 kcal. per 100 ml.) is mixed with only half the usual required amount of water to give a 100 kcal. per 100 ml. formula instead of the usual 67 kcal. per 100 ml. This caloric concentration should be reached gradually over a period of 4 to 5 days. Diarrhea is commonly present in patients with PEM but should not be a reason to stop the feeding. It will probably resolve itself as the nutritional status improves. Some children may not tolerate lactose, in which case milk and other lactose-containing foods will aggra-

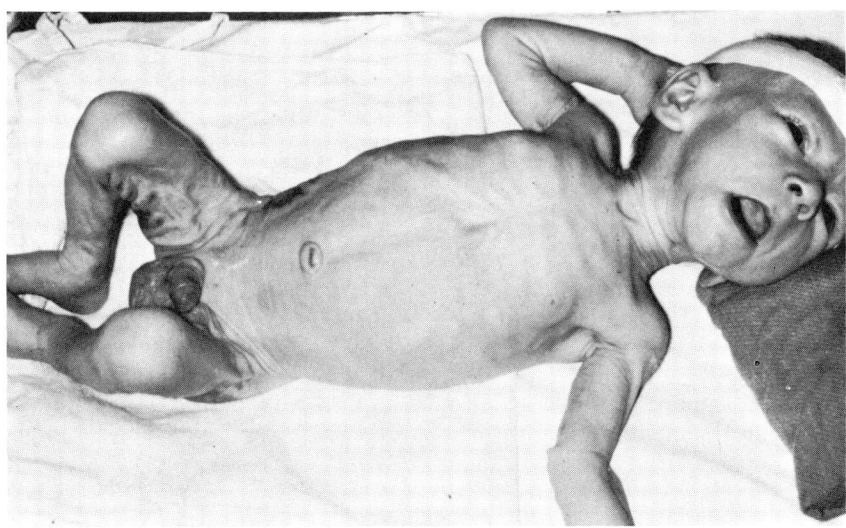

Figure 38–6 Marasmus. This infant shows severe malnutrition resulting from insufficient calories. Note the loose skin and cachectic appearance characteristic of marasmus. (Courtesy of Burtis B. Breeze, M.D., Rochester, New York.)

vate diarrhea. Other high-protein liquids and foods such as a chemically defined liquid diet or lactose-free formula (Prosobee or Neo-Mull-Soy) can be used. Solid foods are added when improvement is noted and appetite increases. Foods are added as tolerated, with emphasis on calories and protein. Frequent small feedings are tolerated better than the customary three daily meals.

Supplementary vitamins are given as indicated. Vitamin A is required to prevent ocular lesions that can occur when children who also have an unsuspected vitamin A deficiency are rehabilitated. De Maeyer recommends an initial intramuscular injection of 100,000 I.U. of a water-miscible preparation. This should be followed by a daily oral supplement (water-miscible or oil-soluble) of 10,000 I.U. until the child is taking adequate amounts of vitamin A in the diet.[8]

Potassium should be supplied daily during the first two weeks of therapy in the form of 1 to 2 gm. of potassium chloride. This is necessary because of the increased potassium uptake that occurs during this period of rapid protein synthesis.

Magnesium (250 mg. to 1 gm. daily, depending on the child's weight) may also be required and is given intramuscularly until the child is able to take it orally.

The continuation of an adequate diet to correct deficiencies is the objective of complete nutritional care. This means that there must be follow-up and that attention must be paid to the home environment to which the child will return when he or she leaves the hospital. This is a difficult task that requires the attention of politicians, educators and health workers in the community.

KWASHIORKOR

Kwashiorkor is protein-calorie malnutrition. This deficiency disease is discussed in Chapter 12.

LINOLEIC ACID DEFICIENCY

Hansen and associates[14] report linoleic acid to be essential in the diet of infants. In a diet adequate except for this fatty acid, dryness of the skin with desquamation, thickening and later intertrigo were the most characteristic features of the deficiency state observed. Unsatisfactory rate of growth was observed in many of the infants. Severe reaction occurred to outbreaks of staphylococcal infection in the hospital. Signs of the deficiency disappeared promptly when 1 per cent or more of calories were provided as linoleic acid. (See page 299 and Fig. 14–1.)

VITAMIN DEFICIENCY DISEASES

Hemorrhagic Disease of the Newborn

This disorder is discussed in Chapter 8 under functions of vitamin K. See also p. 159.

Hemolytic Anemia of the Premature Infant

This disorder is due to a deficiency of vitamin E and is discussed in Chapter 37.

Pyridoxine Deficiency in Infants

In 1954 a formula deficient in pyridoxine (vitamin B_6) was reported[21] to produce epileptiform convulsions in infants 8 to 16 weeks of age. The formula producing the convulsions was a liquid commercial preparation that had been sterilized by autoclave, which had destroyed the pyridoxine. When fed another milk formula or given supplementary vitamin B_6 or foods such as cereals, fruits, meats and vegetables, all of the infants were cured of the convulsions. It was concluded that the convulsions were due to deficiency of pyridoxine. These appear to be the first pyridoxine deficiency states reported in humans and have since been confirmed by other workers. Occurrence of convulsions in rats and pigs fed a diet lacking in this vitamin has been known since 1940. (See pp. 167 to 170 for daily allowance and discussion of pyridoxine.)

Infantile Scurvy

Infantile scurvy occurs usually in artificially fed infants taking evaporated milk formula or whole cow's milk as a result of a deficiency in ascorbic acid. Commercially prepared formulas are all fortified with vitamin C. Normally the fetus receives the vitamin from the maternal blood supply and is born with a satisfactory quantity if the mother had a sufficient amount in her diet. The breast-fed infant receives ascorbic acid that is concentrated in human milk when the mother's diet contains the vitamin, although an infant may receive adequate amounts even when the mother's diet and her blood plasma vitamin C level are inadequate.

Infants taken off the breast and given a starchy diet devoid of fruits and vegetables may develop classic scurvy. This frequently occurs in the developing countries. Clinical manifestations appear slowly after the infant has been deprived of an adequate supply of ascorbic acid. The treatment for scurvy is large doses of ascorbic acid—orange juice (200 to 400 cc.) or 100 to 200 mg. ascorbic acid—given orally or parenterally for several days. (See Chapter 12.)

Rickets

This deficiency disease is also discussed in Chapter 12.

METABOLIC DISORDERS

DIABETES MELLITUS

The etiology of diabetes in children is not clear, but it is thought to be a genetic predisposition aggravated by environmental factors. (See Chapter 25.) It is more severe than adult diabetes and almost always requires insulin therapy, and good nutritional care is very important to maintain blood glucose control and proper growth in the child. The majority of children are undernourished when the disease is first recognized, and the onset of symptoms is relatively sudden.

Treatment

Insulin. The basics of insulin therapy are discussed in Chapter 25, and only comments concerning insulin therapy for children are mentioned here.

About one to three months after beginning insulin therapy, about 90 per cent of juvenile patients appear to have a remission and do not need as much or, in rare cases, any insulin. This *"honeymoon period"* may last for months or years, but it is *always temporary,* and the child and parents should be so informed. This temporary remission is not well understood, but it appears to be a "last ditch" effort by the pancreas to secrete insulin and control the level of blood glucose.

This phenomenon has been the focus of much study, and some physicians have been able to correlate the length of this period with the length of time that elapsed before diagnosis and treatment of the child. Those children diagnosed and treated early, before or soon after the onset of overt diabetes, had lower insulin requirements and a longer period of partial remission, sometimes as long as four years.

Those children diagnosed and treated when they were in severe acidosis had higher insulin requirements and shorter partial remission, some as short as two months.[18] However, these findings are still controversial.

After this "honeymoon period," insulin requirements increase and then remain fairly stable, except during periods of increased growth rate, when they will increase. Requirements also increase after a hypoglycemic attack because the body develops a transitory insulin resistance as a protective mechanism. Insulin resistance and increased insulin requirements also occur during an infection.

As the child reaches adulthood and caloric requirements lessen, it is important to reduce insulin dosage and calorie intake accordingly. The adolescent girl is especially prone to obesity unless insulin and calories are adjusted.

Nutritional Care

The diabetic child's diet follows the same general pattern as that suggested for the adult (Chapter 25). However, a child's calorie and protein requirements per kilogram of body weight are higher, to allow for growth and development. Calories should be the same as those for the normal child (Table 10–1), and protein requirements range from 1.0 to 2.0 gm. per kg. depending on the age of the child. A general starting point for determining daily caloric needs is 1000 kcal. plus 100 kcal. for each year of age of the child. The mineral and vitamin requirements are also increased. Therefore, adjustments from time to time are required to meet the child's changing needs. The increase in dietary intake and insulin dose is calculated in direct proportion to the optimum growth and physical activity needs of the child. Calories should be adequate to maintain the desired weight.

Controversy exists regarding the necessity for strict supervision of the food intake. However, most authorities believe that there is a close relationship between the control of diabetes and the development of complications. Consequently, it is advocated that food intake and insulin distribution be adjusted to avoid insulin reactions and, insofar as practical, to avoid glycosuria.

The diet is adjusted to provide 15 to 20 per cent of the calories from protein, 30 to 35 per cent from fat and 50 to 55 per cent from carbohydrate. The distribution of the carbohydrates and calories throughout the day must be relatively uniform to maintain a high degree of control and prevent dangerous hypoglycemia.

Nutritional Counseling

The interpretation of diets for diabetic children should be particularly liberal. If favorite party dishes are planned occasionally, the child may cooperate more cheerfully and adhere more closely to the established regimen. The many emotional conflicts of childhood and adolescence must be considered in the treatment of the diabetic child and require sympathetic understanding and tact. Some of these problems and ways to deal with them are reviewed by Lum.[19] Planning the diabetic regimen around the usual dietary pattern of the family helps the child to accept it. The child need not appear to be different from other members of the family at the table and can learn to eat at regular intervals and to live a normal life.

Children are apt students and learn quickly how to plan their own diets once they have accepted their disease and are ready to learn. When possible, it is advisable to give diabetic children the responsibility for planning their own diets from the family meals. They are then able to plan their dietary programs to include those foods that will be eaten outside the home. They will appreciate and accept the obligation of the task. (See Chapter 19.)

It is highly important that the diabetic child and the parents be clearly informed concerning the disease and the later complications that inevitably develop to some degree. While there is no known cure at this time, the condition need not interfere with a happy, well-adjusted life, provided the diabetic receives adequate treatment and nutritional care to control the disorder.

HYPERTHYROIDISM (GRAVES' DISEASE)

A discussion of hyperthyroidism appeared in Chapter 26 and will not be repeated here. The treatment for children follows the same general principles outlined for the adult; however, attention is directed to the need for additional calories and protein so the child can meet the requirements for growth and development as well as for the increase in the basal metabolic rate.

HYPOTHYROIDISM (CRETINISM AND JUVENILE MYXEDEMA)

Hypothyroidism, which develops in fetal life or early infancy, is referred to as *cretinism* (Fig. 38–7). The main cause of cretinism is insufficient thyroid hormone in the newborn,

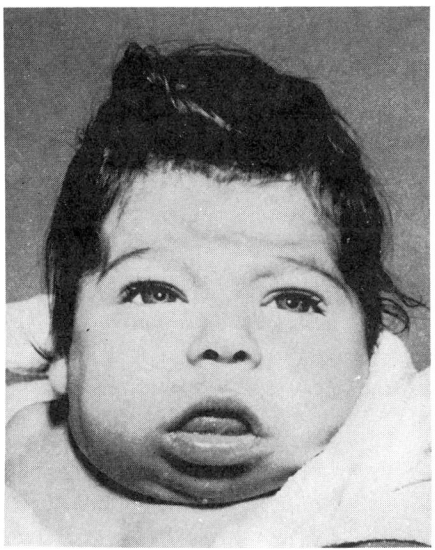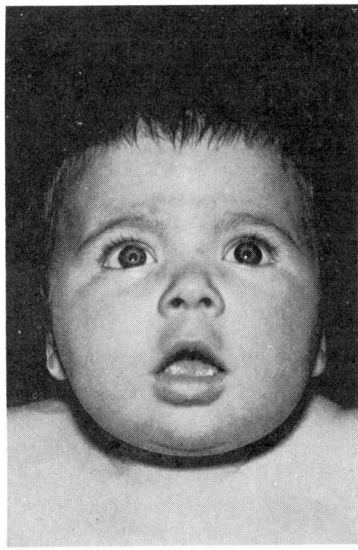

Figure 38–7 Cretinism. Congenitally hypothyroid infant at six months of age. Infant fed poorly in neonatal period and was constipated, had persistent nasal discharge and large tongue, was very lethargic and had no social smile and no head control. *A,* Note puffy face, dull expression, hirsute forehead. Serum cholesterol 172 mg. per 100 ml., alkaline phosphatase 4.8 Bodansky units, negligible uptake to radioiodine. Osseous development that of newborn. *B,* Four months after treatment with U.S.P. thyroid. Note decreased puffiness of face, decreased hirsutism of forehead and alert appearance. (From: Vaughan, V. C., and McKay, R. J.: Nelson Textbook of Pediatrics, 10th ed., Philadelphia, W. B. Saunders Co., 1975, p. 1306.)

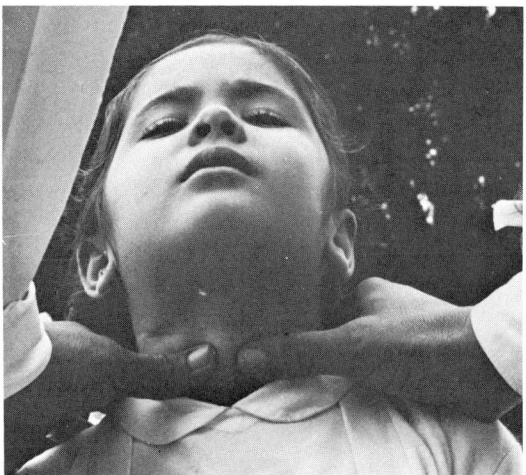

Figure 38–8 Endemic goiter. In certain areas of Ecuador, 70 per cent of the population has been found to have goiter; in some places, the prevalence among schoolchildren is 100 per cent as a result of the iodine deficiency. In the schools of Paraguay, where this photo was taken, children are regularly examined for symptoms of goiter. (Courtesy WHO. Photo by Almasy.)

either because (1) the structure is defective or (2) the iodine intake of the mother has been inadequate. In this country, even in the "goiter belts," the latter is seldom encountered. Distribution of foods that contain iodine and the use of iodized table salt have minimized the danger. In certain areas such as Ecuador, however, the prevalence of endemic goiter as a result of iodine deficiency among school children is 100 per cent (see Fig. 38–8).

Hypothyroidism acquired in childhood is known as *juvenile myxedema*. It usually is suspected in an older child who begins to lag or drop behind in school, loses interest, tires easily and has definitely delayed growth and development.

Treatment

Thyroid tablets by mouth are specific for this condition. Without this therapeutic management the course is regressive, and the physical and mental growth of the child are stunted (Fig. 38–9). When medication is instituted during the first two years, the results are sometimes excellent, although a certain number of children remain slightly subnormal for their age. Signs of improvement may be noted within a few weeks or months, and the dosage is regulated by checking the patient's response to the extract. As a rule, this form of therapy is continued throughout life.

As in all patients who lack thyroid, there is a

tendency toward overweight. The tissues are not firm but flabby, mottled and cool to the touch. The amount of calories in the customary diet is reduced in order to lose and then maintain weight at the desired level. (See Chapter 26 for a more complete discussion of hypothyroidism.)

IMBALANCE OF BODY WEIGHT

OVERWEIGHT

Overnutrition in infants, children and adolescents in this country is a matter of medical and public health concern. The child whose weight is consistently well above normal for age, height and general development should not be classified as "well nourished" but as overweight. This condition requires investigation and treatment.

A pressing reason for paying prompt attention to the overweight child is the evidence which suggests that the number of fat cells in the body is determined in the first few years of life and in a vulnerable period during adoles-

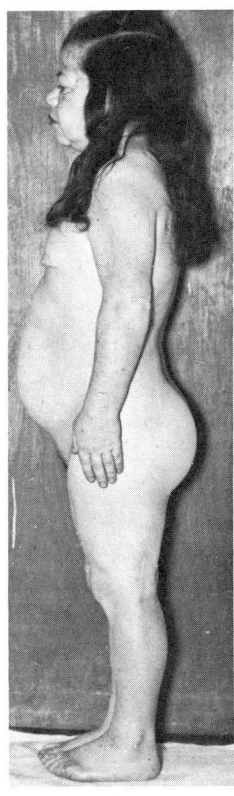

Figure 38–9 Hypothyroidism before full maturity results in cretinism. The cretinous dwarf above shows effects of retardation in growth, with infantile proportions persisting. (Courtesy of the Endocrine Clinic of the Beth Israel Hospital, Boston.)

cence. Overnutrition during these times leads to the formation of an excess number of fat cells. Although the adipose cell *size* can be decreased through weight reduction, the cell *number* cannot, as far as we know. We also know that overweight children tend to become overweight adults.

Heredity may be one of the factors that lead to overweight, but too frequently parents blame family traits rather than make any attempt to correct the situation. Even with a genetic tendency toward obesity, a person's diet can be changed and an exercise program can be started in order to prevent expression of the tendency. In some cases, glandular difficulties may be responsible, but as a rule overeating, accompanied by a minimum amount of exercise, is the chief cause of overweight. If obesity is prevalent among family members, the entire family needs to review their dietary and exercise patterns and change them.

Mild overweight between the ages of 8 and 14 often occurs because of a spurt in body weight gain prior to a rapid gain in height and is simply a brief stage of development. The weight will usually adjust itself automatically through normal appetite and activity, providing there is no abnormality.

Frequently, food is the center of interest at social gatherings. Children, and especially teenagers, meet at favorite places for a soft drink, sandwich, pizza or other snack, and although Type A school lunches provide a well-balanced meal, there is the ever-present distraction on school grounds of vending machines that make high-calorie, low-nutrition foods such as soda pop, candy and pastries easily available. The caloric equivalent of these extra snacks may well exceed energy expenditure and can result in weight gain.

Besides the fact that their social world revolves around food, another frequent reason for obesity development, especially for teenagers, is low activity. Obese adolescents, in general, are less active than non-obese youngsters of the same age group. Bullen and associates[3] compared the activity of obese and non-obese adolescent girls engaged in sports at summer camp by using motion picture sampling. The striking degree of inactivity of the obese girls appears to be a significant factor in their overweight conditions.

Nutritional Care

Unless a child is grossly obese, vigorous reducing is generally not advised. Weight maintenance is the preferable approach with the child "growing into" the present weight. The child's customary food pattern and eating habits are evaluated, and the child is encouraged to become interested in making the necessary changes to improve his or her diet.

For the child who will be following a calorie reduction diet, growth and development must still continue. The essential foods to supply nutritional needs are milk, meat, eggs, fruits, vegetables, breads and cereals. A danger in connection with trying to reduce in a haphazard way is that a child may not get adequate amounts of nutrients, especially of protein. The amount of protein ingested while losing weight should be increased to 1.5 gm. per kg. ideal body weight per day. High-calorie desserts and snacks, sweetened soft drinks and candy between meals are discouraged. Skim milk can be substituted for whole milk if the child drinks milk. (See Chapter 27 for the principles involved in the dietary treatment of obesity.)

Emotional and Social Factors

Understanding a child's weight problem—the reasons for the overweight—is more important than formulating the correct diet for losing weight. The reason for the child's "hunger" must be found and replaced with satisfactions equal to those of eating. It is thought that the obese child cannot accurately recognize hunger and mistakes feelings of guilt, anger or frustration for it. The comfort gained from a full stomach allays the other feelings but reinforces the obesity and the social ostracism felt by the obese child. This leads to depression and then eating to relieve depression, and the vicious cycle continues. (See Fig. 27–4.) Adolescents especially have many physiological and psychological characteristics[13] that must be taken into account, for at this age there is great self-awareness. While girls are sometimes more concerned about their weight than boys are, the markedly obese adolescent of either sex is usually self-conscious and unhappy. Teenagers are great imitators, and here the dietitian-nutritionist or nurse can be of invaluable help by setting a good example for weight control. Adolescents appreciate any interest and understanding about their weight problems. Time spent in counseling is usually rewarding. Acceptance by the "gang" or their peers is vital, because children seek group approval. The feeling that they will be more popular if not overweight is a strong motivation for changing

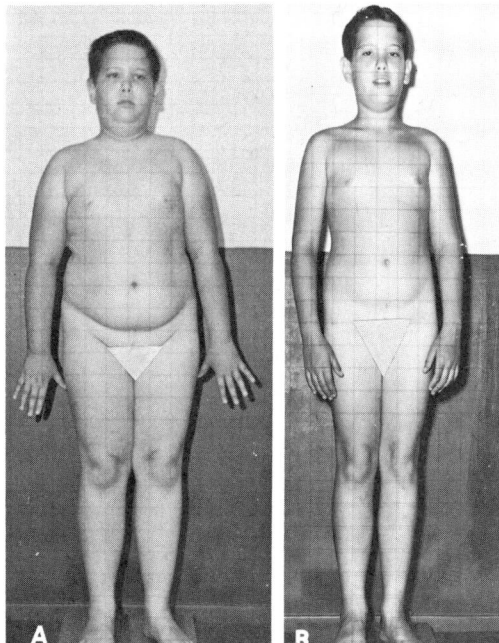

Figure 38–10   Obesity. Before and after 10 months' treatment for obesity in an 11 year old boy. Weight loss was 42½ lb. However, since there was a growth of 1½ inches during this period, the effective weight loss is calculated to be 49½ lb. The change in facial expression is as dramatic as the weight loss, a frequent observation in such cases. (Courtesy of Dr. R. H. Hoffman.)

food habits, but they need tremendous amounts of support. (See Fig. 38–10.)

Group discussions with other overweight adolescents may be useful in helping the obese teenager get involved in new activities, participate in enjoyable sports and get some regular form of exercise. Discussion of common problems is helpful. The focus should be on behavioral change and the learning of new behaviors that promote weight loss instead of weight gain. (See p. 568.)

Family tensions about weight must be avoided. Cooperation of parents and other members of the family is necessary to prevent frustration, and the overall adjustment problems require evaluation to make sure the pressures of obesity are not increased by an impossible regimen. Individual treatment is the keynote of management.

It is easier to prevent obesity than to treat it, and most of our energies should be directed toward that goal. Prevention and even reduction of obesity have been demonstrated through school programs where the activity of the children was significantly increased through daily structured exercise. It is important that health professionals and parents en-

courage and set good examples for regular energy-requiring activity. Obesity is a public health problem that can be solved only through learning on the part of individuals to avoid unwanted weight gain at any time in life.

UNDERWEIGHT

Although slimness in itself does not indicate malnutrition, if a child is more than 10 lb. below the desired optimum weight and fails to grow with regularity, a physical examination is advised. If no disease can be demonstrated, careless eating habits and poor hygiene may be responsible.

In some instances, a scanty breakfast or no breakfast starts the child's day, while others may omit essential foods without suitable substitutes. Some children become tea or coffee addicts at an early age. Many resort to nibbling, which spoils the appetite for regular meals. Some children become so engrossed with the business of play that they eat too rapidly. Adolescents of both sexes are often figure-conscious and skip some nutritious foods in an attempt to keep slim.

The nervous, irritable child with a finicky appetite should receive attractive meals served at regular hours. A glass of milk at midmorning and midafternoon may prove beneficial. A diet high in all the vitamins, especially the B-complex group, usually stimulates the appetite.

The avoidance of fatigue by restricting activity and encouraging additional rest is advised for some children. For others who are kept indoors and have limited activity, plenty of fresh air and sunshine may stimulate the appetite.

The criteria used to calculate the calorie needs of children are different from those for adults. The child requires extra food for growth and for the activity of incessant play. In general, the food allowance for a girl 12 years old averages about 2500 kcal. per day, which is often a greater calorie requirement than that of her mother. An average adolescent boy of 15 to 16 years may use 4000 kcal. daily. Adolescents are not only still growing but are usually extremely active. Consequently, they need more food than do adults of a corresponding size. (See Chapter 27.)

CARDIAC DISEASES

A number of abnormalities of the heart may be present at birth. Some forms are functional

and disappear within months; others are serious and result in early death. Many are benefited by diet therapy and others are successfully treated by surgery.

The most important causes of cardiovascular disease in children are congenital anomalies and rheumatic fever.

CONGENITAL HEART DISEASE

Congenital anomalies of the heart make up 12 per cent of all congenital anomalies. Although most infants with congenital heart anomalies are appropriate size at birth, growth retardation becomes apparent early. This growth retardation can be due to chronic hypoxia, but inadequate nutrition can also be present. One factor that can lead to inadequate nutrition is decreased food intake. Chronic labored respiration and rapid fatigue while feeding can reduce the amount an infant will consume. Such infants also may refuse to nurse or may vomit or spit out food given to them, a tendency that for some unknown reason is resolved by reparative surgery.[9]

Besides decreased food intake in the child with severe heart disease, gastrointestinal absorption is less efficient, which can further prevent the meeting of nutritional requirements. Furthermore, these patients are hypermetabolic and have increased caloric requirements. Other factors that can lead to failure to thrive are congestive heart failure and the increased susceptibility to infections that accompanies congenital heart disease. All these factors act to deter the growth and development of children with severe heart disease, and by nine months of age most have fallen below the 5th percentile for length and weight.[24]

Since surgical correction of the congenital defect is usually attempted when the child is 12 to 15 months of age, it is important that he or she be in the best possible nutritional condition. This requires early initiation of nutritional care.

Nutritional Care

Calories. Most of these infants require more than the usual number of calories for an infant the same age. Their requirement is usually about 120 to 135 kcal. per kg. of body weight per day, and some infants may need as many as 150 to 175 kcal. per kg. per day to gain weight and grow.

Formula. Because of their increased caloric needs and their inability to take more than a small volume of food at one time (many under one year of age can take only 450 ml. per day), these infants should be given calorically dense formulas. Carbohydrate and fat are added to a standard premature infant formula (80 kcal. per 100 ml. or 24 kcal. per oz.) so that it will contain 100 kcal. per 100 ml. (30 kcal. per oz.). This manipulation can be done using standard formula (67 kcal. per 100 ml. or 20 kcal. per oz.), but the protein content may be diluted so much that the infant will not get enough for growth, particularly if he or she can only take a small volume of formula. The formula should not contain butterfat (evaporated milk formula) because of its poor digestibility. The infant will excrete butterfat in the stool, and thus the caloric intake will be decreased.

Later, when the child takes semisolids that are sources of carbohydrate and fat, the carbohydrate and fat added to the formula can be omitted, but the formula should be mixed with a smaller amount of water so that it is still a concentrated source of protein. The commercially prepared concentrated liquid (133 kcal. per 100 ml.) can be mixed with half the usual amount of water to give a formula with a caloric concentration of 100 kcal. per 100 ml. instead of the usual 67 kcal. per 100 ml.

Whenever infants are taking a concentrated food, their fluid balance should be watched closely because of the increased renal solute load presented by the formula and the possibility of excessive renal water loss and dehydration. Careful attention is required to balance the child's water needs and the decreased volume of intake with the increased calorie and protein requirements.

Sodium. Sodium balance is important because excess sodium can precipitate congestive heart failure or disrupt the water balance. Eight mEq. of sodium per day is advised for adequate growth, although the estimated requirement is 2.1 to 2.6 mEq. per day. Standard formulas (e.g. SMA) are usually given, and low-sodium formulas are needed only during periods of severe cardiac failure or excessive sodium retention. Commercially available baby foods that have sodium added should be avoided; some contain as much as 10 mEq. of sodium per 100 kcal. Strained fruits would appear to be a good choice for baby foods because they are low in sodium.

Potassium. Diuretics are used to control congestive heart failure, and if used regularly may cause hypokalemia, digitalis toxicity and impaired renal concentrating ability. Potassium replacements may be necessary.

Table 38–3 ADEQUACY OF SELECTED VITAMINS AND MINERALS IN 450 ML. OF SEVERAL INFANT FORMULAS*

FORMULA (20 kcal./oz.)	CALCIUM (mg./450 ml.)	FOLIC ACID (µg./450 ml.)	SODIUM (mEq./450 ml.)	
Enfamil	260	47	5	
Isomil	315	45	5.8	
PM 60/40	158	22.5	3	
Prosobee	351	45	8	
SMA	179	23	3	
	0–4 MONTHS	4–12 MONTHS	0–12 MONTHS	0–4 MONTHS	4–12 MONTHS
[a]Estimated requirement	388	289	<50	2.5	2.1
[a]Advisable intake	450	350	50	8	6

*From: Rickard, K., Brady, M. S., and Gresham, E. L.: Nutritional management of the chronically ill child. Pediatr. Clin. North Am., 24:157, 1977.

[a]Estimated requirements and advisable intakes during infancy are those suggested by Fomon and associates.[11]

Vitamins and Minerals. Supplements of vitamins, calcium and iron should be given because of possible inadequate intake and inefficient gastrointestinal absorption. For example, an increased prevalence of biochemical riboflavin deficiency has been seen in these children,[27] and folic acid deficiency is frequent.[25] Table 38–3 presents the amounts of calcium, folic acid and sodium in 450 ml. of several infant formulas. This amount is the maximum intake for many infants who have a severe heart problem. Note that the amounts received from this volume of formula are low compared with the estimated requirements and advisable intakes stated by Fomon.[11] Supplementation is therefore necessary.

Nutritional Counseling

The mother must understand the special nutritional needs of her infant in order for the child to grow properly. This may require extensive counseling. A mother may equate weight gain with edema, which she knows is deleterious to her infant's health, and thus feed the child less than he or she needs in order to avoid weight gain. Parents may associate atherosclerotic heart disease with their child's condition and inappropriately modify the diet to lower cholesterol and fat by using skim milk or by omitting all types of fat from the child's diet, with the result that the child's caloric intake is reduced.

When these infants grow older they are frequently the center of the family's attention and can become very manipulative. It is important

that the parents receive adequate counseling and support in their attempts to provide the proper nutritional care.

The children should be followed closely, with regular measurement of growth, serum albumin and urine osmolarity. The urine osmolarity should be maintained below 400 mOsm. per liter. In addition, the osmolarity of the formula can be measured to determine if it is being prepared with the proper dilution. Parents should be instructed carefully in formula preparation and the accurate recording of the infant's fluid intake. They should observe the frequency of urination (number of wet diapers) and the color of the urine.

When the rate of weight gain is less than the twenty-fifth percentile for normal infants, modification of the formula is necessary. If the urine osmolarity is 300 mOsm. per liter or less, the concentration of the formula can be increased by adding less water to the commercially prepared concentrated liquid. However, if the urine osmolarity is greater than 300 mOsm. per liter and the child is not growing, then the concentration of the formula can be increased by adding more carbohydrate and fat without significantly increasing the renal solute load. If an infant still does not grow properly, a fat absorption test should be made to determine if malabsorption exists. If it does, using a formula in which medium-chain triglycerides (MCT) supply the fat or using MCT oil in the diet may be helpful.

After successful surgical repair of the anomaly, the child typically feels better and begins to gain weight. This may partially be due to

increased intestinal absorption due to increased splanchnic blood flow.[20] The absorption rate from the intestine is directly affected by the amount of blood flowing through the intestinal wall.

DISEASES OF THE BLOOD AND BLOOD-FORMING ORGANS

ANEMIA

Nutritional or iron deficiency anemia is the most common form of anemia in infancy and childhood. It affects individuals of all ages, but particularly women and infants, and occurs most frequently among infants 6 to 24 months old. Most of the babies involved received a poor supply of iron from an anemic mother or had fetal blood loss.

Evidence has accumulated to indicate that sensitivity to cow's milk may cause occult loss of significant quantities of blood into the gastrointestinal tracts of some children with hypochromic microcytic anemia.[25] Furthermore, cow's milk is almost devoid of iron, and the anemic infant is not likely to improve unless a supplementary source is administered. In the rapidly growing infant, lack of iron in a milk diet unsupplemented by other foodstuffs is usually the cause of iron deficiency anemia.

Breast-fed infants rarely become anemic, possibly because the iron in breast milk is present in a more easily absorbed form than the iron in cow's milk or cow's milk formula. Other factors in human milk may also be responsible (see Chapter 14).

Introduction of iron-rich supplementary foods, such as egg yolk, strained beef and liver, fortified infant cereals and certain fruits and green vegetables, by the time the infant is five or six months old is helpful. Continuing the child on an iron-fortified formula or on an older infant formula such as Advance (Ross), which contains iron, during the entire first year of life may help to prevent iron deficiency anemia. (See Appendix Table 8 for iron-rich foods.) The iron content of some baby foods and formulas is given in Table 38–4. See Table 10–1 for the recommended allowances for iron at different ages.

There is an almost inevitable development of anemia and iron deficiency in the first year of life of premature infants, whose early birth limits the amount of iron they receive from the mother. In addition, the enormous increase in size during the first two years of life results in increased demands for hemoglobin production. Hence, there is an early requirement for exogenous iron, and iron-fortified formula is recommended from the beginning.

Table 38–4 IRON CONTENT OF SELECTED FOODS FED TO INFANTS IN THE UNITED STATES[*]

FOOD	ELEMENTAL IRON	
	(mg./100 gm. of food)	(mg./100 kcal.)
Milk or formula		
Human milk[a]	0.05	0.07
Cow's milk[a]	0.05	0.07
Iron-fortified formula	0.9–1.3	1.2–1.8
Formula unfortified with iron	<0.05	<0.05
Infant cereals		
Iron-fortified (dry) mixed with milk[b]	4.2	7–14
Wet-packed cereal-fruit	3.3	1.3–7.5
Strained and junior foods		
Meats		
Liver and a few others	4–6	4–6
Most meats	1–2	1–2
Egg yolks	2–3	1.0–1.5
"Dinners"		
High meat	<1	<1
Vegetable-meat	<0.5	<0.5
Vegetables[c]	<0.5	<0.5
Fruits[c]	<0.5	<0.5

[*]From: Fomon, S. J.: Infant Nutrition, 2nd ed. Philadelphia, W. B. Saunders Co., 1974, p. 314.
[a]Data reviewed by Underwood (1971).
[b]Assuming that one part by weight of dry cereal is mixed with six parts of milk.
[c]A few varieties of vegetables and fruits provide 1 to 2 mg. of iron/100 gm. (1 to 3 mg./100 kcal.).

Lowered blood hemoglobin levels are not uncommon among adolescents who consume less iron than is recommended. Iron deficiency anemia is frequently seen in girls at puberty. Growth requires additional iron, and it is easy to understand how some adolescents become anemic when they diet to remain slim at the peak of their adolescent growth spurt and when the girls also begin to menstruate. Additional discussion of the anemias and the nutritional care for them appears in Chapters 12 and 29.

RENAL DISEASES

NEPHRITIS

Clinical manifestations of nephritis may include high fever, headache, malaise, hypertension, oliguria or anuria. Cardiac failure or hypertensive encephalopathy may develop. Anemia may be present. Details of the nutritional care for nephritis are discussed in Chapter 30.

During the acute stage of nephritis a limited amount of protein, depending upon nitrogen retention, is given. The dietary treatment may at first consist chiefly of correcting the electrolyte balance and giving water orally. As the condition improves, calories and protein are added in the form of nutritious liquids. Calorie and protein intakes are increased depending on kidney function. The appetite is usually poor, and every effort should be made to have the child ingest an adequate diet. Familiar foods help to tempt the appetite.

In chronic renal failure, besides controlling symptoms of uremia, special attention must be paid so that the patient receives sufficient calories, calcium, iron and vitamins in an attempt to maintain growth and development. (See Chapter 30, p. 640.)

NEPHROTIC SYNDROME

The nephrotic syndrome is a general metabolic disturbance resulting in continual loss of large amounts of protein, mainly albumin, in the urine. The disease is characterized by edema, marked albuminuria, deficient excretion of urine, a decrease in the total protein content of the blood, with a relative increase in globulin content, an increase in blood lipids and often a low basal metabolic rate. Few, if any, red cells are found in the urine. The disease is not common, occurring chiefly in children in the two to four age group. About 80 per cent of cases occur in children under 15 years of age.

Nutritional Care

In treatment of the nephrotic syndrome, the protein in the diet is increased to a high level (1.5 gm. per kg. body weight, or 60 to 100 gm., per day) in an attempt to make up for the marked loss of albumin in the urine and to restore depleted blood and tissues and maintain nitrogen balance. In practical experience, it is difficult to get a severely and chronically sick child to eat this much food. Fortunately, the appetite frequently improves spontaneously when diuresis begins and edema disappears.

Sodium is restricted to reverse the edematous process through diuresis. The intake is usually restricted to 500 mg. per day, depending on the child's 24-hour urinary excretion of sodium. Fluids are regulated to coincide with the amount of urine excreted and to cover insensible loss.

Amino acids can be given intravenously in the early stages, especially if the patient is experiencing anorexia, nausea and vomiting. Supplementary protein nourishments listed in Table 35–5 are also recommended to increase the protein content of the diet when indicated. Tube feedings may be necessary (see Chapter 35). The nutritional care for nephrotic syndrome is discussed more fully on page 621.

Drugs

Improvement or remission of many of the evidences of the disease has taken place with corticotropin and steroid therapy. When cortisone therapy is used, increase of potassium in the diet may be necessary.

ALLERGY

Food allergies occur quite frequently among formula-fed infants and children. Breast milk is hypoallergenic. A child born into a family where one or both parents have allergies to food stands a 60 per cent chance of following suit. Cow's milk[15] and eggs are common offenders for infants. Changing from cow's milk to goat's milk often solves the problem. A soy-based formula can be used, although 20 per cent of children who are allergic to cow's milk are also allergic to soy protein. Formulas such as Pregestimil or Nutramigen, in which the protein is present as hydrolysate, may be effective. Once a satisfactory milk or milk substitute has been found, cereals such as rice or oatmeal are added. Care is taken to add one at a time in case of a sensitivity. Then single-vegetable purées

are tried, carrots, asparagus, spinach and beets being the least likely to cause symptoms. Fruit purées are then added, beginning with pears and apples.

The most common food allergens in children are milk, eggs, tomatoes, chocolate, legumes, strawberries, wheat, beef, potatoes, cinnamon, fish, pork and corn. Wheat may be replaced by rice, oats and corn cereals. The other foods are often more difficult to replace. Maintaining normal nutrition is something of a problem in instances where the essential foods—milk, eggs and meat—must be eliminated. Careful attention must be given to the individual daily diet to make certain all essential nutrients are included.

A child who is allergic to a specific food or foods during childhood may become desensitized or naturally outgrow the allergy. The common allergens and their treatment are discussed in Chapter 31.

LEAD POISONING

Children with *pica*, an abnormal craving for non-food substances, are particularly prone to chronic lead poisoning, or *plumbism*. The non-food substances they eat are frequently sources of lead, the most common being chips of lead-based paint. Pica may result from nutritional deficiencies or from emotional disorders. Bicknell has presented a thorough discussion of pica.[2]

Most of the paint currently used on children's furniture and toys is free from lead; however, lead-based paints may still be found in many older houses and apartments and on homemade toys and furniture. Infants and young children may chew their cribs, toys or window sills and eat the sweet-tasting chips (see Fig. 38–11). A chip of paint the size of a penny can contain 50 to 100 μg. of lead. Repeated ingestion of this amount daily for a three-month period could easily occur and could result in clinical symptoms. This would mean a daily ingestion of 100 times the adult tolerable intake.[5] Other potential sources of lead are slightly acidic beverages, such as fruit juices, stored in earthenware pitchers painted with lead-based glaze; any air polluted with automotive emission from leaded gasoline; and dirt in city yards or parks.

When an excess amount of lead enters the body, lead poisoning may follow. The normal blood lead level is less than 40 μg. per 100 ml. Children with blood levels of 60 to 80 μg. per 100 ml. usually have symptoms of vomiting,

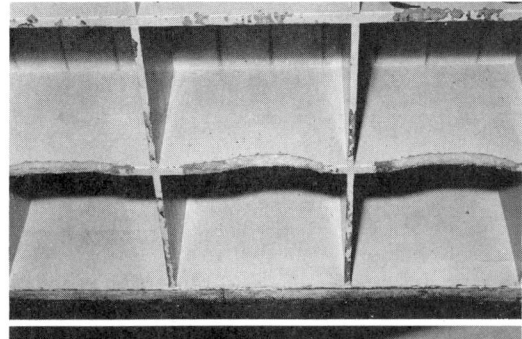
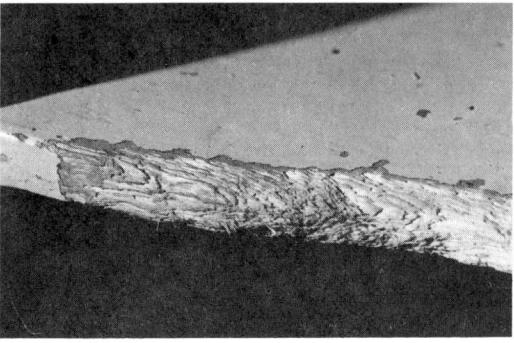

Figure 38–11   A bookshelf and crib with the paint chewed off by an infant. (From: Bicknell, D. J.: Pica, A Childhood Symptom. London, Butterworth and Co., Ltd., 1975, p. 133.)

irritability, loss of weight, weakness, headache, abdominal pain, insomnia and anorexia. These early symptoms after six to eight weeks of lead ingestion are not specific, and the child may be incorrectly diagnosed and treated unless the nurse and physician are alert to the possibility of lead poisoning in the community. With blood lead levels greater than 80 μg. per 100 ml., children exhibit more severe symptoms such as anemia, acute renal tubular injury, peripheral neuritis, muscular incoordination, joint pains and encephalopathy. Eventually death will result. Sometimes chronic nephritis without the acute encephalopathy results from long-term chronic lead poisoning.

Treatment

Since the tubular injury to the kidneys results in Fanconi syndrome—increased urinary loss of amino acids, glucose and phosphate—the first step in treating severe acute lead poisoning is to restore fluid and electrolyte balance, with particular concern to correcting the hypophosphatemia. After fluid and electrolyte balance is restored in the acute phase, the child is started on a regimen of chelating agents, which pick up lead from the tissues and allow its removal by the kidney and liver. A common chelating

agent is *ethylenediaminetetraacetic acid (EDTA)*, which is given intramuscularly along with *British Anti-Lewisite (BAL)* for five days, usually while the child is hospitalized. *Penicillamine* can be used for less severe cases or as follow-up therapy. During chelation therapy it is important for the nurse to maintain the child's fluid intake to allow maximal excretion of the lead. At least 200 ml. of some fluid should be given each hour. Most of the body's burden of lead will have been deposited in the long bones as "lead lines," and some will never be drawn out. However, in the bones it is relatively harmless.

The number of cases of lead toxicity drastically increases during the summer months. Although this observation cannot be explained, it may be that exposure to sunlight during these months and the consequent formation by the skin of vitamin D causes an increased absorption of lead from the gut.[4] Vitamin D appears to enhance lead absorption, and calcium seems to compete with it. Therefore, a diet high in calcium is indicated.

Prognosis

Children with confirmed lead poisoning often have severe neurological and psychological sequelae even after treatment. It has been shown that children with elevated lead levels during the first three years of life had abnormalities of IQ, fine motor coordination and behavior when they were tested at ages seven and eight.[7] Others report that subclinical lead poisoning may lead to a hyperkinetic behavioral pattern, including hyperactivity, impulsiveness and short attention span.[6] Because there seems to be lasting brain damage in 25 per cent of those children who are successfully treated and not re-exposed to lead, it is important to prevent the disease, and treated children should have their blood lead levels tested periodically thereafter, and their environments should be tested for lead.

DENTAL CARIES

A youngster has an excellent chance to develop good teeth if the expectant mother was properly nourished and received adequate calcium and vitamins. Proper nourishment with adequate calcium and vitamin D during the child's early years rates next in importance. Further, prevention of dental caries can be aided by regular brushing of the teeth and by avoidance of sticky foods and sweets, such as cola drinks, candy and sugar.

Fluorides protect against cavities. (See Chapter 7.) If minute amounts are taken daily during the first eight years of life (the growing period when the permanent set of teeth comes through), the incidence of tooth decay has been reported to be reduced 50 per cent. Nutritional care to prevent dental caries is discussed in Chapter 33.

CEREBRAL PALSY

Cerebral palsy, a disturbance of muscular action caused by damage to portions of the brain, is a real challenge to health professionals helping the child who is handicapped since birth to make use of his potential abilities. Difficulty in sucking and swallowing causes feeding problems. The spasticity of the muscles often makes eating and drinking difficult. Observations[26] on cerebral palsy children in a residential school suggest that the extent of "mouth area" involvement is closely associated with poor food intake and, correspondingly, with the general growth curve. The many problems of these individuals—food lost through dribbling due to poor function of mouth, tongue or throat and tiring easily while eating—may contribute to inadequate food intake. The nurse can not only feed these children but can aid in teaching them to feed themselves. Dishes that will not tip over and easy-to-handle cups, glasses and silver should be given to cerebral palsy patients and a great deal of patience should be exercised in helping them to use them.

Nutritional Care

Many of these unfortunate children are underweight and require increased calories to meet the added expenditure of energy produced by the nature of the disease. However, calorie requirement for some spastic patients may be lower than for normal children. Obesity has been observed in some of these children, especially when they reach the early teens. The calorie requirement for athetoid patients, with their involuntary motion, is higher than for spastic patients who expend less energy. The diet should be adequate in all respects, with foods that are easy to handle and eat. Foods that can be held in the hand are easier to manage than those that must be eaten with fork or spoon. In feeding these patients, small amounts of food or fluids should be given at a

time, and enough time should be allowed between bites or drinks for muscles to relax and the nourishment to be swallowed. It is helpful with patients who tend to drool or expectorate to have them hyperextend the neck (head bent backward) when being fed. Chewing is frequently a problem, and dental caries appear to be more prevalent than in the normal child. Drooling is exaggerated by citrus fruits, and if they are avoided, an ascorbic acid supplement may be necessary.

Each patient will have specific problems of eating, and the success in resolving them will be determined by the child's ability and mental capacity.

PROBLEMS AND SUGGESTED TOPICS FOR DISCUSSION

1. Observe the eating habits of the children in your hospital. What considerations should be observed in feeding the sick child?
2. Why is diarrhea so prevalent in the less-developed countries? What is being done to improve the situation?
3. If possible, observe an infant who is suffering with pyloric stenosis. Follow the eating program and evaluate food intake for a day or two. Compare the diet with the accepted nutritional standard allowances for the same age. Observe if any vomiting occurs and estimate the food lost.
4. Study the feeding program prescribed for patients with celiac disease in your hospital. Compare the diets with the nutritional care discussed in this text.
5. Plan a diet with a child who has diabetes. Determine what he or she needs to know about food and meal planning. Involve the child in planning his or her dietary regimen on the basis of family meals.
6. Take a dietary history from an obese adolescent. Be sure to ask about physical activity. Why is he or she overweight? What emotional or social factors are involved? Talk with the teenager about ways that he or she might increase activity and reduce food intake.
7. Plan a diet for a child who is 12 years old and 10 lb. underweight.
8. Describe the nutritional problems of an infant with severe congenital heart disease. With the help of the dietitian-nutritionist, design a diet and counsel the mother about this.
9. In what periods of life does iron deficiency anemia usually occur? What can be done to prevent its occurrence?
10. Talk with a mother whose child has an elevated blood lead level in order to learn about the child's environment. What are the potential sources of lead?
11. How can the nurse help a cerebral palsy patient to feed himself?

CITED REFERENCES

1. Allan, J. D., Mason, A., and Moss, A. D.: Nutritional supplementation in treatment of cystic fibrosis of the pancreas. Am. J. Dis. Child., *126*:22, 1973.
2. Bicknell, D. J.: Pica, A Childhood Symptom. London, Butterworth and Co., Ltd., 1975.
3. Bullen, B. A., et al.: Physical activity of obese and nonobese adolescent girls appraised by motion picture sampling. Am. J. Clin. Nutr., *14*:211, 1964.
4. Chisholm, J. J.: Disturbances in the biosynthesis of heme in lead intoxication. J. Pediatr., *64*:174, 1964.
5. Chisholm, J. J.: Lead Poisoning. Sci. Am., *224*:15, 1971.
6. David, O. J., et al.: Lead and hyperactivity. Behavioral response to chelation: a pilot study. Am J. Psychol., *133*:1155, 1976.
7. de la Burdé, B., and Choate, M. S.: Early asymptomatic lead exposure and development at school age. J. Pediatr., *87*:638, 1975.
8. De Maeyer, E. M.: Protein-energy malnutrition. In: Beaton, G. H., and Bengoa, J. M. (eds.): Nutrition in Preventive Medicine. Geneva, World Health Organization, 1976, p. 40.
9. Dobell, A. R. C., et al.: Severe feeding difficulty in infants with increased pulmonary flow. J. Thorac. Cardiovasc. Surg. *72*:303, 1976.
10. Ellis, C. E., and Hill, E.: Growth, intelligence, and school performances in children with cystic fibrosis who have an episode of malnutrition in infancy. J. Pediatr., *87*:565, 1975.
11. Fomon. S. J.: Infant Nutrition, 2nd ed. Philadelphia, W. B. Saunders Co., 1974, pp. 212, 269.
12. Fomon, S. J., Ziegler, E. E., and O'Donnell, A. M.: Infant feeding in health and disease. In: Fomon, S. J.: Infant Nutrition, 2nd ed. W. B. Saunders Co., 1974, pp. 490–491.
13. Gallagher, J. R.: Weight control in adolescence. J. Am. Diet. Assoc., *40*:519, 1962.
14. Hansen, A. E., et al.: Role of linoleic acid in infant nutrition. Clinical and chemical study of 428 infants fed a milk mixture varying in kind and amount of fat. Pediatrics, *31*:171, 1963.
15. Heiner, C. D., et al.: Sensitivity to cow's milk. JAMA, *189*:563, 568, 1964.
16. Holt, L. E., Jr.: Celiac disease—What is it? J. Pediatr., *46*:369, 1955.
17. Ingelfinger, F. J.: For want of an enzyme. Nutrition Today, *3*:8, 1968.
18. Jackson, R. L., et al.: The Child with Diabetes. Columbus, Mo., University of Missouri, 1973, pp. 18–19.
19. Lum, B. O. L.: Preventing ketoacidosis in the child with juvenile-onset diabetes mellitus. J. Am. Diet. Assoc., *69*:157, 1976.
20. Markiewicz, A., Wajczuk, D., and Iljin, W.: Xylose absorption before and after surgical correction of atrial septal defect (ASD) and ventricular septal defect (VSD). Eur. J. Pediatr., *124*:57, 1976.
21. Molony, C. J., and Parmelee, A. H.: Convulsions in young infants as a result of pyridoxine (vitamin B_6) deficiency. JAMA, *154*:405, 1954.
22. Muller, D. P. R., Harries, J. T., and Lloyd, J. K.: The relative importance of the factors involved in the absorption of vitamin E in children. Gut, *15*:966, 1974.
23. Review: Are peptic ulcers on the increase in children? Food and Nutrition News, *42*(2), 1970. Published by National Live Stock and Meat Board, Chicago, Illinois.)
24. Rickard, K., Brady, M. S., and Gresham, E. L.: Nutritional management of the chronically ill child. Congenital heart disease and myelomeningocele. Pediatr. Clin. North Am., *24*:157, 1977.
25. Rook, G. D., et al.: Folic acid deficiency in infants and children with heart disease. Br. Heart J., *35*:87, 1973.
26. Ruby, D. O., and Matheny, W. D.: Comments on

growth of cerebral palsied children. J. Am. Diet. Assoc., *40*:525, 1962.

27. Steir, M., Lopez, R., and Cooperman, J. M.: Riboflavin deficiency in infants and children with heart disease. Am. Heart J., *92*:139, 1976.

28. Thomson, N. B., Jr., and Jewett, T. C.: Peptic ulcers in infancy and childhood. JAMA, *189*:539, 1964.

ADDITIONAL REFERENCES

Bengoa, J. M., et al.: Some indications for a broad assessment of the magnitude of protein-calorie malnutrition in young children in population groups. Am. J. Clin. Nutr., *7*:714, 1959.

Bullen, B. A., et al.: Attitudes towards physical activity, food and family in obese and nonobese adolescent girls. Am. J. Clin. Nutr., *12*:1, 1963.

Collip, P. J. (ed.): Childhood Obesity. Acton, Mass., Publishing Sciences Group, Inc., 1975.

Committee on Toxicology, Assembly of Life Sciences, National Research Council: Recommendations for the prevention of lead poisoning in children. Nutr. Rev., *34*:321, 1976.

Coursin, D. B.: Convulsive seizures in infants with pyridoxine-deficient diet. JAMA, *154*:406, 1954.

Croft, H., and Frenkel, S.: Children and lead poisoning. Am. J. Nurs., *75*:102, 1975.

di Sant'Agnese, P. A., and Jones, W. O.: The celiac syndrome (malabsorption) in pediatrics. JAMA, *180*:308, 1962.

Drash, A. L.: Diabetes mellitus. In: Vaughan, V. C., and McKay, R. J. (eds.): Nelson Textbook of Pediatrics, 10th ed. Philadelphia, W. B. Saunders Co., 1975, pp. 1259–71.

Etzwiler, D. D., and Sines, L. K.: Juvenile diabetes and its management. JAMA, *181*:304, 1962.

Fajans, S. S., et al.: The various faces of diabetes in the young. Arch. Intern. Med., *136*:194, 1976.

Getty, G., and Hollensworth, M.: Through a child's eye seeing. Nutrition Today, *2*:17, 1967.

Gordon, J. E.: Weaning diarrhea: A synergism of nutrition and infection. Nutr. Rev., *22*:161, 1964.

Green, V. A., Wise, G. W., and Callenbach, J.: Lead poisoning. Clin. Toxicol., *9*:33, 1976.

Griggs, R. C., et al.: Environmental factors in childhood lead poisoning. JAMA, *187*:703, 1964.

Hammond, M. I., et al.: A nutritional study of cerebral palsied children. J. Am. Diet. Assoc., *49*:196, 1966.

Huse, D. M., et al.: Infants with congenital heart disease. Food intake, body weight and energy metabolism. Am. J. Dis. Child., *129*:65, 1975.

Katz, A. J., and Falchuk, Z. M.: Current concepts in gluten-sensitive enteropathy (celiac sprue). Pediatr. Clin. North Am., *22*:767, 1975.

Mahaffey, K. R.: Relations between quantities of lead ingested and health effects of lead in humans. Pediatrics, *59*:448, 1977.

Pratt, E. L.: Food allergy and food intolerance in relation to the development of good eating habits. Pediatrics, *21*:642, 1958.

The rehydration treatment of acute diarrhea with inexpensive oral fluids. Clin. Pediatr., *15*:1095, 1976.

Schizas, A. A., et al.: Medium-chain triglycerides—use in food preparation. J. Am. Diet. Assoc., *51*:228, 1967.

Silver, H. K., and Finkelstein, M.: Deprivation dwarfism. J. Pediatr., *70*:317, 1967.

Soyka, L. F.: Treatment of the nephrotic syndrome in childhood. Am. J. Dis. Child., *113*:693, 1967.

Strangway, A., et al.: Diet and growth in congenital heart disease. Pediatrics, *57*:75, 1976.

White House Conference on Food, Nutrition and Health. Final Report. Washington, D.C., U.S. Government Printing Office, 1970.

Wilson, J. F., et al.: Milk-induced gastrointestinal bleeding in infants with hypochronic microcytic anemia. JAMA, *189*:568, 1964.

Winick, M. (ed.): Childhood Obesity. New York, John Wiley & Sons, 1975.

Yardley, J. H., et al.: Celiac disease: A study of the jejunal epithelium before and after a gluten-free diet. N. Engl. J. Med., *267*:1173, 1962.

Chapter 39

NUTRITIONAL CARE FOR CHILDREN WITH INBORN ERRORS OF METABOLISM

DEBORAH A. ROLAND, M.S., R.D.*

The concept of inborn errors of metabolism was first described by Sir Archibald Garrod in 1906. He observed that four specific conditions—albinism, alkaptonuria, cystinuria and pentosuria—are diseases that are genetically determined.[11] Garrod also recognized that these disorders are congenital, have a familial distribution and are likely to affect one or more siblings. Based on these findings, he developed the concept that certain diseases arise because an enzyme, governing one single metabolic step, is reduced in activity or is missing altogether.[32]

During the past twenty years the rate of discovery of new inborn errors of metabolism has increased as a result of improved technology. To date, approximately 300 genetic defects of metabolism have been described. The focus of this chapter will be directed toward studying those genetic defects that can be treated or ameliorated by specific nutritional therapy.

Metabolic disorders can be categorized according to the nutrient that has the disordered metabolism; for example, inborn errors of amino acid, carbohydrate, lipid, vitamin or mineral metabolism. Only disorders of amino acid and carbohydrate metabolism are discussed in this chapter.

NUTRITIONAL COUNSELING

Nutritional counseling of the patient's parents is an important consideration in the treatment of inborn errors of metabolism. During infancy, when the child is receiving only a special modified formula, the diet is not difficult to implement. Calculating the diet becomes more challenging when solid foods are introduced,

and the actual practice of omitting commonly used foods presents problems and requires effort on the part of the child's family.

There are several common problems that should be anticipated: (1) Other young children in the household may resent the special attention given to the child with the metabolic disorder. (2) Synthetic dietary products may be difficult for the child to consume, especially if they are unpalatable and if he observes his siblings and peers enjoying a complete variety of foods. (3) Expensive dietary products may drain the family's financial resources. (4) Difficulty often arises when the dietary plan is complicated and requires many hours of education and planning. (5) Keeping periodic records of the food their child eats may present a problem for some parents. (6) The parents can become frustrated in their continual monitoring of every food item the child consumes. Counseling should emphasize the importance of the patient's dietary treatment while gradually helping the family make the necessary changes in their lifestyle.

DISORDERS OF AMINO ACID METABOLISM

PHENYLKETONURIA

Metabolic Defect. Phenylketonuria (PKU) is an inerited disorder of phenylalanine catabolism in which the enzyme *phenylalanine hydroxylase* is missing.[37] Phenylalanine hydroxylase normally catalyzes the hydroxylation of the essential amino acid phenylalanine to tyrosine. The enzymatic defect results in an accumulation of phenylalanine and other metabolites, such as phenylpyruvic acid,

*Assistant Professor, Clinical Nutrition, Rush University, Chicago, Illinois.

phenyllactic acid, phenylacetic acid and phenylacetyl glutamine, in the blood and urine[25] (Fig. 39–1).

The designation "phenylketonuria" refers to the urinary excretion of phenylpyruvic acid. Excessive amounts of phenylalanine in the blood prevent normal brain and central nervous system development and lead to mental retardation, convulsions and electroencephalogram abnormalities.[26] The tyrosine deficiency is manifested by a lightening in the pigmentation of the skin, hair and eyes. Eczema, vomiting, irritability and a "musty" odor to the urine are other symptoms of this disease. Current studies show the incidence of PKU to be about one in 15,000 births.[28]

The intrauterine physical growth of the PKU fetus proceeds normally, and there is no appreciable difference between the birthweights of PKU infants and their siblings. However, before clinical expression of the disease is apparent in newborn infants, abnormal intrauterine development may result in a small degree of intellectual damage. Therefore, it is imperative that a prompt diagnosis of this enzyme defect be made.[6]

Diagnosis. Phenylketonuria can be diagnosed in the newborn infant population by using the Guthrie bacterial inhibition assay or the photofluorometric phenylalanine assay. These serum tests provide the earliest reliable qualitative evidence of phenylketonuria.

Most states have mandatory screening laws for the detection of PKU. Since the normal serum phenylalanine level of an infant is below 2 mg. per 100 ml., a test result of 4 mg. per 100 ml. or higher necessitates closer evaluation. If the serum phenylalanine level exceeds 20 mg. per 100 ml. and the serum tyrosine is low (in a ratio of 4:1, phenylalanine to tyrosine), the infant is considered to have phenylketonuria, and treatment is initiated. This type of screening program identifies 95 per cent of all patients with PKU. The other 5 per cent are missed because of inadequate protein intake prior to the test.[33]

Nutritional Care

Nutritional management of the child with PKU should include (1) sharp restriction of the amino acid phenylalanine in the dietary intake, (2) inclusion of limited amounts of phenylalanine, tyrosine and protein for growth and development and (3) the provision of sufficient calories, vitamins and minerals for optimal growth and development.

The first step in dietary regulation is to determine the child's protein and energy needs based on age and weight (Table 39–1). Height, head circumference and general health should also be considered.

Lofenalac (Mead Johnson), an enzymatic hydrolysate of the milk protein casein that is low in phenylalanine, is the most important source of nourishment for infants and children with phenylketonuria (Table 39–2). From 85 to 90 per cent of the total protein consumed must be provided by Lofenalac, because most

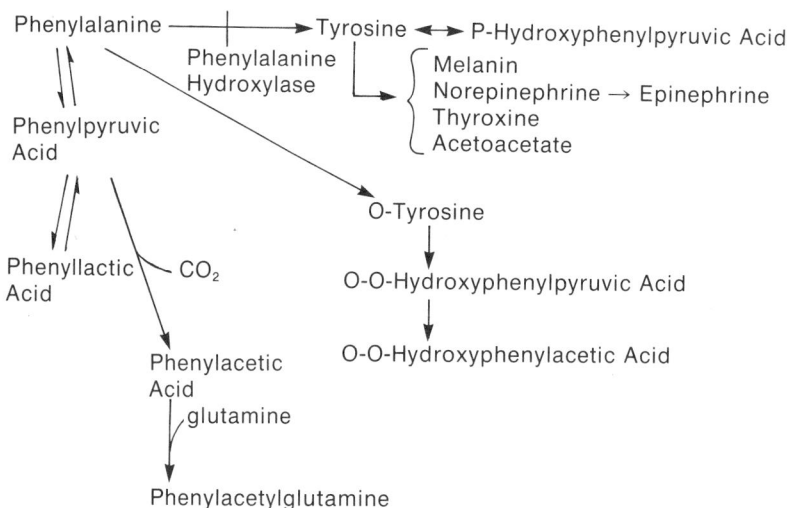

Figure 39–1 Metabolism of phenylalanine in phenylketonuria. Note the blockage in the step from phenylalanine to tyrosine. (Adapted from: Phenylketonuria. Evansville, Indiana, Mead Johnson and Co., 1973, p. 3)

Table 39–1 RECOMMENDED AMOUNTS OF PHENYLALANINE, PROTEIN AND ENERGY FOR PKU INFANTS AND PRESCHOOLERS*

AGE (mo.)	PHENYL- ALANINE (mg./kg./day)	PROTEIN (gm./kg./day)	ENERGY (kcal./kg./day)	PROTEIN FROM LOFENALAC (%)	AMOUNT OF LOFENALAC (ms.[a]/kg.)	AMOUNT OF EVAPO- RATED MILK[b] (oz.)
0–3	88	4.4	120	85	2½–3	1–3
4–6	66	3.3	115	85	2–2½	1–2½
7–9	44	2.5	110	90	1½–2	½–1½
10–12	33	2.5	105	90	1½–2	½–1
		(total gm./day)	(total kcal./day)		(total ms./day)	
13–24	25	25.0	1300	90	16	0–1
25–36	24	25.0	1300	90	16	none
37–48	20	30.0	1300	90	19	none
49–72	18	30.0	1800	90	19	none
73–96	17	35.0	2000	90	24	none
97–120	15	40.0	2200	90	28	none

*Adapted from: Acosta, P., and Elsas, L.: Dietary Management of Inherited Metabolic Disease: Phenylketonuria, Galactosemia, Tyrosinemia, Maple Syrup Urine Disease. Atlanta, Ga., ACELMU Publishers, 1976.
[a]One measure of Lofenalac equals 10 gm. or 1 packed tablespoon.
[b]One ounce of evaporated milk contains 106 mg. phenylalanine, 2.2 gm. protein and 44 calories.

protein-containing foods are too high in pheylalanine content for the PKU infant.

In calculating the diet, the appropriate amount of Lofenalac must be determined for each child. The remaining protein, tyrosine, phenylalanine, energy and other nutrients can then be supplied from regular foods. Although the PKU infant is intolerant to large amounts of phenylalanine, this is still an essential amino acid that is required for growth. Diets based solely on Lofenalac are growth-inhibiting because they contain almost no phenylalanine or tyrosine. Therefore, limited supplementation with whole or evaporated milk as a source of these amino acids is required to balance the dietary amino acid pattern.[1] Table 39–3 illustrates how the diet might be calculated for a child with PKU.

Food exchange lists have been compiled to simplify the inclusion of a variety of foods in the diet. Foods containing similar amounts of phenylalanine have been grouped together and have been given an average phenylalanine value. Foods in the same group can be used interchangeably. For example, three-fourths cup of applesauce and one and one-half apricots each contains 15 mg. of phenylalanine and may be exchanged for each other. Table 39–4 gives the phenylalanine contents of many foods, and Table 39–5 shows a typical day's menu.

The infant's serum phenylalanine level must be monitored frequently to keep it within a safe range. For example, if 88 mg. per kg. per day of phenylalanine is provided in the diet and the daily serum phenylalanine values are consistently greater than the appropriate level, a reduction of dietary phenylalanine must be instituted.

The importance of trace minerals in the diet of the infant with PKU is currently being explored. It is now recognized that dietary mineral components play essential roles in coenzyme and other metabolic functions. Alexander and colleagues have shown that dietary manganese and zinc intakes may be low in individuals whose primary nutritional source is synthetic formulas.[2] Care should be taken in providing and monitoring the trace minerals in the PKU diet and in other diets in which natural foods are restricted.

A major issue in the treatment of phenylketonuria involves the age at which the phenylalanine-restricted diet can be discontinued. A study by Johnson showed that 13 of 14 children who discontinued the restricted diet at six years of age did not demonstrate significant intellectual or behavioral deterioration. Further studies that include data from a larger population and that cover a longer period of time should be carried out before a definite statement can be made on the best age for termination of the diet.[16]

Variant Forms of Hyperphenylalaninemia

Variant forms of hyperphenylalaninemia exist. A transient form must be recognized and

Text continued on page 787

Table 39–2   APPROXIMATE NUTRITIVE COMPOSITION OF SPECIAL DIETARY PRODUCTS*a

NUTRIENT	LOFENA-LAC (MJ)[b]	PKU AID (RL)[b]	LOW-METHIONINE ISOMIL (RL)	3229-A (MJ)	3200-AB (MJ)	MSUD AID (RL)	METHIO-NAID (RL)	3200-K (MJ)	HISTINAID (RL)	80056 (MJ)
Calories	454	240	516	406	460	248	242	464	240	486
Protein (gm.)	15	60	12.5	20.3	15	64.4	63.1	14	61.2	0
Fat (gm.)	18	0	28.1	6.8	18	0	0	19	0	22.5
CHO (gm.)	60	0	57.0	66	60	0	0	60	0	73.5
L-Amino Acids (gm.)										
Essential										
Isoleucine	0.75	2.6	0.56	1.08	0.86	0	2.4	0.67	2.5	0
Leucine	1.41	6.1	1.02	1.70	1.76	0	3.2	1.16	3.8	0
Lysine	1.57	6.1	0.77	1.85	1.91	7.1	6.0	0.87	5.8	0
Methionine	0.45	1.5	0.14	0.62	0.56	1.9	0.2	0.16	1.6	0
Phenylalanine	0.08	<0.07	0.6	0	<0.08	3.8	4.3	0.76	2.2	0
Threonine	0.77	4.8	0.51	0.93	0.65	3.3	3.2	0.52	3.1	0
Tryptophan	0.19	0.9	0.12	0.28	0.20	1.2	0.9	0.16	1.1	0
Valine	1.20	4.6	0.52	1.24	1.38	0	3.2	0.71	3.1	0
Histidine	0.39	1.8	0.28	0.46	0.40	2.7	2.8	0.34	0	0
Non-essential										
Arginine	0.34	3.1	0.83	0.68	0.39	5.1	4.4	0.96	4.6	0
Alanine	0.64	4.1	0.53	NL	0.76	7.1	5.6	0.60	5.9	0
Aspartate	1.34	8.1	1.29	5.15	1.60	12.1	9.5	1.72	10.6	0
Cystine	0.025	1.5	0.15	0.34	0.042	2.1	3.7	0.107	1.8	0
Glutamate	3.78	9.3	2.48	1.85	4.31	13.3	11.0	2.76	12.3	0
Glycine	0.35	3.1	0.52	3.30	0.40	3.9	4.3	0.59	5.9	0
Proline	1.13	3.6	0.6	NL	1.13	2.3	1.6	0.68	1.9	0
Serine	1.02	4.8	0.68	NL	1.09	2.4	1.7	0.72	1.9	0
Tyrosine	0.81	6.0	0.40	0.93	<0.04	3.8	4.3	0.49	4.5	0
Glutamine	NL[b]	NL	NL	4.75	NL	NL	NL	NL	NL	0

Vitamins

Vitamin A (I.U.)	1160	0	2200	2030	1160	0	0	1450	0	1440
Vitamin D (I.U.)	284	0	340	406	284	0	0	290	0	360
Vitamin E (I.U.)	7.1	0	12	10	7.1	0	0	7.2	0	0
Vitamin C (mg.)	37	0	60	53	37	0	0	38	0	45
Thiamin (μg.)	428	2000	0.5	609	438	2000	2000	440	2000	450
Riboflavin (μg.)	714	2000	0.6	1015	714	2000	2000	720	2000	540
Vitamin B6 (μg.)	290	2000	0.5	508	290	2000	2000	360	2000	360
Vitamin B12 (μg.)	1.4	20	35	2.5	1.4	20	20	1.8	20	1.8
Niacin (μg.)	5714	25,000	9	8122	5714	25,000	25,000	5800	25,000	7200
Folic acid (μg.)	72	400	0.12	51	72	400	400	30	400	90
Pantothenic acid (μg.)	2142	20,000	7	3046	2142	20,000	20,000	2200	20,000	2700
Choline (mg.)	61	0	94	86	61	0	0	62	0	76
Biotin (μg.)	36	600	0.13	30	36	600	600	22	600	45
Vitamin K (μg.)	72	0	0.12	102	72	0	0	71	00	90
Inositol (mg.)	72	0	0	102	72	250	100	73	100	90

Minerals

Calcium (mg.)	435	2500	650	634	435	2500	2500	2500	700	540
Phosphorus (mg.)	326	1500	440	508	326	1500	1500	1500	1500	300
Magnesium (mg.)	51	300	40	76	51	300	300	300	80	63
Iron (mg.)	8.6	25	10	12	8.6	50	50	50	4	11
Iodine (μg.)	32	150	120	66	32	150	150	150	60	41
Copper (μg.)	429	2500	500	609	429	2500	2500	2500	500	540
Manganese (mg.)	0.7	3.5	0	2	0.7	3.5	3.5	3.5	0.5	0.9
Zinc (mg.)	2.9	15	4	4.1	2.9	15	15	15	0.9	3.6
Sodium (mEq.)	9	61	10.4	10	9	61	61	61	34	3
Potassium (mEq.)	12	66	10.4	18	12	66	66	66	19	9
Chloride (mEq.)	9	80	12.7	14	9	80	80	80	NL	4

*From: American Academy of Pediatrics Committee on Nutrition: Special diets for infants with inborn errors of amino acid metabolism. Pediatrics, 57:783, 1976.

a Per 100 gm. of powder.

b MJ = Mead Johnson Company; RL = Ross Laboratories; NL = not listed.

Table 39–3   GUIDELINES FOR PKU DIET CALCULATIONS

CASE STUDY

M.S. is a six month old infant with phenylketonuria. The information provided in Tables 39–1, 39–2 and 39–4 can be utilized in planning a diet for this child.

BASELINE DATA

Age	6 months
Sex	Male
Weight (kg.)	7.7
Weight percentile	50th
Height (cm.)	67.8
Height percentile	50th
Head circumference (cm.)	43.3
General Health	Good
Activity	Very active

STEP 1.   Calculate the child's requirement for phenylalanine, protein and kilocalories using Table 39–1.
A. Phenylalanine
7.7 kg. body weight × 66 mg. phenylalanine/kg./day = 508 mg. phenylalanine/day
B. Protein
7.7 kg. body weight × 3.3 gm. protein/kg./day = 25.4 gm. protein/day
For this infant protein is set at 31 gm./day.
C. Kilocalories
7.7 kg. body weight × 115 kcal./kg./day = 885 kcal./day
Because this infant is very active, kcalories are set at 970 kcal./day.

STEP 2.   Determine the amount of Lofenalac required per day. This information is determined from the infant's or child's protein requirement.
7.7 kg. body weight × 2 ms.[a]/kg./day (1 ms. of Lofenalac = 1 packed tablespoon) = 15.4 ms. = 15.4 T., or about 15 T., which is equal to 150 gm. of Lofenalac per day.

STEP 3.   Determine the amount of evaporated milk to be included in the diet, 2 to 2½ oz. of evaporated milk is recommended for an infant 4 to 6 months of age.

STEP 4.   Determine the amount of water to mix with the Lofenalac. The fluid consistency of the formula varies according to the infant's age and fluid requirements. For an infant consuming a formula of 20 kcal./oz., 1 level 8-oz. measuring cup of Lofenalac is mixed with 1 qt. of water.
To prepare formula for the infant described in the case study, mix 15 T. (150 gm.) of Lofenalac and 2½ oz. (75 ml.) of evaporated milk with 4 oz. of water to prevent lumps from forming. Then add water to make a total of 24 oz. of formula. This provides 4 bottles of 6 oz. each.

[a]ms. = measure

Table 39–3   GUIDELINES FOR PKU DIET CALCULATIONS *(Continued)*

STEP 5.   Determine the amounts of phenylalanine, protein and kilocalories in the Lofenalac and evaporated milk.

	Phenylalanine (mg.)	*Protein (gm.)*	*Kcal.*
Lofenalac, 15 T.	120	22.5	681
Evaporated milk, 2½ oz.	265	5.5	97
Total	385	28.0	778

STEP 6.   Determine the amount of phenylalanine, protein and kilocalories to be obtained from foods other than the formula.

Total phenylalanine = 508 mg./day
Phenylalanine in formula = 385 mg./day
Phenylalanine from other foods = 123 mg./day

Total protein	31 gm./day
Protein in formula	28.0 gm./day
Protein from other foods	2.0–3 gm./day

Total kcalories	970 kcal./day
Kcalories in formula	778 kcal./day
Kcalories from other foods	192 kcal./day

STEP 7.   Determine the amount of foods other than formula to be included in the dietary plan. Use exchange lists in Table 39–4.

	Phenylalanine (mg.)	*Protein (gm.)*	*Kcal.*
Oatmeal, dry, 2T.	36	0.8	18
Applesauce & apricots, strained, 6 T.	9	0.2	72
Barley cereal, strained, 2½ T.	37.5	0.8	23
Sweet potatoes, strained, 3 T.	30	0.6	30
Orange-pineapple juice, 6 oz.	6	0.5	59
Total	118.5	2.9	202

STEP 8.   Determine the actual amounts of phenylalanine, protein and kcal. per kg. of body weight by dividing the body weight (in kg.) into the total available nutrients:

Phenylalanine (mg.)
    508 mg. phenylalanine ÷ 7.7 kg. body weight = 66 mg. phenylalanine/kg./day
Protein
    30.9 gm. protein ÷ 7.7 kg. body weight = 4.1 gm. protein/kg./day
Kilocalories
    980 kcal. ÷ 7.7 kg. body weight = 127 kcal./kg./day

Table 39–4   FOOD EXCHANGE LISTS FOR PHENYLALANINE-TYROSINE RESTRICTED DIET*

VEGETABLES

Contain per serving an average of 15 mg. phenylalanine, 10 mg. tyrosine, 0.5 gm. protein and 10 kcal. Protein averages 2.8% phenylalanine and 2% tyrosine.

	PHENYLALANINE (mg.)	TYROSINE (mg.)	PROTEIN (gm.)	ENERGY (kcal.)
Asparagus, raw, 1½ spears (25 gm.)	14	11	0.5	6
Asparagus, canned, green, 1½ spears (28 gm.)	17	12	0.6	5
Beans, snap, green, 4 T. (31 gm.)	11	15	0.4	8
Beets, solids, ¼ c. (42 gm.)	7	14	0.4	15
Cabbage, raw, ⅓ c. (33 gm.)	16	10	0.5	8
Cabbage, cooked, 5 T. (50 gm.)	12	11	0.5	10
Carrots, raw, 1 small (50 gm.)	15	13	0.5	21
Carrots, cooked, ⅔ c. (100 gm.)	18	8	0.5	30
Cauliflower, cooked, 3 T. (25 gm.)	18	8	0.6	5
Cucumber, raw, ½ med. (50 gm.)	12	–	0.5	8
Eggplant, cooked, 2 T. (25 gm.)	11	10	0.2	5
Lettuce, (25 gm.)	17	9	0.3	5
Okra, cooked, 2 pods	18	7	0.5	7
Tomato, raw, ½ small (50 gm.)	16	7	0.6	11
Tomato, canned, ¼ c. (50 gm.)	14	6	0.5	10
Tomato juice, canned, ¼ c. (50 gm.)	13	6	0.4	10
Turnip root, white raw, 6 T. (50 gm.)	9	7	0.4	15
Turnip root, cooked, ⅔ c. (100 gm.)	14	12	0.8	23

GERBER'S STRAINED AND JUNIOR VEGETABLES

	PHENYLALANINE (mg.)	TYROSINE (mg.)	PROTEIN (gm.)	ENERGY (kcal.)
Amounts in 7 T. (100 gm.).				
Beets	17	49	1.3	38
Carrots	22	14	0.7	30
Green beans	63	28	1.3	29
Sweet potatoes	68	35	1.4	69
Amounts in 1 T.				
Beets	2	7	0.2	5
Carrots	3	2	0.1	4
Green beans	9	4	0.2	4
Sweet potatoes	10	5	0.2	10

FRUITS

Contain per serving an average of 10 mg. phenylalanine, 5 mg. tyrosine, 0.4 gm. protein and 55 kcal. Protein averages 2.2% phenylalanine and 1.4% tyrosine.

	PHENYLALANINE (mg.)	TYROSINE (mg.)	PROTEIN (gm.)	ENERGY (kcal.)
Apple, raw, 1 small (100 gm.)	10	6	0.4	58
Applesauce, ⅔ c. (200 gm.)	10	6	0.4	182
Apple juice, 1½ c.	10	6	0.4	174
Apricots, raw, 1½ med. (50 gm.)	6	5	0.4	25
Apricots, canned, 1½ halves (50 gm.)	10	6	0.3	43
Avocado, 2 T. (20 gm.)	9	6	0.3	33
Banana, ¼ small (25 gm.)	11	7	0.3	22
Dates, dried, 1 date (10 gm.)	7	2	0.3	27
Orange, ⅓ small (33 gm.)	10	5	0.3	16
Orange juice, frozen, 3 T. (1½ oz.)	10	5	0.3	22
Peaches, raw, ½ med. (50 gm.)	9	10	0.4	19
Peaches, canned, 2 med. halves (100 gm.)	9	10	0.4	78
Strawberries, raw, 3 large (25 gm.)	6	7	0.2	9

Table 39–4   FOOD EXCHANGE LISTS FOR PHENYLALANINE-TYROSINE
RESTRICTED DIET (*Continued*)

GERBER'S STRAINED AND JUNIOR FRUITS

	PHENYLALANINE *(mg.)*	TYROSINE *(mg.)*	PROTEIN *(gm.)*	ENERGY *(kcal.)*
Per 7 T. (100 gm.)				
Applesauce	10	3	0.2	81
Applesauce & apricots	10	4	0.3	87
Apricots with tapioca	8	8	0.4	80
Bananas with tapioca	14	11	0.5	88
Peaches	22	15	0.6	82
Pears	10	6	0.4	69
Apple juice	<3	2	0.1	49
Orange juice	<3	8	0.5	50
Orange-apple juice	3	5	0.3	54
Orange-apricot juice	3	11	0.6	61
Orange-pineapple juice	6	8	0.5	59
Per Tablespoon				
Applesauce	1.4	0.4	0.03	12
Applesauce & apricots	1.5	0.6	0.04	12
Apricots with tapioca	1.2	1.1	0.06	11
Bananas with tapioca	2.0	1.6	0.07	13
Peaches	3.1	2.1	0.09	12
Pears	1.5	0.9	0.06	10

BREAD AND CEREAL

Contain per serving an average of 18 mg. phenylalanine, 12 mg. tyrosine, 0.4 gm. protein and 15 kcal. Protein averages 4.6% phenylalanine and 3.2% tyrosine.

	PHENYLALANINE *(mg.)*	TYROSINE *(mg.)*	PROTEIN *(gm.)*	ENERGY *(kcal.)*
Dry Cereals				
Bran Flakes, 2 T.	20	14	0.5	16
Bran, Raisin, 2 T.	20	14	0.4	18
Cheerios, 2 T.	22	14	0.4	12
Cornflakes, 3 T.	17	15	0.4	18
Rice Flakes, 3 T.	19	13	0.4	23
Rice Krispies, 4 T.	19	14	0.4	27
Rice, Puffed, 8 T.	19	14	0.4	26
Hot Cereals				
Cream of Wheat, cooked, 1 T.	13	9	0.3	8
Farina, cooked, 2 T.	22	15	0.5	18
Grits, cooked, 2 T.	18	14	0.4	15
Malt-O-Meal, cooked, 1 T.	13	9	0.3	8
Miscellaneous				
Corn, canned, 1 T.	14	10	0.3	9
Macaroni, cooked, tender, 1 T.	16	10	0.3	9
Potatoes, boiled, ¼ med. (25 gm.)	21	13	0.5	16
Rice, brown, cooked, 1 T.	12	9	0.2	11
Rice, white, parboiled, cooked, 2 T.	20	14	0.4	20
Yams, cooked, 1 T.	16	6	0.4	17
Special Products				
Aproten[a]				
Anellini, uncooked, ¾ c. (100 gm.)	12	12	0.5	340
Rigatini, uncooked, 1½ c. (100 gm.)	12	12	0.5	340
Paygel Low Protein Bread, 1 slice (32 gm.)	7	5	0.3	83
Rusks, 1 slice (11.5 gm.)	4	3	0.1	48
Tagliatelle, uncooked, 1¼ c. (100 gm.)	12	12	0.5	340

Table continued on the following page

Table 39–4 FOOD EXCHANGE LISTS FOR PHENYLALANINE-TYROSINE RESTRICTED DIET (*Continued*)

GERBER'S BABY CEREALS (dry)	PHENYLALANINE (mg.)	TYROSINE (mg.)	PROTEIN (gm.)	ENERGY (kcal.)
Per Tablespoon				
Barley cereal	15	9	0.3	9
Mixed cereal	15	9	0.3	9
Oatmeal cereal	18	18	0.4	9
Rice cereal	9	6	0.2	9
Barley with mixed fruit	12	9	0.2	9
Mixed with banana	12	10	0.2	9
Oatmeal with banana	15	12	0.3	9
Rice with strawberries	8	8	0.2	9
Cereals in Jars				
Mixed with applesauce-banana	9	6	0.2	12
Oatmeal with applesauce-banana	7	5	0.1	11
Rice with applesauce-banana	2	2	<0.1	10
Rice with mixed fruit	10	9	0.2	10

FATS

Contain per serving an average of 4 mg. phenylalanine, 6 mg. tyrosine, 0.1 gm. protein and 90 kcal. Protein averages 4.9% phenylalanine and 5.1% tyrosine.

	PHENYLALANINE (mg.)	TYROSINE (mg.)	PROTEIN (gm.)	ENERGY (kcal.)
Butter, 2 tsp.	4	5	0.1	72
Cream, heavy (40% fat), 1 tsp. (5 gm.)	5	5	0.1	17
Italian dressing, 3 T. (14 gm.)	4	4	0.1	231
Margarine, 1 T. (14 gm.)	5	5	0.1	100
Mayonnaise, 1 T. (14 gm.)	5	5	0.1	101
Tartar sauce, ½ T. (10 gm.)	4	4	0.1	47
Thousand Island dressing, 1 T. (14 gm.)	4	4	0.1	57

FREE FOODS

These foods contain little or no protein and may be used as desired in the diet as long as appetite is not depressed by their use and the child is not overweight.

	ENERGY (kcal.)
Candies:	
Butterscotch, 1 piece	20
Cream mints, 1 piece	7
Fondant, patties or mint, 1 piece	40
Gum drops, 1 large	35
Hard candy, 2 pieces	39
Jelly beans, 10	110
Lollipops, 1 med. (2¼" diameter)	108
Corn syrup, 1 T.	58
Danish dessert, ½ c.	123
Fruit ices, ½ c.	69
Kool-Aid, ½ c.	53
Maple syrup, 1 T.	50
Molasses, 1 T.	46
Popsicle, 1 twin bar	95
Prono[a], ⅓ c.	55
Start, liquid, ½ c.	60
Sugar, granulated, 1 T.	43
Tang, liquid, ½ c.	59

*From: Acosta, P., and Elsas, L.: Dietary Management of Inherited Metabolic Disease: Phenylketonuria, Galactosemia, Tyrosinemia, Maple Syrup Urine Disease. Atlanta, Ga., ACELMU Publishers, 1976.

[a]Available from General Mills Chemicals, Inc., Special Dietary Foods, 4620 W. 77th Street, Minneapolis, Minnesota, 55435.

Table 39–5 MENU FOR CHILD WITH PKU

MEAL	PHENYLALANINE (mg.)	PROTEIN (gm.)	ENERGY (kcal.)
Breakfast			
6 oz. Lofenalac	96.3	7.0	194.5
2 T. Baby oatmeal cereal	36	0.8	18
2 T. Strained applesauce and apricots	3	0.06	24
Mid-A.M. Feeding			
6 oz. orange-pineapple juice	6	0.5	59.0
Lunch			
6 oz. Lofenalac	96.3	7.0	194.5
2½ T. Baby barley cereal	37.5	0.8	23
2 T. Strained applesauce and apricots	3	.08	24
Mid-P.M. Feeding			
Water, as desired			
Dinner			
6 oz. Lofenalac	96.3	7.0	194.5
3 T. Strained sweet potatoes	30	0.6	30.0
2 T. Strained applesauce and apricots	3	0.06	24
Evening Feeding			
6 oz. Lofenalac	96.3	7.0	194.5
TOTAL	503.7	30.9	980

treated at birth with a low-phenylalanine diet. Without dietary restriction of phenylalanine, mental retardation can occur.

Another variant form involves a deficiency of *tetrahydropteridine reductase,* which helps to generate a cofactor necessary to activate *phenylalanine hydroxylase.* Unfortunately, it has been demonstrated that dietary treatment alone is not adequate to promote normal intellectual development in children with this disorder.[17]

Maternal Phenylketonuria

As women who have phenylketonuria reach child-bearing age, the issue of their treatment during pregnancy must be considered. Although there is rather limited information about this topic, it is known that these women must follow a low-phenylalanine diet immediately following conception and throughout their entire pregnancy,[3] but they are still likely to have a mentally retarded child. An investigational product, 3229 (Mead Johnson), is currently being utilized to prevent fetal damage (see Table 39–2). The phenylalanine content of 3229 is negligible, and the protein content is more concentrated than Lofenalac in order to provide a larger selection of natural foods. Table 39–6 lists low-protein products that are useful in planning diets for children and adults with phenylketonuria.

TYROSINEMIA

Several disorders of tyrosine metabolism are known to exist. At least two, neonatal

Table 39–6 LOW-PROTEIN SPECIALTY PRODUCTS AND THEIR SOURCES

PRODUCT	SOURCE
Cellu Wheat Starch Lo Pro Pastas Low Protein Baking Mix and Bread	Chicago Dietetic Supply, Inc. 405 East Shawnut Avenue La Grange, Illinois, 60526
Controlyte	D. M. Doyle Pharmaceutical Co. Highway 100 at W. 23rd Street Minneapolis, Minnesota, 55416
Low Protein Bread and Mix Potato Mix Egg Replacer	Ener-G-Foods, Inc. 1526 Utah Avenue, South Seattle, Washington, 98134
Aproten Low Protein Pastas, Rusks, Porridge Cal-Power Beverages Dietetic Paygel Baking Mix Dietetic Paygel Wheat Starch Low Protein Canned Bread Prono (No-Protein Gelatin)	General Mills Chemicals, Inc. 4620 W. 77th Street Minneapolis, Minnesota, 55440

tyrosinemia and hereditary tyrosinemia, are responsive to dietary treatment.

Neonatal Tyrosinemia

Metabolic Defect. Premature infants may be born with insufficient amounts of the liver enzymes *tyrosine aminotransferase, phenylalanine hydroxylase* and *p-hydroxyphenylpyruvic acid oxidase.*[23] (See Fig. 39–2.) The last of these enzymes is required for the conversion of p-hydroxyphenylpyruvic acid to homogentisic acid. This particular enzymatic reaction has an unusually high requirement for ascorbic acid.[19] The manifestation of neonatal tyrosinemia, tyrosyluria, is thought to be aggravated by (1) a limited vitamin C intake, (2) a high-protein diet and (3) limited liver function due to immaturity.[23] The hypertyrosinemia peaks at the end of the first week of life and can persist for several weeks after birth.[8]

It is uncertain at this time whether or not neonatal tyrosinemia is a benign disorder. Gretsky, in a follow-up study of 62 infants when they reached seven years of age, reported that the children affected with neonatal tyrosinemia scored lower on the Wechsler intelligence tests than control children did.[14] However, the lower intelligence scores may not be the result of abnormal tyrosine metabolism. Hyperammonemia, which is a secondary result of high dietary protein intake and the liver's inability to convert it to urea, may be the responsible factor.[23]

Diagnosis. It is necessary to differentiate neonatal tyrosinemia from other types of tyrosinemia before treatment is begun. A convenient method for quantitatively assaying tyrosine in the serum has been described by Fernbach.[10]

Nutritional Care. There is a two-fold goal in the nutritional care of neonatal tyrosinemia: (1) restriction of dietary protein to 2 to 3 gm. per kg. per day to reduce a metabolic overloading of the liver and (2) provision of an adequate amount of ascorbic acid (50 to 100 mg. per day) to serve as cofactor in the conversion of p-hydroxyphenylpyruvic acid to hemogentisic acid.

Hereditary Tyrosinemia

Metabolic Defect. In this more serious type of tyrosinemia, biochemical studies have shown massive tyrosyluria and excessive accumulation of p-hydroxyphenylpyruvic acid and p-hydroxyphenyllactic acid in the urine. Hypermethionemia has been observed in many affected infants and is thought to reflect acute liver failure.[29]

The clinical manifestations of this disease include failure to thrive, progressive liver disease and renal damage that can lead to the Fanconi syndrome, with hypophosphatemic rickets, mental retardation, cataracts, hypoglycemia and hyperpigmentation.

Diagnosis. A diagnosis of hereditary tyrosinemia can be made by *in vitro* assay of the liver enzyme.

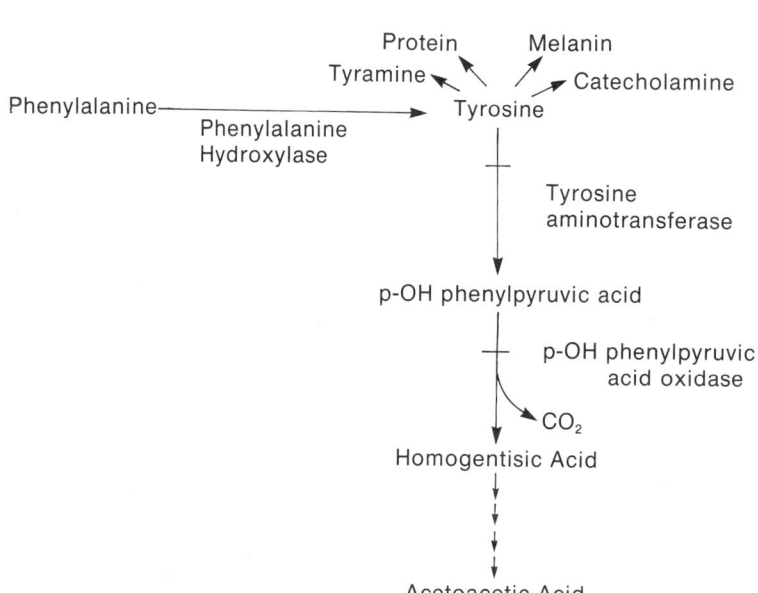

Figure 39–2 Tyrosine metabolism. (Adapted from: Acosta, P., and Elsas, L.: Dietary Management of Inherited Metabolic Disease: Phenylketonuria, Galactosemia, Tyrosinemia, Maple Syrup Urine Disease. Atlanta, Georgia, ACELMU Publishers, 1976.)

Table 39–7 RECOMMENDED PHENYLALANINE, TYROSINE, PROTEIN AND ENERGY INTAKES FOR TYROSINEMIC CHILDREN*†

AGE	PHENYLALANINE (mg./kg.)	TYROSINE (mg./kg.)	PROTEIN (gm./kg.)	ENERGY (kcal.)
0–3 mo.	60–80[a]	60–80[a]	4.4	120
4–6 mo.	58–75[b]	61–82[b]	3.3	115
7–12 mo.	42[c]	42[c]	2.2	110
1–3 yr.	25–85	25–85[e,g]	23 Total	1300 Total
4–8 yr.	22–50[h,i]	8–50[h,i]	30 Total	1800 Total
9–10 yr.	25[i]	25[i]	36 Total	2400 Total
13–14 yr.	1026 Total[j,k]	523 Total[j,k]	44 Total	2400–2800 Total

*From: Acosta, P., and Elsas, L.: Dietary Management of Inherited Metabolic Disease: Phenylketonuria, Galactosemia, Tyrosinemia, Maple Syrup Urine Disease. Atlanta, Ga. ACELMU Publishers, 1976.

†Total phenylalanine plus tyrosine should be considered in the prescription since most phenylalanine is converted to tyrosine.

[a] Acta Paediatr. Scand., 58:37, 1969.
[b] Arch. Dis. Child., 44:258, 1969.
[c] Arch. Dis. Child., 43:540, 1968.
[d] Am. J. Dis. Child., 113:41, 1967.
[e] Am. J. Dis. Child., 113:38, 1967.
[f] Am. J. Dis. Child., 113:47, 1967.
[g] J. Pediatr., 72:620, 1968.
[h] Am. J. Dis. Child., 113:31, 1967.
[i] Can. Med. Assoc. J., 97:1089, 1967.
[j] J. Am. Diet. Assoc., 56:308, 1970.
[k] Can. Med. Assoc. J., 108:477, 1973.

Nutritional Care. A diet that includes the appropriate amounts of tyrosine and phenylalanine must be instituted in order to prevent the clinical disorders of this disease from progressing. Dietary phenylalanine must be monitored in the treatment of hereditary tyrosinemia to prevent a deficiency state from occurring. Table 39–4 lists the tyrosine and phenylalanine values of some commonly used foods. Table 39–7 gives the recommended dietary intakes of phenylalanine, tyrosine and calories for tyrosinemic children.

Mead Johnson's formula 3200-AB (Table 39–2) is available for the treatment of this disease, but it contains a high amount of methionine, which may be inappropriate for individuals who have low levels of the methionine-activating enzyme cystathionine synthetase. A synthetic formula containing specific amounts of dietary phenylalanine, tyrosine, and methionine can be produced in a laboratory.

Guidelines for frequent feedings to prevent the hypoglycemia that may occur when a child is in liver failure should be outlined for the parents. In individuals with hypophosphatemic rickets, large doses of vitamin D (10,000 to 50,000 I.U. per day) should be included, or an analog of the active form of vitamin D ($1\alpha,25$-[OH]$_2D_3$) may be used in much smaller amounts.

HOMOCYSTINURIA

Metabolic Defect. Homocystinuria, a genetic anomaly, results from a defect in the activity of *cystathionine synthetase,* the enzyme responsible for the conversion of methionine to cystine (see Fig. 39–3). Although there are various forms of homocystinuria, only the type described here is amenable to nutritional intervention.

Homocystine and methionine, normally present in trace amounts in the urine, can be found in excessive amounts in individuals with homocystinuria. Increased levels of these amino acids are also present in the serum and cerebrospinal fluid.

A fibrotic change in the intima of the blood vessels is a pathological indication of homocystinuria. This condition causes a fragmentation of the elastic tissue of the large arteries, which is accompanied by a decrease in the protein-polysaccharide matrix. In turn, thromboembolic episodes, which are life-threatening, can occur. The development of these thrombi suggest a hypercoagulability of the blood, which is related to platelet stickiness.[27, 34] However, this clinical finding may not be observed in all cases of homocystinuria.

Another manifestation of homocystinuria is ectopia lentis, a degeneration of the zonular fibers of the eye lens, resulting in a "wandering eye." Studies indicate that the lens of the eye is poorly anchored, a secondary result of the cystine deficiency.[31]

The mental retardation that may occur in the affected child is due either to excessive amounts of methionine and homocystine or to inadequate amounts of cystathionine or cystine. The latter condition could inhibit transport of amino acids to the brain.[8]

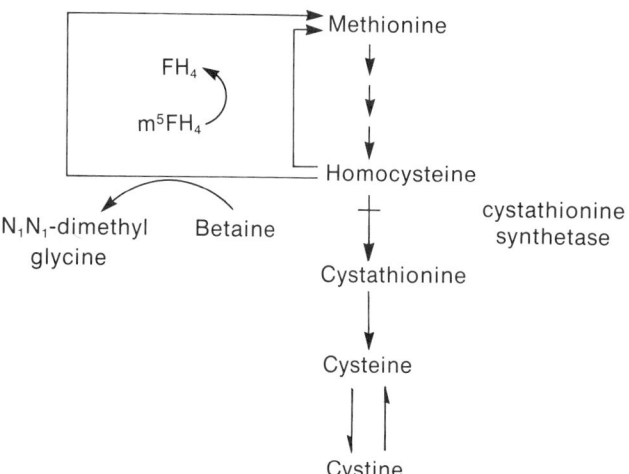

Figure 39–3   Metabolism of methionine.

Diagnosis.   A cyanide-nitroprusside test of the urine can be used as a simple screening method for homocystinuria. However, infants who have this disease may excrete very little homocystine in their urine and thus elude early detection.

Nutritional Care

The aims of dietary treatment are (1) to reduce the potentially toxic levels of methionine and (2) to provide a supplementary allowance of cystine. A low-protein, low-methionine diet should be used to reduce the elevated plasma methionine and homocystine concentrations. This type of diet generally excludes the *animal* forms of protein—meat, fish, egg, milk and dairy products.

Special dietary formulas, such as 3200-K (Mead Johnson), Low Methionine Isomil and Methionaid (both from Ross), have been successfully used in the treatment of this disorder (see Table 39–2).

Table 39–8 outlines the suggested methionine, protein and calorie requirements to be used in the treatment of homocystinuria. Food exchange lists developed by Mahan can be used in planning a diet for a child with this disease. These food groups are presented in Table 39–9.

Controversy exists about whether or not older children and adults with this disorder should adhere to dietary treatment. Some research indicates that lethal vascular occlusions occur less frequently among individuals who maintain a low-methionine diet throughout their lives.[20]

Another issue that must be considered in the nutritional care of homocystinuria is the addition of vitamin B_6 (pyridoxine) to the diet. Spaeth and Barber observed a "complete reversal" of biochemical abnormalities in three children who were treated with 250 to 500 mg. of pyridoxine daily.[31] Results of other studies are not so dramatic and indicate a likelihood that there is more than one mutation of the synthetase enzyme.

HISTIDINEMIA

Metabolic   Defect.   Histidinemia, a metabolic disorder characterized by decreased activity of the enzyme *histidase*, was first described in 1962.[13] Biochemical findings reveal increased amounts of histidine in the blood and urine and impaired formation of urocanic acid, which is easily detected in the sweat. Figure 39–4 illustrates the degradation pathway of histidine.

Table 39–8   SUGGESTED METHIONINE, PROTEIN AND ENERGY REQUIREMENTS FOR USE IN TREATMENT OF HOMOCYSTINURIA*

AGE (years)	METHIONINE (mg./kg./day)	PROTEIN (gm./kg./day)	ENERGY (kcal./kg./day)
0–0.5	42	2.00[a]/4.4[b]	120
0.6–1.0	20	1.50[a]/2.5[b]	110
1–3	10–23	1.25/25 Total	1300 Total
4–6	10–18	1.00/30 Total	1800 Total
7–10	10–13	1.00/35 Total	2400 Total

*From: Acosta, P., and Elsas, L.: Dietary Management of Inherited Metabolic Disease: Phenylketonuria, Galactosemia, Tyrosinemia, Maple Syrup Urine Disease. Atlanta, Ga., ACELMU Publishers, 1976.
[a]Suggested protein level when Isomil is used.
[b]Greater amounts of protein may be offered when Methionaid or 3200-K is used.

Table 39–9 FOOD EXCHANGE LISTS USED IN TREATMENT OF HOMOCYSTINURIA*

BREADS AND CEREALS—10 mg. methionine, 1 gm.
  protein
French or Vienna bread	10 gm.
Rye, American	8 gm.
White, enriched	½ slice
Corn flakes	⅓ cup

SOUPS
Beef broth	65 gm.
Clam chowder	65 gm.

VEGETABLES—5 mg. methionine, 1 gm. protein
Asparagus, canned, white	1 spear
Beans, green, canned	35 gm.
Beets, canned	½ cup diced
Brussels sprouts	1 medium
Cabbage, head	½ cup shredded
Carrots, raw	½ cup diced
Celery, raw	⅓ cup diced
Chard	½ cup cooked
Cucumber	1″ slice
Eggplant, raw	½ cup
Lettuce	100 gm.
Pumpkin, canned	¼ cup
Squash, raw, summer	75 gm.
Tomato	1 small

FRUITS—5 mg. methionine, 0.5 gm. protein
Apple, raw	1 medium
Banana	½ small
Guava	½ medium
Mango	½ small
Orange	1 small
Papaya	⅔ medium
Pineapple	1½ cups

FOODS THAT ARE RELATIVELY FREE OF
  METHIONINE
  Butter
  Candy
    butterscotch
    cream mints
    fondant
    gum drops
    hard candy
    jelly beans
    lollipops
  Carbonated beverages
  Grapefruit
  Guava butter
  Honey
  Jams, jellies, marmalades
  Molasses
  Pineapple (count as fruit if more than 250 gm.)
  Popsicles
  Sugar syrup

FOODS HIGH IN METHIONINE THAT SHOULD
  BE AVOIDED
  Cheese
  Corn
  Cow's milk
  Dried peas and beans
  Eggs
  Flours (white, whole wheat, buckwheat)
  Lima beans
  Meat, poultry, fish
  Nuts and nut butters
  Oatmeal
  Peas, fresh
  Potatoes
  Rice
  Spinach

*Developed by L. K. Mahan.

A unique characteristic of the amino acid histidine is that it is considered an essential amino acid during infancy but not in preadolescence or adulthood. However, the exact age at which liver tissue becomes able to synthesize histidine is still under investigation.[36]

The clinical symptoms present in histidinemia include mental retardation and disordered speech development. The degree of mental retardation or development of a speech defect may be related to the mother's consumption of a high-protein diet during pregnancy or to the infant's consumption of a high-protein diet immediately following birth.[35]

Diagnosis. Successful screening methods have been developed for the detection and diagnosis of histidinemia. Gerber and Gerber have described a technique that measures histidine concentration in the urine. In this test, cupric ions and bis-cyclohexanone react to

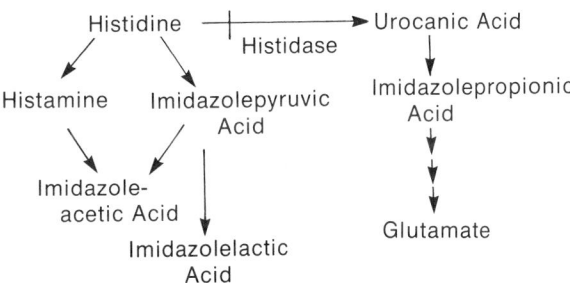

Figure 39–4 Metabolism of histidine.

produce a blue color. The addition of histidine inhibits the color reaction and provides the basis for this simple yet effective test.[12]

Nutritional Care

Although there is limited research concerning the implementation of a low-histidine diet in the treatment of histidinemia, there are indications that dietary control might possibly be effective.[5] Some individuals who have reduced their dietary intake of histidine have reduced the concentration of histidine in their urine and blood. However, clinical manifestations of this disorder are not always improved by adherence to the diet.

Histinaid (Ross), an amino acid mixture (Table 39–2), has been used in the treatment of this disease.

MAPLE SYRUP URINE DISEASE

Metabolic Defect. Maple syrup urine disease (MSUD), also known as *branched-chain alpha-ketoaciduria,* was first described by Menkes in 1954.[21] The metabolic defect is located in the second step of the degradation of valine, leucine and isoleucine. Figure 39–5 demonstrates the catabolism of these three amino acids. It appears that although the transamination reaction proceeds normally in this disorder, there is an impairment in the decarboxylation step. This results in the accumulation of the amino acids and their corresponding keto acids in the blood and urine. The characteristic odor of maple syrup that results from the excess keto acids has been observed in the infant's perspiration, ear wax and urine.

An infant with MSUD may appear normal at birth but begins to eat poorly during the first week of life. It is not unusual for the baby to have severe vomiting and abnormal bowel movements. Neurological symptoms, such as muscle hypertonicity, lethargy, abnormal eye movement and convulsions, may also appear. Respiratory difficulty, which may lead to coma and death if MSUD is not diagnosed and treated, is a grave consequence of this disease.

There are several variant types of maple syrup urine disease. *Intermittent (late-manifesting) branched-chain ketoaciduria* may not be detected until late infancy or early childhood. Affected individuals appear to have a small amount of decarboxylase activity. Clinical symptoms may not appear until a specific stimulus such as an infection precipitates the metabolic abnormality. Dietary intervention may be successful in the treatment of this variant form.

The consistent finding in *mild branched-chain ketoaciduria* is the defective branched-chain keto acid oxidation, which leads to increased concentrations of valine, leucine and isoleucine and their corresponding keto acids in plasma and urine. However, the relationship of enzymatic and environmental factors to the mild and intermittent forms of MSUD is not completely understood. Therefore it is difficult to distinguish between these two variants.

Thiamin-responsive branched-chain ketoaciduria is a variant form of MSUD that is known to improve when supraphysiological amounts of thiamin pyrophosphate (100 to 200 mg. per day) are given. The specific activity of the decarboxylase enzyme is increased by the thiamin, which prolongs its biological half-life.[7]

Diagnosis. A diagnosis of MSUD can be confirmed by measuring the amount of the de-

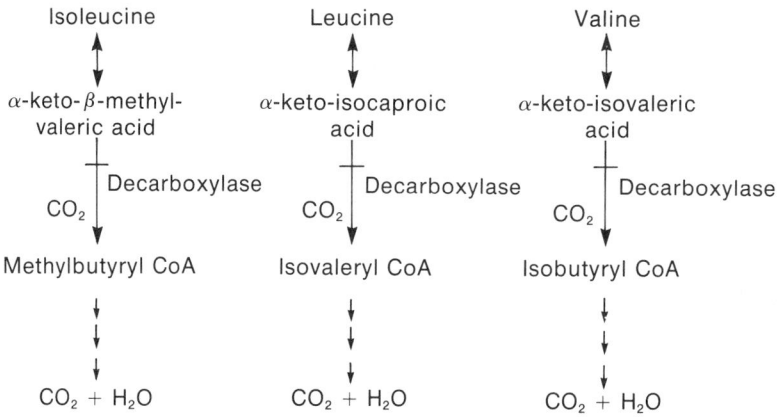

Figure 39–5 Metabolism of isoleucine, leucine and valine.

Table 39–10 RECOMMENDED AMOUNTS OF PROTEIN, ISOLEUCINE, LEUCINE, VALINE AND ENERGY FOR CHILDREN WITH BRANCHED-CHAIN KETOACIDURIA*

AGE	ISOLEUCINE (mg./kg.)	LEUCINE (mg./kg.)	VALINE (mg./kg.)	PROTEIN (gm./kg.)	ENERGY (kcal./kg.)
<3 mo.	70	161	93	2.2[a]/4.4[b]	120
3–6 mo.	70	161	93	2.2/3.3	115
6–9 mo.[c]				2.0/2.5	110
9–11 mo.[c]				2.0/2.5	105
1–3 yr.[c]				25 Total	1300 Total
4–6 yr.[c]				30 Total	1800 Total
7–10 yr.	30	45	33	35 Total	2400 Total

*From: Acosta, P., and Elsas, L.: Dietary Management of Inherited Metabolic Disease: Phenylketonuria, Galactosemia, Tyrosinemia, Maple Syrup Urine Disease. Atlanta, Ga., ACELMU Publishers, 1976.
[a] Amounts to use with gelatin-amino acid mix.
[b] Amounts to use with MSUDAid or pure amino acids.
[c] No data available on amino acid needs for ages 7 mo. to 7 yr. Plasma levels should be used to determine dietary amounts.

carboxylase enzyme present in the infant's skin or blood cells. Cultured skin fibroblasts or leukocyte samples, or both, are used in this determination.

Nutritional Care

Planning a diet for an infant or child with MSUD can be a challenge, as the dietary intake of the three branched-chain amino acids—valine, leucine and isoleucine—must be controlled. The levels of these amino acids in the infant's serum determine the specific amount that must be included in the diet. Recommended amounts of valine, leucine and isoleucine by age category are given in Table 39–10.

Product 80056 (Mead Johnson), a dry blend mixture of carbohydrate, fat, vitamins and minerals, is an appropriate formula base to utilize in this diet (Table 39–2). Since this product does not contain any protein, an additional dry base amino acid mixture must also be provided. Specific amounts of valine, leucine and isoleucine can be supplied in crystalline form. Gelatin can also serve as a source of these and other amino acids.

Food exchange lists that give specific dietary values of valine, leucine and isoleucine are provided in Table 39–11.

OTHER DISORDERS OF AMINO ACID METABOLISM

Table 39–12 outlines some additional amino acid disorders and the enzymatic defect, clinical manifestations and dietary treatment for each.

DISORDERS OF CARBOHYDRATE METABOLISM

GALACTOSEMIA

Metabolic Defect. Galactosemia is the metabolic disorder that results when the enzymatic process fails to convert galactose to glucose. Figure 39–6 describes the enzymatic blocks in the pathway of glucose-galactose interconversion that occur in disorders of galactose metabolism.

In cases of *classical galactosemia,* the enzyme *galactose-1-phosphate uridyl transferase* is deficient or is present in levels too low to allow normal galactose metabolism. (See *B* in Figure 39–6.) This causes galactose-1-phosphate to accumulate in the erythrocytes, liver, spleen, lens of the eye, kidney, heart muscle and cerebral cortex. Shortly after birth the affected infant develops gastrointestinal disturbances, fails to gain weight and frequently becomes jaundiced. If the child is untreated, mental retardation becomes obvious at 6 to 12 months of age.

Hereditary *galactokinase* deficiency, which is a variant of galactosemia, results from a defect in the phosphorylation of galactose to produce galactose-1-phosphate. (See *A* in Figure 39–6.) Since galactose-1-phosphate does not accumulate in this type of galactosemia, the damage results from a high concentration of galactose itself. Clinically, this variant form differs from the classical type in that the gastrointestinal disturbances are absent and mental development appears to be normal. However, if an early diagnosis is not made, cataract

Text continued on page 797

Table 39–11   FOOD EXCHANGE LISTS FOR DIETS RESTRICTED IN ISOLEUCINE, LEUCINE AND VALINE*

VEGETABLES

Contain per serving an average of 23 mg. isoleucine, 30 mg. leucine, 27 mg. valine, 0.7 gm. protein and 15 kcal. Protein is 3.48% isoleucine, 4.55% leucine and 4.09% valine.

	ILEU. (mg.)	LEU. (mg.)	VAL. (mg.)	PRO. (gm.)	ENERGY (kcal.)
Asparagus, raw, 1½–2 spears (33 gm.)	18	32	26	0.7	9
Asparagus, canned, green, 2 med. spears (38 gm.)	26	32	35	0.7	7
Beans, green, raw, cooked in small amount of water, ¼ c. (31 gm.)	22	29	24	0.5	8
Beans, green, canned, drained solids ¼ c. (31 gm.)	20	26	21	0.4	8
Beans, yellow wax, canned, drained solids ¼ c. (50 gm.)	32	40	33	0.7	12
Beets, canned, drained, ½ c. (100 gm.)	29	28	25	0.8	31
Beet greens, cooked, 2 T. (25 gm.)	18	27	21	0.2	4
Brussels sprouts, cooked, drained, 1 sprout (17 gm.)	29	31	31	0.7	6
Cabbage, raw, ½ c. shredded (50 gm.)	26	26	20	0.6	12
Cabbage, cooked in small amount of water, 5 T. (50 gm.)	22	22	16	0.6	10
Carrots, raw, ½ large (50 gm.)	16	25	25	0.55	21
Carrots, canned, drained solids, ½ c.	24	34	30	0.64	24
Chard, frozen cooked, 3 T. (33 gm.)	26	32	23	0.8	8
Collards, frozen cooked, 1½ T. (18 gm.)	16	30	27	0.6	6
Cucumber, not pared, 1 med. (100 gm.)	18	26	20	0.1	16
Eggplant, cooked, drained, ¼ c. (50 gm.)	26	31	30	0.5	10
Kale, frozen cooked, 2 T. (17 gm.)	17	32	24	0.5	5
Lettuce, raw, (25 gm.)	12	21	18	0.3	4
Mustard greens, frozen cooked, ¼ c. (50 gm.)	36	30	52	1.1	10
Okra, cooked, 2 pods (25 gm.)	21	31	28	0.55	10
Onion, raw, 6 T. chopped (60 gm.)	18	30	40	1.2	24
Potato, boiled in skin, ⅓ med. (33 gm.)	31	35	37	0.7	25
Spinach, frozen cooked, 1 T. (12 gm.)	17	28	20	0.4	3
Squash, summer, cooked, drained, ½ c. (100 gm.)	29	41	33	0.9	14
Squash, winter, boiled, 3 T. (50 gm.)	17	25	20	0.55	19
Sweet potato, baked, ¼ small (25 gm.)	25	30	39	0.52	35
Tomato, raw, 1 small (100 gm.)	32	45	31	1.1	22
Tomato, canned, 6 T. (75 gm.)	22	31	21	0.75	16
Tomato juice, canned, ½ c. (100 gm.)	26	37	25	0.9	19
Turnip greens, cooked in small amount of water (12 gm.)	14	27	19	0.37	4

GERBER'S STRAINED AND JUNIOR VEGETABLES

	ILEU. (mg.)	LEU. (mg.)	VAL. (mg.)	PRO. (gm.)	ENERGY (kcal.)
Amounts in 7 T. (100 gm.)					
Beets	47	46	41	1.3	38
Carrots	26	37	33	0.7	30
Green beans	57	75	62	1.3	29
Squash	25	36	29	0.8	27
Sweet potatoes	67	81	105	1.4	69
Amounts in 1 T.					
Beets	6.7	6.6	5.9	0.19	5.4
Carrots	3.7	5.3	4.7	0.1	4.3
Green beans	8.1	10.7	8.9	0.19	4.1
Squash	3.6	5.1	4.1	0.11	3.9
Sweet potatoes	9.6	11.6	15	0.2	9.9

Table 39–11   FOOD EXCHANGE LISTS FOR DIETS RESTRICTED IN ISOLEUCINE, LEUCINE AND VALINE (*Continued*)

FRUITS

Contain per serving an average of 15 mg. isoleucine, 25 mg. leucine, 25 mg. valine, 0.6 gm. protein and 90 kcal. Protein is 2.85% isoleucine, 4.35% leucine and 3.73% valine.

	ILEU. (mg.)	LEU. (mg.)	VAL. (mg.)	PRO. (gm.)	ENERGY (kcal.)
Apple, raw, 1 small 2″ diam. (100 gm.)	13	23	15	0.4	58
Applesauce, canned, sweetened, ⅔ c. (200 gm.)	13	23	15	0.4	182
Apple juice, 1½ c.	13	23	15	0.4	174
Apricot, raw, 2–3 med. (100 gm.)	14	23	19	0.8	51
Apricot, canned, sweetened, 4 med. halves (133 gm.)	14	23	19	0.8	115
Apricots, dried, 3 halves (18 gm.)	14	23	19	0.8	52
Avocado, 3½ T. (33 gm.)	16	25	21	0.5	56
Banana, ½ small (50 gm.)	16	26	22	0.6	42
Dates, domestic natural, 2 med. pitted (20 gm.)	15	15	19	0.4	55
Figs, raw, 1 large (50 gm.)	18	26	23	0.6	40
Orange, raw, 1 small 2½″ diam. (100 gm.)	23	22	31	0.8	49
Orange juice, canned, ²/₅ c. (100 gm.)	23	22	31	0.8	48
Peach, raw, 1 med. (100 gm.)	13	29	30	0.8	38
Peaches, canned, 4 med. halves & 4 T. syrup (200 gm.)	13	29	30	0.8	156
Peach nectar, canned, 1½ c. (370 gm.)	13	29	30	0.8	178
Pear, canned in syrup[a], 6 small halves & 6 T. syrup (300 gm.)	17	26	22	0.6	226
Pear, raw[a], ½ pear (100 gm.)	20	30	26	0.7	61
Pineapple, raw[a], 1½ c. diced (200 gm.)	23	35	30	0.8	104
Pineapple juice[a], 1 c. (240 gm.)	23	35	30	0.8	128
Pumpkin, canned, 3⅓ T. (50 gm.)	19	26	19	0.5	17
Strawberries, fresh, 7½ large (75 gm.)	14	32	17	0.6	28
Strawberries, frozen, & sugar, ½ c. (128 gm.)	14	32	17	0.6	140

GERBER'S STRAINED AND JUNIOR FRUITS

	ILEU. (mg.)	LEU. (mg.)	VAL. (mg.)	PRO. (gm.)	ENERGY (kcal.)
Amounts in 7 T. (100 gm.)					
Applesauce	6	12	8	0.2	81
Applesauce & apricots[b]	7	13	9	0.3	87
Applesauce with pineapple[b]	6	10	7	0.2	77
Apricots with tapioca[a]	6	12	9	0.4	80
Bananas with tapioca[c]	14	23	19	0.5	88
Bananas with pineapple & tapioca[b,c]	8	13	11	0.3	83
Peaches	10	22	22	0.6	82
Pears	11	17	15	0.4	69
Pears & pineapple[b]	11	17	15	0.4	71
Apple juice	3	6	4	0.1	49
Orange juice	14	14	19	0.5	50
Orange-apple juice	9	13	11	0.3	54
Orange-apricot juice	14	17	19	0.6	61
Orange-pineapple juice	14	22	19	0.5	59
Amounts in 1 T.					
Applesauce	<1	1.7	1.1	0.03	11.6
Applesauce & apricots	1	1.9	1.3	0.04	12.4
Applesauce with pineapple	<1	1.4	1	0.03	11.0
Apricots with tapioca	<1	1.7	1.3	0.06	11.4
Bananas with pineapple & tapioca	2	3.3	2.7	0.07	12.6
Peaches	1.4	3.1	3.1	0.09	11.7
Pears	1.6	2.4	2.1	0.06	9.9
Pears & pineapple	1.6	2.4	2.1	0.06	10.1

Table continued on the following page

Table 39–11 FOOD EXCHANGE LISTS FOR DIETS RESTRICTED IN ISOLEUCINE, LEUCINE AND VALINE (*Continued*)

BREAD AND CEREAL

Contain per serving an average of 15 mg. isoleucine, 35 mg. leucine, 20 mg. valine, 0.4 gm. protein and 20 kcal. Protein is 3.83% isoleucine, 8.08% leucine and 5.12% valine.

	ILEU. (mg.)	LEU. (mg.)	VAL. (mg.)	PRO. (gm.)	ENERGY (kcal.)
Ready to Serve					
Bran, All, Kellogg's, 1 T. (3.5 gm.)	13	26	19	0.4	12
Bran Flakes, 40%, 2 T. (4.7 gm.)	16	32	24	0.5	17
Bran, Raisin, Kellogg's, 2 T. (5 gm.)	15	30	22	0.4	18
Cheerios, 2 T. (3 gm.)	17	33	23	0.4	13
Cornflakes, 2 T. (3 gm.)	10	34	12	0.3	12
Rice Krispies, 4 T. (¼ c.) (7 gm.)	18	35	24	0.4	27
Rice, puffed, 8 T. (½ c.) (6 gm.)	18	35	24	0.4	25
Cooked					
Farina, cooked, 2 T.	23	33	21	0.5	18
Rice, brown, cooked, 2 T.	16	30	24	0.4	17
Rice, white, cooked, 2 T.	17	30	25	0.4	17
Special Low Protein Products[d,e]					
Aproten Macaroni Products					
Anellini, uncooked, ¾ c. (100 gm.)	13	26	15	0.5	340
Rigatini, uncooked, 1½ c. (100 gm.)	13	26	15	0.5	340
Tagliatelle, uncooked, 1¼ c. (100 gm.)	13	26	15	0.5	340
Paygel Low Protein Bread, 1 slice (32 gm.)				0.3	83
Aproten Rusks, 1 slice (11.5 gm.)	4	6	4	0.1	48

GERBER'S DRY CEREALS	ILEU. (mg.)	LEU. (mg.)	VAL. (mg.)	PRO. (gm.)	ENERGY (kcal.)
Amounts in 1 T. (2.4 gm.)					
Barley	10	19	14	0.269	9
Oatmeal	14	6	20	0.359	9
Rice	6	12	10	0.159	9

GERBER'S CEREALS IN JARS

Amount in 1 T.					
Mixed with applesauce	6	12	8	0.2	12
Oatmeal with applesauce-bananas	5	9	6	0.2	11
Rice with applesauce-bananas	2	4	2	<0.1	10
Rice with mixed fruit	9	18	12	<0.1	10

FATS

Contain per serving an average of 7 mg. isoleucine, 10 mg. leucine, 8 mg. valine, 0.1 gm. protein and 70 kcal. Protein averages 5.83% isoleucine, 8.33% leucine and 6.67% valine.

Butter, 1 T. (14 gm.)	6	10	7	0.1	100
Cream, whipping (40%), 1 tsp. (5 gm.)	6	10	7	0.1	17
Coffee Rich, liquid, 1 T. (14 gm.)	8	11	8	0.1	24
French dressing, 2 T. (28 gm.)	6	7	7	0.2	114
Margarine, 2 tsp. (10 gm.)	5	7	5	0.1	72
Mayonnaise, 1 T. (14 gm.)	10	13	11	0.15	101
Tartar sauce, ½ T. (10 gm.)	7	9	7	0.1	47
Thousand Island dressing, 1 T. (14 gm.)	7	10	8	0.11	70

*From: Acosta, P., and Elsas, L.: Dietary Management of Inherited Metabolic Disease: Phenylketonuria, Galactosemia, Tyrosinemia, Maple Syrup Urine Disease. Atlanta, Ga., ACELMU Publishers, 1976.

[a] Amino acid content based on mean percentage of protein found in 10 fruits.

[b] Calculated on basis that product is one half of each fruit noted.

[c] Calculated on basis that fruit provides all the protein.

[d] Manufactured by General Mills Chemicals, Inc., Special Dietary Foods, 4620 W. 77th Street, Minneapolis, Minnesota, 55435.

[e] Not calculated in mean figures for amino acid content of Bread and Cereal list.

Table 39–12   SOME AMINO ACID DISORDERS THAT RESPOND TO DIETARY TREATMENT*

DISEASE	AMINO ACID/ ORGANIC ACID	ENZYMATIC DEFECT	CLINICAL MANIFESTATIONS	DIETARY TREATMENT
Hyperprolinemia	Proline	Proline oxidase deficiency. Pyrroline 5-carboxylate dehydrogenase deficiency has also been documented in hyperprolinemia	Mental retardation, renal disease	Effect of proline-restricted diet is not yet proven
Hyperlysinemia	Lysine	Lysine acyclase, lysine dehydrogenase or lysine ketoglutarate reductase deficiency	Convulsions, coma	Lysine-restricted diet
Hypervalinemia	Valine	Unknown	Vomiting, nystagmus, failure to thrive	Valine-restricted diet
Propionicacidemia	Propionic acid	Defective propionyl CoA carboxylase or apoenzyme biotin lipase	Mental retardation, metabolic acidosis, thrombocytopenia	High-calorie, minimum- to low-protein diet, biotin supplements, reduction of leucine, isoleucine & valine during infections
Methylomalonic-acidemia	Methylmalonic acid	Methylomalonyl CoA racemase or coenzyme B_{12} deficiency	Metabolic acidosis, vomiting	High-calorie, low-protein diet. Vitamin B_{12} supplements
Isovalericacidemia	Isovaleric acid	Isovaleric acid CoA dehydrogenase	Smell of sweaty feet, vomiting, lethargy	High-calorie, low-protein diet
Urea Cycle Disorders Arginosuccinic aciduria	Arginosuccinic acid, citrulline	Arginosuccinate lyase deficiency		
Ornithine transcarbamylase deficiency		Ornithine carbamyl transferase deficiency		
Citrullinuria	Citrulline, methionine	Arginosuccinate-synthetase deficiency	Convulsions, coma, ataxia	Protein-restricted diet
Argininuria	Arginine	Liver arginase deficiency		
Carbamyl phosphate synthetase deficiency	Glutamine, ammonia	Carbamyl phosphate synthetase deficiency		
Hyperornithinemia	Ornithine, lysine, ammonia	Unknown		

*Sources: Davidson, S., et al.: Human Nutrition and Dietetics, 6th rev. ed. New York, Longman, 1975; and Francis, D. E. M.: Diets for Sick Children, 3rd ed. Oxford, England, Blackwell Scientific Publications, 1974.

formation leading to blindness can result. Nutritional intervention, when implemented during the first month of life, can prevent cataract formation.

Diagnosis.   The laboratory tests that can be used to confirm a diagnosis of galactosemia include (1) the identification of galactose in the urine, (2) a galactose tolerance test and (3) specific red or white cell enzyme tests.

Ng has demonstrated prenatal diagnosis of galactosemia by studying the enzyme activity of galactokinase and galactose-1-phosphate uridyl transferase in cultures of amniotic cells.

Since there is concern that some degree of irreversible damage may occur to the fetus, prenatal diagnosis of galactosemia can determine the mother's need to restrict her dietary intake of galactose during her pregnancy.[22]

Nutritional Care

Galactose, a simple monosaccharide, is a component of lactose (milk sugar). Since milk is the main source of galactose in the diet, a milk-substitute formula must be used when planning a diet for the infant with galactosemia.

(1) GALACTOSE + ATP ◄——————┤— A ——►GALACTOSE-1-PHOSPHATE + ADP

(2) GALACTOSE-1-PHOSPHATE ◄—┤— B ——►UDP-GALACTOSE + GLUCOSE-1-PHOSPHATE

(3) UDP-GALACTOSE ◄——————┤— C ——► UDP-GLUCOSE

(4) UDP-GLUCOSE + PP ◄——————┤— D ——► UTP + GLUCOSE-1-PHOSPHATE

    A = GALACTOKINASE
    B = GALACTOSE-1-PHOSPHATE
        URIDYLTRANSFERASE
    C = UDP-GALACTOSE-4-EPIMERASE
    D = UDP-GLUCOSE PYROPHOSPHORYLASE

Figure 39–6 Enzymatic blocks in the pathway of galactose-glucose interconversion that occur in disorders of galactose metabolism. (Adapted from: Galactosemia in Infancy. Evansville, Indiana, Mead Johnson and Co., 1976.)

Nutramigen (Mead Johnson), a casein hydrolysate, is the most commonly used formula in the treatment of galactosemia, although the soy milk formulas are also safe to use. (See Table 35–7C.)

As solid foods are introduced into the infant's diet, care must be taken to read the labels on processed food products for lactose-containing ingredients such as non-fat dry milk solids, casein, whey or whey solids. However, foods containing lactate, lactic acid and lactalbumin are safe to include in the diet. See Table 39–13 for a galactose-free diet.

Although some physicians advocate a less stringent galactose-restricted diet as the child reaches puberty, there is evidence that the diet should not be relaxed for older children who have this disorder.[30]

HEREDITARY FRUCTOSE INTOLERANCE

Metabolic Defect. The metabolic disorders associated with abnormal fructose metabolism are (1) essential, or benign, fructosuria, (2) fructose-1,6-diphosphatase deficiency and (3) hereditary fructose intolerance.

In *essential fructosuria,* a relatively rare disorder, the individual is asymptomatic. Although this condition is thought to be harmless, there is a deficiency of the enzyme *fructokinase* (Fig. 39–7). Affected infants, however, appear to have no clinical manifestations.

Fructose-1,6-diphosphatase deficiency, another form of fructose intolerance, can result in hypoglycemia and metabolic acidosis. This disorder is associated with hepatomegaly, but the incidence of liver failure is rare.[35]

In *hereditary fructose intolerance,* the primary enzymatic defect is the absence of *fructose-1-phosphate aldolase* (Fig. 39–7). The symptoms of both this inborn error and the fructose-1,6-diphosphatase deficiency are precipitated after the ingestion of fructose or fructose-containing foods. The clinical manifestations include severe vomiting, hypochromic anemia, hypoglycemia, jaundice and hepatomegaly. The bottle-fed infant who receives a formula containing sucrose, which is hydrolyzed to fructose, develops more severe symptoms of this disorder than the breast-fed infant. Breast-fed infants usually remain asymptomatic, since breast milk contains only lactose, which is not dependent on fructose-1-phosphate aldolase for its catabolism.

Diagnosis. There are several diagnostic tests that can be given to the individual who is suspected of having hereditary fructose intolerance. These procedures include (1) an intravenous fructose tolerance test, (2) an oral fructose tolerance test and (3) analyses of enzyme activity.

Nutritional Care

The exclusion of all sources of fructose and sucrose is essential in the dietary treatment of this disorder. Infant formulas that contain fructose and sucrose must be replaced by formulas that provide an alternate form of carbohydrate. Appropriate products to use include CHO-Free and Pregestimil, which are described in Table 14–3. Table 39–14 outlines those foods that must be eliminated in a fructose-sucrose-free diet. See also Appendix Table 12.

Ascorbic acid supplementation should be provided to compensate for vitamin C de-

Table 39–13   FOOD LIST FOR GALACTOSE-FREE DIET*

FOODS ALLOWED	FOODS NOT ALLOWED
MILK AND MILK SUBSTITUTES	
Isomil	Breast milk
Neo-mull-soy	All forms of animal milk
Nutramigen	Imitation or filled milk
Prosobee	Cream
Soyalac	Cottage cheese
Meat-base formula	Hard cheeses
	Yogurt
	Ice cream, ice milk, sherbet
FRUITS	
All fresh, frozen, canned or dried, except those listed in column two	Fruits processed with unsafe ingredients[a]
	Diabetic or dietetic fruits processed with unsafe ingredients
VEGETABLES	
All fresh, frozen, canned or dried, except those listed in column two	Vegetables processed with unsafe ingredients, seasoned with butter or margarine, breaded or creamed
	Instant mashed potatoes containing lactose or other unsafe ingredients
	Commercially packaged fried potatoes containing lactose or other unsafe ingredients
MEAT, POULTRY, FISH, EGGS AND NUTS	
Plain beef, lamb, veal, pork, ham	Creamed, buttered or breaded meat, fish, eggs or poultry
Plain fish, turkey, chicken, game, fowl	Frankfurters, cold cuts or liver sausage made with milk, lactose or unsafe ingredients
Kosher frankfurters	Organ meats: liver, brains, sweetbreads, kidneys, pancreas, heart
Eggs prepared without milk, cream, butter or margarine	
Nut butters (peanut butter)	
Nuts	
BREADS AND CEREALS	
Cooked and dry cereals without milk or lactose added	Cereals, bread, or crackers that have milk, milk products, or lactose added
Bread or crackers without milk or lactose added (saltines, graham crackers, water breads, hard rolls). Contact bakery if not sure. Read all labels.	Dry cereals
	Cream of wheat or rice
Macaroni, spaghetti, noodles, rice	Pancakes, waffles, French toast
Tortilla, flour, and corn	Zwieback
	Crackers made with butter or margarine
	Prepared muffin or biscuit mixes
FATS	
All vegetable oils (soybean, corn, olive, cottonseed, safflower, peanut)	Butter
All shortening, lard, margarines containing safe ingradients	Cream
	Cream cheese
Bacon	Margarine with lactose
Mayonnaise	Salad dressing with butter, milk or lactose
Olives	
Salad dressings with safe ingredients	

*From: Parents' Guide to the Galactose-Restricted Diet. Davis, California, Maternal and Child Health Branch, California Department of Health Services, Department of Nutrition, University of California. Revised 1976.

[a]Unsafe ingredients would be those containing lactose or galactose.

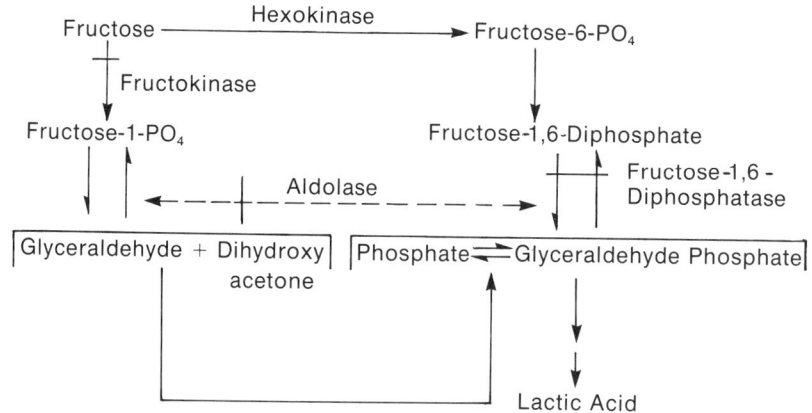

Figure 39–7 Metabolism of fructose. (Adapted from: Wong, P. W., and Hsia, D. Y.: Inborn errors of metabolism. In: Goodhart, R. S., and Shils, M. E. (eds.): Modern Nutrition in Health and Disease, 5th ed., Philadelphia, Lea & Febiger, 1973, p. 1026.)

ficiency caused by the omission of fruit from the diet.

Invert sugar, sorbitol or levulose should never be administered parenterally to individuals affected by hereditary fructose intolerance. In such people, these substances can cause

Table 39–14 FOODS THAT MUST BE ELIMINATED IN A FRUCTOSE-SUCROSE– FREE DIET*

MILK	Infant formulas containing fructose or sucrose; sweetened condensed milk, commercial chocolate milk, milk drinks with added sugar, ice cream or sherbet.
MEATS	Meats processed in sugar brine, such as ham, bacon and luncheon meat.
CEREALS	Sugar-coated cereals, defatted wheat germ, rice, bran.
DESSERTS	Cookies, cakes and other desserts made with sugar, sweet or chocolate milk, syrup or molasses.
POTATOES	Sweet potatoes. (Regular white cooking potatoes may provide a significant source of fructose, depending upon harvesting, storage and cooking techniques.)
VEGETABLES	Broccoli, cucumber, peas, rhubarb, beets, carrots, parsnips, pumpkins, rutabagas, winter squash, turnips, corn and hominy.
FRUITS	ALL FRUITS AND FRUIT JUICES SHOULD BE ELIMINATED.
MISCELLANEOUS	Granulated, powdered and brown sugars; milk and sweet chocolate; honey, jelly, syrup, molasses, sorghum; peanuts and other nuts.

*From: Francis, D. E. M.: Diets for Sick Children, 3rd ed. Oxford, Blackwell Scientific Publications, 1974.

severe vomiting, hypoglycemia and possibly death.

STARCH INTOLERANCE

Metabolic Defect. Newborn infants who have decreased amounts of *pancreatic amylase* exhibit an intolerance for starch. This disorder is sometimes confused with celiac disease, since the symptoms are similar. The stools have the same frothy appearance and foul odor characteristic of steatorrhea. The malabsorption is caused by the undigested carbohydrate, which acts as a substrate for bacterial fermentation. This overgrowth of bacteria in the intestinal tract causes the deconjugation of bile acids. Deconjugated bile acids cannot form micelles; therefore, a fat malabsorption develops. Other symptoms of starch intolerance include abdominal distention and weight loss.

Diagnosis. A starch challenge test can be made to determine starch intolerance. Prior to consumption of the starch load (2 to 3 slices of bread), the individual's fasting blood sugar level should be measured. A glucose tolerance test performed immediately after the consumption of starch should indicate normal or reduced amylase activity. The blood glucose level will not rise normally when reduced amylase activity is present.

Nutritional Care

Diets for infants with this disorder must exclude cereals, flours, root vegetables, potatoes, thickened soups and sauces and any food containing flour or starch. Carbohydrate should be provided in simple forms, such as sugar, honey, corn syrup, dextrose, fruits and fruit

Table 39–15 FOODS TO ELIMINATE IN A
STARCH-FREE DIET*

MILK	Milk substitutes that may contain starch or soy milks.
MEAT	Sausages, processed meats containing starch.
BREAD AND CEREALS	Bread, cakes, biscuits, pastries, wheat, oats, rye, barley, rice flours, tapioca, cornstarch, spaghetti, macaroni and breakfast cereals.
FRUIT	Unripe fruit, bananas, apples.
VEGETABLES	Beans, peas, potatoes, parsnips, corn.
BEVERAGES	Malted milks, cocoa, chocolate.
DESSERTS	Ice cream (unless homemade).
MISCELLA-NEOUS	Nuts, thickened soups, pickles, sauces.

*From: Francis, D. E. M.: Diets for Sick Children, 3rd ed. Oxford, Blackwell Scientific Publications, 1974.

juices. The fat and protein intake of the child should be normal for age, height, weight and activity requirements. See Table 39–15 for foods to avoid when planning a diet for individuals with starch intolerance.

DISACCHARIDASE DEFICIENCIES

Metabolic Defect. In disaccharide intolerance there is a deficiency of one or more of the disaccharide-splitting enzymes, the *disaccharidases* (see Fig. 39–8). The *alpha-disaccharidase lactase* hydrolyzes lactose to glucose and galactose, and maltose and sucrose

are split, respectively, by the *beta-disaccharidases maltase and invertase (sucrase)* into their simple sugars. For further discussion see Chapter 6.

When disaccharidase deficiency occurs, the normal digestion of the disaccharide on the brush border of the intestinal epithelial cells is inhibited. Because of this maldigestion, the disaccharides remain in the gut and exert increased osmotic pressure, resulting in an increased amount of water in the intestinal tract. Cramps, watery diarrhea, flatulence and bloating are symptoms indicative of intestinal disaccharide intolerance. The unabsorbed disaccharides also cause rapid bacterial fermentation and steatorrhea (see Figure 23–6).

Diagnosis. Disaccharidase deficiency is most reliably diagnosed by intestinal biopsy. However, valuable information may also be obtained by disaccharide loading tests. Analysis of the feces for reducing substances and organic acids and determining the pH may also be useful in making a correct diagnosis. The hydrogen breath test is also used in determining lactase deficiency.

Nutritional Care for Lactose Intolerance

Lactose intolerance and its nutritional care are discussed in Chapter 23.

Nutritional Care for Maltose, Isomaltose and Sucrose Intolerance

Those children who are intolerant of maltose or isomaltose must exclude all foods containing

Figure 39–8 Intestinal disaccharidases. (Adapted from: Wong, P. W., and Hsia, D. Y.: Inborn errors of metabolism. In: Goodhart, R. S., and Shils, M. E. (eds.): Modern Nutrition in Health and Disease, 5th ed., Philadelphia, Lea & Febiger, 1973.)

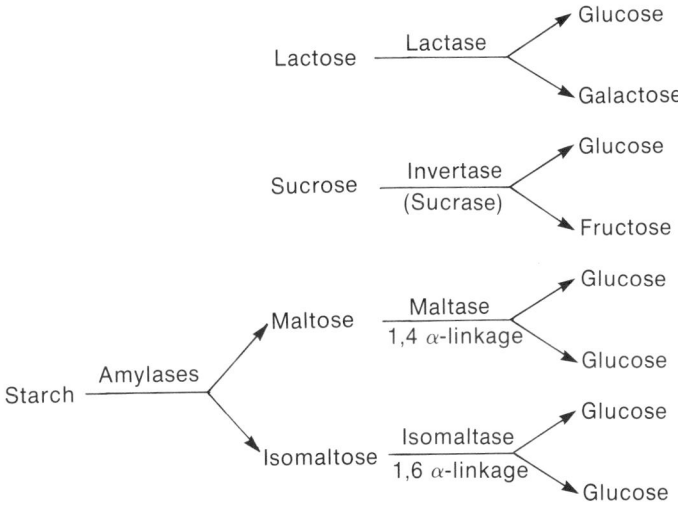

starch or glycogen (liver) from their diets. These foods contain polysaccharides that yield maltose, isomaltose and related oligosaccharides upon hydrolysis by salivary and pancreatic amylase. The diet is similar to that for individuals with starch intolerance (Table 39–15).

Sucrose intolerance due to a deficiency of the enzyme invertase (sucrase) is treated by the exclusion of sucrose from the diet. Sugar (granulated, confectioners and brown), molasses, syrups, jellies, candy, cookies, cakes, pastries, colas, most juices, puddings, fruits and some vegetables high in sugar are omitted or restricted. The diet is the same as that for the fructose-intolerant person. See Table 39–14 for foods that must be eliminated in this diet. Appendix Table 12 is also helpful. A vitamin C supplement is indicated because good sources of this vitamin (fruits and fruit juices) are eliminated.

Nutritional Care for Monosaccharide Intolerance

In *glucose-galactose intolerance,* the infant's gastrointestinal symptoms disappear when all sources of carbohydrate except fructose are excluded from the diet. The appropriate formula for use in controlling this disease is CHO-Free.

GLYCOGEN STORAGE DISEASES

Under normal circumstances, dietary glucose is removed from the portal circulation by the liver. Glycogen is the storage form of glucose that is deposited in liver and muscle tis-

sue. When there is a defect in the pathways of glycogen synthesis or degradation, an abnormal form of glycogen or excessive amounts of glycogen are produced. At present there are ten different known causes of glycogen storage disease. At least one of these, type I, or *von Gierke's disease*, responds to nutritional intervention.

Type I (von Gierke's Disease)

Metabolic Defect. The defective enzyme in von Gierke's disease is *glucose-6-phosphatase,* which is needed to convert liver glycogen to glucose (see Fig. 39–9). The absence of this enzyme deprives the infant of readily available sources of glucose, which results in hypoglycemia. In order to maintain a normal blood glucose level, ketosis and increased gluconeogenesis from protein develop.

Besides severe hypoglycemia, some of the clinical symptoms of this disorder are enlarged liver and kidneys, stunted growth, hypertriglyceridemia, hypercholesterolemia and lowered resistance to infection. In this hepatic type of glycogen storage disease it is not uncommon for the affected infant to die in early childhood.

Diagnosis. Laboratory findings indicative of this disorder are a decreased fasting blood glucose concentration and acidosis. There is also poor response when epinephrine is administered to the affected infant—blood glucose does not measurably increase. Positive diagnosis can be made by confirming the absence of glucose-6-phosphatase in a fresh liver biopsy. This diagnostic procedure, developed by Hers, is accomplished either by open biopsy or punch biopsy.[15]

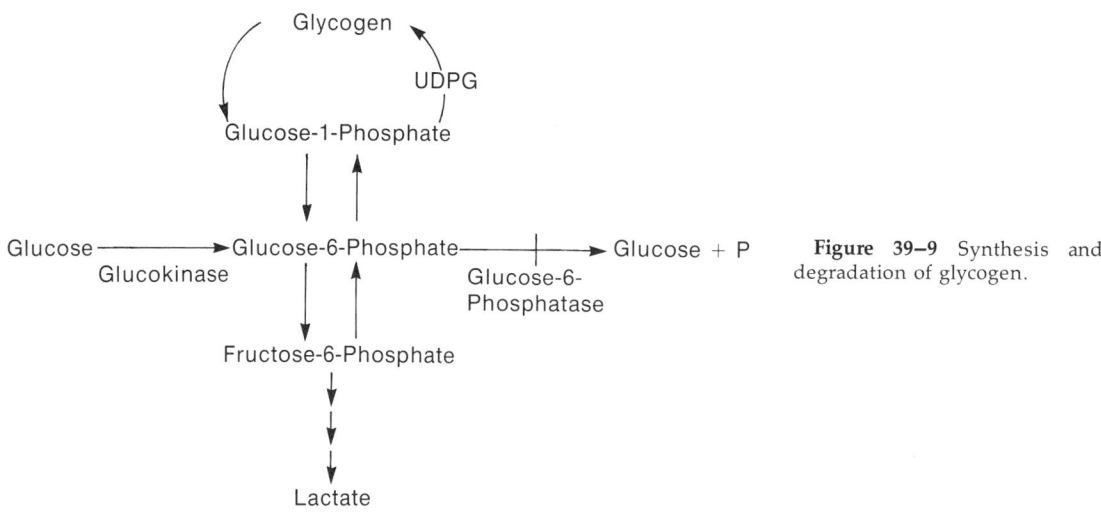

Figure 39–9 Synthesis and degradation of glycogen.

Nutritional Care. The aims of nutritional care are (1) to maintain glucose homeostasis, (2) to avoid the consequences of hypoglycemia and (3) to provide enough protein and calories to maintain positive nitrogen balance and growth.

. The formula for infants with von Gierke's disease should contain only glucose, since the disaccharides sucrose and lactose are digested and absorbed as fructose and galactose. These are then converted to glycogen and lactic acid by the liver and cause increased acidosis. Milk, fruits, table sugar and sugar-containing foods should be avoided.

The product CHO-Free (Syntex), a carbohydrate-free, milk-free liquid, is an appropriate formula to use in the treatment of this disorder. It can be mixed with crystallized glucose to provide the infant with a suitable type and amount of carbohydrate. This is helpful in the maintenance of glucose homeostasis and the prevention of hypoglycemia. Another formula, Pregestimil (nutrient value in Table 35-7C), which contains glucose, casein hydrolysate and medium-chain triglycerides, has also been used in the treatment of von Gierke's disease.

To alleviate the hypoglycemia episodes that may occur, frequent feedings ever three to four hours, day and night, are necessary. Ehrlich has found that providing a 25 per cent glucose solution through an intragastric tube can be an effective method of preventing nocturnal hypoglycemia.[9]

Care must be taken in selecting the diet, because it is important that the infant receive nutrients from all food groups. However, an excessive amount of calories from *any* nutrient (protein, fat or carbohydrate) can result in an accumulation of fat and glycogen in the liver.

PROBLEMS AND SUGGESTED TOPICS FOR DISCUSSION

1. Describe the problems that may be encountered in providing nutritional counseling to parents of children with inborn errors of metabolism.
2. Discuss the nutritional management goals for a child with phenylketonuria.
3. A child with galactosemia is admitted to your outpatient clinic. What information should be obtained before an appropriate diet can be planned?
4. Write a day's menu for a nine month old infant with fructose intolerance.

CITED REFERENCES

1. Acosta, P., and Elsas, L.: Dietary Management of Inherited Disease: Phenylketonuria, Galactosemia, Tyrosinemia, Homocystinuria, Maple Syrup Urine Disease. Atlanta, Georgia, ACELMU Publishers, 1939 Westminster Way, 30307, 1975.
2. Alexander, F. W., Clayton, B. E., and Delves, H. T.: Mineral and trace-metal balances in children receiving normal and synthetic diets. Q. J. Med., *43*:89, 1974.
3. Arthur, L. J. H., and Hulme, J. D.: Intelligent, small for date baby born to oligophrenic phenylketonuric mother after low phenylalanine diet during pregnancy. Pediatrics, *46*:235, 1970.
4. Cornblath, M., and Schwartz, R.: Disorders of Carbohydrate Metabolism in Infancy, 2nd ed. Philadelphia, W. B. Saunders, 1976.
5. Corner, B. D., et al.: A case of histidinemia controlled with a low histidine diet. Pediatrics, *41*:1074, 1968.
6. Dobson, J. C., et al.: Intellectual performance of 36 phenylketonuria patients and their non-affected siblings. Pediatrics, *58*:53, 1976.
7. Donner, P. J., Davidson, E. D., and Elsas, L. J.: Thiamine increase of the specific activity of human liver branched-chain alpha-ketoacid dehydrogenase. Nature, *254*:529, 1975.
8. Duncan, G. G.: Disorders of amino acid metabolism. In: Bondy, P. K., and Rosenberg, L. (eds.): Duncan's Diseases of Metabolism, 7th ed. Philadelphia, W. B. Saunders Co., 1974.
9. Ehrlich, R. M.: Nocturnal feeding for glycogen storage disease. N. Engl. J. Med., *294*:1125, 1976.
10. Fernbach, S. A., et al.: Metabolic studies of transient tyrosinemia in premature infants. Pediatr. Res., *9*:172, 1975.
11. Garrod, A.: Inborn Errors of Metabolism. London, Henry Frowde, 1909.
12. Gerber, M. G., and Gerber, D. G.: A simple screening test for histidinuria. Pediatrics, *43*:40, 1969.
13. Ghadimi, H., Partington, M. W., and Hunter, A.: Inborn error of histidine metabolism. Pediatrics, *29*:714, 1962.
14. Gretsky, N. E.: Relationship of elevated blood tyrosine to the ultimate intellectual performance of premature infants. Pediatrics, *49*:218, 1972.
15. Hers, H. G.: Glycogen storage diseases. In: Levine, R. and Luft, R. (eds.): Advances in Metabolic Disorders, Vol. 1. New York, Academic Press, 1964, pp. 1–44.
16. Johnson, C.: What is the best age to discontinue the low phenylalanine diet in pheylketonuria? Clin. Pediatr., *11*:148, 1972.
17. Kaufman, S., et al.: Phenylketonuria due to a deficiency of dehydropteridine reductase. N. Engl. J. Med., *293*:785, 1975.
18. Kelly, S., and Copeland, W.: A hypothesis on the homocystinuric's response to pyridoxine. Metabolism, *17*:794, 1968.
19. Kretchmer, N.: Enzymatic patterns during development: an approach to a biochemical definition of immaturity. Pediatrics, *23*:606, 1959.
20. McKusick, V. A., Hall, J. G., and Char, F.: The clinical and genetic characteristics of homocystinuria. In: Carson, N. A. J., and Raine, D. N. (eds.): Inherited Disorders of Sulfur Metabolism. Edinburgh, Churchill Livingstone, 1971.
21. Menkes, J. H., Hurst, P. L., and Craig, J. M.: A new syndrome of familial infantile cerebral dysfunction with an unusual urinary substance. Pediatrics, *14*:462, 1954.
22. Ng, W. G., et al.: Prenatal diagnosis of galactosemia. Clin. Chim. Acta, *74*:227, 1977.
23. Nyhan, W. L.: Heritable Disorders of Amino Acid Metabolism: Patterns of Clinical Expression and Ge-

netic Variation. New York, John Wiley & Sons, 1974, p. 165.

24. Parents' Guide to the Galactose-Restricted Diet. Davis, California, Maternal and Child Health Branch, California Department of Health, Department of Nutrition, University of California, October 1976.

25. Phenylketonuria. Evansville, Ind., Mead Johnson Laboratories, 1973.

26. Phenylketonuria: An Inherited Metabolic Disorder Associated with Mental Retardation. Washington, D.C., U.S. Department of Health, Education and Welfare, Health Services and Mental Health Administration, 1972.

27. Ratnoff, O. D.: Activation of Hageman factor by L-homocystine. Science, 162:1007, 1968.

28. A Report to the 1970 (California) Legislature on Medical Tests for Newborn Infants Pursuant to Health and Safety Code, Article 2.5, Chapter 2, Part 1 of Division 1. February 19, 1970.

29. Scriver, C. R.: Hypermethionemia in acute tyrosinosis. Lancet, 1:1319, 1968.

30. Segal, S., Blau, A., and Roth, H.: The metabolism of galactose by patients with congenital galactosemia. Am. J. Med., 38:62, 1965.

31. Spaeth, G. L., and Barber, G. W.: Homocystinuria. Trans. Am. Acad. Ophthalmol. Otolaryngol., 69:912, 1965.

32. Stern, J.: Inborn errors. Nutrition, 28:163, 1974.

33. Tietz, N. (ed.): Fundamentals of Clinical Chemistry, 2nd. ed. Philadelphia, W. B. Saunders Co., 1976.

34. Uhlemann, E. R., et al.: Platelet survival and morphology in homocystinuria due to cystathionine synthetase deficiency. N. Engl. J. Med., 295:1283, 1976.

35. Van Sprang, F. J., and Wadman, S. K.: Treatment of a patient with histidinemia. Acta Paediatr. Scand., 56:493, 1967.

36. Wadman, S. K., et al.: Dietary correction of histidinemia in older children. Clin. Chim. Acta, 49:377, 1973.

37. Wong, P. W. K., and Hsia, D. Y. Y.: Inborn errors of metabolism. In: Goodhart, R. S. and Shils, M. E. (eds.): Modern Nutrition in Health and Disease, 5th ed. Philadelphia, Lea & Febiger, 1973, p. 1012.

ADDITIONAL REFERENCES

Abbott, M. H., and Hussels, I. E.: Ectopia lentis due to homocystinuria. Birth Defects, 7:170, 1971.

Ampola, M. G.: Phenylketonuria and other disorders of amino acid metabolism. Pediatr. Clin. North Am., 20:407, 1973.

Ampola, M. G. (ed.): Symposium on early detection and management of inborn errors. Clin Perinatol., 3(1), 1976.

Bickel, H., Schmidt, H., and Schurrle, L.: Dietary Treatment of inborn errors of amino acid and carbohydrate metabolism. Bibl. Nutr. Dieta, 18:181, 1973.

Brown, E. S., and Warner, R.: Mental development of phenylketonuric children on or off diet after the age of six. Psychol. Med., 6:287, 1976.

Carson, N. A., et al.: Hereditary tyrosinemia. Clinical, enzymatic, and pathological study of an infant with the acute form of the disease. Arch. Dis. Child., 51:106, 1976.

Cohn, R. M., et al.: Phenylalanine-tyrosine deficiency syndrome as a complication of the management of tyrosinemia. Am. J. Clin. Nutr., 30:209, 1977.

Francis, D. E.: Therapeutic special diets. Practitioner, 212 (1270 Spec. No.):545, 1974.

Gershen, J. A.: Galactosemia: a psycho-social perspective. Ment. Retard., 13:20, 1975.

Holtzman, N. A.: Dietary treatment of inborn errors of metabolism. Annu. Rev. Med., 21:335, 1970.

Hsia, D. Y.: Biochemical factors in mental retardation. Proc. Am. Psychopathol. Assoc., 56:28, 1967.

Lombeck, I., et al.: Serum-selenium concentrations in patients with maple syrup urine disease and phenylketonuria under dietotherapy. Clin. Chim. Acta, 64:57, 1975.

Morrow, G.: Nutritional management of infants with inborn metabolic errors. Clin. Perinatol., 2:361, 1975.

Noel, M. B., et al.: Dietary treatment of maple syrup urine disease (branched-chain ketoaciduria). J. Am. Diet. Assoc., 69:62, 1976.

Odieve, M.: The fate of children with galactosemia. Arch. Fr. Pediatr., 33:941, 1976.

Pantarotta, M. F., Zunino, P., and Pecorari, D.: Problem of maternal phenylketonuria. Minerva Ginecol., 27:939, 1975.

Pueschel, S., Yeatman, S., and Hunr, C.: Discontinuing the phenylalanine-restricted diet in young children with PKU. J. Am. Diet. Assoc., 70:506, 1977.

Rickard, K., et al.: Care of children with conditions characterized by high nutritional risks J. Am. Diet. Assoc., 68:546, 1976.

Sansarica, C., et al.: Cystine deficiency during dietotherapy of homocystinemia. Acta Paediatr. Scand., 64:215, 1975.

Saudubray, J. M., and Charpentier, C.: The traps of Guthrie's test. Arch. Fr. Pediatr., 33:915, 1976.

Synderman, S. E.: The dietary therapy of inherited metabolic disease. Prog. Food Nutr. Sci., 1:507, 1975.

Woolf, L. I.: The dietary treatment of inborn errors of metabolism. Proc. Nutr. Soc., 35:31, 1976.

Part Three

FOODS

Chapter 40

CHOOSING FOOD FOR NUTRITION AND HEALTH

In this chapter, the four groups of foods (milk and milk products, meats and meat alternates, grains and cereals, and fruits and vegetables) will be discussed. The nutrient contributions, role in the diet, and techniques for shopping will be presented for each group.

MILK GROUP

The use of milk from cattle goes back to antiquity. It is mentioned in the Bible at least 50 times, and there is evidence of the common use of milk, cheese and butter in Egyptian, Greek and Roman civilizations. A 5000 year old frieze, unearthed in the Euphrates valley, portrays men seated on low stools milking cows. Marco Polo reported in the 13th century that the Asians used dairy products.

Recommended Daily Intake. The following amounts of milk are recommended every day: Children under 9 years of age should drink 2 to 3 cups (1 pt. or more). Children 9 to 12 years old should have 3 or more cups (¾ qt. or more). Teenagers should receive 4 or more cups (1 qt. or more), and the adult requirement is 2 or more cups (1 pt. or more) daily.

Calcium Equivalents

On the basis of calcium content, cheese and ice cream can replace the milk recommended daily. On the basis of the calcium they provide, the following are alternates for 1 cup (8 oz.) of milk:

    1⅓ oz. Cheddar, American or Swiss cheese
16 oz. cream cheese
    1⅓ cups cottage cheese
    1⅔ cups ice cream
    3 cups milk sherbet
    1 cup baked custard
    1 cup non-fat milk
    1 cup buttermilk
    ½ cup undiluted evaporated milk
    ¼ cup dried non-fat milk powder
    ¼ cup dried whole milk powder

MILK BEVERAGES

The most common use of milk is as a drink. It is also the basic ingredient in making many good-tasting, nutritious beverages. Cow's milk is most generally used, although milk from other animals such as goats is consumed in some countries where cows are scarce. Milk is available in whole, skim, evaporated, condensed, dried whole and dried skim (non-fat solids) forms.

Composition of Milk. Milk is a yellowish-white liquid emulsion containing a high-quality protein (mainly casein with small amounts of lactalbumin and lactoglobulin), fat (cream), carbohydrate (lactose or milk sugar), the minerals calcium and phosphorus and the vitamins riboflavin, niacin, vitamin A and (when the milk is fortified) vitamin D.

The composition of milk varies to some degree with the breed of cattle, the season of the year and the feed given to the animal. However, milk purchased in the market is a mixture from different breeds and maintains a fairly constant average composition. Local and state regulations set the required butterfat and solids contents. The average composition of cow's milk is given in Chapter 14, page 302.

Nutritional Value and Digestibility. The value of milk in the diet for all age levels has been repeatedly emphasized throughout this text. It furnishes about a hundred nutrients but is outstanding in importance for calcium, riboflavin, protein, vitamin D (when fortified) and phosphorus. Three-fourths of the calcium, nearly one-half of the riboflavin and one-fourth of the protein in the country's food supply come from milk. If milk is omitted or sparingly used in the diet, it is difficult to meet the requirement for calcium and riboflavin.

A pint of milk in the diet for an adult yields approximately 320 kcal. If calories must be kept down, skim milk can be used to supply all the nutrients in whole milk except fat and vitamin A. (Fortified skim milk provides vitamin A

APPROXIMATE NUMBER OF CALORIES IN MILK AND MILK PRODUCTS

MILK PRODUCT	QUANTITY	KCAL.
Fresh fluid whole milk	1 cup (½ pt.)	160
Fresh fluid skim milk	1 cup	90
Buttermilk (non-fat)	1 cup	90
Half-and-half	1 cup	325
Chocolate-flavored milk drink	1 cup	190
Cocoa	1 cup	235
Malted milk beverage	1 cup	280
Evaporated milk, diluted with equal amount of water	1 cup	173
Non-fat dry milk	4 tblsp. (¼ cup)	63
Ice cream	1 slice (⅛ of qt. brick)	145
Ice milk	½ cup	143
Cheddar cheese	1-in. cube	70
Cottage cheese, creamed	½ cup	120
Cottage cheese, uncreamed	½ cup	98

and usually vitamin D.) One pint of skim milk has 180 kcal.

If calories are to be increased in the diet, ingredients such as cocoa, chocolate, ice cream and malted milk can be added to milk. For example, one pint of malted milk beverage contains approximately 560 kcal.

The protein in milk, casein, is of high quality and is particularly suitable for use by the body in building muscle tissue. It contains all the amino acids needed for body building and tissue repair. The carbohydrate is in the form of lactose, a disaccharide that is not as sweet as cane sugar. Lactose does not ferment readily and does not cause gastric disturbances, as do some sugars. The minerals found in milk, especially calcium and phosphorus, are essential for the structure of bones and teeth for individuals of all ages, especially infants and children. The amount of iron in milk is small, but it is in a form readily used by the body. Milk is a dependable source of vitamin A, thiamin, niacin and riboflavin. Some vitamin C is present but not in adequate quantities. Natural milk does not contain adequate vitamin D to prevent rickets and produce normal growth and tooth development, but it is especially adaptable for fortification with this vitamin. Nearly all homogenized milk, skim milk and non-fat dry milk available today is fortified with vitamin D. The fat (cream) in milk is in an emulsified form that contains vitamin A and is easily digested and well tolerated.

Milk in the Daily Diet. In the amounts recommended, milk contributes more protein to the diet than any other single food. When milk is omitted from the diet, the protein requirement of the child can be met only if special and expert planning is carried out. The mineral and vitamin contributions of milk are equally important.

Adults, especially senior citizens, often feel it is not a necessary food for them, but as a source of calcium it appears to be extremely important in delaying osteoporosis. The objections that it is fattening or not liked can be overcome by encouraging the use of skim milk in reducing diets and incorporating milk in dishes that the person especially enjoys if milk is not liked as a beverage. Milk can be taken in the form of cheese or used in creamed soups, creamed dishes, baked products, vegetables, milk desserts and in beverages made with milk.

Making Milk Safe. Most milk is pasteurized. Pasteurized milk has been heated to destroy pathogenic bacteria and then cooled rapidly, making it safe to drink. In addition to being pasteurized, milk may also be homogenized, a process that reduces the size of the cream particles. As a result, the cream does not rise to the top of the milk but stays suspended. Certified milk is not pasteurized but must meet standards of cleanliness. Federal, state and local public health service legislation protects the public milk supply.

If milk is not pasteurized, a home pasteurizer can be used, or the milk can be heated until it comes to a boil. The latter is a stronger heat treatment than pasteurization; it changes the flavor and destroys all or most of the vitamin C content and some of the thiamin but does render the milk safe to drink.

To protect the nutritive value of milk after it reaches the consumer, the rule of "3 C's and a D" should be followed; that is, keep it clean, cold, covered and dark.

Buyer's Information. Fresh whole or skim milk is purchased pasteurized. If the milk is

"raw" it should be home-pasteurized before being consumed. Evaporated milk is purchased either in tall cans (14½ oz. by weight or 12 fluid oz.) containing 1⅔ cups or in small "baby" cans (6 oz. by weight or 5⅓ fluid oz.) containing ⅔ of a cup. Dried milk is sold in powdered form and packaged in cartons of different sizes. Dry milk costs less than other milk and can be used in place of other milk.

COCOA AND CHOCOLATE

Dried cocoa beans or seeds are imported from Central and South America. Chocolate has a higher fat content, while cocoa has cornstarch incorporated into the defatted powdered form. Theobromine, a substance similar to caffeine, is the stimulant substance present in cocoa and chocolate.

MALTED MILK

The malted milk added to flavor a beverage is a dried and condensed mixture of milk, malt and wheat (which has had the fiber eliminated). Malt is defined as germinated grain, usually sprouted barley, in which the enzyme diastase has changed the starch molecules to maltose. The nutritive value of a malted milk beverage is high. Malted milk is higher in protein, calories, thiamin and vitamin A and has seven times as much iron as whole milk. There is 0.7 mg. of iron in one cup of malted milk, making it a fair source of that mineral. Sometimes ice cream is whipped into the beverage or added as a float.

WHITE SAUCE

White sauce is useful for making a number of cream-style dishes and for adding milk to the diet. Thin white sauce is blended with purée or strained vegetables to make creamed soups; a medium white sauce is blended with meat, fish, fowl or eggs and vegetables to make creamed dishes; a thick white sauce is used as the base for soufflés and a very thick white sauce is blended with other ingredients to make croquettes. To make a white sauce, milk or some other liquid is thickened with flour or another cereal product to the desired consistency.

CREAM SOUPS

Cream soups are blends of vegetable purées or mixtures of chopped, diced or minced vege-

tables and meat, fish or poultry in a white sauce base.

MILK IN SIMPLE DESSERTS

Desserts bring milk to the table in simple and easy-to-digest ways. Milk sherbets, ice cream, custards (baked or soft) and puddings (bread, cornstarch, junket, rice and Bavarian cream) belong on the list.

CHEESE

Dishes prepared with milk, eggs and cheese are sometimes called meat alternates. They can be interchanged in the menu with meat dishes because of the similarity of their nutrients, particularly animal, or complete, proteins.

Buyer's Information. Cheeses are classified into categories of soft, semihard and hard cheeses. Cottage cheese, cream cheese and Neufchatel are unripened soft cheeses. Camembert and Brie are soft cheeses that are ripened by molds; Limburger and Liederkranz are soft cheeses ripened by bacteria. Gorgonzola, Roquefort, bleu and Stilton are semihard cheeses ripened by molds, and brick and Muenster are semihard cheeses ripened by bacteria. Among the hard cheeses without air or "gas" holes are Cheddar, Edam and Gouda, and those with holes include Swiss, Gruyère and Parmesan. Skim milk is the basis for longhorn and cottage cheese, while Cheddar is made from whole milk. A combination of milk and cream is blended into cream cheese. The domestic cheeses are usually less expensive than the imported varieties. See Table 40–1 for information about various cheeses and their uses.

Composition. Cheese of the Cheddar type contains about 25 per cent protein, 32 per cent fat, 2 per cent lactose (milk sugar), minerals (especially calcium and phosphorus), vitamins (especially vitamin A and riboflavin) and 40 per cent water. It retains most of the calcium, phosphorus and iron of milk. Except for cottage cheese, it is high in fat and consequently, a rich source of vitamin A, containing approximately 1700 I.U. per ounce. There is considerable variation in water and fat content, depending upon whether it is made from whole or skim milk. Cottage cheese is lower in fat, with about 4.2 per cent fat if creamed and 0.3 per cent fat if uncreamed.

Nutritive Value. The type of milk used in the manufacture of cheese reflects the nutritive qualities of the cheese. For example, protein,

Table 40–1 GUIDE TO NATURAL CHEESES*

KIND	CHARACTERISTICS	USES
American	See Cheddar.	See Cheddar.
Bel Paese (Bel Pah-A-say)	Mild, sweet flavor; light, creamy yellow interior; slate gray surface; soft to medium firm, creamy texture.	Appetizers, sandwiches, desserts and snacks.
Bleu	Tangy, piquant flavor; semisoft, pasty, sometimes crumbly texture; white interior marbled or streaked with blue veins of mold; resembles Roquefort.	Appetizers, salads and salad dressings, desserts and snacks.
Brick	Mild to moderately sharp flavor; semisoft to medium firm, elastic texture; creamy white to yellow interior; brownish exterior.	Appetizers, sandwiches, desserts and snacks.
Brie (Bree)	Mild to pungent flavor; soft, smooth texture; creamy yellow interior; edible thin brown and white crust.	Appetizers, sandwiches, desserts and snacks.
Caciocavallo (Ca-cheo-ca-VAL-lo)	Piquant, somewhat salty flavor—similar to Provolone, but not smoked; smooth, very firm texture; light or white interior; clay or tan colored surface.	Snacks and desserts. Suitable for grating and cooking when fully cured.
Camembert (KAM-em-bear)	Distinctive mild to tangy flavor; soft, smooth texture—almost fluid when fully ripened; creamy yellow interior; edible thin white or gray-white crust.	Appetizers, desserts and snacks.
Cheddar (often called American)	Mild to very sharp flavor; smooth texture, firm to crumbly; light cream to orange color.	Appetizers, main dishes, sauces, soups, sandwiches, salads, desserts and snacks.
Colby	Mild to mellow flavor, similar to Cheddar; softer body and more open texture than Cheddar; light cream to orange.	Sandwiches and snacks.
Cottage	Mild, slightly acid flavor; soft, open texture with tender curds of varying size; white to creamy white.	Appetizers, salads, used in some cheesecakes.
Cream	Delicate, slightly acid flavor; soft, smooth texture; white.	Appetizers, salads, sandwiches, desserts and snacks.
Edam	Mellow, nutlike, sometimes salty flavor; rather firm, rubbery texture; creamy yellow or medium yellow-orange interior; surface coated with red wax; usually shaped like a flattened ball.	Appetizers, salads, sandwiches, sauces, desserts and snacks.
Gjetost[1] (YET-ost)	Sweetish, caramel flavor; firm, buttery consistency; golden brown.	Desserts and snacks.
Gorgonzola (Gor-gon-ZO-la)	Tangy, rich, spicy flavor; semisoft, pasty, sometimes crumbly texture; creamy white interior, mottled or streaked with blue-green veins of mold; clay colored surface.	Appetizers, salads, desserts and snacks.
Gouda (GOO-da)	Mellow, nutlike, often slightly acid flavor; semisoft to firm, smooth texture, often containing small holes; creamy yellow or medium yellow-orange interior; usually has red wax coating; usually shaped like a flattened ball.	Appetizers, salads, sandwiches, sauces, desserts and snacks.

*From: U.S. Department of Agriculture: Cheese in Family Meals: A Guide for Consumers. Home and Garden Bulletin No. 112. Washington, D.C., U.S. Government Printing Office, 1966.
[1]Imported; not manufactured in the United States.

calcium and vitamin B factors are contributed by the whole milk used in Cheddar cheese.

Cheese is not equal in food value to the milk from which it is made, since some of the protein (lactalbumin), lactose, certain mineral salts (some calcium) and a portion of the vitamins are separated out and left in the whey. The casein of milk is the main constituent of cheese. It is a high biological value protein with a high calcium content, making it a valuable food.

In general, it takes about one-half pound of Cheddar cheese to give the same amount of protein as a pound of meat containing a moderate amount of bone and fat. Cottage

cheese is less concentrated than Cheddar cheese, with about four-fifths as much protein per pound. Cream cheese is almost entirely fat and should not be considered a protein source.

The *sodium content* of milk and milk products is fairly high, and processed cheeses have the highest sodium content. (Sodium is added in processing.) For example, the sodium content of a 1-oz. slice of Cheddar cheese is 168 mg., while that of the same size slice of processed American cheese is 307 mg.

Digestibility. Cheese is easily digested, being rich in easily assimilated fat and in protein of high biological value. In "ripened" cheese, the protein has been partially digested

Table 40–1   GUIDE TO NATURAL CHEESES (*Continued*)

KIND	CHARACTERISTICS	USES
Gruyere (Grew-YARE)	Nutlike, salty flavor, similar to Swiss but sharper; firm, smooth texture with small holes or eyes; light yellow.	Appetizers, desserts and snacks.
Liederkranz (LEE-der-krontz)	Robust flavor, similar to very mild Limburger; soft, smooth texture; creamy yellow interior; russet surface.	Appetizers, desserts and snacks.
Limburger	Highly pungent, very strong flavor and aroma; soft, smooth texture that usually contains small irregular openings; creamy white interior; reddish yellow surface.	Appetizers, desserts and snacks.
Mozzarella (also called Scamorza) (Mottza-REL-la)	Delicate, mild flavor; slightly firm, plastic texture; creamy white.	Main dishes such as pizza or lasagna; sandwiches and snacks.
Muenster (MUN-stir)	Mild to mellow flavor; semisoft texture with numerous small openings; creamy white interior; yellowish tan surface.	Appetizers, sandwiches, desserts and snacks.
Mysost (MEWS-ost)	Sweetish, caramel flavor; firm, buttery consistency; light brown.	Desserts and snacks.
Neufchatal (New-sha-TEL)	Mild, acid flavor; soft, smooth texture similar to cream cheese but lower in fat; white.	Salads, sandwiches, desserts and snacks.
Parmesan	Sharp, distinctive flavor; very hard, granular texture; yellowish white.	Grated for seasoning.
Port du Salut (Pore du sa-LOO)	Mellow to robust flavor similar to Gouda; semisoft, smooth elastic texture; creamy white or yellow.	Appetizers, desserts and snacks.
Provolone (Pro-vo-LO-na)	Mellow to sharp flavor, smoky and salty; firm, smooth texture; cuts without crumbling; light creamy yellow; light brown or golden yellow surface.	Appetizers, main dishes, sandwiches, desserts and snacks.
Ricotta (Ri-COT-ah)	Mild, sweet, nutlike flavor; soft, moist texture with loose curds (fresh ricotta) or dry and suitable for grating; white.	Salads, main dishes such as lasagna and ravioli, and desserts.
Romano	Very sharp, piquant flavor; very hard, granular texture; yellowish-white interior; greenish-black surface.	Seasoning and general table use; when cured one year it is suitable for grating.
Roquefort[1]	Sharp, peppery, piquant flavor; semisoft, pasty, sometimes crumbly texture; white interior streaked with blue-green veins of mold.	Appetizers, salads and salad dressings, desserts and snacks.
Sap Sago[1]	Sharp, pungent, cloverlike flavor; very hard texture suitable for grating; light green or sage green.	Grated for seasoning.
Stilton	Piquant flavor, milder than Gorgonzola or Roquefort; open, flaky texture; creamy white interior streaked with blue-green veins of mold; wrinkled, melon-like rind.	Appetizers, salads, desserts and snacks.
Swiss (also called Emmentaler)	Mild, sweet, nutlike flavor; firm, smooth, elastic body with large round eyes; light yellow.	Sandwiches, salads and snacks.

by bacterial action and made more soluble in the process.

YOGURT

Yogurt is a fermented milk product made from whole, low-fat or skim milk. The bacteria usually used are *Lactobacillus bulgaricus, Streptococcus thermophilus* and possibly *Lactobacillus acidophilus*. Yogurt contains all the food value of the milk from which it was made. The curd is made by the bacteria clotting the milk. There is no evidence to justify the idea that the bacteria in yogurt are needed to maintain healthy gastrointestinal tract flora.

Yogurt is not exceptionally low in calories unless it is made from skim milk and is unsweetened. One cup of this kind of yogurt would contain 90 to 100 kcal. and 8 gm. of protein, a very low kcal.-to-protein ratio. Sweetened, one cup of yogurt can contain as much as 260 kcal. and still only 8 gm. of protein.

MEAT GROUP

Two or more servings from this group are suggested daily. These may consist of meats (beef, veal, pork, lamb), poultry, fish or eggs. Dry beans, dry peas and nuts may be used as alternates.

MEAT

Meat is a popular, high-quality protein food that satisfies the appetites and tastes of many

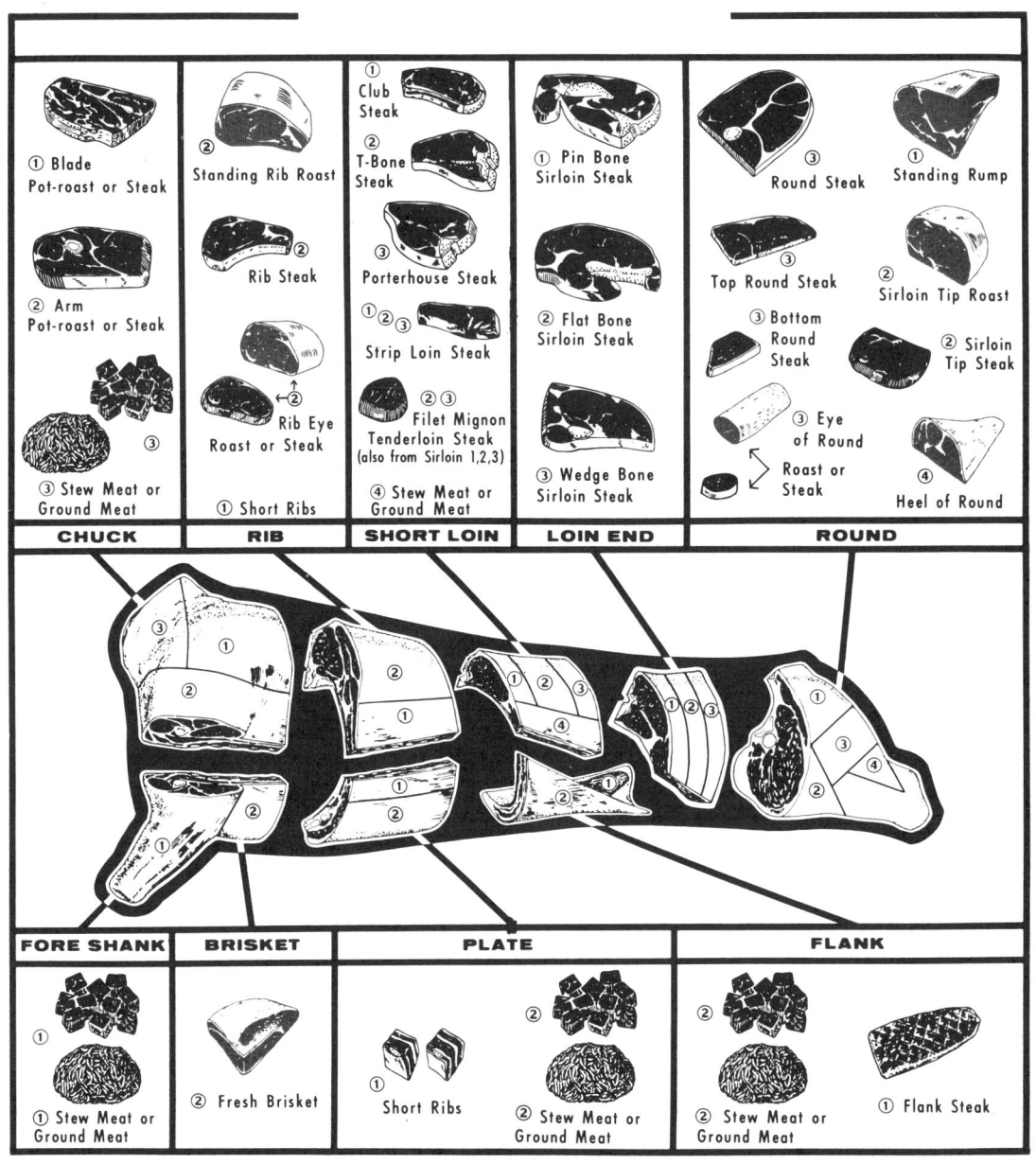

Figure 40–1   Beef chart. (From: Consumer and Marketing Service, U.S. Department of Agriculture: How to Buy Beef Roasts. Home and Garden Bulletin No. 146. Washington, D.C., U.S. Government Printing Office, 1968.)

people. Roasts, steaks and chops are the most popular cuts of meat, and the increased demand seems to put such cuts of meat in the highest price range. With the exception of the organ meats, which are much richer in nutrients, most of the parts of the animal are equally nutritious, although the muscular sections are tougher because of the muscle cells and connective tissue. Therefore, different methods of cooking are employed: dry heat for tender roasts, steaks and chops and moist heat for the tougher cuts.

Beef is the most popular meat eaten in this country, and there is a wide range of cuts (Fig. 40–1) and quality.

Kinds of Meat.   The kinds of meat are *beef* from cattle, *veal* from calves, *pork* from swine and *lamb* (young) and *mutton* (mature) from sheep.

A cut of meat from the market includes muscle tissue, connective tissue, fat and bone. Edible glands and organs, such as liver, heart, kidney, brains, sweetbreads and tongue are classified as glandular, organ, or *variety* meats.

Nutritive Value.   Meat is classified as a protein food with a variable amount of fat. A study by Leverton and Odell[2] of the nutritive value of cooked beef, lamb, veal and pork was made to serve as a guide in the planning and calculation of diets. It was suggested that extremely lean portions average 32 per cent protein and 8 per cent fat and that lean-plus-marble portions contain 28 per cent protein and 16 per cent fat. These figures are of special value in planning a diet of limited fat content.

Yellow connective tissue consists chiefly of the protein *elastin,* and cooking does not make it tender. White connective tissue consists chiefly of the protein *collagen,* and cooking does make it tender and soft.

The age of the animal, the amount and character of connective tissue and the deposits of fat are factors that influence the tenderness of meat. Most meat in this country is produced to contain large amounts of marbling, which Americans seem to like. However, efforts are being made to develop feeding methods that will produce meat with a lower fat content or with fat that has a greater concentration of unsaturated fatty acids. This is a result of our increasing knowledge that relates a high fat intake, especially of saturated fats, to the incidence of atherosclerosis.

Meat is considered a rich source of the minerals iron and phosphorus and contains a variable amount of calcium. *Glycogen* is the type of carbohydrate found in meat. It changes to lactic acid, the non-nitrogenous extractive. The nitrogenous extractives give meat its distinctive flavor. They are the end products of protein metabolism and include such examples as creatine, creatinine, purines and other products.

The hemoglobin present in the tissues and muscles gives the pink or red color to meat. The action of enzymes, alkalies, acids and heat on meat forms new products, such as *hematin* formed by heat, which gives the grayish-brown color of well-done meat.

Vitamin A in the fat of beef and liver and factors of the vitamin B-complex are the vitamins abundant in meat.

The enzymes or ferments in meat are the proteolytic enzymes, which act on protein, the amylolytic enzymes, which act on carbohydrates, and the lipolytic enzymes, which act on fats. The proteolytic enzymes assist in the ripening process, increasing the tenderness and juiciness.

Digestibility.   Meat is almost completely digested—protein 97 per cent and fat 96 per cent—and is well utilized by the body. However, the fat content and method of cooking determine the rate of digestion. Fresh-killed meat is usually indigestible, but after a few days, when the enzymes have had time to "age" or ripen the connective tissue, it becomes tender and easily digested. Veal is digested as easily as beef.

The extractives of meat stimulate the flow of digestive juices, which helps promote the digestion of other foods. However, in certain conditions, such as peptic ulcer, the stimulation of gastric juices may be contraindicated.

Place in the Diet.   Meat has an important place in the menu to supply essential protein of high biological value, the minerals phosphorus and iron, and B-complex vitamins and trace minerals such as zinc. The protein of meat can be compared with that of fish, poultry, eggs and milk.

Meat, or equivalents such as poultry and fish, is included at least once in each day's menus, and is usually the main dish for dinner. The use of organ meats should be encouraged because of the vitamin and mineral content in addition to the high-quality protein. Protein needs are frequently increased in various illnesses and convalescence, and meat may be an important therapeutic part of the diet.

Effect of Cooking on Nutritive Value.   Meat is cooked to destroy microorganisms and tenderize connective tissue. Since it is usually eaten in cooked form, it has been necessary to determine the vitamin content when cooked. Studies have shown that, if properly cooked and with all the drippings used, 30 per cent of the thiamin, 5 per cent of the riboflavin and 5 per cent of the niacin are lost. Excessive heat destroys many nutrients in meat. Roasting and frying, for example, require high temperatures, but the damage to the heat labile substances is counteracted somewhat by the retention of juices.

Buyer's Information.   Meat is sold cut into the standardized pieces for roasts, steaks, chops, stews and other meat dishes. It is sold fresh, frozen, dried, salted, smoked and canned. The cut and variety of meat determine the method of cookery. The more expensive cuts are not necessarily higher in food value than less expensive cuts. The organ meats, such as liver and kidney, are examples of high food value at relatively low cost.

The following are *characteristics of high-quality beef:* the lean meat is light red, appears velvety and is veined liberally with fat; the bones are red, and the fat is flaky and white.

Table 40–2   YIELD OF COOKED MEAT PER POUND OF RAW MEAT*

MEATS AS PURCHASED	MEAT AFTER COOKING (Less Drippings)	
	PARTS WEIGHED	APPROXIMATE WEIGHT OF COOKED PARTS PER LB. OF RAW MEAT (oz.)
Chops or steaks for broiling or frying		
With bone and relatively large amount of fat, such as pork or lamb chops, beef rib, sirloin or porter-house steaks	Lean, bone and fat	10–12
	Lean and fat	7–10
	Lean only	5–7
Without bone and with very little fat, such as round of beef, veal steaks	Lean and fat	12–13
	Lean only	9–12
Ground meat for broiling or frying, such as beef, lamb or pork patties	Patties	9–13
Roasts for oven cooking (no liquid added)		
With bone and relatively large amount of fat, such as beef rib, loin, chuck; lamb shoulder, leg; pork, fresh or cured	Lean, bone and fat	10–12
	Lean and fat	8–10
	Lean only	6–9
Without bone	Lean and fat	10–12
	Lean only	7–10
Cuts for pot-roasting, simmering, braising, stewing With bone and relatively large amount of fat, such as beef chuck, pork shoulder	Lean, bone and fat	10–11
	Lean and fat	8–9
	Lean only	6–8
Without bone and with relatively small amount of fat, such as trimmed beef; veal	Lean with adhering fat	9–11

*From: Nutritive Value of Foods. Home and Garden Bulletin No. 72. Washington, D.C., U.S. Department of Agriculture, 1970.

Two purple stamps usually appear on retail cuts of meat: the U.S. Department of Agriculture stamp indicates the grades U.S. Prime, U.S. Choice, U.S. Good and U.S. Commercial; a round stamp indicates that the meat has been inspected and passed as wholesome food.

The *amount of meat to buy* per serving is: ½ to 1 lb. if the meat has much bone or gristle, ⅓ to ½ lb. if the meat has medium amounts of bone, ¼ to ⅓ lb. if the meat has little bone and ⅕ to ¼ lb. if the meat has no bone. Table 40–2 can be used as a guide to the amount of raw meat to buy in order to have a given amount of cooked meat to serve.

POULTRY

Meat from poultry is a favorite food to include in planned diets. The psychological role of poultry is as important as its nutritive value. Roast chicken, turkey, goose or duck is associated with feast days, holidays, family get-togethers and company meals. The many different kinds and classes of poultry, as well as the many different methods of preparation, offer variety for the main dish the year round.

Nutritive Value.   Like other meats, poultry has protein of high quality and is a good source of iron, phosphorus and the B-complex vitamins, especially niacin. The fat varies with the kind, age and quality of the bird. In addition, the dark meat is slightly higher in fat content than the white meat, while the white meat contains more nicotinic acid.

Poultry, as a rule, is lower in fat than beef is. For instance, 3 oz. of a lean beef cut such as flank steak has about 6 gm. of fat, while the same amount of chicken without the skin (which contains most of the fat) contains about 3 gm. of fat.

Digestibility.   The high coefficient of digestibility, as well as rapidity and ease of digestion, makes poultry a valuable addition to the menu. Since the white meat contains a little less connective tissue and fat than the dark meat, it is slightly easier to digest. Duck and goose are comparatively high in fat. Broilers and fryers, being younger, have less fat than the older roasters and stewing birds. Turkey can be classed with the latter group.

Buyer's Information.   Many factors should be considered when buying poultry.

KINDS OF POULTRY. Chicken, turkey, duck and goose are the kinds of poultry most commonly eaten and, of these, chicken is by far the most plentiful and popular. Less common and more expensive birds enjoyed are Cornish game hen, guinea hen and squab (pigeon).

CLASS. Poultry classes within each kind are based on age, weight and sex and therefore are related to tenderness and suitable methods of cooking. A plump young chicken (usually 9 to 12 weeks of age), selected for broiling, weighs not over 2½ lb. The weight of a frying chicken averages 2½ lb to 3½ lb., and a roasting chicken (usually 3 to 5 months of age) averages 3 to 6 lb. Capons (castrated male birds), deluxe in quality, are usually under 8 months of age and weigh 6 to 9 lb., ready-to-cook weight. They are exceptionally meaty, and the flesh is juicy, tender, and unusually fine in flavor. A capon is usually roasted. Fowls or stewing chickens are mature birds (usually more than 10 months of age) and their weights are variable.

Turkeys are classed as fryers or roasters. Ducks weigh 4 lb. or under for the small size and 5 lb. or more for the large size. Ducks are usually marketed young as ducklings. Geese weigh 8 lb. or under for the small size and 10 lb. or more for the large size. Squabs and guineas are sold in some markets.

STYLE OF PROCESSING. Most poultry is currently marketed ready-to-cook (whole or parts), although live and dressed birds are still available in some markets. Dressed and ready-to-cook poultry is sold fresh-chilled, cold storage or quick-frozen. Cold storage poultry is kept in refrigerated storage for a minimum of 60 days. Dressed poultry indicates that the bird has been bled and the feathers removed, but the head, feet and internal organs remain. The ready-to-cook (eviscerated) poultry has been bled, feathers removed and picked and internal organs, head, feet and oil sac removed.

GOVERNMENT STANDARDS. Some poultry is labeled to show government inspection and grading, some to show inspection only, and some is neither graded nor inspected. The bird that carries an official grade mark has been examined for quality and then assigned a U.S. Grade A, B or C, according to Government standards. The inspection mark refers to the bird's wholesomeness or fitness for food.

The *best quality* poultry show these characteristics: full-fleshed and meaty breast and legs, well-distributed fat, and skin with few blemishes and pinfeathers. Young chickens and turkeys have smooth, tender skin, soft, tender meat and a flexible breastbone. An older chicken or turkey, suitable for stewing or braising, has coarser skin and a firm breastbone.

The *number of servings* obtained from poultry is dependent upon the kind, weight, age, sex, grade and method of cooking. A rough guide of the amount of dressed weight poultry to buy per serving is: ¼ to ½ chicken for broiling, ¾ to 1 lb. chicken for frying and roasting, ⅓ to ¾ lb. chicken for stewing, 1 to 1¼ lb. of duck, ¾ to 1 lb. of goose and ⅔ to ¾ lb. of turkey. Ready-to-cook weight of poultry to buy per serving is: ¼ to ½ chicken for broiling, about ½ lb. of chicken for frying, roasting and stewing, about 1 lb. of duck, about ⅔ lb. of goose and about ¾ lb. of turkey.

The meat of chicken and turkey is sold frozen or canned, and whole small chickens are canned commercially.

FISH

Fish is a high-quality protein food classified into categories of fresh-water fish (caught in fresh-water lakes, rivers and streams), salt-water fish and shellfish.

Composition. Fish and shellfish contain about 19 per cent protein that is similar in amino acid composition to that found in muscle meats. The fat content varies from 1 to 20 per cent, depending upon the species and the season of the year. In general, this is a lower fat content than beef. (See Appendix Table 1.)

Nutritive Value. Fish contains protein of high biological value, essential minerals, vitamins and fats. In general, the nutritive value of fish is similar to that of beef, except that shellfish and salt-water fish are rich in iodine and fluorine, plus appreciable amounts of cobalt, and for that reason make a valuable contribution to the diet. Fish is also a satisfactory source of magnesium, phosphorus, iron and copper. The iron content of fish is lower than that found in meat, but calcium is about equal. Shellfish generally have a higher calcium and iodine content than fish. Herring and oysters are exceptionally high in zinc.

A serving of fat fish, such as salmon or mackerel, will supply about 10 per cent of the daily allowance of vitamin A and all of the vitamin D. The natural oil found in canned fish should be used, since it too is a valuable source of these vitamins. An average serving of either fat or lean fish will supply about 10 per cent of the thiamin, 15 per cent of the riboflavin and 50 per cent of the niacin required daily.

Fish and shellfish have high levels of polyunsaturated fatty acids, which lends to their use in certain dietary regimens. However, the cholesterol content of fish muscle is similar to that of meat and poultry (50 to 70 mg. cholesterol per 100 gm. tissue). Shellfish are low in fat but relatively rich in cholesterol. (See Appendix Table 4.)

Digestibility. Fish and shellfish are excellent sources of easily digestible protein of high nutritional value. Tests have shown that from 85 to 95 per cent of the protein is assimilable. Oyster stew is an especially suitable dish, since it is easily digested, highly nutritious and easy to eat. Some individuals are allergic to shellfish and occasionally to other fish.

Buyer's Information. Fish is sold fresh, frozen, salted, dried and canned.

Certain varieties of fresh fish are more economical when plentiful during specific seasons of the year. When buying whole fresh fish, look for these signs of freshness: eyes are bright, clear and bulging; gills are reddish-pink and free from slime; scales are tight to the skin, bright and shiny; flesh is firm and elastic; and odor is fresh. Fresh fish are marketed (1) whole or round (internal organs, scales, head, tail and fins must be removed at home before cooking), (2) drawn (whole or round fish sold after internal organs are removed), (3) dressed or pan dressed (whole or round fish sold after internal organs and scales are removed), (4) as steaks, which are cross-section slices of the larger dressed fish and are ready to cook as purchased and (5) as fillets, which are the meaty sides of the fish, cut lengthwise away from the bone. These require no preparation for cooking, and there is no waste. Here are the suggested amounts to buy per serving: 1 lb. whole or round fish, ½ lb. large dressed fish and ⅓ lb. steaks and fillets.

Smoked, dried and salted fish are sold either whole (such as herring or small whitefish) or in slices (such as codfish).

Frozen fish consist of steaks and fillets that are quick-frozen and packaged.

Canned fish include tuna, salmon, sardines and other varieties. Some manufacturers are canning fish with less oil or in water for the dietetic market.

The popular varieties of shellfish include oysters, clams, shrimp, crabs and lobsters.

EGGS

Composition. The average hen's egg, without shell, weighs 50 gm. The fat and protein are about equally divided, with 13 per cent protein and 12 per cent fat. The egg yolk contains half of the protein and all of the fat, minerals (except sulfur) and vitamins (except riboflavin). The egg white contains the other half of the protein and riboflavin and part of the sulfur. One egg yields an *average* of 80 kcal., of which 64 are from the yolk and only 16 from the white.

Nutritive Value. Eggs are a good source of complete, high-quality protein, easily assimilated unsaturated fats, iron, copper, phosphorus, vitamin A, riboflavin, vitamin B_{12}, vitamin D, pantothenic acid and thiamin. All the nutritive substances, minerals and vitamins necessary for the development of the chick are furnished by the egg and can be compared in food value with milk and meat. The yolk contains most of the mineral and vitamin activity of whole egg. Eggs lack vitamin C and are a poor source of niacin. Egg protein contains somewhat higher amounts of the sulfur amino acids (methionine and cystine) than does meat. Egg yolk is high in cholesterol; the average egg yolk contains 275 mg.

The color of the shell depends upon the breed of the fowl and does not affect the nutritive value of the egg or the flavor. Neither is it a guide to yolk color. The color of the egg yolk may vary from light to deep yellow. Yolk color is influenced by heredity and diet but does not necessarily affect flavor and nutritive value. The food ration of the hen tends to affect the flavor of the egg and color of the yolk and to influence the vitamin content, especially vitamin A.

Cholesterol-free egg products have been developed for use by those who have been advised to reduce their cholesterol intake. These egg substitutes have no cholesterol, but their sodium content is higher than that of regular eggs.

There is no evidence to say that fertile eggs have more nutritional value than infertile eggs. That the hormones in fertile eggs are needed by human beings is a fallacy.

Place in the Daily Diet. Eggs may be served in innumerable ways for breakfast and as a main dish for luncheon or dinner, or they can be combined with other foods in the preparation of beverages, bread, cake, desserts, salads, salad dressings, sandwiches, sauces, vegetables and countless other dishes.

Fresh eggs are served poached, coddled, scrambled, baked, in omelets and in custards. Cold storage eggs are used in cooking and baking where the flavor of the ingredients helps to mask the taste of "held" eggs. Frozen eggs and

dried or dehydrated eggs can also be used in baked goods.

Eggs are useful in cooking and baking. When air is whipped into whole egg, egg yolk or egg white, the role of leavening agent comes into play. Eggs are used to thicken liquids (custards), to bind ingredients (sauces), to clarify (consommé) and to act as an emulsifying agent (mayonnaise).

Digestibility. Eggs are easily digested and almost completely utilized. The fat in the yolk is of superior quality and is in a finely emulsified form similar to that of milk. Methods of cooking eggs affect their digestibility to some degree but do not affect their total utilization.

Buyer's Information. Large and medium-size eggs are the most common size on the market. Small (pullet) eggs are usually more plentiful in the late summer and fall months. The size does not affect the quality but does affect price. Weight for weight, the nutritive value is the same for small and large eggs of equal quality.

The retail grades for shell eggs are: U.S. Grades A A, A, B and C. Factors that determine the grade are (1) cleanliness and soundness of shell, (2) size of the air cell and (3) condition of the yolk and white, which are judged by candling. Retail cartons of officially graded eggs carry a certificate stating grade, size and the date of grading.

MEAT ALTERNATES

When meat is limited, other foods—macaroni, noodles, spaghetti, rice or legumes (dried peas, beans, lentils)—can be combined with it. This is known as mutual supplementation. Meat loaf, extended with dried milk, oats, wheat germ and grated carrots and bound with egg, is an excellent source of protein. Dried skim milk, split peas or beans flavored with ham bone (or any kind of bone) furnish protein as desirable as that in expensive lamb chops. One half cup of cooked dried peas or beans furnishes about the same amount of protein as 1 oz. of meat.

At a time when famine and malnutrition exist among one eighth of the population of the world, finding less expensive ways of obtaining protein than from animals becomes very important. Grain-fed beef, so popular in the United States, is by far the most expensive form of edible protein, not only in terms of money but in terms of the amounts of protein and energy needed to raise the animal. (See Fig. 40–2.)

Nuts

Nuts are defined as a dry fruit consisting of a kernel in a shell. Since they are generally high in protein and fat, they are sometimes used as meat alternates or extenders. The nuts most commonly used are peanuts (and peanut butter), almonds, filberts, chestnuts, walnuts, cashews and Brazil nuts.

Composition. Except for the chestnut, which is high in carbohydrate and low in protein and fat, nuts are generally high in fat and protein. (See Table 40–3.)

Nutritive Value and Digestibility. Although the protein of nuts is not equal in quality to that of milk, eggs, cheese, meat, fish and poultry, it is of good quality and makes a valuable contribution to the diet. Nuts are a good source of the B-complex vitamins thiamin, riboflavin and niacin and of the minerals iron, copper, phosphorus and manganese. They also contain varying amounts of calcium, depending upon the variety. Since nuts are high in fat (except chestnuts), they digest slowly. Chopped nuts and nut spreads, such as peanut butter, are more easily utilized.

Use in the Diet. Nuts are used as good sources of protein and as meat alternates and extenders, such as in stuffing for poultry, nut loaf, stuffed peppers, potato cakes, fritters and croquettes. In whole or chopped form they are also used as an ingredient in cakes, cookies, pies and various dessert dishes and are also used as a spread for sandwiches in the form of nut butters.

Legumes

Dry beans, peas and lentils are nutritious, low-cost foods that can be used in combination with other foods to provide good quality protein. (See Fig. 10–2 and Table 10–7.) There are many varieties of legumes, including lima beans, split peas, lentils, red kidney beans, pinto beans, and black-eyed peas, chickpeas and many others.

Nutritive Value. Legumes supply important quantities of protein, iron, thiamin, riboflavin and trace minerals and are low in fat. One cup of cooked legumes supplies about 290 kcal., 31 per cent of the protein, 42 per cent of the iron, 26 per cent of the thiamin and 13 per cent of the riboflavin needed by an adult male.

Buyer's Information. Beans, peas and lentils should have a bright, uniform color, be free of visible defects and be of uniform size. Store tightly covered in a cool, dry place. To compare the relative cost of legumes, nuts, peanut

LIVESTOCK PROTEIN CONVERSION EFFICIENCY

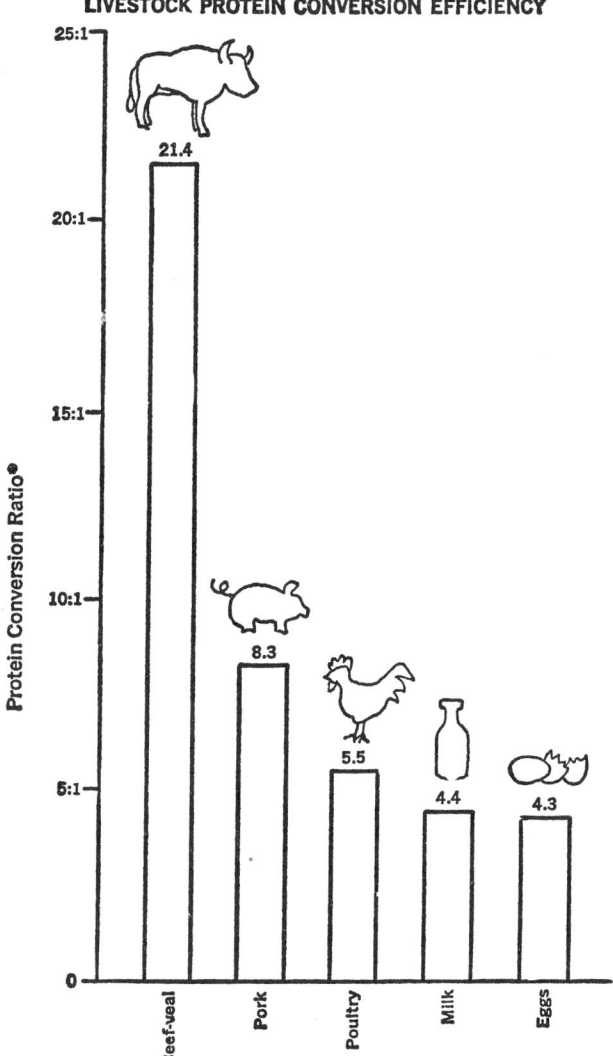

Figure 40–2 Livestock protein conversion efficiency. *Protein conversion ratio is the number of lb. of protein fed to livestock in order to produce 1 lb. of protein for human consumption. (From Lappé, F. M.: Diet for a Small Planet. New York, Ballantine, 1971, p. 7.)

Table 40–3   AVERAGE COMPOSITION OF COMMON NUTS

KIND	WATER (%)	PROTEIN (%)	FAT (%)	CHO (%)	KCAL. (per 100 gm.)
Almonds, dried	5	19	54	20	598
Brazil nuts	5	14	67	11	654
Butternuts	4	24	61	8	629
Cashew nuts	5	17	46	29	561
Chestnuts, fresh	53	3	2	42	194
Chestnuts, dried	8	7	4	79	377
Filberts (hazelnuts)	6	13	62	17	634
Hickory nuts	3	13	69	13	673
Peanuts, roasted	2	26	49	21	582
Pecans	3	9	71	15	687
Pistachio nuts	5	19	54	19	594
Walnuts, black	3	21	59	15	628
Walnuts, English	4	15	64	16	651

butter and meat, quotations of prices can be obtained from a retail store, but they should be evaluated in terms of grams of protein provided. See Table 18–10 for an example of such a comparison. This is based on 1976 prices, but a similar comparison could be made using present prices. This is easier now that nutritional labeling of food products is available. Remember that when a person is consuming most of his protein intake in the form of incomplete proteins, he may require more than the RDA of 0.8 gm. per kg. body weight. (See Chapter 5.)

VEGETABLE AND FRUIT GROUP

Four or more servings from the vegetable and fruit group are recommended daily. These should include citrus fruit or another fruit or vegetable rich in ascorbic acid, a dark green or deep yellow vegetable for vitamin A (at least every other day) and other vegetables and fruits, including potatoes.

VEGETABLES

Vegetables play an important part in the diet. Yellow vegetables provide vitamin A and green vegetables furnish iron and vitamin A, while all of the vegetables are good sources of minerals, vitamins, and fiber.

Appetizing and palatable vegetables depend upon the selection of quality produce and the careful adherence to proper food preparation techniques. Overcooked, woody-textured and soggy vegetables are not appetizing and are usually refused. Rapid transportation facilities and the canning and freezing processes have largely eliminated the regional and seasonal factors in availability. Sources of supply vary with the changing seasons and with crop development in many divergent producing areas. Vegetables are usually lowest in price in any given market area when the local supply is most abundant. Scarcity or abundance of a commodity regulates the price more often than any other factor. Many families obtain fresh vegetables from a garden planted in the back yard, and even apartment dwellers now can rent space in vacant lots for raising vegetables. Home food freezers and refrigerators with enough space for storing frozen foods have changed buying habits. However, the fresh vegetable flavor remains the criterion for judging both frozen and canned vegetables.

Classification by Nutritive Value. Vegetables may be classified according to the part of the plant used for food and according to nutritive value. Vegetables and parts of vegetables vary in nutritive value.

GREEN LEAFY VEGETABLES. Lettuce, romaine, chicory, escarole, endive, cabbage, collards, Chinese cabbage and all greens are examples. They are most valuable for minerals, vitamins and cellulose; they are important sources of the minerals calcium and iron and of the vitamins A, K and riboflavin, and they are valuable sources of ascorbic acid. The young, tender growing leaves contain more ascorbic acid than the mature plants. The green outer leaves of lettuce and cabbage are much richer in vitamin A, calcium and iron than the white inner leaves. The thinner and greener the leaf, the richer in nutritive value. Green leafy vegetables are generally low in calories.

FLOWERING VEGETABLES. Broccoli and cauliflower are the two most commonly used flowering vegetables. Broccoli, being greener, rates higher in nutritive value than cauliflower and is a good source of iron, phosphorus, vitamin A, ascorbic acid and riboflavin. Cauliflower is also a good source of ascorbic acid. One half cup of cooked cauliflower contains about 70 mg. The outer leaves of cauliflower and broccoli are much higher in nutritive value than the flower buds and should be cooked or used in salads.

SEED VEGETABLES. Peas, beans and lentils are classified as seed vegetables or legumes. The more mature legumes provide protein (incomplete) and are frequently supplemented with complete protein foods, such as milk, eggs, meat, cheese, or other incomplete or complementary proteins, such as wheat, rice or corn. (See Fig. 10–2, p. 203.) They may be used as a main dish and are valuable for phosphorus, iron, zinc and thiamin.

ROOT VEGETABLES. Carrots, beets, turnips and white and sweet potatoes are examples of root vegetables, of which the yellow and orange varieties are rich sources of carotene. The deeper the yellow color, the greater the content of carotene, the precursor of vitamin A. Root vegetables in general are good sources of thiamin. White potatoes (modified underground stems) contain some ascorbic acid, and although they are not a rich source, when properly prepared and used in quantity they can add significantly to the total day's allowance.

STEM OR STALK VEGETABLES. Celery and asparagus are examples of stem vegetables. They contain minerals and vitamins in proportion to the green color, similar to that found in green leafy vegetables. Asparagus is a particularly good source of folic acid.

FRUIT VEGETABLES. The tomato and pepper are the outstanding vegetables that are the fruit of the plant. Both are rich in ascorbic acid. Other fruit vegetables are cucumbers, squash, pumpkin and eggplant. Remember, the deeper the green or yellow color, the greater the carotene content.

BULB VEGETABLES. The onion is the outstanding example of a bulb vegetable and is a fair source of ascorbic acid.

Composition of Vegetables. In general, the fresh raw product contains more vitamins and minerals than the processed product. In the raw state, vegetables are also an excellent source of dietary fiber. All vegetables have a high water content and vary in composition, even within one variety, depending upon the species, conditions of growth and method of cooking. Vegetables are composed chiefly of carbohydrates. The carbohydrate content, in general, ranges from 3 per cent—as found in the leafy and stem vegetables—to 27 per cent in sweet potatoes. The root and seed vegetables are among the richest in carbohydrate content. With the exception of legumes, vegetables contain very little protein, averaging from 1 to 3 per cent. There is little or no fat in vegetables. No evidence exists that organically grown vegetables are any richer in nutrients than traditionally grown vegetables, although they will have less pesticide residue. (See Chapter 18.)

Digestibility. The great value of fresh vegetables in keeping the digestive tract functioning normally has been mentioned previously. The bulky, fibrous foods, in contrast with highly refined, concentrated foods, are essential for good digestion and elimination. Adequate bulk makes laxatives generally unnecessary.

There are some conditions, such as diarrhea, peptic ulcers and ulcerative colitis (Chapters 22 and 23), in which the use of bulky vegetables and roughage may be restricted or must be avoided. Furthermore, in conditions such as gallbladder (Chapter 24) and cardiac disease (Chapter 28) certain vegetables, commonly termed "gas-forming," may cause distress and must be used with discretion. However, the normal individual can digest vegetables with ease.

Buyer's Information. Supply, demand and distribution are factors that influence the price of produce. Although practice is the best teacher in the selection of fresh vegetables, here are some suggeseted criteria for judging:

Selecting the fresh and avoiding the shriveled, wilted or decayed is the best rule to follow. Freshness, state of ripeness, firmness, lack of blemishes and no sign of spoilage are some of the guiding factors. Best quality and price are available at the peak of the season.

Canned Vegetables. Commercially canned vegetables offer a large variety of products to choose from the year round, helping to keep the food budget down when certain vegetables are out of season. They are cooked and ready to eat, thus saving time and assuring no waste. The vegetables used for canning are especially grown for that purpose, picked at just the right point of maturity, vacuum sealed and subjected to pressure heat in the briefest possible time after harvesting. The process used in industrial canning does not affect the food value of carbohydrate, protein and fat, and most of the vitamin and mineral nutritive values are retained. Quality canned vegetables are preferable for plain-cooked dishes, salads or serving "as is." Second quality may do for combination dishes such as stews, casseroles, soups or when wholeness or color is not so important.

For those who count calories, limit sodium or potassium intake or are diabetic, there is an increasing number of dietetic-pack canned vegetables.

Frozen Vegetables. Frozen vegetables are becoming increasingly popular and are available all year. They are ready to cook and therefore save labor and time in preparation. The nutritive value is usually equal to that of the fresh product. The best of the crop is harvested at the peak of quality and rapidly frozen within a few hours. Only solid-frozen packages should be selected, never those that are soft and starting to thaw. Refreezing after thawing lowers quality.

Dried Vegetables. Besides fresh, frozen and canned, vegetables are also available in dried or dehydrated form. Legumes are the most popular dried foods and are used as supplementary protein foods. Other dried foods such as soups and seasonings (onion, garlic, parsley) are also available. They take little storage space and have a definite place in the menu.

Maintaining Nutritional Value During Preparation. Cook vegetables quickly (just until tender) in a minimum amount of water (just enough to prevent scorching) in a covered pan and serve immediately. In this respect, steaming and pressure cooking have advantages over boiling. The iron content of broccoli, for example, diminishes 50 per cent after 20 minutes of boiling. Adding bicarbonate of soda to the

water softens the fiber and retains the color of green vegetables but encourages mineral and vitamin loss. Vegetables deteriorate quickly in vitamin value if exposed to air while cooking or if cooked too long. The nutritional content also suffers when vegetables are allowed to stand in the open or are warmed over. This is especially true of the ascorbic acid content of vegetables. Gordon and Noble[1] analyzed ascorbic acid values following three methods of cooking vegetables: in a pressure saucepan, in a "waterless" saucepan, and covered with boiling water. The percentage retention of ascorbic acid was highest with the pesssure saucepan. The "waterless" saucepan ranked second (except for broccoli and Brussels sprouts).

Use the liquid remaining from cooked and canned vegetables to flavor soups, sauces and gravies.

Cook potatoes without peeling to retain more nutrients.

Peel or scrape sparingly any vegetables. The dark outer leaves of cabbage, head lettuce and other greens are rich in iron, calcium and vitamins.

FRUIT

Modern methods of transportation and refrigeration make it possible to have fresh fruits all year. Consumption of citrus fruits has increased greatly in the last century. Even so, clinical studies reveal that many children and adults do not get enough ascorbic acid, often because they lack knowledge about its sources and nutritive value rather than because of cost or availability.

Composition. Fruits provide energy value (through the carbohydrate content), protective vitamins and minerals and cellulose. They contain very little protein and are practically fat-free. Two exceptions to the fat rule are avocados and olives, both of which contain appreciable amounts of fat. Fruits vary widely in their carbohydrate content. The caloric value of fresh and reconstituted dried fruit is comparatively low. Dried fruit, as such, and fruits canned or frozen with sugar have increased calories, depending upon the ingredients used in processing.

Nutritive Value. All fresh fruits contribute some ascorbic acid, but the citrus fruits are outstanding as a source of this vitamin. For example, one medium-size orange will furnish the normal adult daily requirement. Strawberries and cantaloupe are good sources, while apples and peaches are fair sources. However, a fair source can be taken in sufficient quantity to contribute substantially to the diet. (See Table 10–12.)

Most fruits also supply varying amounts of vitamin A and the B-complex vitamins. The yellow fruits, such as peaches, cantaloupe and apricots, are good sources of vitamin A, whereas plums and dried fruits (those not treated with sulfur dioxide) are the best sources of thiamin.

Fruits contribute appreciable amounts of the minerals iron and calcium. Among the fruits richest in iron are dried fruits of all kinds, apricots, peaches, bananas, grapes and berries. Calcium is found in small amounts in the citrus fruits (the whole fruit contains double the amount contained in an equal amount of the juice), strawberries and dried figs. Sodium, magnesium and potassium, which account for the alkaline ash of fruits when metabolized by the body, are also present in varying amounts in most fruits. This is an important therapeutic measure in conditions such as certain types of kidney stones and kidney diseases. (See Chapter 30.)

Careful preparation, storage and service are essential procedures to retain the maximum value of vitamins and minerals. There is some loss of nutritive value in the process of cooking, drying or canning, but losses are not so great as at one time supposed. The frozen fruits compare favorably in vitamin content with fresh ones. See the section on Food Preservation in Chapter 18 for details of vitamin losses in processed foods. Bruising, cutting and allowing fruit and fruit juice to be exposed to the air cause considerable loss of ascorbic acid.

Digestibility. Ripe fruits are easily digested, because the sugar content (glucose and fructose) is in readily absorbable form. Emphasis should be on *ripeness,* since the sugar in green fruits is not fully developed and is therefore difficult to digest. For example, bananas are high in starch when green but when ripe the starch changes to thoroughly digestible sugars. In some conditions, fruits are tolerated better if cooked.

Fruits, like vegetables, contain indigestible cellulose that furnishes bulk necessary for good elimination and intestinal health. Of course, in certain conditions cellulose is to be avoided. (See Chapters 22 and 23.) Prunes and figs are especially valuable as mild laxatives.

Buyer's Information. When selecting fresh fruits, those with no disfigurements or just a few removable blemishes should be picked, while shriveled, wilted and decayed fruit should be rejected.

Bananas are usually purchased by the hand (5 or 6 bananas attached to stem) and by weight, and the color indicates degree of ripeness. The skin of a fully ripened banana shows brown flecks and no green tips.

Among the citrus fruits, the markings on the peel or the color of the peel does not influence the quality. Those with smooth thin skins usually indicate a high juice content. Those that are heavy for size are preferred.

Maintaining Nutritional Value During Preparation. To conserve nutrients, fruits should be peeled thinly. Juice should be extracted from fruit just before serving. Fruit juice should not be allowed to stand long after extraction or after opening the can. If juices (fresh or canned) are stored in the refrigerator, they should be put in covered containers to reduce oxidation and loss of vitamin C. Fresh fruit should be chilled before extraction of the juice.

BREAD AND CEREAL GROUP

Cereal derives its name from the mythological Roman goddess of grains and harvest, Ceres, and furnishes the bulk of the world's food supply. Cereal grains are the source of many food items that are included in normal and modified diet plans. Examples are bread, crackers, cooked cereals, ready-to-eat cereals, macaroni, spaghetti, noodles, rice and barley.

CEREALS AND FLOUR

Composition. Cereal grains furnish an average of 75 per cent carbohydrate, 10 to 15 per cent protein and 2 per cent fat. A cereal grain consists of three parts: the inner germ, the protective endosperm and the outer bran layer, as shown in Figure 3–9. The *germ* is the heart or embryo of the grain, which sprouts when the seed is planted. It is one of the best sources of thiamin and vitamin E, and it contains protein of high quality, other B-complex vitamins, fat, minerals (especialiy iron) and carbohydrate. The *endosperm* makes up by far the largest part of the grain, or approximately 85 per cent, and is chiefly carbohydrate, with some protein in the form of gluten. The *bran,* or outer layer, is chiefly cellulose plus the B-complex vitamins and minerals, especially iron.

Nutritive Value. In Chapter 3 the nutritive value of carbohydrates from grain sources was discussed. Cereal and cereal products furnish approximately 50 per cent of the calories for the people of the world. Whole-grain cereals, or those enriched with vitamins and minerals to whole-grain value, provide significant amounts of iron, thiamin, riboflavin and niacin.

The protein of the germ is a complete protein, but since this is the portion of the grain that spoils first, it is removed in the refining process. The protein in the endosperm is not of such high quality but contributes significantly to the total daily protein requirement. For example, when milk is used with or added to cereals and cereal products such as breakfast cereal and in bread-making, the endosperm proteins complement the protein amino acids in milk and become important and economical sources of protein.

The vitamin and mineral content of cereal grain products depends upon the amount of germ, endosperm and bran present. Whole grains include all three parts, while highly refined cereal grain products contain only the endosperm. Enriched and restored cereal products and flours have had returned some of the vitamins and minerals that were removed during the milling process, namely thiamin, riboflavin, niacin and iron. Table 40–4 reviews the enrichment requirements for flour and cereal grain foods in the United States.

Buyer's Information. There are four different types of wheat flour. (1) Whole-wheat flour, graham flour and entire wheat flour are synonymous. (2) Flour, white flour, wheat flour and plain flour are synonymous terms, and the flour may be either bleached or unbleached. (3) Self-rising flour contains the correct proportions of leavening agent and salt. (4) Enriched flour is white flour with added vitamins and minerals.

Classification of Flours. Flours are identified by the following classification: (1) Macaroni flours are made from durum wheats, high in protein content. (2) Bread flours are milled from blends of hard spring and hard winter wheats, bleached or unbleached. (3) General purpose or all-purpose family flours are milled from hard wheats (nothern areas) and soft wheats (southern areas). (4) Pastry flours are milled usually from soft wheats. (5) Cake flours are milled from soft wheats. Other types of flour are buckwheat flour, corn flour (a by-product of making corn meal), cottonseed flour, lima bean flour, peanut flour, potato flour, soy flour (full-fat and low-fat), rice flour and rye flour.

Cereal Grain Products. A variety of products are manufactured and processed from cereal grains. Corn meal, cornstarch and hominy (pearl, lye, granulated and grits) are

Table 40-4 STANDARDS FOR ENRICHMENT OF CEREAL PRODUCTS

*Minimum and Maximum Amounts of Required and Optimal Nutrients Specified for Foods Labeled "Enriched"*¹

CEREAL PRODUCT	REQUIRED NUTRIENTS											OPTIONAL NUTRIENTS			
	THIAMIN		RIBOFLAVIN		NIACIN		IRON		CALCIUM				CALCIUM		VITAMIN D	
	Min. (mg.)	Max. (mg.)	Min. (mg.)	Max. (mg.)	Min. (mg.)	Max. (mg.)	Min. (mg.)	Max. (mg.)	Min. (mg.)	Max. (mg.)	Min. (mg.)	Max. (mg.)	Min. (I.U.)	Max. (I.U.)
Per Lb. of Product														
Bread, rolls and buns, white	1.1	1.8	0.7	1.6	10.0	15.0	8.0	12.5	–	–	300	800	150	750
Cornmeal; corn grits	2.0	3.0	1.2	1.8	16.0	24.0	13.0	26.0	–	–	500	750	250	1000
Cornmeal, self-rising	2.0	3.0	1.2	1.8	16.0	24.0	13.0	26.0	–	–	500	1750	250	1000
Farina	2.0	2.5	1.2	1.5	16.0	20.0	13.0	(²)	–	–	500	(²)	250	(²)
Flour, white	2.0	2.5	1.2	1.5	16.0	20.0	13.0	16.5	–	–	500³	625³	250	1000
Flour, self-rising	2.0	2.5	1.2	1.5	16.0	20.0	13.0	16.5	500	1500	–	–	250	1000
Macaroni products; noodle products	4.0	5.0	1.7	2.2	27.0	34.0	13.0	16.5	–	–	500	625	250	1000
Rice, milled	2.0	4.0	1.2⁴	2.4⁴	16.0	32.0	13.0	26.0	–	–	500	1000	250	1000
Per 100 Gm. of Product														
Bread, rolls and buns, white	0.24	0.40	0.15	0.35	2.20	3.31	1.76	2.76	–	–	66	176	33	165
Cornmeal; corn grits	0.44	0.66	0.26	0.40	3.53	5.29	2.87	5.73	–	–	110	165	55	220
Cornmeal, self-rising	0.44	0.66	0.26	0.40	3.53	5.29	2.87	5.73	–	386	–	–	55	220
Farina	0.44	0.55	0.26	0.33	3.53	4.41	2.87	(²)	–	–	110	(²)	55	(²)
Flour, white	0.44	0.55	0.26	0.33	3.53	4.41	2.87	3.64	–	–	110³	138	55	220
Flour, self-rising	0.44	0.55	0.26	0.33	3.53	4.41	2.87	3.64	110	331	–	–	55	220
Macaroni products; noodle products	0.88	1.10	0.37	0.48	5.95	7.50	2.87	3.64	–	–	110	138	55	220
Rice, milled	0.44	0.88	0.26⁴	0.53⁴	3.53	7.05	2.87	5.73	–	–	110	220	55	220

*Information here, except for rice and self-rising cornmeal, from: Federal Register, Dec. 20, 1955. Information for rice and self-rising cornmeal from: Federal Register, Aug. 27, 1957 and Aug. 10, 1961 respectively. Standards became effective for latter on Jan. 27, 1962.

¹Standards for enrichment provide for inclusion of calcium and vitamin D within stated limits as optional ingredients for products here, except self-rising cornmeal and self-rising flour; for these items calcium is required as indicated.

²No maximum level established.

³When acidified with monocalcium phosphate at specified range of 0.25 to 0.75 per cent of the finished product, calcium levels may range from 680 to 1165 mg. per lb. (150 to 257 mg. per 100 gm.).

⁴Requirement for riboflavin stayed pending further hearings.

processed from corn. Oatmeal or rolled oats, both regular and quick-cooking, are processed from oats. The varieties of rice include coated (white) or uncoated (brown), long-, medium- and short-grain, rice bran, rice polish and wild rice. Soy grits are obtained from the soybean plant. Tapioca is available in pearl and quick-cooking varieties. Crushed wheat, cracked wheat, farina, macaroni and noodle products are processed from wheat.

SEASONINGS

Seasoning is frequently termed the soul of cooking. The greater the skill in the art of seasoning, the better the cook. While seasonings do not add food value to the diet, they often make a dish that has been unacceptable a desirable food. The main purpose in seasoning foods is to make the product more palatable. Seasonings can do this in several ways: (1) by intensifying the basic flavor of a food, (2) by blending flavors into a more pleasing composite flavor or (3) by changing a flavor or combination of basic flavors to something quite different. Use imagination when adding that extra salt and pepper to cooked vegetables. Experiment by adding garlic or onion salt or herbs to a favorite dish. Sodium-restricted diets can be made palatable by using allowed spices, herbs and other seasonings. In general, seasonings include condiments, spices, herbs and other flavorings. It is difficult to be specific about what should be grouped under each term. They all overlap and can be grouped together roughly as "seasoning."

CONDIMENTS

Salt (sodium chloride) is by far the most commonly used seasoning and is also an essential body mineral. When used in moderation, it gives zest to and brings out the natural flavor of otherwise tasteless food. However, care should be taken not to use excess amounts that mask the natural food flavor and blunt the appetite.

Pepper ranks next to salt as the most common seasoning. It comes in two forms, white and black. Both come from the dried berries of the same tropical vine. The difference is in processing. For white pepper, the outer dark surface of the tiny berries is rubbed off and only the inside is used. White pepper is chiefly valued for its light hue. In creamy sauces, pale soups and other light-colored dishes it leaves none of the dark specks that black pepper does.

It is also somewhat less pungent than black pepper.

Cayenne pepper and *paprika* are members of the pepper family. Cayenne is a pungent chili pepper used in sauces, meat and egg dishes and seafood. Paprika is a mild member of the pepper family, usually sprinkled on and used to add color and flavor to canapes, gravies, salad dressings, certain vegetables, fish and meats.

SPICES

Among the more common spices used to add flavor are cinnamon, ginger, cloves, allspice (resembles a blend of cinnamon, nutmeg and cloves), mace (flavor similar to nutmeg) and aniseed (licorice-like flavor). Table 40–5 lists the more common spices with their sources and uses.

Some spices in large amounts have been found to have pharmacological properties. Nutmeg, for instance, in doses of 1 to 2 tablespoonfuls within 3 to 6 hours, will cause thirst, tachycardia, cutaneous flushing, hallucinations and a feeling of unreality. It has been used for this purpose by prison inmates, among others.

MONOSODIUM GLUTAMATE

Monosodium glutamate (MSG) intensifies taste rather than adding any of its own. It is a fine white powder derived from vegetable protein. Oriental cultures have used it for centuries; in fact, it is sometimes called "Chinese powder." Some people have an adverse reaction to monosodium glutamate and may experience headache, dizziness, a burning sensation in the extremities and chest pain after eating a Chinese meal, since MSG is used so much in this kind of cooking. This is called Chinese restaurant syndrome.

Use monosodium glutamate with chicken and poultry; it probably does more for chicken than for any other food. It also is effective with meat (particularly in overcoming the astringency of beef liver), fish, stews, gravies, soups and vegetables (blots out the raw starch taste of potatoes). Condensed and dried soups probably would be unmarketable without it.

Add about the same amount of monosodium glutamate as you do salt; if a recipe calls for a half teaspoon salt, use an equal measure of this seasoning. Tests show that meat, poultry and vegetables frozen with monosodium glutamate retain quality better than when frozen without it. As yet, however, there is nothing to prove that this seasoning benefits fruits or desserts.

Table 40–5 SPICES—SOURCES AND USES*

NAME	DESCRIPTION AND SOURCE	USES
Allspice	Dried berry of the pimento tree, grown in West Indies. Named allspice because flavor resembled blend of cinnamon, nutmeg and cloves.	Whole: for pickling, spicing meats, seasoning gravies and boiling fish. Ground: for boiled foods, cakes, puddings and relishes.
Caraway seed	Dried seeds of plant grown in Northern Europe, notably Holland.	In rye bread, sauerkraut, new cabbage and on pork, liver and kidney before cooking. In cream and other mild cheeses.
Cayenne	Ground small hot red pepper. Grown in Africa.	With meats, fish, sauces and egg dishes.
Celery seed	Small dried ripe seed-like fruit of celery. Grown in many countries, including France, India, Holland and the United States.	For fish, potato salad, tomato dishes and tomato soup. Used in pickling and salad dressing. Excellent for Irish stews. Gives variety to hamburgers.
Chili powder (blend)	Ground chili peppers (grown in Mexico, California, Carolinas and Louisiana) and blended spices. Two varieties: mild or hot.	For such Mexican dishes as *chili con carne*. Good in shellfish and oyster cocktail sauces; for boiled and scrambled eggs, gravy and stew seasoning, canned corn.
Cinnamon	Dried aromatic bark of cinnamon tree. Major source, Sri Lanka (Ceylon).	Whole pieces of bark: in pickling, preserving and stewed fruits. Ground: in baked goods and to season mincemeat.
Cloves	Nail-shaped flower bud of the clove tree. Imported from Indonesia, the Malagasy Republic and Zanzibar.	Whole: for roast ham garnish, pickling, preserving, spiced syrups and drinks. Ground: for baked goods, puddings and stews.
Curry powder (blend)	Blend of many spices, originating in India.	For curried meat, fish, eggs and chicken, curry sauce, French dressing, scalloped tomatoes and clam and fish chowder.
Ginger	Root stalk of plant grown mainly in Jamaica, West Africa, India and the Orient.	Ground: in cakes, puddings, pumpkin pie and cookies. Whole *fresh* root is used in many oriental dishes. Many canned fruits benefit by a dash of ginger, especially canned pears. Used in preserved, candied (or crystallized) and dried forms.
Mace	Part of nutmeg between shell and outer husk, orange-red in color; flavor resembles nutmeg. From Indonesia and the West Indies.	Blades used in pickling, preserving and fish sauces. Used ground in pound cake, doughnuts, yellow dishes, chocolate dishes and oyster stew. Use sparingly.
Mustard	Seed of mustard plant grown in England and other areas.	Dry ground mustard used as flavoring for sauces and gravy. Prepared mustard (blended with other spices and vinegar) used in salad dressing, with ham, frankfurters and cheese.
Nutmeg	Kernel of a fruit of that name, grown in Indonesia and the West Indies.	Whole: to be grated as needed. Ground: used in baked goods, sauces and puddings. Good sprinkled over certain vegetables, such as cauliflower. Merges well with spinach. Topping for eggnog and custards. Favorite spice for doughnuts.
Paprika	Ground sweet red pepper grown chiefly in Spain and Hungary.	For color and mild flavor in, and sprinkled on, fish, shellfish and salad dressing. Used lavishly as a garnish, also served with sweet corn on the cob. Mixed with butter to make paprika butter.
Pepper	Most generally used of all spices. A small round berry picked before ripe; grows on a climbing vine. Grown in Indonesia and India. White pepper is the mature berry with hull removed.	Whole (black and white): used in pickling, soups and meats. Ground (black and white): used in meat sauces, gravies, vegetables and egg dishes.
Poppy seed	Tiny seeds of poppy plant imported from Holland. About 900,000 seeds to the pound.	Whole: as topping for breads, rolls and cookies. Oil used in salad dressings and margarine.

*Adapted from: U.S. Department of the Navy publication, Navsanda P-277.

Monosodium glutamate used to be added to baby foods to enhance flavor. However, because of the needlessness of this practice and the suspected detrimental effect of high levels of sodium and MSG in baby food on later health, MSG is no longer used in these products.

HERBS

Herbs are different from spices in that spices are plant products while herbs are the non-woody plants themselves. Herbs do wonders for flavoring and seasoning foods. Go slowly at first and use only a small amount. For best results, use one teaspoonful of fresh herbs or a quarter teaspoonful of the dried varieties.

Oregano, imported from Italy and Mexico, is good in or on green salads, tomatoes, cheese dishes, lasagna, omelets, spaghetti sauces, lamb, pork, beef, beef soup, stews and meat balls.

Marjoram is of the mint family, comes from France and Chile and should be used sparingly in or on vegetables such as carrots, greens, asparagus, lima beans and squash; in cheese, egg and chicken dishes, roast lamb, meat pies, hash, stews, stuffings, fish and vegetable sauces.

Tarragon is a leaf with anise flavor and is good added to steaks, chops, chicken, fish, vinegar, French dressing, green salad, duckling, egg dishes, sauces, tomato dishes and vegetables such as beets, greens, peas and mushrooms.

Dill is good added to potato dishes (salad or boiled), cream or cottage cheese mixtures (canapés), fish, fish sauces, gravies, pickles, cucumbers, lamb, vegetable salads, spaghetti and tomato dishes.

Basil is an herb from west Europe that is good cooked with or sprinkled on tomato dishes especially, and on eggplant, salads, green beans, peas, potatoes, squash, meats (especially ham and lamb chops), stew, sausage, eggs, poultry, sauces, salad dressings, soups and spaghetti.

Thyme is especially good in chowder, stuffings, tomatoes, eggplant, carrots, peas, stews, fish and cheese dishes, breads, veal and pork. *Sage* is less subtle and may be substituted for thyme.

Fresh Plant Flavorings

For fresh flavoring, onions, garlic, parsley, shallots, mint, sage, dill and chives are among the more staple and commonly used plants.

DESSERT FLAVORINGS

Flavorings are most often thought of in connection with desserts, cakes, cookies or foods that are enhanced by the addition of extracts to lend a pleasing flavor. Vanilla, almond and fruit extracts are the ones most frequently used. Do not limit the use to one or two flavors. Try new ones or combine flavors such as vanilla and almond or lemon and orange. Coffee and chocolate are also used as flavorings. Flavorings can be purchased in artificial or natural form, and this is always noted on the label.

BUYING AND STORAGE INFORMATION

When buying a spice or an herb, make a note of the purchase date on the label and six months later discard the product if it has not been used. By that time it will have lost its true bouquet and taste. Buy in small amounts. Keep away from heat (do not put a spice shelf over a stove), because heat promotes drying and staling. So does air; hence, a tightly covered container is a must. Shaker tops are approved as long as the openings are closed after the spice has been used. Prepared mustard and horseradish best retain flavor if refrigerated.

No matter what precautions are taken, spices start to lose savor (through evaporation of volatile oils) as soon as they are ground.

CITED REFERENCES

1. Gordon, J., and Noble, I.: "Waterless" vs. boiling water cooking of vegetables. J. Am. Diet. Assoc., 44:378, 1964.
2. Leverton, R. M., and Odell, G. V.: The Nutritive Value of Meat. Miscellaneous Publication MP-49, Stillwater, Oklahoma, Oklahoma Agricultural Experimental Station, Oklahoma State University, 1959.

APPENDIX

GENERAL REFERENCES

JOURNALS

American Journal of Nursing
American Journal of Public Health
Borden's Review of Nutrition Research
Dairy Council Digest
Journal of the American Dietetic Association
Journal of the American Medical Association
Journal of Nutrition
Journal of Nutrition Education
Nursing Outlook
Nutrition Reviews
Nutrition Today
The American Journal of Clinical Nutrition
World Health

RELIABLE RESOURCES FOR NUTRITION INFORMATION AND VISUAL AIDS

American Can Company, 730 Park Avenue, New York 10017.

American Diabetes Association, 18 E. 48th Street, New York 10017.

American Dietetic Association, 430 N. Michigan Avenue, Chicago, Illinois 60611.

American Heart Association, 44 E. 23rd Street, New York 10010.

American Home Economics Association, 1600 20th Street N.W., Washington, D.C. 20009.

American Institute of Baking, Consumer Service Department, 400 E. Ontario Street, Chicago, Illinois 60611.

Borden Company, 350 Madison Avenue, New York 10017.

Cereal Institute, Inc., 135 South LaSalle Street, Chicago, Illinois 60603.

Cooperative Extension Work in Agriculture and Home Economics, Cooperative Extension Services of States. (Contact the services of the State in which you reside.)

Department of Food and Nutrition, American Medical Association, 535 N. Dearborn Street, Chicago, Illinois 60610.

Evaporated Milk Association, 228 North LaSalle Street, Chicago, Illinois 60601.

Extension Service, Department of Home Economics, State Colleges and Universities.

Federal Trade Commission, Bureau of Investigation, Office of Chief Project Attorney, Washington, D.C. 20580.

Fish and Wildlife Service, U.S. Department of Interior, Washington, D.C. 20240.

Food and Nutrition Board, National Research Council, 2101 Constitution Avenue, Washington, D.C. 20237.

Food and Nutrition News, National Live Stock and Meat Board, Chicago, Illinois 60603.

Food and Nutrition Section, American Public Health Association, 1790 Broadway, New York 10019.

General Foods Corporation, 250 North Street, White Plains, New York 10602.

General Mills, Inc., 9200 Wayzata Blvd., Minneapolis, Minnesota 55426.

Gerber Products, Department of Nutrition, Fremont, Michigan 49412.

Home Economics Department, Campbell Soup Company, 385 Memorial Avenue, Camden, New Jersey 08103.

John Hancock Life Insurance Company, 200 Berkley Street, Boston, Massachusetts 02117.

Metropolitan Life Insurance Company, Health and Welfare Division, 1 Madison Avenue, New York 10010.

National Dairy Council, 111 North Canal Street, Chicago, Illinois 60606.

Nutrition Committee News, U.S. Department of Agriculture, Washington, D.C. 20250.

Nutrition Foundation, Inc., 99 Park Avenue, New York 10016.

Nutrition News, National Dairy Council, Chicago, Illinois 60606.

Nutrition Today, Enloe, Stalvey and Associates, Inc., 1140 Connecticut Avenue N.W., Washington, D.C. 20036.

Poultry and Egg National Board, 250 West 57th Street, New York 10010.

State Department of Health, Nutrition Division.

United Fresh Fruit and Vegetable Association, Washington, D.C.

U.S. Department of Agriculture, Institute of Home Economics, Washington, D.C. 20250.

U.S. Department of Health, Education and Welfare: Food and Drug Administration, Public Health Service, Office of Child Development, Washington, D.C. 20204.

APPENDIX TABLE 1   NUTRITIVE VALUES OF THE EDIBLE PART OF FOODS[1]*

[Dashes in the columns for nutrients show that no suitable value could be found although there is reason to believe that a measurable amount of the nutrient may be present]

Food, approximate measure, and weight (in grams)	Water	Food energy	Protein	Fat	Fatty acids			Carbo-hydrate	Cal-cium	Iron	Vita-min A value	Thia-min	Ribo-flavin	Niacin	Ascor-bic acid
					Satu-rated (total)	Unsaturated									
						Oleic	Lin-oleic								
	Per-cent	*Calo-ries*	*Grams*	*Grams*	*Grams*	*Grams*	*Grams*	*Grams*	*Milli-grams*	*Milli-grams*	*Inter-national units*	*Milli-grams*	*Milli-grams*	*Milli-grams*	*Milli-grams*
MILK, CHEESE, CREAM, IMITATION CREAM; RELATED PRODUCTS *Grams*															
Milk:															
Fluid:															
1 Whole, 3.5% fat____ 1 cup_____ 244	87	160	9	9	5	3	Trace	12	288	0.1	350	0.07	0.41	0.2	2
2 Nonfat (skim)_____ 1 cup_____ 245	90	90	9	Trace				12	296	.1	10	.09	.44	.2	2
3 Partly skimmed, 2% nonfat milk solids added. 1 cup_____ 246	87	145	10	5	3	2	Trace	15	352	.1	200	.10	.52	.2	2
Canned, concentrated, undiluted:															
4 Evaporated, un-sweetened. 1 cup_____ 252	74	345	18	20	11	7	1	24	635	.3	810	.10	.86	.5	3
5 Condensed, sweet-ened. 1 cup_____ 306	27	980	25	27	15	9	1	166	802	.3	1,100	.24	1.16	.6	3
Dry, nonfat instant:															
6 Low-density (1⅓ cups needed for re-constitution to 1 qt.). 1 cup_____ 68	4	245	24	Trace				35	879	.4	[1]20	.24	1.21	.6	5
7 High-density (⅞ cup needed for recon-stitution to 1 qt.). 1 cup_____ 104	4	375	37	1				54	1,345	.6	[1]30	.36	1.85	.9	7
Buttermilk:															
8 Fluid, cultured, made from skim milk. 1 cup_____ 245	90	90	9	Trace				12	296	.1	10	.10	.44	.2	2
9 Dried, packaged_____ 1 cup_____ 120	3	465	41	6	3	2	Trace	60	1,498	.7	260	.31	2.06	1.1	----
Cheese:															
Natural:															
Blue or Roquefort type:															
10 Ounce_____ 1 oz._____ 28	40	105	6	9	5	3	Trace	1	89	.1	350	.01	.17	.3	0
11 Cubic inch_____ 1 cu. in._____ 17	40	65	4	5	3	2	Trace	Trace	54	.1	210	.01	.11	.2	0

No.	Food	Measure																
12	Camembert, packaged in 4-oz. pkg. with 3 wedges per pkg.	1 wedge	38	52	115	7	9	5	3	Trace	1	40	0.2	380	0.02	0.29	0.3	0
	Cheddar:																	
13	Ounce	1 oz.	28	37	115	7	9	5	3	Trace	1	213	.3	370	.01	.13	Trace	0
14	Cubic inch	1 cu. in.	17	37	70	4	6	3	2	Trace	Trace	129	.2	230	.01	.08	Trace	0
	Cottage, large or small curd:																	
	Creamed:																	
15	Package of 12-oz., net wt.	1 pkg.	340	78	360	46	14	8	5	Trace	10	320	1.0	580	.10	.85	.3	0
16	Cup, curd pressed down.	1 cup	245	78	260	33	10	6	3	Trace	7	230	.7	420	.07	.61	.2	0
	Uncreamed:																	
17	Package of 12-oz., net wt.	1 pkg.	340	79	290	58	1	1	Trace	Trace	9	306	1.4	30	.10	.95	.3	0
18	Cup, curd pressed down.	1 cup	200	79	170	34	1	Trace	Trace	Trace	5	180	.8	20	.06	.56	.2	0
	Cream:																	
19	Package of 8-oz., net wt.	1 pkg.	227	51	850	18	86	48	28	3	5	141	.5	3,500	.05	.54	.2	0
20	Package of 3-oz., net wt.	1 pkg.	85	51	320	7	32	18	11	1	2	53	.2	1,310	.02	.20	.1	0
21	Cubic inch	1 cu. in.	16	51	60	1	6	3	2	Trace	Trace	10	Trace	250	Trace	.04	Trace	0
	Parmesan, grated:																	
22	Cup, pressed down.	1 cup	140	17	655	60	43	24	14	1	5	1,893	.7	1,760	.03	1.22	.3	0
23	Tablespoon	1 tbsp.	5	17	25	2	2	1	Trace	Trace	Trace	68	Trace	60	Trace	.04	Trace	0
24	Ounce	1 oz.	28	17	130	12	9	5	3	Trace	1	383	.1	360	.01	.25	.1	0
	Swiss:																	
25	Ounce	1 oz.	28	39	105	8	8	4	3	Trace	1	262	.3	320	Trace	.11	Trace	0
26	Cubic inch	1 cu. in.	15	39	55	4	4	2	1	Trace	Trace	139	.1	170	Trace	.06	Trace	0
	Pasteurized processed cheese:																	
	American:																	
27	Ounce	1 oz.	28	40	105	7	9	5	3	Trace	1	198	.3	350	.01	.12	Trace	0
28	Cubic inch	1 cu. in.	18	40	65	4	5	3	2	Trace	Trace	122	.2	210	Trace	.07	Trace	0
	Swiss:																	
29	Ounce	1 oz.	28	40	100	8	8	4	3	Trace	1	251	.3	310	Trace	.11	Trace	0
30	Cubic inch	1 cu. in.	18	40	65	5	5	3	2	Trace	Trace	159	.2	200	Trace	.07	Trace	0
	Pasteurized process cheese food, American:																	
31	Tablespoon	1 tbsp.	14	43	45	3	3	2	1	Trace	1	80	.1	140	Trace	.08	Trace	0
32	Cubic inch	1 cu. in.	18	43	60	4	4	2	1	Trace	1	100	.1	170	Trace	.10	Trace	0
33	Pasteurized process cheese spread, American.	1 oz.	28	49	80	5	6	3	2	Trace	2	160	.2	250	Trace	.15	Trace	0

1 Value applies to unfortified product; value for fortified low-density product would be 1500 I.U. and the fortified high-density product would be 2290 I.U.

*Reprinted from Nutritive Value of Foods, U.S. Dept. of Agriculture, Home and Garden Bulletin No. 72, 1970.

Table continued on the following page

APPENDIX TABLE 1   NUTRITIVE VALUES OF THE EDIBLE PART OF FOODS (Continued)

[Dashes in the columns for nutrients show that no suitable value could be found although there is reason to believe that a measurable amount of the nutrient may be present]

	Food, approximate measure, and weight (in grams)	Water	Food energy	Protein	Fat	Fatty acids Saturated (total)	Fatty acids Unsaturated Oleic	Fatty acids Unsaturated Linoleic	Carbohydrate	Calcium	Iron	Vitamin A value	Thiamin	Riboflavin	Niacin	Ascorbic acid
		Percent	Calories	Grams	Grams	Grams	Grams	Grams	Grams	Milligrams	Milligrams	International units	Milligrams	Milligrams	Milligrams	Milligrams
	MILK, CHEESE, CREAM, IMITATION CREAM; RELATED PRODUCTS—Con. Cream:															
34	Half-and-half (cream and milk). 1 cup — 242	80	325	8	28	15	9	1	11	261	.1	1,160	.07	.39	.1	2
35	1 tbsp — 15	80	20	1	2	1	1	Trace	1	16	Trace	70	Trace	.02	Trace	Trace
36	Light, coffee or table — 1 cup — 240	72	505	7	49	27	16	1	10	245	.1	2,020	.07	.36	.1	2
37	1 tbsp — 15	72	30	1	3	2	1	Trace	1	15	Trace	130	Trace	.02	Trace	Trace
38	Sour — 1 cup — 230	72	485	7	47	26	16	1	10	235	.1	1,930	.07	.35	.1	2
39	1 tbsp — 12	72	25	Trace	2	1	1	Trace	1	12	Trace	100	Trace	.02	Trace	Trace
40	Whipped topping (pressurized). 1 cup — 60	62	155	2	14	8	5	Trace	6	67	---	570	---	.04	---	---
41	Whipping, unwhipped (volume about double when whipped): 1 tbsp — 3	62	10	Trace	1	Trace	Trace	Trace	Trace	3	---	30	---	Trace	---	---
42	Light — 1 cup — 239	62	715	6	75	41	25	2	9	203	.1	3,060	.05	.29	.1	2
43	1 tbsp — 15	62	45	Trace	5	3	2	Trace	1	13	Trace	190	Trace	.02	Trace	Trace
44	Heavy — 1 cup — 238	57	840	5	90	50	30	3	7	179	.1	3,670	.05	.26	.1	2
45	1 tbsp — 15	57	55	Trace	6	3	2	Trace	1	11	Trace	230	Trace	.02	Trace	Trace
	Imitation cream products (made with vegetable fat): Creamers:															
46	Powdered — 1 cup — 94	2	505	4	33	31	1	0	52	21	.6	[2]200	---	---	Trace	---
47	1 tsp — 2	2	10	Trace	1	Trace	Trace	0	1	1	Trace	[2]Trace	---	---	---	---
48	Liquid (frozen) — 1 cup — 245	77	345	3	27	25	1	0	25	29	---	[2]100	0	0	---	---
49	1 tbsp — 15	77	20	Trace	2	1	Trace	0	2	2	---	[2]10	0	0	---	---
50	Sour dressing (imitation sour cream) made with nonfat dry milk. 1 cup — 235	72	440	9	38	35	1	Trace	17	277	.1	10	.07	.38	.2	1
51	1 tbsp — 12	72	20	Trace	2	2	Trace	Trace	1	14	Trace	Trace	Trace	Trace	Trace	---
	Whipped topping:															
52	Pressurized — 1 cup — 70	61	190	1	17	15	1	0	9	5	---	[2]340	---	0	Trace	---
53	1 tbsp — 4	61	10	Trace	1	1	Trace	0	Trace	Trace	---	[2]20	---	0	---	---
54	Frozen — 1 cup — 75	52	230	1	20	18	Trace	0	15	5	---	[2]560	---	0	---	Trace
55	1 tbsp — 4	52	10	Trace	1	1	Trace	0	1	Trace	---	[2]30	---	0	---	---

No.	Food, approximate measure	Grams	Water (%)	Food energy (cal.)	Protein (g)	Fat (g)	Saturated (g)	Oleic (g)	Linoleic (g)	Carbo-hydrate (g)	Calcium (mg)	Iron (mg)	Vitamin A (I.U.)	Thiamine (mg)	Riboflavin (mg)	Niacin (mg)	Ascorbic acid (mg)
56	Powdered, made with whole milk. 1 cup	75	58	175	3	12	10	Trace	1	15	62	Trace	330[2]	.02	.08	.1	Trace
57	1 tbsp.	4	58	10	Trace	1	1	Trace	Trace	1	3	Trace	20[2]	Trace	Trace	Trace	Trace
	Milk beverages:																
58	Cocoa, homemade. 1 cup	250	79	245	10	12	7	4	Trace	27	295	1.0	400	.10	.45	.5	3
59	Chocolate-flavored drink made with skim milk and 2% added butterfat. 1 cup	250	83	190	8	6	3	2	Trace	27	270	.5	210	.10	.40	.3	3
	Malted milk:																
60	Dry powder, approx. 3 heaping teaspoons per ounce. 1 oz.	28	3	115	4	2	----	----	----	20	82	.6	290	.09	.15	.1	0
61	Beverage. 1 cup	235	78	245	11	10	7	5	----	28	317	.7	590	.14	.49	.2	2
	Milk desserts:																
62	Custard, baked. 1 cup	265	77	305	14	15	7	5	1	29	297	1.1	930	.11	.50	.3	1
	Ice cream:																
63	Regular (approx. 10% fat). ½ gal.	1,064	63	2,055	48	113	62	37	3	221	1,553	.5	4,680	.43	2.23	1.1	11
64	1 cup	133	63	255	6	14	8	5	Trace	28	194	.1	590	.05	.28	.1	1
65	3 fl. oz. cup	50	63	95	2	5	3	2	Trace	10	73	Trace	220	.02	.11	.1	1
66	Rich (approx. 16% fat). ½ gal.	1,188	63	2,635	31	191	105	63	6	214	927	.2	7,840	.24	1.31	1.2	12
67	1 cup	148	63	330	4	24	13	8	1	27	115	Trace	980	.03	.16	.1	1
	Ice milk:																
68	Hardened. ½ gal.	1,048	67	1,595	50	53	29	17	2	235	1,635	1.0	2,200	.52	2.31	1.0	10
69	1 cup	131	67	200	6	7	4	2	Trace	29	204	.1	280	.07	.29	.1	1
70	Soft-serve. 1 cup	175	67	265	8	9	5	3	Trace	39	273	.2	370	.09	.39	.2	2
	Yoghurt:																
71	Made from partially skimmed milk. 1 cup	245	89	125	8	4	2	1	Trace	13	294	.1	170	.10	.44	.2	2
72	Made from whole milk. 1 cup	245	88	150	7	8	5	3	Trace	12	272	.1	340	.07	.39	.2	2
	EGGS																
	Eggs, large, 24 ounces per dozen: Raw or cooked in shell or with nothing added:																
73	Whole, without shell. 1 egg	50	74	80	6	6	2	3	Trace	Trace	27	1.1	590	.05	.15	Trace	0
74	White of egg. 1 white	33	88	15	4	Trace	----	----	----	Trace	3	Trace	0	Trace	.09	Trace	0
75	Yolk of egg. 1 yolk	17	51	60	3	5	2	2	Trace	Trace	24	.9	580	.04	.07	Trace	0
76	Scrambled with milk and fat. 1 egg	64	72	110	7	8	3	3	Trace	1	51	1.1	690	.05	.18	Trace	0
	MEAT, POULTRY, FISH, SHELLFISH; RELATED PRODUCTS																
77	Bacon, (20 slices per lb. raw), broiled or fried, crisp. 2 slices	15	8	90	5	8	3	4	1	1	2	.5	0	.08	.05	.8	----

[2] Contributed largely from beta-carotene used for coloring.

Table continued on the following page

APPENDIX TABLE 1   NUTRITIVE VALUES OF THE EDIBLE PART OF FOODS (Continued)

[Dashes in the columns for nutrients show that no suitable value could be found although there is reason to believe that a measurable amount of the nutrient may be present]

	Food, approximate measure, and weight (in grams)	Water	Food energy	Protein	Fat	Fatty acids Saturated (total)	Unsaturated Oleic	Unsaturated Linoleic	Carbohydrate	Calcium	Iron	Vitamin A value	Thiamin	Riboflavin	Niacin	Ascorbic acid
		Grams	Per cent	Calories	Grams	Grams	Grams	Grams	Grams	Grams	Milligrams	Milligrams	International units	Milligrams	Milligrams	Milligrams	Milligrams
	MEAT, POULTRY, FISH, SHELLFISH; RELATED PRODUCTS—Continued																
	Beef,³ cooked:																
	Cuts braised, simmered, or pot-roasted:																
78	Lean and fat____ 3 ounces____ 85	53	245	23	16	8	7	Trace	0	10	2.9	30	.04	.18	3.5	---
79	Lean only_____ 2.5 ounces__ 72	62	140	22	5	2	2	Trace	0	10	2.7	10	.04	.16	3.3	---
	Hamburger (ground beef), broiled:																
80	Lean_____ 3 ounces____ 85	60	185	23	10	5	4	Trace	0	10	3.0	20	.08	.20	5.1	---
81	Regular_____ 3 ounces____ 85	54	245	21	17	8	8	Trace	0	9	2.7	30	.07	.18	4.6	---
	Roast, oven-cooked, no liquid added:																
	Relatively fat, such as rib:																
82	Lean and fat____ 3 ounces____ 85	40	375	17	34	16	15	1	0	8	2.2	70	.05	.13	3.1	---
83	Lean only_____ 1.8 ounces__ 51	57	125	14	7	3	3	Trace	0	6	1.8	10	.04	.11	2.6	---
	Relatively lean, such as heel of round:																
84	Lean and fat____ 3 ounces____ 85	62	165	25	7	3	3	Trace	0	11	3.2	10	.06	.19	4.5	---
85	Lean only_____ 2.7 ounces__ 78	65	125	24	3	1	1	Trace	0	10	3.0	Trace	.06	.18	4.3	---
	Steak, broiled:																
	Relatively fat, such as sirloin:																
86	Lean and fat____ 3 ounces____ 85	44	330	20	27	13	12	1	0	9	2.5	50	.05	.16	4.0	---
87	Lean only_____ 2.0 ounces__ 56	59	115	18	4	2	2	Trace	0	7	2.2	10	.05	.14	3.6	---
	Relatively lean, such as round:																
88	Lean and fat____ 3 ounces____ 85	55	220	24	13	6	6	Trace	0	10	3.0	20	.07	.19	4.8	---
89	Lean only_____ 2.4 ounces__ 68	61	130	21	4	2	2	Trace	0	9	2.5	10	.06	.16	4.1	---
	Beef, canned:																
90	Corned beef_____ 3 ounces____ 85	59	185	22	10	5	4	Trace	0	17	3.7	20	.01	.20	2.9	---
91	Corned beef hash 3 ounces____ 85	67	155	7	10	5	4	Trace	9	11	1.7	---	.01	.08	1.8	---
92	Beef, dried or chipped 2 ounces__ 57	48	115	19	4	2	2	Trace	0	11	2.9	---	.04	.18	2.2	---
93	Beef and vegetable stew 1 cup___ 235	82	210	15	10	5	4	Trace	15	28	2.8	2,310	.13	.17	4.4	15
94	Beef potpie, baked, 4¼-inch diam., weight before baking about 8 ounces. 1 pie____ 227	55	560	23	33	9	20	2	43	32	4.1	1,860	.25	0.27	4.5	7

No.	Food, approximate measure	Grams	Water (%)	Food energy (cal.)	Protein (g)	Fat (g)	Saturated (g)	Oleic (g)	Linoleic (g)	Carbohydrate (g)	Calcium (mg)	Iron (mg)	Vitamin A (I.U.)	Thiamin (mg)	Riboflavin (mg)	Niacin (mg)	Ascorbic acid (mg)
	Chicken, cooked:																
95	Flesh only, broiled — 3 ounces	85	71	115	20	3	1	1	1	0	8	1.4	80	.05	.16	7.4	---
	Breast, fried, ½ breast:																
96	With bone — 3.3 ounces	94	58	155	25	5	1	2	1	1	9	1.3	70	.04	.17	11.2	---
97	Flesh and skin only — 2.7 ounces	76	58	155	25	5	1	2	1	1	9	1.3	70	.04	.17	11.2	---
	Drumstick, fried:																
98	With bone — 2.1 ounces	59	55	90	12	4	1	2	1	Trace	6	.9	50	.03	.15	2.7	---
99	Flesh and skin only — 1.3 ounces	38	55	90	12	4	1	2	1	Trace	6	.9	50	.03	.15	2.7	---
100	Chicken, canned, boneless — 3 ounces	85	65	170	18	10	3	4	2	0	18	1.3	200	.03	.11	3.7	3
101	Chicken potpie, baked 4¼-inch diam., weight before baking about 8 ounces. — 1 pie	227	57	535	23	31	10	15	3	42	68	3.0	3,020	.25	.26	4.1	5
	Chili con carne, canned:																
102	With beans — 1 cup	250	72	335	19	15	7	7	Trace	30	80	4.2	150	.08	.18	3.2	---
103	Without beans — 1 cup	255	67	510	26	38	18	17	1	15	97	3.6	380	.05	.31	5.6	---
104	Heart, beef, lean, braised — 3 ounces	85	61	160	27	5	---	---	---	1	5	5.0	20	.21	1.04	6.5	1
	Lamb,[3] cooked:																
	Chop, thick, with bone, broiled.																
105	1 chop, 4.8 ounces.	137	47	400	25	33	18	12	1	0	10	1.5	---	.14	.25	5.6	---
106	Lean and fat — 4.0 ounces	112	47	400	25	33	18	12	1	0	10	1.5	---	.14	.25	5.6	---
107	Lean only — 2.6 ounces	74	62	140	21	6	3	2	Trace	0	9	1.5	---	.11	.20	4.5	---
	Leg, roasted:																
108	Lean and fat — 3 ounces	85	54	235	22	16	9	6	Trace	0	9	1.4	---	.13	.23	4.7	---
109	Lean only — 2.5 ounces	71	62	130	20	5	3	2	Trace	0	9	1.4	---	.12	.21	4.4	---
	Shoulder, roasted:																
110	Lean and fat — 3 ounces	85	50	285	18	23	13	8	1	0	9	1.0	---	.11	.20	4.0	---
111	Lean only — 2.3 ounces	64	61	130	17	6	3	2	Trace	0	8	1.0	---	.10	.18	3.7	---
112	Liver, beef, fried — 2 ounces	57	57	130	15	6	---	---	---	3	6	5.0	30,280	.15	2.37	9.4	15
	Pork, cured, cooked:																
113	Ham, light cure, lean and fat, roasted. — 3 ounces	85	54	245	18	19	7	8	2	0	8	2.2	0	.40	.16	3.1	---
	Luncheon meat:																
114	Boiled ham, sliced — 2 ounces	57	59	135	11	10	4	4	1	0	6	1.6	0	.25	.09	1.5	---
115	Canned, spiced or unspiced. — 2 ounces	57	55	165	8	14	5	6	1	1	5	1.2	0	.18	.12	1.6	---
	Pork, fresh,[3] cooked:																
116	Chop, thick, with bone — 1 chop, 3.5 ounces.	98	42	260	16	21	8	9	2	0	8	2.2	0	.63	.18	3.8	---
117	Lean and fat — 2.3 ounces	66	42	260	16	21	8	9	2	0	8	2.2	0	.63	.18	3.8	---
118	Lean only — 1.7 ounces	48	53	130	15	7	2	3	1	0	7	1.9	0	.54	.16	3.3	---
	Roast, oven-cooked, no liquid added:																
119	Lean and fat — 3 ounces	85	46	310	21	24	9	10	2	0	9	2.7	0	.78	.22	4.7	---
120	Lean only — 2.4 ounces	68	55	175	20	10	3	4	1	0	9	2.6	0	.73	.21	4.4	---
	Cuts, simmered:																
121	Lean and fat — 3 ounces	85	46	320	20	26	9	11	2	0	8	2.5	0	.46	.21	4.1	---

[3] Outer layer of fat on the cut was removed to within approximately ½-inch of the lean. Deposits of fat within the cut were not removed.

Table continued on the following page

APPENDIX TABLE 1   NUTRITIVE VALUES OF THE EDIBLE PART OF FOODS (Continued)

[Dashes in the columns for nutrients show that no suitable value could be found although there is reason to believe that a measurable amount of the nutrient may be present]

	Food, approximate measure, and weight (in grams)		Water	Food energy	Protein	Fat	Fatty acids Saturated (total)	Fatty acids Unsaturated Oleic	Fatty acids Unsaturated Linoleic	Carbohydrate	Calcium	Iron	Vitamin A value	Thiamin	Riboflavin	Niacin	Ascorbic acid
		Grams	Percent	Calories	Grams	Grams	Grams	Grams	Grams	Grams	Milligrams	Milligrams	International units	Milligrams	Milligrams	Milligrams	Milligrams
	MEAT, POULTRY, FISH, SHELLFISH; RELATED PRODUCTS—Continued																
	Fish and shellfish—Continued																
122	Lean only --- 2.2 ounces --	63	60	135	18	6	2	3	1	0	8	2.3	0	.42	.19	3.7	---
	Sausage:																
123	Bologna, slice, 3-in. diam. by ⅛ inch. 2 slices	26	56	80	3	7	---	---	---	Trace	2	.5	---	.04	.06	.7	---
124	Braunschweiger, slice 2-in. diam. by ¼ inch. 2 slices	20	53	65	3	5	---	---	---	Trace	2	1.2	1,310	.03	.29	1.6	---
125	Deviled ham, canned 1 tbsp.	13	51	45	2	4	2	2	Trace	0	1	.3	---	.02	.01	.2	---
126	Frankfurter, heated (8 per lb. purchased pkg.). 1 frank.	56	57	170	7	15	---	---	---	1	3	.8	---	.08	.11	1.4	---
127	Pork links, cooked (16 links per lb. raw). 2 links	26	35	125	5	11	4	5	1	Trace	2	.6	0	.21	.09	1.0	---
128	Salami, dry type 1 oz.	28	30	130	7	11	---	---	---	Trace	4	1.0	---	.10	.07	1.5	---
129	Salami, cooked 1 oz.	28	51	90	5	7	---	---	---	Trace	3	.7	---	.07	.07	1.2	---
130	Vienna, canned (7 sausages per 5-oz. can). 1 sausage	16	63	40	2	3	---	---	---	Trace	1	.3	---	.01	.02	.4	---
	Veal, medium fat, cooked, bone removed:																
131	Cutlet 3 oz.	85	60	185	23	9	5	4	Trace	---	9	2.7	---	.06	.21	4.6	---
132	Roast 3 oz.	85	55	230	23	14	7	6	Trace	0	10	2.9	---	.11	.26	6.6	---
	Fish and shellfish:																
133	Bluefish, baked with table fat. 3 oz.	85	68	135	22	4	---	---	---	0	25	.6	40	.09	.08	1.6	---
	Clams:																
134	Raw, meat only 3 oz.	85	82	65	11	1	---	---	---	2	59	5.2	90	.08	.15	1.1	8
135	Canned, solids and liquid. 3 oz.	85	86	45	7	1	---	---	---	2	47	3.5	---	.01	.09	.9	---
136	Crabmeat, canned 3 oz.	85	77	85	15	2	---	---	---	1	38	.7	---	.07	.07	1.6	---
137	Fish sticks, breaded, cooked, frozen; stick 3¾ by 1 by ½ inch. 10 sticks or 8 oz. pkg.	227	66	400	38	20	5	4	10	15	25	0.9	---	0.09	0.16	3.6	---
138	Haddock, breaded, fried 3 oz.	85	66	140	17	5	1	3	Trace	5	34	1.0	---	.03	.06	2.7	2

No.	Food, approximate measure, and weight (grams)	Water (%)	Food energy (cal.)	Protein (g)	Fat (g)	Saturated (total) (g)	Oleic (g)	Linoleic (g)	Carbohydrate (g)	Calcium (mg)	Iron (mg)	Vitamin A (I.U.)	Thiamine (mg)	Riboflavin (mg)	Niacin (mg)	Ascorbic acid (mg)
139	Ocean perch, breaded, fried. 3 oz — 85	59	195	16	11	—	—	—	6	28	1.1	—	.08	.09	1.5	—
140	Oysters, raw, meat only (13–19 med. selects). 1 cup — 240	85	160	20	4	—	—	—	8	226	13.2	740	.33	.43	6.0	—
141	Salmon, pink, canned. 3 oz — 85	71	120	17	5	1	1	Trace	0	[4]167	.7	60	.03	.16	6.8	—
142	Sardines, Atlantic, canned in oil, drained solids. 3 oz — 85	62	175	20	9	—	—	—	0	372	2.5	190	.02	.17	4.6	—
143	Shad, baked with table fat and bacon. 3 oz — 85	64	170	20	10	—	—	—	0	20	.5	20	.11	.22	7.3	—
144	Shrimp, canned, meat. 3 oz — 85	70	100	21	1	—	—	—	1	98	2.6	50	.01	.03	1.5	—
145	Swordfish, broiled with butter or margarine. 3 oz — 85	65	150	24	5	—	—	—	0	23	1.1	1,750	.03	.04	9.3	—
146	Tuna, canned in oil, drained solids. 3 oz — 85	61	170	24	7	2	1	1	0	7	1.6	70	.04	.10	10.1	—
	MATURE DRY BEANS AND PEAS, NUTS, PEANUTS; RELATED PRODUCTS															
147	Almonds, shelled, whole kernels. 1 cup — 142	5	850	26	77	6	52	15	28	332	6.7	0	.34	1.31	5.0	Trace
	Beans, dry:															
	Common varieties as Great Northern, navy, and others:															
	Cooked, drained:															
148	Great Northern. 1 cup — 180	69	210	14	1	—	—	—	38	90	4.9	0	.25	.13	1.3	0
149	Navy (pea). 1 cup — 190	69	225	15	1	—	—	—	40	95	5.1	0	.27	.13	1.3	0
	Canned, solids and liquid: White with—															
150	Frankfurters (sliced). 1 cup — 255	71	365	19	18	—	—	—	32	94	4.8	330	.18	.15	3.3	Trace
151	Pork and tomato sauce. 1 cup — 255	71	310	16	7	2	3	1	49	138	4.6	330	.20	.08	1.5	5
152	Pork and sweet sauce. 1 cup — 255	66	385	16	12	4	5	1	54	161	5.9	—	.15	.10	1.3	—
153	Red kidney. 1 cup — 255	76	230	15	1	—	—	—	42	74	4.6	10	.13	.10	1.5	—
154	Lima, cooked, drained. 1 cup — 190	64	260	16	1	—	—	—	49	55	5.9	—	.25	.11	1.3	—
155	Cashew nuts, roasted. 1 cup — 140	5	785	24	64	11	45	4	41	53	5.3	140	.60	.35	2.5	—
	Coconut, fresh, meat only:															
156	Pieces, approx. 2 by 2 by ½ inch. 1 piece — 45	51	155	2	16	14	1	Trace	4	6	.8	0	.02	.01	.2	1
157	Shredded or grated, firmly packed. 1 cup — 130	51	450	5	46	39	3	Trace	12	17	2.2	0	.07	.03	.7	4

[4] If bones are discarded, value will be greatly reduced.

Table continued on the following page

APPENDIX TABLE 1   NUTRITIVE VALUES OF THE EDIBLE PART OF FOODS (Continued)

[Dashes in the columns for nutrients show that no suitable value could be found although there is reason to believe that a measurable amount of the nutrient may be present]

	Food, approximate measure, and weight (in grams)	Water	Food energy	Protein	Fat	Fatty acids Saturated (total)	Fatty acids Unsaturated Oleic	Fatty acids Unsaturated Linoleic	Carbohydrate	Calcium	Iron	Vitamin A value	Thiamin	Riboflavin	Niacin	Ascorbic acid
		Percent	Calories	Grams	Grams	Grams	Grams	Grams	Grams	Milligrams	Milligrams	International units	Milligrams	Milligrams	Milligrams	Milligrams
	MATURE DRY BEANS AND PEAS, NUTS, PEANUTS: RELATED PRODUCTS— Continued															
158	Cowpeas or blackeye peas, dry, cooked. 1 cup — 248 Grams	80	190	13	1	---	---	---	34	42	3.2	20	.41	.11	1.1	Trace
159	Peanuts, roasted, salted, halves. 1 cup — 144	2	840	37	72	16	31	21	27	107	3.0	---	.46	.19	24.7	0
160	Peanut butter. 1 tbsp. — 16	2	95	4	8	2	4	2	3	9	.3	---	.02	.02	2.4	0
161	Peas, split, dry, cooked. 1 cup — 250	70	290	20	1	---	---	---	52	28	4.2	100	.37	.22	2.2	---
162	Pecans, halves. 1 cup — 108	3	740	10	77	5	48	15	16	79	2.6	140	.93	.14	1.0	2
163	Walnuts, black or native, chopped. 1 cup — 126	3	790	26	75	4	26	36	19	Trace	7.6	380	.28	.14	.9	---
	VEGETABLES AND VEGETABLE PRODUCTS															
	Asparagus, green: Cooked, drained:															
164	Spears, ½-in. diam. at base. 4 spears — 60	94	10	1	Trace	---	---	---	2	13	.4	540	.10	.11	.8	16
165	Pieces, 1½ to 2-in. lengths. 1 cup — 145	94	30	3	Trace	---	---	---	5	30	.9	1,310	.23	.26	2.0	38
166	Canned, solids and liquid. 1 cup — 244	94	45	5	1	---	---	---	7	44	4.1	1,240	.15	.22	2.0	37
	Beans:															
167	Lima, immature seeds, cooked, drained. 1 cup — 170	71	190	13	1	---	---	---	34	80	4.3	480	.31	.17	2.2	29
	Snap: Green:															
168	Cooked, drained. 1 cup — 125	92	30	2	Trace	---	---	---	7	63	.8	680	.09	.11	.6	15
169	Canned, solids and liquid. 1 cup — 239	94	45	2	Trace	---	---	---	10	81	2.9	690	.07	.10	.7	10
	Yellow or wax:															
170	Cooked, drained. 1 cup — 125	93	30	2	Trace	---	---	---	6	63	0.8	290	0.09	0.11	0.6	16

No.	Food	Measure	Grams	Water %	Food energy	Protein	Fat				Carbo-hydrate	Calcium	Iron	Vitamin A	Thiamin	Ribo-flavin	Niacin	Ascorbic acid
171	Canned, solids and liquid.	1 cup	239	94	45	2	1	---	---	---	10	81	2.9	140	.07	.10	.7	12
172	Sprouted mung beans, cooked, drained.	1 cup	125	91	35	4	Trace	---	---	---	7	21	1.1	30	.11	.13	.9	8
	Beets: Cooked, drained, peeled:																	
173	Whole beets, 2-in. diam.	2 beets	100	91	30	1	Trace	---	---	---	7	14	.5	20	.03	.04	.3	6
174	Diced or sliced	1 cup	170	91	55	2	Trace	---	---	---	12	24	.9	30	.05	.07	.5	10
175	Canned, solids and liquid.	1 cup	246	90	85	2	Trace	---	---	---	19	34	1.5	20	.02	.05	.2	7
176	Beet greens, leaves and stems, cooked, drained.	1 cup	145	94	25	3	Trace	---	---	---	5	144	2.8	7,400	.10	.22	.4	22
	Blackeye peas. See Cowpeas.																	
	Broccoli, cooked, drained:																	
177	Whole stalks, medium size.	1 stalk	180	91	45	6	1	---	---	---	8	158	1.4	4,500	.16	.36	1.4	162
178	Stalks cut into ½-in. pieces.	1 cup	155	91	40	5	1	---	---	---	7	136	1.2	3,880	.14	.31	1.2	140
179	Chopped, yield from 10-oz. frozen pkg.	1⅜ cups	250	92	65	7	1	---	---	---	12	135	1.8	6,500	.15	.30	1.3	143
180	Brussels sprouts, 7-8 sprouts (1¼ to 1½ in. diam.) per cup, cooked.	1 cup	155	88	55	7	1	---	---	---	10	50	1.7	810	.12	.22	1.2	135
	Cabbage: Common varieties: Raw:																	
181	Coarsely shredded or sliced.	1 cup	70	92	15	1	Trace	---	---	---	4	34	.3	90	.04	.04	.2	33
182	Finely shredded or chopped.	1 cup	90	92	20	1	Trace	---	---	---	5	44	.4	120	.05	.05	.3	42
183	Cooked	1 cup	145	94	30	2	Trace	---	---	---	6	64	.4	190	.06	.06	.4	48
184	Red, raw, coarsely shredded	1 cup	70	90	20	1	Trace	---	---	---	5	29	.6	30	.06	.04	.3	43
185	Savoy, raw, coarsely shredded.	1 cup	70	92	15	2	Trace	---	---	---	3	47	.6	140	.04	.06	.2	39
186	Cabbage, celery or Chinese, raw, cut in 1-in. pieces.	1 cup	75	95	10	1	Trace	---	---	---	2	32	.5	110	.04	.03	.5	19
187	Cabbage, spoon (or pakchoy), cooked.	1 cup	170	95	25	2	Trace	---	---	---	4	252	1.0	5,270	.07	.14	1.2	26
	Carrots: Raw:																	
188	Whole, 5½ by 1 inch, (25 thin strips).	1 carrot	50	88	20	1	Trace	---	---	---	5	18	.4	5,500	.03	.03	.3	4
189	Grated	1 cup	110	88	45	1	Trace	---	---	---	11	41	.8	12,100	.06	.06	.7	9

Table continued on the following page

APPENDIX TABLE 1 — NUTRITIVE VALUES OF THE EDIBLE PART OF FOODS (Continued)

[Dashes in the columns for nutrients show that no suitable value could be found although there is reason to believe that a measurable amount of the nutrient may be present]

	Food, approximate measure, and weight (in grams)		Water	Food energy	Protein	Fat	Fatty acids Saturated (total)	Unsaturated Oleic	Unsaturated Linoleic	Carbohydrate	Calcium	Iron	Vitamin A value	Thiamin	Riboflavin	Niacin	Ascorbic acid
		Grams	Percent	Calories	Grams	Grams	Grams	Grams	Grams	Grams	Milligrams	Milligrams	International units	Milligrams	Milligrams	Milligrams	Milligrams
	VEGETABLES AND VEGETABLE PRODUCTS—Continued																
190	Cooked, diced — 1 cup	145	91	45	1	Trace				10	48	.9	15,220	.08	.07	.7	9
191	Canned, strained or chopped (baby food) — 1 ounce	28	92	10	Trace	Trace				2	7	.1	3,690	.01	.01	.1	1
192	Cauliflower, cooked, flowerbuds — 1 cup	120	93	25	3	Trace				5	25	.8	70	.11	.10	.7	66
	Celery, raw:																
193	Stalk, large outer, 8 by about 1½ inches, at root end — 1 stalk	40	94	5	Trace	Trace				2	16	.1	100	.01	.01	.1	4
194	Pieces, diced — 1 cup	100	94	15	1	Trace				4	39	.3	240	.03	.03	.3	9
195	Collards, cooked — 1 cup	190	91	55	5	1				9	289	1.1	10,260	.27	.37	2.4	87
	Corn, sweet:																
196	Cooked, ear 5 by 1¾ inches.[5] — 1 ear	140	74	70	3	1				16	2	.5	[6]310	.09	.08	1.0	7
197	Canned, solids and liquid — 1 cup	256	81	170	5	2				40	10	1.0	[6]690	.07	.12	2.3	13
198	Cowpeas, cooked, immature seeds — 1 cup	160	72	175	13	1				29	38	3.4	560	.49	.18	2.3	28
	Cucumbers, 10-ounce; 7½ by about 2 inches:																
199	Raw, pared — 1 cucumber	207	96	30	1	Trace				7	35	.6	Trace	.07	.09	.4	23
200	Raw, pared, center slice ⅛-inch thick — 6 slices	50	96	5	Trace	Trace				2	8	.2	Trace	.02	.02	.1	6
201	Dandelion greens, cooked — 1 cup	180	90	60	4	1				12	252	3.2	21,060	.24	.29	----	32
202	Endive, curly (including escarole) — 2 ounces	57	93	10	1	Trace				2	46	1.0	1,870	0.04	0.08	0.3	6
203	Kale, leaves including stems, cooked — 1 cup	110	91	30	4	.1				4	147	1.3	8,140	.14	.13	----	68
	Lettuce, raw:																
204	Butterhead, as Boston types; head, 4-inch diameter — 1 head	220	95	30	3	Trace				6	77	4.4	2,130	.14	.13	.6	18

No.	Food, approximate measure	Grams	Water (%)	Food energy (Cal)	Protein (g)	Fat (g)	Saturated (g)	Oleic (g)	Linoleic (g)	Carbohydrate (g)	Calcium (mg)	Iron (mg)	Vitamin A (IU)	Thiamine (mg)	Riboflavin (mg)	Niacin (mg)	Ascorbic acid (mg)
205	Crisphead, as Iceberg; 1 head, 4¾-inch diameter — 1 head	454	96	60	4	Trace	—	—	—	13	91	2.3	1,500	.29	.27	1.3	29
206	Looseleaf, or bunching varieties, leaves — 2 large	50	94	10	1	Trace	—	—	—	2	34	.7	950	.03	.04	.2	9
207	Mushrooms, canned, solids and liquid — 1 cup	244	93	40	5	Trace	—	—	—	6	15	1.2	Trace	.04	.60	4.8	4
208	Mustard greens, cooked — 1 cup	140	93	35	3	1	—	—	—	6	193	2.5	8,120	.11	.19	.9	68
209	Okra, cooked, pod 3 by ⅝ inch — 8 pods	85	91	25	2	Trace	—	—	—	5	78	.4	420	.11	.15	.8	17
	Onions:																
	Mature:																
210	Raw, onion 2½-inch diameter — 1 onion	110	89	40	2	Trace	—	—	—	10	30	.6	40	.04	.04	.2	11
211	Cooked — 1 cup	210	92	60	3	Trace	—	—	—	14	50	.8	80	.06	.06	.4	14
212	Young green, small, without tops — 6 onions	50	88	20	1	Trace	—	—	—	5	20	.3	Trace	.02	.02	.2	12
213	Parsley, raw, chopped — 1 tablespoon	4	85	Trace	Trace	Trace	—	—	—	Trace	7	.2	340	Trace	.01	Trace	7
214	Parsnips, cooked — 1 cup	155	82	100	2	1	—	—	—	23	70	.9	50	.11	.12	.2	16
	Peas, green:																
215	Cooked — 1 cup	160	82	115	9	1	—	—	—	19	37	2.9	860	.44	.17	3.7	33
216	Canned, solids and liquid — 1 cup	249	83	165	9	1	—	—	—	31	50	4.2	1,120	.23	.13	2.2	22
217	Canned, strained (baby food) — 1 ounce	28	86	15	1	Trace	—	—	—	3	3	.4	140	.02	.02	.4	3
218	Peppers, hot, red, without seeds, dried (ground chili powder, added seasonings). — 1 tablespoon	15	8	50	2	2	—	—	—	8	40	2.3	9,750	.03	.17	1.3	2
	Peppers, sweet:																
	Raw, about 5 per pound:																
219	Green pod without stem and seeds — 1 pod	74	93	15	1	Trace	—	—	—	4	7	.5	310	.06	.06	.4	94
220	Cooked, boiled, drained — 1 pod	73	95	15	1	Trace	—	—	—	3	7	.4	310	.05	.05	.4	70
	Potatoes, medium (about 3 per pound raw):																
221	Baked, peeled after baking — 1 potato	99	75	90	3	Trace	—	—	—	21	9	.7	Trace	.10	.04	1.7	20
	Boiled:																
222	Peeled after boiling — 1 potato	136	80	105	3	Trace	—	—	—	23	10	.8	Trace	.13	.05	2.0	22
223	Peeled before boiling — 1 potato	122	83	80	2	Trace	—	—	—	18	7	.6	Trace	.11	.04	1.4	20
	French-fried, piece 2 by ½ by ½ inch:																
224	Cooked in deep fat — 10 pieces	57	45	155	2	7	2	2	4	20	9	.7	Trace	.07	.04	1.8	12
225	Frozen, heated — 10 pieces	57	53	125	2	5	1	1	2	19	5	1.0	Trace	.08	.01	1.5	12
	Mashed:																
226	Milk added — 1 cup	195	83	125	4	1	—	—	—	25	47	.8	50	.16	.10	2.0	19

[5] Measure and weight apply to entire vegetable or fruit including parts not usually eaten.

[6] Based on yellow varieties; white varieties contain only a trace of cryptoxanthin and carotenes, the pigments in corn that have biological activity.

Table continued on the following page

APPENDIX TABLE 1 NUTRITIVE VALUES OF THE EDIBLE PART OF FOODS (Continued)

[Dashes in the columns for nutrients show that no suitable value could be found although there is reason to believe that a measurable amount of the nutrient may be present]

	Food, approximate measure, and weight (in grams)		Water	Food energy	Protein	Fat	Fatty acids			Carbohydrate	Calcium	Iron	Vitamin A value	Thiamin	Riboflavin	Niacin	Ascorbic acid
							Saturated (total)	Unsaturated Oleic	Unsaturated Linoleic								
		Grams	Percent	Calories	Grams	Grams	Grams	Grams	Grams	Grams	Milligrams	Milligrams	International units	Milligrams	Milligrams	Milligrams	Milligrams
	VEGETABLES AND VEGETABLE PRODUCTS—Continued																
	Potatoes—Continued																
227	Milk and butter added. 1 cup	195	80	185	4	8	4	3	Trace	24	47	.8	330	.16	.10	1.9	18
228	Potato chips, medium, 2-inch diameter. 10 chips	20	2	115	1	8	2	2	4	10	8	.4	Trace	.04	.01	1.0	3
229	Pumpkin, canned 1 cup	228	90	75	2	1				18	57	.9	14,590	.07	.12	1.3	12
230	Radishes, raw, small, without tops. 4 radishes	40	94	5	Trace	Trace				1	12	.4	Trace	.01	.01	.1	10
231	Sauerkraut, canned, solids and liquid. 1 cup	235	93	45	2	Trace				9	85	1.2	120	.07	.09	.4	33
	Spinach:																
232	Cooked 1 cup	180	92	40	5	1				6	167	4.0	14,580	.13	.25	1.0	50
233	Canned, drained solids 1 cup	180	91	45	5	1				6	212	4.7	14,400	.03	.21	.6	24
	Squash:																
	Cooked:																
234	Summer, diced 1 cup	210	96	30	2	Trace				7	52	.8	820	.10	.16	1.6	21
235	Winter, baked, mashed. 1 cup	205	81	130	4	1				32	57	1.6	8,610	.10	.27	1.4	27
	Sweetpotatoes:																
	Cooked, medium, 5 by 2 inches, weight raw about 6 ounces:																
236	Baked, peeled after baking. 1 sweetpotato.	110	64	155	2	1				36	44	1.0	8,910	.10	.07	.7	24
237	Boiled, peeled after boiling. 1 sweetpotato.	147	71	170	2	1				39	47	1.0	11,610	.13	.09	.9	25
238	Candied, 3½ by 2¼ inches. 1 sweetpotato.	175	60	295	2	6	2	3	1	60	65	1.6	11,030	0.10	0.08	0.8	17
239	Canned, vacuum or solid pack. 1 cup	218	72	235	4	Trace				54	54	1.7	17,000	.10	.10	1.4	30
	Tomatoes:																
240	Raw, approx. 3-in. diam. 2⅛ in. high; wt, 7 oz. 1 tomato	200	94	40	2	Trace				9	24	.9	1,640	.11	.07	1.3	[7] 42

No.	Food, approximate measure, and weight	Measure	Grams	Water (%)	Food energy (Cal.)	Protein (g)	Fat (g)	Saturated (g)	Oleic (g)	Linoleic (g)	Carbohydrate (g)	Calcium (mg)	Iron (mg)	Vitamin A (I.U.)	Thiamine (mg)	Riboflavin (mg)	Niacin (mg)	Ascorbic acid (mg)
241	Canned, solids and liquid.	1 cup	241	94	50	2	1	—	—	—	10	14	1.2	2,170	.12	.07	1.7	41
	Tomato catsup:																	
242	Cup	1 cup	273	69	290	6	1	—	—	—	69	60	2.2	3,820	.25	.19	4.4	41
243	Tablespoon	1 tbsp.	15	69	15	Trace	Trace	—	—	—	4	3	.1	210	.01	.01	.2	2
	Tomato juice, canned:																	
244	Cup	1 cup	243	94	45	2	Trace	—	—	—	10	17	2.2	1,940	.12	.07	1.9	39
245	Glass (6 fl. oz.)	1 glass	182	94	35	2	Trace	—	—	—	8	13	1.6	1,460	.09	.05	1.5	29
246	Turnips, cooked, diced	1 cup	155	94	35	1	Trace	—	—	—	8	54	.6	Trace	.06	.08	.5	34
247	Turnip greens, cooked	1 cup	145	94	30	3	Trace	—	—	—	5	252	1.5	8,270	.15	.33	.7	68
	FRUITS AND FRUIT PRODUCTS																	
248	Apples, raw (about 3 per lb.).[5]	1 apple	150	85	70	Trace	Trace	—	—	—	18	8	.4	50	.04	.02	.1	3
249	Apple juice, bottled or canned.	1 cup	248	88	120	Trace	Trace	—	—	—	30	15	1.5	—	.02	.05	.2	2
	Applesauce, canned:																	
250	Sweetened	1 cup	255	76	230	1	Trace	—	—	—	61	10	1.3	100	.05	.03	.1	[8] 3
251	Unsweetened or artificially sweetened.	1 cup	244	88	100	1	Trace	—	—	—	26	10	1.2	100	.05	.02	.1	[8] 2
	Apricots:																	
252	Raw (about 12 per lb.)[5] 3 apricots	3 apricots	114	85	55	1	Trace	—	—	—	14	18	.5	2,890	.03	.04	.7	10
253	Canned in heavy sirup	1 cup	259	77	220	2	Trace	—	—	—	57	28	.8	4,510	.05	.06	.9	10
254	Dried, uncooked (40 halves per cup).	1 cup	150	25	390	8	1	—	—	—	100	100	8.2	16,350	.02	.23	4.9	19
255	Cooked, unsweetened, fruit and liquid.	1 cup	285	76	240	5	1	—	—	—	62	63	5.1	8,550	.01	.13	2.8	8
256	Apricot nectar, canned	1 cup	251	85	140	1	Trace	—	—	—	37	23	.5	2,380	.03	.03	.5	[8] 8
	Avocados, whole fruit, raw:[5]																	
257	California (mid- and late-winter; diam. 3⅛ in.).	1 avocado	284	74	370	5	37	7	17	5	13	22	1.3	630	.24	.43	3.5	30
258	Florida (late summer, fall; diam. 3⅝ in.).	1 avocado	454	78	390	4	33	7	15	4	27	30	1.8	880	.33	.61	4.9	43
259	Bananas, raw, medium size.[5]	1 banana	175	76	100	1	Trace	—	—	—	26	10	.8	230	.06	.07	.8	12
260	Banana flakes	1 cup	100	3	340	4	1	—	—	—	89	32	2.8	760	.18	.24	2.8	7
261	Blackberries, raw	1 cup	144	84	85	2	1	—	—	—	19	46	1.3	290	.05	.06	.5	30
262	Blueberries, raw	1 cup	140	83	85	1	1	—	—	—	21	21	1.4	140	.04	.08	.6	20
263	Cantaloups, raw; medium, 5-inch diameter about 1⅔ pounds.[5]	½ melon	385	91	60	1	Trace	—	—	—	14	27	.8	[9] 6,540	.08	.06	1.2	63

[5] Measure and weight apply to entire vegetable or fruit including parts not usually eaten.

[7] Year-round average. Samples marketed from November through May, average 20 milligrams per 200-gram tomato; from June through October, around 52 milligrams.

[8] This is the amount from the fruit. Additional ascorbic acid may be added by the manufacturer. Refer to the label for this information.

[9] Value for varieties with orange-colored flesh; value for varieties with green flesh would be about 540 I.U.

Table continued on the following page

APPENDIX TABLE 1   NUTRITIVE VALUES OF THE EDIBLE PART OF FOODS (Continued)

[Dashes in the columns for nutrients show that no suitable value could be found although there is reason to believe that a measurable amount of the nutrient may be present]

	Food, approximate measure, and weight (in grams)	Water	Food energy	Protein	Fat	Fatty acids Saturated (total)	Unsaturated Oleic	Unsaturated Linoleic	Carbohydrate	Calcium	Iron	Vitamin A value	Thiamin	Riboflavin	Niacin	Ascorbic acid
		Percent	*Calories*	*Grams*	*Grams*	*Grams*	*Grams*	*Grams*	*Grams*	*Milligrams*	*Milligrams*	*International units*	*Milligrams*	*Milligrams*	*Milligrams*	*Milligrams*
	FRUITS AND FRUIT PRODUCTS—Con.															
264	Cherries, canned, red, sour, pitted, water pack. 1 cup	88	105	2	Trace				26	37	.7	1,660	.07	.05	.5	12
265	Cranberry juice cocktail, canned. 1 cup	83	165	Trace	Trace				42	13	.8	Trace	.03	.03	.1	[10] 40
266	Cranberry sauce, sweetened, canned, strained. 1 cup	62	330	Trace	1				85	14	.5	50	.02	.02	.1	5
267	Dates, pitted, cut. 1 cup	22	490	4	1				130	105	5.3	90	.16	.17	3.9	0
268	Figs, dried, large, 2 by 1 in. 1 fig	23	60	1	Trace				15	26	.6	20	.02	.02	.1	0
269	Fruit cocktail, canned, in heavy sirup. 1 cup	80	195	1	Trace				50	23	1.0	360	.05	.03	1.3	5
	Grapefruit:															
	Raw, medium, 3¾-in. diam.[5]															
270	White. ½ grapefruit.	89	45	1	Trace				12	19	0.5	10	0.05	0.02	0.2	44
271	Pink or red. ½ grapefruit.	89	50	1	Trace				13	20	0.5	540	0.05	0.02	0.2	44
272	Canned, sirup pack. 1 cup	81	180	2	Trace				45	33	.8	30	.08	.05	.5	76
	Grapefruit juice:															
273	Fresh. 1 cup	90	95	1	Trace				23	22	.5	(11)	.09	.04	.4	92
	Canned, white:															
274	Unsweetened. 1 cup	89	100	1	Trace				24	20	1.0	20	.07	.04	.4	84
275	Sweetened. 1 cup	86	130	1	Trace				32	20	1.0	20	.07	.04	.4	78
	Frozen, concentrate, unsweetened:															
276	Undiluted, can, 6 fluid ounces. 1 can	62	300	4	1				72	70	.8	60	.29	.12	1.4	286
277	Diluted with 3 parts water, by volume. 1 cup	89	100	1	Trace				24	25	.2	20	.10	.04	.5	96
278	Dehydrated crystals. 4 oz.	1	410	6	1				102	100	1.2	80	.40	.20	2.0	396
279	Prepared with water 1 cup (1 pound yields about 1 gallon).	90	100	1	Trace				24	22	.2	20	.10	.05	.5	91

No.	Food, approximate measure, and weight (in grams)	Grams	Water (%)	Food energy (cal.)	Protein (g)	Fat (g)	Carbohydrate (g)	Calcium (mg)	Iron (mg)	Vitamin A (I.U.)	Thiamine (mg)	Riboflavin (mg)	Niacin (mg)	Ascorbic acid (mg)
	Grapes, raw:[5]													
280	American type (slip skin). 1 cup	153	82	65	1	1	15	15	.4	100	.05	.03	.2	3
281	European type (adherent skin). 1 cup	160	81	95	1	Trace	25	17	.6	140	.07	.04	.4	6
	Grapejuice:													
282	Canned or bottled. 1 cup	253	83	165	1	Trace	42	28	.8	----	.10	.05	.5	Trace
	Frozen concentrate, sweetened:													
283	Undiluted, can, 6 fluid ounces. 1 can	216	53	395	1	Trace	100	22	.9	40	.13	.22	1.5	(12)
284	Diluted with 3 parts water, by volume. 1 cup	250	86	135	1	Trace	33	8	.3	10	.05	.08	.5	(12)
285	Grapejuice drink, canned. 1 cup	250	86	135	Trace	Trace	35	8	.3	----	.03	.03	.3	(12)
286	Lemons, raw, 2⅛-in. diam., size 165.[5] Used for juice. 1 lemon	110	90	20	1	Trace	6	19	.4	10	.03	.01	.1	39
287	Lemon juice, raw. 1 cup	244	91	60	1	Trace	20	17	.5	50	.07	.02	.2	112
	Lemonade concentrate:													
288	Frozen, 6 fl. oz. per can. 1 can	219	48	430	Trace	Trace	112	9	.4	40	.04	.07	.7	66
289	Diluted with 4⅓ parts water, by volume. 1 cup	248	88	110	Trace	Trace	28	2	Trace	Trace	Trace	.02	.2	17
	Lime juice:													
290	Fresh. 1 cup	246	90	65	1	Trace	22	22	.5	20	.05	.02	.2	79
291	Canned, unsweetened. 1 cup	246	90	65	1	Trace	22	22	.5	20	.05	.02	.2	52
	Limeade concentrate, frozen:													
292	Undiluted, can, 6 fluid ounces. 1 can	218	50	410	Trace	Trace	108	11	.2	Trace	.02	.02	.2	26
293	Diluted with 4⅓ parts water, by volume. 1 cup	247	90	100	Trace	Trace	27	2	Trace	Trace	Trace	Trace	Trace	5
294	Oranges, raw, 2⅝-in. diam., all commercial, varieties.[5] 1 orange	180	86	65	1	Trace	16	54	.5	260	.13	.05	.5	66
295	Orange juice, fresh, all varieties. 1 cup	248	88	110	2	1	26	27	.5	500	.22	.07	1.0	124
296	Canned, unsweetened. 1 cup	249	87	120	2	Trace	28	25	1.0	500	.17	.05	.7	100
	Frozen concentrate:													
297	Undiluted, can, 6 fluid ounces. 1 can	213	55	360	5	Trace	87	75	.9	1,620	.68	.11	2.8	360
298	Diluted with 3 parts water, by volume. 1 cup	249	87	120	2	Trace	29	25	.2	550	.22	.02	1.0	120

[5] Measure and weight apply to entire vegetable or fruit including parts not usually eaten.

[10] Value listed is based on product with label stating 30 milligrams per 6 fl. oz. serving.

[11] For white-fleshed varieties value is about 20 I.U. per cup; for red-fleshed varieties, 1,080 I.U. per cup.

[12] Present only if added by the manufacturer. Refer to the label for this information.

Table continued on the following page

APPENDIX TABLE 1   NUTRITIVE VALUES OF THE EDIBLE PART OF FOODS (Continued)

[Dashes in the columns for nutrients show that no suitable value could be found although there is reason to believe that a measurable amount of the nutrient may be present]

	Food, approximate measure, and weight (in grams)	Water	Food energy	Protein	Fat	Fatty acids Saturated (total)	Unsaturated Oleic	Unsaturated Linoleic	Carbohydrate	Calcium	Iron	Vitamin A value	Thiamin	Riboflavin	Niacin	Ascorbic acid
		Per cent	Calories	Grams	Grams	Grams	Grams	Grams	Grams	Milligrams	Milligrams	International units	Milligrams	Milligrams	Milligrams	Milligrams
	FRUITS AND FRUIT PRODUCTS—Con.															
299	Dehydrated crystals -- 4 oz. -- (113 g)		430	6	2				100	95	1.9	1,900	.76	.24	3.3	408
300	Prepared with water (1 pound yields about 1 gallon). 1 cup (248 g)	88	115	2	1				27	25	.5	500	.20	.07	1.0	109
301	Orange-apricot juice drink 1 cup (249 g)	87	125	1	Trace				32	12	.2	1,440	.05	.02	.5	[10] 40
	Orange and grapefruit juice: Frozen concentrate:															
302	Undiluted, can, 6 fluid ounces. 1 can (210 g)	59	330	4	1				78	61	0.8	800	0.48	0.06	2.3	302
303	Diluted with 3 parts water, by volume. 1 cup (248 g)	88	110	1	Trace				26	20	.2	270	.16	.02	.8	102
304	Papayas, raw, ½-inch cubes. 1 cup (182 g)	89	70	1	Trace				18	36	.5	3,190	.07	.08	.5	102
	Peaches: Raw:															
305	Whole, medium, 2-inch diameter, about 4 per pound.[5] 1 peach (114 g)	89	35	1	Trace				10	9	.5	[13] 1,320	.02	.05	1.0	7
306	Sliced 1 cup (168 g)	89	65	1	Trace				16	15	.8	[13] 2,230	.03	.08	1.6	12
	Canned, yellow-fleshed, solids and liquid: Sirup pack, heavy:															
307	Halves or slices 1 cup (257 g)	79	200	1	Trace				52	10	.8	1,100	.02	.06	1.4	7
308	Water pack 1 cup (245 g)	91	75	1	Trace				20	10	.7	1,100	.02	.06	1.4	7
309	Dried, uncooked 1 cup (160 g)	25	420	5	1				109	77	9.6	6,240	.02	.31	8.5	28
310	Cooked, unsweetened, 10-12 halves and juice. 1 cup (270 g)	77	220	3	1				58	41	5.1	3,290	.01	.15	4.2	6
	Frozen:															
311	Carton, 12 ounces, not thawed. 1 carton (340 g)	76	300	1	Trace				77	14	1.7	2,210	.03	.14	2.4	[14] 135
	Pears:															
312	Raw, 3 by 2½-inch diameter.[5] 1 pear (182 g)	83	100	1	1				25	13	.5	30	.04	.07	.2	7

No.	Food, approximate measure, and weight	Measure	Grams	Water (%)	Food energy (cal.)	Protein (g)	Fat (g)	Fatty acids Saturated	Unsat. Oleic	Unsat. Linoleic	Carbohydrate (g)	Calcium (mg)	Iron (mg)	Vitamin A (I.U.)	Thiamine (mg)	Riboflavin (mg)	Niacin (mg)	Ascorbic acid (mg)
	Canned, solids and liquid: Sirup pack, heavy:																	
313	Halves or slices	1 cup	255	80	195	1	1	---	---	---	50	13	.5	Trace	.03	.05	.3	4
314	Pineapple: Raw, diced	1 cup	140	85	75	1	Trace	---	---	---	19	24	.7	100	.12	.04	.3	24
	Canned, heavy sirup pack, solids and liquid:																	
315	Crushed	1 cup	260	80	195	1	Trace	---	---	---	50	29	.8	120	.20	.06	.5	17
316	Sliced, slices and juice.	2 small or 1 large.	122	80	90	Trace	Trace	---	---	---	24	13	.4	50	.09	.03	.2	8
317	Pineapple juice, canned	1 cup	249	86	135	1	1	---	---	---	34	37	.7	120	.12	.04	.5	[8]22
	Plums, all except prunes:																	
318	Raw, 2-inch diameter, about 2 ounces.[5]	1 plum	60	87	25	Trace	Trace	---	---	---	7	7	.3	140	.02	.02	.3	3
	Canned, sirup pack (Italian prunes):																	
319	Plums (with pits) and juice.[5]	1 cup	256	77	205	1	Trace	---	---	---	53	22	2.2	2,970	.05	.05	.9	4
	Prunes, dried, "softenized", medium:																	
320	Uncooked [5]	4 prunes	32	28	70	1	Trace	---	---	---	18	14	1.1	440	.02	.04	.4	1
321	Cooked, unsweetened, 17–18 prunes and ⅓ cup liquid.[5]	1 cup	270	66	295	2	1	---	---	---	78	60	4.5	1,860	.08	.18	1.7	2
322	Prune juice, canned or bottled.	1 cup	256	80	200	1	Trace	---	---	---	49	36	10.5	---	.03	.03	1.0	[8]5
	Raisins, seedless:																	
323	Packaged, ½ oz. or 1½ tbsp. per pkg.	1 pkg.	14	18	40	Trace	Trace	---	---	---	11	9	.5	Trace	.02	.01	.1	Trace
324	Cup, pressed down	1 cup	165	18	480	4	Trace	---	---	---	128	102	5.8	30	.18	.13	.8	2
	Raspberries, red:																	
325	Raw	1 cup	123	84	70	1	1	---	---	---	17	27	1.1	160	.04	.11	1.1	31
326	Frozen, 10-ounce carton, not thawed.	1 carton	284	74	275	2	1	---	---	---	70	37	1.7	200	.06	.17	1.7	59
327	Rhubarb, cooked, sugar added.	1 cup	272	63	385	1	Trace	---	---	---	98	212	1.6	220	.06	.15	.7	17
	Strawberries:																	
328	Raw, capped	1 cup	149	90	55	1	1	---	---	---	13	31	1.5	90	.04	.10	1.0	88
329	Frozen, 10-ounce carton, not thawed.	1 carton	284	71	310	1	1	---	---	---	79	40	2.0	90	.06	.17	1.5	150
330	Tangerines, raw, medium, 2⅜-in. diam., size 176.[5]	1 tangerine	116	87	40	1	Trace	---	---	---	10	34	.3	360	.05	.02	.1	27
331	Tangerine juice, canned, sweetened.	1 cup	249	87	125	1	1	---	---	---	30	45	.5	1,050	.15	.05	.2	55
332	Watermelon, raw, wedge, 4 by 8 inches (1/16 of 10 by 16-inch melon, about 2 pounds with rind).[5]	1 wedge	925	93	115	2	1	---	---	---	27	30	2.1	2,510	.13	.13	.7	30

[5] Measure and weight apply to entire vegetable or fruit including parts not usually eaten.

[8] This is the amount from the fruit. Additional ascorbic acid may be added by the manufacturer. Refer to the label for this information.

[10] Value listed is based on products with label stating 30 milligrams per 6 fl. oz. serving.

[13] Based on yellow-fleshed varieties; for white-fleshed varieties value is about 50 I.U. per 114-gram peach and 80 I.U. per cup of sliced peaches.

[14] This value includes ascorbic acid added by manufacturer.

Table continued on the following page

APPENDIX TABLE 1 — NUTRITIVE VALUES OF THE EDIBLE PART OF FOODS (Continued)

[Dashes in the columns for nutrients show that no suitable value could be found although there is reason to believe that a measurable amount of the nutrient may be present]

	Food, approximate measure, and weight (in grams)	Water	Food energy	Protein	Fat	Fatty acids			Carbohydrate	Calcium	Iron	Vitamin A value	Thiamin	Riboflavin	Niacin	Ascorbic acid
						Saturated (total)	Unsaturated									
							Oleic	Linoleic								
		Percent	Calories	Grams	Grams	Grams	Grams	Grams	Grams	Milligrams	Milligrams	International units	Milligrams	Milligrams	Milligrams	Milligrams
	GRAIN PRODUCTS															
	Bagel, 3-in. diam.:															
333	Egg --------- 1 bagel ------	32	165	6	2	---	---	---	28	9	1.2	30	0.14	0.10	1.2	0
334	Water ------- 1 bagel ------	29	165	6	2	---	---	---	30	8	1.2	0	.15	.11	1.4	0
335	Barley, pearled, light, uncooked. 1 cup ------	11	700	16	2	Trace	1	1	158	32	4.0	0	.24	.10	6.2	0
336	Biscuits, baking powder from home recipe with enriched flour, 2-in. diam. 1 biscuit ------	27	105	2	5	1	2	1	13	34	.4	Trace	.06	.06	.1	Trace
337	Biscuits, baking powder from mix, 2-in. diam. 1 biscuit ------	28	90	2	3	1	1	1	15	19	.6	Trace	.08	.07	.6	Trace
338	Bran flakes (40% bran), added thiamin and iron. 1 cup ------	3	105	4	1	---			28	25	12.3	0	.14	.06	2.2	0
339	Bran flakes with raisins, added thiamin and iron. 1 cup ------	7	145	4	1	---			40	28	13.5	Trace	.16	.07	2.7	0
	Breads:															
340	Boston brown bread, slice 3 by ¾ in. 1 slice ------	45	100	3	1	---			22	43	.9	0	.05	.03	.6	0
	Cracked-wheat bread:															
341	Loaf, 1 lb ------- 1 loaf ------	35	1,190	40	10	2	5	2	236	399	5.0	Trace	.53	.41	5.9	Trace
342	Slice, 18 slices per loaf. 1 slice ------	35	65	2	1	---			13	22	.3	Trace	.03	.02	.3	Trace
	French or vienna bread:															
343	Enriched, 1 lb. loaf. 1 loaf ------	31	1,315	41	14	3	8	2	251	195	10.0	Trace	1.27	1.00	11.3	Trace
344	Unenriched, 1 lb. 1 loaf ------	31	1,315	41	14	3	8	2	251	195	3.2	Trace	.36	.36	3.6	Trace
	Italian bread:															
345	Enriched, 1 lb. loaf. 1 loaf ------	32	1,250	41	4	Trace	1	2	256	77	10.0	0	1.32	.91	11.8	0
346	Unenriched, 1 lb. loaf. 1 loaf ------	32	1,250	41	4	Trace	1	2	256	77	3.2	0	.41	.27	3.6	0
	Raisin bread:															
347	Loaf, 1 lb ------- 1 loaf ------	35	1,190	30	13	3	8	2	243	322	5.9	Trace	.23	.41	3.2	Trace

No.	Food	Measure																	
348	Slice, 18 slices per loaf	1 slice	25	35	65	2	1	—	—	—	13	18	.3	Trace	.01	.02	.2	Trace
	Rye bread:																	
	American, light (⅓ rye, ⅔ wheat):																	
349	Loaf, 1 lb	1 loaf	454	36	1,100	41	5	—	—	—	236	340	7.3	0	.82	.32	6.4	0
350	Slice, 18 slices per loaf	1 slice	25	36	60	2	Trace	—	—	—	13	19	.4	0	.05	.02	.4	0
351	Pumpernickel, loaf, 1 lb	1 loaf	454	34	1,115	41	5	—	—	—	241	381	10.9	0	1.04	.64	5.4	0
	White bread, enriched:[15]																	
	Soft-crumb type:																	
352	Loaf, 1 lb	1 loaf	454	36	1,225	39	15	3	8	2	229	381	11.3	Trace	1.13	.95	10.9	Trace
353	Slice, 18 slices per loaf	1 slice	25	36	70	2	1	—	—	—	13	21	.6	Trace	.06	.05	.6	Trace
354	Slice, toasted	1 slice	22	25	70	2	1	—	—	—	13	21	.6	Trace	.06	.05	.6	Trace
355	Slice, 22 slices per loaf	1 slice	20	36	55	2	1	—	—	—	10	17	.5	Trace	.05	.04	.5	Trace
356	Slice, toasted	1 slice	17	25	55	2	1	—	—	—	10	17	.5	Trace	.05	.04	.5	Trace
357	Loaf, 1½ lbs	1 loaf	680	36	1,835	59	22	5	12	3	343	571	17.0	Trace	1.70	1.43	16.3	Trace
358	Slice, 24 slices per loaf	1 slice	28	36	75	2	1	—	—	—	14	24	.7	Trace	.07	.06	.7	Trace
359	Slice, toasted	1 slice	24	25	75	2	1	—	—	—	14	24	.7	Trace	.07	.06	.7	Trace
360	Slice, 28 slices per loaf	1 slice	24	36	65	2	1	—	—	—	12	20	.6	Trace	.06	.05	.6	Trace
361	Slice, toasted	1 slice	21	25	65	2	1	—	—	—	12	20	.6	Trace	.06	.05	.6	Trace
	Firm-crumb type:																	
362	Loaf, 1 lb	1 loaf	454	35	1,245	41	17	4	10	2	228	435	11.3	Trace	1.22	.91	10.9	Trace
363	Slice, 20 slices per loaf	1 slice	23	35	65	2	1	—	—	—	12	22	.6	Trace	.06	.05	.6	Trace
364	Slice, toasted	1 slice	20	24	65	2	1	—	—	—	12	22	.6	Trace	.06	.05	.6	Trace
365	Loaf, 2 lbs	1 loaf	907	35	2,495	82	34	8	20	4	455	871	22.7	Trace	2.45	1.81	21.8	Trace
366	Slice, 34 slices per loaf	1 slice	27	35	75	2	1	—	—	—	14	26	.7	Trace	.07	.05	.6	Trace
367	Slice, toasted	1 slice	23	35	75	2	1	—	—	—	14	26	.7	Trace	.07	.05	.6	Trace
	Whole-wheat bread, soft-crumb type:																	
368	Loaf, 1 lb	1 loaf	454	36	1,095	41	12	2	6	2	224	381	13.6	Trace	1.36	.45	12.7	Trace
369	Slice, 16 slices per loaf	1 slice	28	36	65	3	1	—	—	—	14	24	.8	Trace	.09	.03	.8	Trace
370	Slice, toasted	1 slice	24	24	65	3	1	—	—	—	14	24	.8	Trace	.09	.03	.8	Trace

[15] Values for iron, thiamin, riboflavin, and niacin per pound of unenriched white bread would be as follows:

	Iron Milligrams	Thiamin Milligrams	Riboflavin Milligrams	Niacin Milligrams
Soft crumb	3.2	.31	.39	5.0
Firm crumb	3.2	.32	.59	4.1

Table continued on the following page

APPENDIX TABLE 1   NUTRITIVE VALUES OF THE EDIBLE PART OF FOODS (Continued)

[Dashes in the columns for nutrients show that no suitable value could be found although there is reason to believe that a measurable amount of the nutrient may be present]

	Food, approximate measure, and weight (in grams)	Water (Percent)	Food energy (Calories)	Protein (Grams)	Fat (Grams)	Fatty acids — Saturated (total) (Grams)	Fatty acids — Unsaturated Oleic (Grams)	Fatty acids — Unsaturated Linoleic (Grams)	Carbohydrate (Grams)	Calcium (Milligrams)	Iron (Milligrams)	Vitamin A value (International units)	Thiamin (Milligrams)	Riboflavin (Milligrams)	Niacin (Milligrams)	Ascorbic acid (Milligrams)
	GRAIN PRODUCTS—Continued															
	Bread—Continued															
	Whole-wheat bread, firm-crumb type:															
371	Loaf, 1 lb. 1 loaf — 454	36	1,100	48	14	3	6	3	216	449	13.6	Trace	1.18	0.54	12.7	Trace
372	Slice, 18 slices per loaf. 1 slice — 25	36	60	3	1	—	—	—	12	25	.8	Trace	.06	.03	.7	Trace
373	Slice, toasted. 1 slice — 21	24	60	3	1	—	—	—	12	25	.8	Trace	.06	.03	.7	Trace
374	Breadcrumbs, dry, grated. 1 cup — 100	6	390	13	5	1	2	1	73	122	3.6	Trace	.22	.30	3.5	Trace
375	Buckwheat flour, light, sifted. 1 cup — 98	12	340	6	1	—	—	—	78	11	1.0	0	.08	.04	.4	0
376	Bulgur, canned, seasoned. 1 cup — 135	56	245	8	4				44	27	1.9	0	.08	.05	4.1	0
	Cakes made from cake mixes:															
	Angelfood:															
377	Whole cake. 1 cake — 635	34	1,645	36	1				377	603	1.9	0	.03	.70	.6	0
378	Piece, 1/12 of 10-in. diam. cake. 1 piece — 53	34	135	3	Trace				32	50	.2	0	Trace	.06	.1	0
	Cupcakes, small, 2½ in. diam.:															
379	Without icing. 1 cupcake — 25	26	90	1	3	1	1	1	14	40	.1	40	.01	.03	.1	Trace
380	With chocolate icing. 1 cupcake — 36	22	130	2	5	2	2	1	21	47	.3	60	.01	.04	.1	Trace
	Devil's food, 2-layer, with chocolate icing:															
381	Whole cake. 1 cake — 1,107	24	3,755	49	136	54	58	16	645	653	8.9	1,660	.33	.89	3.3	1
382	Piece, 1/16 of 9-in. diam. cake. 1 piece — 69	24	235	3	9	3	4	1	40	41	.6	100	.02	.06	.2	Trace
383	Cupcake, small, 2½ in. diam. 1 cupcake — 35	24	120	2	4	1	2	Trace	20	21	.3	50	.01	.03	.1	Trace
	Gingerbread:															
384	Whole cake. 1 cake — 570	37	1,575	18	39	10	19	9	291	513	9.1	Trace	.17	.51	4.6	2
385	Piece, 1/9 of 8-in. square cake. 1 piece — 63	37	175	2	4	1	2	1	32	57	1.0	Trace	.02	.06	.5	Trace
	White, 2-layer, with chocolate icing:															
386	Whole cake. 1 cake — 1,140	21	4,000	45	122	45	54	17	716	1,129	5.7	680	.23	.91	2.3	2

No.	Food, approximate measure		Weight (g)	Water (%)	Food energy (Cal.)	Protein (g)	Fat (g)	Saturated fatty acids (g)	Oleic (g)	Linoleic (g)	Carbohydrate (g)	Calcium (mg)	Iron (mg)	Vitamin A (I.U.)	Thiamine (mg)	Riboflavin (mg)	Niacin (mg)	Ascorbic acid (mg)
387	Piece, 1/16 of 9-in. diam. cake.	1 piece	71	21	250	3	8	3	3	1	45	70	.4	40	.01	.06	.1	Trace
	Cakes made from home recipes: [16]																	
388	Boston cream pie; piece 1/12 of 8-in. diam.	1 piece	69	35	210	4	6	2	3	1	34	46	.3	140	.02	.08	.1	Trace
	Fruitcake, dark, made with enriched flour:																	
389	Loaf, 1-lb.	1 loaf	454	18	1,720	22	69	15	37	13	271	327	11.8	540	.59	.64	3.6	2
390	Slice, 1/30 of 8-in. loaf.	1 slice	15	18	55	1	2	Trace	1	Trace	9	11	.4	20	.02	.02	.1	Trace
	Plain sheet cake: Without icing:																	
391	Whole cake.	1 cake	777	25	2,830	35	108	30	52	21	434	497	3.1	1,320	.16	.70	1.6	2
392	Piece, 1/9 of 9-in. square cake.	1 piece	86	25	315	4	12	3	6	2	48	55	.3	150	.02	.08	.2	Trace
393	With boiled white icing, piece, 1/9 of 9-in. square cake.	1 piece	114	23	400	4	12	3	6	2	71	56	.3	150	.02	.08	.2	Trace
	Pound:																	
394	Loaf, 8½ by 3½ by 3in.	1 loaf	514	17	2,430	29	152	34	68	17	242	108	4.1	1,440	.15	.46	1.0	0
395	Slice, ½-in. thick.	1 slice	30	17	140	2	9	2	4	1	14	6	.2	80	.01	.03	.1	0
	Sponge:																	
396	Whole cake.	1 cake	790	32	2,345	60	45	14	20	4	427	237	9.5	3,560	.40	1.11	1.6	Trace
397	Piece, 1/12 of 10-in. diam. cake.	1 piece	66	32	195	5	4	1	2	Trace	36	20	.8	300	.03	.09	.1	Trace
	Yellow, 2-layer, without icing:																	
398	Whole cake.	1 cake	870	24	3,160	39	111	31	53	22	506	618	3.5	1,310	.17	.70	1.7	2
399	Piece, 1/16 of 9-in. diam. cake.	1 piece	54	24	200	2	7	2	3	1	32	39	.2	80	.01	.04	.1	Trace
	Yellow, 2-layer, with chocolate icing:																	
400	Whole cake.	1 cake	1,203	21	4,390	51	156	55	69	23	727	818	7.2	1,920	.24	.96	2.4	Trace
401	Piece, 1/16 of 9-in. diam. cake.	1 piece	75	21	275	3	10	3	4	1	45	51	.5	120	.02	.06	.2	Trace
	Cake icings. See Sugars, Sweets. Cookies: Brownies with nuts:																	
402	Made from home recipe with enriched flour.	1 brownie	20	10	95	1	6	1	3	1	10	8	.4	40	.04	.02	.1	Trace
403	Made from mix.	1 brownie	20	11	85	1	4	1	2	1	13	9	.4	20	.03	.02	.1	Trace

[16] Unenriched cake flour used unless otherwise specified.

Table continued on the following page

APPENDIX TABLE 1   NUTRITIVE VALUES OF THE EDIBLE PART OF FOODS *(Continued)*

[Dashes in the columns for nutrients show that no suitable value could be found although there is reason to believe that a measurable amount of the nutrient may be present]

	Food, approximate measure, and weight (in grams)		Water	Food energy	Pro-tein	Fat	Fatty acids			Carbo-hy-drate	Cal-cium	Iron	Vita-min A value	Thia-min	Ribo-flavin	Niacin	Ascor-bic acid
							Satu-rated (total)	Unsaturated Oleic	Unsaturated Lin-oleic								
		Grams	Per cent	Calo-ries	Grams	Grams	Grams	Grams	Grams	Grams	Milli-grams	Milli-grams	Inter-national units	Milli-grams	Milli-grams	Milli-grams	Milli-grams
	GRAIN PRODUCTS—Continued																
	Cookies—Continued																
	Chocolate chip:																
404	Made from home recipe with en-riched flour. 1 cookie	10	3	50	1	3	1	1	1	6	4	0.2	10	0.01	0.01	0.1	Trace
405	Commercial 1 cookie	10	3	50	1	2	1	1	Trace	7	4	.2	10	Trace	Trace	Trace	Trace
406	Fig bars, commercial 1 cookie	14	14	50	1	1	---	---	---	11	11	.2	20	Trace	.01	.1	Trace
407	Sandwich, chocolate or vanilla, commercial. 1 cookie	10	2	50	1	2	1	1	Trace	7	2	.1	0	Trace	Trace	.1	0
	Corn flakes, added nutrients:																
408	Plain 1 cup	25	4	100	2	Trace	---	---	---	21	4	.4	0	.11	.02	.5	0
409	Sugar-covered 1 cup	40	2	155	2	Trace	---	---	---	36	5	.4	0	.16	.02	.8	0
	Corn (hominy) grits, degermed, cooked:																
410	Enriched 1 cup	245	87	125	3	Trace	---	---	---	27	2	.7	[17] 150	.10	.07	1.0	0
411	Unenriched 1 cup	245	87	125	3	Trace	---	---	---	27	2	.2	[17] 150	.05	.02	.5	0
	Cornmeal:																
412	Whole-ground, unbolted, dry. 1 cup	122	12	435	11	5	1	2	2	90	24	2.9	[17] 620	.46	.13	2.4	0
413	Bolted (nearly whole-grain) dry. 1 cup	122	12	440	11	4	Trace	1	2	91	21	2.2	[17] 590	.37	.10	2.3	0
	Degermed, enriched:																
414	Dry form 1 cup	138	12	500	11	2	---	---	---	108	8	4.0	[17] 610	.61	.36	4.8	0
415	Cooked 1 cup	240	88	120	3	1	---	---	---	26	2	1.0	[17] 140	.14	.10	1.2	0
	Degermed, unenriched:																
416	Dry form 1 cup	138	12	500	11	2	---	---	---	108	8	1.5	[17] 610	.19	.07	1.4	0
417	Cooked 1 cup	240	88	120	3	1	---	---	---	26	2	.5	[17] 140	.05	.02	.2	0
418	Corn muffins, made with enriched degermed cornmeal and enriched flour; muffin 2⅜-in. diam. 1 muffin	40	33	125	3	4	2	2	Trace	19	42	.7	[17] 120	.08	.09	.6	Trace

No.	Food	Measure	Weight (g)	Water (%)	Food energy (cal)	Protein (g)	Fat (g)	Saturated (g)	Oleic (g)	Linoleic (g)	Carbohydrate (g)	Calcium (mg)	Iron (mg)	Vitamin A (IU)	Thiamin (mg)	Riboflavin (mg)	Niacin (mg)	Ascorbic acid (mg)
419	Corn muffins, made with mix, egg, and milk; muffin 2⅜-in. diam.	1 muffin	40	30	130	3	4	1	2	1	20	96	.6	100	.07	.08	.6	Trace
420	Corn, puffed, presweetened, added nutrients.	1 cup	30	2	115	1	Trace	—	—	—	27	3	.5	0	.13	.05	.6	0
421	Corn, shredded, added nutrients.	1 cup	25	3	100	2	Trace	—	—	—	22	1	.6	0	.11	.05	.5	0
	Crackers:																	
422	Graham, 2½-in. square	4 crackers	28	6	110	2	3	—	—	—	21	11	.4	0	.01	.06	.4	0
423	Saltines	4 crackers	11	4	50	1	1	—	1	—	8	2	.1	0	Trace	Trace	.1	0
424	Danish pastry, plain (without fruit or nuts): Packaged ring, 12 ounces.	1 ring	340	22	1,435	25	80	24	37	15	155	170	3.1	1,050	.24	.51	2.7	Trace
425	Round piece, approx. 4¼-in. diam. by 1 in.	1 pastry	65	22	275	5	15	5	7	3	30	33	.6	200	.05	.10	.5	Trace
426	Ounce	1 oz.	28	22	120	2	7	2	3	1	13	14	.3	90	.02	.04	.2	Trace
427	Doughnuts, cake type	1 doughnut	32	24	125	1	6	1	4	Trace	16	13	[18].4	30	[18].05	[18].05	[18].4	Trace
428	Farina, quick-cooking, enriched, cooked.	1 cup	245	89	105	3	Trace	—	Trace	—	22	147	[19].7	0	[19].12	[19].07	[19]1.0	0
	Macaroni, cooked: Enriched:																	
429	Cooked, firm stage (undergoes additional cooking in a food mixture).	1 cup	130	64	190	6	1	—	—	—	39	14	[19]1.4	0	[19].23	[19].14	[19]1.8	0
430	Cooked until tender.	1 cup	140	72	155	5	1	—	—	—	32	8	[19]1.3	0	[19].20	[19].11	[19]1.5	0
	Unenriched:																	
431	Cooked, firm stage (undergoes additional cooking in a food mixture).	1 cup	130	64	190	6	1	—	—	—	39	14	.7	0	.03	.03	.5	0
432	Cooked until tender.	1 cup	140	72	155	5	1	1	—	—	32	11	.6	0	.01	.01	.4	0
433	Macaroni (enriched) and cheese, baked.	1 cup	200	58	430	17	22	10	9	2	40	362	1.8	860	.20	.40	1.8	Trace
434	Canned	1 cup	240	80	230	9	10	4	3	1	26	199	1.0	260	.12	.24	1.0	Trace
435	Muffins, with enriched white flour; muffin, 3-inch diam.	1 muffin	40	38	120	3	4	1	2	1	17	42	.6	40	.07	.09	.6	Trace
	Noodles (egg noodles), cooked:																	
436	Enriched	1 cup	160	70	200	7	2	1	1	Trace	37	16	[19]1.4	110	[19].22	[19].13	[19]1.9	0
437	Unenriched	1 cup	160	70	200	7	2	1	1	Trace	37	16	1.0	110	.05	.03	.6	0

[17] This value is based on product made from yellow varieties of corn; white varieties contain only a trace.

[18] Based on product made with enriched flour. With unenriched flour, approximate values per doughnut are: Iron, 0.2 milligram; thiamin, 0.01 milligram; riboflavin, 0.03 milligram; niacin, 0.2 milligram.

[19] Iron, thiamin, riboflavin, and niacin are based on the minimum levels of enrichment specified in standards of identity promulgated under the Federal Food, Drug, and Cosmetic Act.

Table continued on the following page

APPENDIX TABLE 1 NUTRITIVE VALUES OF THE EDIBLE PART OF FOODS (Continued)

[Dashes in the columns for nutrients show that no suitable value could be found although there is reason to believe that a measurable amount of the nutrient may be present]

	Food, approximate measure, and weight (in grams)		Water	Food energy	Protein	Fat	Fatty acids			Carbohydrate	Calcium	Iron	Vitamin A value	Thiamin	Riboflavin	Niacin	Ascorbic acid
							Saturated (total)	Unsaturated Oleic	Unsaturated Linoleic								
		Grams	Percent	Calories	Grams	Grams	Grams	Grams	Grams	Grams	Milligrams	Milligrams	International units	Milligrams	Milligrams	Milligrams	Milligrams
	GRAIN PRODUCTS—Continued																
438	Oats (with or without corn) puffed, added nutrients. 1 cup	25	3	100	3	1	---	---	---	19	44	1.2	0	0.24	0.04	0.5	0
439	Oatmeal or rolled oats, cooked. 1 cup	240	87	130	5	2	---	---	1	23	22	1.4	0	.19	.05	.2	0
	Pancakes, 4-inch diam.:																
440	Wheat, enriched flour (home recipe). 1 cake	27	50	60	2	2	Trace	1	Trace	9	27	.4	30	.05	.06	.4	Trace
441	Buckwheat (made from mix with egg and milk). 1 cake	27	58	55	2	2	1	1	Trace	6	59	.4	60	.03	.04	.2	Trace
442	Plain or buttermilk (made from mix with egg and milk). 1 cake	27	51	60	2	2	1	1	Trace	9	58	.3	70	.04	.06	.2	Trace
	Pie (piecrust made with unenriched flour): Sector, 4-in., 1/7 of 9-in. diam. pie:																
443	Apple (2-crust) 1 sector	135	48	350	3	15	4	7	3	51	11	.4	40	.03	.03	.5	1
444	Butterscotch (1-crust) 1 sector	130	45	350	6	14	5	6	2	50	98	1.2	340	.04	.13	.3	Trace
445	Cherry (2-crust) 1 sector	135	47	350	4	15	4	7	3	52	19	.4	590	.03	.03	.7	Trace
446	Custard (1-crust) 1 sector	130	58	285	8	14	5	6	2	30	125	.8	300	.07	.21	.4	0
447	Lemon meringue (1-crust). 1 sector	120	47	305	4	12	4	6	2	45	17	.6	200	.04	.10	.2	4
448	Mince (2-crust) 1 sector	135	43	365	3	16	4	8	3	56	38	1.4	Trace	.09	.05	.5	1
449	Pecan (1-crust) 1 sector	118	20	490	6	27	4	16	5	60	55	3.3	190	.19	.08	.4	Trace
450	Pineapple chiffon (1-crust). 1 sector	93	41	265	6	11	3	5	2	36	22	.8	320	.04	.08	.4	1
451	Pumpkin (1-crust) 1 sector	130	59	275	5	15	5	6	2	32	66	.7	3,210	.04	.13	.7	Trace
	Piecrust, baked shell for pie made with:																
452	Enriched flour 1 shell	180	15	900	11	60	16	28	12	79	25	3.1	0	.36	.25	3.2	0
453	Unenriched flour 1 shell	180	15	900	11	60	16	28	12	79	25	.9	0	.05	.05	.9	0

No.	Food	Measure	Grams	Water (%)	Food energy (cal)	Protein (g)	Fat (g)	Saturated (g)	Oleic (g)	Linoleic (g)	Carbohydrate (g)	Calcium (mg)	Iron (mg)	Vitamin A (I.U.)	Thiamin (mg)	Riboflavin (mg)	Niacin (mg)	Ascorbic acid (mg)
	Piecrust mix including stick form:																	
454	Package, 10-oz., for double crust.	1 pkg	284	9	1,480	20	93	23	46	21	141	131	1.4	0	.11	.11	2.0	0
455	Pizza (cheese) 5½-in. sector; ⅛ of 14-in. diam. pie.	1 sector	75	45	185	7	6	2	3	Trace	27	107	.7	290	.04	.12	.7	4
	Popcorn, popped:																	
456	Plain, large kernel	1 cup	6	4	25	1	Trace	---	---	---	5	1	.2	---	---	.01	.1	0
457	With oil and salt	1 cup	9	3	40	1	2	Trace	1	Trace	5	1	.2	---	---	.01	.2	0
458	Sugar coated	1 cup	35	4	135	2	1	---	---	---	30	2	.5	---	---	.02	.4	0
	Pretzels:																	
459	Dutch, twisted	1 pretzel	16	5	60	2	1	---	---	---	12	4	.2	0	Trace	Trace	.1	0
460	Thin, twisted	1 pretzel	6	5	25	1	Trace	---	---	---	5	1	.1	0	Trace	Trace	Trace	0
461	Stick, small, 2¼ inches	10 sticks	3	5	10	Trace	Trace	---	---	---	2	1	Trace	0	Trace	Trace	Trace	0
462	Stick, regular, 3⅛ inches	5 sticks	3	5	10	Trace	Trace	---	---	---	2	1	Trace	0	Trace	Trace	Trace	0
	Rice, white:																	
	Enriched:																	
463	Raw	1 cup	185	12	670	12	1	---	---	---	149	44	[20]5.4	0	[20].81	[20].06	[20]6.5	0
464	Cooked	1 cup	205	73	225	4	Trace	---	---	---	50	21	[20]1.8	0	[20].23	[20].02	[20]2.1	0
465	Instant, ready-to-serve	1 cup	165	73	180	4	Trace	---	---	---	40	5	[20]1.3	0	[20].21	[20]--	[20]1.7	0
466	Unenriched, cooked	1 cup	205	73	225	4	Trace	---	---	---	50	21	.4	0	.04	.02	.8	0
467	Parboiled, cooked	1 cup	175	73	185	4	Trace	---	---	---	41	33	[20]1.4	0	[20].19	[20]--	[20]2.1	0
468	Rice, puffed, added nutrients.	1 cup	15	4	60	1	Trace	---	---	---	13	3	.3	0	.07	.01	.7	0
	Rolls, enriched:																	
	Cloverleaf or pan:																	
469	Home recipe	1 roll	35	26	120	3	3	1	1	1	20	16	.7	30	.09	.09	.8	Trace
470	Commercial	1 roll	28	31	85	2	2	Trace	1	Trace	15	21	.5	Trace	.08	.05	.6	Trace
471	Frankfurter or hamburger.	1 roll	40	31	120	3	2	1	1	1	21	30	.8	Trace	.11	.07	.9	Trace
472	Hard, round or rectangular.	1 roll	50	25	155	5	2	Trace	1	Trace	30	24	1.2	Trace	.13	.12	1.4	Trace
473	Rye wafers, whole-grain, 1⅞ by 3½ inches.	2 wafers	13	6	45	2	Trace	---	---	---	10	7	.5	0	.04	.03	.2	0
474	Spaghetti, cooked, tender stage, enriched.	1 cup	140	72	155	5	1	---	---	---	32	11	[19]1.3	0	[19].20	[19].11	[19]1.5	0

[19] Iron, thiamin, riboflavin, and niacin are based on the minimum levels of enrichment specified in standards of identity promulgated under the Federal Food, Drug, and Cosmetic Act.

[20] Iron, thiamin, and niacin are based on the minimum levels of enrichment specified in standards of identity promulgated under the Federal Food, Drug, and Cosmetic Act. Riboflavin is based on unenriched rice. When the minimum level of enrichment for riboflavin specified in the standards of identity becomes effective the value will be 0.12 milligram per cup of parboiled rice and of white rice.

Table continued on the following page

APPENDIX TABLE 1   NUTRITIVE VALUES OF THE EDIBLE PART OF FOODS (Continued)

[Dashes show that no basis could be found for imputing a value although there was some reason to believe that a measurable amount of the constituent might be present]

	Food, approximate measure, and weight (in grams)	Water	Food energy	Protein	Fat	Fatty acids Saturated (total)	Unsaturated Oleic	Unsaturated Linoleic	Carbohydrate	Calcium	Iron	Vitamin A value	Thiamin	Riboflavin	Niacin	Ascorbic acid
		Per cent	Calories	Grams	Grams	Grams	Grams	Grams	Grams	Milligrams	Milligrams	International units	Milligrams	Milligrams	Milligrams	Milligrams
	GRAIN PRODUCTS—Continued															
	Spaghetti with meat balls, and tomato sauce:															
475	Home recipe — 1 cup — 248	70	330	19	12	4	6	1	39	124	3.7	1,590	0.25	0.30	4.0	22
476	Canned — 1 cup — 250	78	260	12	10	2	3	4	28	53	3.3	1,000	.15	.18	2.3	5
	Spaghetti in tomato sauce with cheese:															
477	Home recipe — 1 cup — 250	77	260	9	9	2	5	1	37	80	2.3	1,080	.25	.18	2.3	13
478	Canned — 1 cup — 250	80	190	6	2	1	1	1	38	40	2.8	930	.35	.28	4.5	10
479	Waffles, with enriched flour, 7-in. diam. 1 waffle — 75	41	210	7	7	2	4	1	28	85	1.3	250	.13	.19	1.0	Trace
480	Waffles, made from mix, enriched, egg and milk added, 7-in. diam. 1 waffle — 75	42	205	7	8	3	3	1	27	179	1.0	170	.11	.17	.7	Trace
481	Wheat, puffed, added nutrients. 1 cup — 15	3	55	2	Trace	—	—	—	12	4	.6	0	.08	.03	1.2	0
482	Wheat, shredded, plain— 1 biscuit— 25	7	90	2	1	—	—	—	20	11	.9	0	.06	.03	1.1	0
483	Wheat flakes, added nutrients. 1 cup — 30	4	105	3	Trace	—	—	—	24	12	1.3	0	.19	.04	1.5	0
	Wheat flours:															
484	Whole-wheat, from hard wheats, stirred. 1 cup — 120	12	400	16	2	Trace	1	1	85	49	4.0	0	.66	.14	5.2	0
	All-purpose or family flour, enriched:															
485	Sifted — 1 cup — 115	12	420	12	1	—	—	—	88	18	[19]3.3	0	[19].51	[19].30	[19]4.0	0
486	Unsifted — 1 cup — 125	12	455	13	1	—	—	—	95	20	[19]3.6	0	[19].55	[19].33	[19]4.4	0
487	Self-rising, enriched— 1 cup — 125	12	440	12	1	—	—	—	93	331	[19]3.6	0	[19].55	[19].33	[19]4.4	0
488	Cake or pastry flour, sifted. 1 cup — 96	12	350	7	1	—	—	—	76	16	.5	0	.03	.03	.7	0
	FATS, OILS															
	Butter:															
	Regular, 4 sticks per pound:															
489	Stick — ½ cup — 113	16	810	1	92	51	30	3	1	23	0	[21]3,750	—	—	—	0

Item No.	Food, approximate measure	Weight (grams)	Water (percent)	Food energy (calories)	Protein (grams)	Fat (grams)	Saturated (total)	Oleic	Linoleic	Carbohydrate (grams)	Calcium (mg)	Iron (mg)	Vitamin A (I.U.)	Thiamin (mg)	Riboflavin (mg)	Niacin (mg)	Ascorbic acid (mg)
490	Tablespoon (approx. ⅛ stick). 1 tbsp	14	16	100	Trace	12	6	4	Trace	Trace	3	0	[21]470	—	—	—	0
491	Pat (1-in. sq. ⅓-in. high; 90 per lb.). 1 pat	5	16	35	Trace	4	2	1	Trace	Trace	1	0	[21]170	—	—	—	0
	Whipped, 6 sticks or 2, 8-oz. containers per pound:																
492	Stick. ½ cup	76	16	540	1	61	34	20	2	Trace	15	0	[21]2,500	—	—	—	0
493	Tablespoon (approx. ⅛ stick). 1 tbsp	9	16	65	Trace	8	4	3	Trace	Trace	2	0	[21]310	—	—	—	0
494	Pat (1¼-in. sq. ⅓-in. high; 120 per lb.). 1 pat	4	16	25	Trace	3	2	1	Trace	Trace	1	0	[21]130	—	—	—	0
	Fats, cooking:																
495	Lard. 1 cup	205	0	1,850	0	205	78	94	20	0	0	0	0	0	0	0	0
496	Lard. 1 tbsp	13	0	115	0	13	5	6	1	0	0	0	0	0	0	0	0
497	Vegetable fats. 1 cup	200	0	1,770	0	200	50	100	44	0	0	0	—	0	0	0	0
498	Vegetable fats. 1 tbsp	13	0	110	0	13	3	6	3	0	0	0	—	0	0	0	0
	Margarine: Regular, 4 sticks per pound:																
499	Stick. ½ cup	113	16	815	1	92	17	46	25	Trace	23	0	[22]3,750	—	—	—	0
500	Tablespoon (approx. ⅛ stick). 1 tbsp	14	16	100	Trace	12	2	6	3	Trace	3	0	[22]470	—	—	—	0
501	Pat (1-in. sq. ⅓-in. high; 90 per lb.). 1 pat	5	16	35	Trace	4	1	2	1	Trace	1	0	[22]170	—	—	—	0
	Whipped, 6 sticks per pound:																
502	Stick. ½ cup	76	16	545	1	61	11	31	17	Trace	15	0	[22]2,500	—	—	—	0
	Soft, 2 8-oz. tubs per pound:																
503	Tub. 1 tub	227	16	1,635	1	184	34	68	68	1	45	0	[22]7,500	—	—	—	0
504	Tablespoon. 1 tbsp	14	16	100	Trace	11	2	4	4	Trace	3	0	[22]470	—	—	—	0
	Oils, salad or cooking:																
505	Corn. 1 cup	220	0	1,945	0	220	22	62	117	0	0	0	—	0	0	0	0
506	1 tbsp	14	0	125	0	14	1	4	7	0	0	0	—	0	0	0	0
507	Cottonseed. 1 cup	220	0	1,945	0	220	55	46	110	0	0	0	—	0	0	0	0
508	1 tbsp	14	0	125	0	14	4	3	7	0	0	0	—	0	0	0	0
509	Olive. 1 cup	220	0	1,945	0	220	24	167	15	0	0	0	—	0	0	0	0
510	1 tbsp	14	0	125	0	14	2	11	10	0	0	0	—	0	0	0	0
511	Peanut. 1 cup	220	0	1,945	0	220	40	103	64	0	0	0	—	0	0	0	0
512	1 tbsp	14	0	125	0	14	3	7	4	0	0	0	—	0	0	0	0
513	Safflower. 1 cup	220	0	1,945	0	220	18	37	165	0	0	0	—	0	0	0	0
514	1 tbsp	14	0	125	0	14	1	2	10	0	0	0	—	0	0	0	0
515	Soybean. 1 cup	220	0	1,945	0	220	33	44	114	0	0	0	—	0	0	0	0
516	1 tbsp	14	0	125	0	14	2	3	7	0	0	0	—	0	0	0	0

[19] Iron, thiamin, riboflavin, and niacin are based on the minimum levels of enrichment specified in standards of identity promulgated under the Federal Food, Drug, and Cosmetic Act.

[21] Year-round average.

[22] Based on the average vitamin A content of fortified margarine. Federal specifications for fortified margarine require a minimum of 15,000 I.U. of vitamin A per pound.

Table continued on the following page

APPENDIX TABLE 1 NUTRITIVE VALUES OF THE EDIBLE PART OF FOODS (Continued)

[Dashes in the columns for nutrients show that no suitable value could be found although there is reason to believe that a measurable amount of the nutrient may be present]

	Food, approximate measure, and weight (in grams)	Water	Food energy	Protein	Fat	Fatty acids			Carbohydrate	Calcium	Iron	Vitamin A value	Thiamin	Riboflavin	Niacin	Ascorbic acid
						Saturated (total)	Unsaturated									
							Oleic	Linoleic								
		Per cent	Calories	Grams	Grams	Grams	Grams	Grams	Grams	Milligrams	Milligrams	International units	Milligrams	Milligrams	Milligrams	Milligrams
	FATS, OILS—Continued															
	Salad dressings:															
517	Blue cheese -------- 1 tbsp. ----	15	32	75	1	8	2	2	4	1	12	Trace	30	Trace	0.02	Trace	Trace
	Commercial, mayonnaise type:															
518	Regular ---- 1 tbsp. ----	15	41	65	Trace	6	1	1	3	2	2	Trace	30	Trace	Trace	Trace	----
519	Special dietary, low-calorie. 1 tbsp. ----	16	81	20	Trace	2	Trace	Trace	1	1	3	Trace	40	Trace	Trace	Trace	----
	French:															
520	Regular ---- 1 tbsp. ----	16	39	65	Trace	6	1	1	3	3	2	.1	----	----	----	----	----
521	Special dietary, low-fat with artificial sweeteners. 1 tbsp. ----	15	95	Trace	Trace	Trace	----	----	----	Trace	2	.1	----	----	----	----	----
522	Home cooked, boiled---- 1 tbsp. ----	16	68	25	1	2	1	1	Trace	2	14	.1	80	.01	.03	Trace	Trace
523	Mayonnaise ---- 1 tbsp. ----	14	15	100	Trace	11	2	2	6	Trace	3	.1	40	Trace	.01	Trace	Trace
524	Thousand island ---- 1 tbsp. ----	16	32	80	Trace	8	1	2	4	3	2	.1	50	Trace	Trace	Trace	Trace
	SUGARS, SWEETS															
	Cake icings:															
525	Chocolate made with milk and table fat. 1 cup ----	275	14	1,035	9	38	21	14	1	185	165	3.3	580	.06	.28	.6	1
526	Coconut (with boiled icing). 1 cup ----	166	15	605	3	13	11	1	Trace	124	10	.8	0	.02	.07	.3	0
527	Creamy fudge from mix with water only. 1 cup ----	245	15	830	7	16	5	8	3	183	96	2.7	Trace	.05	.20	.7	Trace
528	White, boiled ---- 1 cup ----	94	18	300	1	0	----	----	----	76	2	Trace	0	Trace	.03	Trace	0
	Candy:															
529	Caramels, plain or chocolate. 1 oz. ----	28	8	115	1	3	2	1	Trace	22	42	.4	Trace	.01	.05	.1	Trace
530	Chocolate, milk, plain-- 1 oz. ----	28	1	145	2	9	5	3	Trace	16	65	.3	80	.02	.10	.1	Trace
531	Chocolate-coated peanuts. 1 oz. ----	28	1	160	5	12	3	6	2	11	33	.4	Trace	.10	.05	2.1	Trace

No.	Food	Measure																
532	Fondant; mints, uncoated; candy corn.	1 oz.	28	8	105	Trace	Trace	—	—	—	25	4	.3	0	0	Trace	Trace	0
533	Fudge, plain.	1 oz.	28	8	115	1	4	2	1	Trace	21	22	.3	Trace	.01	.03	.1	Trace
534	Gum drops.	1 oz.	28	12	100	Trace	Trace	—	—	—	25	2	.1	0	Trace	Trace	Trace	0
535	Hard.	1 oz.	28	1	110	0	Trace	—	—	—	28	6	.5	0	0	0	0	0
536	Marshmallows.	1 oz.	28	17	90	1	Trace	—	—	—	23	5	.5	0	0	Trace	Trace	0
	Chocolate-flavored sirup or topping:																	
537	Thin type.	1 fl. oz.	38	32	90	1	1	Trace	Trace	Trace	24	6	.6	Trace	.01	.03	.2	0
538	Fudge type.	1 fl. oz.	38	25	125	2	5	3	2	Trace	20	48	.5	60	.02	.08	.2	Trace
	Chocolate-flavored beverage powder (approx. 4 heaping teaspoons per oz.):																	
539	With nonfat dry milk.	1 oz.	28	2	100	5	1	Trace	Trace	Trace	20	167	.5	10	.04	.21	.2	1
540	Without nonfat dry milk.	1 oz.	28	1	100	1	1	Trace	Trace	Trace	25	9	.6	—	.01	.03	.1	0
541	Honey, strained or extracted.	1 tbsp.	21	17	65	Trace	0	—	—	—	17	1	.1	0	Trace	.01	.1	Trace
542	Jams and preserves.	1 tbsp.	20	29	55	Trace	Trace	—	—	—	14	4	.2	Trace	Trace	.01	Trace	Trace
543	Jellies.	1 tbsp.	18	29	50	Trace	Trace	—	—	—	13	4	.3	Trace	Trace	.01	Trace	1
	Molasses, cane:																	
544	Light (first extraction).	1 tbsp.	20	24	50	—	—	—	—	—	13	33	.9	—	.01	.01	Trace	—
545	Blackstrap (third extraction).	1 tbsp.	20	24	45	—	—	—	—	—	11	137	3.2	—	.02	.04	.4	—
	Sirups:																	
546	Sorghum.	1 tbsp.	21	23	55	—	—	—	—	—	14	35	2.6	0	0	.02	Trace	0
547	Table blends, chiefly corn, light and dark.	1 tbsp.	21	24	60	0	0	—	—	—	15	9	.8	0	0	0	0	0
	Sugars:																	
548	Brown, firm packed.	1 cup.	220	2	820	0	0	—	—	—	212	187	7.5	0	.02	.07	.4	0
	White:																	
549	Granulated.	1 cup.	200	Trace	770	0	0	—	—	—	199	0	.2	0	0	0	0	0
550		1 tbsp.	11	Trace	40	0	0	—	—	—	11	0	Trace	0	0	0	0	0
551	Powdered, stirred before measuring.	1 cup.	120	Trace	460	0	0	—	—	—	119	0	.1	0	0	0	0	0
	MISCELLANEOUS ITEMS																	
552	Barbecue sauce.	1 cup.	250	81	230	4	17	2	5	9	20	53	2.0	900	.03	.03	.8	13
	Beverages, alcoholic:																	
553	Beer.	12 fl. oz.	360	92	150	1	0	—	—	—	14	18	Trace	—	.01	.11	2.2	—
	Gin, rum, vodka, whiskey:																	
554	80-proof.	1½ fl. oz. jigger.	42	67	100	—	—	—	—	—	Trace	—	—	—	—	—	—	—
555	86-proof.	1½ fl. oz. jigger.	42	64	105	—	—	—	—	—	Trace	—	—	—	—	—	—	—
556	90-proof.	1½ fl. oz. jigger.	42	62	110	—	—	—	—	—	Trace	—	—	—	—	—	—	—

Table continued on the following page

APPENDIX TABLE 1   NUTRITIVE VALUES OF THE EDIBLE PART OF FOODS *(Continued)*

[Dashes in the columns for nutrients show that no suitable value could be found although there is reason to believe that a measurable amount of the nutrient may be present]

	Food, approximate measure, and weight (in grams)		Water	Food energy	Protein	Fat	Fatty acids			Carbohydrate	Calcium	Iron	Vitamin A value	Thiamin	Riboflavin	Niacin	Ascorbic acid
							Saturated (total)	Unsaturated									
								Oleic	Linoleic								
			Percent	Calories	Grams	Grams	Grams	Grams	Grams	Grams	Milligrams	Milligrams	International units	Milligrams	Milligrams	Milligrams	Milligrams
	MISCELLANEOUS ITEMS—Continued																
	Beverages, alcoholic—Continued																
	Gin, rum, vodka, whiskey—Con.																
557	94-proof	1½ fl. oz. jigger.	60	115	---	---				Trace		---					---
558	100-proof	1½ fl. oz. jigger.	58	125	---	---				Trace		---					---
	Wines:																
559	Dessert	3½ fl. oz. glass.	77	140	Trace	0				8	8	---		.01	.02	.2	---
560	Table	3½ fl. oz. glass.	86	85	Trace	0				4	9	.4		Trace	.01	.1	---
	Beverages, carbonated, sweetened, nonalcoholic:																
561	Carbonated water	12 fl. oz.	92	115	0	0				29	---	---	0	0	0	0	0
562	Cola type	12 fl. oz.	90	145	0	0				37	---	---	0	0	0	0	0
563	Fruit-flavored sodas and Tom Collins mixes.	12 fl. oz.	88	170	0	0				45	---	---	0	0	0	0	0
564	Ginger ale	12 fl. oz.	92	115	0	0				29	---	---	0	0	0	0	0
565	Root beer	12 fl. oz.	90	150	0	0				39	---	---	0	0	0	0	0
566	Bouillon cubes, approx. ½ in.	1 cube	4	5	1	Trace				Trace							
	Chocolate:																
567	Bitter or baking	1 oz.	2	145	3	15	8	6	Trace	8	22	1.9	20	.01	.07	.4	0
568	Semi-sweet, small pieces.	1 cup	1	860	7	61	34	22	1	97	51	4.4	30	.02	.14	.9	0
	Gelatin:																
569	Plain, dry powder in envelope.	1 envelope	13	25	6	Trace				0							
570	Dessert powder, 3-oz. package.	1 pkg.	2	315	8	0				75							
571	Gelatin dessert, prepared with water.	1 cup	84	140	4	0				34							

No.	Food, approximate measure	Measure	Grams	Water (%)	Food energy (cal.)	Protein (g)	Fat (g)	Fatty acids, Saturated (g)	Oleic (g)	Linoleic (g)	Carbohydrate (g)	Calcium (mg)	Iron (mg)	Vitamin A (I.U.)	Thiamin (mg)	Riboflavin (mg)	Niacin (mg)	Ascorbic acid (mg)
572	Olives, pickled: Green	4 medium or 3 extra large or 2 giant.	16	78	15	Trace	2	Trace	2	Trace	Trace	8	.2	40	—	—	—	—
573	Ripe: Mission	3 small or 2 large.	10	73	15	Trace	2	Trace	2	Trace	Trace	9	.1	10	Trace	Trace	—	—
	Pickles, cucumber:																	
574	Dill, medium, whole, 3¾ in. long, 1¼ in. diam.	1 pickle	65	93	10	1	Trace	—	—	—	1	17	.7	70	Trace	.01	Trace	4
575	Fresh, sliced, 1½ in. diam., ¼ in. thick.	2 slices	15	79	10	Trace	Trace	—	—	—	3	5	.3	20	Trace	Trace	Trace	1
576	Sweet, gherkin, small, whole, approx. 2½ in. long, ¾ in. diam.	1 pickle	15	61	20	Trace	Trace	—	—	—	6	2	.2	10	Trace	Trace	Trace	1
577	Relish, finely chopped, sweet.	1 tbsp.	15	63	20	Trace	Trace	—	—	—	5	3	.1	—	—	—	—	1
	Popcorn. See Grain Products.																	
578	Popsicle, 3 fl. oz. size.	1 popsicle	95	80	70	0	0	0	0	0	18	0	Trace	0	0	0	0	0
	Pudding, home recipe with starch base:																	
579	Chocolate	1 cup	260	66	385	8	12	7	4	Trace	67	250	1.3	390	.05	.36	.3	1
580	Vanilla (blanc mange)	1 cup	255	76	285	9	10	5	3	Trace	41	298	Trace	410	.08	.41	.3	2
581	Pudding mix, dry form, 4-oz. package.	1 pkg.	113	2	410	3	2	1	1	Trace	103	23	1.8	Trace	.02	.08	.5	0
582	Sherbet	1 cup	193	67	260	2	2	—	—	—	59	31	Trace	120	.02	.06	Trace	4
	Soups: Canned, condensed, ready-to-serve: Prepared with an equal volume of milk:																	
583	Cream of chicken	1 cup	245	85	180	7	10	3	3	3	15	172	.5	610	.05	.27	.7	2
584	Cream of mushroom	1 cup	245	83	215	7	14	4	4	5	16	191	.5	250	.05	.34	.7	1
585	Tomato	1 cup	250	84	175	7	7	3	2	1	23	168	.8	1,200	.10	.25	1.3	15
	Prepared with an equal volume of water:																	
586	Bean with pork	1 cup	250	84	170	8	6	1	2	2	22	63	2.3	650	.13	.08	1.0	3
587	Beef broth, bouillon consomme.	1 cup	240	96	30	5	0	—	—	—	3	Trace	.5	Trace	Trace	.02	1.2	—
588	Beef noodle	1 cup	240	93	70	4	3	1	1	1	7	7	1.0	50	.05	.07	1.0	Trace
589	Clam chowder, Manhattan type (with tomatoes, without milk).	1 cup	245	92	80	2	3	1	1	1	12	34	1.0	880	.02	.02	1.0	—
590	Cream of chicken	1 cup	240	92	95	3	6	1	2	3	8	24	.5	410	.02	.05	.5	Trace
591	Cream of mushroom	1 cup	240	90	135	2	10	1	3	5	10	41	.5	70	.02	.12	.7	Trace
592	Minestrone	1 cup	245	90	105	5	3	—	—	1	14	37	1.0	2,350	.07	.05	1.0	—

Table continued on the following page

APPENDIX TABLE 1   NUTRITIVE VALUES OF THE EDIBLE PART OF FOODS *(Continued)*

[Dashes in the columns for nutrients show that no suitable value could be found although there is reason to believe that a measurable amount of the nutrient may be present]

MISCELLANEOUS ITEMS—Continued

Soups—Continued

Canned, condensed, ready-to-serve—Con.

Prepared with an equal volume of water—Con.

Food, approximate measure, and weight (in grams)	Water	Food energy	Protein	Fat	Fatty acids Saturated (total)	Fatty acids Unsaturated Oleic	Fatty acids Unsaturated Linoleic	Carbohydrate	Calcium	Iron	Vitamin A value	Thiamin	Riboflavin	Niacin	Ascorbic acid
	Percent	*Calories*	*Grams*	*Grams*	*Grams*	*Grams*	*Grams*	*Grams*	*Milligrams*	*Milligrams*	*International units*	*Milligrams*	*Milligrams*	*Milligrams*	*Milligrams*
593 Split pea ___ 1 cup ___ *245 Grams*	85	145	9	3	1	2	Trace	21	29	1.5	440	0.25	0.15	1.5	1
594 Tomato ___ 1 cup ___ 245	90	90	2	3	Trace	1	1	16	15	.7	1,000	.05	.05	1.2	12
595 Vegetable beef ___ 1 cup ___ 245	92	80	5	2	---	---	---	10	12	.7	2,700	.05	.05	1.0	---
596 Vegetarian ___ 1 cup ___ 245	92	80	2	2	---	---	---	13	20	1.0	2,940	.05	.05	1.0	---
Dehydrated, dry form:															
597 Chicken noodle (2-oz. package). 1 pkg ___ 57	6	220	8	6	2	3	1	33	34	1.4	190	.30	.15	2.4	3
598 Onion mix (1½-oz. package). 1 pkg ___ 43	3	150	6	5	1	2	1	23	42	.6	30	.05	.03	.3	6
599 Tomato vegetable with noodles (2½-oz. pkg.). 1 pkg ___ 71	4	245	6	6	2	3	1	45	33	1.4	1,700	.21	.13	1.8	18
Frozen, condensed:															
Clam chowder, New England type (with milk, without tomatoes):															
600 Prepared with equal volume of milk. 1 cup ___ 245	83	210	9	12	---	---	---	16	240	1.0	250	.07	.29	.5	Trace
601 Prepared with equal volume of water. 1 cup ___ 240	89	130	4	8	---	---	---	11	91	1.0	50	.05	.10	.5	---
Cream of potato:															
602 Prepared with equal volume of milk. 1 cup ___ 245	83	185	8	10	5	3	Trace	18	208	1.0	590	.10	.27	.5	Trace
603 Prepared with equal volume of water. 1 cup ___ 240	90	105	3	5	3	2	Trace	12	58	1.0	410	.05	.05	.5	---

No.	Food, approximate measure, and weight	Measure	Grams	Water (%)	Food energy (Cal.)	Protein (g)	Fat (g)	Saturated (g)	Oleic (g)	Linoleic (g)	Carbohydrate (g)	Calcium (mg)	Iron (mg)	Vitamin A (I.U.)	Thiamine (mg)	Riboflavin (mg)	Niacin (mg)	Ascorbic acid (mg)
	Cream of shrimp:																	
604	Prepared with equal volume of milk.	1 cup	245	82	245	9	16	---	---	---	15	189	.5	290	.07	.27	.5	Trace
605	Prepared with equal volume of water.	1 cup	240	88	160	5	12	---	---	---	8	38	.5	120	.05	.05	.5	---
	Oyster stew:																	
606	Prepared with equal volume of milk.	1 cup	240	83	200	10	12	---	---	---	14	305	1.4	410	.12	.41	.5	Trace
607	Prepared with equal volume of water.	1 cup	240	90	120	6	8	---	---	---	8	158	1.4	240	.07	.19	.5	---
608	Tapioca, dry, quick-cooking.	1 cup	152	13	535	1	Trace	---	---	---	131	15	.6	0	0	0	0	0
	Tapioca desserts:																	
609	Apple	1 cup	250	70	295	1	Trace	---	---	---	74	8	.5	30	Trace	Trace	Trace	Trace
610	Cream pudding	1 cup	165	72	220	8	8	4	3	Trace	28	173	.7	480	.07	.30	.2	2
611	Tartar sauce	1 tbsp	14	34	75	Trace	8	1	1	4	1	3	.1	30	Trace	Trace	Trace	Trace
612	Vinegar	1 tbsp	15	94	Trace	Trace	0	---	---	---	1	1	.1	---	Trace	Trace	---	---
613	White sauce, medium	1 cup	250	73	405	10	31	16	10	1	22	288	.5	1,150	.10	.43	.5	2
	Yeast:																	
614	Baker's, dry, active	1 pkg	7	5	20	3	Trace	---	---	---	3	3	1.1	Trace	.16	.38	2.6	Trace
615	Brewer's, dry	1 tbsp	8	5	25	3	Trace	---	---	---	3	17	1.4	Trace	1.25	.34	3.0	Trace
	Yoghurt. See Milk, Cheese, Cream, Imitation Cream.																	

APPENDIX TABLE 2   FOOD COMPOSITION TABLE FOR SHORT METHOD OF DIETARY ANALYSIS (3RD REVISION)

Food and Approximate Measure	Weight, gm	Food Energy, Cal.	Protein, gm	Fat, gm	Carbohydrate, gm	Calcium, mg	Iron, mg	Vitamin A Value, IU	Thiamine, mg	Riboflavin, mg	Niacin, mg	Ascorbic Acid, mg
Milk, cheese, cream; related products												
Cheese: blue, cheddar (1 cu in., 17 gm), cheddar process (1 oz), Swiss (1 oz)	30	105	6	9	1	165	0.2	345	0.01	0.12	trace	0
cottage (from skim) creamed (½ c)	115	120	16	5	3	105	0.4	190	0.04	0.28	0.1	0
Cream: half-and-half (cream and milk) (2 tbsp)												
For light whipping add 1 pat butter	30	40	1	4	2	30	trace	145	0.01	0.04	trace	trace
Milk: whole (3.5% fat) (1 c)	245	160	9	9	12	285	0.1	350	0.08	0.42	0.1	2
fluid, nonfat (skim) and buttermilk (from skim)	245	90	9	trace	13	300	trace	—	0.10	0.44	0.2	2
milk beverages, (1 c) cocoa, chocolate drink made with skim milk. For malted milk add 4 tbsp half-and-half (270 gm)	245	210	8	8	26	280	0.6	300	0.09	0.43	0.3	trace
milk desserts, custard (1 c) 248 gm, ice cream (8 fl oz) 142 gm	245	290	8	17	29	210	0.4	785	0.07	0.34	0.1	1
cornstarch pudding (248 gm), ice milk (1 c) 187 gm		280	9	10	40	290	0.1	390	0.08	0.41	0.3	2
White sauce, med (½ c)	130	215	5	16	12	150	0.2	610	0.06	0.22	0.3	trace
Egg: 1 large	50	80	6	6	trace	25	1.2	590	0.06	0.15	trace	0
Meat, poultry, fish, shellfish, related products												
Beef, lamb, veal: lean and fat, cooked, inc. corned beef (3 oz) (all cuts)	85	245	22	16	0	10	2.9	25	0.06	0.19	4.2	0
lean only, cooked; dried beef (2 + oz) (all cuts)	65	140	20	5	0	10	2.4	10	0.05	0.16	3.4	0
Beef, relatively fat, such as steak and rib, cooked (3 oz)	85	350	18	30	0	10	2.4	60	0.05	0.14	3.5	0
Liver: beef, fried (2 oz)	55	130	15	6	3	5	5.0	30,280	0.15	2.37	9.4	15
Pork, lean & fat, cooked (3 oz) (all cuts)	85	325	20	24	0	10	2.6	0	0.62	0.20	4.2	0
lean only, cooked (2 + oz) (all cuts)	60	150	18	8	0	5	2.2	0	0.57	0.19	3.2	0
ham, light cure, lean & fat, roasted (3 oz)	85	245	18	19	0	10	2.2	0	0.40	0.16	3.1	0
Luncheon meats: bologna (2 sl), pork sausage, cooked (2 oz), frankfurter (1), bacon, broiled or fried crisp (3 sl)		185	9	16	-	5	1.3	—	0.21	0.12	1.7	0
Poultry												
chicken: flesh only, broiled (3 oz)	85	115	20	3	0	10	1.4	80	0.05	0.16	7.4	0
fried (2 + oz)	75	170	24	6	1	10	1.6	85	0.05	0.23	8.3	0
turkey, light & dark, roasted (3 oz)	85	160	27	5	0	—	1.5	—	0.03	0.15	6.5	0
Fish and shellfish												
salmon (3 oz) (canned)	85	130	17	5	0	165	0.7	60	0.03	0.16	6.8	0
fish sticks, breaded, cooked (3-4)	75	130	13	7	5	10	0.3	—	0.03	0.05	1.2	0
mackerel, halibut, cooked	85	175	19	10	0	10	0.8	515	0.08	0.15	6.8	0
blue fish, haddock, herring, perch, shad, cooked (tuna canned in oil, 20 gm)	85	*160	19	8	2	20	1.0	60	0.06	0.11	4.4	0
clams, canned; crab meat, canned; lobster; oyster, raw; scallop; shrimp, canned	85	75	14	1	2	65	2.5	65	0.10	0.08	1.5	0

Mature dry beans and peas, nuts, peanuts, related products												
Beans: white with pork & tomato, canned (1 c)	260	320	16	7	50	140	4.7	340	0.20	0.08	1.5	5
red (128 gm), Lima (96 gm), cowpeas (125 gm), cooked (½ c)		125	8	—	25	35	2.5	5	0.13	0.06	0.7	—
Nuts: almonds (12), cashews (8), peanuts (1 tbsp), peanut butter (1 tbsp), pecans (12), English walnuts (2 tbsp), coconut (¼ c)	15	95	3	8	4	15	0.5	5	0.05	0.04	0.9	—
Vegetables and vegetable products												
Asparagus, cooked, cut spears (⅔ c)	115	25	3	trace	4	25	0.7	1,055	0.19	0.20	1.6	30
Beans: green (½ c) cooked 60 gm; canned 120 gm		15	1	trace	3	30	0.4	340	0.04	0.06	0.3	8
Lima, immature, cooked (½ c)	80	90	6	1	16	40	2.0	225	0.14	0.08	1.0	14
Broccoli spears, cooked (⅔ c)	100	25	3	trace	4	90	0.8	2,500	0.09	0.20	0.8	90
Brussels sprouts, cooked (⅔ c)	85	30	3	trace	5	30	1.0	450	0.07	0.12	0.7	75
Cabbage (110 gm); cauliflower, cooked (80 gm); and sauerkraut, canned (150 gm) (reduce ascorbic acid value by one-third for kraut) (⅔ c)		20	1	trace	4	35	0.5	80	0.05	0.05	0.3	37
Carrots, cooked (⅔ c)	95	30	1	trace	7	30	0.6	10,145	0.05	0.05	0.5	6
Corn, 1 ear, cooked (140 gm); canned (130 gm) (½ c)		75	2	trace	18	5	0.4	315	0.06	0.06	1.1	6
Leafy greens: collards (125 gm), dandelions (120 gm), kale (75 gm), mustard (95 gm), spinach (120 gm), turnip (100 gm cooked, 150 gm canned) (⅔ c cooked and canned) (reduce ascorbic acid one-half for canned)		30	3	trace	5	175	1.8	8,570	0.11	0.18	0.8	45
Peas, green (½ c)	80	60	4	1	10	20	1.4	430	0.22	0.09	1.8	16
Potatoes-baked, boiled (100 gm), 10 pc French fried (55 gm) (for fried, add 1 tbsp cooking oil)		85	3	trace	30	10	0.7	trace	0.08	0.04	1.5	16
Pumpkin, canned (½ c)	115	40	1	1	9	30	0.5	7,295	0.03	0.06	0.6	6
Squash, winter, canned (½ c)	100	65	2	1	16	30	0.8	4,305	0.05	0.14	0.7	14
Sweetpotato, canned (½ c)	110	120	2	—	27	25	0.8	8,500	0.05	0.05	0.7	15
Tomato, 1 raw, ⅔ c canned, ⅔ c juice	150	35	2	trace	7	14	0.8	1,350	0.10	0.06	1.0	29
Tomato catsup (2 tbsp)	35	30	1	trace	8	10	0.2	480	0.04	0.02	0.6	6
Other, cooked (beets, mushrooms, onions, turnips) (½ c)	95	25	1	—	5	20	0.5	15	0.02	0.10	0.7	7
Others commonly served raw, cabbage (½ c, 50 gm), celery (3 sm stalks, 40 gm), cucumber (¼ med, 50 gm), green pepper (½, 30 gm), radishes (5, 40 gm)		10	trace	trace	2	15	0.3	100	0.03	0.03	0.2	20
carrots, raw (½ carrot)	25	10	trace	trace	2	10	0.2	2,750	0.02	0.02	0.2	2
lettuce leaves (2 lg)	50	10	1	trace	2	34	0.7	950	0.03	0.04	0.2	9
Fruits and fruit products												
Cantaloup (½ med)	385	60	1	trace	14	25	0.8	6,540	0.08	0.06	1.2	63
Citrus and strawberries: orange (1), grapefruit (½), juice (½ c), strawberries (½ c), lemon (1), tangerine (1)		50	1	—	13	25	0.4	165	0.08	0.03	0.3	55
Yellow, fresh: apricots (3), peach (2 med); canned fruit and juice (½ c) or dried, cooked, unsweetened: apricot, peaches (½ c)		85	—	—	22	10	1.1	1,005	0.01	0.05	1.0	5
Other, dried: dates, pitted (4), figs (2), raisins (¼ c)	40	120	1	—	31	35	1.4	20	0.04	0.04	0.5	—
Other, fresh: apple (1), banana (1), figs (3), pear (1)		80	—	—	21	15	0.5	140	0.04	0.03	0.2	6
Fruit pie: to 1 serving fruit add 1 tbsp flour, 2 tbsp sugar, 1 tbsp fat												

Table continued on the following page

APPENDIX TABLE 2   FOOD COMPOSITION TABLE FOR SHORT METHOD OF DIETARY ANALYSIS (3RD REVISION) (Continued)

Food and Approximate Measure	Weight, gm	Food Energy, Cal.	Protein, gm	Fat, gm	Carbohydrate, gm	Calcium, mg	Iron, mg	Vitamin A Value, IU	Thiamine, mg	Riboflavin, mg	Niacin, mg	Ascorbic Acid, mg
Grain products												
Enriched and whole grain: bread (1 sl, 23 gm), biscuit (½), cooked cereals (½ c), prepared cereals (1 oz), Graham crackers (2 lg), macaroni, noodles, spaghetti (½ c, cooked), pancake (1, 27 gm), roll (½), waffle (½, 38 gm)		65	2	1	16	20	0.6	10	0.09	0.05	0.7	—
Unenriched: bread (1 sl, 23 gm), cooked cereal (½ c), macaroni, noodles, spaghetti (½ c), popcorn (½ c), pretzel sticks, small (15), roll (½)		65	2	1	16	10	0.3	5	0.02	0.02	0.3	—
Desserts												
Cake, plain (1 pc), doughnut (1). For iced cake or doughnut add value for sugar (1 tbsp). For chocolate cake add chocolate (30 gm)	45	145	2	5	24	30	0.4	65	0.02	0.05	0.2	—
Cookies, plain (1)	25	120	1	5	18	10	0.2	20	0.01	0.01	0.1	—
Pie crust, single crust (¼ shell)	20	95	1	6	8	3	0.3	0	0.04	0.03	0.3	0
Flour, white, enriched (1 tbsp)	7	25	1	trace	5	1	0.2	0	0.03	0.02	0.2	0
Fats and Oils												
Butter, margarine (1 pat, ½ tbsp)	7	50	trace	6	trace	1	0	230	—	—	—	—
Fats and oils, cooking (1 tbsp), French dressing (2 tbsp)	14	125	0	14	0	0	0	0	0	0	0	0
Salad dressing, mayonnaise type (1 tbsp)	15	80	trace	9	1	2	0.1	45	trace	trace	trace	0
Sugars, sweets												
Candy, plain (½ oz), jam and jelly (1 tbsp), sirup (1 tbsp), gelatin dessert, plain (½ c), beverages, carbonated (1 c)		60	0	0	14	3	0.1	trace	trace	trace	trace	trace
Chocolate fudge (1 oz), chocolate sirup (3 tbsp)		125	1	2	30	15	0.6	10	trace	0.02	0.1	trace
Molasses (1 tbsp), caramel (⅔ oz)		40	trace	trace	8	20	0.3	trace	trace	trace	trace	trace
Sugar (1 tbsp)	12	45	0	0	12	0	trace	0	0	0	0	0
Miscellaneous												
Chocolate, bitter (1 oz)	30	145	3	15	8	20	1.9	20	0.01	0.07	0.4	0
Sherbet (½ c)	96	130	1	1	30	15	trace	55	0.01	0.03	trace	2
Soups: bean, pea (green) (1 c)		150	7	4	22	50	1.6	495	0.09	0.06	1.0	4
noodle, beef, chicken (1 c)		65	4	2	7	10	0.7	50	0.03	0.04	0.9	trace
clam chowder, minestrone, tomato, vegetable (1 c)		90	3	2	14	25	0.9	1,880	0.05	0.04	1.1	3

The use of the short method of dietary analysis reduces the time required to compute the nutritive value of a diet. In the evaluation of a mixed dietary using this method the accuracy approximates that of computations using the conventional food table.

The values in Table 2 were computed chiefly from the figures compiled by Watt and Merrill in Agriculture Handbook 8, *Composition of Foods—Raw, Processed, Prepared*, revised 1963.

Courtesy of Wilson, E. D., et al.: Principles of Nutrition, 2nd ed. New York, John Wiley & Sons, 1965.

APPENDIX TABLE 3   CALORIE VALUES OF BEVERAGES AND SNACK FOODS

FOOD	WEIGHT (gm.)	APPROXIMATE MEASURE	KCALORIES	FOOD	WEIGHT (gm.)	APPROXIMATE MEASURE	KCALORIES
Beverages				Doughnut, cake type,			
Carbonated, cola type	369	1 bottle, 12 ounces	145	plain	32	1 average	125
Malted milk	235	1 regular (1 cup)	245	Doughnut, jelly	65	1 average	226
Chocolate milk				Doughnut, raised	30	1 average	120
(made with skim milk)	250	1 cup	190				
Cocoa	250	1 cup	245	Fruits			
soda, vanilla ice cream	242	1 regular	60	Apple	150	1 medium, 2¹/₂ in. diameter	70
				Banana	100	1 medium, 6 by 1¹/₂ in.	85
Beverages, alcoholic				Grapes, European type	160	1 cup	95
Beer	360	1 bottle, 12 ounces	150	Orange	180	1 medium, 2⁵/₈ in.	65
Brandy	30	1 brandy glass	75			diameter	
Gin	43	1 jigger	107	Pear	182	1 medium, 3 by 2¹/₂ in.	100
Liqueurs (average)	20	1 cordial glass	165			diameter	
Martini		1 cocktail glass	145				
Manhattan		1 cocktail glass	165	Miscellaneous			
Rum	43	1 jigger	105	Hamburger and bun	96	1 average	334
Whiskey	43	1 jigger	107	Ice cream, vanilla	62	3-ounce container	95
Wine, port	100	1 wine glass	160	Sherbet	96	¹/₂ cup	130
Wine, sauterne	100	1 wine glass	85	Jams, jellies,			
				marmalades, preserves	21	1 tablespoon	55
Cake				Syrup, blended	21	1 tablespoon	60
Angel food	53	1 piece	135	Waffles	75	1 waffle, 4¹/₂ by 5¹/₂ by	210
Cupcake, chocolate, iced	36	1 cake, 2³/₄ in.	130			¹/₂ inch	
		diameter					
Fruit cake	30	1 piece, 2 by 2 by ¹/₂ in.	110	Nuts			
				Mixed, shelled	15	8 to 12	94
Candy and Popcorn				Peanut butter	16	1 tablespoon	95
Butterscotch	15	3 pieces	60	Peanuts, shelled,			
Candy bar, plain	28	1 bar	145	roasted	144	1 cup	840
Caramels	28	3 medium	115				
Choc. coated peanuts	28	1 ounce	160	Pie			
Fudge	28	1 piece	115	Apple	135	4-inch sector	350
Peanut brittle	30	1 ounce	128	Cherry	135	4-inch sector	350
Popcorn with oil added	9	1 cup	40	Custard	130	4-inch sector	285
				Lemon meringue	120	4-inch sector	305
Cheese				Mince	135	4-inch sector	365
Camembert	38	1 wedge	115	Pumpkin	130	4-inch sector	275
Cheddar	28	1 ounce	115				
Cream	28	1 ounce	106	Potato chips			
Swiss (domestic)	28	1 ounce	100	Potato chips	20	10 chips, 2 inches in	115
						diameter	
Cookies							
Brownies, made with				Sandwiches			
mix	20	1 piece	85	Bacon, lettuce, tomato	148	1 sandwich	282
Cookies, plain and		1 cooky, 3 in.		Egg salad	138	1 sandwich	279
assorted	25	diameter	120	Ham	81	1 sandwich	281
				Liverwurst	91	1 sandwich	251
Crackers				Peanut butter	83	1 sandwich	328
Cheese	18	5 crackers	86				
Graham	14	2 medium	55	Soups, commercial canned			
Saltines	11	4 crackers	50	Bean with pork	250	1 cup	170
Rye	26	4 crackers	85	Beef noodle	250	1 cup	70
				Chicken noodle	198	1 cup	51
Dessert type cream puff				Cream (mushroom)	241	1 cup	215
and doughnuts				Tomato	198	1 cup	73
Cream puff – custard				Vegetable with beef			
filling	100	1 average	233	broth	241	1 cup	80

APPENDIX TABLE 4   FATTY ACID AND CHOLESTEROL CONTENT OF FOODS*

| Food | Approximate amount | Weight | Total fat | Saturated fat | Unsaturated fatty acids | | Choles-terol |
| | | | | | Oleic | Linoleic | |
		gm	*gm*	*gm*	*gm*	*gm*	*mg*
Meat Group							
Beef	1 oz	30	7.5	3.6	3.3	Trace	27
Veal	1 oz	30	3.6	1.8	1.5	Trace	27
Lamb	1 oz	30	6.3	3.6	2.4	Trace	27
Pork, ham	1 oz	30	7.8	3.0	3.3	Trace	27
Liver	1 oz	30	1.5	0.4	Trace	Trace	75
Beef, dried	2 slices	20	1.2	0.6	0.6	...	18
Pork sausage	2 links	40	17.6	6.4	7.6	1.6	45
Cold cuts	1 slice	45	9.7	2.4	2.7	0.6	30
Frankfurters	1	50	17.4	9.0	8.0	0.4	50
Fowl	1 oz	30	3.6	1.2	1.2	0.6	23
Eggs	1	50	6.0	2.0	2.5	0.5	253
Fish	1 oz	30	2.7	0.5	1.7	0.5	21
Salmon and tuna	1/4 cup	30	5.1	1.4	1.5	1.2	...
Shellfish	1 oz	30	1.9	0.6	1.0	0.3	45
Cheese	1 oz	30	9.0	5.1	3.0	...	45
Cottage cheese	1/4 cup	50	2.1	1.0	0.5	...	5
Peanut butter	2 T	30	15.0	2.7	7.5	4.2	...
Peanuts	25	25	12.0	2.5	5.0	3.2	...
Fat Group							
Avocado	1/8	30	5.1	0.9	2.4	0.6	...
Bacon	1 strip	5	2.6	0.9	1.0	0.3	5
Butter	1 tsp	5	4.0	2.3	1.2	...	12
Margarine	1 tsp	5	4.0	1.1	2.5	0.4	...
Special margarine	1 tsp	5	4.0	0.6	2.3	1.1	...
Coconut oil	1 tsp	5	5.0	4.4	0.5	0.1	...
Corn oil	1 tsp	5	5.0	0.5	1.8	2.7	...
Cottonseed oil	1 tsp	5	5.0	1.3	1.2	2.5	...
Olive oil	1 tsp	5	5.0	0.6	4.0	0.4	...
Peanut oil	1 tsp	5	5.0	0.9	1.6	1.5	...
Safflower oil	1 tsp	5	5.0	0.4	1.0	3.6	...
Sesame oil	1 tsp	5	5.0	0.9	1.0	2.1	...
Soybean oil	1 tsp	5	5.0	0.8	1.6	2.6	...
Vegetable fat	1 tsp	5	5.0	1.0	2.6	0.4	...
Half and half	2 T	30	3.6	1.8	1.8	...	12
Cream substitute, dried	1 T	2	0.5	0.3	0.2	...	...
Whipping cream	1 T	15	5.6	3.2	2.2	0.2	18
Cream cheese	1 T	15	5.3	3.0	2.2	0.1	18
Mayonnaise	1 tsp	5	4.0	0.7	1.3	2.0	8
French dressing	1 T	15	5.0	1.1	1.1	3.0	...
Nuts							
Almonds	5	6	3.5	0.3	2.5	0.7	...
Pecans	4	5	3.6	0.3	2.6	0.7	...
Walnuts	5	10	6.5	0.4	2.0	4.0	...
Olives	3	30	4.2	0.6	3.0	0.3	...

*From Mayo Clinic Diet Manual, 4th Ed. Philadelphia, W. B. Saunders Co., 1971.

APPENDIX TABLE 4   FATTY ACID AND CHOLESTEROL CONTENT OF FOODS *(Continued)*

Food	Approximate amount	Weight	Total fat	Saturated fat	Unsaturated fatty acids		Choles-terol
					Oleic	Linoleic	
		gm	*gm*	*gm*	*gm*	*gm*	*mg*
Milk Group							
Milk, whole	1 cup	240	8.5	4.9	3.6	...	27
2% milk	1 cup	240	4.9	2.4	2.5	...	15
Skim milk	1 cup	240	...	...	...	...	7
Cocoa (skim milk)	1 cup	240	1.9	0.7	1.2	...	...
Chocolate milk	1 cup	240	8.5	2.5	6.0	...	...
Bread Group							
Bread	1 slice	25	0.8	0.3	0.5	...	...
Biscuit	1	35	6.5	2.3	3.4	0.8	17
Muffin	1	35	3.5	0.7	2.4	0.4	16
Cornbread	1 (1 1/2″ cube)	35	4.0	1.4	2.1	0.4	16
Roll	1	28	1.3	0.3	0.7	0.3	...
Pancake	1 (4″ diam)	45	3.2	0.9	1.9	0.4	38
Waffle	1	35	3.4	1.0	2.1	0.4	28
Sweet roll	1	35	8.2	2.4	5.1	0.7	25
French toast	1 slice	65	8.1	3.9	3.4	0.8	130
Doughnut	1	30	6.0	1.3	4.4	0.3	27
Cereal, cooked	2/3 cup	140	1.4	...	1.4	0.3	...
Crackers (saltines)	6	20	2.4	0.6	1.4	...	...
Popcorn (unbuttered)	1 cup	15	0.7	0.1	0.2	0.4	...
Potatoes							
Potato chips	1–oz bag	30	12.0	3.0	4.0	6.0	...
French fried							
In corn oil	10	50	6.2	0.4	2.3	3.5	...
In hydroge-nated fat	10	50	6.2	1.6	4.0	0.6	...
Mashed potato	1/2 cup	100	4.3	2.0	2.3	...	...
Soup, cream	1/2 cup	100	4.2	1.0	2.2	1.0	9
Dessert							
Ice milk	1/2 cup	75	2.5	1.5	...	...	5
Ice cream	1/2 cup	75	9.0	5.0	3.9	...	43
Sherbet	1/3 cup	50	0.6	0.4	0.2	...	...
Low fat cookies	5	15	1.8	0.3	...	...	...
Cake	1 piece	50	14.0	2.0	...	0.5	45
Fruit pie	1/6 pie (9″)	160	15.0	4.0	9.5	1.4	11
Miscellaneous							
Gravy	1/4 cup	60	13.8	6.8	6.6	0.4	18
White sauce	1/4 cup	60	8.2	4.6	3.6	...	29
Coconut	1 oz	28	10.9	9.5	1.4	...	...
Chocolate sauce	1 oz	30	3.8	2.0	1.8	...	...

APPENDIX TABLE 5   FOLACIN CONTENT OF FOODS

In Terms of 100 Gm. Edible Portion and of Specified Units[*,a,b]

ITEM NUMBER	FOOD AND DESCRIPTION	Free Folacin (μg.)	Total Folacin[c] (μg.)	Approximate Measure	Weight (gm.)	Free Folacin (μg.)	Total Folacin[c] (μg.)
		PER 100 GM. EDIBLE PORTION		*PER SPECIFIED UNIT*			
CEREAL GRAINS AND THEIR PRODUCTS							
1	barley, pot	9	20	1 c.	200	18	40
2	corn, whole-grain	15	19				
3	cornmeal, degermed	9	24	1 c.	122	11	29
4	macaroni, dry	4	12	8-oz. pkg.	227	9	27
	rice						
5	brown	12	16	1 c.	185	22	30
6	white	–[d]	10	1 c.	185	–	18
7	parboiled	9	11	1 c.	185	17	20
8	rice bran	–	39				
9	rice germ	–	64				
10	rice flour, sifted	31	78	1 c.	88	27	69
11	sorghum, grain	18	27				
12	spaghetti, dry	4	12	8-oz. pkg.	227	9	27
13	wheat, whole-grain	39	52				
	wheat flour						
14	whole	40	54	1 c.	120	48	65
15	clear	29	32				
	patent						
16	bread, sifted	19	25	1 c.	115	22	29
17	all-purpose, sifted	18	21	1 c.	115	21	24
18	wheat bran	134	258				
19	wheat germ	257	328				
	breakfast cereals, dry						
20	farina	–	24	1 c.	180	–	43
21	farina, wheat germ added	17	34	1 c.	180	31	61
22	oatmeal	16	52	1 c.	80	13	42
	breakfast cereals, ready-to-eat; not fortified with folacin						
23	cornflakes	9	12	1 oz.	28	3	3
24	oats, with added wheat gluten	8	22	1 oz.	28	2	6
25	rice, puffed	8	23	1 oz.	28	2	6
26	rice, with added protein concentrate and wheat gluten	14	31		28	4	9
27	wheat germ, toasted	125	420	1 oz.	28	35	118
28	wheat and malted barley granules	15	54	1 oz.	28	4	15
29	wheat, shredded	10	50	1 oz.	28	3	14
	bakery products						
	bread						
30	rye	6	23	1 slice	25	2	6
31	white	13	39	1 slice	25	3	10
32	whole-wheat	27	58	1 slice	28	8	16
	cakes						
33	chocolate with icing	4	6	1 slice (3″ high; 2⅜″ arc)	99	4	6
34	sponge	3	7	1 slice (3″ high; 2¼″ arc)	44	1	3
	cookies						
35	chocolate chip	4	9	1 cookie	10	<0.5	1
36	shortbread	4	9	1 cookie	8	<0.5	1

*From: Perloff, B. P., and Butrum, R. R.: Folacin in selected foods. J. Am. Diet. Assoc., *70*:161, 1977.

[a] Measure and weight apply to edible part of food only.

[b] Assays using *L. casei* except when studies using *L. casei* could not be found. Reducing agent such as ascorbic acid used except for items 100, 107, 111, 140, 187 and 197.

[c] Recommend using total folacin for diet calculations.

[d] Dash denotes value not available.

APPENDIX TABLE 5   FOLACIN CONTENT OF FOODS (*Continued*)

		PER 100 GM. EDIBLE PORTION		PER SPECIFIED UNIT			
ITEM NUM-BER	FOOD AND DESCRIPTION	*Free Folacin* ($\mu g.$)	*Total Folacin* ($\mu g.$)	*Approximate Measure*	*Weight* ($gm.$)	*Free Folacin* ($\mu g.$)	*Total Folacin* ($\mu g.$)
CEREAL GRAINS AND THEIR PRODUCTS (*Continued*)							
	doughnuts						
37	cake type	5	8	1 doughnut	32	2	3
38	yeast-leavened	5	22	1 doughnut	35	2	8
39	pie, apple	2	4	$^1/_6$ of pie	158	3	6
LEGUMINOUS SEEDS AND THEIR PRODUCTS							
	beans, common, mature seeds						
	white						
40	raw, dry	25	129	1 c.	205	51	264
41	canned, baked with tomato						
	sauce	8	24	1 c.	255	20	61
	red						
42	raw, dry	24	133	1 c.	185	44	246
43	cooked	–	37	1 c.	185	–	68
	pinto, mature seeds, dry						
44	raw, dry	57	216	1 c.	190	108	410
45	cooked	–	59	1 c.	190	–	112
46	canned, drained	–	51	1 c.	190	–	97
	beans, Lima, mature seeds						
47	raw, dry	25	113	1 c.	190	48	215
48	cooked	–	43	1 c.	190	–	82
49	beans, mung, mature seeds, dry	26	133	1 c.	210	55	279
50	beans, mungo, mature seeds, dry	28	108				
	chickpeas or garbanzos, mature seeds						
51	raw, dry	32	199	1 c.	200	64	398
52	roasted	22	139				
53	canned, drained	–	102				
	cowpeas, mature seeds						
54	raw, dry	69	133	1 c.	170	117	226
55	canned, drained	–	80	1 c.	165	–	132
56	lentils, mature seeds, dry	19	36	1 c.	190	36	68
57	peanuts, roasted	24	106	1 c.	144	35	153
58	peanut butter	20	79	1 tbsp.	16	3	13
59	pigeon peas, mature seeds, dry	20	110				
60	soybeans, mature seeds, dry	75	171	1 c.	210	158	359
	soybean products, fermented						
61	natto	95	126				
62	tempeh	12	156				
63	soy sauce	8	28	1 tbsp.	18	1	5
NUTS AND SEEDS (OTHER THAN LEGUMINOUS SEEDS)							
64	almonds	33	96	1 c.	142	47	136
65	Brazil nuts, shelled	1	4	1 c.	140	1	6
66	cashew nuts, roasted	8	68	1 c.	140	11	95
67	coconut, shredded	10	24	1 c.	130	13	31
68	filberts (hazelnuts), shelled	23	72	1 c.	135	31	97
69	pecans, shelled	13	24	1 c.	108	14	26
70	pistachio nuts	10	58				
71	sesame seeds	49	96	1 tbsp.	8	4	8
72	walnuts, English, shelled	52	66	1 c.	100	52	66
VEGETABLES							
73	asparagus, raw	58	64	1 c.	135	78	86
74	bean sprouts, canned	7	10	1 c.	125	9	12
	beans, snap						
	green						
75	raw	33	44	1 c.	110	36	48
76	cooked, drained	–	40	1 c.	125	–	50

Table continued on the following page

APPENDIX TABLE 5   FOLACIN CONTENT OF FOODS (*Continued*)

ITEM NUM-BER	FOOD AND DESCRIPTION	Free Folacin (μg.)	Total Folacin (μg.)	Approximate Measure	Weight (gm.)	Free Folacin (μg.)	Total Folacin (μg.)
		PER 100 GM. EDIBLE PORTION		PER SPECIFIED UNIT			
	VEGETABLES (*Continued*)						
	beans, snap (*Continued*)						
77	frozen	8	33	1 c.	125	10	41
	yellow or wax						
78	raw	32	40	1 c.	110	35	44
79	frozen	8	34	1 c.	125	10	42
80	beans, Lima, frozen	9	31	1 c.	160	14	50
	beets, common, red						
81	raw	69	93	1 c.	135	93	126
82	cooked	38	78	1 c.	170	65	133
	broccoli						
	spears						
83	raw	51	69	3 med.	354	181	244
84	cooked	27	56	1 med.	180	49	101
85	flower, raw	102	105				
86	stem, raw	35	59				
	Brussels sprouts						
87	raw	55	78	6 med.	114	63	89
88	cooked	6	36	1 c. (7–8	155	9	56
	cabbage						
	common varieties						
89	raw	33	66	1 c.	90	30	59
90	cooked	2	18	1 c.	145	3	26
91	red, raw	23	34	1 c.	90	21	31
	cabbage, Chinese (also called celery cabbage or petsai)						
92	raw	42	83	1 c.	75	32	62
93	cooked	5	19				
	carrots						
94	raw	14	32	1 med.	59	8	19
95	cooked	2	24	1 c.	155	3	37
	cauliflower						
96	raw	31	55	1 c.	100	31	55
97	cooked	2	34	1 c.	125	2	42
98	celery, raw	6	12	1 c.	100	6	12
99	chicory greens, raw	33	52				
100	collards, raw	–	102	1 c.	55	–	56
	corn, sweet						
101	raw, whole-kernel	27	33	1 c.	165	45	54
102	frozen	2	21	1 c.	162	3	35
103	cucumber, raw, pared	12	15	1 small	128	15	19
	eggplant						
104	raw	9	31				
105	cooked	2	16	1 c.	200	4	32
106	endive, raw	–	49	1 c.	50	–	24
107	kale, raw	44	60	1 c.	110	48	66
	lettuce, raw						
108	leaf or head	34	37	1 c.	55	19	20
109	romaine	60	179	1 c.	55	33	98
110	mushrooms, raw	20	23	1 c.	68	14	16
111	okra, raw	10	24	1 c.	100	10	24
112	onion, mature, dry	10	25				
112a	onion, mature, chopped			1 c.	170	17	42
112b	onion, mature, chopped			1 tbsp.	10	1	2
	onion, young green, raw						
113	bulbs and white portion of top	40	36	1 tbsp.	6	2	2
114	tops only (green portion), chopped	52	80	1 tbsp.	6	3	5
	onion, Welsh, raw						
115	bulbs and white portion of top	16	66				
116	tops only (green portion)	49	105				

APPENDIX TABLE 5   FOLACIN CONTENT OF FOODS (*Continued*)

ITEM NUM-BER	FOOD AND DESCRIPTION	PER 100 GM. EDIBLE PORTION		PER SPECIFIED UNIT			
		Free Folacin (μg.)	*Total Folacin* (μg.)	*Approximate Measure*	*Weight* (gm.)	*Free Folacin* (μg.)	*Total Folacin* (μg.)
VEGETABLES (*Continued*)							
117	parsnips, raw	57	67	1 c.	130	74	87
118	parsley, raw	41	116	1 tbsp.	4	2	5
119	peas, green, frozen	17	53	1 c.	145	25	77
120	peppers, hot, mature, red, raw	23	52				
121	peppers, sweet, immature, green, raw	8	19	1 med.	164	13	31
	potatoes						
122	raw	11	19	1 med.	122	13	23
	cooked						
123	French-fried	8	22	10 pieces	50	4	11
124	hashed brown	3	17	1 c.	155	5	26
125	mashed	5	10	1 c.	210	10	21
	pumpkin						
126	raw	5	36				
127	cooked	2	19	1 c.	245	5	47
128	radishes, common, raw	18	24	4 small	36	6	9
	rutabagas						
129	raw	23	27	1 c.	140	32	38
130	cooked	9	21				
130a	cooked, cubed			1 c.	170	15	36
130b	cooked, mashed			1 c.	240	22	50
	spinach						
131	raw	119	193	1 c.	55	65	106
132	cooked	60	91	1 c.	180	108	164
	squash, summer						
133	raw	23	•31	1 c.	130	30	40
134	frozen, cooked	2	10	1 c.	210	4	21
	sweet potatoes						
135	raw	33	50	1 med.	146	48	73
136	cooked	7	18	1 med.	146	10	26
137	tomatoes, raw	21	39	1 med.	135	28	53
138	tomato juice, canned	10	26	1 c.	243	24	63
139	turnips, raw	17	20	1 c.	130	22	26
140	turnip greens, raw	–	95	1 c.	55	–	52
FRUITS							
141	apples, raw	3	8	1 med.	166	5	13
142	applesauce, sweetened	1	1	1 c.	255	3	3
143	apricots, dried	10	14	1 c.	130	13	18
143a	apricots, dried			10 halves	35	4	5
144	avocados, raw	31	51	½ med.	115	36	59
145	bananas, raw	22	28	1 med.	119	26	33
146	blueberries, raw	2	6	1 c.	145	3	9
	cantaloupe, *see* muskmelon						
147	cherries, raw	6	8	1 c.	117	7	9
147a	cherries, raw			10 cherries	68	4	5
148	cranberries, raw	1	2	1 c.	91	1	2
149	currants, dried	4	11				
150	dates, dried	14	21	1 c.	178	25	37
150a	dates, dried			10 dates	80	11	17
151	figs, dried	3	9	1 large	21	1	2
152	grapefruit, raw	8	11	½ med.	98	8	11
153	grapefruit juice, fresh or frozen reconstituted	8	21	1 c.	247	20	52
154	grapes, red or white, raw	4	7	1 c.	152	6	11
155	grape juice, canned or frozen reconstituted	2	2	1 c.	253	5	5
156	lemon, raw	12	12	1 med.	74	9	9
157	lemonade	2	5	1 c.	248	5	12

Table continued on the following page

APPENDIX TABLE 5   FOLACIN CONTENT OF FOODS (*Continued*)

ITEM NUM-BER	FOOD AND DESCRIPTION	PER 100 GM. EDIBLE PORTION		PER SPECIFIED UNIT			
		Free Folacin (μg.)	Total Folacin (μg.)	Approximate Measure	Weight (gm.)	Free Folacin (μg.)	Total Folacin (μg.)
FRUITS (*Continued*)							
158	limes, raw	6	4	1 lime	67	4	3
159	muskmelon or cantaloupe	30	30	½ med.	272	82	82
160	nectarines, raw	7	5	1 med.	138	10	7
161	oranges, raw	32	46	1 med.	141	45	65
162	orange juice, fresh or frozen reconstituted	34	55	1 c.	248	84	136
163	peaches, raw	2	8	1 med.	100	2	8
164	pears, raw	5	14	1 med.	164	8	23
165	pineapple, raw	9	11	1 c.	155	14	17
166	plantain (baking banana), raw	2	16	1 med.	263	5	42
167	plums, raw	4	6	1 med.	55	2	3
168	prunes, dried, softenized, raw	1	4	1 med.	26	<0.5	1
169	raisins, natural (unbleached), raw	3	4	1 c.	145	4	6
170	rhubarb, raw	9	7	1 c.	122	11	9
171	strawberries, raw	15	16	1 c.	149	22	24
172	tangerines, raw	19	21	1 med.	86	16	18
173	watermelon, raw	2	8	1 wedge, 4″ × 8″	426	9	34
MEAT							
	beef, separable lean						
174	raw	4	7				
175	cooked	–	4	3 oz.	85	–	3
	beef, ground						
176	raw	3*	7				
177	cooked	–	4	3 oz.	85	–	3
	kidney						
178	beef, raw	63	80				
	lamb						
179	raw	24	42				
180	cooked	–	32	3 oz.	85	–	27
	lamb						
181	raw	1	4				
182	cooked	–	3	3 oz.	85	–	3
	liver						
	beef, lamb, or pork						
183	raw	80	219				
184	cooked	–	145	3 oz.	85	–	123
	pork						
	separable lean						
185	raw	3	8				
186	cooked	–	5	3 oz.	85	–	4
187	ham, smoked	–	11	3 oz.	85	–	9
	veal						
188	raw	4	5				
189	cooked	–	3	3 oz.	85	–	3
	sausages, cold cuts, and luncheon meats						
190	beerwurst	1	3	1 slice (1 oz.)	28	<0.5	1
191	bologna	2	5	1 slice (1 oz.)	28	1	1
192	frankfurters, unheated	2	4	1 (5″ long, ¾″ diam.)	45	1	2
193	head cheese	1	2	1 slice (1 oz.)	28	<0.5	1
194	liverwurst	20	30	1 slice (1 oz.)	28	6	8
	luncheon meats						
195	boiled ham	1	4	1 slice (1 oz.)	28	<0.5	1
196	pork, spiced	1	3	1 slice (1 oz.)	28	<0.5	1
197	sausage, pork, raw	–	14	3 oz.	85	–	12

APPENDIX TABLE 5   FOLACIN CONTENT OF FOODS (*Continued*)

ITEM NUM-BER	FOOD AND DESCRIPTION	PER 100 GM. EDIBLE PORTION		PER SPECIFIED UNIT			
		Free Folacin (μg.)	*Total Folacin (μg.)*	*Approximate Measure*	*Weight (gm.)*	*Free Folacin (μg.)*	*Total Folacin (μg.)*
	POULTRY						
	chicken, without skin						
	dark meat						
198	raw	5	11				
199	cooked	–	7	3 oz.	85	–	6
	light meat						
200	raw	3	6				
201	cooked	–	4	3 oz.	85	–	3
	liver, chicken						
202	raw	–	364				
203	cooked	–	240	3 oz.	85	–	204
	turkey, without skin						
	dark meat						
204	raw	8	11				
205	cooked	–	7	3 oz.	85	–	6
	light meat						
206	raw	4	9				
207	cooked	–	5	3 oz.	85	–	4
	FISH AND SHELLFISH						
208	cod, frozen	6	18	3 oz.	85	5	15
209	crab, frozen	2	20	3 oz.	85	2	17
210	haddock, frozen	4	10	3 oz.	85	3	8
211	halibut, frozen	4	12	3 oz.	85	3	10
212	lobster, canned	8	17	3 oz.	85	7	14
213	ocean perch, frozen	5	9	3 oz.	85	4	8
	salmon						
214	canned	10	20	3 oz.	85	8	17
215	frozen	4	26	3 oz.	85	3	22
216	sardines, canned	13	16	1 fish	12	2	2
217	scallops, frozen	18	16	3 oz.	85	15	14
	shrimp						
218	canned	8	15	3 oz.	85	7	13
219	frozen	8	11	3 oz.	85	7	9
220	smelt, frozen	6	16	3 oz.	85	5	14
221	sole, frozen	5	11	3 oz.	85	4	9
222	tuna, canned	8	15	3 oz.	85	7	13
	EGGS AND EGG PRODUCTS						
	eggs						
	whole						
223	raw	46	65	1 med.	44	20	29
224	hard-cooked	–	49	1 med.	44	–	22
225	white, raw	3	16	1 med.	29	1	5
226	yolk, raw	121	152	1 med.	15	18	23
227	eggnog	<0.5	1	½ c.	128	–	1
	DAIRY PRODUCTS						
228	butter	1	3	1 tbsp.	14	<0.5	<0.5
	cheeses, natural						
229	Cheddar	1	18	1 c. shredded	113	1	20
229a	Cheddar			1 oz.	28	<0.5	5
230	cottage	–	12	1 c. packed	245	–	29
231	cream	–	13	3-oz. pkg.	85	–	11
231a	cream			1 cu. in.	16	–	2
232	cheese spread, pasteurized process	3	7	1 oz.	28	1	2
	cream, fluid						
233	half-and-half	2	2	1 c.	242	5	5
234	light coffee or table	1	2	1 c.	240	2	5
235	sour, cultured	–	11	1 c.	230	–	25
236	whipping, light	2	4	1 c.	239	5	10

Table continued on the following page

APPENDIX TABLE 5   FOLACIN CONTENT OF FOODS (Continued)

ITEM NUM-BER	FOOD AND DESCRIPTION	PER 100 GM. EDIBLE PORTION		PER SPECIFIED UNIT			
		Free Folacin (µg.)	Total Folacin (µg.)	Approximate Measure	Weight (gm.)	Free Folacin (µg.)	Total Folacin (µg.)
DAIRY PRODUCTS (Continued)							
237	ice cream, vanilla	2	2	1 c.	133	3	3
	milk, cow's, fluid						
238	whole, pasteurized	5	5	1 c.	244	12	12
239	skim, raw	3	–	1 c.	245	1	–
240	evaporated	4	8	1 c.	252	10	20
241	milk, goat's	1	1	1 c.	244	2	2
242	milk, human	3	5	1 fl. oz.	31	1	2
243	yogurt	<0.5	11	1 c.	245	–	27
MIXED DISHES, FROZEN							
244	beef with one vegetable	2	5	1 pkg.	254	5	13
245	beef with two vegetables, soup, dessert	5	12	1 pkg.	456	23	55
246	beef with three vegetables	8	24	1 pkg.	327	26	78
247	chicken, fried, with one vegetable	6	12	1 pkg.	205	12	25
248	chicken, fried, with two vegetables, dessert	6	18	1 pkg.	315	19	57
249	haddock with one vegetable	6	18	1 pkg.	273	16	49
250	ham with two vegetables, dessert	5	15	1 pkg.	314	16	47
251	lasagna	–	22	10-oz. portion	280	–	62
	pizza						
252	cheese	–	37	⅛ pie, 13¾" diam.	65	–	24
253	pepperoni	–	38	⅛ pie, 13¾" diam.	67	–	25
254	sausage	–	35	⅛ pie, 13¾" diam.	67	–	23
255	pork with one vegetable, one fruit, dessert	2	7	1 pkg.	303	6	21
256	poultry, Oriental style with rice, vegetables	2	4	1 pkg.	415	8	17
257	shrimp, Oriental style with rice, vegetables	4	13	1 pkg.	388	16	50
258	shrimp with one vegetable	8	14	1 pkg.	264	21	37
259	shrimp with two vegetables	9	22	1 pkg.	234	21	51
260	spaghetti with meatballs, one vegetable, dessert	6	18	1 pkg.	354	21	64
261	turkey with one vegetable	4	11	1 pkg.	264	11	29
262	turkey with two vegetables, dessert	6	14	1 pkg.	346	21	48
BABY FOODS—STRAINED, CANNED							
263	applesauce	<0.5	1				
263a	applesauce			1 jar	134	–	1
263b	applesauce			1 oz.	28	–	<0.5
264	apricots	<0.5	1				
264a	apricots			1 jar	134	–	1
264b	apricots			1 oz.	28	–	<0.5
265	bananas	1	2				
265a	bananas			1 jar	134	1	3
265b	bananas			1 oz.	28	<0.5	1
266	beans, green or wax	1	6				
266a	beans, green or wax			1 jar	128	1	8
266b	beans, green or wax			1 oz.	28	<0.5	2
267	beef with broth	1	6				
267a	beef with broth			1 jar	99	1	6
267b	beef with broth			1 oz.	28	<0.5	2
268	beets	2	10				
268a	beets			1 jar	128	3	13

APPENDIX TABLE 5   FOLACIN CONTENT OF FOODS (*Continued*)

| ITEM NUM-BER | FOOD AND DESCRIPTION | PER 100 GM. EDIBLE PORTION | | PER SPECIFIED UNIT | | | |
		Free Folacin (μg.)	Total Folacin (μg.)	Approximate Measure	Weight (gm.)	Free Folacin (μg.)	Total Folacin (μg.)
	BABY FOODS—STRAINED, CANNED (*Continued*)						
268b	beets			1 oz.	28	1	3
269	carrots	1	2				
269a	carrots			1 jar	128	1	3
269b	carrots			1 oz.	28	<0.5	1
270	chicken with broth	1	2				
270a	chicken with broth			1 jar	99	1	2
270b	chicken with broth			1 oz.	28	<0.5	1
271	corn, creamed	1	3				
271a	corn, creamed			1 jar	128	1	4
271b	corn, creamed			1 oz.	28	<0.5	1
272	egg yolk	8	20				
272a	egg yolk			1 jar	94	8	19
272b	egg yolk			1 oz.	28	2	6
273	fruit, mixed	1	1				
273a	fruit, mixed			1 jar	134	1	1
273b	fruit, mixed			1 oz.	28	<0.5	<0.5
274	ham with broth	<0.5	6				
274a	ham with broth			1 jar	99	<0.5	6
274b	ham with broth			1 oz.	28	<0.5	2
275	lamb with vegetables	1	8				
275a	lamb with vegetables			1 jar	99	1	8
275b	lamb with vegetables			1 oz.	28	<0.5	2
276	oatmeal	–	4				
276a	oatmeal			1 jar	135	–	5
276b	oatmeal			1 oz.	28	–	1
277	peas	1	7				
277a	peas			1 jar	128	1	9
277b	peas			1 oz.	28	<0.5	2
278	spinach, creamed	2	4				
278a	spinach, creamed			1 jar	128	3	5
278b	spinach, creamed			1 oz.	28	1	1
279	squash	1	6				
279a	squash			1 jar	128	1	8
279b	squash			1 oz.	28	<0.5	2
280	sweet potatoes	1	3				
280a	sweet potatoes			1 jar	128	1	4
280b	sweet potatoes			1 oz.	28	<0.5	1
281	turkey with broth	2	4				
281a	turkey with broth			1 jar	99	2	4
281b	turkey with broth			1 oz.	28	1	1
282	veal with broth	2	7				
282a	veal with broth			1 jar	99	2	7
282b	veal with broth			1 oz.	28	1	2
283	vegetables, mixed	1	4				
283a	vegetables, mixed			1 jar	128	1	5
283b	vegetables, mixed			1 oz.	28	<0.5	1
	MISCELLANEOUS						
284	barbecue sauce	3	4	1 c.	250	8	10
285	candy, milk chocolate, plain	4	7	1 oz.	28	1	2
286	margarine	2	2				
286a	margarine			1 c.	227	5	5
286b	margarine			1 tbsp.	14	<0.5	<0.5
287	mayonnaise	1	3	1 tbsp.	14	<0.5	<0.5
288	rice pudding	5	–	1 c.	255	13	–
	soups, commercial, canned						
289	asparagus, cream of	5	19	1 c.	245	12	47
290	beef broth	1	4	1 c.	240	2	10
291	clam chowder	3	7	1 c.	250	8	18

Table continued on the following page

APPENDIX TABLE 5   FOLACIN CONTENT OF FOODS (*Continued*)

ITEM NUM-BER	FOOD AND DESCRIPTION	PER 100 GM. EDIBLE PORTION		PER SPECIFIED UNIT			
		Free Folacin (μg.)	*Total Folacin* (μg.)	*Approximate Measure*	*Weight* (gm.)	*Free Folacin* (μg.)	*Total Folacin* (μg.)
MISCELLANEOUS (*Continued*)							
292	mushroom, cream of	1	3	1 c.	245	2	7
293	vegetable beef	2	6	1 c.	250	5	15
294	strawberry jam	7	8	1 tbsp.	20	1	2
295	tapioca, dry	2	8				
295a	tapioca, dry			1 c.	152	3	12
295b	tapioca, dry			1 tbsp.	8	<0.5	1
296	tapioca pudding	2	–	1 c.	255	5	–
297	tomato catsup	2	5				
297a	tomato catsup			1 c.	273	5	14
297b	tomato catsup			1 tbsp.	15	<0.5	1
	yeast						
298	baker's dry, active	140	4090	1 pkg.	7	10	286
299	brewer's, debittered	175	3909	1 tbsp.	8	14	313

APPENDIX TABLE 6 — AMINO ACID CONTENT OF FOODS, 100 GRAMS, EDIBLE PORTION*

ITEM, PROTEIN CONTENT, AND NITROGEN CONVERSION FACTOR	TRYPTO-PHAN	THREO-NINE	ISO-LEUCINE	LEUCINE	LYSINE	SULFUR CONTAINING			PHENYL-ALANINE	TYRO-SINE†	VALINE	ARGININE	HISTIDINE
						Meth-ionine†	Cystine†	Total					
	Gm.	Gm.	Gm.	Gm.	Gm.	Gm.	Gm.	Gm.	Gm.	Gm.	Gm.	Gm.	Gm.
Milk; Milk Products:													
Milk (Protein, N x 6.38):													
Cow:													
Fluid, whole and nonfat (3.5% protein)	0.049	0.161	0.223	0.344	0.272	0.086	0.031	0.117	0.170	0.178	0.240	0.128	0.092
Canned:													
Evaporated, unsweetened (7.0% protein)	.099	.323	.447	.688	.545	.171	.063	.234	.340	.357	.481	.256	.185
Condensed, sweetened (8.1% protein)	.114	.374	.518	.796	.631	.198	.072	.271	.393	.413	.557	.296	.214
Dried:													
Whole (25.8% protein)	.364	1.191	1.648	2.535	2.009	.632	.231	.863	1.251	1.316	1.774	.944	.680
Nonfat (35.6% protein)	.502	1.641	2.271	3.493	2.768	.870	.318	1.188	1.724	1.814	2.444	1.300	.937
Goat (3.3% protein)	.039	.217	.087	.278	.312	.065	.027		.121		.139	.174	.068
Human (1.4% protein)	.023	.062	.075	.124	.090	.028	.058		.060	.071	.086	.055	.030
Indian buffalo (4.2% protein)	.059	.212	.204	.420	.331	.112		.170	.177		.255	.136	.086
Milk Products:													
Buttermilk (3.5% protein, N x 6.38)	.038	.165	.219	.348	.291	.082	.032	.114	.186	.137	.262	.168	.099
Casein (100.0% protein, N x 6.29)	1.335	4.277	6.550	10.048	8.013	3.084	.382	3.466	5.389	5.819	7.393	4.070	3.021
Cheese (protein, N x 6.38):													
Blue mold (21.5% protein)	.293	.799	1.449	2.096	1.577	.559	.121	.680	1.153	1.028	1.543	.785	.701
Camembert (17.5% protein)	.239	.650	1.179	1.706	1.284	.455	.099	.554	.938	.837	1.256	.639	.571
Cheddar (25.0% protein)	.341	.929	1.685	2.437	1.834	.650	.141	.791	1.340	1.195	1.794	.913	.815
Cheddar processed (23.2% protein)	.316	.862	1.563	2.262	1.702	.604	.131	.735	1.244	1.109	1.665	.847	.756
Cheese foods, cheddar (20.5% protein)	.280	.761	1.382	1.998	1.504	.533	.116	.649	1.099	.980	1.472	.749	.668
Cottage (17.0% protein)	.179	.794	.989	1.826	1.428	.469	.147	.616	.917	.917	.978	.802	.549
Cream cheese (9.0% protein)	.080	.408	.519	.923	.721	.229	.085	.314	.547	.408	.538	.313	.278
Limburger (21.2% protein)	.289	.788	1.429	2.067	1.555	.552	.120	.672	1.136	1.014	1.522	.774	.691
Parmesan (36.0% protein)	.491	1.337	2.426	3.510	2.641	.937	.203	1.140	1.930	1.721	2.584	1.315	1.174
Swiss (27.5% protein)	.375	1.021	1.853	2.681	2.017	.715	.155	.870	1.474	1.315	1.974	1.004	.896
Swiss processed (26.4% protein)	.360	.981	1.779	2.574	1.937	.687	.149	.836	1.415	1.262	1.895	.964	.861
Lactalbumin (100.0% protein, N x 6.49)	2.203	5.239	6.209	12.342	9.060	2.250	3.405	5.655	4.360	3.806	5.686	3.498	1.911
Whey (Protein, N x 6.49):													
Fluid (0.9% protein)	.010	.048	.052	.074	.055	.013	.018	.031	.023	.009	.045	.017	.011
Dried (12.7% protein)	.147	.677	.734	1.043	.769	.188	.250	.438	.323	.131	.640	.235	.159

* Adapted from the more comprehensive Table 2 compiled by M. L. Orr and B. K. Watt in "Amino Acid Content of Foods," Home Economics Research Report No. 4. U. S. Dept. of Agriculture. Washington, D. C., U. S. Govt. Printing Office, 1968.

† All amino acids except those designated with † are essential to man. Histidine is essential for the human infant only.

Table continued on the following page

APPENDIX TABLE 6   AMINO ACID CONTENT OF FOODS, 100 GRAMS, EDIBLE PORTION (Continued)

ITEM, PROTEIN CONTENT, AND NITROGEN CONVERSION FACTOR	TRYPTOPHAN	THREONINE	ISO-LEUCINE	LEUCINE	LYSINE	SULFUR CONTAINING			PHENYL-ALANINE	TYROSINE	VALINE	ARGININE	HISTIDINE
						Methionine	Cystine	Total					
	Gm.	Gm.	Gm.	Gm.	Gm.	Gm.	Gm.	Gm.	Gm.	Gm.	Gm.	Gm.	Gm.
Eggs, Chicken (Protein, N x 6.25):													
Fresh or stored:													
Whole (12.8% protein)	0.211	0.637	0.850	1.126	0.819	0.401	0.299	0.700	0.739	0.551	0.950	0.840	0.307
Whites (10.8% protein)	.164	.477	.698	.950	.648	.420	.263	.683	.689	.449	.842	.634	.233
Yolks (16.3% protein)	.235	.827	.996	1.372	1.074	.417	.274	.691	.717	.756	1.121	1.132	.368
Dried:													
Whole (46.8% protein)	.771	2.329	3.108	4.118	2.995	1.468	1.093	2.561	2.703	2.014	3.474	3.070	1.123
Whites (85.9% protein)	1.306	3.793	5.553	7.559	5.154	3.340	2.089	5.429	5.484	3.573	6.693	5.044	1.855
Yolks (31.2% protein)	.449	1.582	1.907	2.626	2.057	.799	.524	1.323	1.373	1.448	2.147	2.167	.704
Meat; Poultry; Fish and Shellfish; Their Products:													
Meat (Protein, N x 6.25):													
Beef carcass or side:													
Thin (18.8% protein)	.220	.830	.984	1.540	1.642	.466	.238	.704	.773	.638	1.044	1.212	.653
Medium fat (17.5% protein)	.204	.773	.916	1.434	1.529	.434	.221	.655	.720	.594	.972	1.128	.608
Fat (16.3% protein)	.190	.720	.853	1.335	1.424	.404	.206	.610	.670	.553	.905	1.051	.566
Very fat (13.7% protein)	.160	.605	.717	1.122	1.197	.340	.173	.513	.563	.465	.761	.883	.476
Medium fat, trimmed to retail basis (18.2% protein)	.213	.804	.952	1.491	1.590	.451	.230	.681	.748	.617	1.010	1.174	.632
Beef cuts, medium fat:													
Chuck (18.6% protein)	.217	.821	.973	1.524	1.625	.461	.235	.696	.765	.631	1.033	1.199	.646
Flank (19.9% protein)	.232	.879	1.041	1.630	1.738	.494	.252	.746	.818	.675	1.105	1.283	.691
Hamburger (16.0% protein)	.187	.707	.837	1.311	1.398	.397	.202	.599	.658	.543	.888	1.032	.556
Porterhouse (16.4% protein)	.192	.724	.858	1.343	1.433	.407	.207	.614	.674	.556	.911	1.057	.569
Rib roast (17.4% protein)	.203	.768	.910	1.425	1.520	.432	.220	.652	.715	.590	.966	1.122	.604
Round (19.5% protein)	.228	.861	1.020	1.597	1.704	.484	.246	.730	.802	.661	1.083	1.257	.677
Rump (16.2% protein)	.189	.715	.848	1.327	1.415	.402	.205	.607	.666	.550	.899	1.045	.562
Sirloin (17.3% protein)	.202	.764	.905	1.417	1.511	.429	.219	.648	.711	.587	.960	1.116	.601
Beef, canned (25.0% protein)	.292	1.104	1.308	2.048	2.184	.620	.316	.936	1.028	.848	1.388	1.612	.868
Beef, dried or chipped (34.3% protein)	.401	1.515	1.795	2.810	2.996	.851	.434	1.285	1.410	1.163	1.904	2.212	1.191
Lamb carcass or side:													
Thin (17.1% protein)	.222	.782	.886	1.324	1.384	.410	.224	.634	.695	.594	.843	1.114	.476
Medium fat (15.7% protein)	.203	.718	.814	1.216	1.271	.377	.206	.583	.638	.545	.774	1.022	.437
Fat (13.0% protein)	.168	.595	.674	1.007	1.052	.312	.171	.483	.528	.451	.641	.847	.362
Lamb cuts, medium fat:													
Leg (18.0% protein)	.233	.824	.933	1.394	1.457	.432	.236	.668	.732	.625	.887	1.172	.501
Rib (14.9% protein)	.193	.682	.772	1.154	1.206	.358	.195	.553	.606	.517	.734	.970	.415
Shoulder (15.6% protein)	.202	.714	8.09	1.208	1.263	.374	.205	.579	.634	.542	.769	1.016	.434

Meat; Poultry; Fish and Shellfish; Their Products—Continued
Meat (Protein, N x 6.25)—Continued

	Gm.	Gm.	Gm.	Gm.	Gm.	Gm.	Gm.	Gm.	Gm.	Gm.	Gm.	Gm.	Gm.
Pork, packer's carcass or side:													
Thin (14.1% protein)	0.183	0.654	0.724	1.038	1.157	0.352	0.165	0.517	0.555	0.503	0.733	0.864	0.487
Medium fat (11.9% protein)	.154	.552	.611	.876	.977	.297	.139	.436	.468	.425	.619	.729	.411
Fat (9.8% protein)	.127	.455	.503	.721	.804	.245	.114	.359	.386	.350	.510	.601	.339
Pork cuts, medium fat, fresh:													
Ham (15.2% protein)	.197	.705	.781	1.119	1.248	.379	.178	.557	.598	.542	.790	.931	.525
Loin (16.4% protein)	.213	.761	.842	1.207	1.346	.409	.192	.601	.646	.585	.853	1.005	.567
Miscellaneous lean cuts (14.5% protein)	.188	.673	.745	1.067	1.190	.362	.169	.531	.571	.517	.754	.889	.501
Pork, cured:													
Bacon, medium fat (9.1% protein)	.095	.306	.399	.728	.587	.141	.106	.247	.434	.234	.434	.622	.246
Fat back or salt pork (3.9% protein)	.006	.141	.110	.367	.317	.055	.043	.098	.157	.052	.168	.379	.035
Ham (16.9% protein)	.162	.692	.841	1.306	1.420	.411	.273	.684	.646	.652	.879	1.068	.544
Luncheon meat:													
Boiled ham (22.8% protein)	.219	.934	1.135	1.762	1.915	.554	.368	.923	.872	.879	1.186	1.441	.733
Canned, spiced (14.9% protein)	.143	.610	.741	1.151	1.252	.362	.241	.603	.570	.575	.775	.942	.479
Rabbit, domesticated, flesh only (21.0% protein)		1.021	1.082	1.636	1.818	.541			.793		1.021	1.176	.474
Veal, carcass or side:													
Thin (19.7% protein)	.258	.854	1.040	1.444	1.645	.451	.233	.684	.801	.709	1.018	1.283	.634
Medium fat (19.1% protein)	.251	.828	1.008	1.400	1.595	.437	.226	.663	.776	.688	.987	1.244	.614
Fat (18.5% protein)	.243	.802	.977	1.356	1.545	.423	.219	.642	.752	.666	.956	1.205	.595
Veal cuts, medium fat:													
Round (19.5% protein)	.256	.846	1.030	1.429	1.629	.446	.231	.677	.792	.702	1.008	1.270	.627
Shoulder (19.4% protein)	.255	.841	1.024	1.422	1.620	.444	.230	.674	.788	.698	1.003	1.263	.624
Stew meat (18.3% protein)	.240	.793	.966	1.341	1.528	.419	.217	.636	.744	.659	.946	1.192	.589
Poultry (Protein, N x 6.25):													
Chicken, flesh only:													
Broilers or fryers (20.6% protein)	.250	.877	1.088	1.490	1.810	.537	.277	.814	.811	.725	1.012	1.302	.593
Hens (21.3% protein)	.259	.907	1.125	1.540	1.871	.556	.286	.842	.838	.750	1.046	1.346	.613
Ducks, domesticated, flesh only (21.4% protein)		.935	1.109	1.657	1.842	.531			.842		1.027	1.301	.486
Turkey, flesh only (24.0% protein)		1.014	1.260	1.836	2.173	.664	.330	.994	.960		1.187	1.513	.649
Fish and Shellfish (Protein, N x 6.25):													
Blue fish (20.5% protein)	.203	.889	1.040	1.548	1.797	.597	.276	.873	.761	.554	1.092	1.155	
Cod:													
Fresh (16.5% protein)	.164	.715	.837	1.246	1.447	.480	.222	.702	.612	.446	.879	.929	
Dried (81.8% protein)	.811	3.547	4.149	6.178	7.172	2.383	1.099	3.481	3.036	2.212	4.358	4.607	

Table continued on the following page

APPENDIX TABLE 6　AMINO ACID CONTENT OF FOODS, 100 GRAMS, EDIBLE PORTION (Continued)

ITEM, PROTEIN CONTENT, AND NITROGEN CONVERSION FACTOR	TRYPTO-PHAN	THREO-NINE	ISO-LEUCINE	LEUCINE	LYSINE	SULFUR CONTAINING			PHENYL-ALANINE	TYRO-SINE	VALINE	ARGININE	HISTIDINE
						Meth-ionine	Cystine	Total					
	Gm.	Gm.	Gm.	Gm.	Gm.	Gm.	Gm.	Gm.	Gm.	Gm.	Gm.	Gm.	Gm.
*Meat; Poultry; Fish and Shellfish; Their Products—*Continued													
*Fish and Shellfish; Their Products—*Continued													
Croaker (17.8% protein)	0.177	0.772	0.903	1.344	1.561	0.518	0.239	0.757	0.661	0.481	0.948	1.002	—
Eel (18.6% protein)	.185	.806	.943	1.405	1.631	.542	.250	.792	.690	.503	.991	1.048	—
Flounder (14.9% protein)	.148	.646	.756	1.125	1.306	.434	.200	.634	.553	.403	.794	.839	—
Haddock (18.2% protein)	.181	.789	.923	1.374	1.596	.530	.245	.775	.676	.492	.970	1.025	—
Halibut (18.6% protein)	.185	.806	.943	1.405	1.631	.542	.250	.792	.690	.503	.991	1.048	—
Herring:													
Atlantic (18.3% protein)	.182	.793	.928	1.382	1.605	.533	.246	.779	.679	.495	.975	1.031	—
Lake (18.5% protein)	.184	.802	.938	1.397	1.622	.539	.249	.788	.687	.500	.986	1.042	—
Pacific (16.6% protein)	.165	.720	.842	1.254	1.455	.483	.223	.706	.616	.449	.884	.935	—
Mackerel:													
Raw, common Atlantic (18.7% protein)	.186	.811	.948	1.412	1.640	.545	.251	.796	.694	.506	.996	1.053	—
Canned, solids and liquid:													
Atlantic (19.3% protein)	.191	.837	.979	1.458	1.692	.562	.259	.821	.716	.522	1.028	1.087	—
Pacific (21.1% protein)	.209	.915	1.070	1.593	1.850	.614	.284	.898	.783	.571	1.124	1.188	—
Salmon:													
Raw, Pacific (Chinook or King) (17.4% protein)	.173	.754	.883	1.314	1.526	.507	.234	.741	.646	.470	.927	.980	—
Canned, solids and liquid (Sockeye or red) (20.2% protein)	.200	.876	1.025	1.526	1.771	.588	.271	.859	.750	.546	1.076	1.138	—
Sardines, canned, solids and liquid:													
Atlantic type (21.1% protein)	.209	.915	1.070	1.593	1.850	.614	.284	.898	.783	.571	1.124	1.188	—
Pacific type (17.7% protein)	.176	.767	.898	1.337	1.552	.515	.238	.753	.657	.479	.943	.997	—
Shrimp, canned, solids and liquid (18.7% protein)	.186	.811	.948	1.412	1.640	.545	.251	.796	.694	.506	.996	1.053	—
Products from Meat, Poultry, and Fish (Protein, N x 6.25):													
Brains (10.4% protein)	.138	.494	.504	.845	.760	.220	.145	.365	.506	.433	.536	.614	0.278
Chitterlings (8.6% protein)	.094	.398	.308	.457	.670	.193	.109	.302	.359	.228	.462	1.406	.169
Fish flour (76.0% protein)	.754	4.378	4.232	6.189	7.381	2.019			2.845		3.916	5.204	1.289
Gelatin (85.6% protein, N x 5.55)	.006	1.912	1.357	2.930	4.226	.787	.077	.864	2.036	.401	2.421	7.866	.771
Gizzard, chicken (23.1% protein)	.207	1.072	1.094	1.689	1.567	.554	.218	.772	.968	.680	1.116	1.741	.480
Heart:													
Beef or pork (16.9% protein)	.219	.776	.857	1.509	1.387	.403	.168	.571	.765	.627	.973	1.068	.433
Chicken (20.5% protein)	.266	.941	1.040	1.830	1.683	.489	.203	.692	.928	.761	1.181	1.296	.525

	Gm.	Gm.	Gm.	Gm.	Gm.	Gm.	Gm.	Gm.	Gm.	Gm.	Gm.	Gm.	Gm.
Meat; Poultry; Fish and Shellfish; Their Products— Continued													
Products from Meat, Poultry, and Fish (Protein N x 6.25)—Continued													
Kidney:													
Beef (15.0% protein)	0.221	0.665	0.730	1.301	1.087	0.307	0.182	0.489	0.706	0.557	0.876	0.934	0.377
Pork (16.3% protein)	.240	.722	.793	1.414	1.181	.334	.198	.532	.767	.605	.952	1.015	.409
Sheep (16.6% protein)	.244	.736	.807	1.440	1.203	.340	.202	.542	.781	.616	.969	1.033	.417
Liver:													
Beef or pork (19.7% protein)	.296	.936	1.031	1.819	1.475	.463	.243	.706	.993	.738	1.239	1.201	.523
Calf (19.0% protein)	.286	.903	.994	1.754	1.423	.447	.234	.681	.958	.711	1.195	1.158	.505
Chicken (22.1% protein)	.332	1.050	1.156	2.040	1.655	.520	.272	.792	1.114	.827	1.390	1.347	.587
Sheep or lamb (21.0% protein)	.316	.998	1.099	1.939	1.572	.494	.259	.753	1.058	.786	1.320	1.280	.558
Pancreas:													
Beef (13.5% protein)	.175	.626	.683	1.054	.996	.244	—	—	.562	.590	.724	.771	.266
Pork (14.5% protein)	.188	.673	.733	1.132	1.070	.262	—	—	.603	.633	.777	.828	.285
Pork and beef, canned (14.3% protein)	.151	.618	.730	1.190	1.345	.327	.261	.588	.579	.570	.810	1.050	.460
Potted meat (16.1% protein)	.149	.662	.641	1.203	1.061	.361	—	—	.641	—	.943	1.002	.322
Sausage:													
Bologna (14.8% protein)	.126	.606	.718	1.061	1.191	.313	.185	.498	.540	.481	.744	1.028	.398
Braunschweiger (15.4% protein)	.172	.668	.754	1.291	1.200	.320	.187	.507	.700	.471	.956	.954	.458
Frankfurters (14.2% protein)	.120	.582	.688	1.018	1.143	.300	.177	.477	.518	.461	.713	.986	.382
Head cheese (15.0% protein)	.079	.418	.509	.946	.907	.250	.209	.459	.569	.569	.617	1.075	.278
Liverwurst (16.7% protein)	.187	.724	.818	1.400	1.301	.347	.203	.550	.759	.510	1.037	1.034	.497
Pork, links or bulk, raw (10.8% protein)	.092	.442	.524	.774	.869	.228	.135	.363	.394	.351	.543	.750	.290
Pork, bulk, canned (15.4% protein)	.131	.631	.747	1.104	1.239	.325	.192	.517	.562	.500	.774	1.069	.414
Salami (23.9% protein)	.203	.979	1.159	1.713	1.923	.505	.298	.803	.872	.776	1.201	1.660	.642
Vienna sausage, canned (15.8% protein)	.134	.647	.766	1.133	1.272	.334	.197	.531	.576	.513	.794	1.097	.425
Tongue:													
Beef (16.4% protein)	.197	.708	.792	1.286	1.364	.357	.207	.564	.661	.548	.840	1.065	.412
Pork (16.8% protein)	.202	.726	.812	1.317	1.398	.366	.212	.578	.677	.562	.860	1.091	.422
Veal and pork loaf, canned (17.2% protein)	.198	.627	.859	1.236	1.258	.418	.209	.627	.619	.468	.958	.916	.388
Legumes (Dry Seed); Common Nuts; Other Nuts and Dry Seeds; Their Products:													
Legume Seeds and Their Products:													
Beans (Phaseolus vulgaris) (N x 6.25):													
Pinto and red Mexican (23.0% protein)	.213	.997	1.306	1.976	1.708	.232	.228	.460	1.270	.887	1.395	1.384	.655

Table continued on the following page

APPENDIX TABLE 6   AMINO ACID CONTENT OF FOODS, 100 GRAMS, EDIBLE PORTION (Continued)

ITEM, PROTEIN CONTENT, AND NITROGEN CONVERSION FACTOR	TRYPTO-PHAN	THREO-NINE	ISO-LEUCINE	LEUCINE	LYSINE	SULFUR CONTAINING			PHENYL-ALANINE	TYRO-SINE	VALINE	ARGININE	HISTIDINE
						Meth-ionine	Cystine	Total					
	Gm.	Gm.	Gm.	Gm.	Gm.	Gm.	Gm.	Gm.	Gm	Gm.	Gm.	Gm.	Gm.
Legumes (Dry Seed); Common Nuts; Other Nuts and Dry Seeds; Their Products—Continued													
Legume Seeds and Their Products—Continued													
Beans (Phaseolus vulgaris) (N x 6.25)—Continued													
Red kidney:													
Raw (23.1% protein)	0.214	1.002	1.312	1.985	1.715	0.233	0.229	0.462	1.275	0.891	1.401	1.390	0.658
Canned, solids and liquid (5.7% protein)	.053	.247	.324	.490	.423	.057	.057	.114	.315	.220	.346	.343	.162
Other common beans including navy, peabean, white marrow:													
Raw (21.4% protein)	.199	.928	1.216	1.839	1.589	.216	.212	.428	1.181	.825	1.298	1.287	.609
Baked with pork, canned (5.8% protein)	.057	.274	.291	.486	.354	.059	.018	.077	.333	.165	.312	.251	.186
Black gram, raw (23.6% protein, N x 6.25)	.242	.801	1.390	2.062	1.510	.332	.287	.619	1.242	.551	1.450	1.552	.559
Broadbeans, raw (25.4% protein, N x 6.25)	.236	.829	1.593	2.211	1.426	.106	.179	.285	1.057	.687	1.276	1.780	.748
Chickpeas (20.8% protein, N x 6.25)	.170	.739	1.195	1.538	1.434	.276	.296	.572	1.012	.692	1.025	1.551	.559
Cowpeas (22.9% protein, N x 6.25)	.220	.901	1.110	1.715	1.491	.352	.297	.649	1.198	.678	1.293	1.473	.692
Dolichos, twinflower (21.6% protein, N x 6.25)	.221	.836	1.448	1.707	1.700	.294	.480	.774	1.486	.560	1.286	1.230	.650
Lentils, whole (25.0% protein, N x 6.25)	.216	.896	1.316	1.760	1.528	.180	.204	.384	1.104	.664	1.360	1.908	.548
Lima beans (20.7% protein, N x 6.25)	.195	.980	1.199	1.722	1.378	.331	.311	.642	1.222	.543	1.298	1.315	.669
Lupine (32.3% protein, N x 6.25)		1.101	1.618	1.964	1.447	.114			1.271		1.328	2.718	.811
Moth beans (24.4% protein, N x 6.25)	.164		1.093	1.484	1.202	.191	.109	.300	1.003	1.245	.695		.722
Mung beans (24.4% protein, N x 6.25)	.180	.765	1.351	2.202	1.667	.265	.152	.417	1.167	.390	1.444	1.370	.543
Peanuts (26.9% protein, N x 5.46)	.340	.828	1.266	1.872	1.099	.271	.463	.734	1.557	1.104	1.532	3.296	.749
Peanut flour (51.2% protein, N x 5.46)	.647	1.575	2.410	3.563	2.091	.516	.881	1.397	2.963	2.100	2.916	6.273	1.425
Peanut butter (26.1% protein, N x 5.46)	.330	.803	1.228	1.816	1.066	.263	.449	.712	1.510	1.071	1.487	3.198	.727
Peas (Pisum sativum) (N x 6.25):													
Entire seeds (23.8% protein)	.251	.918	1.340	1.969	1.744	.286	.308	.594	1.200	.960	1.333	2.102	.651
Split (24.5% protein)	.259	.945	1.380	2.027	1.795	.294	.318	.612	1.235	.988	1.372	2.164	.670
Pigeonpeas, without seed coat (21.9% protein, N x 6.25)	.119	.834	1.346	1.717	1.580	.256	.308	.564	1.875	.725	1.153	1.489	.617
Soybeans, whole (34.9% protein, N x 5.71)	.526	1.504	2.054	2.946	2.414	.513	.678	1.191	1.889	1.216	2.005	2.763	.911
Soybean flour, flakes, and grits (protein, N x 5.71):													
Low fat (44.7% protein)	.673	1.926	2.630	3.773	3.092	.658	.869	1.527	2.419	1.558	2.568	3.538	1.166
Medium fat (42.5% protein)	.640	1.831	2.501	3.588	2.940	.625	.826	1.451	2.300	1.481	2.441	3.364	1.109
Full fat (35.9% protein)	.541	1.547	2.112	3.030	2.483	.528	.698	1.226	1.943	1.251	2.062	2.842	.937
Soybean curd (7.0% protein, N x 6.25)						.081	.091	.172					
Soybean milk (3.4% protein, N x 5.71)	.051	.176	.175	.305	.269	.054	.071	.125	.195	.193	.186	.302	.121
Vetch (28.8% protein, N x 6.25)	.203	.899	2.198	2.290	1.898	.346	.336	.682	1.014	.369	1.442	2.249	.659

Legumes (Dry Seed); Common Nuts; Other Nuts and Dry Seeds; Their Products:—Continued

	Gm.	Gm.	Gm.	Gm.	Gm.	Gm.	Gm.	Gm.	Gm.	Gm.	Gm.	Gm.	Gm.
Common Nuts and Their Products:													
Almonds (18.6% protein, N x 5.18)........	0.176	0.610	0.873	1.454	0.582	0.259	0.377	0.636	1.146	0.618	1.124	2.729	0.517
Brazil nuts (14.4% protein, N x 5.46)......	.187	.422	.593	1.129	.443	.941	.504	1.445	.617	.483	.823	2.247	.367
Cashews (18.5% protein, N x 5.30)........	.471	.737	1.222	1.522	.792	.353	.527	.880	.946	.712	1.592	2.098	.415
Coconut (3.4% protein, N x 5.30)........	.033	.129	.180	.269	.152	.071	.062	.133	.174	.101	.212	.486	.069
Coconut meal (20.3% protein, N x 5.30)...	.199	.770	1.076	1.605	.908	.421	.372	.793	1.038	.605	1.268	2.899	.414
Filberts (12.7% protein, N x 5.30)........	.211	.415	.853	.939	.417	.139	.165	.304	.537	.434	.934	2.171	.288
Peanuts. See Legumes.													
Pecans (9.4% protein, N x 5.30)	.138	.389	.553	.773	.435	.153	.216	.369	.564	.316	.525	1.185	.273
Walnuts (English or Persian) (15.0% protein, N x 5.30)........	.175	.589	.767	1.228	.441	.306	.320	.626	.767	.583	.974	2.287	.405
Other Nuts and Seeds and Their Products (Protein, N x 5.30):													
Acorns (10.4% protein)........	.126	.434	.561	.808	.636	.139	.184	.323	.473	—	.718	.722	.251
Amaranth (14.6% protein)........	.149	.832	.882	1.209	1.074	.372	.521	.893	1.141	—	.849	1.747	.441
Balsampear seed meal (41.9% protein)....					1.265	.056	.142		2.609	.617		5.914	.917
Breadnuttree, Ramon (9.6% protein)......	.261	.373	.543	1.041	.418				.453		.927	.884	.147
Chinese tallow tree-nut flour (57.6% protein)...	.837	2.174	3.510	4.347	1.587	.924	.696	1.620	2.847	2.011	4.510	10.031	1.587
Chocolatetree, Nicaragua (38.5% protein)....	.588	1.496	2.092	3.952	2.223	.276	—	—	2.630	—	2.404	4.220	.683
Cottonseed flour (42.3% protein)....	.591	1.764	1.884	2.945	2.139	.686	.814	1.500	2.610	1.365	2.458	5.603	1.325
Earpodtree, Guanacaste (34.1% protein)....	.444	1.165	2.213	4.581	1.930	.360	—	—	1.325	—	1.570	2.857	1.004
Leadtree (24.1% protein)........	.191	.828	1.651	1.787	1.164	.055	—	—	.855	—	.864	2.410	.564
Pumpkin seed (30.9% protein)........	.560	.933	1.737	2.437	1.411	.577	—	—	1.749	—	1.679	4.810	.711
Safflower seed meal (42.1% protein)........	.675	1.462	1.914	2.740	1.525	.731	—	—	2.605	—	2.446	4.623	.985
Sesame:													
Seed (19.3% protein)........	.331	.707	.951	1.679	.583	.637	.495	1.132	1.457	.951	.885	1.992	.441
Meal (33.4% protein)........	.573	1.223	1.645	2.905	1.008	1.103	.857	1.960	2.521	1.645	1.531	3.447	.763
Sunflower:													
Kernel (23.0% protein)........	.343	.911	1.276	1.736	.868	.443	.464	.907	1.220	.647	1.354	2.370	.586
Meal (39.5% protein)........	.589	1.565	2.191	2.981	1.491	.760	.797	1.557	2.094	1.110	2.325	4.069	1.006
Grains and Their Products:													
Barley (12.8% protein, N x 5.83)........	.160	.433	.545	.889	.433	.184	.257	.441	.661	.466	.643	.659	.239
Bread, white (4% nonfat dry milk, flour basis) (8.5% protein, N x 5.70)........	.091	.282	.429	.668	.225	.142	.200	.342	.465	.243	.435	.340	.192

Table continued on the following page

APPENDIX TABLE 6   AMINO ACID CONTENT OF FOODS, 100 GRAMS, EDIBLE PORTION (Continued)

ITEM, PROTEIN CONTENT, AND NITROGEN CONVERSION FACTOR	TRYPTOPHAN	THREONINE	ISO-LEUCINE	LEUCINE	LYSINE	SULFUR CONTAINING			PHENYL-ALANINE	TYRO-SINE	VALINE	ARGININE	HISTIDINE
						Meth-ionine	Cystine	Total					
	Gm.	Gm.	Gm.	Gm.	Gm.	Gm.	Gm.	Gm.	Gm.	Gm.	Gm.	Gm.	Gm.
Grains and Their Products—Continued													
Buckwheat flour:													
Dark (11.7% protein, N x 6.25)	0.165	0.461	0.440	0.683	0.687	0.206	0.228	0.434	0.442	0.240	0.607	0.930	0.256
Light (6.4% protein, N x 6.25)	.090	.252	.241	.374	.376	.113	.125	.238	.242	.131	.332	.509	.140
Cañihua (14.7% protein, N x 6.25)	.118	.706	1.000	.851	.882	.263	.162	.425	.529	.294	.677	1.162	.367
Cereal combinations:													
Corn and soy grits (18.0% protein, N x 6.25)	.161	.792	.841	1.656	.772	.271	.311	.582	.832	.562	1.054	.982	.472
Infant food, precooked, mixed cereals with non-fat dry milk and yeast (19.4% protein, N x 6.25)	.118				.273	.310	.137	.447	.543	.447		.447	.233
Oat-corn-rye mixture, puffed (14.5% protein, N x 5.83)	.172	.545	.841	1.368	.343	.388	.234	.622	.933	.622	.900	.776	.326
Corn, field (10.0% protein, N x 6.25)	.061	.398	.462	1.296	.288	.186	.130	.316	.454	.611	.510	.352	.206
Corn flour (7.8% protein, N x 6.25)	.047	.311	.361	1.011	.225	.145	.101	.246	.354	.477	.398	.275	.161
Corn grits (8.7% protein, N x 6.25)	.053	.347	.402	1.128	.251	.161	.113	.274	.395	.532	.444	.306	.180
Cornmeal:													
Whole ground (9.2% protein, N x 6.25)	.056	.367	.425	1.192	.265	.171	.119	.290	.418	.562	.470	.324	.190
Degermed (7.9% protein, N x 6.25)	.048	.315	.365	1.024	.228	.147	.102	.249	.359	.483	.403	.278	.163
Corn products:													
Flakes (8.1% protein, N x 6.25)	.052	.275	.306	1.047	.154	.135	.152	.157	.354	.283	.386	.231	.226
Germ (14.5% protein, N x 6.25)	.144	.622	.578	1.030	.791	.232	.130	.362	.483	.343	.789	1.134	.464
Gluten (10.0% protein, N x 6.25)	.059	.344	.443	1.563	.179	.282	.141	.423	.558	.582	.512	.322	.200
Hominy (8.7% protein, N x 6.25)	.084	.316	.349	.810	.358	.099			.333	.331	.398	.444	.203
Masa (2.8% protein, N x 6.25)	.010				.103	.108	.030	.138					
Pozol (5.9% protein, N x 6.25)	.042	.336	.304	.591	.234	.087			.254		.267	.197	.122
Tortilla (5.8% protein, N x 6.25)	.031	.235	.345	.939	.145	.111			.252		.304	.223	.128
Zein (16.1% protein, N x 6.25)	.010	.495	.822	3.184		.281	.162	.443	1.664	.981	.654	.286	.216
Job's tears (13.8% protein, N x 5.83)	.066	.620	1.065	3.506	.362	.459	.265	.724	.703			.518	.317
Millets:													
Foxtail millet (9.7% protein, N x 5.83)	.103	.323	7.90	1.737	.218	.291			.697		.717	.374	.218
Little millet (7.2% protein, N x 5.83)	.047	.262	.517	.841	.138	.178		.422	.370		.471	.363	.147
Pearlmillet (11.4% protein, N x 5.83)	.248	.456	.635	1.746	.383	.270	.152	.422	.506		.682	.524	.240
Ragimillet (6.2% protein, N x 5.83)	.085	.270	.398	.620	.202	.270	.187	.457	.263		.473	.100	.079
Oatmeal and rolled oats (14.2% protein, N x 5.83)	.183	.470	.733	1.065	.521	.209	.309	.518	.758	.524	.845	.935	.261
Quinoa (11.0% protein, N x 6.25)	.120	.523	.722	.781	.729	.278	.107	.385	.394	.253	.447	.820	.297
Rice:													
Brown (7.5% protein, N x 5.95)	.081	.294	.352	.646	.296	.135	.102	.237	.377	.343	.524	.432	.126
White and converted (7.6% protein, N x 5.95)	.082	.298	.356	.655	.300	.137	.103	.240	.382	.347	.531	.438	.128

ITEM, PROTEIN CONTENT, AND NITROGEN CONVERSION FACTOR	TRYPTOPHAN	THREONINE	ISOLEUCINE	LEUCINE	LYSINE	SULFUR CONTAINING			PHENYLALANINE	TYROSINE	VALINE	ARGININE	HISTIDINE
						Methionine	Cystine	Total					
	Gm.	Gm.	Gm.	Gm.	Gm.	Gm.	Gm.	Gm.	Gm.	Gm.	Gm.	Gm.	Gm.
Fruits (Protein, N x 6.25):													
Abiu (1.7% protein)	0.028				0.085	0.013							
Avocados (1.3% protein)	.014				.074	.012							
Bananas, ripe:													
Common (1.2% protein)	.018				.055	.011				.031			
Dwarf (1.2% protein)	.012				.049	.04							
Dates (2.2% protein)	.061	.061	.074	.077	.065	.027			.063		.094	.049	
Grapefruit (0.5% protein)	.001				.006	.000							
Guavas, common (1.0% protein)	.010				.030	.010							.049
Limes (0.8% protein)	.003				.015	.002							
Mamey (0.5% protein)	.006				.040	.007							
Mangos (0.7% protein)	.014				.093	.008							
Muskmelons (0.6% protein)	.001				.015	.002							
Oranges, sweet (0.9% protein)	.003				.024	.003							
Orange juice (0.8% protein)	.003				.021	.002							
Oranges, mandarin including tangerines (0.8% protein)	.005				.028	.004							
Papayas (0.6% protein)	.012				.038	.002							
Pineapple (0.4% protein)	.005				.009	.001	.016	.021					
Plantain or baking banana (1.1% protein)	.010	.027	.056	.059	.050	.005							
Soursop (1.0% protein)	.011				.060	.007					.065	.045	
Sugarapple (1.8% protein)	.009				.071	.008			.049				
Vegetables:													
Immature Seeds (Protein, N x 6.25):													
Corn, sweet, white or yellow:													
Raw (3.7% protein)	.023	.151	.137	.407	.137	.072	.062	.134	.207	.124	.231	.174	.095
Canned, solids and liquid (2.0% protein)	.012	.082	.074	.220	.074	.039	.033	.072	.112	.067	.125	.094	.052
Cowpeas (9.4% protein)	.099	.353	.465	.653	.617	.131			.523		.513	.615	.310
Lima beans:													
Raw (7.5% protein)	.097	.338	.460	.605	.474	.080	.083	.163	.389	.259	.485	.454	.247
Canned, solids and liquid (3.8% protein)	.049	.171	.233	.306	.240	.041	.042	.083	.197	.131	.246	.230	.125
Peas:													
Raw (6.7% protein)	.056	.245	.308	.418	.316	.054	.073	.127	.257	.163	.274	.595	.109
Canned, solids and liquid (3.4% protein)	.028	.125	.156	.212	.160	.027	.037	.064	.131	.083	.139	.302	.055

Table continued on the following page

APPENDIX TABLE 6   AMINO ACID CONTENT OF FOODS, 100 GRAMS, EDIBLE PORTION *(Continued)*

	Gm.	Gm.	Gm.	Gm.	Gm.	Gm.	Gm.	Gm.	Gm.	Gm.	Gm.	Gm.	Gm.
Grains and Their Products—Continued													
Rice products:													
Flakes or puffed (5.9% protein, N x 5.95)	0.046				0.056	.420	0.044	.589	0.286	0.124		0.137	0.137
Germ (14.2% protein, N x 5.95)	.270	2.177	.630	.838	1.707	.191	.169	.432	.750	.929	.938	1.559	.430
Rye (12.1% protein, N x 5.83)	.137	.448	.515	.813	.494	.148	.241	.335	.571	.390	.631	.591	.276
Rye flour:													
Light (9.4% protein, N x 5.83)	.106	.348	.400	.632	.384	.180	.187	.407	.443	.303	.490	.459	.214
Medium (11.4% protein, N x 5.83)	.129	.422	.485	.766	.465	.190	.227	.373	.538	.368	.594	.557	.260
Sorghum (11.0% protein, N x 6.25)	.123	.394	.598	1.767	.299	.496	.183	.521	.547	.303	.628	.417	.211
Teosinte (22.0% protein, N x 6.25)	.049				.348								
Wheat, whole grain:													
Hard red spring (14.0% protein, N x 5.83)	.173	.403	.607	.939	.384	.214	.307	.458	.691	.523	.648	.670	.286
Hard red winter (12.3% protein, N x 5.83)	.152	.354	.534	.825	.338	.188	.270	.380	.608	.460	.570	.589	.251
Soft red winter (10.2% protein, N x 5.83)	.126	.294	.443	.684	.280	.156	.224	.349	.504	.382	.472	.488	.208
White (9.4% protein, N x 5.83)	.116	.271	.408	.630	.258	.143	.206	.473	.464	.351	.435	.450	.192
Durum (12.7% protein, N x 5.83)	.157	.366	.551	.852	.348	.194	.279	.495	.627	.475	.588	.608	.259
Wheat flour:													
Whole grain (13.3% protein, N x 5.83)	.164	.383	.577	.892	.365	.203	.292	.518	.657	.497	.616	.636	.271
Intermediate extraction (12.0% protein, N x 5.70)					.356	.198	.320	.348	.732	.335		.549	.286
White (10.5% protein, N x 5.70)	.129	.392	.619	.924	.239	.138	.210	.415	.577	.359	.583	.466	.210
Wheat products:													
Bran (12.0% protein, N x 6.31)	.196	.302	.483	.809	.491	.145	.270	.619	.434	.259	.453	.742	.280
Burghul (12.4% protein, N x 5.83)	.070	.342	.485	.717	.430	.300	.319		.579	.447	.552		.268
Farina (10.9% protein, N x 5.70)	.124	.356	.496	.891	.199	.143	.184	.327	.478	.311	.572	.424	.231
Flakes (10.8% protein, N x 5.70)	.121				.360	.127	.191	.318				.559	
Germ (25.2% protein, N x 5.80)	.265	1.343	1.177	1.708	1.534	.404	.287	.691	.908	.882	1.364	1.825	.687
Gluten, commercial (80.0% protein, N x 5.70)	.856	2.119	3.677	5.993	1.530	1.389	1.726	3.115	4.351	2.596	3.789	3.481	1.825
Gluten flour (41.4% protein, N x 5.70)	.443	1.097	1.903	3.101	.792	.719	.893	1.612	2.252	1.344	1.961	1.801	.944
Macaroni or spaghetti (12.8% protein, N x 5.70)	.150	.499	.642	.849	.413	.193	.243	.436	.669	.422	.728	.582	.303
Noodles, contain egg solids (12.6% protein, N x 5.70)	.133	.533	.621	.834	.411	.212	.245	.457	.610	.312	.745	.621	.301
Shredded wheat (10.1% protein, N x 5.83)	.085	.405	.449	.684	.331	.139	.204	.343	.481	.236	.577	.523	.236
Whole wheat with added germ (12.8% protein, N x 5.83)	.136				.466		.246		.755	.481		.742	.371

Vegetables—Continued

Leafy Vegetables, Raw (Protein, N x 6.25):

	Gm.	Gm.	Gm.	Gm.	Gm.	Gm.	Gm.	Gm.	Gm.	Gm.	Gm.	Gm.	Gm.
Amaranth (3.5% protein)	0.038	0.056	0.164	0.206	0.141	0.025	0.024	0.049	0.096	0.105	0.136	0.134	0.069
Beet greens (2.0% protein)	.024	.076	.084	.129	.108	.034			.116		.101	.083	.026
Brussels sprouts (4.4% protein)	.044	.153	.186	.194	.197	.046	.028	.041	.148	.030	.193	.279	.106
Cabbage (1.4% protein)	.011	.039	.040	.057	.066	.013			.030		.043	.105	.025
Chard (1.4% protein)	.014	.058	.060	.076	.055	.004	.006	.022	.046		.055	.035	.018
Chicory (1.6% protein)	.024	.114	.121	.218	.052	.016	.059	.105	.124	.040	.195	.258	.024
Collards (3.9% protein)	.055	.139	.133	.252	.202	.046	.036	.071	.158	.151	.184	.202	.087
Kale (3.9% protein)	.042				.121	.035							.062
Lettuce (1.2% protein)	.012	.060	.075	.062	.070	.004	.035	.059	.074	.121	.108	.167	.041
Mustard greens (2.3% protein)	.037				.111	.024							
Parsley, curly garden (2.5% protein)	.050				.160	.012							
Spinach (2.3% protein)	.037	.102	.107	.176	.142	.039	.046	.085	.099	.073	.126	.116	.049
Turnip greens (2.9% protein)	.045	.125	.107	.207	.129	.052	.045	.097	.146	.105	.149	.167	.051
Watercress (1.7% protein)	.028	.084	.076	.131	.091	.010			.062	.036	.084	.053	.034

Starchy Roots and Tubers (Protein, N x 6.25):

	Gm.	Gm.	Gm.	Gm.	Gm.	Gm.	Gm.	Gm.	Gm.	Gm.	Gm.	Gm.	Gm.
Apio arracacia (1.2% protein)	.008				.042	.003							
Cassava:													
Flour (1.6% protein)	.021	.044	.045	.066	.066	.010	.018	.028	.045	.030	.049	.159	.025
Root (1.1% protein)	.014	.030	.031	.045	.045	.007	.012	.019	.031	.021	.033	.110	.017
Potatoes:													
Raw (2.0% protein)	.021	.079	.088	.100	.107	.025	.019	.044	.088	.036	.107	.099	.029
Canned, solids and liquid (1.7% protein)	.018	.067	.075	.085	.091	.021	.016	.037	.075	.030	.091	.084	.024
Flour (7.1% protein)	.076	.279	.311	.353	.378	.089	.068	.157	.314	.127	.379	.350	.102
Sweetpotatoes (Ipomaea batatas):													
Raw (1.8% protein)	.031	.085	.087	.103	.085	.033	.029	.062	.100	.081	.135	.094	.036
Dehydrated (5.0% protein)	.087	.235	.241	.286	.236	.093	.080	.173	.278	.225	.374	.261	.099
Taro (1.9% protein)	.035	.089	.099	.169	.110	.021			.099		.114	.118	.032
Yam (Dioscorea spp.) (2.1% protein)	.035				.110	.034							
Yautia malanga (1.7% protein)	.023				.067	.016							

Other Vegetables (Protein, N x 6.25):

	Gm.	Gm.	Gm.	Gm.	Gm.	Gm.	Gm.	Gm.	Gm.	Gm.	Gm.	Gm.	Gm.
Asparagus:													
Raw (2.2% protein)	.027	.066	.080	.096	.103	.032			.069		.106	.123	.036
Canned, solids and liquid (1.9% protein)	.023	.057	.069	.083	.089	.027			.060		.092	.106	.031

Table continued on the following page

APPENDIX TABLE 6 AMINO ACID CONTENT OF FOODS, 100 GRAMS, EDIBLE PORTION (Continued)

ITEM, PROTEIN CONTENT, AND NITROGEN CONVERSION FACTOR	TRYPTO-PHAN	THREO-NINE	ISO-LEUCINE	LEUCINE	LYSINE	SULFUR CONTAINING			PHENYL-ALANINE	TYRO-SINE	VALINE	ARGININE	HISTIDINE
						Meth-ionine	Cystine	Total					
	Gm.	Gm.	Gm.	Gm.	Gm.	Gm.	Gm.	Gm.	Gm.	Gm.	Gm.	Gm.	Gm.
Vegetables—Continued													
Other Vegetables (Protein, N x 6.25)—Continued													
Beans, snap:													
Raw (2.4% protein)	0.033	0.091	0.109	0.139	0.126	0.035	0.024	0.059	0.057	0.050	0.115	0.101	0.045
Canned, solids and liquid (1.0% protein)	.014	.038	.045	.058	.052	.014	.010	.024	.024	.021	.048	.042	.019
Beets:													
Raw (1 6% protein)	.014	.034	.051	.055	.086	.006			.027		.049	.028	.022
Canned, solids and liquid (0.9% protein)	.008	.019	.029	.031	.048	.003			.015		.028	.016	.012
Broccoli (3.3% protein)	.037	.122	.126	.163	.147	.050			.119		.170	.192	.063
Carrots:													
Raw (1.2% protein)	.010	.043	.046	.065	.052	.010	.029	.039	.042	.020	.056	.041	.017
Canned, solids and liquid (0.5% protein)	.004	.018	.019	.027	.022	.004	.012	.016	.018	.008	.023	.017	.007
Cauliflower (2.4% protein)	.033	.102	.104	.162	.134	.047			.075	.034	.144	.110	.048
Celery (1.3% protein)	.012				.021	.015	.006	.021		.016			
Chayote (0.6% protein)	.008				.038	.001							
Cowpeas, yardlong, immature pod (3.4% protein)	.034				.203	.021							
Cucumbers (0.7% protein)	.005	.019	.022	.030	.031	.007			.016		.024	.053	.001
Cushaw (1.5% protein)	.014				.044	.008							
Eggplant (1.1% protein)	.010	.038	.056	.068	.030	.006			.048		.065	.037	.019
Mallow (3.7% protein)	.144	.155		.259	.155	.030			.166		.181	.189	.063
Mushrooms:													
(Agaricus campestris)[1]	.006	.156	.532	.281	.088	.167			.018		.378	.235	.027
(Lactarius spp.)[2]	.006		.201	.139		.021					.116	.021	
Okra (1.8% protein)	.018	.066	.069	.101	.076	.022	.017	.039	.065	.079	.091	.093	.030
Onions, mature (1.4% protein)	.021	.022	.021	.037	.064	.013			.039	.046	.031	.180	.014
Peppers (1.2% protein)	.009	.050	.046	.046	.051	.016			.055		.033	.024	.014
Pricklypears (1.1% protein)	.009	.053	.044	.057	.044	.008			.059		.041	.032	.016
Pumpkin (1.2% protein)	.016	.028	.044	.063	.058	.011			.032	.016	.045	.043	.019
Radishes (1.2% protein)	.005	.059			.034	.002					.030		
Seepweed (2.6% protein)	.027	.089	.113	.152	.089	.013			.116		.091	.062	.036
Soybean sprouts (6.2% protein)		.159	.225	.265	.211	.045			.186		.225	.225	.133
Squash, summer (0.6% protein)	.005	.014	.019	.027	.023	.008			.016		.022	.027	.009

[1] Total nitrogen is 0.58%. This is equivalent to 2.4% protein on the basis that ⅔ of the nitrogen is protein nitrogen. If total nitrogen is used for the calculation, the protein content is 3.6%.

[2] Total nitrogen is 0.69%. This is equivalent to 2.9% protein on the basis that ⅔ of the nitrogen is protein nitrogen. If total nitrogen is used for the calculation, the protein content is 4.3%.

	Gm.	Gm.	Gm.	Gm.	Gm.	Gm.	Gm.	Gm.	Gm.	Gm.	Gm.	Gm.	Gm.
Vegetables—Continued													
Other Vegetable (Protein, N x 6.25)—Continued													
Tomatoes and cherry tomatoes (1.0% protein)..	0.009	0.033	0.029	0.041	0.042	0.007	—	—	0.028	0.014	0.028	0.029	0.015
Turnips (1.1% protein).............	—	—	.020	—	.057	.012	—	—	.020	.029	—	—	—
Waxgourd, Chinese (0.4% protein).............	.002	—	—	—	.009	.003	—	—	—	—	—	—	—
Miscellaneous Food Items:													
Vegetable patty or steak (principally wheat protein) (15% protein, N x 5.70).............	.142	.411	.884	1.079	.321	.253	—	—	.811	—	.705	.597	.321
Yeast:													
Baker's, compressed (3, N x 6.25).............	.122	.655	.655	1.151	.914	.248	0.120	0.368	.607	.580	.840	.536	.353
Brewer's, dried (4, N x 6.25).............	.710	2.353	2.398	3.226	3.300	.836	.548	1.384	1.902	1.902	2.723	2.250	1.251
Primary, dried:													
(Saccharomyces cerevisiae) (4, N x 6.25).............	.636	2.353	2.708	3.300	3.337	.851	.444	1.295	1.813	2.472	2.553	1.931	1.103
(Torulopsis utilis) (4, N x 6.25).............	.636	2.331	3.323	3.707	3.648	.710	.422	1.132	2.361	2.464	2.901	3.337	1.251

[3] Total nitrogen is 2.1%. This is equivalent to 10.6% protein on the basis that 4/5 of the nitrogen is protein nitrogen. If total nitrogen is used for the calculation, the protein content is 13.1%.

[4] Total nitrogen is 7.4%. This is equivalent to 36.9% protein on the basis that 4/5 of the nitrogen is protein nitrogen. If total nitrogen is used for the calculation, the protein content is 46.1%.

APPENDIX TABLE 7   FOODS HIGH IN CALCIUM*
(More Than 25 Milligrams Calcium per Serving)

Food	Approximate amount	Weight *gm*	Calcium *mg*
Meat Group			
Egg	1	50	27
Fish			
Salmon (with bones)	1 oz	30	51
Sardines	1 oz	30	115
Clams	1 oz	30	29
Oysters	1 oz	30	31
Shrimp	1 oz	30	35
Cheese			
Cheddar	1 oz	30	218
Cheese foods	1 oz	30	160
Cheese spread	1 oz	30	158
Cottage cheese	1/4 cup	50	53
Fat			
Cream			
Half and half	2 T	30	32
Sour	2 T	30	31
Bread Group			
Bread			
Biscuit	2″ diameter	35	42
Muffin	2″ diameter	35	36
Cornbread	1 1/2 cube	35	36
Pancake	4″ diameter	45	45
Waffle	1/2 square	35	39
Beans, dry (canned or cooked)	1/2 cup	90	45
Lima beans	1/2 cup	100	42
Parsnips	2/3 cup	100	45
Milk			
Whole	1 cup	240	288
Evaporated whole milk	1/2 cup	120	302
Powdered whole milk	1/2 cup	30	252
Buttermilk	1 cup	240	296
Skim milk	1 cup	240	298
Powdered skim milk, dry	1/4 cup	30	367
Fruit			
Blackberries	3/4 cup	100	32
Orange	1 medium	100	41
Raspberries	3/4 cup	100	30
Rhubarb	1 cup	100	96
Tangerine	2 small	100	40

*From Mayo Clinic Diet Manual, 4th Ed. Philadelphia, W. B. Saunders Co., 1971.

APPENDIX TABLE 7   FOODS HIGH IN CALCIUM   *(Continued)*

Food	Approximate amount	Weight *gm*	Calcium *mg*
Vegetable A, cooked			
Beans, green or wax	1/2 cup	100	50
Beet greens	1/2 cup	100	99
Broccoli	1/2 cup	100	88
Cabbage	1/2 cup	100	49
Cabbage, Chinese	1/2 cup	100	43
Celery	1/2 cup	100	39
Chard	1/2 cup	100	73
Collards	1/2 cup	100	188
Cress	1/2 cup	100	81
Dandelion greens	1/2 cup	100	140
Mustard greens	1/2 cup	100	138
Sauerkraut	1/2 cup	100	36
Spinach	1/2 cup	100	93
Squash, summer	1/2 cup	100	25
Turnip greens	1/2 cup	100	184
Turnips	1/2 cup	100	35
Vegetable B, cooked			
Artichokes	1/2 cup	100	51
Brussels sprouts	1/2 cup	100	32
Carrots	1/2 cup	100	33
Kale	1/2 cup	100	187
Kohlrabi	1/2 cup	100	33
Leeks, raw	3–4	100	52
Okra	1/2 cup	100	92
Pumpkin	1/2 cup	100	25
Rutabagas	1/2 cup	100	59
Squash, winter	1/2 cup	100	28
Dessert			
Cake, white	1 piece	50	32
Custard, baked	1/3 cup	100	112
Ice cream	1/2 cup	75	110
Ice milk	1/2 cup	75	118
Pie, cream	1/6 of 9″ pie	160	120
Pudding	1/2 cup	100	117
Sherbet	1/3 cup	50	25

APPENDIX TABLE 8   FOODS HIGH IN IRON*

FOOD	AVERAGE SERVING Weight Gm.	AVERAGE SERVING Approximate Measure	IRON, MG. Per Serving	IRON, MG. Per 100 Gm.
Almonds	15	12–15	0.7	4.4
Apricots, dried	30	5 halves	1.5	4.9
Bacon, cooked	25	4–5 slices	0.8	3.3
Beans, dried	30 (dry)	½ cup (cooked)	2.1	6.9
Lima, dried	30 (dry)	½ cup (cooked)	2.3	7.5
Beef, rib roast, cooked	60	2 ounces	1.8	3.0
Corned, medium fat	60	2 ounces	2.6	4.3
Dried	30	1 ounce	1.5	5.1
Beet greens, cooked	75	½ cup	2.4	3.2
Bologna	30	1 slice	0.7	2.2
Bran flakes, 40 per cent	15	½ cup	0.8	5.1
Brazil nuts	15	2 medium	0.5	3.4
Breaded, whole wheat	25	1 slice	0.6	2.2
Cashews	15	6–8	0.8	5.0
Chard	75	½ cup	1.9	2.5
Chocolate, bitter	30	1 square	1.3	4.4
Sweetened, plain	30	1 square	0.8	2.8
Clams	60	2 ounces	4.2	7.0
Cocoa	7	1 tablespoon	0.8	11.6
Coconut, fresh	15	½ ounce	0.3	2.0
Dried	15	2 tablespoons	0.5	3.6
Cornmeal, degermed, enriched	15 (dry)	½ cup (cooked)	0.4	2.9
Cress, garden	10	5–8 sprigs	0.3	2.9
Currants, dried	30	2 tablespoons	0.8	2.7
Dandelion greens	75	½ cup	2.3	3.1
Dates	30	3–4	0.6	2.1
Egg, whole	50	1	1.4	2.7
Yolk	20	1	1.4	7.2
Figs, dried	30	2 small	0.9	3.0
Flour, all-purpose, enriched	15	2 tablespoons	0.4	2.9
Flour, whole wheat	15	2 tablespoons	0.5	3.3
Ham, smoked	60	2 ounces	1.7	2.9
Hazelnuts	15	10–12	0.6	4.1
Heart, beef	60	2 ounces	2.8	4.6
Kale	75	¾ cup	1.7	2.2
Kidney, beef	60	2 ounces	4.7	7.9
Lamb, leg	60	2 ounces	1.9	3.1
Lentils, dry	30 (dry)	½ cup (cooked)	2.2	7.4
Liver, beef	60	2 ounces	4.7	7.8
Liver sausage	30	1 slice	1.6	5.4
Molasses, light	20	1 tablespoon	0.9	4.3
Oatmeal	15 (dry)	½ cup (cooked)	0.7	4.5
Oysters, raw	60	2 ounces	3.4	5.6
Parsley	10	10 small sprigs	0.4	4.3
Peaches, dried	30	3 halves	1.9	6.9
Peas, dry	30 (dry)	½ cup (cooked)	1.4	4.7
Pecans	15	12 halves	0.4	2.4
Popcorn	15	1 cup, popped	0.4	2.7
Pork loin, cooked	60	2 ounces	1.8	3.0
Pork sausage	60	2 ounces	1.4	2.3
Prunes, dried	30	4 prunes	1.2	3.9
Raisins, dried	50	5 tablespoons	1.7	3.3
Rice, brown	15 (dry)	½ cup (cooked)	0.3	2.0
Rye, whole meal	15	1 tablespoon	0.6	3.7
Sardines	60	2 ounces	1.6	2.7
Shrimp, canned	60	2 ounces	1.9	3.1

*From Mayo Clinic Diet Manual. 3rd Ed. Philadelphia, W. B. Saunders Company, 1961, pp. 188–189.

APPENDIX TABLE 8   FOODS HIGH IN IRON *(Continued)*

FOOD	AVERAGE SERVING		IRON, MG.	
	Weight Gm.	*Approximate Measure*	*Per Serving*	*Per 100 Gm.*
Syrup, table blends	20	1 tablespoon	0.8	4.1
Soybeans, dried	25	2 tablespoons	2.0	8.0
Flour, medium fat	15	3 tablespoons	2.0	13.0
Spinach, cooked	75	½ cup	1.5	2.0
Sugar, brown	15	1 tablespoon	0.4	2.6
Tongue, beef	60	2 ounces	1.7	2.8
Turkey	60	2 ounces	2.3	3.8
Turnip greens	75	½ cup	1.8	2.4
Veal roast, cooked	60	2 ounces	2.2	3.6
Walnuts	15	8 to 15 halves	0.3	2.1
Wheat flakes	15	½ cup	0.5	3.0
Shredded, plain	30	1 biscuit	1.1	3.5
Whole meal	15	½ cup (cooked)	0.5	3.4
Yeast, compressed	30	1 ounce	1.5	4.9
Dried brewer's	15	2 tablespoons	2.7	18.2

APPENDIX TABLE 9   SODIUM AND POTASSIUM CONTENT OF FOODS**

Food	Approximate amount	Weight gm	Sodium mEq	Potassium mEq
Meat				
Meat (cooked)				
Beef	1 ounce	30	0.8	2.8
Ham	1 ounce	30	14.3	2.6
Lamb	1 ounce	30	0.9	2.2
Pork	1 ounce	30	0.9	3.0
Veal	1 ounce	30	1.0	3.8
Liver	1 ounce	30	2.4	3.2
Sausage, pork	2 links	40	16.5	2.8
Beef, dried	2 slices	20	37.0	1.0
Cold cuts	1 slice	45	25.0	2.7
Frankfurters	1	50	24.0	3.0
Fowl				
Chicken	1 ounce	30	1.0	3.0
Goose	1 ounce	30	1.6	4.6
Duck	1 ounce	30	1.0	2.2
Turkey	1 ounce	30	1.2	2.8
Egg	1	50	2.7	1.8
Fish	1 ounce	30	1.0	2.5
Salmon				
Fresh	1/4 cup	30	0.6	2.3
Canned	1/4 cup	30	4.6	2.6
Tuna				
Fresh	1/4 cup	30	0.5	2.2
Canned	1/4 cup	30	10.4	2.3
Sardines	3 medium	35	12.5	4.5
Shellfish				
Clams	5 small	50	2.6	2.3
Lobster	1 small tail	40	3.7	1.8
Oysters	5 small	70	2.1	1.5
Scallops	1 large	50	5.7	6.0
Shrimp	5 small	30	1.8	1.7
Cheese				
Cheese, American or Cheddar type	1 slice	30	9.1	0.6
Cheese foods	1 slice	30	15.0	0.8
Cheese spreads	2 tablespoons	30	15.0	0.8
Cottage cheese	1/4 cup	50	5.0	1.1
Peanut butter	2 tablespoons	30	7.8	5.0
Peanuts, unsalted	25	25	...	4.5
Fat				
Avocado	1/8	30	...	4.6
Bacon	1 slice	5	2.2	0.6
Butter or margarine	1 teaspoon	5	2.2	...
Cooking fat	1 teaspoon	5	...	...

**From: Mayo Clinic Diet Manual, 4th ed. Philadelphia, W. B. Saunders Co., 1971, pp. 144–149.

Food	Approximate amount	Weight *gm*	Sodium *mEq*	Potassium *mEq*
Fat (*Continued*)				
Cream				
Half and half	2 tablespoons	30	0.6	1.0
Sour	2 tablespoons	30	0.4	...
Whipped	1 tablespoon	15	0.3	1.0
Cream cheese	1 tablespoon	15	1.7	...
Mayonnaise	1 teaspoon	5	1.3	...
Nuts				
Almonds, slivered	5 (2 teaspoons)	6	...	0.8
Pecans	4 halves	5	...	0.8
Walnuts	5 halves	10	...	1.0
Oil, salad	1 teaspoon	5	...	...
Olives, green	3 medium	30	31.3	0.4
Bread				
Bread	1 slice	25	5.5	0.7
Biscuit	1 (2″ diameter)	35	9.6	0.7
Muffin	1 (2″ diameter)	35	7.3	1.2
Cornbread	1 (1 1/2″ cube)	35	11.3	1.7
Roll	1 (2″ diameter)	25	5.5	0.6
Bun	1	30	6.6	0.7
Pancake	1 (4″ diameter)	45	8.8	1.1
Waffle	1/2 square	35	8.5	1.0
Cereals				
Cooked	2/3 cup	140	8.7	2.0
Dry, flake	2/3 cup	20	8.7	0.6
Dry, puffed	1 1/2 cups	20	...	1.5
Shredded wheat	1 biscuit	20	...	2.2
Crackers				
Graham	3	20	5.8	2.0
Melba toast	4	20	5.5	0.7
Oyster	20	20	9.6	0.6
Ritz	6	20	9.5	0.5
Rye-Krisp	3	30	11.5	3.0
Saltines	6	20	9.6	0.6
Soda	3	20	9.6	0.6
Dessert				
Commercial gelatin	1/2 cup	100	2.2	...
Ice cream	1/2 cup	75	2.0	3.0
Sherbet	1/3 cup	50	...	...
Angel food cake	1 1/2″ × 1 1/2″	25	3.0	0.6
Sponge cake	1 1/2″ × 1 1/2″	25	1.8	0.6
Vanilla wafers	5	15	1.7	...
Flour products*				
Cornstarch	2 tablespoons	15	...	...
Macaroni	1/4 cup	50	...	0.8
Noodles	1/4 cup	50	...	0.6
Rice	1/4 cup	50	...	0.9
Spaghetti	1/4 cup	50	...	0.8
Tapioca	2 tablespoons	15	...	...
Vegetable*				
Beans, dried (cooked)	1/2 cup	90	...	10.0
Beans, lima	1/2 cup	90	...	9.5

Table continued on the following page

Food	Approximate amount	Weight gm	Sodium mEq	Potassium mEq
Vegetable (*Continued*)				
Corn				
Canned[†]	1/3 cup	80	8.0	2.0
Fresh	1/2 ear	100	...	2.0
Frozen	1/3 cup	80	...	3.7
Hominy (dry)	1/4 cup	36	4.1	...
Parsnips	2/3 cup	100	0.3	9.7
Peas				
Canned[†]	1/2 cup	100	10.0	1.2
Dried	1/2 cup	90	1.5	6.8
Fresh	1/2 cup	100	...	2.5
Frozen	1/2 cup	100	2.5	1.7
Popcorn	1 cup	15	...	...
Potato				
Potato chips	1 oz	30	13.0	3.7
White, baked	1/2 cup	100	...	13.0
White, boiled	1/2 cup	100	...	7.3
Sweet, baked	1/4 cup	50	0.4	4.0
Milk				
Whole milk	1 cup	240	5.2	8.8
Evaporated whole milk	1/2 cup	120	6.0	9.2
Powdered whole milk	1/4 cup	30	5.2	10.0
Buttermilk	1 cup	240	13.6	8.5
Skim milk	1 cup	240	5.2	8.8
Powdered skim milk	1/4 cup	30	6.9	13.5
Vegetable A[*]				
Asparagus				
Cooked	1/2 cup	100	...	4.7
Canned[†]	1/2 cup	100	10.0	3.6
Frozen	1/2 cup	100	...	5.5
Bean sprouts	1/2 cup	100	...	4.0
Beans, green or wax				
Fresh or frozen	1/2 cup	100	...	4.0
Canned[†]	1/2 cup	100	10.0	2.5
Beet greens	1/2 cup	100	3.0	8.5
Broccoli	1/2 cup	100	...	7.0
Cabbage, cooked	1/2 cup	100	0.6	4.2
Raw	1 cup	100	0.9	6.0
Cauliflower, cooked	1 cup	100	0.4	5.2
Celery, raw	1 cup	100	5.4	9.0
Chard, Swiss	3/5 cup	100	3.7	8.0
Collards	1/2 cup	100	0.8	6.0
Cress, garden (cooked)	1/2 cup	100	0.5	7.2
Cucumber	1 medium	100	0.3	4.0
Eggplant	1/2 cup	100	...	3.8
Lettuce	Varies	100	0.4	4.5
Mushrooms, raw	4 large	100	0.7	10.6
Mustard greens	1/2 cup	100	0.8	5.5
Pepper, green or red				
Cooked	1/2 cup	100	...	5.5
Raw	1	100	0.5	4.0

Food	Approximate amount	Weight *gm*	Sodium *mEq*	Potassium *mEq*
Vegetable A (*Continued*)				
Radishes	10	100	0.8	8.0
Sauerkraut	2/3 cup	100	32.0	3.5
Spinach	1/2 cup	100	2.2	8.5
Squash	1/2 cup	100	...	3.5
Tomatoes	1/2 cup	100	...	6.5
Tomato juice†	1/2 cup	100	9.0	5.8
Turnip greens	1/2 cup	100	0.7	3.8
Turnips	1/2 cup	100	1.5	4.8
Vegetable B*				
Artichokes	1 large bud	100	1.3	7.7
Beets	1/2 cup	100	1.8	5.0
Brussels sprouts	2/3 cup	100	...	7.6
Carrots, cooked	1/2 cup	100	1.4	5.7
Raw	1 large	100	2.0	8.8
Dandelion greens	1/2 cup	100	2.0	6.0
Kale, cooked	3/4 cup	100	2.0	5.6
Frozen	1/2 cup	100	1.0	5.0
Kohlrabi	2/3 cup	100	...	6.6
Leeks, raw	3–4	100	...	9.0
Okra	1/2 cup	100	...	4.4
Onions, cooked	1/2 cup	100	...	2.8
Pumpkin	1/2 cup	100	...	6.3
Rutabagas	1/2 cup	100	...	4.4
Squash, winter				
Baked	1/2 cup	100	...	12.0
Boiled	1/2 cup	100	...	6.5
Fruit				
Apple				
Fresh	1 small	80	...	2.3
Sauce	1/2 cup	120	...	2.5
Juice	1/2 cup	120	...	3.1
Apricots				
Canned	1/2 cup	120	...	6.0
Dried	4 halves	20	...	5.0
Fresh	3 small	120	...	8.0
Nectar	1/3 cup	80	...	3.0
Banana	1/2 small	60	...	4.8
Berries, fresh				
Blackberries	3/4 cup	100	...	3.0
Blueberries	1/2 cup	80	...	1.5
Boysenberries	1 cup	120	...	3.2
Gooseberries	3/4 cup	120	...	4.0
Loganberries	3/4 cup	100	...	4.4
Raspberries	3/4 cup	100	...	4.5
Strawberries	1 cup	150	...	6.3
Cherries				
Canned	1/2 cup	120	...	4.0
Fresh	15 small	80	...	2.7
Dates				
Pitted	2	15	...	2.5

Table continued on the following page

Food	Approximate amount	Weight gm	Sodium mEq	Potassium mEq
Fruit (*Continued*)				
Figs				
Canned	1/2 cup	120	...	4.6
Dried	1 small	15	...	2.5
Fresh	1 large	60	...	3.0
Fruit cocktail	1/2 cup	120	...	5.0
Grapes				
Canned	1/3 cup	80	...	2.2
Fresh	15	80	...	3.2
Juice				
Bottled	1/4 cup	60	...	2.8
Frozen	1/3 cup	80	...	2.4
Grapefruit				
Fresh	1/2 medium	120	...	3.6
Juice	1/2 cup	120	...	4.1
Sections	3/4 cup	150	...	5.1
Mandarin orange	3/4 cup	200	...	6.5
Mango	1/2 small	70	...	3.4
Melon				
Cantaloupe	1/2 small	200	...	13.0
Honeydew	1/4 medium	200	...	13.0
Watermelon	1/2 slice	200	...	5.0
Nectarine	1 medium	80	...	6.0
Orange				
Fresh	1 medium	100	...	5.1
Juice	1/2 cup	120		5.7
Sections	1/2 cup	100	...	5.1
Papaya	1/2 cup	120	...	7.0
Peach				
Canned	1/2 cup	120	...	4.0
Dried	2 halves	20	...	5.0
Fresh	1 medium	120	...	6.2
Nectar	1/2 cup	120	...	2.4
Pear				
Canned	1/2 cup	120	...	2.5
Dried	2 halves	20	...	3.0
Fresh	1 small	80	...	2.6
Nectar	1/3 cup	80	...	0.9
Pineapple				
Canned	1/2 cup	120	...	3.0
Fresh	1/2 cup	80	...	3.0
Juice	1/3 cup	80	...	3.0
Plums				
Canned	1/2 cup	120	...	4.5
Fresh	2 medium	80	...	4.1
Prunes	2 medium	15	...	2.6
Juice	1/4 cup	60	...	3.6
Raisins	1 tablespoon	15	...	2.9
Rhubarb ·	1/2 cup	100	...	6.5
Tangerines				
Fresh	2 small	100	...	3.2
Juice	1/2 cup	120	...	5.5
Sections	1/2 cup	100	...	3.2

*Value for products without added salt.
†Estimated average based on addition of salt, approximately 0.6% of the finished product.

TO CONVERT MILLIGRAMS TO MILLIEQUIVALENTS

1. Divide milligrams by atomic weight

Example: 1,000 mg sodium $= \dfrac{1,000}{23} = 43.5$ mEq sodium

Mineral	Atomic weight
Sodium	23
Potassium	39

TO CONVERT SPECIFIC WEIGHT OF SODIUM TO SODIUM CHLORIDE

1. Multiply by 2.54

Example: 1,000 mg sodium $= 1,000 \times 2.54 = 2,540$ mg sodium chloride (2.5 gm)

TO CONVERT SPECIFIC WEIGHT OF SODIUM CHLORIDE TO SODIUM

1. Multiply by 0.393

Example: 2.5 gm sodium chloride $= 2.5 \times 0.393 = 1,000$ mg sodium

| | **Sodium Values** | |
Milligrams	Milliequivalents	Grams of Sodium Chloride
500	21.8	1.3
1,000	43.5	2.5
1,500	75.3	3.8
2,000	87.0	5.0

APPENDIX TABLE 10   CALCULATION OF THE CALORIC DISTRIBUTION OF A DIET

To calculate the number of grams of carbohydrate, protein and fat needed to make up a diet that has a particular distribution of calories:

total kcal. in the diet × % of kcal. desired from a particular nutrient = number of kcal. to come from that nutrient

$$\frac{\text{number of kcal. from a nutrient}}{\text{number of kcal. per gm. of that nutrient}} = \text{grams of nutrient required}$$

For example, to calculate the required number of grams of protein, carbohydrate and fat for this diet:
total kcal. = 2400
20% of kcal. = protein
50% of kcal. = carbohydrate
30% of kcal. = fat
2400 kcal. × 20% = 480 kcal. from protein

$$\frac{480 \text{ kcal. from protein}}{4 \text{ kcal./gm. of protein}} = 120 \text{ gm. of protein}$$

2400 kcal. × 50% = 1200 kcal. from carbohydrate

$$\frac{1200 \text{ kcal. from carbohydrate}}{4 \text{ kcal./gm. of carbohydrate}} = 300 \text{ gm. carbohydrate}$$

2400 kcal. × 30% = 720 kcal. from fat

$$\frac{720 \text{ kcal. from fat}}{9 \text{ kcal./gm. of fat}} = 80 \text{ gm. of fat}$$

The final diet contains 120 gm. protein, 300 gm. carbohydrate and 80 gm. fat.

To calculate the caloric distribution of a diet of known composition:
gm. protein in diet × 4 kcal./gm. protein = number of kcal. from protein
gm. carbohydrate in diet × 4 kcal./gm. carbohydrate = number of kcal. from carbohydrate
gm. fat in diet × 9 kcal./gm. fat = number of kcal. from fat
kcal. from protein + kcal. from carbohydrate + kcal. from fat = total kcal. in the diet

$$\frac{\text{kcal. from nutrient}}{\text{total kcal. in the diet}} \times 100 = \% \text{ of total kcal. from nutrient}$$

For example, to calculate the caloric distribution of a diet that contains 100 gm. fat, 100 gm. protein and 300 gm. carbohydrate:
100 gm. protein × 4 kcal./gm. protein = 400 kcal. from protein
300 gm. carbohydrate × 4 kcal./gm. carbohydrate = 1200 kcal. from carbohydrate
100 gm. fat × 9 kcal./gm. fat = 900 kcal. from fat
400 kcal. + 1200 kcal. + 900 kcal. = 2500 kcal. = total kcal. in diet

$$\frac{400 \text{ kcal. from protein}}{2500 \text{ total kcal. in diet}} \times 100 = 16\% \text{ of kcal. from protein}$$

$$\frac{1200 \text{ kcal. from carbohydrate}}{2500 \text{ total kcal. in diet}} \times 100 = 48\% \text{ of kcal. from carbohydrate}$$

$$\frac{900 \text{ kcal. from fat}}{2500 \text{ total kcal. in diet}} \times 100 = 36\% \text{ of kcal. from fat}$$

APPENDIX TABLE 11   EXCESS OF ACIDITY OR ALKALINITY IN FOODS*

NEUTRAL FOODS

Butter	Lard	Sugar, white
Candy, plain	Oil, olive and salad	Tapioca
Coffee	Postum	Tea
Cornstarch		

FOODS WITH ACID ASH

FOOD	SIZE OF SERVING		NORMAL ACID, CC.	
	Weight Gm.	Approximate Measure	Per Serving	Per 100 Gm.
Bread				
White	25	1 slice	1.2	4.8
Whole Wheat	25	1 slice	1.5	6.1
Rye	25	1 slice	1.3	5.2
Cake, plain	75	1 piece	1.7	2.3
Cereal				
Cornflakes	15	½ cup	0.3	2.1
Farina	15 (dry)	½ cup (cooked)	1.4	9.6
Macaroni	15 (dry)	½ cup (cooked)	1.8	12.0
Oatmeal	15 (dry)	½ cup (cooked)	2.0	13.1
Puffed wheat	15	1 cup	1.6	10.8
Puffed rice	15	1 cup	1.4	9.0
Rice	15 (dry)	½ cup (cooked)	1.2	7.8
Shredded wheat	15	½ biscuit	1.8	12.2
Fat, mayonnaise	15	1 tablespoon	0.3	2.3
Fruit				
Cranberries	100	½ cup	+	+
Plums	100	½ cup	+	+
Prunes	100	½ cup	+	+
Meat				
Bacon	30	5 strips	5.9	19.6
Beef, roast	60	2 ounces	10.6	17.7
Cheese, Cheddar	30	1 ounce	1.7	5.5
Cheese, cottage	70	2 heaping tablespoons	3.2	4.5
Chicken	60	2 ounces	10.7	17.8
Eggs	50	1	7.7	15.4
Fish, halibut	60	2 ounces	12.4	20.7
Ham	60	2 ounces	9.1	15.2
Lamb	60	2 ounces	11.1	18.5
Pork	60	2 ounces	9.8	16.3
Veal	60	2 ounces	11.3	18.8
Nuts				
Brazil nuts	15	2 medium	1.7	11.0
Peanut butter	15	1 tablespoon	0.7	4.7
Peanuts	15	16–17 nuts	0.9	6.0
Walnuts, English	15	4–8 nuts	1.3	8.4
Vegetables				
Corn	100	½ cup	3.6	3.6
Lentils, dried	30	½ cup (cooked)	1.8	6.0

*From Mayo Clinic Diet Manual. 3rd ed. Philadelphia, W. B. Saunders Company, 1961, pp. 182–184.

Table continued on the following page

APPENDIX TABLE 11   EXCESS OF ACIDITY OR ALKALINITY IN FOODS
(Continued)

FOODS WITH ALKALINE ASH

| | | SIZE OF SERVING | NORMAL BASE, CC. | |
FOOD	Weight Gm.	Approximate Measure	Per Serving	Per 100 Gm.
Cream	75	⅓ cup	0.8	1.0
Fruit				
Apple	100	1 small	3.8	3.8
Apricots, raw	100	2–3	6.8	6.8
Apricots, dried	30	4–6 halves	10.9	36.3
Banana	100	1 small	7.9	7.9
Blackberries, raw	100	⅝ cup	5.0	5.0
Blueberries, raw	100	⅝ cup	2.7	2.7
Cantaloupe	150	½ melon	9.0	6.0
Cherries, fresh	100	15 large	7.0	7.0
Currants, fresh	100	¾ cup	7.5	7.5
Dates, dried	30	3–4	2.9	9.7
Figs, dried	30	2 small	10.8	36.0
Gooseberries	100	⅔ cup	4.1	4.1
Grapefruit	100	½ medium	6.0	6.0
Grapes	100	1 bunch	6.0	6.0
Lemon	30	1 ounce	1.2	4.0
Lime	30	1 ounce	1.2	4.0
Loganberries	100	⅔ cup	5.0	5.0
Mango	100	1 small	5.0	5.0
Nectarines	100	2 small	6.2	6.2
Olives, green. and ripe	30	3 medium	6.5	21.5
Orange	100	1 small	5.0	5.0
Peach, raw	100	1 medium	7.0	7.0
Pear, raw	100	1 medium	3.3	3.3
Persimmon	100	1 medium	7.5	7.5
Pineapple, raw	100	½ cup	6.5	6.5
Pineapple juice	200	1 cup, scant	6.0	3.0
Raisins	30	3 tablespoons	4.5	15.0
Raspberries, black and red	100	¾ cup	6.0	6.0
Strawberries	100	10 large	3.5	3.5
Tangerine	100	1 large	5.5	5.5
Watermelon	600	1 slice	22.8	3.8
Ice cream	70	⅓ cup	0.5	0.7
Jam	20	1 rounded teaspoon	0.7	3.3
Milk	240	½ pint	4.8	2.0
Nuts				
Almonds	15	12–15 nuts	1.8	12.0
Chestnuts	15	2 large	1.5	10.0
Coconut, fresh	15	1 piece	0.6	4.0
Sweets				
Molasses, medium	20	1 tablespoon	7.0	35.0
Vegetables				
Asparagus	75	6–8 tips	2.3	3.0
Beans, baked	100	½ cup	2.8	2.8
Beans, lima	75	⅓ cup	9.8	13.1
Beans, navy, pea	30	½ cup (cooked)	5.4	18.0
Beans, snap	75	⅓ cup	2.5	3.3
Beets	75	⅓ cup	7.9	10.5
Beet greens	75	⅓ cup	20.3	27.0
Broccoli	75	½ cup	3.0	4.0

APPENDIX TABLE 11 EXCESS OF ACIDITY OR ALKALINITY IN FOODS
(Continued)

FOODS WITH ALKALINE ASH (Continued)

FOOD	SIZE OF SERVING		NORMAL BASE, CC.	
	Weight Gm.	Approximate Measure	Per Serving	Per 100 Gm.
Vegetables (continued)				
Cabbage, cooked	75	⅓ cup	3.3	4.4
Carrots	75	½ cup	5.2	6.9
Cauliflower	75	½ cup	1.5	2.0
Celery	30	3 strips	2.5	8.4
Chard, Swiss	75	½ cup	12.0	16.0
Cucumber	50	½ medium	4.0	8.0
Dandelion greens	75	⅓ cup	14.7	19.6
Eggplant	75	⅓ cup	3.0	4.0
Endive, curly	50	10 leaves	4.5	9.0
Kale	75	⅓ cup	7.4	9.8
Kohlrabi	75	⅓ cup	8.3	11.1
Lettuce	50	5 leaves	3.0	6.0
Mushrooms	75	⅓ cup	2.3	3.1
Okra	75	⅓ cup	2.0	2.6
Onions	75	⅓ cup	0.1	0.1
Parsnips	75	⅓ cup	6.0	8.0
Peas	75	⅓ cup	0.7	0.9
Peppers	30	3 strips	0.6	2.0
Potato, white	100	1 small	9.0	9.0
Potato, baked	100	1 small	10.6	10.6
Potato, mashed	100	½ cup	9.6	9.6
Pumpkin	75	⅓ cup	5.9	7.8
Radish	50	5	1.5	3.0
Rutabagas	75	⅓ cup	6.4	8.5
Salsify	75	½ cup	2.2	2.9
Sauerkraut	75	½ cup	4.3	5.7
Squash, summer	75	⅓ cup	0.8	1.0
Squash, winter	75	⅓ cup	2.3	3.0
Sweet potato	100	1 small	6.0	6.0
Tomatoes or juice	75	½ large or ⅓ cup	3.8	5.0
Turnip greens	75	⅓ cup	1.7	2.3
Turnip	75	⅓ cup	1.7	2.3
Water cress	50	10 leaves	4.0	8.0

APPENDIX TABLE 12   COMMON CARBOHYDRATES IN FOODS PER 100 GM. EDIBLE PORTION**

FOOD	MONO-SACCHARIDES		REDUC-ING SUGARS*	DISACCHARIDES			POLYSACCHARIDES					
	Fructose	Glucose		Lactose	Maltose	Sucrose	Cellu-lose	Dextrins	Hemi-cellu-lose	Pectin	Pento-sans	Starch
Fruits												
	gm.	gm.	gm.	gm.	gm.	gm.	gm.	gm.	gm.	gm.	gm.	gm.
Agave juice	17.0		19.0	†								
Apple	5.0	1.7	8.3			3.1	0.4		0.7	0.6		0.6
Apple juice			8.0			4.2						
Apricots	0.4	1.9				5.5	0.8		1.2	1.0		
Banana												
Yellow green			5.0			5.1						8.8
Yellow			8.4			8.9						1.9
Flecked	3.5	4.5				11.9						1.2
Powder			32.6			33.2		9.6				7.8
Blackberries	2.9	3.2				0.2						
Blueberry juice, com-mercial			9.6			0.2						
Boysenberries			5.3			1.1				0.3		
Breadfruit												
Hawaiian			1.8			7.7						
Samoan			4.9			9.7						
Cherries												
Eating	7.2	4.7	12.5			0.1				0.3		
Cooking	6.1	5.5	11.6			0.1						
Cranberries	0.7	2.7				0.1						
Currants												
Black	3.7	2.4				0.6						
Red	1.9	2.3				0.2						
White	2.6	3.0										
Dates												
Invert sugar, seedling type	23.9	24.9				0.3						
Deglet Noor			16.2			45.4						
Egyptian			35.8			48.5						3.0
Figs, Kadota												
Fresh	8.2	9.6				0.9						0.1
Dried	30.9	42.0				0.1						0.3
Gooseberries	4.1	4.4				0.7						
Grapes												
Black	7.3	8.2										
Concord	4.3	4.8	9.5			0.2						
Malaga			22.2			0.2						
White	8.0	8.1										
Grapefruit	1.2	2.0				2.9					1.3	
Guava			4.4			1.9						
Lemon												
Edible portion			1.3			0.2				3.0	0.7	
Whole	1.4	1.4				0.4						
Juice	0.9	0.5				0.1						
Peel			3.4			0.1						
Loganberries	1.3	1.9				0.2						
Loquat												
Champagne		12.0				0.8						
Thales		9.0				0.9						
Mango			3.4			11.6						0.3
Melon												
Cantaloupe	0.9	1.2	2.3			4.4				0.3		
Cassaba,												
Vine ripened			2.8			6.2						
Picked green			3.2			3.9						
Honeydew												
Vine ripened			3.3			7.4						
Picked green			3.6			3.3						
Yellow	1.5	2.1				1.4						
Mulberries	3.6	4.4										
Orange												
Valencia (Calif.)	2.3	2.4	4.7			4.2						
Composite values	1.8	2.5	5.0			4.6	0.3		0.3	1.3	0.3	
Juice												
Fresh	2.4	2.4	5.1			4.7						
Frozen, reconstituted			4.6			3.2						

**From: Hardinge, M. G., et al.: Carbohydrate in foods. J. Am. Diet. Assoc., *46*:197, 1965.

APPENDIX TABLE 12   COMMON CARBOHYDRATES IN FOODS PER 100 GM.
EDIBLE PORTION (Continued)

FOOD	MONO-SACCHARIDES		REDUC-ING SUGARS*	DISACCHARIDES			POLYSACCHARIDES					
	Fructose	Glucose		Lactose	Maltose	Sucrose	Cellu-lose	Dextrins	Hemi-Cellu-lose	Pectin	Pento-sans	Starch
FRUITS, continued												
	gm.	gm.	gm.	gm.	gm.	gm.	gm.	gm.	gm.	gm.	gm.	gm.
Palmyra palm, tender kernel	1.5	3.2				0.4						
Papaw (Asimina triloba) (North America)			5.9			2.7						
Papaya (Carica papaya) (tropics)			9.0			0.5						
Pashion fruit juice	3.6	3.6				3.8						1.8
Peaches	1.6	1.5	3.1			6.6		0.7		0.7		
Pears												
Anjou			7.6			1.9				0.7		
Bartlett	5.0	2.5	8.0			1.5				0.6		
Bosc	6.5	2.6				1.7				0.6		
Persimmon			17.7									
Pineapple												
Ripened on plant	1.4	2.3	4.2			7.9						
Picked green			1.3			2.4						
Plums												
Damson	3.4	5.2	8.4			1.0						
Green Gage	4.0	5.5				2.9						
Italian prunes			4.6			5.4				0.9		
Sweet	2.9	4.5	7.4			4.4		0.5		1.0	0.1	
Sour	1.3	3.5				1.5				1.0		
Pomegranate			12.0			0.6						
Prunes, uncooked	15.0	30.0	47.0			2.0	2.8		10.7	0.9	2.0	0.7
Raisins, Thompson seedless			70.0							1.0		
Raspberries	2.4	2.3	5.0			1.0				0.8		
Sapote	3.8	4.2		0.7								
Strawberries												
Ripe	2.3	2.6				1.4						
Medium ripe			3.8			0.3						
Tangerine			4.8			9.0						
Tomatoes	1.2	1.6	3.4				0.2			0.3	0.3	
Canned			3.0			0.3						
Seedless pulp			6.5			0.4	0.4			0.5		
Watermelon												
Flesh red and firm, ripe			3.8			4.0				0.1		
Red, mealy, overripe			3.0			4.9				0.1		
Vegetables												
Asparagus, raw			1.2						0.3			
Bamboo shoots			0.5			0.2	1.2					
Beans												
Lima												
Canned						1.4						
Fresh						1.4						
Snap, fresh			1.7			0.5	0.5	0.3	1.0	0.5	1.2	2.0
Beets, sugar						12.9	0.9		0.8			
Broccoli							0.9		0.9		0.9	1.3
Brussel Sprouts							1.1		1.5			
Cabbage, raw			3.4			0.3	0.8		1.0			
Carrots, raw			5.8			1.7	1.0		1.7	0.9		
Cauliflower		2.8				0.3	0.7		0.6			
Celery												
Fresh			0.3			0.3						
Hearts			1.7			0.2						
Corn												
Fresh		0.5				0.3	0.6	0.1	0.9		1.3	14.5
Bran									77.1		4.0	
Cucumber			2.5			0.1						
Eggplant			2.1			0.6			0.5			
Lettuce			1.4			0.2	0.4		0.6			
Licorice root		1.4				3.2						22.0
Mushrooms, fresh			0.1				0.9		0.7			2.5
Onions, raw			5.4			2.9			0.3	0.6		
Parsnips, fresh						3.5						7.0
Peas, green						5.5	1.1		2.2			4.1

Table continued on the following page

APPENDIX TABLE 12   COMMON CARBOHYDRATES IN FOODS PER 100 GM.
EDIBLE PORTION (*Continued*)

FOOD	MONO-SACCHARIDES		REDUC-ING SUGARS*	DISACCHARIDES			POLYSACCHARIDES					
	Fructose	Glucose		Lactose	Maltose	Sucrose	Cellu-lose	Dextrins	Hemi-Cellu-lose	Pectin	Pento-sans	Starch
VEGETABLES, continued												
	gm.	gm.	gm.	gm.	gm.	gm.	gm.	gm.	gm.	gm.	gm.	gm.
Potatoes, white	0.1	0.1	0.8			0.1	0.4		0.3			17.0
Pumpkin			2.2			0.6			0.5			0.1
Radishes			3.1			0.3			0.3	0.4		
Rutabagas		5.0				1.3					0.8	
Spinach			0.2				0.4		0.8			
Squash												
Butternut	0.2	0.1				0.4						2.6
Blue Hubbard	1.2	1.1				0.4	0.7					4.8
Golden Crookneck			2.8			1.0						
Sweet potato												
Raw	0.3	0.4	0.8		1.6	4.1	0.6		1.4	2.2		16.5
Baked			14.5			7.2						4.0
Mature Dry Legumes												
Beans												
Mung												
Black gram						1.6						
Green gram						1.8						
Navy							3.1	3.7	6.4		8.2	35.2
Soy			1.6			7.2	2.6	1.4	6.6		4.0	1.9
Cow pea						1.5	5.4		4.8			
Garbanzo (chick peas)						2.4						
Garden pea (*Pisum sativum*)‡						6.7	5.0		5.1			38.0
Horse gram (*Dolichos biplorus*)						2.7						
Lentils						2.1						28.5
Pigeon pea (red gram)						1.6						
Soybean												
Flour						6.8						
Meal						6.8						
Milk and Milk Products												
Buttermilk												
Dry				39.9								
Fluid, genuine and cultured				5.0								
Casein		0.1		4.9								
Ice cream (14.5% cream)				3.6		16.6						
Milk												
Ass				6.0								
Cow				4.9								
Dried												
Skim				52.0								
Whole				38.1								
Fluid												
Skim				5.0								
Whole				4.9								
Sweetened, condensed				14.1		43.5						
Ewe				4.9								
Goat				4.7								
Human												
Colostrum				5.3								
Mature				6.9								
Whey				4.9								
Yogurt				3.8								
Nuts and Nut Products												
Almonds, blanched			0.2			2.3					2.1	
Chestnuts			2.2			3.6					1.2	18.0
Virginia			1.2			8.1		0.3			2.8	18.6
French			3.3			3.6					2.5	33.1
Coconut milk, ripe						2.6						
Copra meal, dried	1.2	1.2				14.3	15.6	0.6			2.2	0.9
Macadamia nut			0.3			5.5						

APPENDIX TABLE 12   COMMON CARBOHYDRATES IN FOODS PER 100 GM. EDIBLE PORTION (*Continued*)

FOOD	MONO-SACCHARIDES		REDUC-ING SUGARS*	DISACCHARIDES			POLYSACCHARIDES					
	Fructose	Glucose		Lactose	Maltose	Sucrose	Cellulose	Dextrins	Hemi-cellulose	Pectin	Pento-sans	Starch
Nuts and Nut Products, continued												
	gm.	gm.	gm.	gm.	gm.	gm.	gm.	gm.	gm.	gm.	gm.	gm.
Peanuts			0.2			4.5	2.4	2.5	3.8			4.0
Peanut butter			0.9									5.9
Pecans						1.1					0.2	
Cereals and Cereal Products												
Barley												
Grain, hulled							2.6		6.0		8.5	62.0
Flour						3.1					1.2	69.0
Corn, yellow							4.5		4.9		6.2	62.0
Flaxseed							1.8		5.2			
Millet grain									0.9		6.5	56.0
Oats, hulled											6.4	56.4
Rice												
Bran			1.4			10.6	11.4		7.0		7.4	
Brown, raw			0.1			0.8		2.1			2.1	69.7
Polished, raw		2.0	trace#			0.4	0.3	0.9			1.8	72.9
Polish			0.7								3.8	
Rye												
Grain							3.8		5.6		6.8	57.0
Flour											4.1	71.4
Sorghum grain											2.5	70.2
Soya-wheat (cereal)											3.3	46.4
Wheat												
Germ, defatted						8.3					6.2	
Grain			2.0			1.5	2.0	2.5	5.8		6.6	59.0
Flour, patent			2.0		0.1	0.2		5.5			2.1	68.8
Spices and Condiments												
Allspice (pimenta)			18.0			3.0						
Cassia			23.3									
Cinnamon			19.3									
Cloves			9.0									2.7
Nutmeg			17.2									14.6
Pepper, black			38.6									34.2
Sirups and Other Sweets												
Corn sirup		21.2			26.4			34.7				
High conversion		33.0			23.0			19.0				
Medium conversion		26.0			21.0			23.0				
Corn sugar		87.5			3.5			0.5				
Chocolate, sweet dry						56.4						
Golden sirup			37.5			31.0						
Honey	40.5	34.2				1.9		1.5				
Invert sugar			74.0			6.0						
Jellies, pectin						40-65						
Royal jelly	11.3	9.8				0.9						
Jellies, starch						25-60						7 = 12
Maple sirup			1.5			62.9						
Milk chocolate				8.1		43.0						
Molasses	8.0	8.8				53.6						
Blackstrap	6.8	6.8	26.9			36.9						
Sorghum sirup			27.0			36.0						
Miscellaneous												
Beer			1.5					2.8			0.3	
Cacao beans, raw, Arriba	0.6	0.5	1.1			1.9						
Carob bean												
Pod			11.2			23.2				1.4		
Pod and seeds			11.1			19.4						
Soy sauce	0.9											

Mainly monosaccharides plus the disaccharides, maltose and lactose.
†Blanks indicate lack of acceptable data.
‡Also known as Alaska pea, field pea, and common pea.
#Trace = less than 0.05 gm.

APPENDIX TABLE 13 INORGANIC ELEMENTS IN COMMON FOODS**

(Milligrams per 100 Grams Food)

mg./100 gm.

FOOD	DESCRIPTION	PHOS-PHORUS	POTAS-SIUM	CAL-CIUM	MAGNE-SIUM	SODIUM	ALUMI-NUM	BARIUM	IRON	STRON-TIUM	BORON	COPPER	ZINC	MANGA-NESE	CHRO-MIUM
Beverages and Dietary Concentrates															
Chocolate sirup		88	183	15	64	57	<0.2	0.17	1.4	0.13	0.3	0.43	1.1	0.23	<0.06
Coffee															
Instant	dry	367	1,103	156	380	56	<1.0	0.36	5.5	0.16	1.6	0.28	1.2	2.1	0.79
Ground	dry	119	2,045	98	179	<1.0	1.1	0.32	3.1	0.61	0.79	1.3	0.36	1.5	<0.06
Beverage	brewed	2.4	65	7	6.7	0.86	<0.04	<0.008	<0.02	<0.004	0.016	<0.004	0.042	0.014	<0.012
Cocoa	dry	526	1,990	100	442	89	4.5	1.2	8	1.7	2.2	5	5.4	2.5	0.06
Drinking and cooking water		0.5	2.0	8.8	4.5	3.8	<0.02	<0.004	0.011	<0.002	0.0035	<0.002	0.015	<0.004	<0.006
Meritene, plain flavor	dry	664	2,020	846	89	588	1.5	0.11	12	0.38	0.37	0.09	3.3	<0.04	<0.06
Sustagen, imitation vanilla flavor	dry	425	750	663	58	285	1.6	0.056	1.02	0.28	0.26	0.085	2.9	0.04	<0.06
Tea, orange pekoe															
Bag	dry	277	1,795	465	192	37	128	2.7	33	1.3	2.6	4.8	5.4	71	0.3
Beverage	steeped	<0.5	9.3	7.3	4.2	0.7	0.28	<0.004	<0.01	0.002	0.002	0.007	0.037	0.22	<0.006
Breads, Cereal Products, Crackers, and Pastas															
Bread															
Rye		145	183	96	42	873	<0.2	0.062	1.5	0.3	0.042	0.17	1.2	0.5	<0.06
White	enriched, 4% nonfat milk solids; calcium propionate added	105	154	128	25	863	0.3	0.051	1.9	0.31	0.069	0.11	0.75	0.25	<0.06
Whole wheat		192	176	74	59	752	0.54	0.11	3.8	0.15	0.048	0.17	1.7	1.2	<0.06
Bran flakes, 40%		483	730	34	175	923	<0.2	0.39	15	0.15	0.23	0.64	3.9	4.1	<0.06
Cheerios		359	353	147	106	1,150	0.47	0.13	3.9	0.18	0.13	0.34	3	2.7	<0.06
Corn flakes		31	111	<10	8.7	1,000	<0.2	0.04	1.4	0.024	<0.02	0.023	0.13	<0.04	<0.06
Crackers															
Graham		80	100	12	18	725	<0.2	0.11	0.55	0.066	<0.02	0.04	0.76	0.43	<0.06
Saltines		85	100	15	18	1,335	<0.2	0.04	1.7	0.14	<0.02	0.09	0.7	0.39	<0.06
Egg noodles	uncooked	242	266	31	74	30	<0.2	0.16	4.6	0.06	0.105	0.17	2.2	0.78	<0.06
Macaroni	uncooked	181	233	15	50	5.7	<0.2	0.11	3.1	0.024	0.063	0.13	1.6	0.5	<0.06
Oatmeal, rolled oats (quick)	uncooked	368	390	39	128	4.7	<0.2	0.11	3.7	0.024	0.13	0.022	3.4	3.7	<0.06
Puffed Rice		154	229	15	40	6.7	<0.2	<0.04	0.21	<0.02	0.15	0.17	1.3	1.5	<0.06
Quick Cream of Wheat															
Enriched	uncooked	1,028	388	1,010	41	345	2.5	0.2	84	0.55	0.65	0.12	2.2	1.1	<0.3
Regular	uncooked	441	149	403	17	267	0.8	0.15	34	0.16	0.2	0.11	1.1	0.58	<0.06
Rice Krispies		102	89	<10	30	1,100	<0.2	<0.04	2.2	0.024	0.024	0.085	1.4	0.99	<0.06
Rice, white	uncooked	120	89	14	28	1.4	<0.2	<0.04	0.27	<0.02	0.024	<0.02	1.8	1.5	<0.06
Shredded Wheat		355	390	26	109	25	<0.2	0.22	2.7	0.024	0.24	0.17	3.2	2.9	<0.06
Spaghetti	uncooked	169	183	18	61	4.7	<0.2	0.11	2.4	0.066	0.069	0.068	1.7	0.54	<0.06
Wheaties		297	390	30	89	1,400	<0.2	0.14	3.0	0.15	0.048	0.34	2.4	1.5	<0.06

**From Gormican, A.: Inorganic lesions in foods used in hospital menus. J. Am. Diet. Assoc., 56:397, 1970.

Eggs and Dairy Products

mg./100 gm.

Cheese															
American		795	167	545	20	1,770	69.5	0.12	0.63	0.29	0.24	0.11	4.1	<0.4	0.17
Cottage	creamed	159	89	74	5.5	444	<0.2	<0.04	<0.1	<0.02	<0.02	<0.02	0.4	<0.04	<0.06
Swiss		530	180	843	34	297	1.9	0.22	0.46	0.26	0.13	0.11	4.6	<0.04	<0.06
Eggs															
Whole		191	100	48	9.8	147	0.14	0.76	2.1	0.02	0.063	0.053	1.8	<0.02	0.052
White		10	140	3.6	9.9	180	<0.05	<0.01	<0.025	0.024	0.013	0.005	0.009	<0.01	<0.015
Yolk		255	89	72	4.0	20	<0.1	0.058	2.1	0.027	0.066	0.01	1.5	<0.02	<0.03
Milk															
Nonfat solids		710	1,940	991	94	561	1.7	<0.08	<0.2	0.24	0.29	<0.04	4.4	<0.08	<0.16
Fluid Whole	3.5% butterfat; vitamin D enriched, 400 U.S.P. units/qt.)	85	145	105	9	50	0.2	<0.01	0.028	0.022	0.028	0.005	0.43	<0.01	<0.015
Skim	0% butterfat; 2,000 U.S.P. units vitamin A and 400 U.S.P. units vitamin D added/qt.	82	170	108	9.2	56	0.2	<0.01	0.027	0.017	0.029	0.005	0.46	<0.01	<0.015
Buttermilk	Grade A, cultured	75	190	98	8.4	238	0.2	<0.01	0.028	0.028	0.027	<0.005	0.37	<0.01	<0.015
Ice cream	vanilla	96	210	120	12	87	0.26	<0.01	0.037	0.033	0.033	0.005	0.53	<0.01	<0.015
Sherbet	orange	46	90	59	6.7	39	0.14	<0.01	0.067	0.019	0.053	0.022	0.24	<0.01	<0.015
Fruits and Fruit Juices															
Apple															
Raw	with peel	6.9	95	7.1	4.8	0.5	<0.05	0.075	2.0	0.008	0.37	0.014	0.012	0.035	<0.015
Juice	canned	4.2	85	3.1	3.2	2.2	0.08	<0.002	0.4	<0.001	0.12	0.023	0.043	0.21	<0.006
Sauce	canned, drained	5.6	70	2.9	2.0	16	<0.05	<0.01	0.24	<0.005	0.19	0.01	0.013	<0.01	<0.015
Apricots	canned, drained	16	170	8.3	6.4	22	<0.05	<0.01	0.23	0.063	0.58	0.041	0.085	<0.01	<0.015
Banana	ripe	17	405	<2.5	26	2.9	<0.05	<0.01	0.17	0.024	0.074	0.11	0.15	0.13	<0.015
Blueberries	water-pack, drained	14	45	6.2	3.8	0.9	0.26	0.014	9.2	<0.005	0.12	0.027	0.085	0.15	<0.015
Cantaloupe		10	295	9	8.4	33	<0.05	<0.01	0.6	0.05	0.24	0.014	0.14	<0.01	<0.015
Cherries, Royal Anne	canned, drained	20	155	12	8.4	1.2	<0.05	0.029	1.7	0.041	0.57	0.061	0.11	0.029	<0.015
Grapes															
Fresh	with peel	29	230	12	5.8	<0.5	<0.05	<0.05	1.1	0.064	0.45	0.035	0.035	0.065	<0.015
Juice	canned	10.3	125	4.8	7.3	2.2	0.11	0.023	0.15	0.017	0.23	0.009	0.04	0.36	<0.006
Grapefruit															
Juice	canned	11	125	7	7.7	2.2	<0.04	<0.008	0.27	0.13	0.026	0.008	0.03	<0.008	<0.012
Sections Fresh	skinless	23	170	18	12	<0.5	<0.05	<0.01	0.17	0.071	0.15	0.041	0.10	<0.01	<0.015
Canned	drained	10	100	20	7.2	3.6	<0.05	<0.01	0.35	0.61	0.059	0.014	0.04	<0.01	<0.015

Table continued on the following page

APPENDIX TABLE 13　　INORGANIC ELEMENTS IN COMMON FOODS (Continued)

(Milligrams per 100 Grams Food)

mg/100 gm.

FOOD	DESCRIPTION	PHOSPHORUS	POTASSIUM	CALCIUM	MAGNESIUM	SODIUM	ALUMINUM	BARIUM	IRON	STRONTIUM	BORON	COPPER	ZINC	MANGANESE	CHROMIUM
						Fruit and Fruit Juices—Concluded									
Orange															
Juice	frozen, reconstituted	10.2	185	10	8.2	1.8	<0.04	<0.008	0.042	0.011	0.055	0.0075	0.015	<0.008	0.012
Sections	skinless	14	135	6.2	6.7	<0.4	<0.04	<0.003	0.042	0.019	0.18	0.004	0.02	<0.008	<0.012
Pineapple															
Crushed	canned, drained	6.9	95	16	14	3.6	<0.05	0.014	0.2	0.17	0.085	0.15	0.08	1.16	<0.015
Juice	canned	6.9	145	11	11	0.9	<0.04	0.008	0.119	0.025	0.067	0.04	0.07	0.99	<0.012
Peach, cling	canned, drained	12	100	<2.5	3.8	1.6	<0.05	<0.01	1.0	<0.005	0.28	0.041	0.05	<0.01	<0.015
Pear	canned, drained	6.9	73	3.6	3.8	9.0	<0.05	0.047	0.04	0.026	0.15	0.041	0.055	<0.01	<0.015
Prunes															
Cooked		35	340	28	24	3.6	0.62	0.064	1.3	0.19	0.71	0.25	0.33	0.078	<0.015
Juice	canned	8.3	170	5.1	5.8	1.3	<0.04	0.014	0.35	0.025	0.28	0.018	0.12	0.02	0.012
Watermelon		5.6	95	14	10.2	1.6	<0.05	0.022	0.25	0.014	0.108	0.017	0.085	0.026	<0.015
						Meat, Poultry, Fish, and Shellfish									
Beef, fresh, uncooked															
Flank	U. S. Good	148	365	<5	16	73	<0.1	<0.02	1.4	<0.01	<0.01	0.02	3.6	<0.02	<0.03
Ground	U. S. Cutter	182	350	<5	17	65	<0.1	<0.02	2.6	0.012	0.034	0.061	3.4	<0.02	<0.03
Liver		355	323	<10	8.2	77	<0.2	<0.04	2.9	<0.02	0.054	4.6	4.2	0.17	<0.06
Round	U. S. Good	160	285	<5	16	63	<0.1	<0.02	2	0.012	0.044	0.045	3	<0.02	<0.03
Rump	U. S. Good	172	370	<5	18	67	<0.1	<0.02	2.1	<0.01	<0.01	0.077	3.3	<0.02	<0.03
Sirloin	U. S. Good, medium fat	159	395	<5	16	53	<0.1	<0.02	1.4	<0.01	0.21	0.042	3.1	<0.02	<0.03
Tenderloin	U. S. Prime	153	330	<5	16	55	<0.1	<0.02	1.5	<0.01	<0.01	0.012	2.5	<0.02	<0.03
Lamb, fresh, uncooked															
Chop	medium fat	145	325	6.8	16	83	<0.1	<0.02	1.3	<0.01	<0.01	0.045	2.4	<0.02	<0.03
Leg	medium fat	159	350	<5	17	107	<0.1	<0.02	1	<0.01	<0.01	0.063	3.2	<0.02	<0.03
Luncheon meat, big bologna		77	148	8.5	8.9	2,275	<0.1	<0.02	1.6	0.078	<0.01	0.02	1.5	<0.02	<0.03
Pork, fresh, uncooked															
Bacon	medium fat	131	122	<10	6.9	979	<0.2	<0.04	0.81	0.1	<0.02	0.023	1.4	<0.04	<0.06
Ham	cured	217	350	10	14	2,505	<0.1	<0.02	0.71	0.081	0.024	0.034	1.7	<0.02	<0.03
Liver		366	296	<10	14	118	<0.2	<0.04	3.8	<0.02	0.069	0.55	6.7	0.23	<0.06
Loin	medium fat	141	300	<5	15	35	<0.1	<0.02	0.8	<0.01	<0.01	0.011	1.4	<0.02	<0.03
Veal, fresh, uncooked															
Round	medium fat	136	245	7.4	11	124	<0.1	<0.02	1.5	<0.01	0.01	0.043	2.3	<0.02	<0.03
Steak	medium fat	160	295	<5	15	92	<0.1	<0.02	0.8	<0.01	<0.01	0.052	2.9	<0.02	<0.03
Poultry, uncooked															
Chicken, roaster															
Dark meat		137	240	7.4	16	81	<0.1	<0.02	1.1	0.011	0.014	0.02	1.5	<0.02	<0.03
White meat		152	225	8.7	17	49	<0.1	<0.02	0.8	<0.01	0.024	0.011	0.59	<0.02	<0.03
Turkey, roaster															
Dark meat		175	330	<5	17	69	<0.1	<0.02	1.5	<0.01	0.024	0.037	2.4	<0.02	<0.03
White meat		185	235	<5	20	48	<0.1	<0.02	0.73	0.012	0.024	0.037	1.8	<0.02	<0.03

Meat, Poultry, Fish, and Shellfish—Concluded

mg./100 gm.

Fish and shell fish															
Crab	canned, salted	147	265	25	41	500	<0.1	<0.02	0.48	0.37	0.01	0.27	3.6	<0.02	<0.03
Haddock	uncooked, frozen	164	370	10	24	202	<0.1	<0.02	1.4	0.031	0.021	0.011	0.32	<0.02	<0.03
Salmon, Sockeye	canned, salt-free	312	400	272	29	51	0.82	<0.02	1.4	1.0	0.064	0.076	1.1	<0.02	<0.03
Shrimp	canned, salted	141	163	18	23	2,300	<0.1	<0.02	1.6	0.17	0.022	0.17	1.9	<0.02	<0.03
Sole	uncooked, frozen	110	220	25	44	397	<0.1	0.02	0.33	0.2	0.062	0.011	0.31	<0.02	<0.03
Tuna	canned, salt-free, water pack	184	330	<5	23	44	<0.1	<0.02	3.2	<0.01	0.054	0.011	0.44	<0.02	<0.03
						Nuts									
Peanuts															
Butter	smooth	314	790	34	172	602	<0.2	<0.04	1.8	0.127	0.03	0.61	2.9	1.9	<0.06
Salted, blanched		326	830	36	160	324	<0.2	0.21	1.2	0.14	1.7	0.43	2.9	1.5	<0.06
Pecans	unsalted	281	368	76	110	11	<0.2	0.67	1.7	0.36	0.76	1.1	4.1	1.5	<0.06
Walnuts	unsalted	337	530	103	144	6.4	<0.2	0.072	4.2	<0.02	<0.059	1.4	3.2	2.1	<0.06
						Sugars and Flours									
Sugar															
Brown		<5	640	68	62	44	<0.2	<0.04	1.8	0.127	0.03	<0.02	0.029	<0.04	<0.06
Powdered		<5	<20	<10	<1	1.4	<0.2	<0.04	<0.1	<0.02	<0.02	<0.02	<0.02	<0.04	<0.06
White		5	<20	<10	<1	1.2	<0.2	<0.04	<0.1	<0.02	<0.02	<0.02	<0.02	<0.04	<0.06
Flour	bleached, enriched	121	117	14	27	6.1	<0.2	0.072	4.2	<0.02	0.059	0.13	0.93	0.4	0.06
						Vegetables									
Asparagus spears	frozen, uncooked	91	300	32	14	3.3	<0.1	<0.02	2.1	0.012	0.26	0.21	0.76	0.18	<0.03
Beans															
Baked with pork		85	240	50	28	427	<0.1	<0.02	2.5	0.073	0.18	0.17	1.7	0.2	<0.06
Green	frozen, uncooked	30	148	38	21	0.9	<0.1	0.16	1.5	0.2	0.19	0.04	0.31	0.27	<0.06
Lima, baby	frozen, uncooked	116	560	34	57	136	<0.1	0.031	2.6	0.31	0.31	0.18	0.77	0.54	<0.06
Wax	canned, salt-free, drained	20	90	40	11	7	0.28	0.11	3.5	0.065	0.064	0.02	0.23	0.21	<0.06
Beets	canned, salt-free, drained	22	148	13	23	69	<0.1	0.26	1	0.14	0.14	0.2	0.3	0.082	<0.03
Broccoli	frozen, uncooked	52	220	34	15	25	<0.1	<0.02	0.75	0.101	0.16	0.011	0.27	0.056	<0.03
Brussels sprouts	frozen, uncooked	65	475	29	21	14	<0.1	<0.02	1.5	0.075	0.23	0.011	0.37	0.11	<0.03
Cabbage	uncooked	31	199	46	16	6.9	<0.1	<0.02	2.4	0.023	0.34	0.06	0.14	0.063	<0.03
Carrots	uncooked	36	315	28	9.4	109	<0.1	0.052	1.6	0.2	0.21	0.011	0.12	<0.02	<0.03
Cauliflower	frozen, uncooked	66	310	18	14	12	<0.1	<0.02	1.4	0.068	0.17	0.011	0.46	0.16	<0.03
Celery	fresh	20	245	23	8.7	87	<0.1	<0.02	1.1	0.069	0.14	<0.01	0.065	<0.02	<0.03
Corn, whole kernel	canned, salt-free, drained	44	117	<5	11	<0.5	<0.1	<0.02	0.26	<0.01	0.021	0.011	0.33	<0.02	<0.03
Cucumber		13	148	18	10	0.7	<0.1	<0.02	0.59	0.12	0.044	<0.01	0.1	0.056	<0.03
Lettuce		31	139	22	12	7.6	<0.1	<0.02	0.53	0.078	0.082	0.037	0.25	0.069	<0.03
Mushrooms, stems and pieces	canned	66	98	13	6.5	355	0.4	<0.02	2.3	0.067	<0.01	0.26	1.1	0.033	<0.03
Onions	fresh, mature	33	141	22	10.1	2.2	<0.1	0.053	0.75	0.2	0.17	0.097	0.11	0.078	<0.03

Table continued on the following page

APPENDIX TABLE 13 INORGANIC ELEMENTS IN COMMON FOODS (Continued)

(Milligrams per 100 Grams Food)

mg./100 gm.

Vegetables—Concluded

FOOD	DESCRIPTION	PHOSPHORUS	POTASSIUM	CALCIUM	MAGNESIUM	SODIUM	ALUMINUM	BARIUM	IRON	STRONTIUM	BORON	COPPER	ZINC	MANGANESE	CHROMIUM
Peas	canned, salt-free, drained	71	118	23	22	5.4	<0.1	<0.02	1.2	0.012	0.16	0.13	1.3	0.11	<0.03
Potato															
Fresh	uncooked	44	280	6.7	14	1.45	<0.1	<0.02	0.58	0.012	0.052	0.052	0.2	0.042	<0.03
Instant	uncooked	179	625	66	68	124	<0.2	0.056	0.97	0.18	0.26	0.17	0.56	0.16	0.06
Pumpkin	canned	38	176	36	18	0.7	0.26	0.053	16	0.056	0.27	0.054	0.19	0.11	<0.03
Spinach	frozen, uncooked	40	575	139	104	140	2.2	0.04	3.3	0.48	0.33	0.083	0.37	0.56	<0.03
Squash	frozen, cooked	28	172	32	26	0.9	0.34	0.082	1.1	0.15	0.2	0.14	0.3	0.096	<0.03
Sweet potatoes	canned	22	164	22	18	16	<0.1	0.22	0.47	0.23	0.08	0.063	0.16	0.62	<0.03
Tomato															
Fresh	canned, salt-free	13	178	<5	4.3	1.45	<0.1	<0.02	0.53	0.012	0.014	<0.01	0.046	<0.02	<0.03
Juice		8.3	250	2.9	4.1	2.2	0.04	0.008	0.053	<0.004	0.023	0.004	0.065	0.013	<0.012

Analyzed values for inorganic elements in representative hospital menus

mg./day

MENU	PHOSPHORUS*	POTASSIUM	CALCIUM*	MAGNESIUM*	SODIUM	ALUMINUM	BARIUM	IRON	STRONTIUM	BORON	COPPER	ZINC*	MANGANESE	CHROMIUM
General														
Summer	1,486	3,942	1,304	294	5,912	6.974	<0.303	7.6	1.243	1.577	0.425	13.34	0.88	<0.455
Winter	2,041	4,881	1,390	385	7,158	5.324	0.592	9.2	1.893	1.154	<0.296	14.49	1.78	0.887
Mechanical soft														
Summer	1,153	3,436	1,031	226	4,221	5.644	<0.245	6.6	0.810	1.055	0.466	12.52	0.66	<0.368
Winter	1,591	4,473	1,291	330	4,263	9.006	0.721	11.1	0.360	0.600	0.600	16.81	1.38	0.901
Low (1 gm.)-sodium														
Summer	1,180	3,934	1,124	250	1,377	3.934	0.337	9.0	0.871	1.461	0.731	12.08	0.76	<0.422
Winter	1,323	3,737	986	311	960	<2.595	0.519	12.2	0.260	0.467	<0.260	18.43	1.43	0.779
40-gm. protein														
Summer	776	2,209	716	191	3,343	<1.990	<0.398	3.6	0.856	0.935	<0.199	7.56	0.40	<0.597
Winter	635	1,813	505	142	1,420	1.869	0.374	5.2	0.262	0.561	<0.187	6.36	0.38	0.561
1,000-calorie														
Summer	1,179	3,237	1,064	277	3,491	4.393	0.324	16.2	0.948	1.272	0.532	16.65	0.95	<0.347
Winter	1,231	2,904	999	200	4,251	<2.323	<0.465	6.0	0.372	0.465	<0.232	11.38	0.47	0.697
1,500-calorie														
Summer	909	2,751	765	220	3,755	3.349	0.431	13.2	0.622	0.789	0.455	13.40	1.24	<0.359
Winter	1,224	3,492	867	219	5,327	4.843	<0.510	6.6	0.357	0.510	<0.255	12.24	1.17	<0.765
Giovanetti†	846	1,481	1,058	134	150	634.5	0.752	25.9	1.105	0.917	<0.235	<3.29	0.85	<0.705
20-gm. protein (no salt added)†	430	1,328	359	110	323	<1.795	<0.359	2.3	<0.180	0.539	<0.180	1.98	<0.36	<0.539
Full liquid†	1,354	3,745	1,815	242	3,832	4.033	<0.288	2.9	0.807	0.951	0.288	8.64	1.18	<0.432
Clear liquid†	<21	736	57	57	2,618	2.290	0.164	1.1	<0.082	0.164	0.082	0.33	0.92	<0.245
Estimated daily intake of Americans (1, 13)	800-1,200	2,000-6,000	800-1,200	300-450	2,300-6,900	36.4	16.0	15.0	2.0	10.0	2.0	12.0	5.0	0.06

*A daily allowance is recommended by Food and Nutrition Board.
†Winter menu only.

APPENDIX TABLE 14   DESIRABLE WEIGHTS FOR MEN

(Ages 25 and Over)*

HEIGHT (WITH SHOES, 1-INCH HEELS)		WEIGHT IN POUNDS ACCORDING TO FRAME (IN INDOOR CLOTHING)		
		Small Frame	*Medium Frame*	*Large Frame*
Feet	Inches			
5	2	112–120	118–129	126–141
5	3	115–123	121–133	129–144
5	4	118–126	124–136	132–148
5	5	121–129	127–139	135–152
5	6	124–133	130–143	138–156
5	7	128–137	134–147	142–161
5	8	132–141	138–152	147–166
5	9	136–145	142–156	151–170
5	10	140–150	146–160	155–174
5	11	144–154	150–165	159–179
6	0	148–158	154–170	164–184
6	1	152–162	158–175	168–189
6	2	156–167	162–180	173–194
6	3	160–171	167–185	178–199
6	4	164–175	172–190	182–204

*Courtesy of the Metropolitan Life Insurance Company, New York, N.Y. Derived from data of the 1959 Build and Blood Pressure Study, Society of Actuaries.

APPENDIX TABLE 15   DESIRABLE WEIGHTS FOR WOMEN
*(Ages 25 and Over)**

HEIGHT (WITH SHOES, 2-INCH HEELS)		WEIGHT IN POUNDS ACCORDING TO FRAME (IN INDOOR CLOTHING)		
		Small Frame	*Medium Frame*	*Large Frame*
Feet	Inches			
4	10	92– 98	96–107	104–119
4	11	94–101	98–110	106–122
5	0	96–104	101–113	109–125
5	1	99–107	104–116	112–128
5	2	102–110	107–119	115–131
5	3	105–113	110–122	118–134
5	4	108–116	113–126	121–138
5	5	111–119	116–130	125–142
5	6	114–123	120–135	129–146
5	7	118–127	124–139	133–150
5	8	122–131	128–143	137–154
5	9	126–135	132–147	141–158
5	10	130–140	136–151	145–163
5	11	134–144	140–155	149–168
6	0	138–148	144–159	153–173

*Note: for girls between 18 and 25, subtract 1 pound for each year under 25. Courtesy of the Metropolitan Life Insurance Company, New York, N.Y. Derived from data of the 1959 Build and Blood Pressure Study, Society of Actuaries.

APPENDIX 16   NCHS GROWTH CHART FOR HEIGHT AND WEIGHT FOR
BOYS AGE 2 TO 18 YEARS

**BOYS: 2 TO 18 YEARS
PHYSICAL GROWTH
NCHS PERCENTILES***

NAME _____   RECORD # _____

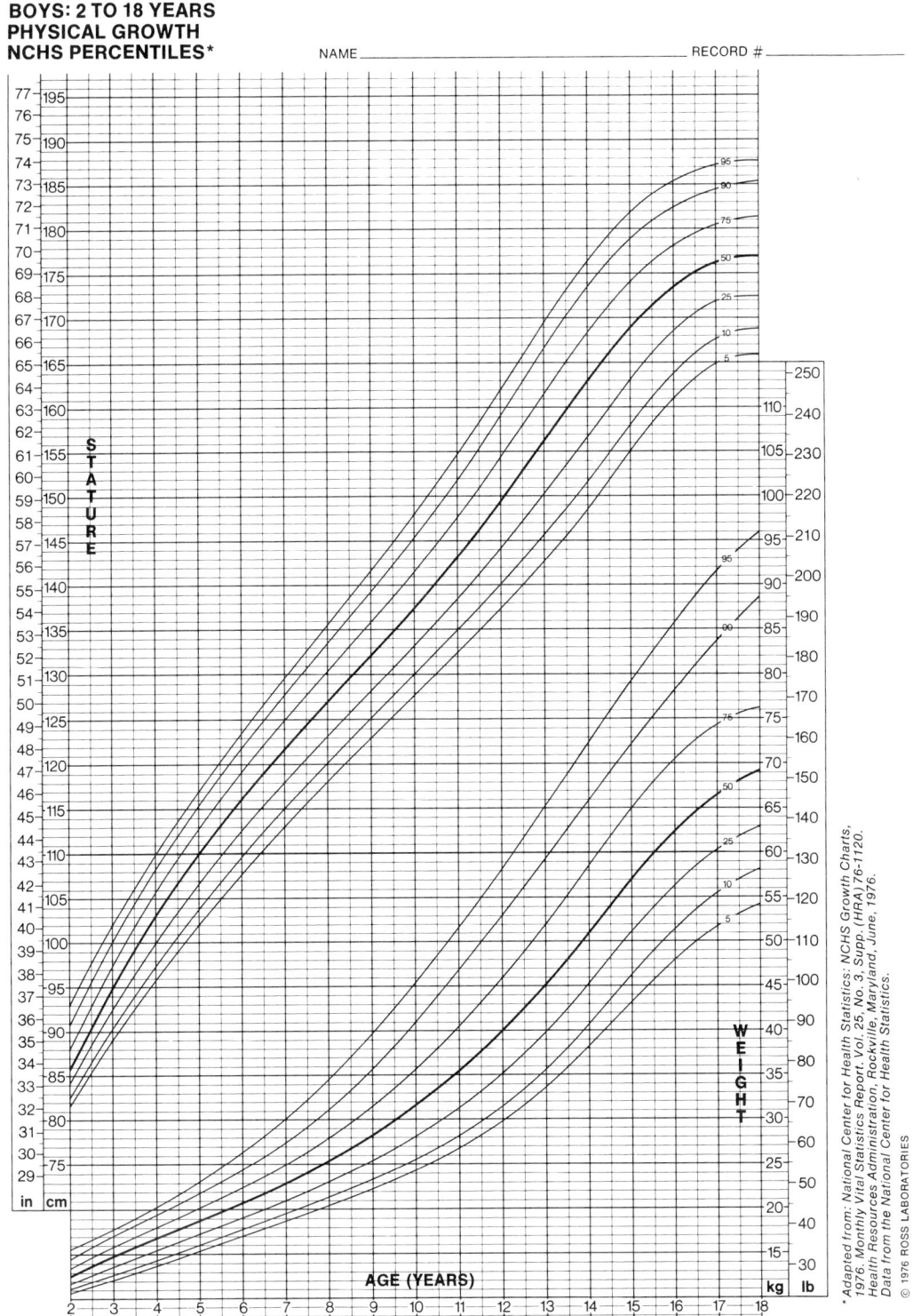

* Adapted from: National Center for Health Statistics: NCHS Growth Charts,
1976. Monthly Vital Statistics Report. Vol. 25, No. 3, Supp. (HRA) 76-1120.
Health Resources Administration, Rockville, Maryland, June, 1976.
Data from the National Center for Health Statistics.

© 1976 ROSS LABORATORIES

APPENDIX 17   NCHS GROWTH CHART FOR HEIGHT AND WEIGHT FOR
GIRLS AGE 2 TO 18 YEARS

GIRLS: 2 TO 18 YEARS
PHYSICAL GROWTH
NCHS PERCENTILES*

NAME _____ RECORD # _____

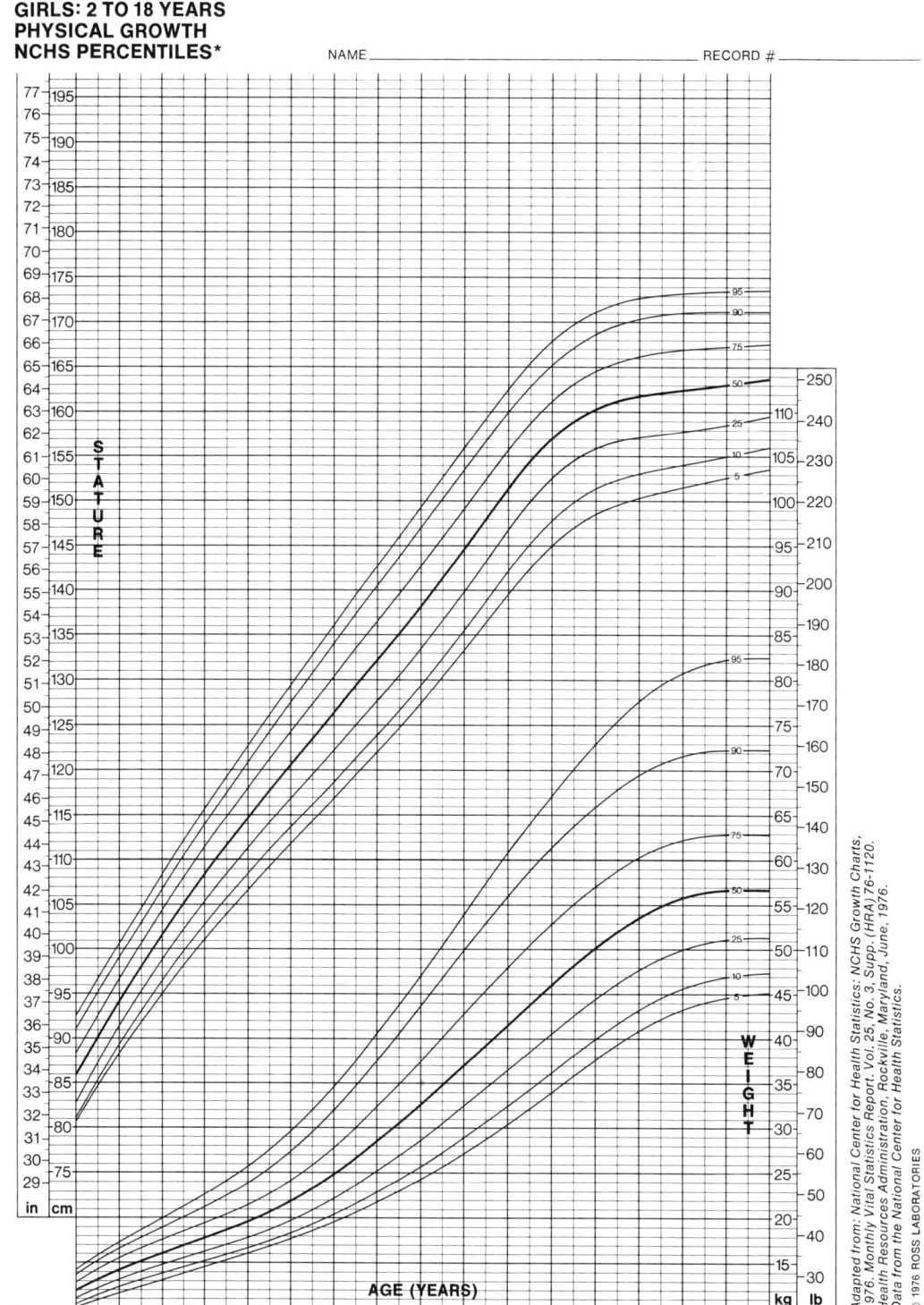

* Adapted from: National Center for Health Statistics: NCHS Growth Charts, 1976. Monthly Vital Statistics Report. Vol. 25, No. 3, Supp. (HRA) 76-1120. Health Resources Administration, Rockville, Maryland, June, 1976. Data from the National Center for Health Statistics.

© 1976 ROSS LABORATORIES

APPENDIX TABLE 18   CURRENT GUIDELINES FOR MEASUREMENTS OF NUTRITIONAL STATUS

NUTRIENT	DETERMINATION	CLASSIFICATION CATEGORY		
		LESS THAN ACCEPTABLE		ACCEPTA-BLE[a]
		Deficient	Low	
	Serum protein (gm./100 ml.[b])			
	0–11 mo.		<5.0	≧5.0
	1–5 yr.		<5.5	≧5.5
	6–17 yr.		<6.0	≧6.0
	Adult	<6.0	6.0–6.4	≧6.5
	Pregnant, 2nd and 3rd trimester	<5.5	5.5–5.9	≧6.0
Protein				
	Serum albumin (gm./100 ml.[b])			
	0–11 mo.		<2.5	≧2.5
	1–5 yr.		<3.0	≧3.0
	6–17 yr.		<3.5	≧3.5
	Adult	<2.8	2.8–3.4	≧3.5
	Pregnant, 1st trimester	<3.0	3.0–3.9	≧4.0
	Pregnant, 2nd and 3rd trimester	<3.0	3.0–3.4	≧3.5
	Serum triglycerides (mg./100 ml.)			
	1–19 yr.			≦150
	20 yr.			≦200
Lipids				
	Serum cholesterol (mg./100 ml.)			
	1–19 yr.			≦230
	20 yr.			≦240
Iodine	Urinary iodine (μg./gm. creatinine[b])	<25	25–49	≧50
	Hemoglobin (gm./100 ml.[b])			
	6–23 mo.	<9.0	9.0–9.9	≧10.0
	2–5 yr.	<10	10.0–10.9	≧11.0
	6–12 yr.	<10	10.0–11.4	≧11.5
	13–16 yr., male	<12	12.0–12.9	≧13.0
	13–16 yr., female	<10	10.0–11.4	≧11.5
	>16 yr., male	<12	12.0–13.9	≧14.0
	>16 yr., female	<10	10.0–11.9	≧12.0
	Pregnant, 2nd trimester	<9.5	9.5–10.9	≧11.0
	Pregnant, 3rd trimester	<9.0	9.0–10.4	≧10.5
	Hematocrit (%[b])			
	6–23 mo.	<28	28–30	≧31
	2–5 yr.	<30	30–33	≧34
	6–12 yr.	<30	30–35	≧36
	13–16 yr., male	<37	37–39	≧40
	13–16 yr., female	<31	31–35	≧36
Iron	>16 yr., male	<37	37–43	≧44
	>16 yr., female	<31	31–37	≧38
	Pregnant, 2nd trimester	<30	30–34	≧35
	Pregnant, 3rd trimester	<30	30–32	≧33
	Serum iron (μg./100 ml.[b])			
	0–5 mo.		–	–
	6–23 mo.		<30	≧30
	2–5 yr.		<40	≧40
	6–12 yr.		<50	≧50
	>12 yr., male		<60	≧60
	>12 yr., female		<40	≧40

[a]Excessively high levels may indicate abnormal clinical status or toxicity.
[b]From the Ten-State Nutrition Survey, 1968–70.

Table continued on the following page

APPENDIX TABLE 18   CURRENT GUIDELINES FOR MEASUREMENTS OF
NUTRITIONAL STATUS (*Continued*)

NUTRIENT	DETERMINATION	CLASSIFICATION CATEGORY		
		LESS THAN ACCEPTABLE		ACCEPTA-BLE[a]
		Deficient	*Low*	
Iron (*Continued*)				
	Transferrin saturation (%[b])			
	0–5 mo.		–	–
	6–23 mo.		<15	≧15
	2–12 yr.		<20	≧20
	>12 yr., male		<20	≧20
	>12 yr., female		<15	≧15
Vitamin A	Plasma carotene (μg./100 ml.[b])			
	0–5 mo.		<10	≧10
	6–11 mo.		<30	≧30
	1–17 yr.		<40	≧40
	Adult	<20[c]	20–39	≧40
	Pregnant, 2nd trimester		30–79	≧80
	Pregnant, 3rd trimester		40–79	≧80
	Plasma vitamin A (μg./100 ml.[b])			
	All ages	<20	20–29	≧30
Vitamin E	Serum vitamin E (mg./100 ml.[d,e])			
	All ages	<0.5	0.5–0.7	>0.7
	Red cell hemolysis in H_2O_2[d]			
	All ages	>20	10–20	<10
Thiamin	Urinary thiamin (μg./gm. creatinine[b])			
	1–3 yr.	<120	120–175	≧176
	4–6 yr.	<85	85–120	≧121
	7–9 yr.	<70	70–180	≧181
	10–12 yr.	<60	60–180	≧181
	13–15 yr.	<50	50–150	≧151
	Adult	<27	27–65	≧66
	Pregnant, 2nd trimester	<23	23–54	≧55
	Pregnant, 3rd trimester	<21	21–49	≧50
	RBC transketolase-TPP-effect (ratio)[d,e]			
	All ages	≧25	15–25	<15
Riboflavin	Urinary riboflavin (μg./gm. creatinine[b])			
	1–3 yr.	<150	150–499	≧500
	4–6 yr.	<100	100–299	≧300
	7–9 yr.	<85	85–269	≧270
	10–15 yr.	<70	70–199	≧200
	Adult	<27	27–79	≧80
	Pregnant, 2nd trimester	<39	39–119	≧120
	Pregnant, 3rd trimester	<30	30–89	≧90
	RBC glutathione reductase-FAD-effect (ratio)[d]			
	All ages	>1.4	1.2–1.4	<1.2

[c]May indicate unusual diet or malabsorption.

[d]From: Sauberlich, H. E., Dowdy, R. P., and Skala, J. H.: Laboratory Tests for Assessment of Nutritional Status. Cleveland, Ohio, CRC Press, 1973.

[e]Criteria may vary with different methodology.

APPENDIX TABLE 18   CURRENT GUIDELINES FOR MEASUREMENTS OF
NUTRITIONAL STATUS (*Continued*)

| NUTRIENT | DETERMINATION | CLASSIFICATION CATEGORY | | |
| | | LESS THAN ACCEPTABLE | | ACCEPTA-BLE[a] |
		Deficient	*Low*	
Niacin	Urinary *N*-methylnicotinamide (mg./gm. creatinine[f])			
	Adult	<0.5	0.5–1.59	≥1.6
	Pregnant, 2nd trimester	<0.6	0.6–1.99	≥2.0
	Pregnant, 3rd trimester	<0.8	0.8–2.49	≥2.5
Folacin	Red cell folacin (ng./ml.[b])			
	All ages	<140	140–159	≥160–650
	Serum folacin (ng./ml.[b])	<3.0	3.0–5.9	≥6.0
Pyridoxine	Tryptophan load (mg. xanthurenic acid excreted[d,e])			
	Adult	>50	–	<25
	Urinary pyridoxine (μg./gm. creatinine[d,e])			
	1–3 yr.	<90	–	≥90
	4–6 yr.	<80	–	≥75
	7–9 yr.	<50	–	≥50
	10–12 yr.	<40	–	≥40
	13–15 yr.	<30	–	≥30
	16+	<20	–	≥20
	Transaminase index (ratio)[d,e]			
	EGOT[g]			
	Adult	>1.5	–	≤1.5
	EGPT[h]			
	Adult	>1.25	–	≤1.25
Vitamin B$_{12}$	Serum vitamin B$_{12}$ (pg./ml.[d,e])			
	All ages	<100	100–149	≥150+
Vitamin C	Serum vitamin C (mg./100 ml.[d])			
	≥1 yr.	<0.20	0.2–0.29	≥0.3

[f] From: ICNND Manual for Nutrition Surveys, 2nd ed. Washington, D.C., U.S. Government Printing Office, 1963.
[g] Erythrocyte glutamic oxalacetic transaminase.
[h] Erythrocyte glutamic pyruvic transaminase.

APPENDIX TABLE 19   TRICEPS SKINFOLD THICKNESS STANDARDS

(A) Triceps Skinfold, Birth to 60 Months, Sexes Separate*

TRICEPS SKINFOLD *(mm.)*

AGE *(mo.)*	STANDARD M	STANDARD F	90% STANDARD M	90% STANDARD F	80% STANDARD M	80% STANDARD F	70% STANDARD M	70% STANDARD F	60% STANDARD M	60% STANDARD F
Birth	6.0	6.5	5.4	5.9	4.8	5.2	4.2	4.6	3.6	3.9
6	10.0	10.0	9.0	9.0	8.0	8.0	7.0	7.0	6.0	6.0
12	10.3	10.2	9.3	9.2	8.2	8.2	7.2	7.1	6.2	6.1
18	10.3	10.2	9.3	9.2	8.2	8.2	7.2	7.1	6.2	6.1
24	10.0	10.1	9.0	9.1	8.0	8.1	7.0	7.1	6.0	6.1
36	9.3	9.7	8.4	8.7	7.5	7.8	6.5	6.8	5.6	5.8
48	9.3	10.2	8.4	9.2	7.5	8.2	6.5	7.2	5.6	6.1
60	9.1	9.4	8.2	8.5	7.3	7.5	6.4	6.6	5.5	5.7

(B) Triceps Skinfold, 5–15 Years, Sexes Separate*

TRICEPS SKINFOLD *(mm.)*

AGE *(yr.)*	STANDARD M	STANDARD F	90% STANDARD M	90% STANDARD F	80% STANDARD M	80% STANDARD F	70% STANDARD M	70% STANDARD F	60% STANDARD M	60% STANDARD F
5	9.1	9.4	8.2	8.5	7.3	7.5	6.4	6.6	5.5	5.7
6	8.2	9.6	7.4	8.6	6.6	7.7	5.8	6.7	4.9	5.8
7	7.9	9.4	7.1	8.5	6.3	7.5	5.5	6.6	4.7	5.7
8	7.6	10.1	6.8	9.1	6.1	8.1	5.3	7.1	4.5	6.1
9	8.2	10.3	7.4	9.2	6.6	8.2	5.8	7.2	4.9	6.2
10	8.2	10.4	7.4	9.3	6.6	8.3	5.7	7.3	4.9	6.2
11	8.9	10.6	8.1	9.6	7.2	8.5	6.3	7.5	5.4	6.4
12	8.5	10.1	7.6	9.1	6.8	8.1	5.9	7.0	5.1	6.0
13	8.1	10.4	7.3	9.4	6.5	8.3	5.7	7.3	4.9	6.2
14	7.9	11.3	7.1	10.1	6.3	9.0	5.5	7.9	4.8	6.8
15	6.3	11.4	5.7	10.2	5.0	9.1	4.4	8.0	3.8	6.8

(C) Triceps Skinfold, Adults, Sexes Separate**

TRICEPS SKINFOLD *(mm.)*

SEX	STANDARD	90% STANDARD	80% STANDARD	70% STANDARD	60% STANDARD
Male	12.5	11.3	10.0	8.8	7.5
Female	16.5	14.9	13.2	11.6	9.9

*From: Hammond, W. H.: Body measurements of pre-school children. Br. J. Prev. Soc. Med., *9*:152, 1955; and Tanner, J. M., and Whitehouse, R. H.: Standards for subcutaneous fat in British children. Br. Med. J., *1*:446, 1962.

**From: Jelliffe, D. B.: The Assessment of the Nutritional Status of the Community. WHO Monograph No. 53. Geneva, WHO, 1966, p. 227.

APPENDIX TABLE 20   ARM CIRCUMFERENCE STANDARDS

(A) Arm Circumference, 1–60 Months, Sexes Separate*

ARM CIRCUMFERENCE (cm.)

AGE (mo.)	STANDARD M	F	90% STANDARD M	F	80% STANDARD M	F	70% STANDARD M	F	60% STANDARD M	F
1	11.5	11.1	10.3	10.0	9.2	8.9	8.0	7.8	6.9	6.7
2	12.5	12.0	11.2	10.8	10.0	9.6	8.7	8.4	7.5	7.2
3	12.7	13.3	11.4	12.0	10.2	10.6	8.9	9.3	7.6	8.0
4	14.6	13.5	13.2	12.1	11.7	10.8	10.2	9.4	8.8	8.1
5	14.7	13.9	13.2	12.5	11.7	11.1	10.3	9.7	8.8	8.3
6	14.5	14.3	13.1	12.9	11.6	11.5	10.2	10.0	8.7	8.6
7	15.0	14.6	13.5	13.2	12.0	11.7	10.5	10.2	9.0	8.8
8	15.5	15.0	14.0	13.5	12.4	12.0	10.9	10.5	9.3	9.0
9	15.8	15.3	14.2	13.7	12.6	12.2	11.0	10.7	9.5	9.2
10	15.8	15.4	14.2	13.8	12.6	12.3	11.1	10.8	9.5	9.2
11	15.8	15.5	14.3	14.0	12.7	12.4	11.1	10.9	9.5	9.3
12	16.0	15.6	14.4	14.0	12.8	12.5	11.2	10.9	9.6	9.4
15	16.1	15.7	14.5	14.1	12.9	12.5	11.3	11.0	9.7	9.4
18	15.7	16.1	14.1	14.5	12.5	12.9	11.0	11.3	9.4	9.7
21	16.2	15.9	14.6	14.3	13.0	12.7	11.4	11.1	9.7	9.6
24	16.3	15.9	14.7	14.4	13.0	12.8	11.4	11.2	9.8	9.6
27	16.6	16.4	15.0	14.7	13.3	13.1	11.7	11.5	10.0	9.8
30	16.4	16.4	14.8	14.8	13.1	13.1	11.5	11.5	9.9	9.8
33	16.4	16.1	14.8	14.5	13.1	12.9	11.5	11.3	9.8	9.7
36	16.2	15.9	14.6	14.3	13.0	12.7	11.3	11.1	9.7	9.6
39	16.9	17.4	15.2	15.7	13.5	14.0	11.8	12.2	10.1	10.5
42	16.5	16.3	15.0	14.7	13.2	13.1	11.6	11.4	9.9	9.8
45	16.7	16.8	15.0	15.1	13.4	13.5	11.7	11.8	10.0	10.1
48	16.9	16.9	15.2	15.2	13.5	13.5	11.8	11.8	10.1	10.2
51	17.2	16.8	15.5	15.1	13.8	13.4	12.0	11.7	10.3	10.1
54	17.5	16.6	15.7	15.0	14.0	13.3	12.2	11.7	10.5	10.0
57	17.2	16.8	15.5	15.1	13.8	13.4	12.1	11.7	10.4	10.1
60	17.0	16.9	15.3	15.2	13.6	13.5	11.9	11.8	10.2	10.1

(B) Arm Circumference, 6–17 Years, Sexes Separate**

ARM CIRCUMFERENCE (cm.)

AGE (yr.)	STANDARD M	F	90% STANDARD M	F	80% STANDARD M	F	70% STANDARD M	F	60% STANDARD M	F
6	17.3	17.3	15.6	15.5	13.8	13.8	12.1	12.1	10.4	10.4
7	17.8	17.8	16.0	16.0	14.2	14.2	12.5	12.5	10.7	10.7
8	18.4	18.4	16.5	16.6	14.7	14.7	12.9	12.9	11.0	11.1
9	19.0	19.1	17.1	17.2	15.2	15.3	13.3	13.4	11.4	11.5
10	19.7	19.9	17.7	17.9	15.8	15.9	13.8	13.9	11.8	11.9
11	20.4	20.7	18.4	18.6	16.3	16.5	14.3	14.5	12.2	12.4
12	21.2	21.5	19.1	19.3	16.9	17.2	14.8	15.0	12.7	12.9
13	22.2	22.4	20.0	20.2	17.7	17.9	15.5	15.7	13.3	13.4
14	23.2	23.2	20.9	20.9	18.6	18.5	16.3	16.2	13.9	13.9
15	25.0	24.4	22.5	22.0	20.0	19.5	17.5	17.1	15.0	14.6
16	26.0	24.7	23.4	22.2	20.8	19.7	18.2	17.3	15.6	14.8
17	26.8	24.9	24.1	22.3	21.4	19.9	18.8	17.4	16.1	14.9

*From: Wolanski (personal communication with D. B. Jelliffe), 1964. In: Jelliffe, D. B.: The Assessment of the Nutritional Status of the Community. WHO Monograph No. 53. Geneva, WHO, 1966.

**Adapted from: O'Brien, R., Girshik, M. A., and Hunt, E. D.: Body Measurements of American Boys and Girls for Garment and Pattern Construction. USDA Misc. Publ. No. 454. Washington, D.C., U.S. Government Printing Office, 1941.

Table continued on the following page

APPENDIX TABLE 20   ARM CIRCUMFERENCE STANDARDS (*Continued*)

*(C) Arm Circumference, Adults, Sexes Separate***

	ARM CIRCUMFERENCE (*cm.*)				
SEX	STANDARD	90% STANDARD	80% STANDARD	70% STANDARD	60% STANDARD
Male	29.3	26.3	23.4	20.5	17.6
Female	28.5	25.7	22.8	20.0	17.1

***Adapted from: Hertzberg, H. T., et al.: Anthropometric Survey of Turkey and Greece. Oxford, England, Pergamon Press, 1963.

APPENDIX TABLE 21   MID-ARM MUSCLE CIRCUMFERENCE STANDARDS*

(A) Mid-Arm Muscle Circumference, 6–60 Months, Sexes Separate

MID-ARM MUSCLE CIRCUMFERENCE (cm.)

AGE (mo.)	STANDARD M	STANDARD F	90% STANDARD M	90% STANDARD F	80% STANDARD M	80% STANDARD F	70% STANDARD M	70% STANDARD F	60% STANDARD M	60% STANDARD F
6	11.4	11.2	10.3	10.1	9.1	9.0	8.0	7.8	6.8	6.7
12	12.7	12.4	11.4	11.2	10.2	9.9	8.9	8.7	7.6	7.4
18	12.9	12.5	11.6	11.3	10.3	10.1	9.0	8.8	7.7	7.6
24	13.1	12.8	11.8	11.5	10.5	10.2	9.2	9.0	7.9	7.7
36	13.3	12.9	12.0	11.6	10.3	10.3	9.3	9.0	8.0	7.7
48	14.0	13.7	12.6	12.3	11.2	11.0	9.8	9.6	8.4	8.2
60	14.1	13.9	12.7	12.5	11.3	11.1	9.9	9.7	8.5	8.3

(B) Mid-Arm Muscle Circumference, 6–15 Years, Sexes Separate

MUSCLE CIRCUMFERENCE (cm.)

AGE (yr.)	STANDARD M	STANDARD F	90% STANDARD M	90% STANDARD F	80% STANDARD M	80% STANDARD F	70% STANDARD M	70% STANDARD F	60% STANDARD M	60% STANDARD F
6	14.7	14.2	13.2	12.8	11.8	11.4	10.3	9.9	8.8	8.5
7	15.3	14.8	13.8	13.3	12.2	11.8	10.7	10.4	9.2	8.9
8	16.0	15.3	14.4	13.8	12.8	12.2	11.2	10.7	9.6	9.2
9	16.5	15.9	14.9	14.3	13.2	12.7	11.6	11.1	9.9	9.5
10	17.1	16.6	15.4	14.9	13.7	13.3	12.0	11.6	10.3	10.0
11	17.6	17.3	15.8	15.6	14.1	14.1	12.3	12.1	10.6	10.4
12	18.5	18.3	16.6	16.5	14.8	14.6	12.9	12.8	11.1	11.0
13	19.6	19.1	17.6	17.2	15.7	15.3	13.7	13.4	11.8	11.5
14	20.8	19.6	18.7	17.6	16.6	15.7	14.6	13.7	12.5	11.8
15	23.0	20.8	20.7	18.7	18.4	16.6	16.1	14.6	13.8	12.5

(C) Mid-Arm Muscle Circumference, Adults, Sexes Separate

MUSCLE CIRCUMFERENCE (cm.)

SEX	STANDARD	90% STANDARD	80% STANDARD	70% STANDARD	60% STANDARD
Male	25.3	22.8	20.2	17.7	15.2
Female	23.2	20.9	18.6	16.2	13.9

*From: Jelliffe, D. B.: The Assessment of the Nutritional Status of the Community. WHO Monograph No. 53. Geneva, WHO, 1966.

APPENDIX TABLE 22   LEVELS OF NUTRITIONAL ASSESSMENT FOR ADULTS*

LEVEL OF AP-PROACH	HISTORY			CLINICAL EVALUATION	LABORATORY EVALUATION
	DIETARY	MEDICAL AND SOCIOECONOMIC			
Minimal	1. Meals eaten per day, week; regularity 2. Frequency of ingestion of protective foods (four food groups) 3. Supplemental vitamins, protein concentrates, mineral mixes 4. General knowledge of nutrition, sources of information	1. Chronic illness and/or disability; occupational hazard exposure; use of tobacco, alcohol, drugs 2. Symptoms such as bleeding, fainting, loss of memory, dyspnea, headache, pain, changed bowel and/or bladder habits, altered sight and/or hearing, condition of teeth and/or dentures 3. Therapy (prescribed or self-administered) such as drugs, alcohol, vitamins, food fads, prescription items, eyeglasses, hearing aids 4. Names, addresses and phone numbers of persons providing medical or health care; close family or friends 5. Lives alone, with spouse or with companion 6. Sources of income		1. Height and weight; cachexia; obesity 2. Blood pressure, pulse rate and rhythm 3. Pallor, skin color and texture 4. Condition of teeth and/or dentures and oral hygiene 5. Affect during interview and examination 6. Vision and hearing appraised subjectively and objectively by examiner 7. Any gross evidence of neglect	1. Hemoglobin 2. Blood and/or urine sugar levels 3. Urinalysis (color, odor, bile and sediment by gross inspection; pH, glucose, albumin blood, and ketones by stick test) 4. Feces (color, texture, gross blood; occult blood by guaiac test)
Mid-level	In addition to the above: 1. Food preferences and rejections 2. Overt food fads 3. Meal preparation facilities and knowledge 4. Food budget 5. Usual daily diet: Protective foods (meats, dairy products, fruits and vegetables, cereals); Nutrients (protein, fat, carbohydrates, iron, water and fat-soluble vitamins, min-	In addition to the above: 1. Family history of spouse, parents and siblings, other relatives, persons living in same household 2. Pain: location, frequency, character, duration 3. Mental status: attitudes, fears, prejudices, symptoms of psychoses, possible psychosomatic symptoms and signs 4. Income: amount and adequacy for nutrition, housing,		In addition include: 1. Head and neck examinations (otoscopic, opthalmoscopic, dental and oral cavity, nose and throat) 2. Chest (inspection, palpation, auscultation and percussion, bi-manual examination of breast tissue) 3. Abdomen (inspection, auscultation, percussion and palpation) 4. Rectal and pelvic	In addition include: 1. Serum lipids (including beta-lipoproteins) 2. Serum iron and iron-binding capacity 3. Urinalysis 4. Electrocardiogram 5. Peripheral blood smear for differential white blood cell count and red cell morphology 6. Chest film 7. Post-voiding residual urine by catheterization (if indicated)

erals, trace elements and water); *Empty-calorie food* (alcohol, candy, sucrose)	health, utilities, clothing, transportation, etc.	5. Inspection and palpation of extremities (evaluation for temperature, edema, pulse, discoloration, ulcers) 6. Gross neurological evaluation; motor and sensory	If indicated, include: 1. Serum total protein and albumin; serum creatinine and/or blood urea nitrogen (BUN) levels 2. Roentgenographic evaluation of bones and joints suspected of being fractured, harboring infection and affected by rheumatic and/or metabolic bone disease and/or metastatic or primary neoplastic disease 3. Glucose tolerance tests 4. Blood and/or urine vitamin assays for water-soluble and fat-soluble vitamins 5. Trace element assays of blood, urine, and/or tissue 6. Kidney-ureter-bladder (KUB) film for stones in urinary tract or gallbladder 7. Bacteriological cultures of any chronic infections 8. Barium enema, upper gastrointestinal series, gallbladder series and intravenous pyelography 9. Fluoroscopy of chest 10. Angiography for coronary arteries, aorta, peripheral vessels 11. Bone marrow for unexplained anemia 12. Renal clearance studies 13. Histological evaluation of biopsies of tissue suspected of being neoplastic
In-depth	In addition include: 1. 24-hour dietary recall, preferably for each of several widely separated days; analysis of nutrient intake; evaluation of adequacy, e.g., relate to activity, body weight, laboratory data, affect, etc. 2. History of past and present food preparation and practices 3. History of dining practices and facilities, including companionship	In addition include: 1. System review 2. Social history 3. Economic history including specifics on sources and amounts of income 4. Mental evaluation (attitudes toward aging)	If indicated, include: 1. Complete sensory and motor neurological examination 2. Sigmoidoscopy 3. Ophthalmologic examination (ophthalmoscopic examination with pupils dilated, refraction, dark adaptation, color perception, visual field examination) 4. Audiometry	

*From Christakis, G. (ed.): Nutritional Assessment in Health Programs. Washington, D.C., American Public Health Association, Inc. 1973, p. 34.

APPENDIX TABLE 23   LEVELS OF NUTRITIONAL ASSESSMENT FOR INFANTS AND CHILDREN*

(A) Birth to 24 Months

| LEVEL OF AP-PROACH[a] | HISTORY | | CLINICAL EVALUATION | LABORATORY EVALUATION |
	DIETARY	MEDICAL AND SOCIOECONOMIC		
Minimal	1. Source of iron 2. Vitamin supplement 3. Milk intake (type and amount)	1. Birth weight 2. Length of gestation 3. Serious or chronic illness 4. Use of medicines	1. Body weight and length 2. Gross defects	1. Hematocrit 2. Hemoglobin
Mid-level	1. Semi-quantitative a) Iron-cereal, meat, egg yolks, supplement b) Energy nutrients c) Micronutrients—calcium, niacin, riboflavin, vitamin C d) Protein 2. Food intolerances 3. Baby foods—processed commercially; home cooked	1. Family history: Diabetes Tuberculosis 2. Maternal: Height Prenatal care 3. Infant: Immunizations Tuberculin test	1. Head circumference 2. Skin color, pallor, turgor 3. Subcutaneous tissue paucity, excess	1. RBC morphology 2. Serum iron 3. Total iron-binding capacity 4. Sickle cell testing
In depth	1. Quantitative 24-hour recall 2. Dietary history	1. Prenatal details 2. Complications of delivery 3. Regular health supervision	1. Cranial bossing 2. Epiphyseal enlargement 3. Costochondral beading 4. Ecchymoses	Same as above, plus vitamin and appropriate enzyme assays; protein and amino acids; hydroxyproline, etc., should be available

(B) Ages 2 to 5 Years

	Determine amount of intake	Probe about pica; medications	Add height at all levels Add arm circumference at all levels Add triceps skinfolds at in-depth level	Add serum lead at mid-level; Add serum micronutrients (vitamins A, C, folate, etc.) at in-depth level

(C) Ages 6 to 12 Years

	Probe about snack foods; determine whether salt intake is excessive	Ask about medications taken; drug abuse	Add blood pressure at mid-level Add description of changes in tongue, skin, eyes for in-depth level	All of above plus BUN level

*From: Christakis, G. (ed.): Nutritional Assessment in Health Programs, Washington, D.C., American Public Health Association, Inc., 1973, p. 46.

[a]It is understood that what is included at a minimal level would also be included or represented at successively more sophisticated levels of approach. However, it may be entirely appropriate to use a minimal level of approach to clinical evaluations and a maximal approach to laboratory evaluations.

APPENDIX 24

BOYS: BIRTH TO 36 MONTHS
PHYSICAL GROWTH
NCHS PERCENTILES*

NAME _____   RECORD # _____

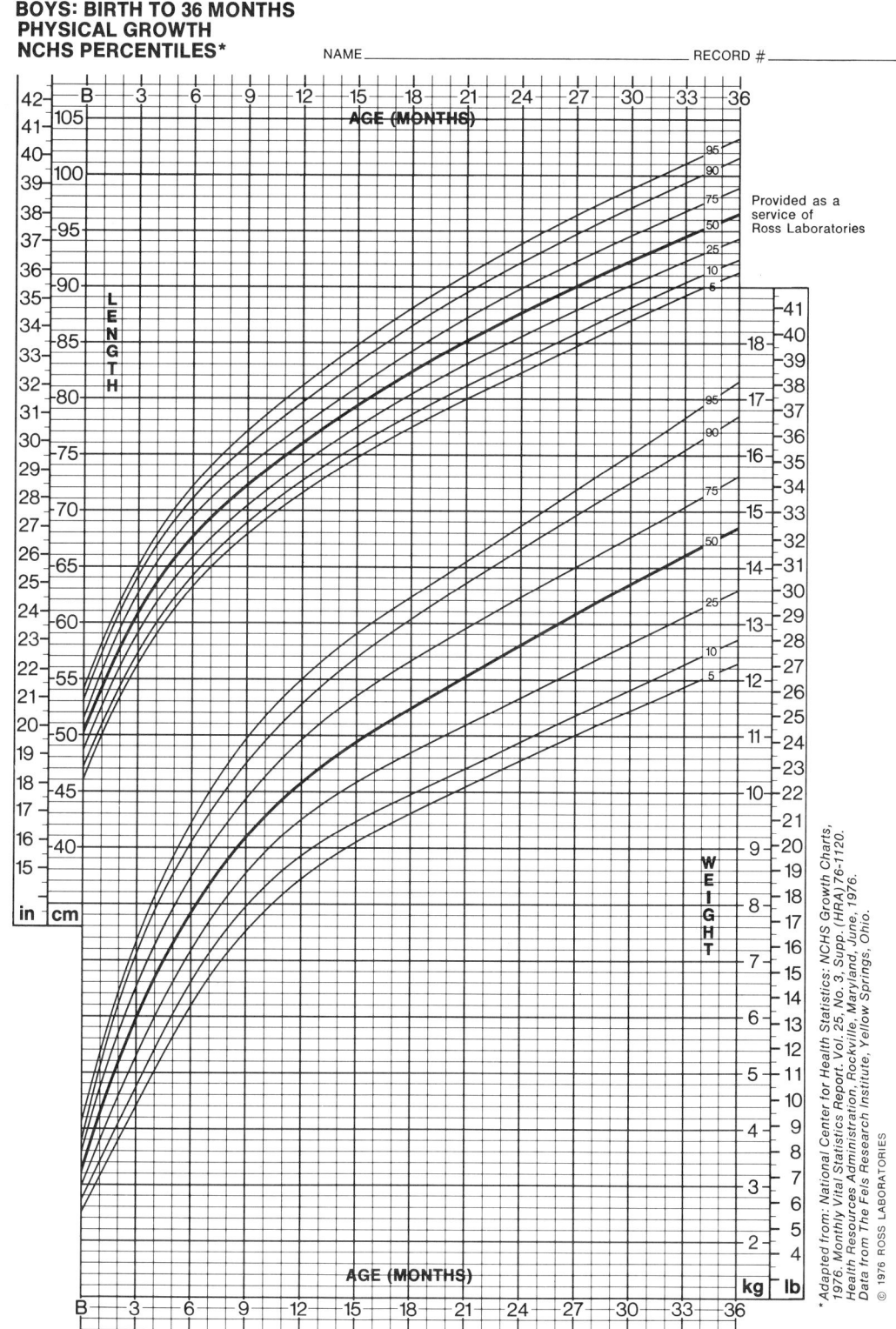

Provided as a
service of
Ross Laboratories

* Adapted from: National Center for Health Statistics: NCHS Growth Charts,
1976. Monthly Vital Statistics Report. Vol. 25, No. 3, Supp. (HRA) 76-1120.
Health Resources Administration, Rockville, Maryland, June, 1976.
Data from The Fels Research Institute, Yellow Springs, Ohio.

APPENDIX 25

BOYS: BIRTH TO 36 MONTHS
PHYSICAL GROWTH
NCHS PERCENTILES* NAME _____ RECORD # _____

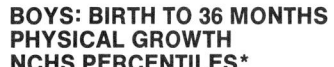

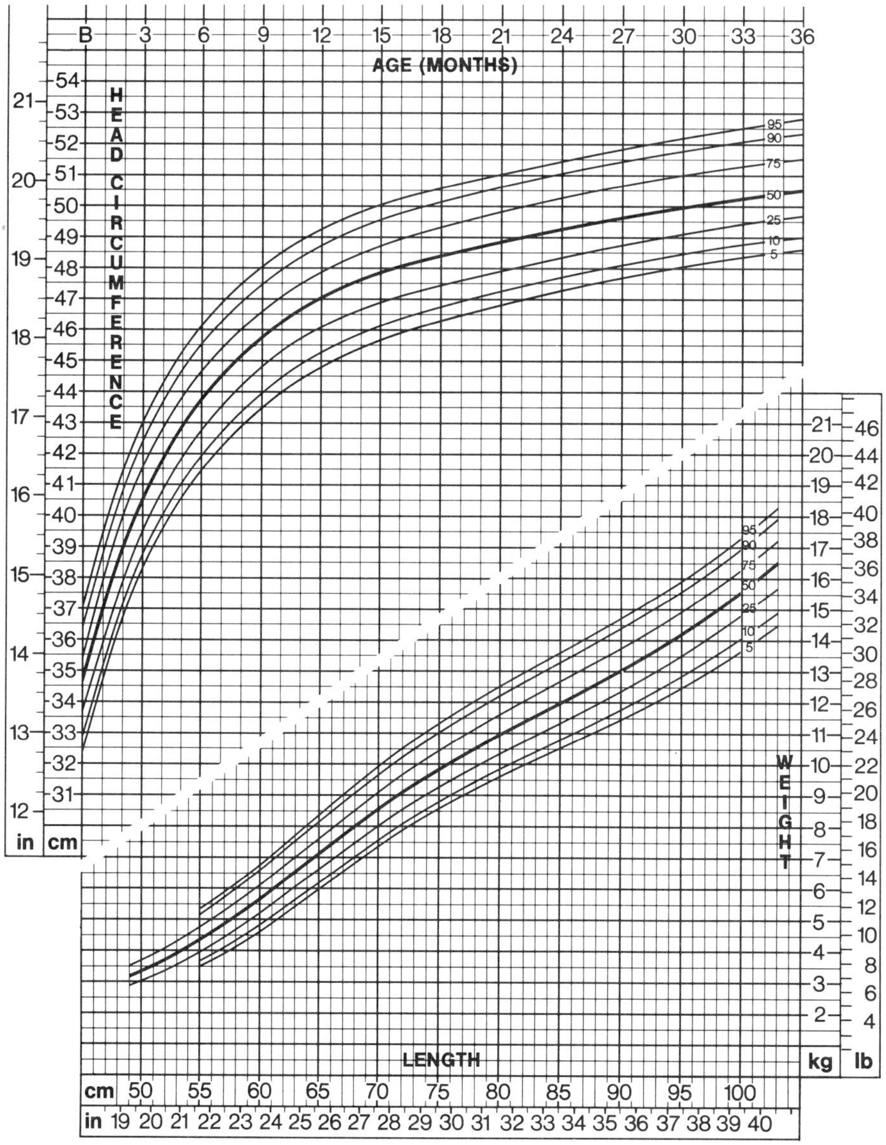

AGE (MONTHS)

HEAD CIRCUMFERENCE

LENGTH

WEIGHT

*Adapted from: National Center for Health Statistics: NCHS Growth Charts, 1976. Monthly Vital Statistics Report. Vol. 25, No. 3, Supp. (HRA)76-1120. Health Resources Administration, Rockville, Maryland, June, 1976. Data from The Fels Research Institute, Yellow Springs, Ohio.

© 1976 ROSS LABORATORIES

DATE	AGE	LENGTH	WEIGHT	HEAD C.
	BIRTH			

DATE	AGE	LENGTH	WEIGHT	HEAD C.

APPENDIX 26

**GIRLS: BIRTH TO 36 MONTHS
PHYSICAL GROWTH
NCHS PERCENTILES***

NAME_____ RECORD #_____

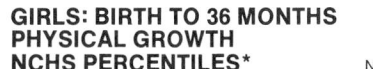

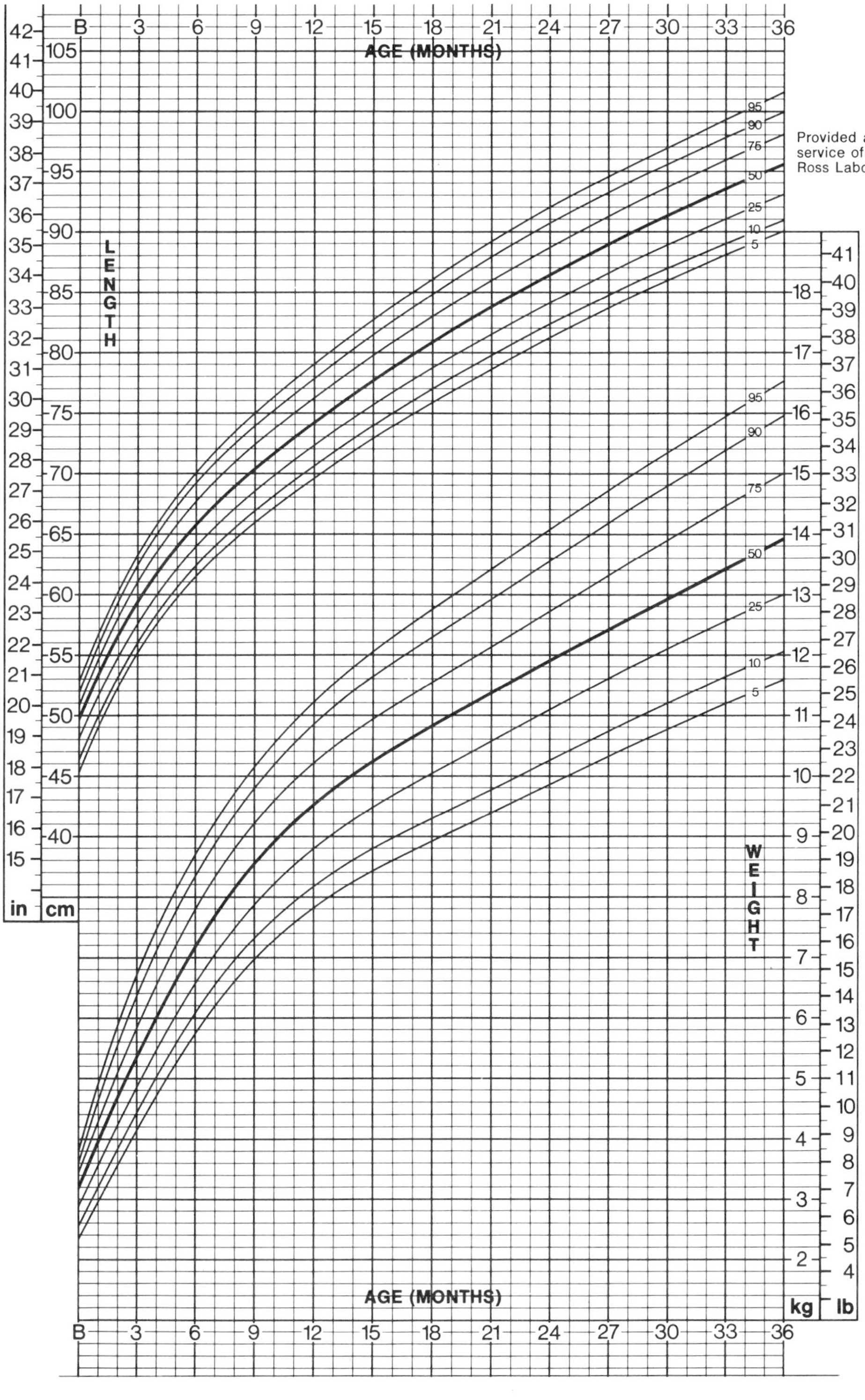

Provided as a
service of
Ross Laboratories

*Adapted from: National Center for Health Statistics: NCHS Growth Charts, 1976. Monthly Vital Statistics Report. Vol. 25, No. 3, Supp. (HRA) 76-1120. Health Resources Administration, Rockville, Maryland, June, 1976. Data from The Fels Research Institute, Yellow Springs, Ohio.

APPENDIX 27

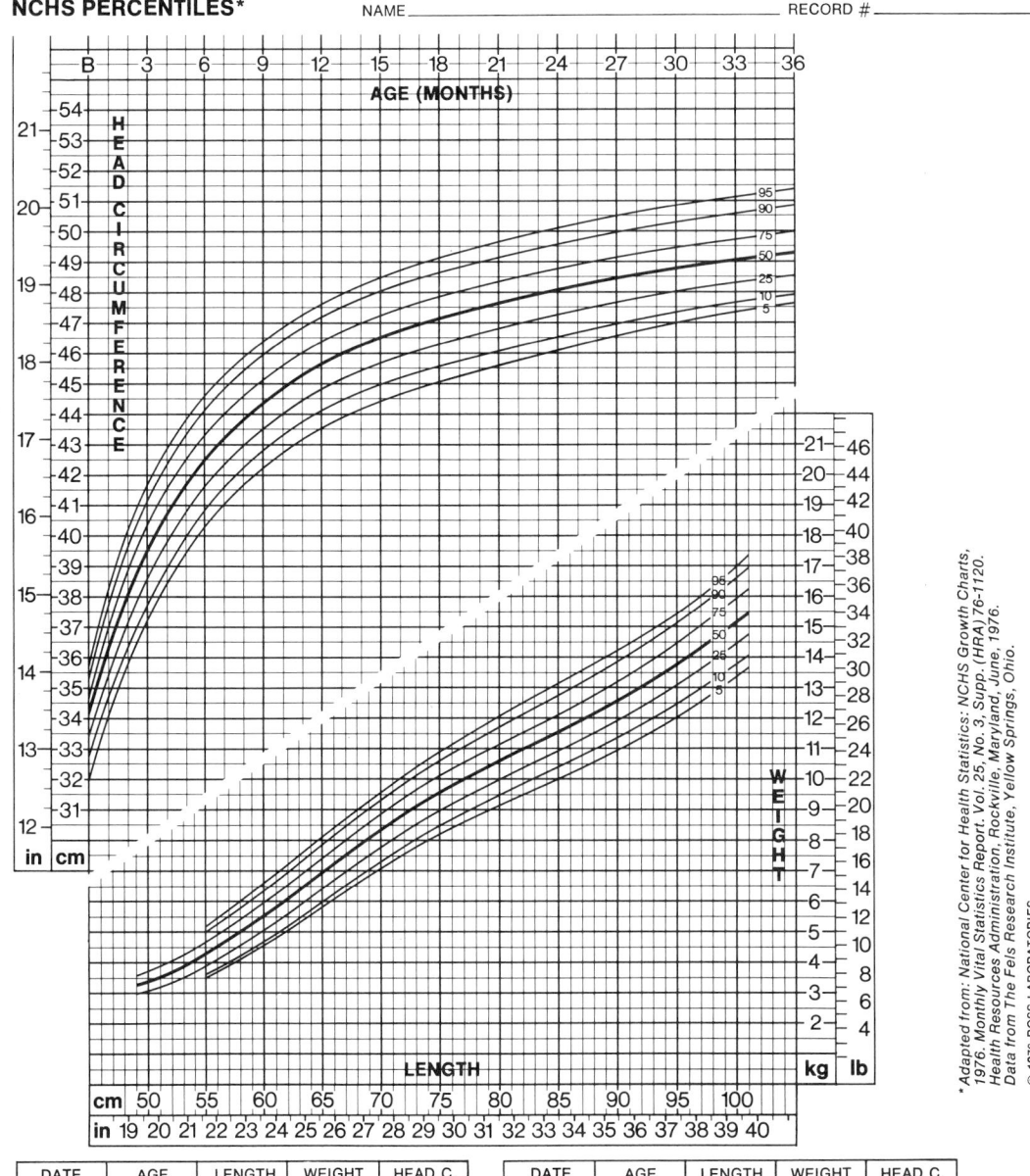

**GIRLS: BIRTH TO 36 MONTHS
PHYSICAL GROWTH
NCHS PERCENTILES***

NAME_____ RECORD #_____

*Adapted from: National Center for Health Statistics: NCHS Growth Charts, 1976. Monthly Vital Statistics Report. Vol. 25, No. 3, Supp. (HRA) 76-1120. Health Resources Administration, Rockville, Maryland, June, 1976. Data from The Fels Research Institute, Yellow Springs, Ohio.

© 1976 ROSS LABORATORIES

DATE	AGE	LENGTH	WEIGHT	HEAD C.		DATE	AGE	LENGTH	WEIGHT	HEAD C.
	BIRTH									

APPENDIX 28 ARM ANTHROPOMETRY FOR ADULTS

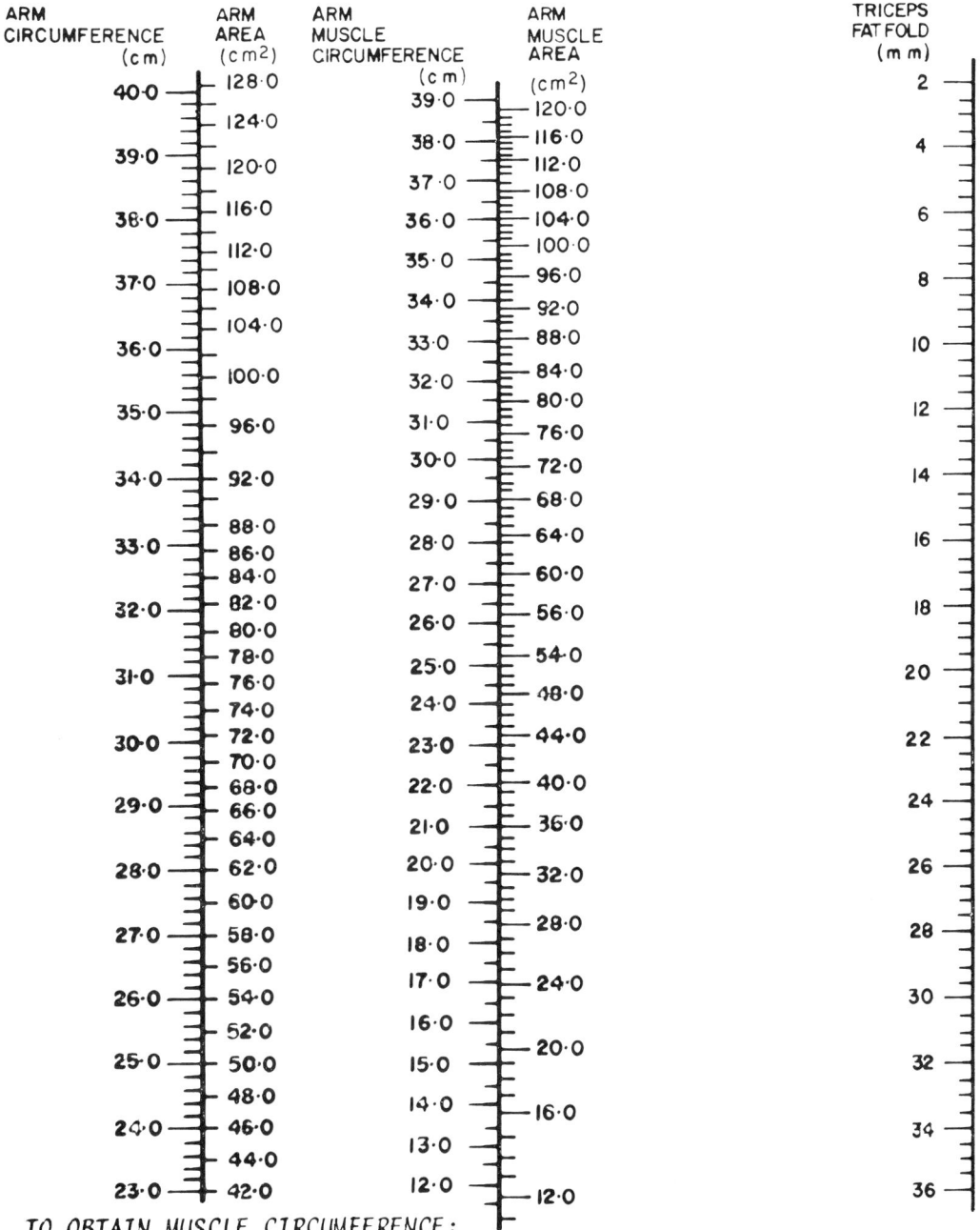

TO OBTAIN MUSCLE CIRCUMFERENCE:
1. LAY RULER BETWEEN VALUE OF ARM CIRCUMFERENCE AND FATFOLD
2. READ OFF MUSCLE CIRCUMFERENCE ON MIDDLE LINE

TO OBTAIN TISSUE AREAS:
1. THE ARM AREA AND MUSCLE AREA ARE ALONGSIDE THEIR
   RESPECTIVE CIRCUMFERENCES
2. FAT AREA = ARM AREA-MUSCLE AREA

(From: Gurney, J. M., and Jelliffe, D. B.: Arm anthropometry in nutritional assessment: nomogram for rapid calculation of muscle circumference and cross-sectional muscle fat areas. Am. J. Clin. Nutr., 26:912, 1973.)

APPENDIX 29   ARM ANTHROPOMETRY FOR CHILDREN

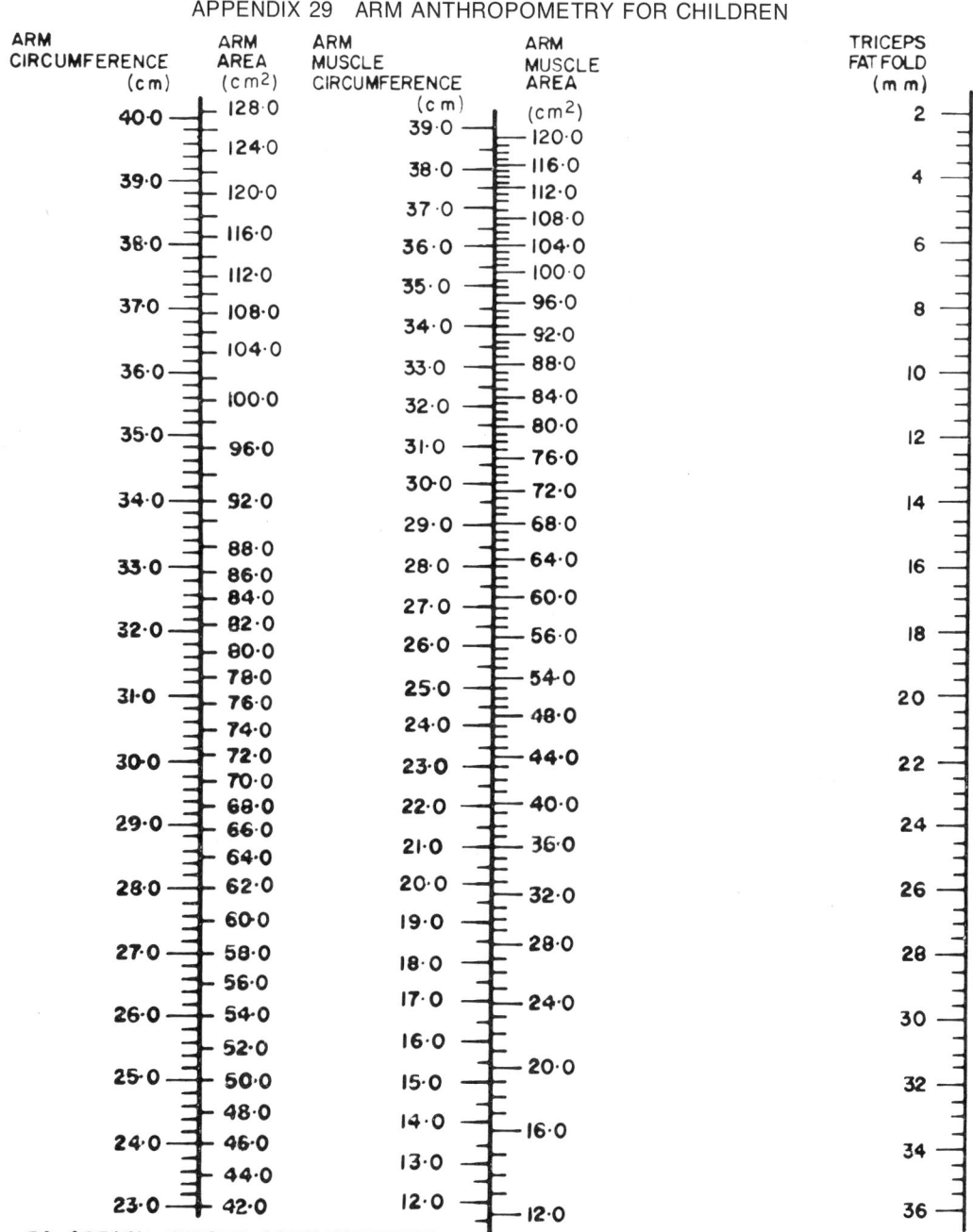

| ARM CIRCUMFERENCE (cm) | ARM AREA (cm²) | ARM MUSCLE CIRCUMFERENCE (cm) | ARM MUSCLE AREA (cm²) | TRICEPS FAT FOLD (mm) |

TO OBTAIN MUSCLE CIRCUMFERENCE:
1. LAY RULER BETWEEN VALUE OF ARM CIRCUMFERENCE AND FATFOLD
2. READ OFF MUSCLE CIRCUMFERENCE ON MIDDLE LINE

TO OBTAIN TISSUE AREAS:
1. THE ARM AREA AND MUSCLE AREA ARE ALONGSIDE THEIR RESPECTIVE CIRCUMFERENCES
2. FAT AREA = ARM AREA-MUSCLE AREA

(From: Gurney, J. M., and Jelliffe, D. B.: Arm anthropometry in nutritional assessment: nomogram for rapid calculation of muscle circumference and cross-sectional muscle fat areas. Am. J. Clin. Nutr., 26:912, 1973.)

APPENDIX 30   PHYSICAL SIGNS AND NUTRITIONAL TERMS ASSOCIATED WITH MALNUTRITION*

GENERAL APPEARANCE

Apathy. Unreactive, unresponsive, disinterested and inattentive to surroundings.

Clinical Marasmus. Evidence of pronounced wasting of subcutaneous fat without edema. Significant apathy may be present. Frequently the face and eyes of the child may appear unusually bright due to the combination of wasting and prominence of the eyes. The child is usually considerably underdeveloped in relation to age, and there may or may not be associated hair changes such as dyspigmentation, thinness, ease in plucking or signs of avitaminosis.

Irritability. Hyperresponsive; excessive or overreaction to minor stimuli, particularly manifest through crying or unusual indication of fear as a result of minor or relatively insignificant happenings.

Kwashiorkor. Pitting edema at least on the pretibial region; underweight, undersize, underdeveloped for age. Muscular wasting may be present but masked by edema. Apathy of some degree is present. Changes in the hair are usually noted, such as thinning, easily pluckable with dyspigmentation or flag sign, and change in texture to silken, sparse hair. Dermatosis with desquamation of the so-called flaky-paint type, with or without hyperpigmentation. In severe cases the dermatosis may resemble a relatively severe burn but lacks erythema.

Pallor. Paleness and loss of color of skin, nail beds, mucosa and lips.

Pre-kwashiorkor. An underweight, undersized, underdeveloped child, without the evident pronounced wasting present in marasmus. Child is thin and undersized but has relatively normal body proportions and rather poor muscle tone, and hair changes may be present. Not apathetic, though would not be described as alert.

HAIR

Dry Staring. Dry, wirelike, unkempt, stiff hair, often brittle, sometimes may exhibit some bleaching of the normal color.

Dyspigmentation. Definite change from normal pigment of the hair, most usually evident distally and best seen by carefully combing hair strands upward and viewing the orderly array of hair in good light. Dyspigmentation includes both change of pigment (usually lightening of color) and depigmentation. Not to be confused with dyed or tinted hair. Dyspigmentation is often bandlike in character and usually is associated with some change in texture

of hair in the depigmented band. In some ethnic groups, particularly among Negroid groups, the pigment may be slightly reddish in color. In others, especially among straight black-haired peoples, the bandlike depigmentation (''flag sign'') is common.

Easily Pluckable. Easily pluckable hair is that in which the shafts are readily removed with minimum tug when a few strands are grasped between the finger and thumb and gently pulled. In such cases there is a lack of reaction of the child, indicating a lack of pain associated with removing of the hair.

SKIN

Crackled Skin. Definite scales larger in size than those seen in xerosis. It is often congenital and is most prominent in cool weather. It is non-nutritional in origin.

Dependent Edema. The presence of abnormally large amounts of fluid in the intercellular tissue spaces of the body; usually applied to demonstrable accumulation of excessive fluid in the subcutaneous tissues that are dependent upon position and gravity.

Dermatitis with Desquamation, or Crazy-pavement Type. Under this heading should be recorded those desquamating changes of the skin, usually with increased pigmentation, that occur on the extremities, especially legs, thighs and buttocks, but may occur over the trunk in association with kwashiorkor. (These have been termed ''flaky-paint'' dermatoses.) Small, circumscribed bleblike lesions are sometimes seen in association with kwashiorkor and on occasion may precede the desquamation. In addition, any ''crazy-pavement'' type of lesions observed should be noted. These are characterized by a thin-appearing epithelium marked by striations usually resembling in outline the microscopic picture of epithelial cells. Not to be confused, however, with ichthyosis (scaly skin).

Follicular Hyperkeratosis. This lesion has been likened to the ''gooseflesh'' that is seen on chilling, but it is not generalized and does not disappear with brisk rubbing of the skin. Readily felt, as it presents a ''nutmeg grater'' feel. Follicular hyperkeratosis is more readily detected by the sense of touch than by the eye. The skin is rough, with papillae formed by keratotic plugs that project from the hair follicles. The surrounding skin is dry and lacks the usual amount of moisture or oiliness. Differentiation from adolescent folliculosis can usually be made through recognition of the normal skin between the follicles in the adolescent disorder. It is distinguished from perifolliculosis by the ring of capillary congestion that occurs about each follicle in scorbutic perifolliculosis.

Pellagrous Dermatitis. Symmetrical lesions typical of acute or chronic, mild or severe pellagra are observed; lesions are usually red, often swollen or blistered like sunburn, pigmented, scaly over

---

*From: Christakis, G. (ed.): Nutritional Assessment in Health Programs. Washington, D.C., American Public Health Association, Inc., 1973, pp. 26–27.

exposed areas, clearly demarcated from normal skin.

Purpura or Petechia. Small localized extravasations of blood, red or purplish in color, depending on time elapsed since formation. Usually distributed at sites of pressure, and may be perifollicular.

Xerosis. Xerosis is a clinical term used to describe a dry and crinkled skin that is accentuated by pushing the skin parallel to its surface. In more pronounced cases it is often mottled and pigmented and may appear as scaly or alligator-like pseudoplaques, usually not greater than 0.5 cm. in diameter. Nutritional significance is not established. Differential diagnosis must be made from changes due to dirt and exposure and ichthyosis.

SKELETAL

Bowleg. An outward curve of one or both legs at or below the knee (genu varum).

Costochondral Beading. Palpable and visible enlargement of the costochondral junctions.

Cranial Bossing. Abnormal prominence or protrusion of frontal or parietal areas.

Enlarged Joints. When the more obvious ends of long bones are enlarged; i.e., the wrist, ankles, knees.

Winged Scapula. A scapula having a prominent vertebral border.

MUSCLE

Muscle Wasting. Appearance indicates abnormal loss of muscle substance, as exhibited by unusual prominence of bony skeleton, undue degree of folding of the skin of the buttocks, or the abnormal flabby feel (sometimes described as jellylike) of the child with poor muscle tone.

EYES

Bitot's Spots. Bitot's spots are small, circumscribed grayish or yellowish gray, dull, dry, foamy superficial lesions of the conjunctiva. They most often occur on the lateral aspect of the bulbar conjunctiva in the interpalpebral area. Do not confuse with pterygium.

Blepharitis. Inflammation of eyelids.

Keratomalacia. Softening of the cornea.

Thickened Opaque Bulbar Conjunctivae. All degrees of thickening may occur. The blueness of the sclera may disappear and the bulbar conjunctivae develop a wrinkled appearance with increase in vascularity. The thickened conjunctivae may result in a glazed, porcelain-like appearance, obscuring the vascularity.

Xerosis Conjunctivae. The conjunctivae, upon exposure by holding the lids open and having the subject rotate the eyes, appear dull and lusterless and exhibit a striated or roughened surface.

FACE

Angular Lesions. Present bilaterally when mouth is held half open. May appear as pink or moist whitish macerated angular lesions that blur the mucocutaneous junction. Angular fissures are recorded when there is definite break in continuity of epithelium at the angles of the mouth.

Angular Scars. Scars at the angles that, if recent, may be pink; if old, may appear blanched.

Cheilosis. Cheilosis is present when the lips are swollen, tense or puffy and, where it appears, the buccal mucosa extends out onto the lips. These lesions are also denuded. This category may be used to record vertical fissuring of the lips but not for lesions of the angles of the mouth only.

Nasolabial Seborrhea. Definite greasy yellowish scaling or filiform excrescences in the nasolabial area that become more pronounced on slight scratching with the fingernail or a tongue blade.

MOUTH

Filiform Papillary Atrophy. Filiform papillae exceedingly low or absent, giving the tongue a smooth appearance that remains after scraping slightly with an applicator stick. "Mild" involves less than one fourth of the tongue (tip and lateral margins only); "moderate" involves one fourth to three fourths of the tongue; "severe" involves over three fourths of the tongue.

Glossitis. Glossitis is any increase in redness, fissuring or swelling with color change (break in lingual mucosa) or diffuse involvement of mucosa. Geographic tongue has the typical irregularly shaped and distributed areas of atrophy with irregular white patches resembling leukoplakia. Glossitis is usually associated with some sensation of pain or burning, particularly upon eating.

Magenta Color. The color of alkaline phenolphthalein.

Swollen Gums. Swollen, red interdental papillae, with more than one papilla involved.

TEETH

Carious Teeth. Molecular decay of a bone, in which it becomes friable, thinned and dark and gradually breaks down, with the formation of pus.

Fluorosis. Opaque paper-white areas in the enamel of the tooth, ranging in size from a few flecks to entire enamel surface. In the latter case brown stain is a frequent accompaniment, as is attrition of opposing surfaces. The most severe forms of fluorosis include discrete or confluent

APPENDIX 30   PHYSICAL SIGNS AND NUTRITIONAL TERMS ASSOCIATED WITH MALNUTRITION (*Continued*)

pitting, with widespread brown staining and a general corroded appearance.

GLANDS

Parotid Enlargement.   Because of various types of facial configuration, parotid enlargement may be easily missed in certain populations. Check by palpation, moving the gland with fingers upward and backward toward the ear. Check if bilateral.

Thyroid Enlargement.   Thyroid enlargement is when a visually perceptible enlargement that is definitely palpable with or without swallowing is noted. It is preferable to examine the subject with his head slightly extended in order to detect thyroid enlargements.

ORGANS

Hepatomegaly.   Liver edges more than 2 cm. below the costal margin. (In children, the liver edge may normally be palpable.)

Splenomegaly.   Spleen is palpable.

APPENDIX 31   ABBREVIATIONS

Along with the specialized vocabulary that is employed in the medical, dietetic and nursing fields, there are acceptable forms of abbreviations. Here is a list of abbreviations commonly used.

aa: Gr. *ana;* of each
a.c.: L. *ante cibum;* before meals
ad., add: L. *adde, addatur,* or *addantur;* add or added
ad. lib.: L. *ad libitum;* at pleasure, as desired
aq.: L. *aqua;* water
aq. dest.: L. *aqua destillata;* distilled water
b.i.d., bis in d.: L. *bis in die;* twice a day
c.: L. *cum;* with
c.: cup
cc.: cubic centimeter
Cent.; cent.; C.: centigrade, Celsius
cm.: centimeter
dilut.: L. *dilutus;* dilute
div.: L. *divide;* divide
fac.: make
gm.: gram
gr.: L. *granum;* grain
gtt.: L. *guttae;* drops
h.s.: L. *hora somni;* at hour of sleep, 8 P.M.
I.U.: international unit
kcal.: kilocalorie
kg.: kilogram

kJ.: kilojoule
lb.: pound
μg.: microgram
mcg.: microgram
μU.: microunit
mEq.: milliequivalent
mg.: milligram
mil. or ml.: milliliter
mM.: millimole
mOsm.: milliosmole
oz.: ounce
p.r.n.: L. *pro re nata;* may be repeated according to instructions
pt.: pint
pulv.: L. *pulvis;* powder
q.d.: L. *quaque die;* every day
Q.I.D., q.i.d.: L. *quater in die;* four times daily
q. 3h.: every three hours
q.s.: L. *quantum satis;* a sufficient quantity
qt.: quart
R.E.: retinol equivalent
s.: L. *sine;* without
sol.: solution
ss.: L. *semis;* half
stat.: L. *statim;* immediately
t., tsp.: teaspoon
T., tbsp.: tablespoon
t.i.d.: L. *ter in die;* three times a day

APPENDIX 32   THE METRIC SYSTEM AND EQUIVALENTS

The metric system is a standardized system of measurement that is used internationally. However, the United States also employs another system of measurement based on the old English system. In the field of dietetics, both systems are used. The following charts give equivalents for common household measures. With this information it is possible to calculate measure and weigh in either system.

EQUIVALENT LEVEL MEASURES AND WEIGHTS

60 drops	=	1 tsp.
		5 cc.
		5 gm.
1 tsp.	=	5 gm.
3 tsp.	=	1 tbsp.
		15 cc.
		15 gm.
1 dessert spoon	=	10 cc.
2 tbsp.	=	30 cc.
		30 gm.
		1 oz. (fluid)
4 tbsp.	=	¼ cup
		60 cc.
		60 gm.
8 tbsp.	=	½ cup
		120 cc.
		120 gm.
16 tbsp.	=	1 cup
		240 gm.
		250 ml.
		8 oz. (fluid)
		½ lb.

2 cups	=	1 pt.
		480 gm.
		500 ml.
		16 oz. (fluid)
		1 lb.
4 cups	=	2 pt.
		1 qt.
		1000 or 960 cc.
		1000 ml.
		1 kg.
		2.2 lb.

4 qt.	=	1 gal.
8 qt.	=	1 peck
2 gal.	=	1 peck
4 pecks	=	1 bushel
8 gal.	=	1 bushel

EQUIVALENTS IN GRAMS

For easy computing purposes, the cubic centimeter (cc.) is considered equivalent to 1 gram:

$$1 \text{ cc.} = 1 \text{ gm.}$$

Also for easy computing purposes, one ounce equals 30 gm. or 30 cc.

1 qt.	=	960 gm.
1 pt.	=	480 gm.
1 cup	=	240 gm.
½ cup	=	120 gm.
1 soup cup	=	120 gm.
1 glass (8 oz.)	=	240 gm.
½ glass (4 oz.)	=	120 gm.
1 orange juice glass	=	100 to 120 gm.
1 tbsp.	=	15 gm.
1 tsp.	=	5 gm.

INDEX

Note: Page numbers in *italics* refer to illustrations. Page numbers followed by the letter *t* refer to tables.